Alfredo Berardelli

NEUROLOGY OF SAPIENZA

Società Editrice
ESCULAPIO

ISBN 978-88-9385-419-1

Società Editrice Esculapio s.r.l.
Via Terracini, 30 – 40131 Bologna
www.editrice-esculapio.com – info@editrice-esculapio.it

On the front cover: Diagram of a frontal section performed through a cerebral hemisphere from the book by G. Mingazzini, "Clinical Anatomy of Nervous Centers," Turin, Unione Tipografica – Editrice Torinese, 1913.

Layout: Laura Tondelli, Laura Brugnoli, Carlotta Lenzi
Cover Layout: Laura Tondelli
Editing supervisor: Ivana Barberini

Printed in Italy by Legodigit - Lavis (TN)

Società Editrice
ESCULAPIO

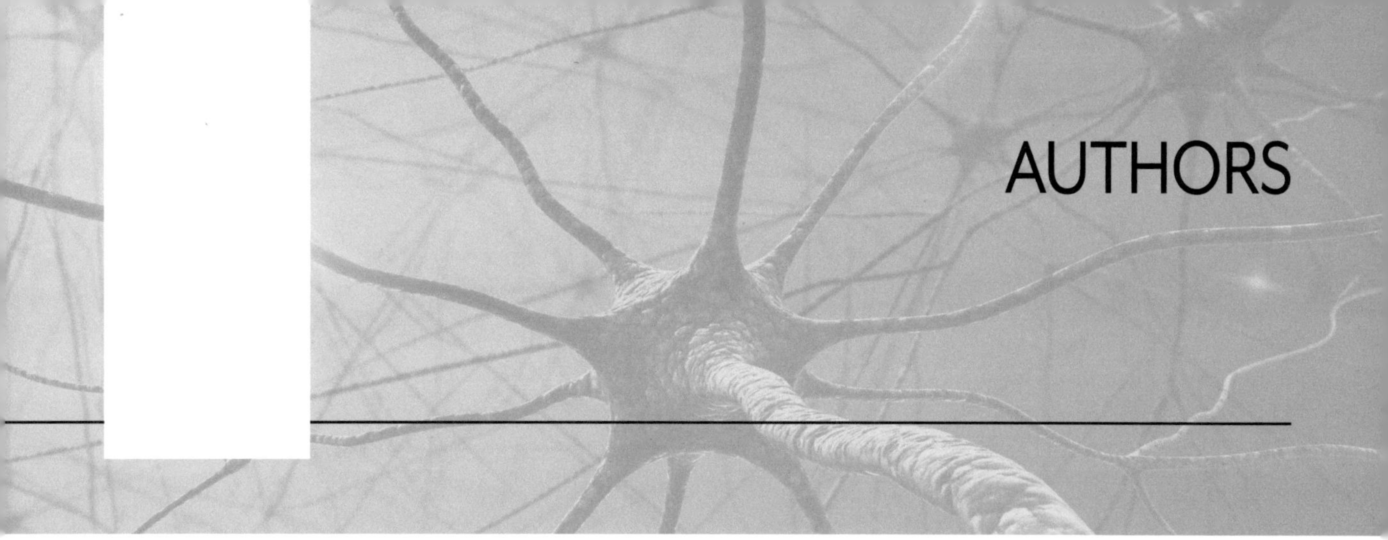

AUTHORS

Alfredo BERARDELLI

Marta ALTIERI
Giovanni ANTONINI
Michelangelo BARTOLO
Daniele BELVISI
Isabella BERARDELLI
Luigi Valentino BERRA
Massimo BIONDI
Matteo BOLOGNA
Giuseppe BRUNO
Chiara CAMBIERI
Marco CANEVELLI
Stefano Filippo CASTIGLIA
Michele CAVALLARI
Marco CECCANTI
Maria CIARDI
Giulia COARELLI
Claudio COLONNESE
Antonella CONTE
Giorgio CRUCCU
Antonio CURRÀ
Luca D'ANGELO
Fabrizia D'ANTONIO
Carlo DE LENA
Roberto DELFINI
Carlo DI BONAVENTURA
Laura DI CLEMENTE
Vittorio DI PIERO
Giulia DI STEFANO
Vincenzo ESPOSITO
Giovanni FABBRINI
Francesco FATTAPPOSTA
Jinane FATTOUCH
Laura FIONDA
Marco FIORELLI
Serena GALOSI
Matteo GARIBALDI
Anna Teresa GIALLONARDO
Costanza GIANNÌ
Renzo GUGLIELMI
Maurizio INGHILLERI
Giorgio LEODORI
Vincenzo LEUZZI
Laura LIBONATI
Mario MANFREDI
Francesco MARZETTI
Mario MASTRANGELO
Oriano MECARELLI
Paolo MISSORI
Alessandra MORANO
Stefania MORINO
Francesca NARDECCHIA
Francesco ORZI
Patrizia PANTANO
Sergio PAOLINI

Massimo PASQUINI
Francesco PIERELLI
Francesco PISANI
Patrizia PULITANO
Silvia ROMANO
Marco SALVETTI
Antonio SANTORO
Mariano SERRAO
Antonio SUPPA
Danilo TONI
Alessandro TREBBASTONI
Andrea TRUINI
Paolo VASSALINI
Edoardo VICENZINI

FOREWORD

The teaching of Neurology in Rome boasts a glorious tradition, which began with Sciamanna in 1883 and continued with Mingazzini in 1905 at the Umberto I Policlinic (inaugurated in 1904). In 1924, it relocated to the current neoclassical building at Viale dell'Università 30.

The establishment of the Clinic of Nervous and Mental Diseases dates back to 1921, with Mingazzini as the first Director of the Clinic. Mingazzini was succeeded by Sante De Sanctis, Vittorio Challiol, Mario Gozzano in the 1950s, and in the 1970s, Cornelio Fazio and Vincenzo Floris. Since the early 1980s, the teaching of Neurology has been carried out by their disciples.

The authors of the Manual "La Neurologia della Sapienza" represent the continuation of the neurologic school of Cornelio Fazio and Vincenzo Floris.

The Manual has been written by neurologists from the Sapienza University of Rome, experts in various fields of Neurology. The editor has promoted stylistic coherence and uniformity in the approach to the subject with the aim of providing a concise and effective tool for knowledge and consultation.

Particular attention has been devoted to the diagnostic, clinical, and therapeutic aspects of various neurological diseases, also highlighting recent scientific advances.

The volume consists of 33 chapters (covering topics in Neurology, Neuroradiology, and Neurosurgery), including a chapter on Neurorehabilitation, one on Child Neurology, and one on the Principles of Psychiatry. We believe that these last three chapters, despite their diversity, are essential for a better and comprehensive understanding of Neurology.

The Manual is a valuable tool primarily for medical students, including students in healthcare professions, but also for Neurology residents. Indeed, the utmost space has been dedicated to symptoms of possible neurological origin encountered in general clinical practice and the neurological pathologies that clinicians must be acquainted with.

We would like to express our gratitude for the dedication and professionalism of all the authors who have contributed to the current edition of the Manual, as well as the authors who contributed to previous editions. Special thanks go to Prof. Mario Manfredi for contributing to the chapter on Cranial Nerves and allowing us to use many of the illustrations from his renowned Neurology volume. Thanks also to Prof. Giorgio Cruccu for his role as editor in previous editions of the volume.

The Manual "La Neurologia della Sapienza" is not an endpoint but a starting point. Our intention is to update and make the volume more comprehensive with successive editions. Research, indeed, continues, and in this 4th Edition, nearly all chapters have been updated, demonstrating the vitality of the neurologic scientific community at Sapienza and the need for constant updates for students and residents

Prof. Alfredo Berardelli

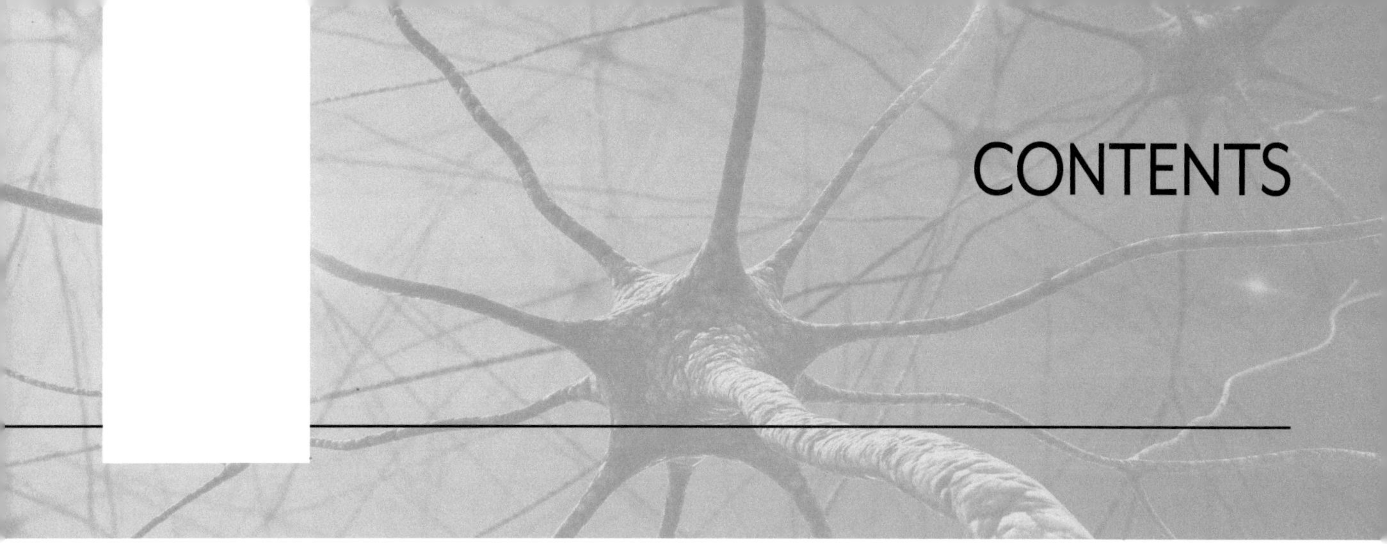

CONTENTS

1 MOTOR SYSTEM 1

Matteo Bologna, Antonio Suppa, Alfredo Berardelli

2 SENSITIVITY 31

Giulia Di Stefano, Andrea Truini, Giorgio Cruccu

3 CRANIAL NERVES 43

Mario Manfredi

4 ANATOMICAL BASES OF COGNITIVE PROCESSES 101

Marco Canevelli, Fabrizia D'Antonio, Alessandro Trebbastoni, Giuseppe Bruno

5 NEURORADIOLOGY DIAGNOSTICS AND THERAPEUTICS 117

Patrizia Pantano, Costanza Giannì, Claudio Colonnese, Marco Fiorelli

19 MOTOR NEURON DISEASES (MND) 411

Marco Ceccanti, Chiara Cambieri, Laura Libonati, Maurizio Inghilleri

20 PERIPHERAL NERVOUS SYSTEM DISEASES 423

Andrea Truini, Giulia Di Stefano, Giorgio Cruccu

21 MYOPATHIES AND DISEASES OF THE NEUROMUSCULAR JUNCTION 455

Matteo Garibaldi, Laura Fionda, Stefania Morino, Giovanni Antonini

22 DISEASES OF THE AUTONOMIC NERVOUS SYSTEM 499

Antonella Conte, Alfredo Berardelli

23 CEPHALALGIAS 513

Laura Di Clemente, Marta Altieri, Vittorio Di Piero

24 MENINGITIS AND OTHER INFECTIONS OF THE NERVOUS SYSTEM 531

Giovanni Fabbrini, Maria Ciardi, Paolo Vassalini, Alfredo Berardelli

27 TRAUMATIC BRAIN INJURY 585

Luca D'Angelo, Roberto Delfini, Antonio Santoro

28 ARTHRITIC, TRAUMATIC AND ONCOLOGICAL PATHOLOGY OF THE SPINE 603

Francesco Marzetti, Luigi Valentino Berra, Luca D'Angelo, Antonio Santoro

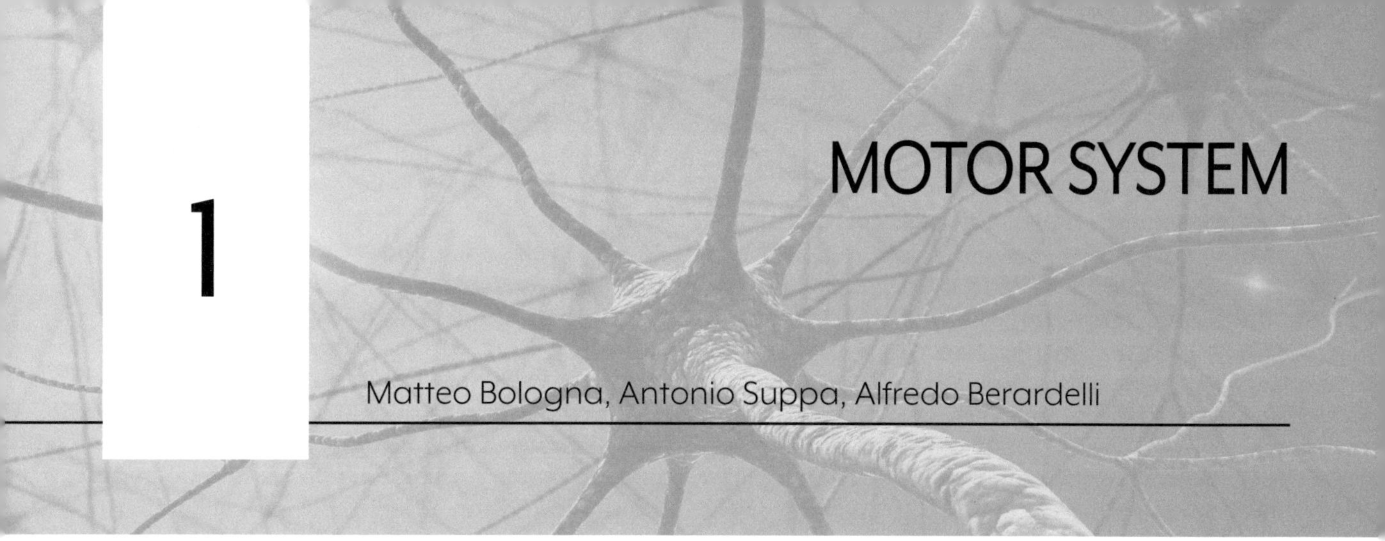

1 MOTOR SYSTEM

Matteo Bologna, Antonio Suppa, Alfredo Berardelli

In this chapter, the anatomical and functional properties of the different components of the motor system are summarized, from muscles to spinal circuits, to suprasegmental movement control systems, namely motor cortical areas (primary and non-primary), basal ganglia, and cerebellum. These three systems directly or indirectly regulate the activation of lower motor neurons (spinal and cranial) through descending motor pathways, which represent the common final pathway of the motor system. The axons of the lower motor neurons run in peripheral nerves and innervate the skeletal muscles of the limbs, trunk, and head through the neuromuscular junction. Motor function, in terms of movement ideation, planning, and execution, is therefore the result of a complex functional integration at multiple levels of the nervous system. In the concluding part of the chapter, the characteristic signs and symptoms resulting from dysfunction of the different components of the motor system are illustrated, as well as the main examination maneuvers. For further details on muscles, the neuromuscular junction, peripheral nerves, and lower motor neurons, refer to the chapters on neuromuscular diseases. For further details on basal ganglia and cerebellum, refer to the chapter on movement disorders.

1.1 The skeletal muscle and the neuromuscular junction

Skeletal muscle is composed of muscle fibers enclosed within a connective tissue sheath that extends deeply to create additional compartments. The epimysium is the outermost connective tissue membrane, the perimysium is the intermediate one, and the endomysium is the innermost membrane that lines individual muscle fibers. The innervation and vascularization of the muscle are mediated by nerves and blood vessels that penetrate deeply, piercing the connective membranes. Muscle fibers are made up of myofibrils containing actin and myosin filaments that cyclically interact in the presence of ATP and calcium, resulting in muscle contraction.

The *neuromuscular junction* or motor end plate represents the point of contact between the axon terminal of the motor neuron and the muscle fiber. The action potential that propagates along the motor axon to the presynaptic terminal causes the opening of voltage-gated calcium channels and an increase in calcium ion concentration, facilitating the adhesion of acetylcholine-containing vesicles to the presynaptic membrane and the release of this neurotransmitter into the synaptic space. Acetylcholine binds to postsynaptic nicotinic receptors, leading to the influx of sodium ions and depolarization of the muscle membrane. Changes in the muscle potential (muscle fiber's electric potential) that exceed the threshold value induce an action potential that rapidly propagates along the muscle fiber, promoting the release of calcium from the sarcoplasmic reticulum and initiating the sliding of actin and myosin filaments, leading to muscle contraction.

Muscle contraction is defined as isotonic when muscle tension remains constant during muscle shortening. *Isotonic contraction* (constant-tension contraction) is commonly divided into two phases: 1) *Concentric or positive phase*, when the muscle shortens while developing tension (e.g., lifting a weight), and 2) *Eccentric or negative phase*, when the muscle lengthens while developing tension (e.g., slowly lowering the same weight). *Isometric contraction* is characterized by an increase in muscle tension generated without changes in muscle length. Among the main factors influencing muscle mechanical properties, muscle length is particularly noteworthy. The muscle can generate variable force depending on the starting length. The tension developed by a muscle can be divided into two components: 1) *Passive tension*, which depends on the viscoelastic components of the muscle, and; 2) *Active tension*, which is developed by the muscle during voluntary contraction. The total tension developed by the muscle reflects the sum of these two components (passive tension + active tension). By varying the initial length of the muscle, different values of passive and active tension are obtained, creating the length-tension relationship curve. Within physiological limits, the greater the muscle stretch (*passive tension*), the greater the force the muscle can generate. Finally, the total tension developed during muscle contraction is also related to the velocity of muscle fiber shortening, following the force-velocity relationship curve. These biomechanical properties of the muscle are utilized by the motor system to produce the appropriate muscle tension necessary for performing the desired task.

1.2 The peripheral nerve

The *peripheral nerve* originates from the fusion of nerve roots that arise from the spinal cord and brainstem, where there is a replacement of astrocytes and oligodendrocytes by Schwann cells, which form the protective sheath of the nerve fibers muscles, the peripheral nerve is surrounded by connective tissue bundles, namely epineurium, perineurium, and endoneurium, which provide elasticity and strength to the nerve. The epineurium represents the outermost connective tissue layer adhering to the surrounding connective tissue. Deeper connective tissue bundles (perineurium) isolate the fibers into fascicles. From the perineurium, the endoneurial connective tissue bundles originate, enclosing the individual axons. The trophism of the axon depends on its continuity with the respective cell body, from which it receives proteins and enzymes necessary for its metabolism through anterograde axoplasmic flow. The axon returns the residues and degradation products of its metabolism to the cell body through retrograde axoplasmic flow. The peripheral nerve can consist of motor, sensory, and autonomic fibers, myelinated and/or unmyelinated. The motor and sensory fibers that contribute to motor control are predominantly myelinated. Lower motor neurons (α and γ) originate in the spinal cord (innervating extrafusal and intrafusal muscle fibers, respectively), while sensory afferents originate from neuromuscular spindles and Golgi tendon organs.

1.3 The lower motor neurons (spinal and cranial)

The *spinal motor neurons* (α motor neurons) innervate the skeletal musculature and are in the anterior horns of the spinal cord. The spinal motor neurons situated in the medial portion of the anterior horns predominantly innervate the musculature of the trunk, while the spinal motor neurons located more laterally (especially in the cervical and lumbosacral segments) predominantly innervate the musculature of the limbs. The motor neurons located in the dorsal or ventral portion of the anterior horns innervate the extensor or flexor muscles, respectively. Cranial motor neurons originate in the motor nuclei of the cranial nerves (see also the Cranial Nerves chapter) such as the oculomotor nucleus (III) at the rostral mesencephalic level near the superior colliculus, the trochlear nucleus (IV) caudally in the midbrain at the level of the inferior colliculus, the motor nucleus of the trigeminal nerve (V), the abducens nucleus (VI), and the facial motor nucleus (VII) located in the pons. Finally, the ambiguous nucleus (IX and X) and the hypoglossal nucleus (XII) are in the medulla. Additionally, the spinal accessory nucleus (XI) extends caudally in the medulla to the cervical spinal cord. Cranial motor neurons innervate the extraocular and intraocular muscles, the muscles of mastication and facial motility, the muscles of the larynx, pharynx, and tongue, and finally the sternocleidomastoid and upper trapezius muscles.

The set of muscle fibers innervated by a single α motor neuron constitutes the motor unit. The innervation ratio is defined as the number of muscle fibers innervated by a single motor neuron. This ratio is variable and inversely proportional to the muscles' ability to perform fine movements. Based on their contractile properties, motor units can be classified as either phasic or tonic. Motor units also differ in terms of the caliber of the motor neurons that characterize them. The caliber of the α motor neurons innervating phasic motor units is greater than that of the α motor neurons innervating tonic motor units. Additionally, the caliber of a motor neuron's axon is proportional to the diameter of its corresponding cell body. Motor units are commonly classified into three types: slow - S motor units (Type I), fast fatigable - FF motor units (Type IIa), and fast fatigue-resistant - FR motor units (Type IIb). S motor units (the most numerous) are characterized by the ability to exert relatively low levels of muscle force, slow contractions, and high resistance to fatigue. S motor units include small-sized motor neurons with slow conduction velocities that innervate a reduced number of muscle fibers. On the other hand, FF motor units (Type IIa) (the least numerous) are capable of exerting high levels of force, very rapid muscle contractions but with low fatigue resistance, and are therefore involved in movements characterized by maximum speed and force but short duration. FF motor units include large-sized motor neurons with high conduction velocities that innervate many muscle fibers. FR motor units (Type IIb) are characterized by intermediate levels of force, contraction speed, and fatigue resistance. FR motor units consist of motor neurons with intermediate characteristics that innervate a variable number of muscle fibers. The relative proportion of each type of motor unit (S, FF, and FR) in a muscle determines its physiological action. A phasic muscle such as the medial rectus of the eye is predominantly composed of fast fibers, while a tonic muscle such as the soleus, with anti-gravity function, is mainly composed of slow fibers. The recruitment order of motor units depends on the size of the motor neuron that comprises them. According to this principle, a motor command transmitted by descending pathways initially activates motor units of smaller caliber and subsequently those of larger caliber. Therefore, the force exerted by skeletal muscles depends not only on the mechanical properties of the muscle (muscle length, etc.) but also on the number of recruited motor units and their discharge frequency. Proper muscle innervation by lower motor neurons ensures the maintenance of physiological muscle trophism.

A specific subpopulation of spinal motor neurons is that of γ motor neurons, characterized by smaller sizes and axons of smaller caliber compared to α motor neurons. γ motor neurons innervate the neuromuscular spindles in their most eccentric part (spindle poles) and are classified as static and dynamic γ motor neurons, which respectively increase the sensitivity of the spindle to muscle length and stretch velocity. γ motor neurons play a fundamental role in reflexes and segmental control of movement.

1.4 Spinal Circuits and reflexes

Reflex refers to an involuntary response mediated by a circuit, consisting of a receptor, an afferent branch, one or more central synapses (at the level of the spinal cord or brainstem), an efferent branch, and an effector. Depending on the type of afferent branch that characterizes them, reflexes are divided into proprioceptive or deep (muscle receptors, tendon receptors, etc.), exteroceptive or superficial (cutaneous receptors), and enteroreceptive (visceral receptors) reflexes (see Table 1.1). Based on the number of central synapses involved in the reflex circuit, reflexes can also be classified as monosynaptic (e.g., stretch reflex) or polysynaptic (e.g., abdominal reflexes). Monosynaptic spinal reflexes reflect the division of the spinal cord into segments called myelomers, from which nerve roots originate to connect the spinal cord with the peripheral nerve and muscles. The circuit of proprioceptive or deep reflexes (also known as stretch or myotatic reflexes) originates from muscle spindles that contain intrafusal muscle fibers

Table 1.1 DEEP, CUTANEOUS, AND MUCOSAL REFLEXES

Reflex	Nerve	Reflex Center	Muscles	Tapping / Stimulation	Response
		DEEP REFLEXES			
Masseter	Trigeminal	Pons	Masseter and temporal muscles	Mandible	Jaw closure
Biceps	Musculocutaneous	C5-C6	Brachial biceps	Biceps tendon	Elbow flexion
Brachioradialis or Radial flexor	Radial	C5-C6	Brachioradialis	Distal portion of the radius	Elbow flexion
Triceps	Radial	C6-C7	Brachial triceps	Triceps tendon	Elbow extension
Pronator or cubitopronator	Median	C6-C7 e C8-T1	Pronator teres and quadratus	Volar surface of the distal radius	Forearm pronation
Finger Flexor	Median and Ulnar	C7-C8	Finger flexors	Flexor tendons	Finger flexion
Patellar	Femoral	L2-L3-L4	Femoral quadriceps	Quadriceps tendon	Knee extension.
Adductor	Obturator and sciatic	L2-L3-L4	Adductors, semitendinosus, and semimembranosus	Medial condyle of the tibia	Thigh adduction
Achilles (ankle jerk)	Tibial branch of the sciatic	S1-S2	Gastrocnemius and soleus	Achilles tendon	Plantar flexion of the foot
Medioplantar	Tibial branch of the sciatic	S1-S2	Gastrocnemius and soleus	Sole of the foot	Plantar flexion of the foot
		CUTANEOUS SUPERFICIAL REFLEXES			
Upper abdominal or epigastric	Intercostal	T7-T8	External and internal oblique	Upper quadrant of the abdomen	Contraction of the abdominal wall
Middle abdominal or mesogastric	Intercostal	T9-T10	External and internal oblique	Middle region of the abdomen	"
Lower abdominal or hypogastric	Intercostal and Iliohypogastric	T11-T12	External and internal oblique	Lower quadrant of the abdomen	"
Cremasteric	Ilioinguinal, femoral, genitofemoral, and obturator	L1-L2	Cremaster	Upper inner surface of the thigh	Testicle elevation
Plantar	Tibial branch of the sciatic	L5-S1	Toe flexors	Outer surface of the sole and the outer edge of the foot	Toe flexion
Anal	Anococcygeal	S4-S5	External sphincter	Perianal skin	Contraction of the external sphincter
		SUPERFICIAL MUCOSAL REFLEXES			
Corneal	First branch of the trigeminal and facial	Bulb and pons	Orbicularis oculi	Cornea	Eyelid closure
Palatal	Second branch and motor branch of the trigeminal and vagus	Bulb	Palatal elevators	Soft palate	Palate elevation
Pharyngeal	Glossopharyngeal and vagus	Bulb	Pharyngeal constrictors	Posterior wall of the pharynx	Constriction of the pharynx

arranged in parallel with extrafusal muscle fibers. Muscle spindles are characterized by a connective tissue sheath that encloses some muscle fibers (intrafusal fibers). Sensory afferents originate from the central portion of muscle spindles, organized into primary endings (annulospiral endings) and secondary endings (flower-spray endings), represented respectively by group Ia and II axons (see Figure 1.1). The activation state of muscle spindles is regulated by muscle stretch, which can be modified either by passive mobilization (e.g., through tendon percussion with a reflex hammer) or by voluntary activation of the muscle itself. Passive muscle stretch activates the sensory endings of the muscle spindle. In contrast, voluntary muscle activation reduces the tension in muscle spindles, leading to a decrease in afferent discharge from intrafusal sensory endings. Furthermore, muscle spindles are innervated, in their most eccentric part, by γ motor neurons. During voluntary muscle activation, the so-called α/γ coactivation occurs. However, γ motor neurons can be activated independently of α motor neurons. Activation of γ motor neurons constantly adjusts the length of the muscle spindle to the length of the muscle. If a γ motor neuron induces contraction of the eccentric component (poles) of the spindle, the central component of the spindle will be stretched, thus increasing fusimotor afferents. Physiologically, the activation of γ motor neurons allows for the regulation of the stretch reflex. Both static and dynamic γ motor neurons are increasingly activated with an increase in the speed and difficulty of the motor task required (increased γ activity corresponds to increased fusimotor responsiveness). Primary spindle endings respond to both phasic and tonic muscle stretch. Secondary endings predominantly respond to tonic muscle stretch (see Figure 1.1). The afferent discharge from Ia endings directly activates α motor neurons of the agonist muscle, inducing the stretch reflex, and reciprocally inhibits antagonist muscle groups through an inhibitory interneuron, a circuit known as “reciprocal inhibition” (see Figure 1.2). The afferent discharge from secondary endings contributes to the tonic regulation of the stretch reflex, primarily involved in postural tone control. Stretch reflexes therefore represent a system that contributes to muscle length control. Muscle stretch or direct nerve stimulation can activate not only the segmental spinal circuit but also reflex circuits that, through the dorsal columns, activate suprasegmental structures such as cortical areas (long-latency or transcortical reflexes). It is believed that such reflexes may play a role in the pathophysiology of certain movement

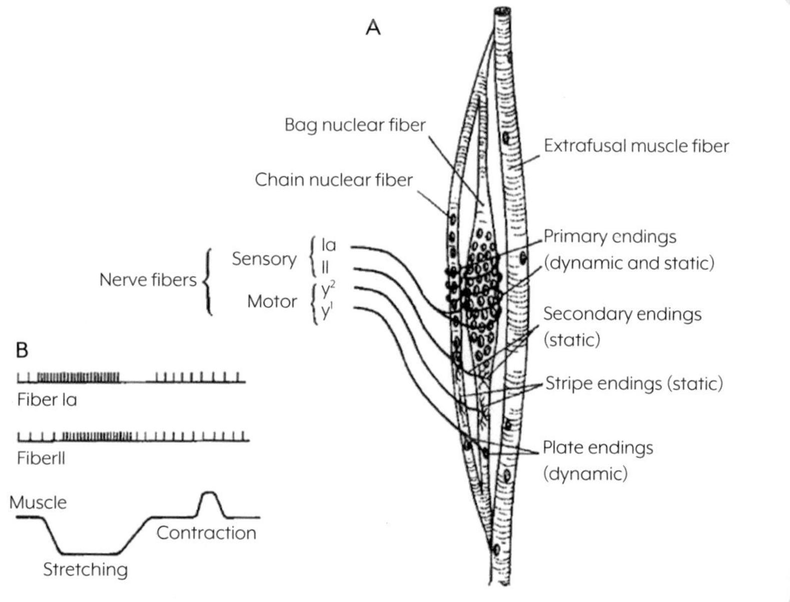

Figure 1.1

Neuromuscular spindle. A) Morphology and sensory and motor innervation. B) Discharge of afferent fibers during muscle stretching and contraction. The endings respond to both dynamic and static stretching, while the type II endings mainly respond during static stretching. γ innervation keeps the afferent spindle discharge active even during contraction (with kind permission from Prof. Mario Manfredi).

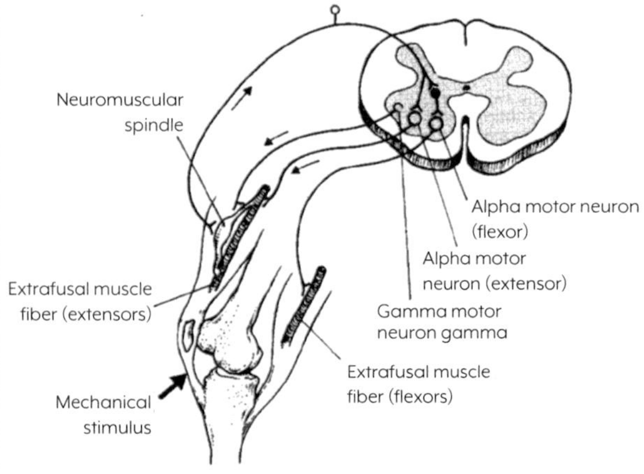

Figure 1.2

Deep reflex or stretch circuit and reciprocal inhibition. Afferent fibers from the spindles activate, through a monosynaptic pathway, the α motor neurons of the agonist muscle (in this case an extensor), and, via an inhibitory interneuron (in black), inhibit the α motor neurons of the antagonist muscle (flexor). The spindle tension is regulated by the γ motor neurons (kindly provided by Prof. Mario Manfredi).

disorders, particularly muscle rigidity in Parkinson's disease and spasticity secondary to central motor pathway lesions.

The excitability of the motor neuron is also regulated by the circuits mediating tendon inhibition and recurrent inhibition. The circuit of tendon inhibition consists of afferents from type Ib fibers originating from Golgi tendon organs, muscle tension receptors, inserted in series at the junction between the muscle component and the tendon component of the muscle (see Figure 1.3). The activation state of the Golgi tendon organs is predominantly influenced by voluntary contraction, while it is minimally influenced by passive stretching of the muscle itself. Finally, the circuit of recurrent inhibition consists of recurrent collaterals of motor axons that synapse with Renshaw interneurons (located in the spinal cord), which in turn exert an inhibitory action on the spinal motor neuron from which the motor command originated. Recurrent inhibition prevents excessive recruitment of the agonist and synergist muscles targeted by the motor command.

Among the exteroceptive or superficial (polysynaptic) reflexes activated by cutaneous receptors, the cutaneous avoidance, or defensive reflexes is included. This reflex is mediated by a network of spinal interneurons and spinal motor neurons that control the flexor musculature of the ipsilateral limbs to the nociceptive stimulation and the extensor musculature of the contralateral limbs to the stimulated side (see

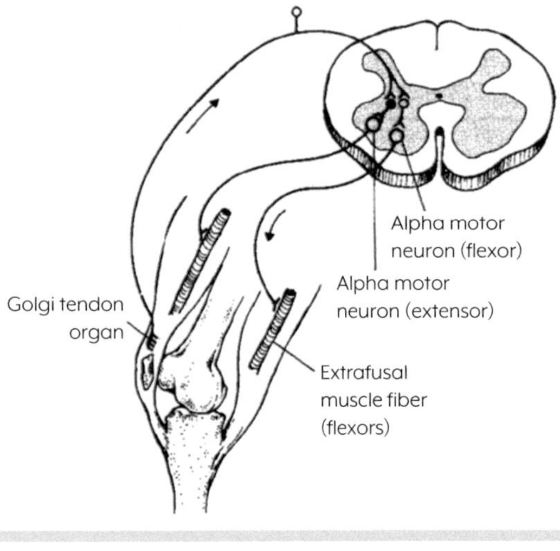

Figure 1.3

Golgi tendon organ action. When the tendon is excessively stretched, the afferent discharge from the Golgi tendon organs inhibits, through an inhibitory interneuron (in black), the α motor neurons of the agonist muscle (in this case an extensor), and activates, through an excitatory interneuron (in white), the α motor neurons of the antagonist muscle (flexor) (reproduced with permission from Prof. Mario Manfredi).

Figure 1.4). The defensive reflexes moves the limb away from a potentially harmful stimulus (by flexing the stimulated limb) and at the same time evoke a series of postural adjustments to maintain balance. Among the superficial reflexes are the abdominal reflexes (upper, middle, and lower) elicited by stimulation of the skin (in the corresponding abdominal regions) using a blunt tip. The afferent cutaneous stimulus results in the reflexive contraction of the ipsilateral abdominal musculature with ipsilateral deviation of the navel. In the lower limbs, the cutaneous plantar reflex can be tested by rubbing the sole of the foot. From 18 months of age onwards, such stimulation results in plantar flexion of the foot and toes. Other superficial reflexes include the corneal reflex and the cremasteric reflex (see Table 1.1).

Spinal reflexes are subject to suprasegmental control exerted by descending projections. For examination purposes, the suprasegmental influence on the circuits of deep reflexes can be demonstrated by the Jendrassik maneuver. This manoeuvre involves asking the patient to perform a voluntary movement, such as clenching the teeth or squeezing the hands, while the examiner performs the manoeuvre to evoke deep reflexes in the upper or lower limbs. The Jendrassik manoeuvre results in facilitation of the stretch reflex.

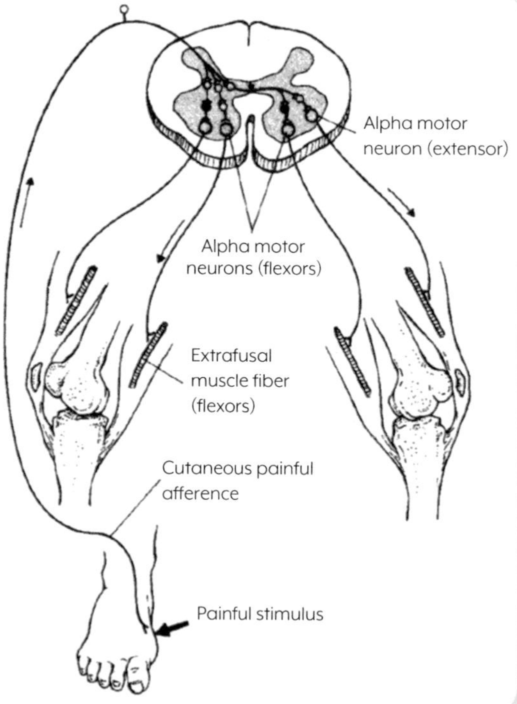

Figure 1.4

Cutaneous Avoidance or Defense Reflex Circuit. Painful afferent fibers from the skin activate, through excitatory interneurons (in white), the α-motoneurons of the flexor muscles and inhibit, through inhibitory neurons (in black), the α-motoneurons of the extensor muscles, causing limb retraction. Simultaneously, they induce extension of the contralateral limb (courtesy of Prof. Mario Manfredi).

1.5 Motor control systems of the brainstem

The *brainstem contains* numerous nuclei and descending nerve tracts that are involved in the control of movement. It consists of three regions, which are arranged in a caudal-to-cranial direction: the medulla, the pons, and the midbrain. The motor descending tracts destined for the spinal cord originate from the *vestibular nuclei* and the *reticular formation* at the *bulbar-pontine* level, and from the *tectal nuclei* and the *red nucleus* at the *midbrain level* (see Figures 1.5 e 1.6). The vestibular nuclei integrate vestibular, visual, and cerebellar inputs and send direct efferent projections to the cerebellum itself and the reticular formation. From the vestibular nuclei, descending tracts also originate, namely the medial and lateral vestibulospinal tracts, as well as a projection to the *oculomotor nuclei* via the medial *longitudinal fasciculus*. The reticular formation is composed of a network of interneurons located in the brainstem. It receives sensory inputs through the spinoreticular tracts, projections from the sensory structures of the brainstem, particularly the vestibular nuclei, cerebellar inputs, and inputs from the motor cortex. The mesencephalic portion of the reticular formation (ascending reticular formation) modulates cortical activity, while the bulbar-pontine portion (descending reticular formation) sends *the medial* (*pontine*) and *lateral* (*bulbar*) reticulospinal tracts.

The tectal nuclei of the midbrain (superior colliculi) integrate visual, auditory, and somatic inputs and give rise to the *tectospinal tract*, which directly influences the ocular

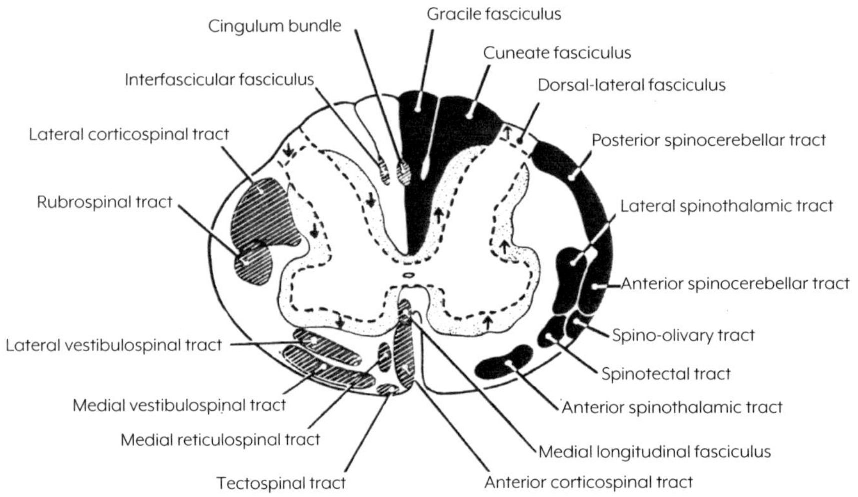

Figure 1.5

Diagram of ascending (in black) and descending (dashed) pathways of the spinal cord. The propriospinal system (dotted) and the dorsolateral fasciculus contain both ascending and descending fibers (adapted from R.C. Truex and M.B. Carpenter: Human Neuroanatomy. The Williams and Wilkins Company, Baltimore, 1969).

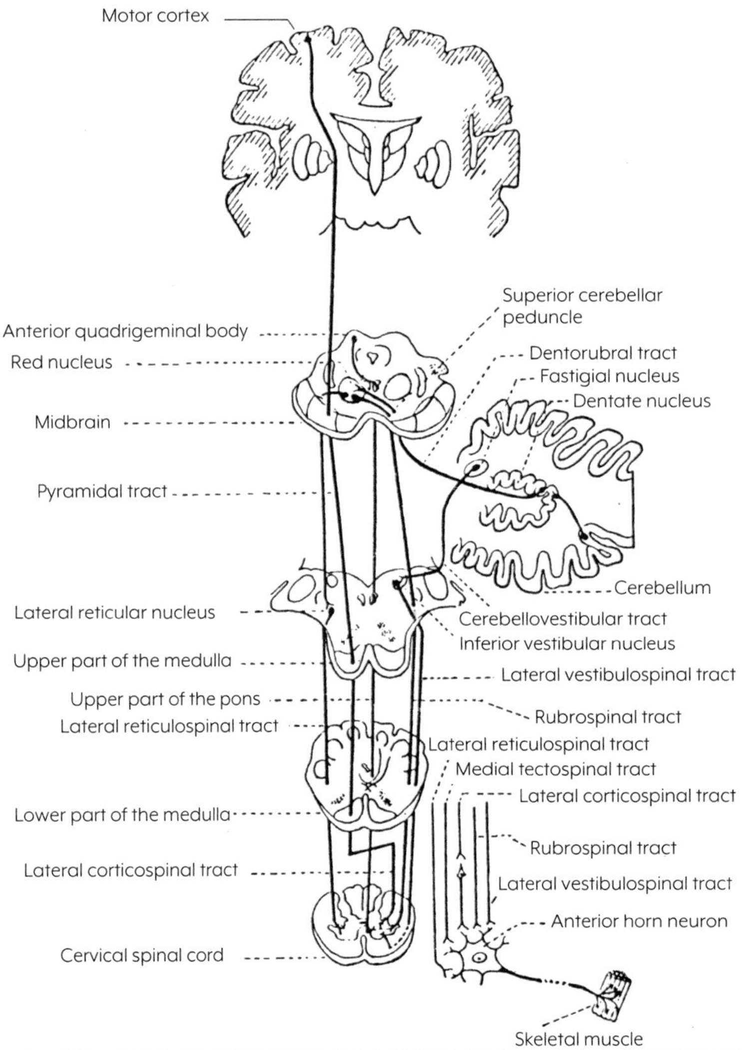

Figure 1.6

The most important descending motor pathways and their relationships with a cell in the anterior horn of the spinal cord (final common pathway) (from De Jong A.: The Neurological Examination Haeber Medical Division, Harper and Ron, New York, 1967).

motor systems, as well as the *tectopontine tract*, which crosses and terminates in the cervical spinal cord for the control of neck movements.

The red nucleus, located in the midbrain, receives inputs from the cerebellum and the cortex and gives rise to the *rubrospinal tract*, which is, however, poorly developed in humans (see Figures 1.5 and 1.6).

From a physiological standpoint, the descending pathways can be grouped into a dorsolateral system, which includes the rubrospinal pathway destined for the distal muscles of the limbs, and a ventromedial system, primarily involved in the control of axial and proximal muscles. The ventromedial system includes the medial and lateral vestibulospinal tracts, responsible for balance and posture control, the tectospinal tracts that coordinate conjugate movements of the head, eyes, and trunk, and finally, the medial and lateral reticulospinal tracts that control upright stance and antigravity movements.

In summary, the function of the brainstem's motor control systems is to regulate muscle tone and balance. The regulation of muscle tone is achieved by modulating the excitability level of the monosynaptic reflex arc, while balance and posture control involve the integration of labyrinthine, somatic, and visual sensory inputs with cerebellar motor inputs, inputs from the basal nuclei, and the pyramidal system.

Finally, the brainstem gives rise to the *monoaminergic pathways*, which, unlike the motor pathways of the dorsolateral and ventromedial systems, have a less specific topographic organization. The *monoaminergic pathways* include descending projections originating from the *Locus Coeruleus* (*noradrenergic projections*) and the *Raphe Nuclei* (*serotonergic projections*). These pathways run through the dorsolateral funiculus and terminate diffusely in the spinal cord, where they synapse onto interneurons of the dorsal horns and the motoneurons of the ventral horns. From a physiological standpoint, the noradrenergic (ceruleospinal tract) and serotonergic (rafespinal tract) projections exert primarily inhibitory effects on the interneurons of the dorsal horn, allowing for fine modulation of somatosensory and nociceptive inputs, and a predominantly excitatory effect on the motoneurons of the ventral horns, leading to increased excitability of spinal reflexes.

1.5.1 The primary motor area and the corticospinal tract

The *primary motor area* (*M1*) is located at the level of the precentral gyrus or precentral convolution (Brodmann's area 4). M1 is also called the agranular cortex because the cortical layer IV (granular layer), the main layer where afferents reaching the cerebral cortex terminate, is almost absent in this area. Moreover, it is characterized by the presence of giant pyramidal neurons (Betz cells) in layer V, which contribute to the main contingent of the corticospinal tract. In M1, there is a complete motor representation or map of the contralateral hemisoma (*motor homunculus*) (Figure 1.7 and 1.8). In the *motor homunculus*, the face is represented at the level of the lateral sulcus, while the representation areas of the upper limb and trunk are located superiorly. Finally, the representation of the lower limb is located at the hemispheric convexity and in the medial region, specifically at the interhemispheric fissure, corresponding to the precentral gyrus. In the *motor homunculus*, the face and hands have a wide cortical representation, more extensive than the cortical representation areas of the trunk and limbs (Figure 1.8). Recently, it has been demonstrated that the organization of M1 is more complex than previously thought and that a somato-cognitive action network alternates with effector regions in M1, which is relevant for integrating goals, physiology and body movement.

M1 receives afferents from both subcortical structures, such as the thalamus, and cortical structures. An important thalamic afferent to M1 is represented by the pallidum (internal segment)-thalamo-cortical projection, which functionally belongs to the basal ganglia circuit. Through the thalamus, M1 also receives afferents from the cerebellum through the cerebello-thalamo-cortical circuit. Furthermore, M1 receives afferents from the premotor cortical areas (premotor area - PM and supplementary motor area - SMA), primary somatosensory areas (S1 or postcentral gyrus or post-rolandic gyrus or Brodmann's areas 3, 2, 1) and secondary somatosensory areas (S2, anterior insula), as well as from associative areas (e.g., prefrontal and parietal).

M1 represents the cortical region where the motor schema, elaborated in higher-

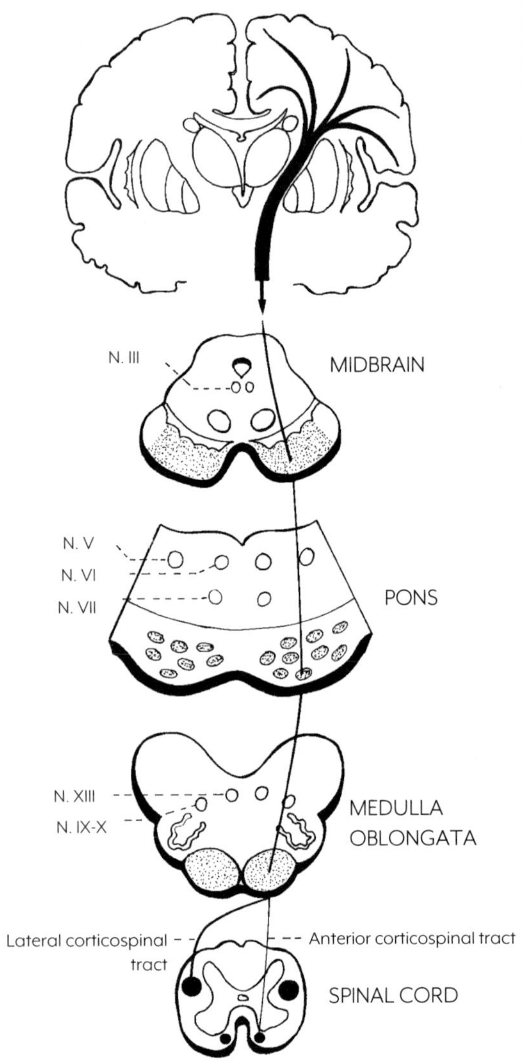

Figure 1.7

Pyramidal tract (in black). The nuclei of the motor cranial nerves are depicted, receiving contralateral pyramidal fibers (cortico-nuclear) of origin.

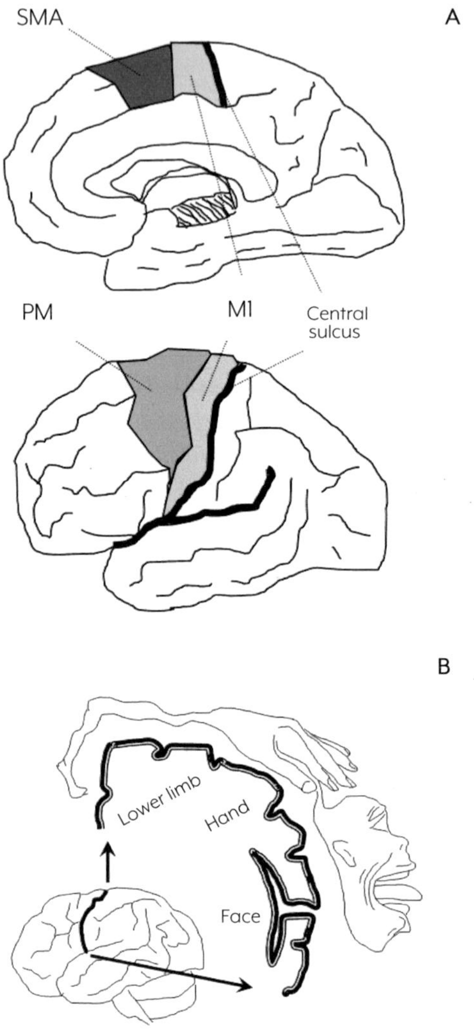

Figure 1.8

Motor Areas. A) Localization of the primary motor area (M1), premotor area (PM), and supplementary motor area (SMA) on the medial surface (top) and lateral surface (bottom) of the hemisphere. B) *Motor homunculus.*

order motor areas, is converted into static and dynamic parameters, i.e., the force and direction of the movement to be executed. The *corticospinal tract* originates predominantly from M1 and, to a lesser extent, from the premotor areas (PM and SMA) and the primary somatosensory cortex (S1) (Figure 1.7). The fibers of the corticospinal tract converge in the corona radiata, run through the genu and posterior limb of the internal capsule, and pass through the midbrain at the level of the cerebral peduncle, ventral to the substantia nigra. At the level of the pons, the fibers of the corticospinal tract run between the pontine nuclei. In the medulla, the corticospinal fibers come together to form the pyramids, which represent the only anatomical site where the corticospinal tracts are not mixed with other descending tracts. At the junction between the medulla and the spinal cord, most of the fibers of the corticospinal tract cross the midline, forming the pyramidal decussation. The crossed fibers descend in the lateral column of the spinal cord and form the lateral corticospinal tracts, while the uncrossed fibers descend in the anterior column and form the ventral corticospinal tracts. The lateral corticospinal tract terminates primarily in the lateral parts of the anterior horns, while the ventral corticospinal tract projects bilaterally to the medial component of the anterior horns, which contains the motoneurons innervating the axial and proximal musculature of the limbs. Corticospinal axons establish direct excitatory connections with α motoneurons in the anterior horns, particularly with the motoneurons innervating the distal muscles of the limbs. The corticobulbar tract consists of projections to the brainstem motor nuclei of the V, VII, IX, X, XI, and XII cranial nerves (Figure 1.7). The component of the motor nucleus of the VII cranial nerve that is responsible for innervating the upper facial musculature receives innervation from both ipsilateral and contralateral hemispheres. Conversely, the component of the motor nucleus of the VII cranial nerve that innervates the lower facial musculature receives motor fibers exclusively from the contralateral cortex. This explains the relative sparing of the upper facial musculature in central lesions of the motor pathways that converge at the facial nerve nucleus.

In summary, M1 directly modulates the excitability of spinal and cranial α motoneurons through the corticospinal and corticobulbar tracts, and it exerts control over spinal segmental circuits both directly (e.g., presynaptic inhibition phenomenon) and indirectly through the modulation of brainstem descending systems. The main functional role of M1 is to control fine finger movements. Neurons in M1 encode the key parameters of voluntary movement, such as *force*, *speed*, and *direction*. Additionally, M1 contributes to the maintenance and regulation of muscle tone, and therefore to the maintenance of balance and postural control.

1.5.2 The non-primary motor areas

The control of voluntary movement is integrated by two main non-primary motor cortical areas (Figure 1.8). The *premotor area* (PM) receives inputs from the posterior parietal areas (areas 5 and 7, 39 and 40 of Broadmann) that contribute to the processing of visual information and the processing of spatial relationships necessary for the proper execution of movements directed towards a target. The PM area projects, in turn, to M1 and specific regions of the brainstem and spinal cord involved in the control of axial musculature. Therefore, the PM area plays a role in the coordination and preparation of voluntary movement and in the control of axial musculature, with a more relevant role in the programming of movements that arise in response to external stimuli.

The supplementary motor area (SMA) plays a fundamental role in the programming and coordination of complex motor sequences. The SMA generates motor commands that initiate voluntary movement and coordinate the postural activities necessary for the correct execution of the movement itself, through projections from the basal nuclei and specific regions of the frontal lobe (dorsolateral prefrontal area and anterior cingulate cortex). Furthermore, the extensive connectivity between motor areas of the two cerebral hemispheres through the corpus callosum and between non-primary motor areas and non-motor areas (sensory and associative) allows for sensorimotor integration phenomena at the basis of precision voluntary movements guided by sensory information (e.g., grasping and manipulation movements with the upper limb). The SMA would play a more relevant role in the planning of spontaneous movements, regardless of external stimuli.

1.5.3 The basal ganglia nuclei

The term ganglia or basal nuclei is commonly used to indicate areas of gray matter located at the subcortical level. The basal nuclei consist of the Striatum, Globus Pallidus (GP), Subthalamic Nucleus of Luys (STN), and Substantia Nigra (SN). The striatum consists of two nuclei with a common embryological origin: the caudate nucleus and the putamen. The GP is composed of an internal part - GPi, and an external part - GPe, both derived from the diencephalic embryonic origin. The term *lenticular nucleus* refers to the combination of the putamen and globus pallidus. Finally, the SN (*substantia nigra*) is a mesencephalic neuronal aggregate divided into a ventral area (pars reticulata or SNr) and a dorsal area characterized by the presence of dopaminergic neurons (pars compacta or SNc) and pigmented due to the presence of neuromelanin (Figure 1.9).

The basal nuclei integrate afferents from the cerebral cortex and project back to the cerebral cortex itself, constituting a network of parallel reverberating circuits. The cortico-nucleobasal circuits are predominantly organized in a topographic and somatotopic manner, meaning specific cortical areas project to specific striatal motor areas and receive afferent projections from them. It is believed that a similar organization largely characterizes the non-motor circuits of the basal nuclei as well.

The Striatum receives afferents from motor, sensory, associative, and limbic cortical areas through excitatory glutamatergic cortico-striatal projections. The Striatum also receives important dopaminergic afferents from the SNc (nigro-striatal projections) and from thalamic nuclei (such as the intralaminar nuclei of the thalamus and the centromedian/parafascicular nucleus) through excitatory glutamatergic thalamo-striatal projections. The caudate nucleus receives projections from associative areas. The ventral striatum and nucleus accumbens receive afferents from the amygdala and hippocampus and are involved in impulse control, emotions, and memory.

From a microstructural point of view, the Striatum is organized into functionally separate neural systems called striosomes (also referred to as striatal patches) and a matrix. Motor, sensory, and associative areas predominantly project at the level of the matrix, while limbic areas terminate in the striosomes.

The intrinsic basal ganglia circuits are traditionally distinguished into the so-called direct pathway and indirect pathway circuits (Figure 1.10 and 1.11). The direct pathway consists of monosynaptic inhibitory projections from the Striatum to the GPi and SNr. The indirect pathway consists of a circuit that includes efferent projections from the Striatum to the GPe, which in turn influences the activity of the GPi and SNr through direct or indirect projections, consisting of inhibitory projections from the GPe to the STN, and excitatory projections originating from the STN and directed to the GPi and SNr. Additionally, there is a "hyperdirect" pathway that connects cortical areas to the STN. From a neurochemical point of view, striatal neurons in the direct pathway contain GABA, dynorphin, and substance P, while striatal neurons in the indirect pathway contain

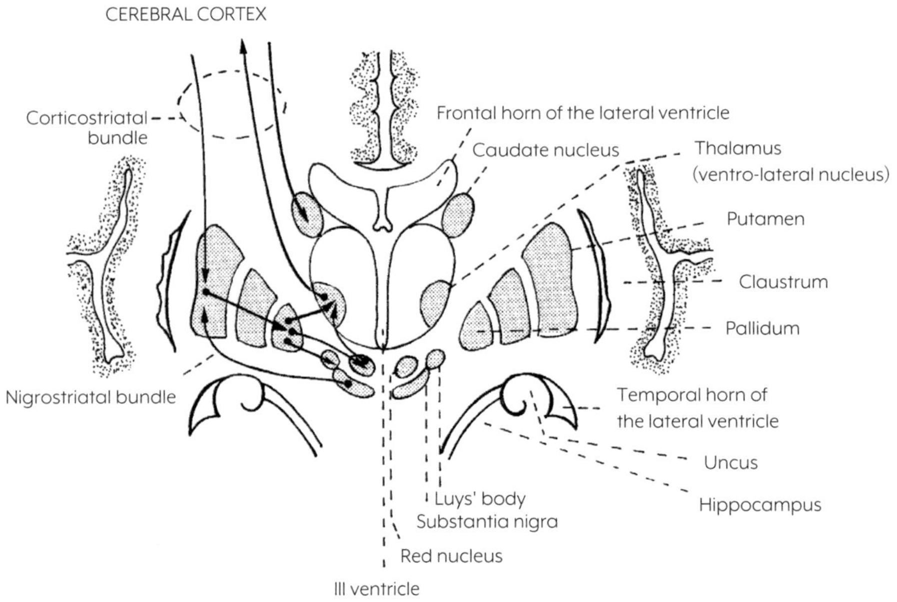

Figure 1.9

Nuclei and extrapyramidal pathways.

GABA and enkephalin. The striatum is also characterized by the presence of cholinergic and GABAergic interneurons. The possible role of endogenous opioids, serotonin, and adenosine in the basal nuclei circuits is still debated.

The GPi (internal globus pallidus) and SNr (substantia nigra pars reticulata) are the main structures from which efferent projections originate, predominantly directed towards the thalamus (specifically the ventral lateral, ventral anterior, dorsomedial, and centromedian nuclei) and brainstem structures. The efferent projections from the GPi and SNr inhibit the activity of thalamic neurons, thus reducing the facilitatory effect that thalamic neurons exert on cortical areas, including the primary and non-primary motor areas. In terms of projections to the brainstem, the GPi and SNr exert an inhibitory effect on the superior colliculus and the pedunculopontine nucleus (PPN). The superior colliculus contributes to regulating the excitability of the blink reflex trigeminal circuits. The PPN plays an important role in locomotion and muscle tone control.

The motor thalamus represents the site where afferents from cortico-striato-pallido-thalamo-cortical and cerebello-ponto-thalamo-cortical circuits converge (see the next paragraph). The thalamus, therefore, represents an important nervous center where signals processed by both basal ganglia nuclei and the cerebellum are integrated.

To date, five main cortico-nucleobasal circuits have been identified:

1) The *motor circuit*, primarily involved in the control of voluntary movement, muscle tone, and posture. The direct pathway facilitates selected voluntary movements, while simultaneous activation of the indirect pathway has an inhibitory effect on involuntary or undesired movements, thus improving the specificity of motor commands. Dopamine released by nigrostriatal projections has an excitatory effect on neurons in the direct

Figure 1.10

Schematic diagram of the main cortico-basal motor circuits. The Striatum (caudate + putamen) represents the primary input structure of the basal ganglia system and receives excitatory afferents (glutamatergic) from the cerebral cortex and thalamus. The Striatum also receives dopaminergic projections from the substantia nigra pars compacta (SNc) that exert inhibitory effects on D1 receptors and excitatory effects on D2 receptors. From the Striatum, inhibitory monosynaptic projections (GABAergic) of the 'direct pathway' originate, reaching the globus pallidus pars interna (GPi) and the substantia nigra pars reticulata (SNr), the main output structures of the basal ganglia system. The GPi and SNr also receive projections from the striatum via the so-called 'indirect pathway,' consisting of the globus pallidus pars externa (GPe) and the subthalamic nucleus (STN). The STN receives excitatory glutamatergic afferents from the cerebral cortex through the so-called "hyperdirect pathway." The GPi and SNr exert inhibitory influence on the thalamus and brainstem structures through inhibitory GABAergic projections. The thalamus exerts a facilitatory effect on cortical areas through glutamatergic projections. Various descending systems originating from the brainstem play a role in regulating the excitability of spinal cord circuits.

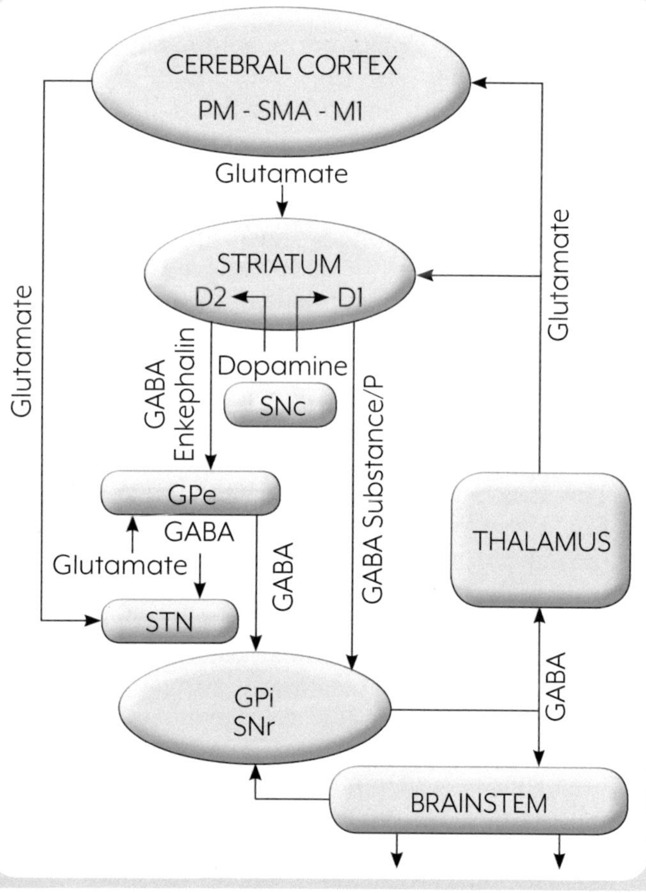

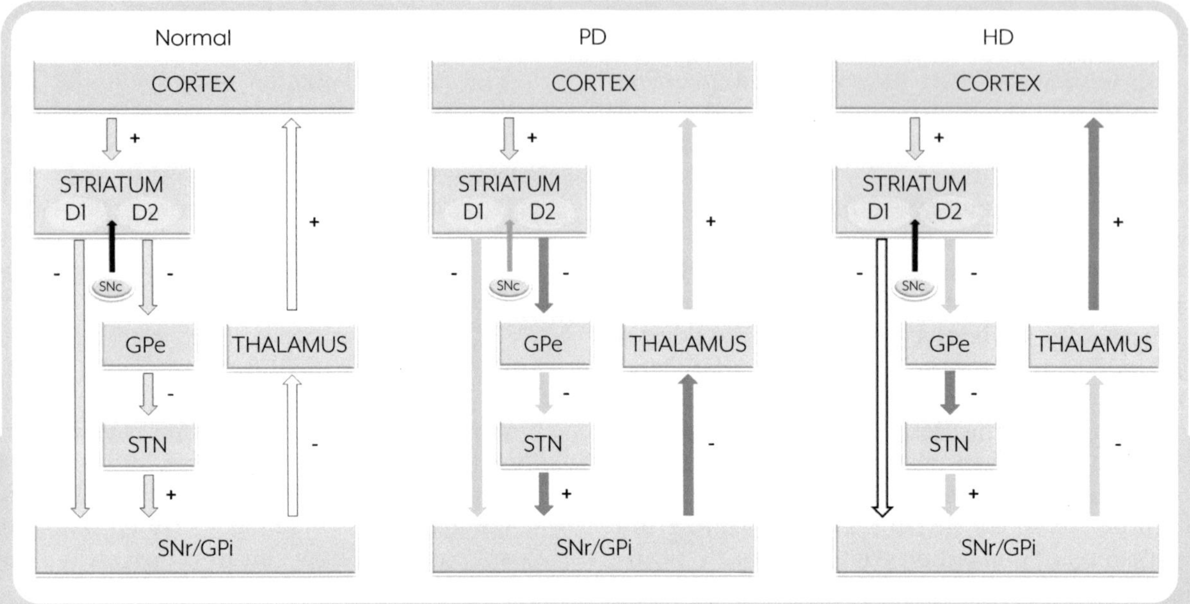

Figure 1.11

Functional organization schema of the basal ganglia nuclei and their major internuclear connections under normal conditions, in Parkinson's disease - PD (an example of hypokinetic syndrome), and in Huntington's disease - HD (an example of hyperkinetic syndrome).

pathway via D1 dopamine receptors, while simultaneously exerting an inhibitory effect on the indirect pathway through D2 dopamine receptors. Dopamine, therefore, facilitates the execution of voluntary movement by enhancing the activation of the direct pathway and inhibiting the indirect pathway. It is believed that activation of the subthalamic nucleus (STN), mediated by the hyperdirect pathway, leads to a global improvement in the balance between the activation of the direct and indirect pathways and the subsequent activation of thalamic neurons.

2) The *oculomotor circuit* originates from the *frontal eye fields* (FEF) in the frontal lobes (Brodmann area 8), which project to the body of the caudate nucleus, which in turn projects directly to the superior colliculus and, through the thalamus, back to the frontal eye fields. This circuit is involved in the control of saccadic eye movements.
3) The *dorsolateral prefrontal cortex circuit* originates from projections of the dorsolateral prefrontal cortex and other associative areas directed towards the dorsolateral head of the caudate nucleus, which in turn projects through the ventral anterior and dorsomedial thalamus to the dorsolateral prefrontal cortex. This circuit is involved in higher-order motor and non-motor tasks (cognitive and associative functions), including the planning of complex motor patterns and sequences, as well as visuospatial memory.
4) The *lateral orbitofrontal cortex circuit* connects the lateral orbitofrontal cortex with the ventromedial region of the caudate nucleus, which in turn projects through the ventral anterior and dorsomedial thalamus to the lateral orbitofrontal cortex. It is believed to be involved in the control of behavior and its appropriateness in relation to the environmental context.
5) The *anterior cingulate cortex circuit connects the anterior* cingulate cortex with the ventral striatum, which in turn projects through the dorsomedial thalamus to the anterior cingulate cortex. This circuit is implicated in behavioral aspects, including impulse control, emotion, and memory.

It is believed that the functional role of the basal ganglia nuclei is to assist and focus motor commands by selectively facilitating desired movements and inhibiting undesired ones (*surround inhibition*). The direct pathway is involved in activating the selected motor program (*go* signal), while the indirect pathway functions to increase inhibition of motor generators (*no-go* signal). The hyperdirect pathway is thought to inhibit all motor responses until the correct response is selected. The circuitry of the basal ganglia contributes to modulating the exerted force according to the desired motor task (*scaling effect*), particularly during complex voluntary movements characterized by sequential and simultaneous motor acts. Experimental evidence suggests that the basal ganglia nuclei may be involved in the initiation of internally generated movements (*motor initiation*). The basal ganglia nuclei are also implicated in the control of muscle tone, posture, and automatic and reflexive involuntary motility. The latter includes automatic movements of certain body segments occurring during movements of other segments (e.g., pendulum-like motion of the upper limbs during walking) as well as facial and gestural expressiveness. The basal ganglia nuclei compare motor commands generated at the level of the cerebral cortex with proprioceptive sensory afferents providing feedback from the movement itself. These functions imply an important role of the basal ganglia nuclei in motor learning mechanisms. Additionally, the basal ganglia nuclei play a role in encoding complex cognitive-motor sequences and patterns.

1.5.4 The cerebellum

From an anatomical-topographical point of view, the cerebellum lies in the posterior cranial fossa, posterior to the brainstem (to which it is connected through the inferior, middle, and superior cerebellar peduncles) and inferior to the occipital lobes, from which it is separated by an extension of the dura mater called the tentorium cerebelli. Anatomically, the cerebellum is organized into a longitudinal median structure, i.e. the *cerebellar vermis*, and two *cerebellar hemispheres*. From a microanatomical perspective, the cerebellum is characterized by a uniformly structured cortex, divided into a molecular layer (the most superficial layer) and the underlying layers of *Purkinje cells* (intermediate layer) and granule cells (the deepest layer). Additionally, the cerebellum consists of four deep nuclei located in each cerebellar hemisphere: dentate nucleus, emboliform nucleus, globose nucleus, and fastigial nucleus (from lateral to medial).

The cerebellar surface is characterized by numerous transverse grooves and fissures, giving the organ a lamellar appearance, and defining three cerebellar lobes: anterior, posterior, and flocculonodular. The transverse fissure runs along the upper surface of the cerebellum, separating the anterior lobe from the posterior lobe. The posterior lobe, in turn, is separated from the flocculonodular lobe by the posterolateral fissure, which is observed on the lower surface of the cerebellum. The three cerebellar lobes are further subdivided into lobules by secondary fissures. From a phylogenetic perspective, the cerebellum can be divided into three areas known as the archicerebellum, paleocerebellum, and neocerebellum. The archicerebellum corresponds to the flocculonodular lobe, the paleocerebellum corresponds to the cerebellar vermis and the paravermian portion of the cerebellar hemispheres, and the neocerebellum corresponds to the lateral portion of the cerebellar hemispheres.

The cerebellum integrates various afferent inputs and gives rise to efferent outputs to brainstem, spinal, and cerebral structures. The main cerebellar afferents can be divided into mossy *fibers and climbing fibers*. Mossy fibers represent the main type of afferent cerebellar fibers originating from brainstem nuclei and the spinal cord, converging at the granular layer. Climbing fibers originate from the inferior olivary nuclei and reach the cerebellum via the contralateral inferior cerebellar peduncle, forming synapses directly with Purkinje cells. The cerebellum also receives monoaminergic afferents, such as noradrenergic fibers from the *Locus Coeruleus* and serotonergic fibers from the Dorsal Raphe Nuclei, the effects of which are still not fully understood. Both mossy and climbing cerebellar afferents exert an excitatory effect on Purkinje cells. Purkinje cells project to the deep cerebellar nuclei, where they exert an inhibitory effect (mediated by the neurotransmitter GABA). The cerebellar cortex of the vermis projects to the fastigial nucleus, the intermediate part of the hemispheres to the globose and emboliform nuclei, and the lateral part of the hemispheres to the dentate nucleus. Efferent fibers originating from the cerebellar nuclei project to structures in the brainstem, spinal cord, and cerebral cortex, where they predominantly exert an excitatory effect (mediated by the neurotransmitter glutamate).

The *cerebellar system* can be divided into the vestibulocerebellar, spinocerebellar, and cerebrocerebellar (or pontocerebellar) systems, as well as the bulbar olivary system (Figure 1.12). The vestibulocerebellar system consists of afferents that originate from the inner ear and the vestibular nuclei, and they are directed, through the vestibulocerebellar tracts, to the flocculonodular lobe. The flocculonodular lobe projects to the vestibular nuclei via the cerebellovestibular pathway. Descending projections from the vestibular nuclei originate and directly target the motor structures of the spinal cord, gathered in the vestibulospinal tracts, and the brainstem oculomotor nuclei, collected in the medial longitudinal fasciculus. *The vestibulocerebellar system* mediates the regulation of balance and eye movements.

The *spinocerebellar system* consists of somatosensory afferents directed to the vermis and the paravermian portion of the cerebellar hemispheres. The somatosensory afferents are collected in the dorsal, ventral, rostral spinocerebellar tracts, the cuneocerebellar tract, and the trigeminocerebellar tract. Efferent projections from the vermis and the paravermian portion of the cerebellar hemispheres directly target the fastigial, globular, and emboliform nuclei, whose projections, in turn, are directed to the red nucleus (magnocellular portion) and other motor structures of the brainstem, including the reticular formation, from which the reticulospinal tracts and the vestibular nuclei, from which the vestibulospinal tracts originate. The spinocerebellar system is involved in the regulation of ipsilateral appendicular and axial movements.

The *cerebrocerebellar* (or pontocerebellar) system derives its name from the cerebral afferents originating from the contralateral motor cortex and directed to the lateral portion of the cerebellar hemispheres through the pontine nuclei. Efferent projections from the lateral portion of the cerebellar hemispheres directly target the dentate nucleus, from which projections are further directed to the red nucleus (parvicellular portion), the thalamus (ventrolateral nucleus), and from there to the motor cortex. The cerebrocerebellar system is predominantly involved in the planning and execution of voluntary movement.

The system of the *bulbar olives* consists of the bulbar olives, which serve as an integration center for somatic, visual, and auditory afferents, and a system of fibers that project diffusely to the entire cerebellar cortex. The bulbar olives receive afferents from the cerebellar cortex and deep cerebellar nuclei through the parvicellular portion of the red nucleus, known as the cerebello-rubro-olivary pathway. It is believed that the system of bulbar olives may play a role in motor learning.

Recent evidence has shown that the cerebellum is directly interconnected with the basal ganglia. For example, it has been observed that the subthalamic nucleus of Luys is a source of disynaptic projection to the cerebellar cortex. Similarly, the dentate nucleus in the cerebellum is a source of disynaptic projection to the Striatum (see Figure 1.13).These observations offer a new perspective and suggest that the cerebellum, basal ganglia, and cortical areas form a functionally integrated network. This network is organized topographically in such a way that the motor, cognitive, and affective territories of each node are interconnected. Consequently, modifications in a particular node can have functional effects on the entire network. Recent theories suggest that various movement disorders, such as hyperkinetic disorders (e.g., dystonia and tremor) or hypokinetic disorders, could be interpreted based on a network dysfunction.

1.6 Motor syndromes

1.6.1 Signs and symptoms secondary to muscle and neuromuscular junction disorders

The structural or functional alterations of the striated muscle in myopaties result in muscle weakness with a variable topographic distribution, but more frequently affecting the proximal musculature of the shoulder and

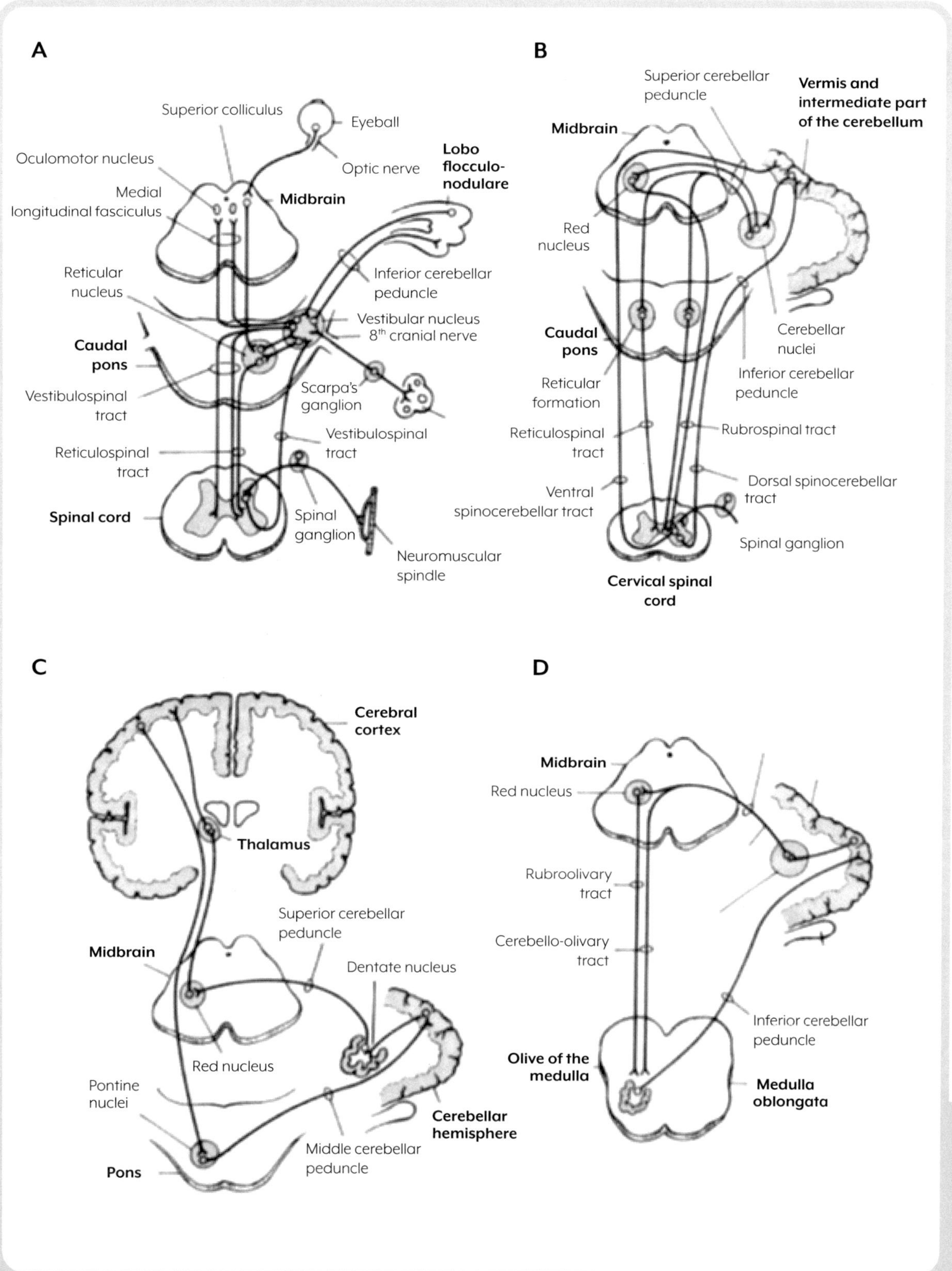

Figure 1.12

A) Vestibulocerebellar System. B) Spinocerebellar System. C) Cerebrocerebellar System. D) Inferior Olivary System.

pelvic girdles and the cranial region. In most cases, myopathies lead to a reduction in muscle trophism, namely hypotrophy or atrophy. On the other hand, certain muscle diseases, such as dystrophies, may present pseudohypertrophy, which is an increase in volume of certain muscle groups (most commonly affecting the lower limbs) associated with a reduction in strength. The neuromuscular junction or myasthenic syndrome is characterized by a progressive reduction in muscle strength during the execution of repeated muscle contractions over time (fatigability). Patients with myasthenic syndrome report fatigue and muscle exhaustibility. Finally, disorders of muscle excitability can result in delayed muscle relaxation (myotonia) in response to a specific stimulus, such as voluntary contraction or mechanical percussion of the muscle.

1.6.2 Signs and symptoms of peripheral paralysis (lower motor neuron syndrome)

Peripheral paralysis or lower motor neuron syndrome is secondary to the damage of the peripheral nerve, nerve roots, and lower motor neuron at the level of the anterior horns of the spinal cord or motor nuclei of the brainstem. It is mainly characterized by a deficit in voluntary movements. Strength is commonly assessed by opposing the action of gravity and the active resistance of the examiner against the muscle's pushing direction. The muscle strength grading scale (MRC - Medical Research Council) is commonly divided into 6 grades, where 0 indicates no contraction and 5 indicates normal strength (see Table 1.2). The term "paresis" refers to muscle weakness, while "plegia" refers to complete loss of muscle strength. In peripheral nerve disorders (neuropathies), the strength deficit affects one or more muscles, depending on the type of neuropathy (mononeuropathies or multineuropathies). In polyneuropathies, a strength deficit with a characteristic distal and symmetrical distribution is observed. A strength deficit resulting from an injury to one or more roots or spinal motor neurons manifests in all muscles innervated by the affected roots or corresponding myelomers. For examination purposes, it can sometimes be difficult to distinguish signs of lower motor neuron damage from a radicular syndrome, and therefore, the assistance of neurophysiological techniques such as motor and sensory conduction velocity studies and electromyography is used. A focal strength deficit at the cranial level may result from cranial mononeuropathy or isolated damage to the motor neurons of the brainstem nuclei, as observed in mononeuropathies of the third,

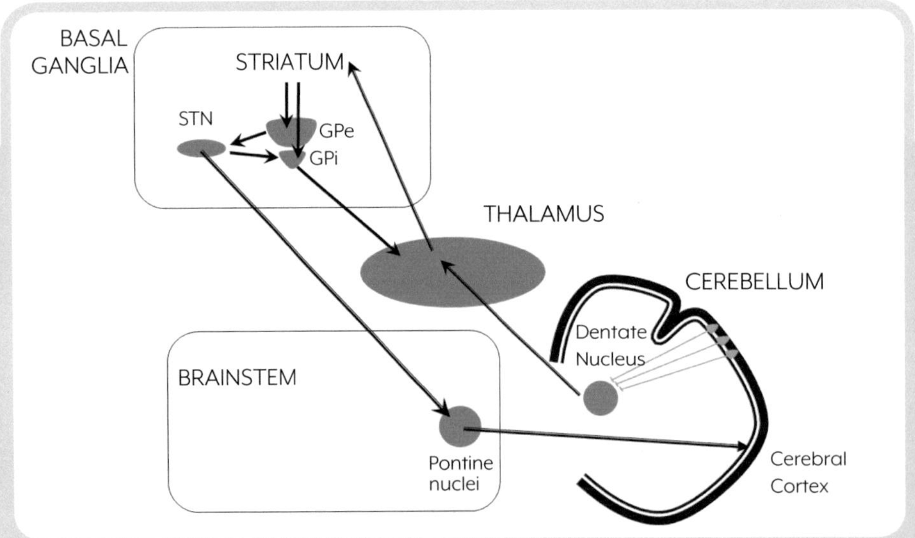

Figure 1.13

Schematic diagram of the connections between basal ganglia and cerebellum. The striatum receives inputs from the cerebellar cortex via the dentate nucleus and thalamic nuclei. Direct projections from the subthalamic nucleus of Luys originate to the cerebellar cortex through the pontine nuclei.

fourth, and sixth cranial nerves, causing nuclear gaze paralysis, or in the case of damage to the seventh cranial nerve, as in Bell's palsy. Finally, degeneration of the motor neurons of the cranial nerve nuclei (V, VII, IX, X, and XI) can manifest as bulbar paralysis characterized by dysarthria (difficulty in articulating speech), dysphagia (difficulty in swallowing), and dysphonia (difficulty in phonation). Degeneration of bulbar motor neurons is one of the most typical clinical signs of motor neuron disease.

Peripheral paralysis is also characterized by an alteration of muscle trophism, a reduction in muscle tone, and deep reflexes. Muscle trophism is assessed by observing, palpating, and measuring the circumference of a muscle or muscle groups. The decrease in muscle trophism is called *hypotrophy* or *atrophy* (in the case of extreme reduction in trophism). Muscle tone refers to the resistance to passive mobilization of a limb performed by the examiner and the bouncing manoeuvre, which involves applying oscillation to body segments and observing their excursions. Additionally, muscle tone should also be examined at the level of the head (axial tone). If the resistance to passive movement is reduced, it is referred to as *hypotonia* or *atonia* (in the case of marked reduction or complete absence of tone). Peripheral paralysis is also associated with a reduction in deep reflexes, known as *hyporeflexia* or *areflexia* (in the case of reflex absence). The examination of proprioceptive reflexes can be performed by striking a muscle tendon with a reflex hammer. In response to stretching, the muscle contracts. The examination of muscle tone, trophism, and reflexes should always be performed by comparing the same body segment on both sides. The commonly evaluated deep reflexes are listed in Table 1.1.

Additional signs and symptoms accompanying peripheral paralysis include the appearance of fibrillations, fasciculations, muscle cramps, myokymia, spasms, and myoclonus (see below). *Fibrillations* consist of involuntary activation of individual muscle fibers (detectable only through electromyographic techniques), while *fasciculations* are involuntary contractions of a single motor unit or part of it that do not cause movement of the affected body segment and are often clinically visible. Fibrillations and fasciculations result from irritative activity of the lower motor neuron due to cellular or axonal damage. Fasciculations can, however, be benign in nature (e.g., in neuromuscular hyperexcitability syndromes). *Muscle cramps* are considered a consequence of irritative activity in the terminal branches of axons, the proximal portion of axons, or the cell body of lower motor neurons in diseases of the anterior horns, radiculopathy, neuropathy, and myopathy. However, there are benign muscle cramps due to dehydration and electrolyte depletion, as well as benign familial forms, such as in idiopathic cramp or pseudotetanus syndrome. *Myokymia* is described as involuntary muscle contractions that can be observed subcutaneously, continuous, or sub-continuous, originating from the same motor unit and resulting from irritative activity in more distal axon branches. A benign form of myokymia is represented by eyelid myokymia, often present in anxious states. *Spasms* are involuntary, tonic, often painful muscle contractions with co-contraction of agonist and antagonist muscles. Spasms likely originate from irritative activity in the axon associated with muscle fiber instability. Spasms are also present in tetany and can affect the cranial muscles, particularly the masticatory muscles (trismus), or the limbs in the stiff-person syndrome and in cases of dehydration with electrolyte.

Table 1.2 MUSCLE STRENGTH GRADING SCALE FOR CLINICAL EXAMINATION

0	Absence of muscle contraction
1	Muscle contraction without body segment movement
2	Body segment movement against gravity eliminated
3	Body segment movement against gravity
4	Body segment movement against resistance
5	Normal strength

1.6.3 Signs and symptoms of central paralysis (upper motor neuron syndrome)

The *upper motor neuron syndrome* (pyramidal syndrome) is caused by a lesion or dysfunction of M1 or the corticospinal tract and is characterized by a deficit in strength and a reduction or loss of voluntary movements of the limbs (especially fine finger movements), increased muscle tone (spasticity), hyperactive deep tendon reflexes, and the occurrence of pathological reflexes.

The terms *monoparesis* and *monoplegia* refer to a strength deficit in a single limb. *Hemiparesis* and *hemiplegia* refer to a strength deficit in one entire half of the body, while paraparesis and paraplegia refer to a bilateral strength deficit in the lower limbs. Finally, *tetraparesis* and *tetraplegia* refer to a strength deficit in all four limbs. Brachial or crural monoparesis and monoplegia reflect a unilateral lesion of M1 or the corticospinal tract contralateral to the affected limb or a homolateral spinal cord lesion. Hemiparesis and hemiplegia with facio-brachial-crural distribution result from a unilateral lesion of M1 or the corticospinal tract above the brainstem (e.g., internal capsule), while hemiparesis and hemiplegia sparing the face result from lesions of the corticospinal tract located between the medulla and the upper cervical spinal cord. If the lesion is located above the pyramidal decussation, the strength deficit will be contralateral to the lesion, while a lesion at the cervical spinal cord level will affect the ipsilateral limbs to the lesion. A characteristic feature of the upper motor neuron syndrome is the loss of voluntary movements of the lower part of the face with preservation of movements of the upper half of the face and emotional expressions. Paraparesis and paraplegia are secondary to a bilateral lesion of the thoracic or lumbar spinal cord. In the presence of paraparesis, a scissor gait characterized by crossing of the lower limbs maintained in adduction and extension (spastic paraparesis or diplegia) may occur. Lastly, tetraparesis and tetraplegia result from a transverse lesion of the cervical spinal cord. The strength deficit is assessed at the level of an individual muscle by asking the patient to voluntarily contract the examined muscle against the resistance of the examiner (see Table 1.2). The strength deficit secondary to a lesion of M1 or the corticospinal tracts is evaluated with specific functional tests in an anti-gravity position (see Table 1.3). For the upper limbs, the *Mingazzini's test* (see Figure 1.14) involves maintaining the upper limbs extended in a parallel position. If one upper limb is lower than the contralateral limb, it indicates weakness in the upper limb. Another test consists of asking the patient to extend the upper limbs in a parallel position with the palms facing upward. In the case of a strength deficit, the affected limb will manifest hand and forearm pronation. The Mingazzini's test for the lower limbs involves asking the patient, lying in a supine position, to lift the flexed lower limbs at a 90-degree angle and parallel to the ground. If one lower limb is lower than the contralateral limb, it indicates weakness in the limb. A subsequent test to assess segmental strength in the lower limbs is the *Barré's test*, which requires the patient to lift the flexed lower limbs while in a prone position. If one lower limb is lower than the contralateral limb, it indicates weakness in the limb.

The increased muscle tone during the upper motor neuron syndrome is defined *spastic hypertonia* or *spasticity*. Spasticity is examined by mobilising the patient's limb and assessing the resistance the limb involuntarily opposes to passive movement applied by the examiner. Spasticity primarily affects antigravity muscles (flexor muscles in the upper limbs and extensor muscles in the lower limbs) and increases proportionally to the speed of limb stretching until a sudden reduction in muscle tone is observed (the *"clasp-knife" phenomenon*). Spasticity is caused by an alteration of the stretch reflex, resulting from impaired suprasegmental control of spinal motor neurons excitability in response to Ia afferent input. From a pathophysiological perspective, it is believed that spasticity depends on the impairment of spinal inhibitory systems that act on the stretch reflex (reciprocal inhibition, Ib inhibition mediated by Golgi tendon organs, and recurrent inhibition mediated by Renshaw cells) due to altered descending influence from suprasegmental systems. However, an isolated and selective lesion of the direct corticospinal tract (at the level of the bulbar

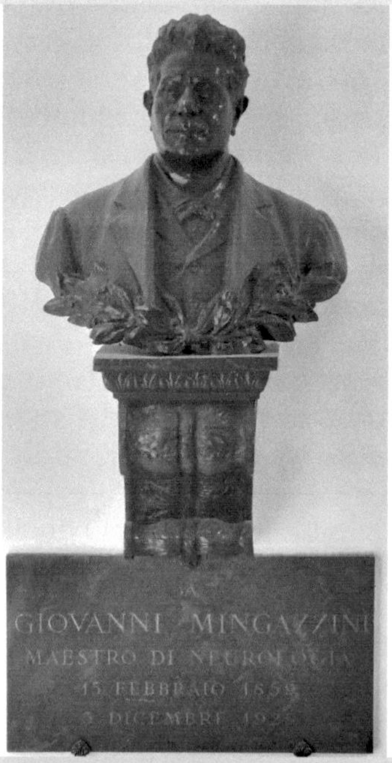

Figure 1.14

pyramids) does not result in spasticity but rather causes selective impairment in fine finger movements. Therefore, it is believed that spasticity is not solely the consequence of an isolated lesion of the corticospinal tract but rather reflects an imbalance between facilitatory and inhibitory mechanisms at the level of cortical projections to brainstem nuclei, where the motor descending pathways originate (reticulospinal and vestibulospinal tracts) that project to α and γ motor neurons. Specifically, spasticity is secondary to a reduction in reticulospinal projections, which normally have the physiological function of inhibiting α and γ motor neurons innervating antigravity muscles (or physiological extensor muscles).

In upper motor neuron syndrome, deep reflexes are brisk (*hyperreflexia*). The evaluation of tendon reflexes should always be done comparatively between the two sides of the body. Hyperreflexia is characterized by the presence of both ipsilateral and contralateral spread of responses and the extension of the reflexogenic area. Hyperreflexia can also be associated with the presence of a polysynaptic response, which is a repetitive response evoked by a single impulse. Of particular importance is the phenomenon of clonus, which consists of a sequence of rhythmic and involuntary contractions, either spontaneous or induced by a sudden and continuous passive stretching of a muscle and its tendon, often at the level of the patella or the ankle (patellar and Achilles clonus). Clonus can be either exhaustible or sustained. Also of semiotic interest are the *Hoffmann* and *Tromner signs*, which consist of hyperreflexia of the flexor reflexes of the fingers and hand. Hyperreflexia and spasticity gradually occur after damage to the corticospinal tract. Following an acute lesion of the corticospinal pathway, a paralysis with reduced muscle tone (flaccid paralysis) is observed, associated with transient areflexia below the level of the lesion; this condition is defined as *spinal shock* or *diaschisis*. Hyperreflexia shares, at least in part, the pathophysiological mechanisms underlying spasticity.

Table 1.3 MANEUVERS FOR THE CLINICAL EXAMINATION OF MUSCLE STRENGTH: ANTI-GRAVITY TESTS

Segment	Naming	Initial position	Deficit
Upper limbs	Mingazzini's test	Upper limbs maintained in horizontal position and the palm of the hand facing downwards	Flattening or dropping of the hand and limb
	Pronation	Upper limbs maintained in horizontal position and the palm of the hand facing upwards	Pronation of the forearm and elbow flexion
	Hollow hand	Flexed limbs with the palm facing forward and fingers spread and extended	Flexion and adduction of the fingers with the palm hollowed
Lower limbs	Mingazzini's test	Supine position with hips and knees flexed	Flattening or dropping of the limb
	Barrè's test	Prone position with knees flexed	Flattening or dropping of the leg

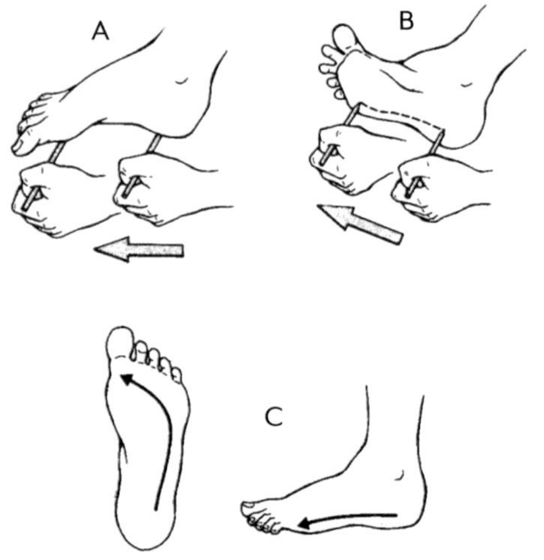

Figure 1.15

Plantar Reflex. A) Normal flexion response. B) Pathological extension response (Babinski sign). C) Optimal stimulation sites to evoke the plantar reflex, according to Babinski (left) and according to Chaddock (right) (courtesy of Prof. Mario Manfredi).

Other indicative signs of corticospinal tract impairment are *Babinski's sign* and *Chaddock's sign*, which consist of the appearance of an extensor response in the cutaneous-plantar reflex. This reflex is usually elicited by stroking the plantar or outer surface of the foot, from the heel forward in a curvilinear path (see Figure 1.15). The presence of a slow tonic dorsiflexion response of the big toe with fan-shaped opening or spreading of the other toes (*Babinski's sign*) indicates impairment of the corticospinal tract, which physiologically exerts tonic inhibition of the reflex. An abnormal response of the *cutaneous-plantar reflex* is sometimes associated with spinal automatism reflexes such as the triple flexion reflex, which consists of a slow withdrawal movement from the stimulus of the lower limb and sometimes also of the contralateral limb (crossed flexor reflex). If these reflexes are accompanied by tonic contractions of the abdominal muscles, bladder, and intestines, as well as other autonomic phenomena, *the Riddoch's mass reflex appears*. Repetitive and prolonged stimulation can lead to a fixed posture of triple flexion. The triple flexion reflex can be interpreted at least in part because of abnormal regulation of spinal mechanisms controlling the superficial avoidance or defensive reflexes. Another sign of pyramidal syndrome is the appearance of pathological synkinesis due to disinhibition, which refers to involuntary contraction concomitant with voluntary or reflex movements that are usually not present in healthy individuals. For example, an attempt to flex the thigh on the pelvis and the leg on the thigh in a patient with homolateral foot palsy results in the involuntary dorsiflexion of the foot (*shortening synkinesis of the lower limb or Strumpell's phenomenon*). Finally, in the upper motor neuron syndrome, superficial reflexes are reduced or abolished (e.g., abdominal reflexes and corneal reflex).

The disconnection between cortical motor areas and brainstem nuclei (usually due to bilateral vascular lesions) leads to pseudobulbar syndrome characterized by the appearance of dysarthria, dysphagia, and dysphonia. This syndrome is also characterized by the presence of signs of emotional lability (spastic crying and laughing) and motor alterations secondary to bilateral pyramidal syndrome.

A lesion that disconnects the brainstem from the cortex also results in characteristic changes in tone and posture secondary to brainstem control of muscle tone. In such cases, if the lesion spares the midbrain, the modulatory influence of the red nucleus on vestibular extensor tone determines a relatively

Table 1.4 MAIN CHARACTERISTICS OF PERIPHERAL AND CENTRAL PARALYSIS

Peripheral paralysis	Central paralysis
Reduced strength	Reduced strength
Reduced muscle trophism	Preserved muscle trophism
Reduced muscle tone (hypotonia)	Increased muscle tone (spasticity)
Reduced deep tendon reflexes (hyporeflexia)	Increased deep tendon reflexes (hyperreflexia)
	Presence of pathological reflexes (Babinski sign) and possible clonus

physiological distribution of tone with extension of the lower limbs and flexion of the upper limbs (decerebrate rigidity). However, if the lesion involves the midbrain and damages the red nucleus, the vestibular integrative level emerges, leading to an increased overall extensor tone and forced extensor posture (decerebrate rigidity).

The main semeiological signs that allow distinguishing peripheral paralysis from central paralysis are summarized in Table 1.4.

1.6.4 Signs and symptoms of non-primary motor area dysfunction

Apraxia

The injuries to non-primary (or premotor) and parietal motor areas (particularly in the left hemisphere), and in some cases, injuries to the corpus callosum and interhemispheric connections, result in an impaired ability to plan and execute motor acts and complex motor sequences, a condition known as apraxia (see also Chapter 4). Patients with apraxia do not exhibit motor, sensory, or attention deficits that would independently compromise motor performance. The assessment of apraxia involves requesting the patient to perform gestures based on verbal commands, imitate gestures performed by the examiner, use, or imitate the use of common objects, and execute complex motor sequences. This allows for the classification of apraxia into several main categories. Motor apraxia involves the inability to smoothly perform simple and habitual motor acts and is associated with reduced motor initiative. Ideomotor apraxia is the most observed form and is characterized by impaired execution of a gesture upon command, such as pantomiming the use of an object or imitating a gesture performed by the examiner, even though it is understood. Ideomotor apraxia primarily manifests when movements are generated from mental images (i.e., the inability to translate such mental images into appropriate motor actions), and interaction with external objects improves the execution of the movements. Ideational apraxia involves the alteration of the mental representation of a gesture or sequence of movements to be performed and manifests as an inability to understand and plan the movement, execute motor sequences correctly, and use common objects.

Other higher-order motor disorders

These are abnormal motor behaviors that result from dysfunction in the cortical processes preceding the execution of the motor action itself. Higher-order motor disorders typically reflect dysfunction in the frontal lobes, particularly the medial frontal areas and the cingulate gyrus (usually affecting both hands even with unilateral lesions, without hemispheric preferences). Among the most representative higher-order motor disorders are disinhibition disorders. These include, for example, the grasping reflex, which consists of an automatic tendency to grasp objects, characterized by a forced closure of the hand on the object, triggered by pressure on the palm of the hand. The behavior of grasping is a more elaborate phenomenon than grasping, in which the patient's hand follows a presented object, such as a tactile or visual stimulus, to grasp it. Utilization behavior is an automatic tendency to manipulate surrounding objects; in this case, patients use objects appropriately but in inappropriate contexts. Another disinhibition motor disorder is imitation behavior, where the patient imitates the gestures and behavior of others. Motor perseverations are inappropriate repetitions of a movement. A useful clinical test is the "clapping sign" (in this case, the subject is asked to clap three times after demonstration by the examiner. The sign is positive if the subject claps more than three times). Finally, paratonia, involuntary resistance to passive movement due to the apparent inability of the subject to relax, is also included among the so-called disinhibition disorders. The examiner come away with the impression that the patient actively resists passive movement (e.g., the patient's limb remains elevated after being lifted and then released by the examiner, even after repeated relaxation instructions).

Another category of higher-order motor disorders is represented by the so-called disorders of motor intention, namely *neglect* and motor impersistence. Motor *neglect* refers to the underutilization of the contralateral limb to the brain lesion (usually of the right hemisphere), which cannot be fully explained by sensory and motor deficits. Patients with motor *neglect* are not aware of their deficit, but if prompted by the examiner, they can perform the movement of the neglected limb. Motor impersistence is the inability to sustain a motor act (movement or posture) unless repeatedly requested by the examiner. Disorders of motor intention can have a significant impact on the patient's performance and recovery, although they generally tend to improve over time.

1.6.5 Signs and symptoms of basal ganglia dysfunction

In case of basal ganglia dysfunction, signs and symptoms can be classified into two main categories. The first is the hypokinetic or parkinsonian syndrome, a clinical condition characterized by bradykinesia, hypokinesia, akinesia, rigidity, and tremor. The second category is represented by the hyperkinetic syndrome, characterized by the presence of involuntary movements such as dystonia, chorea, tics, and other dyskinesias.

Bradykinesia refers to the slowness of voluntary movements, *hypokinesia* refers to the reduction in the amplitude of the movement performed, and *akinesia* refers to the inability to initiate the movement itself, in the absence of central motor pathway alterations. Bradykinesia, hypokinesia, and akinesia can affect movements of the limbs, trunk, and face. Therefore, the patient should be examined using specific functional tests (such as rapid repetitive opening and closing of the hands, rapid repetitive movements between the thumb and index finger, flexion-extension movements of the foot at the ankle, etc.) to assess the limbs. In particular, the bradykinesia present in Parkinson's disease is characterized by the progressive reduction in amplitude and speed of repetitive movements (sequence effect). This characteristic allows differentiation of the bradykinesia typical of Parkinson's disease from the slowing of voluntary movement observed in other motor syndromes, cerebellar disorders, and upper motor neuron syndrome. Bradykinesia, hypokinesia, and akinesia can also manifest as reduced and impoverished handwriting (micrographia) and automatic movements (e.g., facial hypomimia, reduced frequency of blinking, and reduced swinging of the upper limbs during walking).

Rigidity is characterized by an increase in muscle tone and is assessed by mobilizing the patient's limb and evaluating the resistance that the limb opposes to passive movement imposed by the examiner. Rigidity is generally constant during the passive mobilization of the limb under examination. It is independent of the speed of muscle stretching and is similar in both extension and flexion movements. These characteristics allow differentiation between the typical rigidity of Parkinson's syndrome and the characteristic spastic hypertonia of the upper motor neuron syndrome. One characteristic of rigidity is the *cogwheel phenomenon* or *trochlea*, which consists of sudden increases and reductions in muscle tone during passive extension or flexion of the limb. Rigidity should also be differentiated from paratonia, which is the inability to voluntarily relax muscles and is often found in the elderly but can sometimes be evident following diffuse brain injuries.

Tremor refers to the rhythmic oscillation of one or more body segments. Tremor is classified based on the frequency and amplitude of the oscillations. Tremor can occur at rest, during the execution of voluntary movements (action or intentional tremor), or during the voluntary maintenance of postures (postural tremor). Tremors disappear during sleep. Resting tremor is typically observed in Parkinson's syndrome and tends to decrease or disappear during voluntary movements. Postural tremor is typical of essential tremor. In rare cases, tremor manifests during the execution of specific motor tasks (e.g. primary writing tremor).

From a pathophysiological perspective, basal ganglia disorders reflect the alteration of motor and non-motor circuits connecting the basal nuclei and thalamus to cortical motor areas. Parkinson's syndrome is believed to be secondary to dysfunction of the direct pathway, resulting in increased pallido-thalamic inhibition and reduced activity of thalamo-cortical excitatory projections. Since the direct pathway plays a role in facilitating desired voluntary movement, an alteration in this pathway leads to reduced facilitation of cortical motor areas (see Figure 1.11). Consequently, bradykinesia, altered control of movement amplitude and velocity (*scaling effect*), particularly during the execution of sequential, simultaneous, and bilateral movements, reduced motor initiative, altered motor and postural adjustments during voluntary movement, diminished facial and gestural expressiveness, alterations in motor learning and complex cognitive-motor sequences and patterns can be observed. Rigidity reflects an alteration of suprasegmental mechanisms controlling muscle tone due to increased pallido-thalamic inhibition, as evidenced by changes in long-latency reflexes, or it may be secondary to a specific alteration in group II spindle afferents.

Tremor is the result of activity in one or more neuronal oscillators located in the central nervous system (basal nuclei, thalamus, brainstem, and cerebellum).

The involvement of basal nuclei in the extensive neural *network* that controls balance and posture justifies the appearance of postural instability in Parkinsonian syndromes. Postural instability is commonly assessed in a clinical setting using the pull test, which evaluates the motor response to a sudden backward pull exerted on the patient's shoulders while in an upright position with eyes open. Spontaneous loss of balance or only a slight backward pull indicates severe impairment of physiological postural responses, resulting in an increased risk of patient falls and associated comorbidities (fractures, hospitalization, immobility, etc.).

Hyperkinetic movement disorders

Dystonia is an involuntary and prolonged muscle contraction that results in repetitive twisting movements and/or abnormal postures. It can affect a single body part (focal dystonia), adjacent or non-adjacent muscle groups (segmental and multifocal dystonia, respectively), or the entire body (generalized dystonia). The term hemi-dystonia is used to indicate dystonia that affects one half of the body. Dystonia can occur at rest or during voluntary muscle activation. Sometimes dystonia manifests during the performance of specific motor tasks (task-specific dystonia). Often, dystonia can be associated with tremor.

Chorea consists of rapid, irregular, arrhythmic, and purposeless involuntary movements with variable amplitude and location. Choreic movements can randomly involve the muscles of the limbs, trunk, and face; they can occur at rest and typically accentuate during the execution of voluntary motor acts. The term *ballism* refers to a clinical condition characterized by the presence of involuntary movements of significant intensity and amplitude, primarily involving the proximal segment of the limbs. It is typically unilateral (hemiballismus) and often due to an acute ischemic lesion of the subthalamic nucleus and other medical conditions. Finally, *athetosis* refers to slow, sinuous, tentacle-like, continuous, or sub-continuous involuntary movements localized distally in the limbs and face. The term *dyskinesia* is used to indicate involuntary movements, generally of the choreiform, athetoid, or dystonic type. Dyskinesias are typically observed in patients undergoing chronic treatment with L-dopa (L-dopa-induced dyskinesias) or with dopamine D2 receptor-blocking drugs (tardive dyskinesias).

Tics are rapid involuntary movements, classified as simple if they consist of brief and stereotyped movements of a body part, or complex if they consist of sequences of movements. They reproduce movements or gestures from daily life (blowing, clicking the tongue, turning the head, touching the nose, etc.). Tics typically predominate in the face, upper limbs, and neck. One of the main clinical characteristics of tics is that they are partially controlled (reduced) by willpower and are preceded by an internal sense of urgency to move, which diminishes with the execution of the movement. Tics can manifest as sudden emission of sounds, words, or complete phrases (vocal tics). Motor tics can occur as isolated manifestations or represent one of the clinical signs of Gilles de la Tourette syndrome.

It is believed that hyperkinesias (dystonia, chorea, levodopa-induced dyskinesias) are determined by an increase in the activity of the indirect pathway, resulting in pallido-thalamic disinhibition and abnormal facilitation of thalamo-cortical activity. Since the indirect pathway is responsible for suppressing unwanted movements, alterations in the indirect pathway led to abnormal facilitation of cortical motor areas, resulting in the appearance of involuntary movements (see Figure 1.11). In dystonia, the most important pathophysiological alterations are represented by abnormalities in segmental control mechanisms (reciprocal inhibition, inhibitory brainstem circuits) and cortical mechanisms, which mainly involve alterations in synaptic plasticity mechanisms. Lastly, in dystonia and other movement disorders, there is an alteration in sensorimotor integration, a function necessary for the proper execution of voluntary movements.

Myoclonus consists of rapid and sudden movements, typically expressed as brief muscular contractions, but it can also involve a sudden absence of contraction, resulting in the so-called negative myoclonus (asterixis). Myoclonus can be classified based on spatial distribution (focal, segmental, multifocal, generalized), temporal distribution (rhythmic/arrhythmic, synchronous/asynchronous), and mode of appearance (spontaneous, action-induced, reflex stimulus-dependent). Myoclonus is typically accompanied by movements of the affected muscle region, unlike fasciculations and myokymia, where the muscular contraction remains localized without causing movement. Modern neurophysiological techniques allow for the classification of myoclonus as peripheral, spinal, subcortical, or cortical, depending on the site of origin. Peripheral, spinal, and segmental myoclonus stem from continuous or sub-continuous activity secondary to impairment or instability of excitability in the lower motor neurons or their axons. The topographic distribution of myoclonus helps differentiate peripheral myoclonus from spinal or segmental myoclonus. A particular example of spinal myoclonus is propriospinal myoclonus, which often originates at the level of thoracic segments and then spreads cranially and caudally to cervical and lumbar segments through the slow-conducting propriospinal fiber system. Patients with propriospinal myoclonus frequently present with continuous or sub-continuous myoclonus, causing flexion of the trunk onto the abdomen and the cervical region onto the trunk. Recent evidence suggests that some cases where involuntary movements suggestive of propriospinal myoclonus are observed may have a psychogenic origin. Finally, in some cases, myoclonic movements can be entirely physiological, such as during the falling asleep phase or in response to unexpected acoustic stimuli (e.g., the *startle reflex*).

1.6.6 Signs and symptoms of cerebellar disorders

The alterations of the cerebellar system result in a set of characteristic neurological signs and symptoms that constitute the cerebellar syndrome. The key elements of *cerebellar syndrome* are ataxia, hypotonia, and tremor.

Ataxia represents the impaired ability to coordinate the sequential activation of muscle groups involved in the movement of different body segments (limbs, trunk, oculomotor system, and speech), in maintaining posture, and in walking. It manifests in the limbs as altered amplitude and directionality of movement (dysmetria: hypermetria/hypometria), altered uniformity of movement due to disharmonious activation of muscle groups involved in movement (asynergia), and impaired ability to perform rapid and regular alternating movements repetitively (adiadocokinesia). Ataxia can also manifest as difficulty maintaining posture and the presence of rhythmic oscillatory movements of the trunk or head on the trunk (titubation) at a frequency of 3-5Hz.

Cerebellar alterations also result in dysarthria, which can manifest as slowed speech, alteration of prosody, and fragmentation of words into syllables (scanning speech).

The main alterations in oculomotion observed in cerebellar syndrome involve slow pursuit movements, which lose their characteristic fluidity and are replaced by movements with a characteristic cogwheel appearance. Saccadic eye movements generally overshoot the target (ocular hypermetria). Finally, maintaining gaze in an eccentric position (in all directions of gaze) leads to nystagmus.

Upper limb ataxia can be examined using the finger-to-nose test, in which the patient, starting from an abducted position of the arm with the elbow extended, is asked to reach the tip of the nose with their index finger and quickly return to the starting position (see Figure 1.16). Alternatively, ataxia

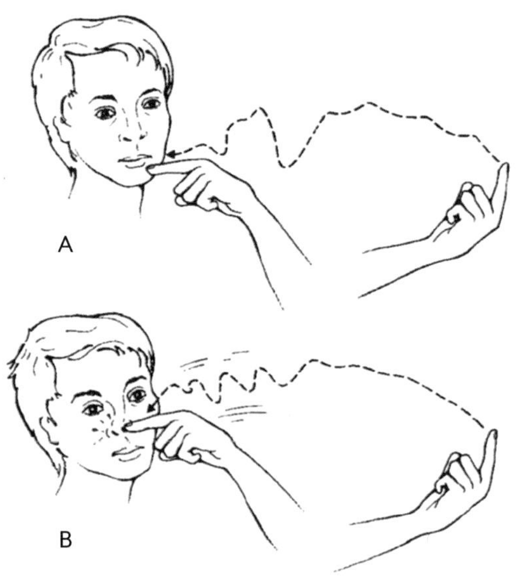

Figure 1.16

Finger-to-Nose test. A) Intentional tremor with dysmetria. B) Terminal tremor with hypermetria (courtesy of Prof. Mario Manfredi).

can be assessed by instructing the patient to alternatively touch their own nose and the examiner's index finger with their own index finger. Other tests involve evaluating rapid pronation-supination movements of the forearm (marionette test). Similarly, regarding the lower limb, the most performed test is the heel-knee test, which involves flexing the lower limb to position the heel on the knee of the contralateral limb and sliding the heel downward along the anterior surface of the leg and the back of the foot.

Postural control is evaluated by asking the patient to maintain an upright stance with feet together and upper limbs close to the trunk, or to maintain balance on one foot. Posture is initially assessed with eyes open and then with eyes closed. In cases of cerebellar dysfunction, instability is observed, characterized by difficulty in maintaining an upright stance and a tendency to widen the base of support by spreading the lower limbs apart. Additionally, multidirectional oscillations (lateral and/or anteroposterior) of the trunk are observed. The closure of the eyes is generally insignificant (negative *Romberg test*). The Romberg test is positive when significant deterioration in maintaining an upright stance is observed upon eye closure and indicates sensory ataxia, resulting from lesions of the posterior spinal cord (e.g., in tabes dorsalis) or peripheral nerve dysfunction.

Dysarthria is assessed by asking the patient to repeat words of increasing difficulty (e.g., territory, territoriality, extra-territoriality).

The slow pursuit eye movements are examined by inviting the patient to track a target that is moved in space by the examiner. Saccadic movements are examined by asking the patient to fixate on fixed targets placed in different positions in space. Nystagmus is evaluated by asking the patient to maintain gaze on an eccentrically positioned target.

The tremor that characterizes cerebellar syndrome can be either intentional, observed during the execution of voluntary movements approaching a target, or postural, manifesting when attempting to maintain a fixed position. Cerebellar tremor is a wide, coarse, irregular tremor of low frequency (3-5 Hz). It predominantly affects the limbs but can also involve the head and trunk. When present in the upper limbs, it is observed during the execution of goal-directed movements, such as the finger-to-nose test.

Cerebellar syndrome can clinically manifest with different characteristics depending on the location and type of damage. In general, lesions involving the midline structures, particularly the flocculonodular lobe, result in a syndrome predominantly characterized by altered eye movement, impaired upright stance maintenance, and gait disturbance, with minimal involvement of limb movement (archicerebellar or vestibulocerebellar syndrome). Lesions localized in the midline, primarily affecting the vermis, lead to a syndrome mainly characterized by trunk ataxia or impaired upright stance maintenance (like that observed in vestibulocerebellar syndrome) and gait disturbance (paleocerebellar or spinocerebellar syndrome). Finally, lesions predominantly located in the cerebellar hemispheres or cerebellar peduncles exhibit neocerebellar syndrome (or corticocerebellar syndrome), characterized by ataxia of the ipsilateral limbs; additionally, action tremor and lateral pulsion during gait towards the affected side may be observed. Regarding eye movement, there may be fragmentation of slow pursuit movements towards the side of the lesion, along with alteration of saccadic movements, which are hypometric towards the side of the lesion and hypermetric towards the opposite side; nystagmus may occasionally be present. Lastly, dysarthria is frequently observed in cerebellar syndrome. In cases of lesion in the olivopontocerebellar pathway, there is ataxia of voluntary movement in the upper limb like the impairment observed in lesions of the cerebellar hemispheres. Lesions of the rubro-olivary pathway, typical in brainstem lesions, result in the so-called myoclonus or more accurately (according to recent interpretations) palatal tremor, which is a rhythmic movement of the ipsilateral or bilateral palate to the side of the lesion.

In addition to motor symptoms and signs, it is now known that various neurological disorders characterized by cerebellar dysfunction can present the so-called *cerebellar cognitive affective syndrome* (CCAS) or *Schmahmann syndrome*, characterized by deficits in executive functions, language processing, spatial cognition, and affective disorders. The diagnosis of this syndrome relies on detailed neuropsychological assessments.

1.6.7 Additional signs of motor system involvement

Posture, facial expression and gait

The *attitude* concerns peculiar aspects of the body seen as a whole, with a global semiotic meaning. The *attitude* includes alterations in the appearance or posture of limited body regions such as the trunk, limbs (for example, hand and foot posture), and face.

Myopathies assume different aspects. For example, atrophy of the posterior spinal muscles and the pelvic girdle causes marked lordosis, delineating the *myopathic lordotic attitude*. Atrophy of the upper dorsal muscles results in the picture of *myopathic winged scapula*, in which the lower edge of the scapula becomes pronounced, especially when the upper limbs are extended.In specific cases of peripheral paralysis, peculiar attitudes related to different sites of injury can manifest. The *wrist drop* is defined as such due to its inert downward slope with flexion at the wrist, which occurs when the patient holds the forearm horizontally raised in pronation. It is mostly an expression of radial nerve involvement, root lesions, or lower motor neurons located in the anterior horns of the C6-C7-C8 myotomes, although sometimes this phenomenon may be a consequence of a lesion of the direct corticospinal tract (*central dropped hand*). Similarly, the *foot drop*, secondary to deficits in the extensor muscles of the anterior compartment of the leg, is positioned in plantar flexion both at the tibiotalar and midtarsal joints due to gravity. It originates from a lesion of the common peroneal nerve, root lesions, or lower motor neurons located in the anterior horns of the L4-L5-S1 myotomes. For further details on specific segmental attitudes, please refer to the chapter on neuromuscular diseases and neuropathies.

Hemiplegia is characterized by the upper limb in adduction and internal rotation at the shoulder and semi-flexion at the elbow, the hand pronated, flexed at the wrist, and with ulnar deviation of the fingers (hemiplegic hand). Additionally, in this condition, the lower limb is in extension at the thigh and leg with the foot hyperextended in supination and internal rotation.

Spastic-paraplegia is similar to the hemiplegic attitude but with bilateral distribution in the lower limbs, with pronounced adduction of the thighs, causing the knees to be in close contact and the foot in varus equinus.

In the *decerebrate rigidity*, the head is erect, the jaw is clenched, the trunk is in opisthotonos, the upper limbs are extended with the arm internally rotated and adducted, the forearm is pronated, the lower limbs are hyperextended and internally rotated, with the feet in equinism and varus, and the toes in plantar flexion.

The *decorticate rigidity* presents with an extended trunk, the upper limbs flexed at the elbow and wrist, the lower limbs internally rotated with leg extension and plantar flexion of the feet.

The *parkinsonian posturing* (Parkinson's disease) is typically characterized by a flexed head and trunk (camptocormia generally refers to severe cases of trunk flexion that disappears when the patient assumes a horizontal position), and sometimes on one side (Pisa syndrome).

The upper limbs are slightly adducted, with the forearm in partial flexion and slight pronation, the thighs in slight flexion on the trunk, and the legs in partial flexion on the thighs. The extensor type of parkinsonian attitude affects the upper and lower limbs and characterizes some forms of atypical or secondary parkinsonism (see Chapter on Movement Disorders).

Catatonia manifests as the persistence of sometimes bizarre and uncomfortable positions for a long period of time.

Hyperkinesia refer to abnormal and variable involuntary movements in terms of extension, affected area, range, intensity, rhythm, and frequency (choreiform and dystonic movements). For further details on tremor, chorea and athetosis, dyskinesias, dystonia, ballism, tics, myoclonus, fasciculations, and spasms, please refer to the respective chapters.

Different neurological conditions can determine characteristic *facial features*. *Myopathic facies*, observed in muscular disorders, present with a fixed and indifferent appearance, flattening of prominences and grooves, and a reduction or absence of facial muscle movements with difficulty or inability to speak, whistle, and blow. *Myasthenic facies*, seen in neuromuscular junction disorders, are characterized by smoothing of wrinkles, generally bilateral drooping of the eyelids (ptosis), compensatory overextension of the head, and possible strabismus. In the presence of a lesion of the seventh cranial nerve, there are facies characterized by flattened forehead wrinkles, wide-eyed appearance without blinking, flattened nasolabial groove, partially open mouth, and ultimately absent voluntary and reflexive facial mobility. In the case of lesions of the central motor pathways, the *facies* is characterized by oral asymmetry, with the affected side having a lower angle of the labial corner compared to the unaffected side, and reduced mobility during voluntary contraction. The different direct corticobulbar innervation of the facial motor neurons in the nucleus of the seventh cranial nerve, projecting to the upper facial muscles (bilateral and ipsilateral innervation) and lower facial muscles (exclusively contralateral innervation), explains the different clinical picture that *characterizes peripheral* and *central paralysis facies*. Moreover, in *central-type facies*, emotional expressiveness is preserved. *Hypomimic facies*, typical of Parkinson's syndrome, is defined by the fixed gaze associated with infrequent blinking, swallowing acts, and expressive oral language manifestations. *Hypermimic facies*, on the other hand, is characterized by involuntary movements that can take on grotesque aspects or grimaces, as in the case of choreic facies. *Wilsonian facies* is distinguished by a peculiar persistent and expressionless smile or a sardonic expression known as risus sardonicus. Similarly, tic-like facies is characterized by the presence of rapid, sudden, repetitive, stereotyped, gestural involuntary movements.

Walking is a complex motor act, mostly automatic, which requires the functional integration of segmental and suprasegmental motor systems. From an anatomical and functional perspective, locomotion is generated at the spinal level by the presence of distributed circuits at a multi-segmental level that are interconnected, capable of generating coordinated and automatic limb movements (*central pattern generators* - CPG). The activity of spinal CPGs responsible for locomotion is modulated by the activity of suprasegmental structures such as the reticular formation at the brainstem level, sensory and motor cortical areas (primary and non-primary), basal nuclei, and the cerebellum. In particular, the *mesencephalic locomotor region* (MLR), which includes the pedunculopontine, cuneiform, and subcuneiform nuclei, represents the most important suprasegmental structure for the control of walking and posture. The MLR constantly monitors the relationship between the body and gravity, allowing for the regulation of muscle tone and postural adjustments necessary for adapting walking to environmental and motivational circumstances. Deficits in any component of the motor system, from the muscle effector to the cortical control systems, result in an alteration of walking that often assumes localized and, in some cases, diagnostic characteristics. Neurological disorders of walking are observed in various clinical conditions characterized by peripheral and central nervous system impairment.

Gait disturbances occurring in myopathy involving the pelvic girdle muscles are characterized by the presence of a *waddling gait*, in which the pelvis, not being sufficiently anchored by the gluteal muscles to the supporting limb, tilts with each step. In the case of unilateral or bilateral paresis or paralysis of the muscles in the anterior compartment of the leg, secondary to peripheral nerve damage (common peroneal nerve) or lower motor neuron injury, a foot drop is observed, resulting in a steppage gait characterized by thigh elevation to avoid dragging and foot drop when the lower limb is projected forward.

In case of basal ganglia dysfunction, it is possible to observe *parkinsonian gait* characterized by slow walking, small steps, reduced arm swinging, and sometimes sudden accelerations (festination) and episodic *freezing of gait*.

In case of corticospinal tract or M1 impairment, a patient with hemiplegia presents a gait with the upper limb flexed at the elbow and adducted, in pronation with wrist and fingers flexed, while the lower limb is extended and adducted, with the foot in equinovarus position, that is, plantar flexion and inversion. This gait is called "paretic-spastic" and is due to the circumduction movement of the lower limb at the hip level (see Figure 1.17). Finally, bilateral involvement of non-primary motor areas can result in a gait characterized by a wide base, small hesitant steps, and is known as "*frontal gait*" or *gait apraxia*.

In case of cerebellar dysfunction, walking appears unsteady and irregular (ataxic gait) and is characterized by an expanded base of support; it is called "cerebellar ataxic gait." When the impairment is mild, it may only be evident during tandem walking. Like assessing maintaining an upright stance, walking is evaluated with both eyes open and closed. Cerebellar ataxic gait differs from sensory and vestibular ataxic gait as it does not significantly worsen with eye closure.

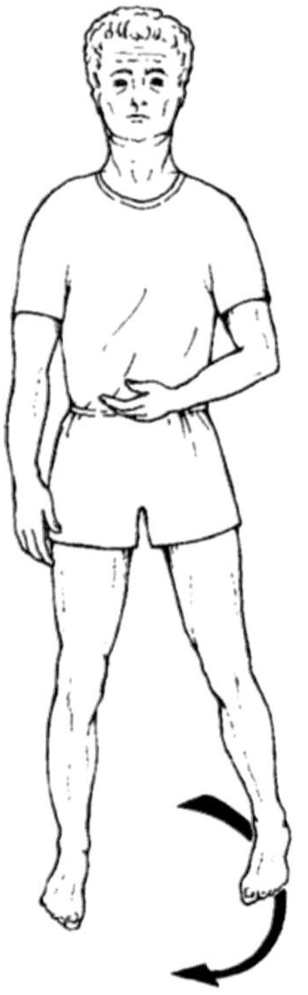

Figure 1.17

Paretic-spastic or hemiplegic gait. Note, in a patient with left hemiplegia, the flexed posture of the upper limb and the circumduction of the lower limb (with kind permission from Prof. Mario Manfredi).

Bibliography

Berardelli A., Neurophysiology of basal ganglia diseases. In Handbook of Clinical Neurology. Parkinson's disease and related disorders. Part I. Edited by W.C. Koller e E. Melamed, Elsevier, Vol. 83, 2007.

Brodal A., Neuroanatomia clinica. Edizioni Ermes, 1983.

Currà A., Agostino R., Berardelli A., Neurophysiology of Parkinson's disease, levodopa induced dyskinesias, dystonia, Huntington's disease and myoclonus. In Neurodegenerative diseases. Neurobiology, pathogenesis and therapeutics. Edited by M. Flint Beal, A.E. Lang e A. Ludolph, Cambridge University Press, 2005.

Fahn S., Jankovic J., Hallett M., Principles and Practice of Movement Disorders. Elsevier, 2011.

Gordon EM, Chauvin RJ, Van AN, et al. A somato-cognitive action network alternates with effector regions in motor cortex. Nature. 2023 May;617(7960):351-359.

Rothwell J., Control of Human Voluntary Movement. Chapman & Hill, 1994.

2 SENSITIVITY

Giulia Di Stefano, Andrea Truini, Giorgio Cruccu

The sensitivity can be distinguished into somatic and visceral. Somatic sensitivity pertains to the afferents originating from the skin, muscles, and joints. Visceral sensitivity, mostly not reaching consciousness, involves the afferents that come from the internal organs.

2.1 Somatic sensitivity

2.1.1 Functional organization

Somatic sensory information is transmitted to the cortex through afferent pathways consisting of a receptor, a peripheral neuron, and central neurons (Figure 2.1). Somatic sensitivities include tactile, vibratory, proprioceptive (sense of position and movement), thermal (warm and cold), and nociceptive (pain) sensitivities. The receptor selectively sensitive to a specific stimulus converts the energy contained in the stimulus into a change in membrane potential (receptor potential). When the membrane potential reaches a critical level, it generates a nerve impulse that is transmitted along the nerve fiber.

The peripheral sensory neuron consists of a pseudounipolar cell, with its cell body located in the sensory ganglia attached to the dorsal

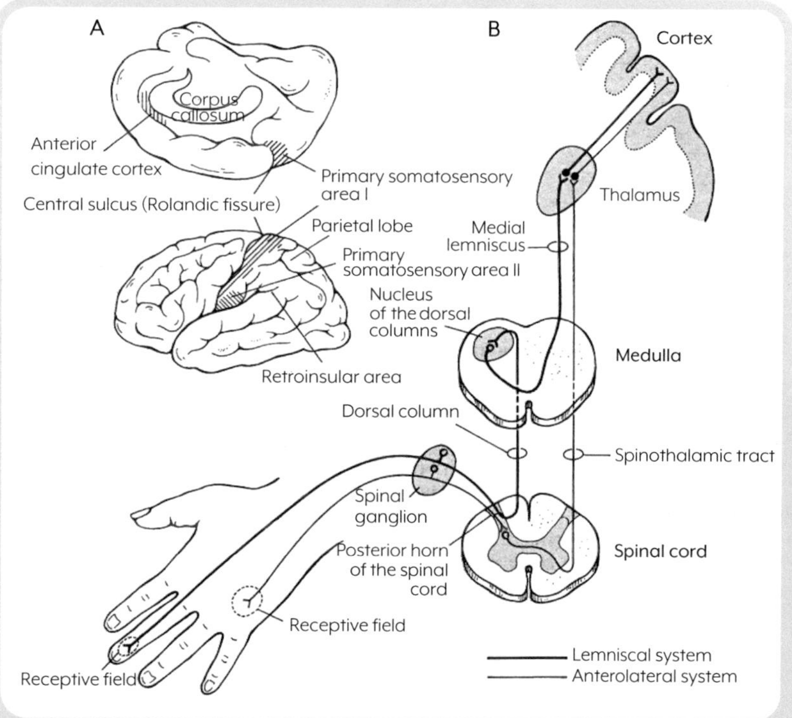

Figure 2.1

Somatic Sensory System.
A. Cortical areas.
B. Main ascending pathways.
Diagram of the neuronal chain that projects sensory input from the skin to the cortex. In both the anterolateral system and the lemniscal system, decussation occurs after the second neuron of the sensory pathway (courtesy of Prof. Mario Manfredi).

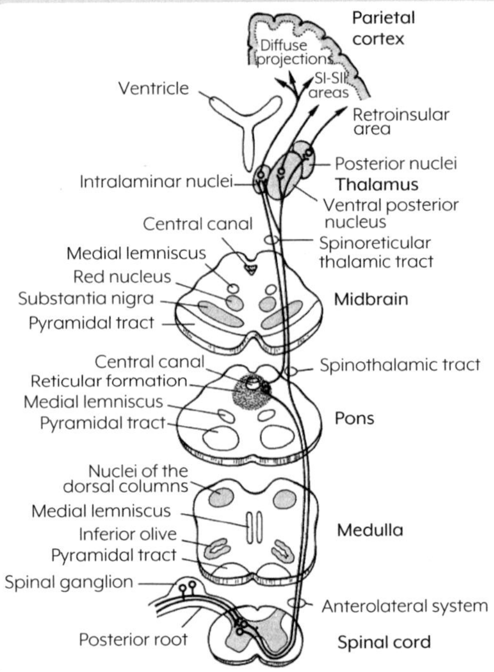

Figure 2.2

Anterolateral System. Spinotalamic and spinoreticulothalamic tracts (courtesy of Prof. Mario Manfredi).

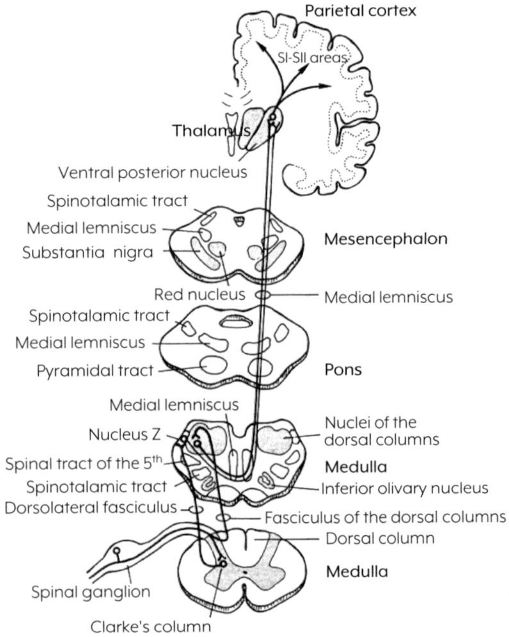

Figure 2.3

Lemniscal System. Bundle of dorsal columns, dorsolateral fasciculus, and medial lemniscus (courtesy of Prof. Mario Manfredi).

roots of spinal nerves or cranial nerves; the axon divides into two branches, a peripheral branch and a central one. The peripheral branch terminates with the receptor organ, while the central branch, through the posterior roots and sensory roots of cranial nerves, enters the spinal cord and forms synapses with the second neuron, located ipsilaterally in sensory nuclei of the spinal cord and cranial nerves. The axon of the second neuron forms synapses with the third neuron, located contralaterally in a thalamic sensory nucleus, from which cortical projections originate and terminate in sensory areas.

The somatosensory system is capable of detecting the modality, location, intensity, and duration of sensory stimuli. Modal discrimination arises from the receptor's specificity for a single form of energy and the presence of selective afferent pathways for specific sensations. Spatial discrimination, on the other hand, arises from the activation of specific receptive fields, which are regions that activate a particular sensory neuron, and from somatotopic organization from the periphery to the cerebral cortex. The various body territories are represented by a precise cortical map, albeit different depending on the receptor density. For example, the cortical area for the perioral region and the fingers of the hand are much larger than the cortical areas for body regions with lower receptor density, such as the chest. The intensity of the stimulus is encoded by the frequency of action potentials originating from the receptor (temporal summation) and the number of receptors that are activated (spatial summation). The minimum stimulus intensity capable of eliciting an action potential in an afferent fiber is defined as the "receptor threshold." Temporal discrimination is determined by the adaptation rate of the receptors. Receptors that respond to prolonged stimulation are called "slowly adapting," while those that are only activated at the onset and end of a stimulus, signaling its frequency and velocity, are called "rapidly adapting."

Somatic sensitivities can be classified into two distinct systems: the anterolateral system and the lemniscal system. The anterolateral system (so named for the localization of ascending fibers along the spinal cord) conveys pain sensations, thermal sensations (warm and cold), itch, and orgasm (Figure 2.2). It comprises small-diameter nerve fibers (Aδ and C fibers) with slow conduction velocity, wide and largely overlapping receptive fields. The spinothalamic, spinoreticular, and spinomesencephalic tracts belong to the anterolateral system.

The lemniscal system (so named for the pathway of ascending fibers within the medial lemniscus) conveys information related to touch, vibration, proprioception (sense of position and movement) (Figure 2.3). It consists of large-diameter fibers, Aα fibers and Aβ fibers, with fast conduction velocity. The dorsal column pathway and the dorsolateral pathway belong to the lemniscal system.

Thermal Sensitivity | Receptors for temperature consist of free nerve endings of Aδ and C fibers and are distinguished into receptors for warmth and cold. Cold receptors begin firing from 34°C, proportional to the rate of temperature reduction and the magnitude of the stimulus. Warm receptors begin firing from 32°C and increase their firing frequency with increasing thermal stimuli. When the temperature remains constant, thermoreceptors exhibit tonic activity, generating action potentials at a constant frequency depending on the detected temperature. If the temperature changes, the firing frequency of warm and cold receptors is altered, reaching their maximum level at temperatures of approximately 45°C and 25°C, respectively. Above 45°C, warm receptors cease firing, and a painful sensation is perceived due to nociceptor activation.

Pain Sensitivity | Pain sensitivity is mediated by mechanothermal receptors and polymodal receptors. Mechanothermal receptors linked to A fibers are activated in response to intense mechanical stimuli, increasing their firing frequency with the intensity of the stimulus. They mediate the sensation of acute and/or pricking pain that occurs following a noxious stimulus. These receptors also respond to temperatures above 45°C. Two main types of mechanothermal receptors linked to Aδ fibers are distinguished: Type I and Type II. Type I receptors, distributed in glabrous and hairy skin, have a higher thermal activation threshold and a lower mechanical activation threshold compared to Type II receptors, which are concentrated in hairy skin. Polymodal nociceptors, linked to C fibers, respond to painful thermal (starting from 39°C and 24°C), mechanical, and chemical (bradykinin, histamine, etc.) stimuli. They mediate the sensation of burning, prolonged pain that follows a certain latency after a noxious stimulus (delayed pain). C fibers also provide receptors that selectively mediate itch (Figure 2.4).

Tactile Sensitivity | Unlike thermal and pain sensitivity, tactile sensitivity is served by encapsulated receptors (mechanoreceptors) located in the dermis. In glabrous skin, Meissner's corpuscles, rapidly adapting, and Merkel's disks, slowly adapting, are responsible

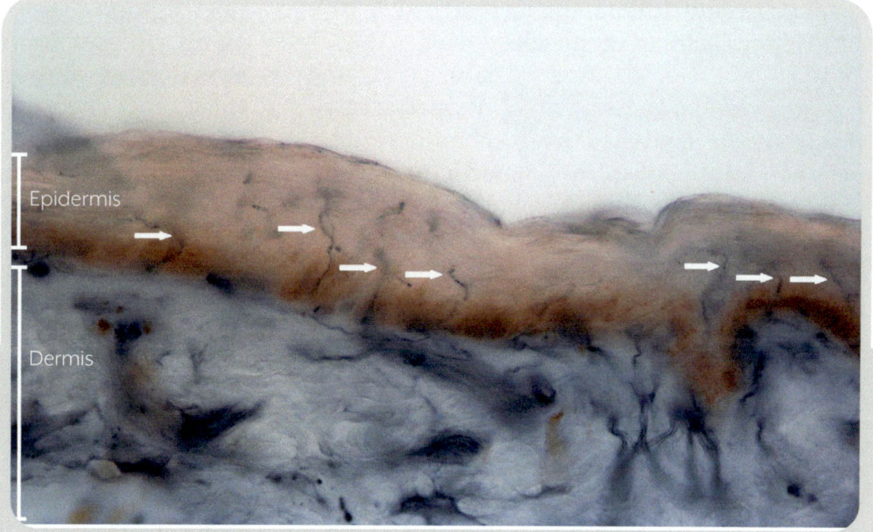

Figure 2.4

Photo under the optical microscope (40X) of a skin biopsy. The arrows indicate the free endings of Aδ and C fibers.

for discriminative tactile sensitivity. Meissner's corpuscles are small globular structures innervated by about ten axonal endings, located at the apex of dermal papillae. Merkel's disks appear as terminals of branching single axons, located in the center of the dermal ridge. They are often grouped together to form a single receptor organ called "Iggo's dome receptor." Epithelial cells transduce mechanical stimuli by establishing synaptic contact with nerve fiber endings. Both types of receptors have very narrow receptive fields (24 mm).

In hairy skin, the most represented mechanoreceptor is the follicular receptor, rapidly adapting and sensitive to hair movement. Deeper in the subcutaneous tissue of both glabrous and hairy skin, Pacinian corpuscles, rapidly adapting, are located. They consist of a capsule with multiple concentric layers of collagen fibers and specialized fibroblasts that envelop the fiber. Ruffini corpuscles, fusiform structures consisting of capsulated and multi-branched slow-adapting endings, are also present. These receptors are responsible for pressure sensation, contribute to the detection of more global properties of objects, and have much larger receptive fields than Meissner's and Merkel's corpuscles. Vibratory sensitivity, of great importance in clinical examination, is mediated by rapidly adapting mechanoreceptors (Meissner's corpuscles, Pacinian corpuscles, and follicular receptors). The preferred frequency of response occurs for stimuli of 10-100 Hz for Meissner's corpuscles and follicular receptors, and 100-400 Hz for Pacinian corpuscles.

Proprioceptive Sensitivity | Proprioceptive sensitivity is mediated by mechanoreceptors in the joint capsules, periarticular skin, and muscle spindles. Mechanoreceptors in the joint capsules are predominantly of the Ruffini type and signal the extreme degrees of joint excursion. Mechanoreceptors in the periarticular skin also signal the smallest joint movements and are involved primarily in the sensitivity of the small joints of the fingers.

Muscle spindles are provided with two types of sensory endings: primary or annulospiral endings innervated by Aα fibers, and secondary or flower-spray endings innervated by Aβ fibers. They signal muscle elongation and absolute muscle length and are responsible for the sense of position and movement. They also play a key role in the regulation of postural tone.

2.1.2 Peripheral sensory fibers

Peripheral sensory fibers are classified on the basis of their diameter, thickness of the myelin sheath, and conduction velocity. There are four categories of nerve fibers. Aα fibers are large-myelinated fibers (12-20 μm), with a conduction velocity of 50-120 m/s and are destined for the primary or annulospiral endings of neuromuscular spindles.

Aβ fibers are intermediate-sized myelinated fibers (6-12 μm), with a conduction velocity of 30-70 m/s, and are destined for the secondary or flower-spray endings of neuromuscular spindles and low-threshold mechanoreceptors in the skin, subcutaneous tissue, and joint capsules.

Aδ fibers are small myelinated fibers (1-6 μm), and C fibers are unmyelinated fibers (0,2-1,5 μm), with conduction velocities of 5-30 e 0.4-2 m/s, respectively. They innervate high-threshold mechanoreceptors, nociceptors, and thermoreceptors.

2.1.3 Spinotalamic tract

It is composed of Aδ and C fibers originating from thermoreceptors and nociceptors. The central branches of the axons of pseudounipolar neurons enter the spinal cord through the lateral aspects of the dorsal roots, run for a short segment in the Lissauer›s tract, and make contact with the second-order neuron located in laminae I, II, and V of the ipsilateral posterior horn. Synaptic transmission at this level occurs through the release of glutamate and peptide neurotransmitters from the central terminals of the sensory fibers. The axons of the second-order neurons decussate at the midline in the ventral white commissure and ascend in the anterolateral column of the spinal cord. They are arranged somatotopically, with fibers from lower segments located laterally compared to those from thoracic and cervical segments, which assume a more medial position. At the bulb level, the spinotalamic tract is accompanied by the trigeminothalamic tract, originating from the spinal nucleus of the trigeminal nerve and responsible for thermal and pain sensitivity of the contralateral half of the face. The spinotalamic tract terminates in three thalamic structures: the ventral posterior complex (ventroposteromedial and ventroposterolateral nuclei), which projects to the primary and secondary somatosensory cortex, the posterior complex, which projects to the retroinsular cortex, and the intralaminar complex, with diffuse projections to the cortex. The anterolateral system consists of pathways that project to the thalamus not only directly but also indirectly via the spinoreticular and spinomesencephalic tracts. Peripheral fibers belonging to the spinoreticular tract make contact with second-order neurons in laminae I, V, VII, and VIII. Some of the axons decussate at the level of the anterior white commissure to run in the contralateral anterolateral column, while others run in the ipsilateral propriospinal tracts. Finally, the axons project to the neurons in the brainstem reticular formation, which in turn project to the intralaminar and posterior nuclei of the thalamus and the hypothalamus. The spinomesencephalic tract from laminae I and V connects with various nuclei in the mesencephalic tectum, the periaqueductal gray, and the cuneiform nucleus. The periaqueductal gray and other brainstem structures, such as the raphe magnus nucleus, *locus coeruleus*, and ventral rostral region of the bulb, are involved in the descending modulation system of pain. Descending projections originating from these nuclei reach the dorsal horn and utilize opioids and monoamines (norepinephrine and serotonin) as neuromodulators, regulating the input of nociceptive information.

2.1.4 Dorsal Column Pathway and Dorsolateral Pathway

The Dorsal Column Pathway is composed of large-diameter myelinated fibers (Aβ fibers) originating from mechanoreceptors, as well as Aα fibers from neuromuscular spindles in the upper limbs. The axons of first-order neurons enter the spinal cord through the medial portion of the dorsal roots and then run in the ipsilateral posterior column. The axons in the dorsal columns also exhibit a precise somatotopic arrangement: fibers from the lower half of the trunk and the lower limb converge to form the medial gracile fasciculus of Goll, while fibers from the remaining rostral regions are arranged laterally and form the lateral cuneate fasciculus of Burdach. These fibers synapse with second-order neurons in the gracile and cuneate nuclei at the dorsal portion of the medulla. The axons of these second-order neurons decussate and run as the dorsal medial lemniscus dorsally to the pyramidal tract, and then reach the ventral posterior complex of the thalamus. In the pons, the medial lemniscus is joined by the trigeminal lemniscus, consisting of fibers from the principal nucleus of the trigeminal nerve, which carries discriminative touch sensations from the contralateral half of the face. At the ventral posterior complex of the thalamus, the ventroposteromedial (VPM) nucleus (VPL) receives mainly trigeminal afferents, while the ventroposterolateral (VPL) nucleus receives afferents from the remaining body regions. From the thalamus, direct projections to the primary somatosensory area originate.

The dorsolateral pathway carries muscle afferents from the lower limb. The afferent fibers separate from the gracile fasciculus and establish connections at the level of Clarke's column with second-order neurons, whose axons run in the dorsal spinocerebellar fasciculus. These fibers connect with the Z nucleus, located cranially to the gracile and cuneate nuclei. From here, some fibers reach the cerebellum, while another contingent projects to the thalamus via the medial lemniscus.

2.1.5 Cortical areas

Somatic information is processed at the cortical level through multiple levels of integration. The involved cortical areas include the primary somatosensory cortex (S1) or Brodmann areas 3, 1, 2 in the postcentral gyrus of the parietal lobe, the secondary somatosensory cortex (S2), and areas 5 and 7 in the posterior parietal cortex. S1 primarily receives tactile and proprioceptive information, mainly responsible for discriminative sensitivity, which involves recognizing the elementary characteristics of sensations. The subsequent processing of the message, carried out by neurons at higher integrative levels within S1, involves recognizing object shapes or sizes. Finally, a third integrative level occurs in areas 5 and 7, where mnemonic images of objects are formed. A lesion in each of these three levels will result in anesthesia (loss of sensitivity), astereognosis (inability to assess object shapes and sizes, despite maintaining the ability to recognize individual elementary sensations), and tactile asymbolia (the object is described in its physical characteristics but cannot be "recognized" as belonging to the same category).

Thermo-nociceptive afferents are transmitted to multiple cortical areas. Experimental studies have shown that the main areas related to pain perception are S1, S2, the insula, and the cingulate gyrus. It is hypothesized that while S1 and S2 are involved in discriminative processes, the insula and cingulate gyrus are involved in attentional and affective processes related to pain. As known, pain corresponds to a sensory and emotional "experience," associated with tissue damage or described by the patient in such terms.

2.2 Visceral sensitivity

Visceral sensitivity includes both painful and non-painful afferents, with the latter only partially reaching consciousness. Both types of signals are generally conveyed by unmyelinated peripheral nerve fibers, whose cell bodies are located in the dorsal ganglia. Some of these nerve fibers synapse with spinal neurons and form the basis of visceral reflexes. Others form synapses with neurons in the dorsal horn, and the afferent input is then transmitted via the spinothalamic tract to the thalamus and the nucleus of the solitary tract. The thalamus subsequently projects to the main somatosensory areas to provide, at least partially, conscious perception of visceral afferents. The nucleus of the solitary tract directly and indirectly projects to the hypothalamus, which represents one of the higher integrative levels of autonomic functions.

Compared to somatic sensitivity, visceral sensitivity exhibits a significantly lower level of topographic accuracy. A common example is referred pain. In the dorsal horn, the second-order neurons that receive visceral afferent fibers are shared with thermosensitive and nociceptive somatic sensitivity, and they project to the same thalamic and cortical neurons. For this reason, during a myocardial infarction, for example, the pain is felt in the shoulder or arm and is not precisely localized to the heart.

2.2.1 Sensory examination

Sensory examination requires adequate cooperation and attention from the patient. Stimuli applied to the patient for sensory testing should be administered irregularly, with the patient's eyes closed, comparing the affected area with a normal reference area (adjacent or contralateral symmetrical areas). It should also be noted that the somatosensory system undergoes physiological deterioration with advancing age. Therefore, sensory thresholds, as well as osteotendinous reflexes, particularly in the extremities, should always be considered in relation to the age-specific normal standards for the patient.

Thermal Sensitivity | The examination of thermal sensitivity is performed using two tubes: one containing warm water and the other containing cold water. The tubes are brought close to the subject's skin, alternated, and the patient is asked to recognize warm and cold sensations and assess the different intensities of warmth and coldness between affected and unaffected areas. In patients with neuropathic pain secondary to thalamic lesion, thermal hypoesthesia (especially to cold) is the most frequent and severe sensory disturbance.

Pain Sensitivity | For the examination of pain sensitivity, a pinprick stimulus is used. The patient is asked to report any differences in the intensity of perception between the affected area and a healthy area. It is also important to assess the preservation of pain sensitivity by alternating the punctate stimulus with a tactile stimulus. Since the overlap of adjacent dermatomes for small-caliber myelinated fibers (which mediate pain sensitivity to puncture) is much more limited than that of larger-caliber myelinated fibers, the study of pain sensitivity allows for relatively accurate delimitation of the hypoesthetic region (e.g., in radiculopathies). Although pain sensitivity can also be evaluated using other tools, such as the cutaneous or subcutaneous application of capsaicin (which activates polymodal nociceptors) or compression of muscle masses, these maneuvers are not commonly used in daily clinical practice.

Tactile and vibratory Sensitivity | Tactile sensitivity is assessed using a cotton swab or gauze, comparing the sensitivity of the affected area with a symmetrical normal reference area. Various tools can be used to evaluate the discriminative aspects of tactile sensitivity. Blunt-tipped calipers (Weber compass) can be used, or symbols (such as numbers) can be drawn on the skin with a blunt object for the patient to recognize. An alternative method for assessing spatial discrimination ability is the identification of the direction of stroking by a blunt object on the skin.

Vibratory sensitivity is examined using a 128 Hz tuning fork, with its base placed on bony prominences. The patient is asked to indicate the absence or reduction of vibration. Distal reduction of vibration (ankle, big toe) compared to more proximal territories is one of the typical signs in patients with distal axonopathy.

Sense of Position and Movement | The patient is asked to identify the movement or position applied by the examiner to the fingers of the hands and feet. Alternatively, the patient can be asked to reproduce a position imposed by the examiner using the contralateral limb. If there is a significant deficit in the sense of position, slow involuntary movements of the fingers (pseudoathetotic movements) and swaying in the upright stance (Romberg's sign) may occur.

Elementary Disturbances of Sensation | These include deficient sensory disorders such as hypoesthesia and anesthesia, as well as "positive" sensory disorders such as paresthesia, dysesthesia, and neuropathic pain. Hypoesthesia and anesthesia refer to reduced and complete loss of sensation, respectively. They can be either global, involving all sensory modalities, or dissociated, affecting only tactile and proprioceptive or thermal and pain sensation. Paresthesia refers to abnormal spontaneous non-painful sensations, often described as tingling or numbness. Dysesthesia refers to spontaneous or evoked unpleasant (but not painful) sensations, often described as pins and needles. Neuropathic pain refers to pain directly resulting from a lesion in the somatosensory system.

In addition to neuropathic pain, nociceptive pain and nociplastic pain are distinguished. Nociceptive pain is due to the physiological activation of nociceptors signaling actual or potential tissue damage. Therefore, all conditions that cause organ damage can produce nociceptive pain. Nociplastic pain, on the other hand, originates from altered nociception in the absence of evidence of actual or potential tissue damage or lesion in the somatosensory system. This category tends to include conditions such as fibromyalgia, a condition of chronic pain currently without a known cause.

2.3 Neuropathic Pain

The International Association for the Study of Pain (IASP) defines neuropathic pain as pain that arises as a direct consequence of a lesion or disease of the nervous system. A definitive diagnosis of neuropathic pain is based on the presence of a clinical history suggestive of damage to the somatosensory system, the presence of sensory deficits or positive symptoms with a congruent neuroanatomical distribution on clinical examination, and the presence of abnormalities in diagnostic tests confirming damage to the somatosensory pathway. Neuropathic pain is a commonly encountered condition in many peripheral and central nervous system disorders. Peripheral nervous system disorders, which are more frequently associated with neuropathic pain, include polyneuropathies (such as diabetic neuropathy), focal neuropathies of traumatic origin (such as brachial plexus injuries), and those following surgical interventions (such as intercostobrachial nerve neuropathy following breast surgery). Central nervous system disorders that are commonly associated with neuropathic pain include multiple sclerosis, post-traumatic myelopathies, and cerebrovascular disorders. This wide spectrum of etiologies explains the high prevalence of neuropathic pain in the population, estimated at 7-8%, with significant medical, social, and economic implications. Neuropathic pain encompasses two main types of pain: spontaneous pain, which is independent of stimuli, and evoked pain, which occurs in response to certain stimuli. Spontaneous pain can present as continuous pain, such as burning or compressive pain, or as paroxysmal pain, described as stabbing or electric shock-like pain. Evoked pain (allodynia and hyperalgesia), on the other hand, occurs in response to stimuli that under normal conditions would not activate the pain pathway, such as light touch on the skin (dynamic mechanical allodynia) or thermal stimuli (thermal allodynia). Evoked pain can also occur in response to stimuli that physiologically activate the pain pathway, such as mechanical stimuli that cause pain (hyperalgesia). The most common and characteristic forms of neuropathic pain include continuous burning pain, paroxysmal pain, and dynamic mechanical allodynia.

Burning pain is the most common form of neuropathic pain. Clinical studies report that the percentage of patients with neuropathy experiencing burning pain ranges from 50 to 90%. This type of pain is dependent on damage to the afferent pain pathway. In distal axonopathies, the damaged Aδ and C pain afferents of the peripheral nerve emit regenerative "sprouts" that are spontaneously hyperactive (a phenomenon known as "peripheral sensitization"). This spontaneous hyperactivity results in the sensation of burning pain reported by the patient. However, the mechanism underlying burning pain varies depending on the site of damage. In central nervous system disorders, this type of pain is more dependent on deafferentation. For example, damage to the spinotalamic tract in traumatic myelopathies causes spontaneous hyperactivity in deafferented thalamic neurons. Similarly, in patients with multiple sclerosis, burning pain is a consequence of deafferentation of thalamic and cortical neurons secondary to the presence of demyelinating plaques along the spinotalamic pathway.

The most common form of paroxysmal spontaneous pain is electric shock-like pain. Recent evidence suggests that this form of neuropathic pain is likely secondary to focal damage to large-caliber non-painful myelinated Aβ fibers. Specifically, following focal demyelination, Aβ fibers generate high-frequency action potential discharges, resulting in the perception of electric shock-like pain by the patient. Trigeminal neuralgia represents an exemplary condition of paroxysmal pain involving the facial region, characterized by intense and brief episodes of electric shock-like pain in the territory supplied by one or more contiguous trigeminal divisions, triggered by innocuous tactile stimulation of specific trigger zones. This particular type of neuropathic pain is caused by focal demyelination of the primary trigeminal afferents near the entry zone of the trigeminal root into the pons, either in an extracranial location as seen in neurovascular conflicts or benign tumors of the cerebellopontine angle, or in an intracranial location such as demyelinating plaques in the pons in patients with trigeminal neuralgia associated with multiple sclerosis.

Dynamic mechanical allodynia (pain with light touch) is one of the most characteristic forms of neuropathic pain. Stimuli capable of producing dynamic mechanical allodynia include the touch of a shirt on the chest in patients with post-herpetic thoracic neuralgia, or the touch of sheets on the feet in patients with diabetic neuropathy. There are two main mechanisms underlying dynamic mechanical allodynia, one peripheral and one central. In patients with neuropathy, peripheral sensitization of primary pain afferents, in addition to spontaneous hyperactivity, also involves an increased response to stimuli, including mechanical stimuli, by nociceptors. In patients with neuropathy, therefore, mild mechanical stimulation can activate nociceptors, whose mechanical activation threshold is abnormally reduced due to peripheral sensitization. An alternative mechanism of dynamic mechanical allodynia is central sensitization. According to this mechanism, the spontaneous hyperactivity of first-order pain afferents affects second-order pain neurons, resulting in sensitization. This central sensitization manifests as both spontaneous hyperactivity and a reduction in the activation threshold. This reduction means that even usually ineffective synapses, such as those with first-order tactile afferents, will be able to activate the pain afferent pathway. As a result of these phenomena, even stimuli that are not normally able to activate the pain pathway will be able to activate the spinotalamic system, generating pain. Both peripheral and central mechanisms can contribute to the development of dynamic mechanical allodynia.

Although in some conditions, a certain type of pain may be more common or characteristic (for example, burning pain in diabetic polyneuropathy, electric shock-like pain in trigeminal neuralgia, or dynamic mechanical allodynia in patients with post-herpetic neuralgia), in most patients, various types of pain and other sensory disturbances such as sensory deficits, paresthesias, and dysesthesias combine in different ways, producing different sensory phenotypes.

Different categories of drugs have proven to be effective in the treatment of neuropathic pain. These drugs can have different mechanisms of action. Topical drugs such as lidocaine or capsaicin reduce nociceptor activation, thereby reducing the phenomena of peripheral sensitization involving the receptor. Drugs like gabapentin or pregabalin bind to the $\alpha 2\delta$ subunit of voltage-gated calcium channels in the presynaptic terminal of the pain afferent pathway, reducing their conductance. This reduces the amount of neurotransmitter released from the first-order pain neuron and reduces activation of the pain afferent pathway. Tricyclic antidepressants or Serotonin-Noradrenaline Reuptake Inhibitors (SNRIs) or opioids, on the other hand, potentiate the descending modulation pathways of the pain afferent pathway. Drugs that block voltage-gated sodium channels (such as carbamazepine and oxcarbazepine) work by stabilizing neuronal membranes and inhibiting high-frequency discharges responsible for paroxysmal pain.

2.4 Sensory syndromes

They are classified, based on the site of the damage, into peripheral (see Figure 2.5) and central syndromes.

2.4.1 Peripheral syndromes

Nerve injuries | All sensory modalities are generally uniformly affected, and the sensory deficit involves the territory of the damaged nerve. Motor and autonomic fibers may also be involved.

Plexus injury | It presents with a similar pattern as the previous one but involves the territories of multiple contiguous nerves, resulting in variable hypoesthesia or anesthesia depending on the affected plexus and the extent of the damage.

Ganglion pathologies | They can be focal, as in the case of herpetic neuropathy, affecting one or more dermatomes, or they can be diffuse, predominantly affecting large-caliber fibers and causing a polyneuropathic distribution (as in the case of ganglionopathy caused by platinum derivatives or in Sjögren's syndrome).

Root lesions | They manifest with sensory disturbances in the territory of the affected root. Typical features include pain radiating in longitudinal bands along the limbs and transverse bands along the trunk, which is exacerbated by maneuvers that stretch the roots (e.g., neck flexion, thigh flexion with extended leg) or by increased endolymphatic pressure (e.g., coughing, sneezing).

Distal axonopathies | These are characterized by sensory disturbances with a distal and symmetric distribution (stocking-and-

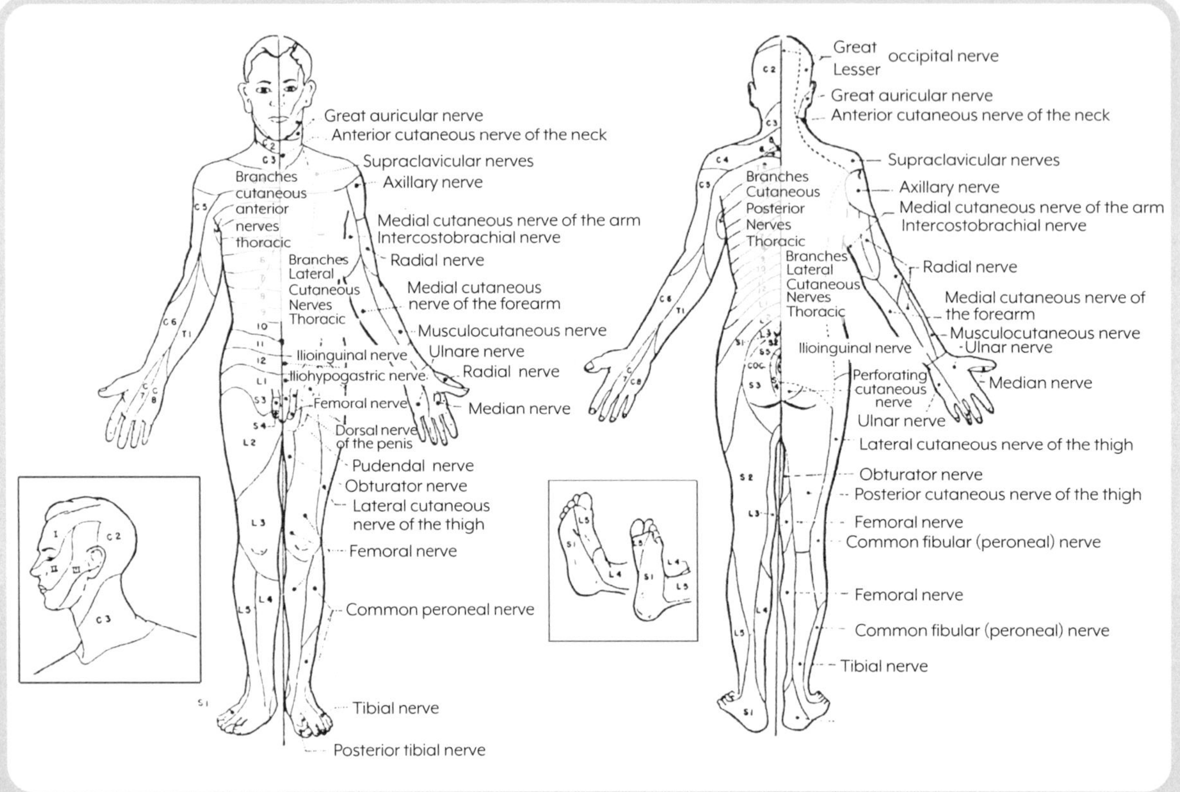

Figure 2.5

Skin distribution areas of the posterior roots and individual nerves. A) Lower left: distribution of the C2-C3 roots (Cl does not have a posterior root); B) left: distribution to the foot of the last lumbar and first sacral posterior roots.

glove hypoesthesia). This distribution is due to the fact that the pathological process primarily affects the portions of the axon farthest from the cell body, which are the first to suffer from reduced axoplasmic transport efficiency.

2.4.2 Central syndromes

Spinotalamic tract lesion | It presents as a dissociated sensory deficit with contralateral involvement of only thermal and pain sensations below the level of the lesion. Tactile sensitivity, proprioception, and the sense of movement are spared. This dissociation of sensations is known as syringomyelic. Due to the ascension of peripheral fibers in Lissauer's tract before synapsing in the posterior horn and before crossing over, the deficit spares 2-3 dermatomes immediately below the lesion.

Posterior column lesion | It causes impairment of discriminative touch, vibratory sensation, and proprioception on the same side as the lesion (because the crossing of the sensory pathway occurs rostrally, after the synapse with the second neuron). This type of sensory dissociation is known as "tabetic" because it was originally described in tabes dorsalis. A lesion of the posterior columns at the cervical level, with demyelination of large-caliber fibers, can lead to the formation of high-frequency ectopic discharges along the fibers, resulting in Lhermitte's sign (a lightning-like sensation or electric shock associated with movements involving neck flexion and radiation along the trunk and limbs).

Brown-Séquard syndrome | It is caused by a hemisection of the spinal cord. It manifests in the areas of the body below the lesion, with contralateral involvement of the anterolateral sensations and deficits in lemniscal sensations and pyramidal signs ipsilaterally.

Syringomyelic syndrome | It is caused by a lesion at the level of the anterior white commissure, where the thermoreceptive and nociceptive fibers destined for the contralateral spinotalamic tract decussate. It results in a dissociated and suspended hypoanesthesia selectively affecting thermal sensations in the cutaneous territories of the affected metameres. If the lesion extends to the descending trigeminal root nucleus, the sensory disturbance affects the face from the periphery, with an extension in concentric circles.

Transverse section of the spinal cord | All sensory modalities are compromised below the lesion. The level of thermal and nociceptive sensations is 2-3 dermatomes below the level of the lesion.

Lesion of the lateral portion of the medulla | It involves the spinotalamic tract and the spinal trigeminal nucleus, resulting in an alternate sensory syndrome with thermal and pain anesthesia in the contralateral hemisoma and in the ipsilateral facial side, relative to the site of the lesion. The involvement of other structures such as the spinocerebellar and olivocerebellar tracts, the direct pathway to the ciliospinal nucleus, vestibular nuclei, and vagal fibers constitutes Wallenberg's syndrome. In addition to the alternate sensory syndrome, it is accompanied by vertigo and ipsilateral cerebellar alterations, Horner's syndrome, and paralysis of the pharyngeal muscles, palatal muscles, and vocal cords.

Thalamic lesions | They cause sensory deficits extending to the contralateral hemisoma. They may be associated with hyperpathia, hemiparesis, hemiataxia, hemitremor, choreoathetoid movements, and homonymous lateral hemianopsia (Déjerine-Roussy syndrome).

Subcortical lesions | Similarly to thalamic lesions, they manifest with sensory deficits in the contralateral hemisoma.

Postrolandic cortex lesions | They present with deficits in sensation in a circumscribed territory of the contralateral hemisoma, corresponding to the cortical area of somatotopic representation involved. The proximity between the face area and the hand area explains the frequent association of deficits in these two areas (cheiro-oral distribution). Discriminative aspects of sensation, such as tactile localization and graphesthesia, are particularly affected. A characteristic manifestation of lesions in the parietal lobe is the phenomenon of extinction, which refers to the inability to perceive a stimulus presented simultaneously on both sides when there is a lesion in the cortical area. Irritative lesions can produce paroxysmal sensory symptoms during a partial epileptic seizure with elementary sensory symptoms.

Bibliography

Cruccu G, Di Stefano G, Truini A. Trigeminal Neuralgia. N Engl J Med.; 383(8):754-762, 2020.

Kandel E.R., Schwartz J.H., Jessell T.M., Principi di neuroscienze. Casa Editrice Ambrosiana, 2003.

Pertovaara A., Almeida A., Chapter 13 Descending inhibitory systems. Handb Clin Neurol; 81:179-92, 2006.

Truini A., Leone C., Di Stefano G., Biasiotta A., La Cesa S., Teofoli P., Padua L., Cruccu G., Topographical distribution of warmth, burning and itch sensations in healthy humans. Neurosci Lett; 494(2):165-8, 2011.

Truini A., Garcia-Larrea L., Cruccu G. Reappraising neuropathic pain in humans-how symptoms help disclose mechanisms. Nat Rev Neurol; 9(10):572-82, 2013.

Villanueva L., LopezAvila A., Monconduit L., Chapter 8 Ascending nociceptive pathways. Handb Clin Neurol; 81:93-102, 2006.

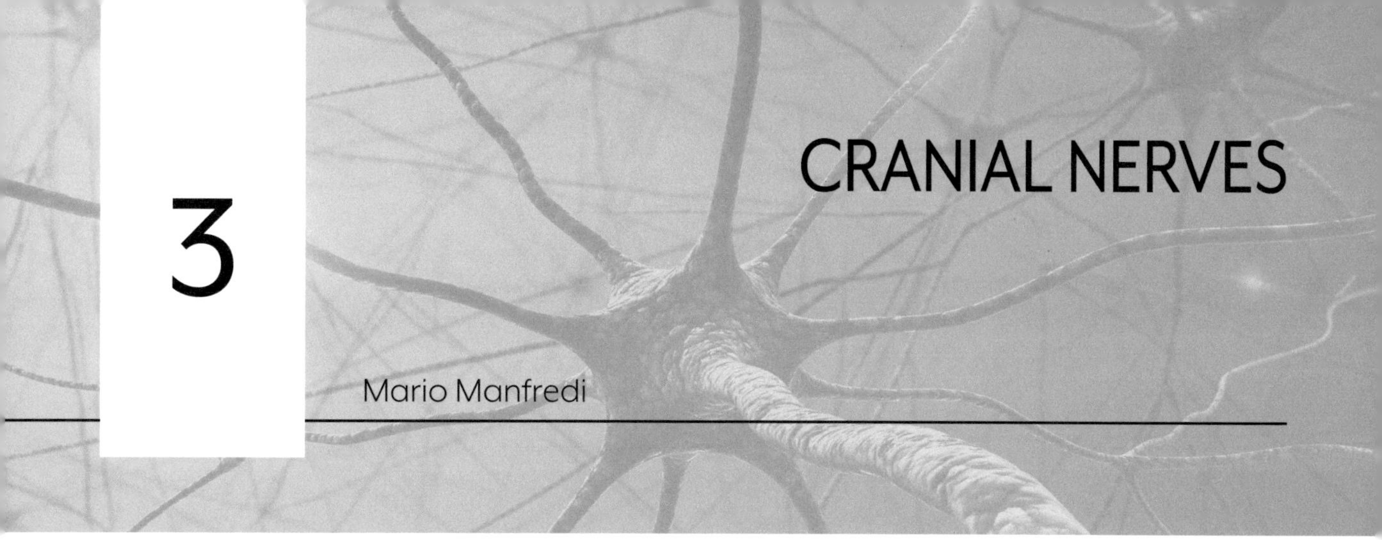

3 CRANIAL NERVES

Mario Manfredi

The cranial nerves are 12 and they share the common feature of exiting through the bony channels of the skull. They are numbered in a cranio-caudal sequence.

Table 3.1 CRANIAL NERVES

Denomination	Exit canal
1st Olfactory	Cribriform plate of the ethmoid bone
2nd Optic	Optic canal
3rd Oculomotor	Superior orbital fissure
4th Trochlear	Superior orbital fissure
5th Trigeminal	Superior orbital fissure (1st branch, ophthalmic) Foramen rotundum (2nd branch, maxillary) Foramen ovale (3rd branch, mandibular)
6th Abducens	Superior orbital fissure
7th Facial	Internal acoustic meatus
8th Acoustic (Vestibular and Cochlear)	Internal acoustic meatus
9th Glossopharyngeal	Posterior lacero foramen
10th Vagus	Posterior lacero foramen
11th Spinal Accessory (Accessory Nerve)	Posterior lacero foramen
12th Hypoglossal	Hypoglossal canal

3.1 Functional organization of the cranial nerves

Like the spinal nerves, the cranial nerves are composed of *afferent* (*sensory*) and efferent (motor and autonomic) axons.

The *afferent axons* originate from neurons in the sensory ganglia along the course of the nerves. Their extension divides into two branches: the peripheral branch travels along the nerve to the periphery, while the central branch terminates in a sensory nucleus in the brainstem. They possess *general somatic components*, such as the skin of the face, and *special somatic components*, such as hearing. They also have *general visceral components for the sensitivity of internal organs and special components, such as taste* (Figure 3.1A).

The *afferent axons* originate from nuclei in the brainstem and also have *somatic components* (e.g., those destined for the lingual muscles) and *visceral components* (responsible for autonomic functions, such as salivary gland secretion) Somatic efferents terminate directly on muscles, while visceral efferents terminate in autonomic ganglia located near the viscera. There is also a *special component* for efferent axons, consisting of muscles derived from branchial arches (e.g., swallowing muscles), which is considered visceral (lacking the special somatic efferent component) (Figure 3.1A).

Apart from the olfactory and optic nerves, which have a peculiar origin, the sensory, motor, and autonomic nuclei of the brainstem are organized into vertical columns derived from the primitive neural tube. This arrangement is maintained in the spinal cord, where the *sensory cell columns* are located posteriorly and the motor columns are located anteriorly. The autonomic nuclear column develops in the intermediate position.

The *visceral structures* (intermediate structures), consist of the sensory column of the solitary nucleus (glossopharyngeal, vagus, and accessory) laterally and the motor column of the dorsal motor nuclei (vagus), inferior salivatory (glossopharyngeal), superior

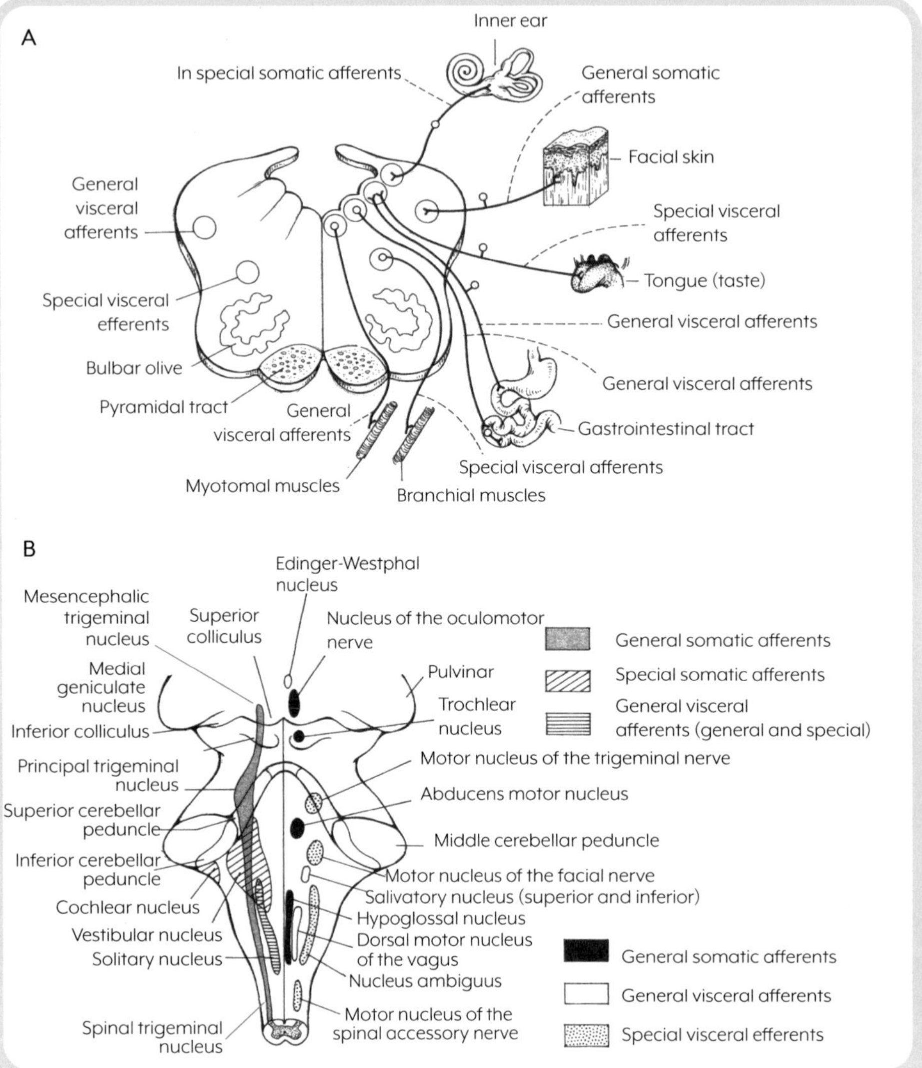

Figure 3.1

Cranial Nerve Nuclei. A) Cross-section of the brainstem with functional components and main functions. B) Top view of the brainstem with sensory nuclei (on the left) and motor nuclei (on the right). (Modified from Ranson and Clark, 1959, and Brodal, 1965).

salivatory (facial), and Edinger-Westphal (oculomotor) medially.

The olfactory (1st) and optic (2nd) nerves are unique. They do not originate from the brainstem but develop from the telencephalon. The olfactory nerve arises from neurons in the olfactory mucosa, while the optic nerve arises from ganglion cells in the retina and is considered a central tract. They can be regarded as special senses, with the olfactory nerve being visceral and the optic nerve being somatic.

The *functional components* of the cranial nerves are as follows:

a) *General somatic afferent fibers*: They originate from the jugular (vagus), superior (glossopharyngeal), geniculate (facial), and Gasser's semilunar ganglia (trigeminal). They innervate a small part of the skin of the auricle, the mucous membranes of the mouth, nose, paranasal sinuses, pharynx, larynx, the facial skin, and the cranial meninges. The central axons terminate in the complex of the trigeminal nuclei.
b) *Special somatic afferent fibers*: They originate from the Scarpa's vestibular ganglion and Corti's cochlear ganglion (acoustic nerve). They innervate the labyrinth and cochlea and underlie the senses of balance and hearing. The central axons terminate in the vestibular and cochlear nuclei. The optic nerve is included in this component.

c) *General visceral afferent fibers*: They originate from the nodose (vagus) and petrosal (glossopharyngeal) ganglia for the sensitivity of the thoracic and abdominal viscera and carotid baroreceptors. The central axons terminate in the solitary nucleus.
d) *Special visceral afferent fibers*: They originate from the neurons of the nodose (vagus), petrosal (glossopharyngeal), and geniculate (facial) ganglia and underlie gustatory sensitivity. The central axons terminate in the solitary nucleus. The olfactory nerve is included in this component.
e) *General somatic efferent fibers*: They originate from the hypoglossal nucleus and the three oculomotor nuclei (abducens, trochlear, and oculomotor). They innervate the tongue muscles and the extrinsic ocular muscles.
f) *General visceral efferent fibers*: They originate from the dorsal motor nucleus (vagus), inferior salivatory nucleus (glossopharyngeal), superior salivatory nucleus (facial), and Edinger-Westphal nucleus (oculomotor). They provide parasympathetic innervation to the thoracic and abdominal viscera, salivary and lacrimal glands, and the intrinsic eye muscles.
g) *Special visceral efferent fibers*: They originate from the accessory nucleus (spinal accessory), ambiguous nucleus (accessory of the vagus, vagus, and glossopharyngeal), facial motor nucleus, and trigeminal motor nucleus. They innervate the musculature derived from branchial arches, including the sternocleidomastoid and trapezius muscles, muscles of phonation, swallowing, facial expression, and mastication.

The nerves will be discussed based on their functional affinities:

- Olfaction and taste (olfactory nerve; special visceral afferent fibers of the glossopharyngeal, vagus, and accessory nerves);
- Sensation and motor function of the face (trigeminal and facial nerves);
- Neuro-ophthalmology: vision (optic nerve and visual pathways) and extrinsic and intrinsic ocular motility (oculomotor, trochlear, and abducens nerves);
- Neurotology: balance and hearing (acoustic nerve);
- Bulbar functions (glossopharyngeal, vagus, accessory, and hypoglossal nerves).

3.2 Olfaction and taste

They are chemical senses, based on the contact between the molecules of the stimulus substance and the receptor, and they underlie common functions related to food and reproduction. Additionally, they constitute a defensive mechanism against many respiratory and food-related intoxications. Odors are perceived without involving taste, while tastes have an important olfactory component, and the loss of smell also compromises taste sensitivity

3.2.1 Smell (olfactory nerve, 1st cranial nerve)

The *olfactory epithelium* occupies the apex of the nasal cavities. It *contains olfactory* neurons, bipolar cells with peripheral extensions that serve as receptors and central unmyelinated extensions, gathered in approximately 20 nerve bundles (the olfactory nerve). These bundles pass through the cribriform plate of the ethmoid bone and terminate in the olfactory bulb, where they make contact with the dendrites of *mitral cells* in the olfactory glomeruli (Figure 3.2).

The axons of mitral cells form the olfactory tract, which travels through the *olfactory sulcus* of the frontal bone and projects to the anterior olfactory nucleus, the olfactory tubercle, the amygdala, and the piriform and entorhinal cortices, where conscious perception of odors occurs. Secondary projections reach the medial dorsal nucleus of the thalamus, the orbitofrontal cortex, and the hippocampus, and are involved in odor memory and the emotional component of odors. Projections to the hypothalamus and the autonomic nuclei of the brainstem support autonomic reactions to odors (salivary and gastric secretion, nausea, etc.).

Molecules of odorants, carried by the air, diffuse into the mucus and activate the receptor cells. To assess the *sense of smell*, it is necessary to use pure and non-irritating odors

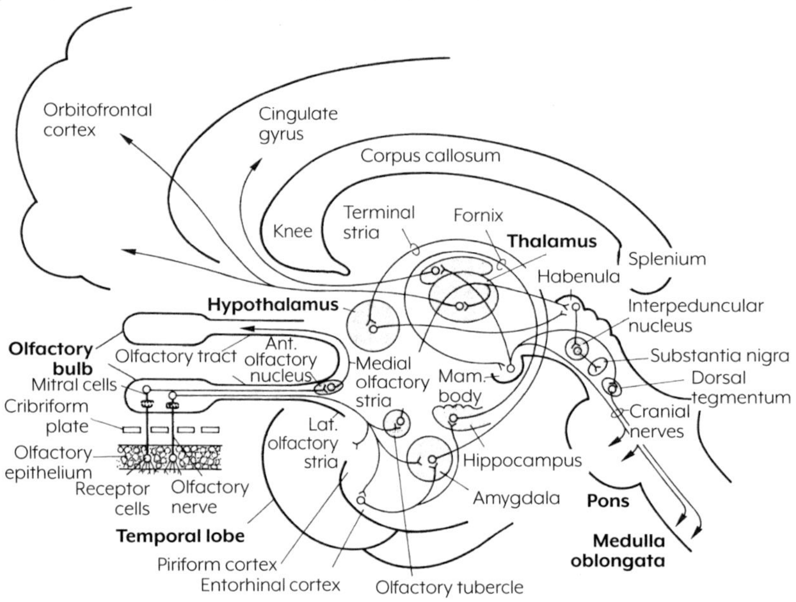

Figure 3.2

Olfactory System Connections. The central extensions of the receptor cells located in the olfactory mucosa constitute the olfactory nerve. The central pathway originates from the mitral cells of the olfactory bulb and terminates in the primary olfactory areas (temporal cortex and frontal orbit), directly and through the olfactory tubercle and the dorsomedial nucleus of the thalamus, for conscious perception of odors; in the amygdala, hippocampus, and hypothalamus for emotional and vegetative reactions to odors.

(such as coffee, orange peel, dried mushrooms, vanilla sugar, commercial perfumes, laundry soap, etc.). The substance is inhaled through one nostril, while manually occluding the other nostril, which can be tested after half a minute. For specific studies, "scratch-and-sniff" cards with encapsulated odors in microcrystals are used.

Disorders of the sense of smell include *hyposmia* and *anosmia* (reduced and loss of smell), *dysosmia* (distorted sense of smell) and *olfactory hallucinations*. Anosmia, often unnoticed when unilateral, becomes significantly bothersome when bilateral, as it greatly diminishes the pleasure of food and exposes individuals to occasional risks in contaminated environments (such as gas leaks). The main causes are listed in Table 3.2.

Certain nasal pathologies, identifiable through local examination, can cause anosmia due to direct damage to the olfactory epithelium. The most common cause of persistent anosmia is head trauma, which mechanically damages the bundles of the olfactory nerve anchored to the ethmoid bone, the fracture of which can be indicated by cerebrospinal fluid leakage from the nose. Traumas in the occipital region pose a higher risk, while recovery, which is common in mild traumas, occurs within the first few weeks.

Table 3.2 CAUSES OF HYPOSMIA AND ANOSMIA

Nasal issues	
Bilateral obstructions of the airways	Acute viral or allergic rhinitis Intranasal polyps Ethmoidal sinusitis Paranasal and nasopharyngeal carcinomas
Olfactory mucosa injuries	Chronic rhinitis Excessive smoking
Olfactory neuron injuries	Viral infections
Intracranial	
Cranial traumas	Strain or tearing of the olfactory nerves Fractures of the cribriform plate Hematomas at the base of the anterior cranial fossa
Tumors	Meningiomas of the olfactory groove, tuberculum sellae, and sphenoid wing Craniopharyngiomas Tumors of the frontal lobe
Infections	Meningitis of the anterior cranial fossa base Abscesses from osteomyelitis of the frontal bones
Vascular diseases	Giant aneurysms of the anterior communicating and anterior cerebral arteries Obstruction of the anterior cerebral arteries
Degenerative diseases	Parkinson's disease Parkinsonisms Alzheimer's disease
Congenital conditions	
Pandysautonomia	
Hysterical or simulated	

Some neurodegenerative diseases, such as Parkinson's disease, parkinsonism, and Alzheimer's disease, often present with a loss of smell, which should be specifically investigated. In *hysterical or feigned anosmia*, it can be useful to expose patients to impure odors, such as ammonia, which activates trigeminal pain receptors and is always detected in organic forms but may be denied in factitious disorders.

Dysosmia can occur in all nasal pathologies that cause anosmia. *Olfactory hallucinations* can occur during epileptic seizures involving the olfactory cortex.

3.2.2 Taste (facial, glossopharyngeal, and vagus nerves; 7th, 9th, and 10th cranial nerves)

Taste buds are formed by receptor cells arranged like segments of an orange and equipped with cilia that protrude towards a pore at the apex of the taste bud, which opens onto the lingual mucosa. They are concentrated on the tip of the tongue, corresponding to the fungiform papillae, along the edges in the foliate papillae, and at the base in the vallate papillae. There are also receptors on the soft palate and in the pharyngeal wall. The receptor cells are continuously regenerated but decrease with aging. They are innervated by three nerves (Figure 3.3): the *facial nerve* (7th) for the anterior two-thirds of the tongue, the *glossopharyngeal nerve* (9th) for the posterior one-third, and the vagus nerve (10th) for the palate and pharynx.

The *fibers of the facial nerve* originate from the geniculate ganglion. The peripheral extensions travel along the nerve until the descending portion of the intrapetrous canal, where they separate with the chorda tympani and reach the lingual branch of the trigeminal nerve, through which they reach the lingual mucosa. The central extensions enter the brainstem with the intermediate branch of the facial nerve. The *fibers of the glossopharyngeal nerve* originate from the petrous ganglion and travel along the nerve both peripherally and centrally to the brainstem. *The fibers of the vagus nerve* originate from the nodose ganglion: the peripheral extensions leave the main

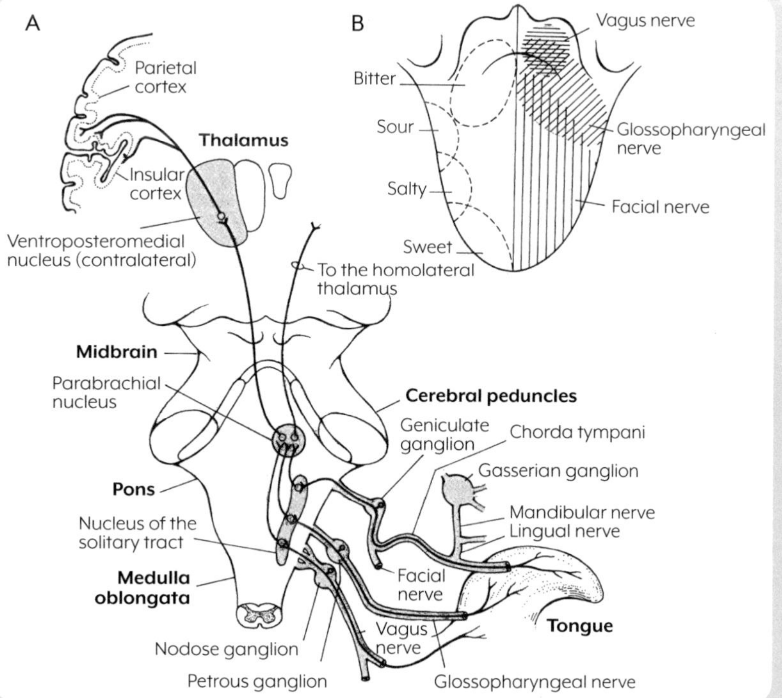

Figure 3.3

Gustatory Innervation of the Tongue. A) Gustatory Pathways. Afferent fibers from the geniculate, petrous, and nodose ganglia terminate in the nucleus of the solitary tract; from there, the pathway ascends to the parabrachial nucleus of the pons and then to the ventroposteromedial nucleus of the thalamus on both sides, projecting to the parietal and insular cortices. B) Tongue Surface (left: taste localization, right: nerve distribution territory).

branch at the level of the pharyngeal plexus, while the central ones enter the brainstem. The gustatory fibers of the three nerves terminate in the solitary nucleus, located in the medulla, below the floor of the fourth ventricle, laterally to the nucleus of the dorsal motor vagus. From the solitary nucleus, there are projections to the autonomic nuclei of the brainstem and the hypothalamus for autonomic reflexes. An ascending projection for conscious sensation ascends bilaterally in close proximity to the trigeminothalamic tract, reaches the *parabrachial nucleus* of the brainstem, and terminates in the *ventroposteromedial thalamic nucleus*. The cortical projection area is adjacent to the *somatosensory area* of the tongue in the post-rolandic parietal cortex.

Taste provides four flavors (sweet, salty, sour, and bitter; Figure 3.3B),and the complex sensations generated by food arise from a combination of the four flavors, general trigeminal sensations in the mouth, and especially olfactory sensations. Taste buds are relatively specific, with the tip of the tongue housing receptors most sensitive to sweet, the edges to salty and sour, and the base to bitter flavors.

The taste examination is performed using a cotton swab or a pipette with the sample solution (5% sucrose, 2.5% sodium chloride, 1% acetic acid, and 0.075% quinine hydrochloride), which is placed on a protruded area of the tongue. The patient indicates on a sheet of paper which taste they perceived, without retracting the tongue to avoid spreading the taste. The mouth should be rinsed between different tastes.

Disorders of *taste* include *hypogeusia* and *ageusia* (reduction and loss of taste), *dysgeusia* (distortion of taste) and *gustatory hallucinations*. Local irradiation for tumor treatment can destroy the receptors, which need to regenerate, and cause temporary ageusia. In hereditary autonomic neuropathies, similar to the sense of smell, taste buds and the sense of taste are absent. Loss of taste in the anterior two-thirds of one side of the tongue occurs in a *Bell's palsy*, when the nerve damage extends proximally and involves the taste fibers of the chorda tympani (Figure 3.4), but it usually goes unnoticed. The deficit regresses along with motor recovery.

Since saliva brings taste substances into contact with the receptors, disturbances of taste

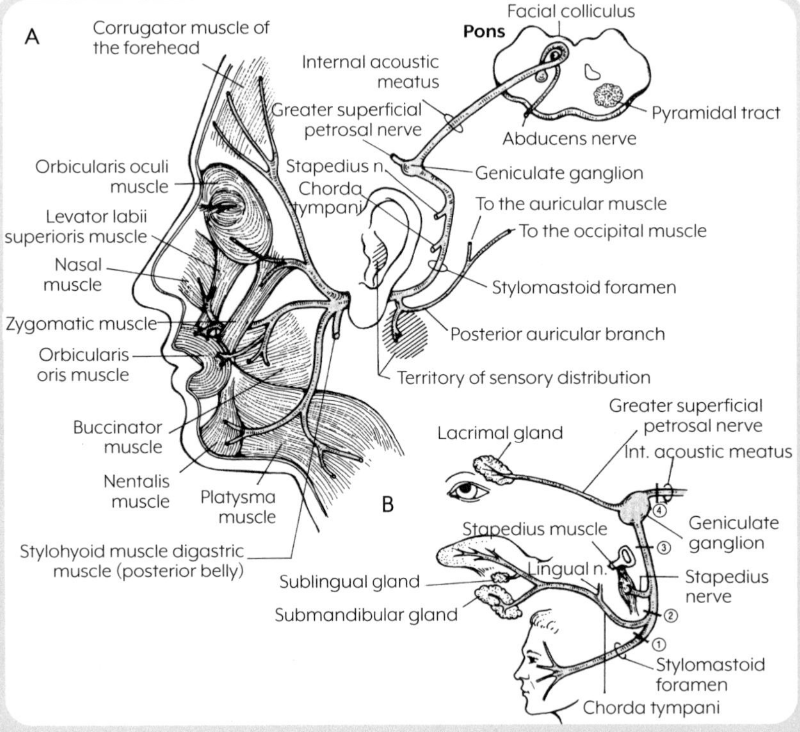

Figure 3.4

Origin and distribution of the facial nerve. A) Motor distribution (branches and main muscles are marked) and sensory distribution. B) Useful branches for localizing nerve lesions. Lesion at (1) only affects motor functions, lesion at (2) before the tympanic nerve compromises taste in the anterior half of the tongue, lesion at (3) also results in hyperacusis, and lesion at (4) abolishes tear secretion.

sensitivity can occur when salivary secretion is reduced (*xerostomia*), as seen during treatments with anticholinergic drugs, autoimmune lymphocytic infiltration of salivary glands (*Sjögren's syndrome*) or after irradiation of the lateral neck region. Influenza and other viral illnesses, as well as certain systemic diseases (scleroderma, hepatitis, myxedema, tumors), can cause *ageusia* and, particularly, *dysgeusia* due to damage to the receptor cells, similar to that in olfactory dysfunction. The most frequent cause of *dysgeusia* is medication (especially tricyclic antidepressants, but also antiepileptics, statins, anticancer drugs, triptans). Finally, *gustatory hallucinations* can occur in parietal and temporal lobe epileptic seizures.

3.3 Sensibility and motility of the face

The face is innervated by the t*rigeminal and facial nerves*. The trigeminal nerve is responsible for the general sensitivity of the skin of the anterior half of the head and the mucous membranes of the cornea, conjunctiva, nose, and mouth, as well as the pain sensitivity of the meninges. It has an important motor component for the muscles of mastication. The facial nerve is responsible for the motility of the facial muscles and the secretion of the lacrimal, nasal, submandibular, and sublingual glands. It also contributes, through the intermediate branch, to the general sensitivity of the auricle and the gustatory sensitivity.

3.3.1 Trigeminal (5th cranial nerve)

It emerges from the ventrolateral wall of the pons with two roots, the sensory root, which enlarges into the Gasserian ganglion, and the motor root, which bypasses the ganglion and joins the mandibular branch.

Sensory contingent

Comprised of general somatic afferent fibers, it originates from the *semilunar ganglion of Gasser*, located in Meckel's cave at the apex of the petrous ridge (Figure 3.5). The peripheral extensions of the ganglion's pseudounipolar neurons are distributed into the three branches: ophthalmic, maxillary, and mandibular; while the central extensions gather in the sensory root (*portio major*), which crosses the cerebellopontine angle and enters the brainstem. The sensory distribution is strictly unilateral.

The 1st *branch, ophthalmic*, traverses the lateral wall of the cavernous sinus and divides

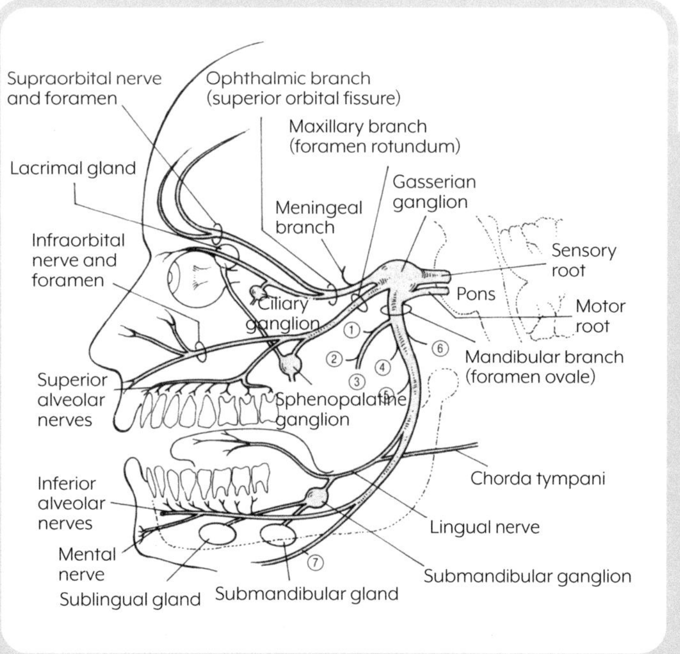

Figure 3.5

Trigeminal Nerve Course and Distribution. The sensory and motor roots that emerge from the lateral surface of the pons, the Gasserian ganglion, and the three branches—ophthalmic, maxillary, and mandibular—with their main divisions, are represented. The mandibular branch carries the motor fibers for the muscles of mastication. The ciliary, sphenopalatine, and submandibular ganglia (adjacent to the ophthalmic, maxillary, and mandibular branches, respectively) have autonomic functions. (1) Temporal muscle; (2) External pterygoid muscle; (3) Masseter muscle; (4) Tensor veli palatini muscle; (5) Internal pterygoid muscle; (6) Tensor tympani muscle; (7) Mylohyoid muscle and anterior belly of the digastric muscle.

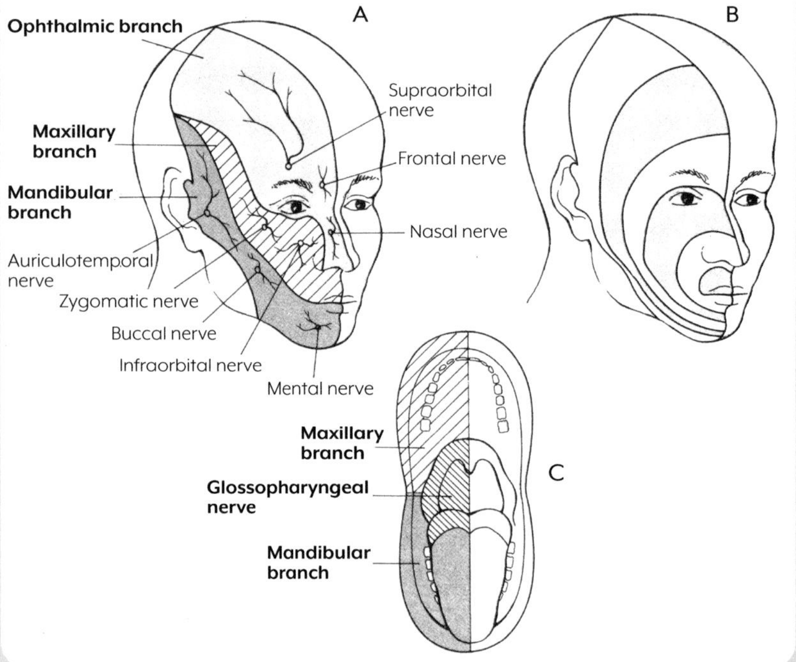

Figure 3.6

Sensory distribution of the trigeminal nerve. A) Distribution of the three branches and terminal branches for the facial skin. B) 'Onion leaf' representation of the painful and thermal sensory territories of the face in the spinal nucleus of the trigeminal nerve. C) General sensory innervation of the oropharyngeal mucosa (maxillary and mandibular branches of the trigeminal nerve and glossopharyngeal nerve).

into the lacrimal, frontal, and nasociliary branches, which exit the skull through the superior orbital fissure and reach the orbit. The terminal branch (*supraorbital nerve*) emerges beneath the skin of the eyebrow. It innervates the skin of the head up to a line connecting the ears, the forehead, upper eyelid, and dorsum of the nose (Figure 3.6A). Additionally, it innervates the mucosa of the conjunctiva and cornea, the sphenoidal, frontal, and ethmoidal sinuses, the anterior part of the nasal fossae, and the dura mater of the upper surface of the tentorium and the anterior cranial fossa.

The 2nd branch, *maxillary*, runs along the wall of the cavernous sinus and exits the skull through the foramen rotundum. It travels through the infraorbital canal and gives off the zygomatic, superior dental, and pterygopalatine branches. It emerges with the terminal branch (*infraorbital nerve*) beneath the skin of the cheek. It innervates the skin of the ala of the nose, lower eyelid, temple, cheek, and upper lip (Figure 3.6B), as well as the mucosa of the septum and the posterior part of the nasal fossae, the maxillary sinus, the upper palate, and the upper gum with the teeth of the upper arch (Figure 3.6C), and the dura mater of the middle cranial fossa.

The 3rd branch mandibular, exits through the foramen ovale, next to Meckel's cave, and divides into the branches: masticatory, auriculotemporal, lingual, buccal, and inferior dental. The terminal branch (*mental nerve*) emerges beneath the anterior skin of the chin. It innervates the skin of the lower lip, chin, cheek, temple, and ear. (Figure 3.6A). Furthermore, it innervates the mucosa of the tongue, cheek, floor of the mouth, and lower gum with the teeth of the lower arch (Figure 3.6C). It also participates in the innervation of the meninges of the middle cranial fossa (the posterior fossa is innervated by the cervical branches and the vagus nerve).

Central trigeminal pathways

The fibers of the sensory root, upon entering the brainstem, divide according to their functional significance (Figure 3.7). *Thermal* and *nociceptive afferents* converge in the *spinal tract* and terminate in the caudal portion of the *spinal trigeminal nucleus* (an elongated nuclear formation that extends up to the second cervical segment), equivalent to the posterior horn of the spinal cord. They are arranged orderly based on the position of their receptive fields: neurons with lateral receptive fields adjacent to cervical innervation territories project to the most caudal portion of the nucleus, which continues into the posterior horn of the spinal cord, while neurons with perioral fields project more cranially. This arrangement underlies the distribution of "onion skin" anesthesia in syringobulbia (Figure 3.6B). The spinal nucleus also receives thermal and nociceptive afferents from the facial, glossopharyngeal, and vagus nerves and serves as a second-order station for all cranial thermal and nociceptive afferents. It gives rise to the *trigeminothalamic tract*, which crosses over and ascends along with the spinothalamic tract to the ventroposteromedial, intralaminar, and posterior thalamic nuclei.

The *discriminative touch afferents* terminate in the *principal nucleus*, the trigeminal equivalent of the nuclei of the dorsal columns. The principal nucleus also receives tactile afferents from the facial, glossopharyngeal, and vagus nerves from the concha of the ear; it gives rise to a projection (*trigeminal lemniscus*) that crosses over and merges with the medial lemniscus, terminating in the ventroposteromedial nucleus of the thalamus. The subsequent cortical projection follows the general arrangement of lemniscal afferents.

Afferents from neuromuscular spindles of the masticatory muscles reach the mesencephalic nucleus. This nucleus constitutes an exception: it is composed of neurons similar to those in the Gasserian ganglion that have not migrated outward but remained in anomalous positions within the central nervous system. Collaterals of its fibers reach the trigeminal motor nucleus and form the monosynaptic circuit of the *jaw jerk reflex*. It also sends fibers to periodontal mechanoreceptors, dental alveoli for pressure sensitivity and bite force regulation, and oculomotor nerves for muscle spindles of the ocular muscles.

Motor Component

It is composed of special visceral efferent fibers that originate from the *motor nucleus* located in the lateral segment of the pons, beneath the floor of the fourth ventricle (Figure 3.7). It exits with the *motor root* (*portio minor*), which joins the sensory root, bypasses the Gasserian ganglion, and reaches the mandibular branch, exiting the skull

Figure 3.7

Central projections of the trigeminal system. A) Trigeminal pathways. The thermo-nociceptive pathway ascends from the spinal nucleus through the trigeminothalamic tract (directly or after synapses in the reticular formation) and reaches three thalamic structures (intralaminar nuclei, ventroposteromedial nucleus, and posterior nuclei); the tactile pathway ascends from the principal nucleus through the trigeminal lemniscus to the ventroposteromedial nucleus of the thalamus (cortical projections from the mesencephalic nucleus are poorly understood). B) Areas of cortical projection.

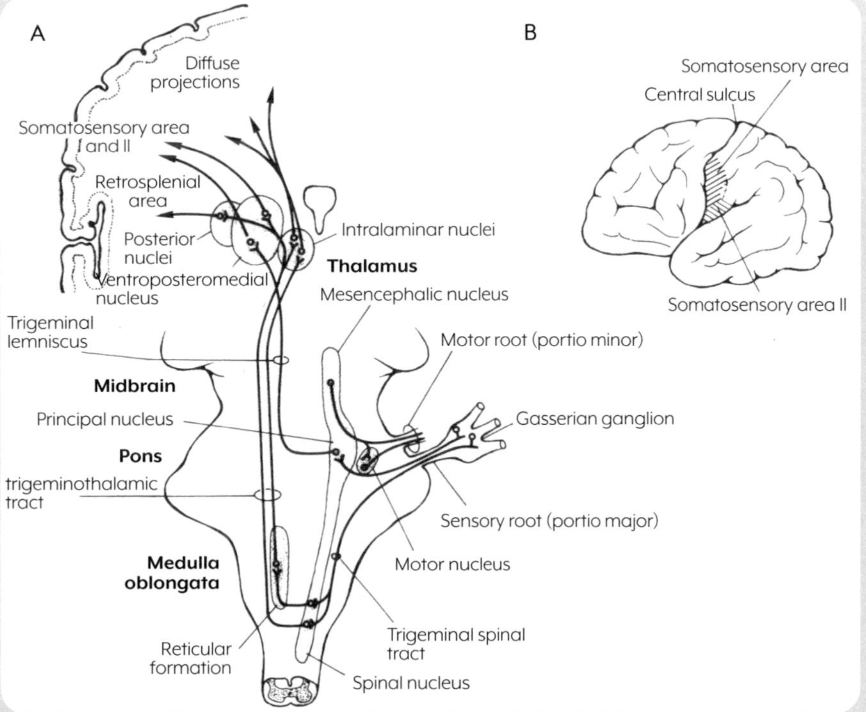

Table 3.3 MUSCLES INNERVATED BY THE TRIGEMINAL NERVE

Muscle	Function
Temporalis	Elevates and retracts the mandible
External Pterygoid	Opens the mouth and assists in lateral jaw movement
Masseter	Elevates the mandible and assists in closing the mouth
Tensor Veli Palatini	Laterally moves and elevates the palate
Internal pterygoid	It adducts, elevates, and protrudes the mandible
Tensor tympani	Stiffens the ossicular chain
Mylohyoid and anterior belly of digastric	They lower the mandible and elevate the hyoid bone

through the foramen ovale. It innervates the masticatory muscles (temporalis, masseter, external and internal pterygoids), mylohyoid muscle, anterior belly of the digastric muscle, as well as the tensor veli palatini and tensor tympani muscles (Figure 3.4). The motor projections onto the motor nucleus are predominantly crossed.

Examination of Trigeminal Functions

The cutaneous sensitivity of the face is examined as in the rest of the body. The skin of the angle of the mandible belongs to the C2-C3 territory and is spared in trigeminal anesthesia (Figure 3.6A). Corneal sensitivity is tested by lightly touching it with a cotton wisp, avoiding visual control, and evaluating subjective sensation and the corneal reflex. The mucosa of the tongue is examined with the tongue protruded, agreeing with the patient on a responsive gesture.

To assess the *motor function* of the masticatory muscles, the patient is asked to forcefully clench their teeth, comparing the prominence of the masseter and temporalis muscle bellies, which may be reduced on the affected side. When the patient forcefully opens their mouth, the mandible deviates toward the affected side due to the unopposed action of the healthy side's pterygoid muscles, particularly the external pterygoid (*oval mouth*); The same deviation occurs during mandibular protrusion. The weakness of the mylohyoid and digastric muscles is difficult to appreciate by palpating the reduced resistance of the floor of the mouth on the affected side. Similarly, the weakness of the tensor veli palatini slightly lowers the arch of the palate on the affected side. The tensor tympani muscle cannot be examined directly, but the patient may report hyperacusis. Motor functions are impaired in lesions affecting the nucleus, motor root, and the third branch of the nerve. There are usually no significant deficits in the masticatory muscles in unilateral pyramidal lesions, except during the acute phase of hemiplegia. In bilateral pyramidal deficits (*pseudobulbar syndrome*), the masseter reflex, usually weak or absent, becomes brisk.

Trigeminal Nerve Lesions

They mainly manifest with paresthesia and pain. The most common pathology is *trigeminal neuralgia*, which presents with a characteristic, intense, brief (often described as electric shock or stabbing) and recurrent pain affecting the territory of one or more branches of the nerve, with precise territorial boundaries (it never extends to the opposite side). The pain can be spontaneous or triggered by tactile stimuli on specific areas of the cutaneous or mucosal territory of the nerve ("trigger zones"). Two forms of trigeminal neuralgia are distinguished: idiopathic and symptomatic. Idiopathic trigeminal neuralgia is caused by a conflict between the trigeminal root and an arterial vessel (most commonly the superior cerebellar artery) or, more rarely, a venous vessel. It usually begins after the age of 50, typically involving the second or third branch. Symptomatic forms can onset in young age and are caused by multiple sclerosis plaques at the nerve entry point in the pons and tumors of the cerebellopontine angle compressing the trigeminal root. In both idiopathic and symptomatic forms, the cause of the pain is focal demyelination of the nerve, resulting from compression exerted by a vessel or tumor, or from demyelination of an inflammatory nature. In the area of focal demyelination, ectopic high-frequency action potentials are generated in the demyelinated nerve fibers, transmitted ephaptically to the non-myelinated pain fibers, and perceived as pain.

The diagnosis of trigeminal neuralgia is clinical and is based on the distribution and characteristics of the pain. It is more difficult to distinguish between idiopathic and symptomatic forms based solely on clinical symptoms, as they are usually indistinguishable. Features suggestive of a symptomatic form include the presence of sensory deficits, involvement of the tongue, and especially young age. Trigeminal reflexes and auditory evoked potentials (altered in the symptomatic form, normal in the idiopathic form) are the simplest, quickest, and most effective diagnostic tools for differential diagnosis, with a sensitivity and specificity of approximately 90%. MRI allows for accurate identification of the cause of symptomatic trigeminal neuralgia (cerebellopontine angle tumor or multiple sclerosis plaque).

Pharmacological treatment of trigeminal neuralgia is based on the use of antiepileptic drugs such as carbamazepine and oxcarbazepine, which block the activity of voltage-gated sodium channels in a "frequency-dependent" manner (the higher the discharge frequency, the greater the blockade). This reduces the discharge frequency of the trigeminal afferent fibers involved in focal demyelination. Treatment with carbamazepine and oxcarbazepine is effective in almost all patients with trigeminal neuralgia. If pharmacological treatment does not provide adequate pain control, the patient should undergo surgical treatment. There are several effective surgical procedures with varying degrees of invasiveness. One non-invasive surgical procedure is gamma-knife, which involves stereotactic irradiation of the trigeminal root. Alternative procedures include gangliolysis maneuvers, performed percutaneously through a needle inserted into the foramen ovale, producing a controlled lesion of the Gasserian ganglion by injecting glycerol, applying mechanical compression with a balloon, or creating a thermal lesion using radiofrequency. The most invasive surgical procedure, involving craniotomy, is microvascular decompression in the posterior cranial fossa. Unlike other procedures, the goal of this intervention is to resolve the cause of trigeminal neuralgia by eliminating neurovascular conflict through the insertion of an inert material like Teflon between the vessel and the nerve. It is a relatively safe and effective procedure and should therefore be the intervention of choice for patients without significant surgical risk. In symptomatic forms, concurrent treatment of the underlying pathology (such as multiple sclerosis or cerebellopontine angle tumors) is necessary alongside pain pharmacotherapy.

The trigeminal nerve can be compressed or invaded by skull base tumors (meningiomas, cholesteatomas, chordomas, dermoids), aneurysms, or basilar artery tortuosity. In the cerebellopontine angle, the most common pathology is acoustic neuroma, which initially presents with unilateral hearing loss. Trigeminal neuroma, which causes early trigeminal signs, is much rarer.

The *Gasserian ganglion* can be compressed by *infraclinoid internal carotid artery* aneurysms and can be involved in *purulent otitis media* extending to the cells of the temporal pyramid, along with the abducens nerve (Gradenigo's syndrome). *Herpes zoster* of the ganglion manifests as pain followed by vesicular eruption in the territory of one or more branches, most commonly the ophthalmic branch. Corneal vesicles can leave opaque scars or become infected, leading to serious complications. Immediate therapy with acyclovir (800 mg five times a day for one week) is required, which reduces the risk of residual and difficult-to-control pain (*post-herpetic neuralgia*).

The trigeminal nerve can be the site of an *isolated idiopathic neuropathy*, either monolateral or bilateral, with a chronic course, sometimes accompanied by nasal ulcers. Some cases develop within the context of scleroderma or other autoimmune diseases such as Sjogren's syndrome or lupus erythematosus. Biopsy of a nerve branch is required.

Finally, it is responsible for a dysesthetic syndrome (burning mouth syndrome or *burning mouth disorder*) that mainly affects elderly women and is characterized by a burning pain, hyperesthesia, and dysesthesias of the tongue, palate, lips, and gums, as well as taste alterations and reduced salivary secretion. Symptoms worsen towards the evening. It can occur in an idiopathic form or in the course of diabetes, nutritional deficiencies, dental treatments, as well as psychological disorders.

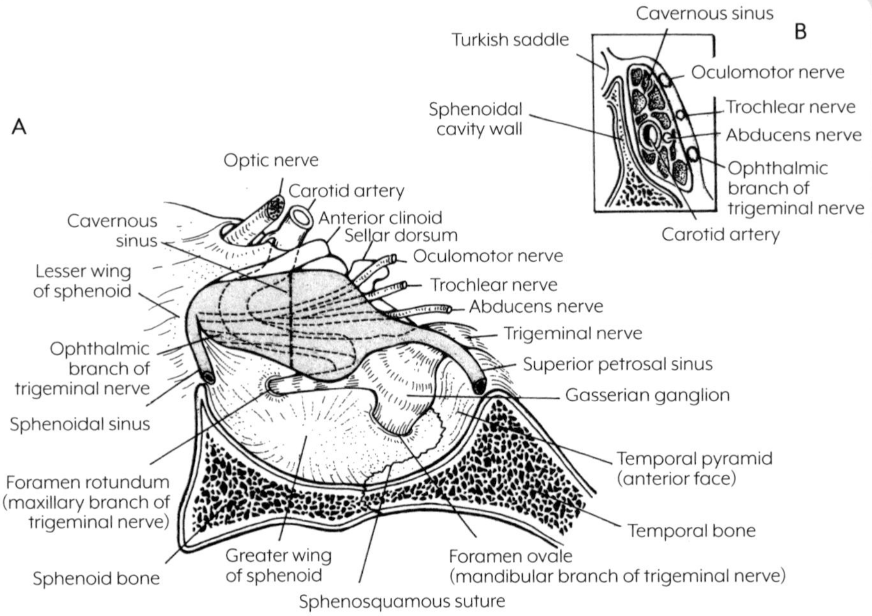

Figure 3.8

Relationships between the cavernous sinus and the nerves of the middle cranial fossa. A) Lateral view of the left middle cranial fossa; the cavernous sinus contains within it the three oculomotor nerves, the ophthalmic branch of the trigeminal nerve, and the carotid artery, and communicates anteriorly with the spheno-parietal sinus and posteriorly with the superior petrosal sinus. B) Section of the cavernous sinus along the dashed vertical line in A, to highlight the position of the nerves and the carotid artery. (Redrawn from Spector and Fiandaca, 1986).

Lingual biopsy and trigeminal potentials suggest a neuropathy of the small fibers of the third branch. Therapy is disappointing.

Injuries to individual branches occur in the course of cranial base and paranasal sinus neoplasms, purulent sinusitis, and facial bone fractures. *Tolosa-Hunt syndrome* is a granulomatous inflammation that affects the first branch along with the oculomotor nerves at the level of the superior orbital fissure or cavernous sinus (Figure 3.8). *Raeder's paratrigeminal syndrome* is characterized by a dull and continuous pain in the territory of the first branch, associated with miosis and conjunctival congestion, and it depends on the involvement of the first branch and the pupillary dilator fibers. Some cases are caused by aneurysms or dissections of the terminal segment of the internal carotid artery or parasellar pathologies, while others are idiopathic. The mental nerve can sometimes be affected in breast and prostate tumors and multiple myeloma, causing a sensation of numbness in the chin and lower lip.

At *the central level*, the trigeminal tract and spinal nucleus are included in the ischemic zone in *lateral medullary infarctions*, along with the vestibular nuclei, spinothalamic tract, inferior and olivocerebellar spinocerebellar tracts, descending pupillary dilator pathway, and vagal fibers. The lesion results from occlusions of the vertebral artery or posterior inferior cerebellar artery and is one of the most common neurovascular syndromes. It presents acutely with vertigo, followed by alternating sensory deficits (homolateral thermopainful anesthesia of the face and contralateral body) and ipsilateral cerebellar signs, Bernard-Horner syndrome, and paresis of the larynx and pharynx, accompanied by excessive mucosal secretion and dysarthria (*Wallenberg's syndrome*).

The spinal nucleus is sometimes involved in *syringomyelia* when the syrinx cavity ascends towards the first cervical segments (*syringobulbia*). A dissociated thermopainful anesthesia of the face appears, starting in the peripheral trigeminal territory and gradually extending towards the oral region (onion bulb distribution- Figure 3.6B).

3.3.2 Facial (7th cranial nerve)

The nerve leaves the brainstem at the level of the caudal border of the pons (Figure 3.4A), It crosses the pontocerebellar angle, enters the internal acoustic meatus alongside the *vestibulocochlear nerve,* and continues on its own within the *facial canal* inside the petrous pyramid. The canal runs laterally and, bending backward, forms an initial curve (*knee of the canal*), where the nerve presents the swelling of the *geniculate ganglion* and gives off the *greater petrosal nerve*; it then forms a second curve, bending downward: in this segment, the *stapedial nerve* and *chorda tympani* branch off. It terminates at the stylomastoid foramen, medially to the mastoid, where the nerve exits, travels forward, passes through the parotid gland, and divides into its terminal branches.

The nerve has a motor component, a sensory component, and an autonomic component.

The *motor component* (composed of special visceral efferent fibers) originates from the *motor nucleus* located in the caudal portion of the pons, rostral to the nucleus ambiguus. It forms a loop around the abducens nucleus, creating an elevation on the floor of the 4th ventricle (*facial colliculus*), and exits as the *motor root* or facial nerve proper. The fibers for the stapedius muscle separate with the stapedial nerve, while the remaining fibers continue to the terminal branches, which reach the facial and neck mimic muscles, the stylohyoid muscle, and the posterior belly of the digastric muscle. The *pyramidal projections* onto the motor nucleus are distributed differently between the motoneurons of the muscles in the upper half of the face (which receive roughly equal numbers of direct and crossed pyramidal fibers) and the motoneurons of the muscles in the lower half of the face (which receive a predominance of crossed fibers). This distribution explains the central facial palsy, which affects the lower half of the face.

The *sensory component originates* from the geniculate ganglion. It consists of *special visceral afferent fibers* for the gustatory sensation of the anterior two-thirds of the tongue, as previously described. These fibers leave the nerve with the chorda tympani, reach the tongue through the lingual branch of the trigeminal nerve's third division, and project centrally to the solitary nucleus. Additionally, there are *general somatic afferent fibers* for the concha of the auricle, which are reached through the posterior auricular branch. These fibers enter the nerve trunk with the *sensory root or intermediate nerve,* laterally to the motor root, and terminate centrally in the sensory nuclei of the trigeminal nerve. They are responsible for the pain accompanying peripheral facial paralysis.

The autonomic component is composed of *general visceral efferent fibers* of parasympathetic nature, involved in secretory functions. These fibers originate from the superior *salivatory nucleus* located in the paramedian pontine tegmentum, beneath the floor of the fourth ventricle. They exit with the intermediate nerve. A portion of these fibers, destined for the lacrimal and nasal glands, follows the greater petrosal nerve, reaches the pterygopalatine ganglion, and postganglionic fibers, through trigeminal branches, reach the lacrimal, nasal, and palatal glands. The remaining fibers, for the submandibular and sublingual salivary glands, follow the chorda tympani, the lingual nerve, and the submandibular ganglion. From there, the postganglionic fibers reach the two salivary glands. The most important clinical examination concerns facial motility. Attention is given to the symmetry of the resting and involuntary mimetic expressions while the subject speaks and laughs. Kinetic tests are then performed, such as frowning, tightly closing the eyes, wrinkling the nose, showing the teeth by stretching the corner of the mouth on one side and the other, puffing the cheeks, and stretching the neck skin through forced mouth opening (platysma muscle). In comatose patients, mimetic responses are provoked with moderately intense painful stimuli, such as compressing the eyeball (*Modonesi-De Lisi sign*), the supraorbital arch, the area behind the angle of the mandible, etc. Stapedial deficit results in hyperacusis, which can be objectively assessed with tympanometry in response to a sound (*stapedial reflex*). The cutaneous sensory component is difficult to explore due to the overlap of territories from multiple nerves, but it becomes evident with the appearance of vesicles in the concha of the auricle in cases of geniculate ganglion herpes zoster. Taste examination has already been described. Tear secretion is evaluated by placing a thin strip of filter paper between the lower eyelid and the eyeball and comparing the moistened area by tears on both sides.

Facial Pathology

The most common condition is *idiopathic facial paralysis* (also known as *"Bell's palsy"*), an inflammatory disorder that affects a variable length segment of the nerve, typically within the canal. It is more common in middle-aged individuals and has a higher incidence during pregnancy and in diabetic subjects. It is believed that the *herpes simplex virus* is involved in the majority of cases. Exposure to cold, which is present in a significant number of patients, acts as a predisposing factor. The onset is acute, with retroauricular pain. The paralysis appears suddenly or evolves over hours or days. The deficit is of peripheral type and equally affects the upper and lower half of the face on one side; usually, it is complete. The forehead wrinkles appear smoothed, the eyebrow is lowered, the eye does not wink, the groove between the cheek and the lip is flattened, and the corner of the mouth is drooped. During kinetic tests, half of the face remains immobile or moves noticeably less than the unaffected side. In the attempt to forcefully close the eye, it remains open, and the automatic upward rotation of the eyeballs exposes the sclera (Bell's sign). When showing the teeth, the oral fissure is stretched towards the healthy side. When blowing or whistling, air escapes from the deficient corner of the mouth, and if the skin of the neck is stretched, no fold lifts the skin. The detachment of the lower eyelid from the conjunctiva allows tears to flow down the face, and saliva drools from the corner of the mouth.

The lesion usually affects the nerve at the level of the stylomastoid foramen. If the damage extends proximally, it can involve the gustatory fibers (ageusia of the anterior part of the tongue, in half of the cases), the fibers of the stapedius muscle (hyperacusis, 30% of the cases), and the lacrimal fibers (reduced tear secretion, 20% of the cases) (■ Figure 3.4B).

The prognosis is generally good, as spontaneous recovery occurs in almost 90% of cases, either completely or with a high level of satisfaction. The recovery depends on the extent of the lesion, which can block conduction or interrupt the continuity of the axons: in the former case, the axon recovers within a few weeks, while in the latter case, it needs to regenerate, a process that takes months and is not always successful. Clinical and neurophysiological findings at one week from the onset provide prognostic indications. An incomplete motor deficit and a motor evoked potential of normal amplitude in response to electrical stimulation of the nerve at the angle of the mandible predict good recovery within 3-6 weeks. If the motor potential shows increased latency and reduced amplitude, recovery will take several months. If the nerve is unexcitable, the recovery will be incomplete.

The outcomes can include permanent deficit, contractions (which initially improve the appearance of the face but can deform facial expressions in the opposite direction), and axonal confusion phenomena. The latter are errors in the target selection of the axons, which, during regeneration, take wrong directions. As a result, synkinesias of the mouth may appear during eye closure and vice versa. The *crocodile tears syndrome* is caused by salivary fibers that erroneously innervate the lacrimal gland, leading to tear secretion during meals.

The therapy is based on corticosteroids to reduce nerve edema and fiber compression within the canal. It should be initiated immediately and continued at full doses for one week (prednisone 1 mg per kilogram per day; betamethasone 0.1 mg per kilogram per day). An antiviral agent (acyclovir, 200-400 mg five times a day) is usually added. The eye, exposed to trauma due to incomplete eyelid closure, should be protected with wraparound glasses or a prosthesis.

In addition to the idiopathic form, the facial nerve is involved in many other pathologies.

Herpes zoster of the geniculate ganglion manifests with intense pain and, after 3-5 days, vesicular eruption in the concha of the ear and usually complete paralysis. Treatment with full doses of acyclovir is mandatory (800 mg five times a day), combined with steroids.

The nerve is compressed in the cerebellopontine angle and the internal acoustic meatus by *acoustic neurinomas* and other tumors of the region (meningiomas of the petrous bone, acoustic neurofibromas, dermoids, cholesteatomas). It is also susceptible to injury in *aneurysms of the vertebral* or *basilar artery* and can be easily damaged during surgical removal of large tumors (4 cm). It is vascularized at the base of the skull, along with the 2nd and 3rd branches of the trigeminal nerve, by branches of the *middle meningeal artery*, and these three branches can suffer ischemic damage. It is involved in *fractures of the petrous pyramid and middle ear infections*. It can be injured by tumors of the parotid gland as it passes through the gland. In Guillain-Barré syndrome (acute inflammatory polyneuropathy), the oculomotor nerves (*Fisher syndrome*) can be involved bilaterally along with the facial nerve. Another cause of bilateral involvement is base *meningitis* (due to Borrelia, tuberculosis, fungal, carcinomatous, lymphomatous).

Lastly, intrinsic lesions of the brainstem (ischemic infarcts, infiltrating gliomas, cavernous angiomas with hemorrhagic foci) can damage the nerve at the pontine level, along with the 6th cranial nerve and the pyramidal tract, causing an alternating syndrome with ipsilateral facial and abducens nerve paralysis and contralateral brachiocrural hemiparesis (*Millard-Gubler syndrome*).

In all pathologies involving the nerve or the motor nucleus, the deficit presents with the characteristics of peripheral paralysis. In pyramidal lesions, however, the deficit is of a central type and spares the upper half of the face. Facial muscles frequently experience *pathological involuntary movements*, with the most common being *hemifacial spasm* and *blepharospasm*.

3.4 Neuroophthalmology

Neuroophthalmology is the study of the neurological aspects of visual function. The main aspects involve: vision, which depends on the optic nerve (2nd cranial nerve) and the visual pathways; extrinsic ocular motility, which depends on three nerves (3rd cranial nerve, oculomotor; 4th cranial nerve, trochlear; 6th cranial nerve, abducens); and intrinsic ocular motility, which depends on the 3rd cranial nerve and the cervicothoracic sympathetic system.

3.4.1 Vision

Functional organization of the visual pathways

From a phylogenetic perspective, the retina is a direct extension of the central nervous system. Light receptors (cones and rods) are located in the outer layers, within a niche of the pigmented epithelium, and light must pass through all retinal layers before reaching them. Cones and rods are connected to bipolar cells (equivalent to neurons in a sensory ganglion), which in turn are connected to ganglion cells (equivalent to neurons in the first central station

Figure 3.9

Visual pathways. A) Top view; note the projections from the two left hemi-retinas (right visual field) to the striate cortex (area 17) through the lateral geniculate nucleus (geniculostriate system), and to the peristriate areas (areas 18 and 19) through the superior colliculus and pulvinar (colliculoperistriate system); projections to the pretectal region are also indicated (for light reflex). B) Side view, showing the projection from the upper retina (lower visual field) to the upper lip of the calcarine fissure, and from the lower retina (upper visual field) to the lower lip of the calcarine fissure.

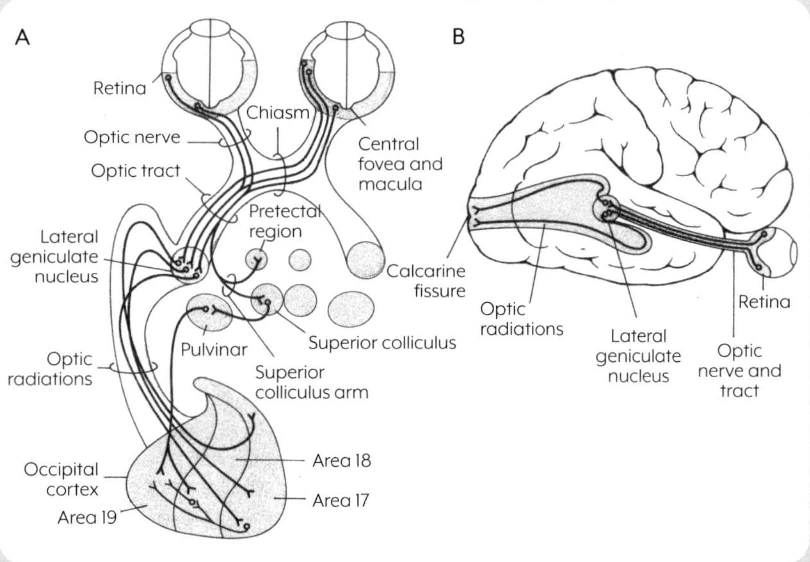

of a sensory pathway). Cones are responsible for high-intensity vision and form the basis of color detection and detail discrimination, i.e., visual acuity. They are concentrated in the macula, especially in its central region called the fovea, which contains only cones and lacks ganglion cells, which are displaced to its periphery. Rods, on the other hand, are responsible for low-light vision and are more numerous than cones in the rest of the retina.

Axons of ganglion cells converge at the optic disc or optic disk, where they acquire myelin sheaths and form the optic nerve, which is equivalent to a central sensory pathway. The optic nerve traverses the sclera, passes through the orbital cavity and the optic canal, enters the cranial cavity, and, upon merging with the contralateral nerve, forms the optic chiasm. Fibers originating from the macula, primarily from cones, exit from the temporal side of the optic disc and gather at the center of the nerve (*maculopapillary bundle*). The optic nerve is surrounded by meninges, which continue anteriorly with the sclera and posteriorly with the meninges of the brain.

The *optic chiasm* is located in the subarachnoid space (chiasmatic cistern), above the diaphragm of the sella turcica and in front of the pituitary stalk, adjacent to the thin lamina of the hypothalamus, forming the wall of the third ventricle.

The chiasm continues into the *optic tracts*: axons from the nasal half of the retina cross over and pass into the optic tract of the opposite side, while those from the temporal half continue without crossing into the optic tract of the same side (Figure 3.9A). The nasal and temporal fibers of the maculopapillary bundle undergo a similar distribution and position themselves in the posterior part of the chiasm. The optic fibers maintain their respective altitudinal relationships, with the upper half of the retina corresponding to the upper part of the chiasm, and the lower half to the lower part.

As a result of the decussation, the optic tract of one side contains fibers from both homologous hemiretinas, the nasal half from the opposite side, and the temporal half from the same side. Due to the crossing of light rays, both hemiretinas "look" towards the contralateral space. Therefore, the optic tract and all posterior structures process visual information from the contralateral half of space, similar to how the somatosensory cortex processes information from the opposite half of the body.

The optic tract extends backward, surrounding the midbrain peduncle. Its fibers undergo different destinations (Figure 3.9A):

a) The overwhelmingly largest contingent terminates in the *six layers of the lateral geniculate nucleus* (three layers, 2-3-5, receive fibers from the ipsilateral temporal retina, and three layers, 2-4-6, receive fibers from the contralateral nasal retina). From the neurons of the geniculate nucleus, optic radiations originate, reaching the striate area (primary visual area or area 17), located on the borders of the calcarine fissure, in the medial aspect of the occipital lobe. Fibers from the lower quadrants of the retina fan out in the temporal pole before converging toward the occipital cortex and projecting below the calcarine fissure, while fibers from the upper quadrants remain compact and project above the calcarine. The maculopapillary bundle follows a relatively straight path at the center of the radiation and projects to the occipital pole; peripheral retinal areas project to increasingly anterior concentric circles of the striate cortex (Figure 3.9B). In the striate area, the afferents from homologous hemiretinas (temporal on one side and nasal on the opposite side) merge, and conscious discrimination of visual reality begins, continuing in the peristriate areas (areas 18 and 19) to which the striate area is connected.
b) A second contingent bypasses the lateral geniculate nucleus and terminates in the *superior colliculus*, located in the roof of the midbrain, a layered structure involved in visuomotor integration, where, in addition to retinal projections, somatic and acoustic afferents converge. It sends ascending projections to the pulvinar of the thalamus, and from there to the peristriate visual areas and frontal oculomotor fields. It also sends descending projections to brainstem and spinal structures that control eye and head movements. It plays a role in gaze fixation and the latency and accuracy of eye movements towards a region of space.

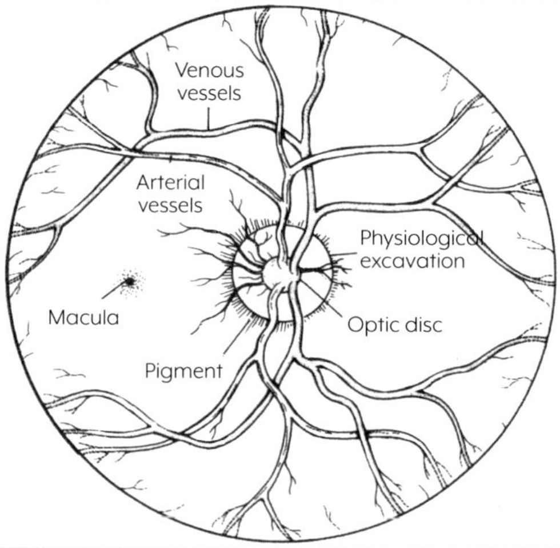

Figure 3.10

Right eye fundus. The fundus is viewed using direct ophthalmoscopy.

c) A third contingent also bypasses the geniculate nucleus and terminates in the *pretectal region*, located at the junction between the midbrain and thalamus, from which connections originate with the Edinger-Westphal nuclei on both sides. It underlies the pupillary light reflex and regulates pupillary motility.

Examination of the visual pathways

The clinical examination consists of exploring the fundus of the eye, visual acuity, and visual field.

Fundus examination (fundus oculi) is performed using direct imaging ophthalmoscopy, which provides an enlarged image of approximately 20 times and allows examination of the optic disc and the central area of the retina, and with more difficulty, the macula, located on the temporal side of the optic disc. Illumination during the examination enhances the pupillary light reflex and causes miosis (Figure 3.10). The examination should be conducted in a low-light environment while the subject fixates on a distant object. In elderly individuals who typically have miotic pupils, it may be necessary to dilate the pupils with eye drops to examine the peripheral retina. However, this should be avoided in an outpatient setting since even a short-acting medication (e.g., 0.5% tropicamide) can trigger an acute glaucoma attack and disturb vision for at least an hour. Pharmacological mydriasis should be avoided in individuals with altered consciousness to avoid losing information about the pupillary status.

When describing an ophthalmoscopic finding, the fundus is read like the quadrants of a clock, using the diameter of the optic disc as the unit of measurement (e.g., "hemorrhage at 12 o'clock, two disc diameters from the optic disc"). The use of green light allows for a more precise visualization of vessels and hemorrhages.

Visual acuity (visus) is examined using the Snellen chart or optotype chart. Refractive errors are corrected with lenses or by having the person look through a pinpoint hole (pinhole examination). Indications can be obtained by having the person read a text with characters of different sizes while wearing their usual glasses.

With optimal lighting and correction of refractive errors, the visual acuity of a normal individual is 10/10. Lower values are

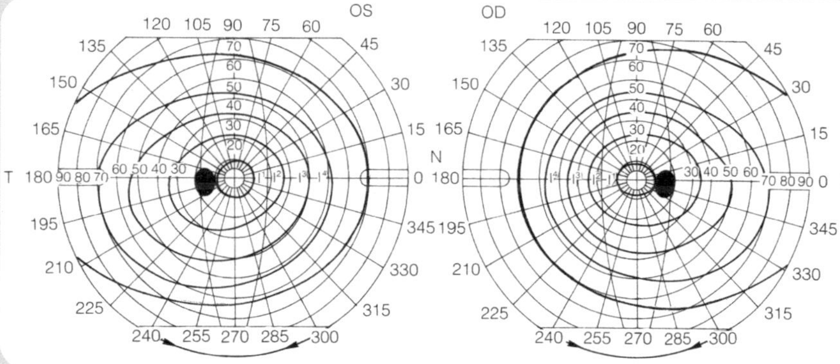

Figure 3.11

Normal Visual Field. Dynamic perimetry of the two eyes. The isopters I1, I2, I3, I4, and I5 are obtained with increasingly larger target diameters. The macula is located at the center; the black area corresponds to the blind spot.

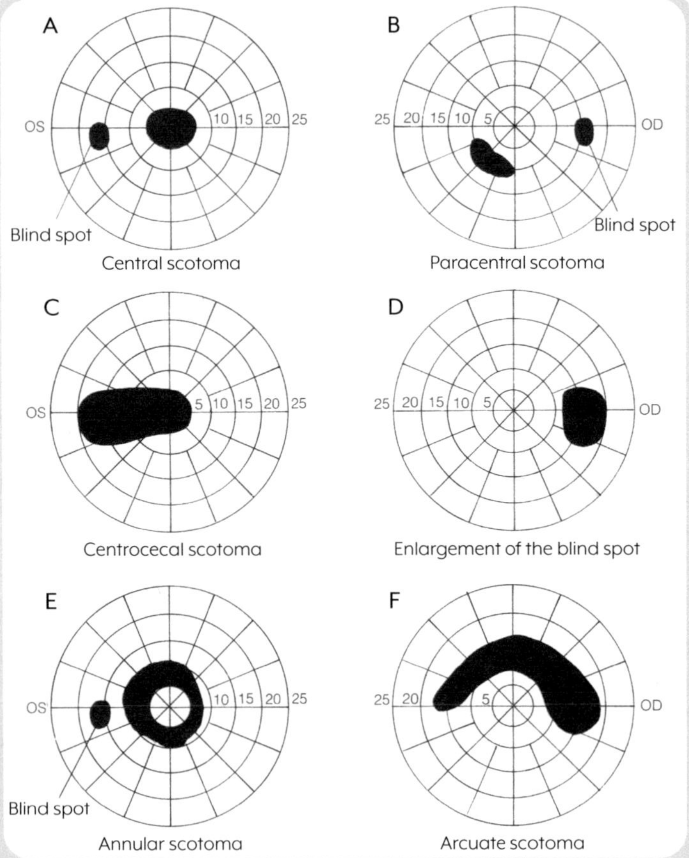

Figure 3.12

Defects of the central visual field with the Bjerrum tangent screen. On the left, the left eye; on the right, the right eye. The blind spot is a physiological scotoma. A, B, C, D: see text. E: annular scotoma in retinitis pigmentosa. F: arcuate scotoma in glaucoma.

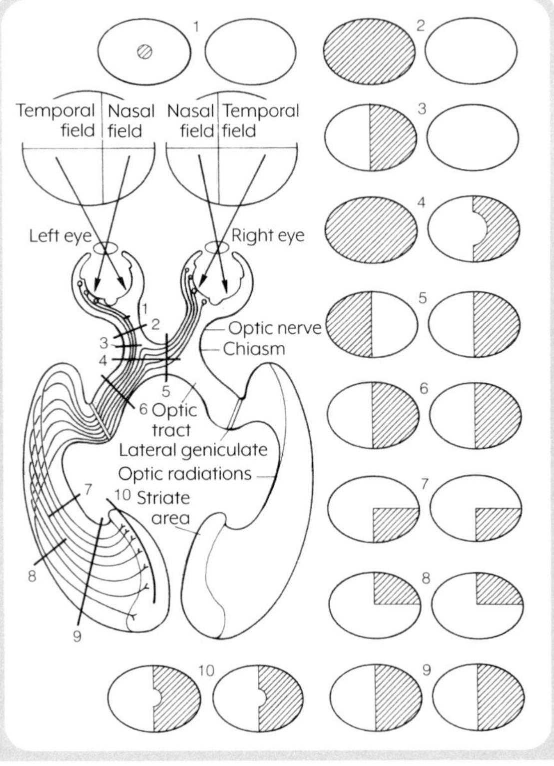

Figure 3.13

Defects of the visual field with static perimetry. The lesion is indicated by a line and the corresponding number in the visual pathway diagram; the blind spot appears hatched. 1 = Central scotoma in the left eye (lesion of the maculopapillary bundle); 2 = Blindness in the left eye (total lesion of the optic nerve); 3 = Nasal hemianopia in the left eye (partial lesion of the left side of the chiasm); 4 = Blindness in the left eye, temporal hemianopia with macular sparing in the right eye (subtotal chiasm lesion starting from the left side); 5 = Bitemporal hemianopia (total chiasm lesion); 6 = Right homonymous hemianopia (lesion of the optic tract); 7 = Right inferior homonymous quadrantanopia (lesion of the upper portion of the optic radiations); 8 = Right superior homonymous quadrantanopia (lesion of the lower portion of the optic radiations); 9 = Right homonymous hemianopia (total lesion of the optic radiations); 10 = Right homonymous hemianopia with macular sparing (lesion of the striate area with sparing of the posterior pole).

pathological and, if not explained by opacities of the refractive media, depend on lesions of the macula or macular projections to the striate area. It is sufficient for one of the contingents of the maculopapillary bundle (nasal or temporal) to project onto the striate cortex to ensure a visual acuity of 10/10. Visual acuity, along with color vision, is therefore compromised in lesions of the macula and optic nerve, while remaining normal in lesions of the chiasm and unilateral lesions of the retrochiasmatic pathways.

Examination of the visual field (perimetry or campimetry) | Provides a map of the visual defects in each eye. It can be performed manually (confrontation examination) but should be supplemented by examination with a perimeter.

The *confrontation examination* involves comparing the patient's visual field to the examiner's own visual field. The examiner and patient face each other at a distance of about one meter, with one eye closed and the corresponding eyes fixated on each other. The examiner moves their hand halfway between themselves and the patient along various meridians, and the patient signals when they perceive the stimulus. Another method is to ask the patient to quickly count the fingers that the examiner presents in one of the four quadrants of the visual field, avoiding the horizontal and vertical meridians. Alternatively, the patient can compare the sharpness of fingers or a red object simultaneously presented in the nasal and temporal quadrants. A coarser method is to present both hands in the area under investigation, alternately moving a finger and asking the patient to indicate which one is moving.

The *Goldmann perimeter* is a hemispherical dome with controlled brightness onto which adjustable targets of various sizes and luminosity are projected. The subject fixates on a central target. By adjusting the brightness or moving the targets, a map of the static or dynamic visual field is constructed (Figure 3.11). *Computerized perimeters* allow detailed mapping up to 30° from the macula and are particularly used in ophthalmology to map central defects. They have replaced the Bjerrum screen, a simple black cloth placed one meter from the patient, which expands the central area of the field for cartographic reasons (Figure 3.12). In neurology departments, the *Foerster perimeter* may still be found, which includes a chin rest and an orientable graduated semicircle in various meridians, onto which the target is manually shifted.

Defects in the visual field are called scotomas. The blind spot is a physiological scotoma of which one has no awareness, corresponding to the optic disc, which lacks receptors. Pathological scotomas are blind areas that the patient only notices when they affect the macular region or when they become very extensive.

Scotomas can be classified as follows (in Figures 3.12 e 3.13):

a) *Central*: occupies the central portion of the visual field and causes a decrease in visual acuity; occurs in lesions of the macular region and the optic nerve that affect the maculopapillary bundle.
b) *Paracentral*: occupies the immediate vicinity of the central region and is usually due to lesions of the perimacular retina; a particular type of paracentral scotoma is the enlargement of the blind spot, which occurs in optic disc edema.
c) *Centrocecal*: occupies the central region, encompassing the blind spot within the defective area, usually enlarged; it is typical of inflammatory or ischemic lesions of the optic nerve head, which damage the maculopapillary bundle and cause optic disc edema.
d) *Peripheral*: occupies a peripheral zone, usually due to focal pathologies of the retina.
e) *Concentric*: observed in retinitis pigmentosa but is not uncommon in psychogenic visual defects.
f) *Altitudinal*: occupies the upper or lower half of the visual field on one side, along the horizontal meridian passing through the fovea, and is caused by occlusion of the ciliary vessels or the superior or inferior branches of the central retinal artery; bilateral deficits result from bilateral lesions of the striate cortex above or below the calcarine fissure.
g) *Hemianoptic*: occupies half of the visual field in both eyes; the blind zone is

separated from the normal zone along the vertical meridian passing through the center. The scotoma can affect the two temporal halves (bitemporal hemianopsia) due to a midline lesion of the chiasm, or the two homonymous portions (temporal and nasal) on the right or left side (homonymous hemianopsia) due to retrochiasmal lesions. The defect can be complete and occupy both hemifields entirely or incomplete, affecting only a portion. Quadrantanopsia is an incomplete defect in the symmetric quadrants of both eyes. If the lesion spares the macular projections, the central region remains excluded from the blind area (macular sparing), as can occur in retrochiasmal lesions. An incomplete defect can be incongruous, meaning it is more extensive in one eye, as seen in lesions of the optic tract and lateral geniculate nucleus, where the inputs from the two eyes are not uniformly mixed, or congruous, meaning it is symmetrical in both eyes, as seen in lesions of the optic radiations and striate cortex where the projections from the two eyes are fused, as shown in Figure 3.13.

Pathology of the visual pathways

Retina | The retinal receptors are vascularized by the choroidal vessels, while the inner layers of the retina receive blood from the central retinal artery.

Hypertensive retinopathy. It is a consequence of systemic arterial hypertension. The retinal arterioles appear narrowed, irregular in caliber, and stretched in appearance; in the macular region, they assume a serpentine (corkscrew) course. The reflection of light projected by the ophthalmoscope onto the vessel surface increases in intensity. At the point of crossing with an arteriole, the course of the vein appears deviated or the venous blood column interrupted (arteriovenous nicking). In severe forms, the arterioles take on a silvery-white appearance (silver-wire), whitish cotton-wool exudates and punctate areas of retinal degeneration appear, which in the macular region assume a radial arrangement (macular star degeneration). Hemorrhages also occur, flame-shaped in the superficial layers, and round in the deep layers of the retina, and finally, papillary edema.

Diabetic retinopathy. It is characterized by tortuosity of arterial vessels, focal dilations of capillaries appearing as red dots (microaneurysms), retinal and preretinal hemorrhages, including large ones, punctate or cotton-wool exudates, more abundant in the macular region. In the proliferative form, the hemorrhages are invaded by fibrous strands with neovascularization, a source of new hemorrhages and a precursor to retinal detachment. In both hypertensive and diabetic forms, the decrease in visual acuity is related to macular pathology.

Chorioretinitis. It manifests as round scarred foci with a pearly appearance, with irregular accumulations of pigment at the margins. They cause scotomas and a decrease in visual acuity when they involve the macular region. The most common etiologies are toxoplasmosis, cytomegalovirus, syphilis, sarcoidosis, and tuberculosis.

Retinitis pigmentosa. It is an inherited disease with recessive transmission, characterized by the degeneration of the retinal receptors and pigment epithelium, starting from the perimacular or peripheral areas. Retinal pigment forms irregular accumulations of black color, similar to osteoblasts; the blood vessels become impoverished, and the optic disc becomes atrophic. The first symptom is a loss of vision in low light conditions (nyctalopia or night blindness); the visual field shows a ring scotoma (Figure 3.12E) or concentric narrowing, with relative sparing of central vision. The electroretinogram is depressed at an early stage. It is frequently associated with degenerative and metabolic disorders of the nervous system (cerebellar degenerations, ceroid lipofuscinosis, Refsum's disease, Bassen-Kornzweig disease, Kearns-Sayre syndrome, etc.). Non-pigmented retinal degeneration with concentric narrowing can be observed with prolonged use of drugs such as phenothiazines (antipsychotics), chloroquine (antimalarial), and vigabatrin (antiepileptic).

Macular degeneration. It is a degenerative process affecting the pigment epithelium and photoreceptors in the central retina, very common in old age. The macula takes on a granular appearance with wax-like accumulations of lipoprotein material (drusen) and punctate pigmentary clumps between the retina and the choroid. In the rarer wet form, new blood vessels form with exudates and small hemorrhagic deposits. There is a decline in visual acuity, earlier in the wet form, with a central scotoma. Associations are similar to retinitis pigmentosa.

Other ophthalmoscopic findings that may be observed by a neurologist consulted for a decrease in vision include *central vein occlusion*, with hemorrhagic flooding of the retina, and occlusion of the central artery or its branches, with retinal pallor and fragmentation of the blood column. The macula allows the choroidal vessels to show through and appears red (cherry-red spot). A similar appearance occurs in childhood due to sphingolipid accumulation.

Optic Nerve | *Papilledema* (or *stasis papilla*). It is the consequence of intracranial hypertension. The increased cerebrospinal fluid pressure is transmitted to the subarachnoid spaces surrounding the optic nerve, impeding venous return. The optic nerve head, unaffected by the increased intracranial pressure, swells due to transudation and protrudes into the eyeball. Axonal swelling contributes to the swelling as it impedes orthograde axoplasmic flow. The edema is usually bilateral but can be asymmetric. On ophthalmoscopic examination, the optic disc margins appear indistinct from the surrounding retina, the physiological cup is obscured, venous vessels are congested, and venous pulsation, which is not always present in a normal individual, disappears early. Subsequently, the optic nerve head protrudes into the eyeball, flame-shaped peripapillary venous hemorrhages and white exudate patches appear. Visual acuity and the light reflex remain normal for an extended period, and the visual field shows an enlargement of the blind spot. However, with the development of atrophy, visual acuity is also compromised. Papilledema develops in tumors and other causes of subacute and chronic intracranial hypertension such as meningitis, venous sinus occlusion, obstructive hydrocephalus, subdural hematomas, respiratory encephalopathy with hypercapnia, etc.

Pseudotumor cerebri consists of bilateral papillary edema in the absence of space-occupying masses. It almost always occurs in young obese women; it can sometimes be caused by excessive intake of vitamin A (animal oils) or prolonged use of tetracyclines. Symptoms are minimal; there may be headaches, and in the long term, a decrease in visual acuity, even rapidly, preceded by episodes of transient visual loss. Visual field testing shows a centrocecal scotoma with concentric narrowing of the visual field.

Retrobulbar optic neuritis. It is an acute condition of the optic nerve that occurs in adolescents or young adults. It rapidly compromises visual acuity and color discrimination. The pupillary light reflex, both direct and consensual, is decreased. The visual field shows a central scotoma, while the *fundus of the eye* appears normal. Pain upon eye movement or compression is often present. It consists of acute demyelination with perivascular inflammatory reaction affecting the retrobulbar segment of the nerve, compromising the maculopapillary bundle without altering the appearance of the optic disc. A glial scar may remain. In most cases, it is the initial manifestation of multiple sclerosis; it can remain an isolated manifestation, although it may affect the other eye at a later time. There remains a suspicion of isolated demyelinating pathology that does not progress further.

The condition can resolve without damage and with complete regression of the deficit within days or weeks; favorable outcomes are more common in cases with lesser initial visual impairment. In other cases, the fibers of the maculopapillary bundle undergo axonal degeneration, and the visual deficit is permanent. Ophthalmoscopic findings consist of pallor of the temporal half of the optic disc (where the maculopapillary bundle enters) and slowed nerve conduction as evidenced by visual evoked potentials. The diagnosis is straightforward: acute visual loss, central scotoma, normal fundus. In cases where multiple sclerosis will develop, magnetic resonance imaging usually reveals other previous lesions.

Treatment is based on corticosteroid therapy, as in acute episodes of multiple sclerosis.

Bulbar optic neuritis. Rarely, the optic nerve is affected at the level of the optic disc

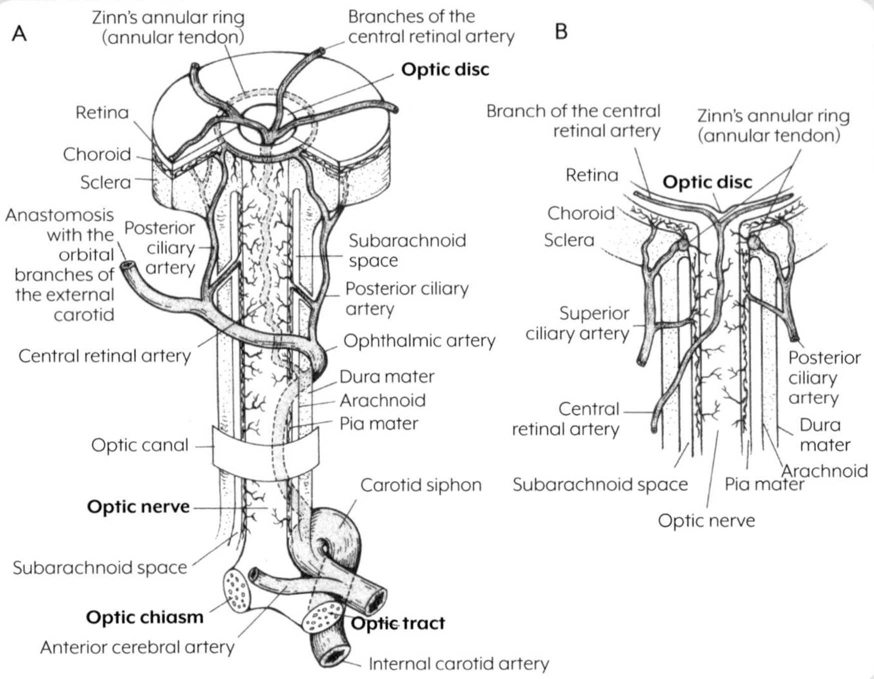

Figure 3.14

Vascularization of the optic nerve. A) Right optic nerve seen from above and anteriorly; the posterior pole of the eye has been sectioned to show the origin of the nerve from the optic disc. B) Longitudinal section of the optic disc and the distal portion of the nerve.

(bulbar optic neuritis or papillitis). Alternative causes to multiple sclerosis include Lyme disease, lupus, antiphospholipid syndrome, drug-induced vasculitis, Crohn's disease, and sphenoid and ethmoid sinusitis. It manifests, similar to retrobulbar neuritis, with rapid visual loss, but ophthalmoscopic examination reveals edema and swelling of the optic disc, and the visual field detects enlargement of the blind spot with a centrocecal scotoma. Distinguishing papilledema from papillitis, early visual loss, is not easy on ophthalmoscopic examination. The outcomes are less favorable than for the retrobulbar form, and residual visual impairment with secondary optic atrophy may remain (see below).

Anterior ischemic optic neuropathy. is a common condition in adulthood characterized by ischemic infarction of the optic nerve head. The anterior portion of the nerve (Figure 3.14) is supplied by the posterior ciliary arteries, which provide blood to the choroid and deep layers of the retina. The inner part of the nerve and the superficial layers of the retina are supplied by the central retinal artery, which enters the distal third of the nerve. The vessels originate from the ophthalmic artery. Within the globe, perfusion pressure is counteracted by intraocular pressure, and flow can be disrupted by both a drop in perfusion pressure and an increase in intraocular pressure.

Ischemic optic neuropathy is caused by a decrease in blood flow in the ciliary vessels due to atherosclerotic stenosis or vasculitis. In atherosclerosis, the damage usually occurs during a general drop in blood pressure, shock, or simply due to the physiological hypotension during sleep, facilitated by the evening intake of antihypertensive or erectile dysfunction drugs (sildenafil). The onset is typically in the morning, ischemia mainly affects the upper half of the optic disc, and it may be reversible. In vasculitis, the most common neurological form being giant cell arteritis or Horton's arteritis, symptoms such as fever, migratory arthralgia, polymyalgia, tenderness and palpable hardening of the temporal arteries, *claudication* of the jaw muscles, and increased erythrocyte sedimentation rate appear. Optic ischemia is massive and causes a sudden and painless loss of vision in one eye, sometimes preceded by episodes of transient amaurosis. It becomes irreversible if rapid intervention with corticosteroid therapy is not initiated. The other eye may be affected at a later time. The visual field usually exhibits inferior altitudinal defects. Ophthalmoscopic examination reveals disc edema with hemorrhages, which progress to atrophy within 4-8 weeks. Fluorescein angiography of retinal vessels can help delineate the ischemic territory and differentiate between the two etiologies in the early days, but the diagnosis of giant cell arteritis requires arterial biopsy.

The differential diagnosis from optic neuritis is based on advanced age, absence of pain, and the type of visual field defect (altitudinal scotoma in ischemic neuropathy, central or centrocecal scotoma in neuritis); differentiation from central retinal artery and branch occlusions is based on ophthalmoscopy and fluorescein angiography. Treatment for forms associated with vasculitis (also useful in non-arteritic form) involves corticosteroids. Therapy should be continued to prevent involvement of the other eye.

Leber hereditary optic neuropathy. It is an inherited mitochondrial disorder affecting the ganglion cells and axons of the retina, particularly the maculopapillary bundle. It predominantly develops in males in the 2nd and 3rd decade of life, with a subacute or acute onset of visual impairment that progresses and leads to severe loss of visual acuity over several months. The disorder is bilateral, either from the beginning or within a few weeks. The visual field exhibits a large central scotoma, and even in advanced stages, some visual perception may persist in the peripheral field. Ophthalmoscopic examination initially shows transient bilateral papillary edema with peripapillary telangiectasia, followed by optic atrophy. Degeneration of other neuronal systems (cerebellar signs, spasticity, mental retardation), and cardiac arrhythmia can also be associated. Treatment with idebenone, which reactivates mitochondrial respiration, has been shown to be beneficial.

Nutritional and toxic optic neuropathies. They are almost always bilateral and develop as a result of vitamin deficiencies (B1 and B12), malnutrition, intoxication from methanol produced in illicit distillation (sometimes in epidemic form), and the use of certain substances (ethambutol, chloroquine, streptomycin, chloramphenicol, etc.). Visual impairment develops within a few weeks and is accompanied by central scotoma and temporal pallor of the optic disc.

Tumors and compressions of the optic nerve. Tumors, more common in females, can be intrinsic (gliomas) or extrinsic (meningiomas). Gliomas appear in the first two decades of life, in approximately 10% of cases within the context of neurofibromatosis type I; they are usually low-grade and have a benign course. Meningiomas appear after the age of 30, originating from the optic nerve itself or more commonly from the optic canal, olfactory groove, or sphenoid wing. They cause progressive loss of visual acuity that develops over months or years, with an ophthalmoscopic picture of primary optic atrophy or, more rarely, unilateral stasis, later accompanied by exophthalmos. Their slow progression differentiates them from neuritis and optic neuropathies. The nerve can also be compressed by internal carotid, anterior cerebral, anterior communicating, and ophthalmic aneurysms.

Traumatic injuries. They occur due to penetrating orbital wounds or fractures of the skull base involving the optic canal. The impairment is immediate and is followed within a few weeks by primary optic atrophy.

Optic atrophy. It is a terminal aspect of the optic disc resulting from the degeneration of optic nerve axons. There are two ophthalmoscopic patterns of atrophy: primary and secondary. *Primary atrophy* is the expression of primitive degeneration, sometimes associated with degenerative or metabolic pathologies of the retina or other neuronal systems (such as cerebellar), or it follows pathologies of the retrobulbar portion of the optic nerve, up to the optic tract. The disc appears pale, with a mother-of-pearl-like appearance, poor in vessels; the physiological cupping is wider, the margins are sharp and stand out against the surrounding retina, and the retinal vessels are narrowed. If the degenerative process is limited to the maculopapillary bundle, as in retrobulbar neuritis, atrophy affects only the temporal half of the optic disc. Since this portion is always paler than the nasal portion, judgment is delicate; however, in atrophy, the peripheral zone of the disc also appears pale, whereas it is pink in normal subjects.

Secondary atrophy is the consequence of prolonged optic disc edema. It develops after long-lasting papilledema, in cases of bulbar optic neuritis and anterior ischemic optic neuritis. The optic disc takes on a grayish color, the physiological cupping is obscured, the margins are indistinct, and convoluted newly formed vessels are often observed around the disc.

In all atrophic processes, there is a severe impairment of vision and the visual field, leading to blindness, with loss of the pupillary light reflex.

Foster Kennedy syndrome. It develops in the course of large-sized meningiomas of the olfactory groove and sphenoid wing, which cause primary optic atrophy due to compression in one eye and edema due to stasis in the other eye. Neuritis and ischemic neuropathies, which affect the two eyes at different times, result in a similar ophthalmoscopic picture.

The chiasma | is almost always affected by compressive pathologies. Intrinsic tumors (gliomas) or more commonly extrinsic tumors (pituitary adenomas, craniopharyngiomas, and meningiomas) are very common. Adenomas, when they become large (macroadenomas), compress the chiasm from below; craniopharyngiomas (and Rathke's cleft cysts, which originate from embryonic remnants in the pituitary gland) develop above the sella turcica and compress the chiasm from behind and above. Meningiomas are frequent and often of considerable size: they originate from the tuberculum sellae and sellar diaphragm and compress the chiasm from below and posteriorly, from the sphenoid wing, and grow laterally. Common compressive pathologies include aneurysms of the anterior cerebral artery, anterior communicating artery, and supraclinoid segment of the internal carotid artery, as well as hydrocephalus of the third ventricle. Rarely, the pathology is ischemic (chiasmal apoplexy) and/or demyelinating (chiasmal optic neuritis). Arachnoiditis of the base and sphenoid sinus mucocele are also rare. Finally, the chiasm can be drawn towards the sella turcica in the so-called "empty sella" condition.

The visual field deficit is highly variable as anterior lesions tend to involve the optic nerve, and posterior lesions involve the optic tract. The classic bitemporal hemianopsia from a lesion of the decussation is observed in lesions of the central portion of the chiasm. Anterior lesions are accompanied by a unilateral central scotoma due to damage to one optic nerve, while posterior lesions involve the decussation of the maculopapillary bundle fibers and cause paracentral temporal scotomas. They can affect the optic tract and result in a homonymous

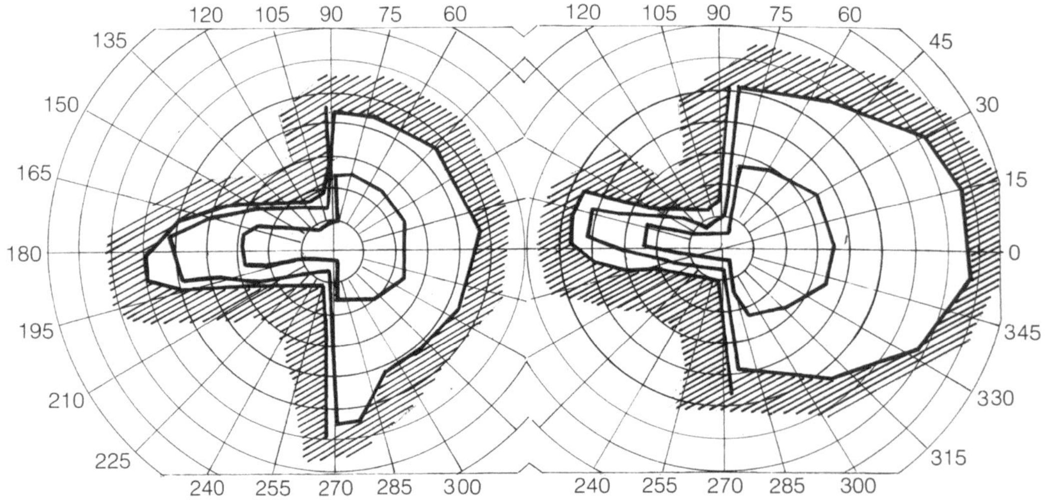

Figure 3.15

Campimetric defect in a case of ischemic lesion of the right lateral geniculate nucleus. Surgical ligation of the right carotid artery. (From Frisen, 1979).

lateral hemianopsia. Visual acuity, color discrimination, and pupillary reflexes can be preserved due to the temporal maculopapillary fibers, which do not cross over. Atrophy of the nasal half of the optic disc may develop.

Retrochiasmatic pathways | *Isolated unilateral lesions of the optic tract* are very rare and result in an incomplete and incongruous contralateral homonymous hemianopsia. Atrophy of the nasal half of the optic discs may become evident. *Lesions of the geniculate body*, usually ischemic in nature, cause a hemianopsia involving the upper and lower quadrants of the contralateral hemifields and may spare vision along the horizontal meridian (Figure 3.15). *Lesions of the optic radiations* lead to a usually incongruous contralateral homonymous hemianopsia due to fiber dispersion.

Lesions of the occipital cortex, on the other hand, typically result in a congruous hemianopsia. If the occipital pole remains intact, macular sparing occurs, and in the recovery phase, central vision resumes earlier. The hemianopsia can assume an altitudinal distribution in both eyes due to bilateral lesions affecting the upper or lower lips of the calcarine fissure.

In *bilateral lesions*, where the striate and peristriate areas can be affected together, complex neuropsychological conditions arise, such as cortical blindness, blindness with denial of visual defect (Anton syndrome), inability to recognize faces (prosopagnosia) or colors (achromatopsia), inability to direct gaze and fixate on the examiner's eyes (psychic paralysis of gaze), and inability to visually control and grasp an object (optic ataxia). Some of these deficits are encompassed in Balint's syndrome.

The etiologies differ in various segments of the retrochiasmatic pathways:

a) In the optic tract: occlusions of the anterior choroidal artery, multiple sclerosis plaques;
b) In the lateral geniculate body: occlusions of the anterior choroidal artery, glial tumors;
c) In the optic radiations: occlusion of the temporal or parietal branches of the middle cerebral artery, hematomas at the temporo-parieto-occipital junction, vascular malformations, glial or metastatic tumors, abscesses, demyelination plaques, leukodystrophies, venous sinus thrombosis;
d) In the striate and peristriate cortex: tumors, hematomas, and occlusions of the posterior cerebral artery (often bilateral due to the common origin from the basilar artery), post-traumatic contusional foci, and all degenerative pathologies of the posterior cortical areas, starting with Alzheimer's disease.

Some patients with geniculostriate lesions seem to retain a vague visual sensitivity in the hemianopic field: for example, they can direct their hand and react to objects and lights they do not consciously see ("*blind sight*"). It is likely supported by visual projections to the superior colliculus, pulvinar, and peristriate areas ("second visual system").

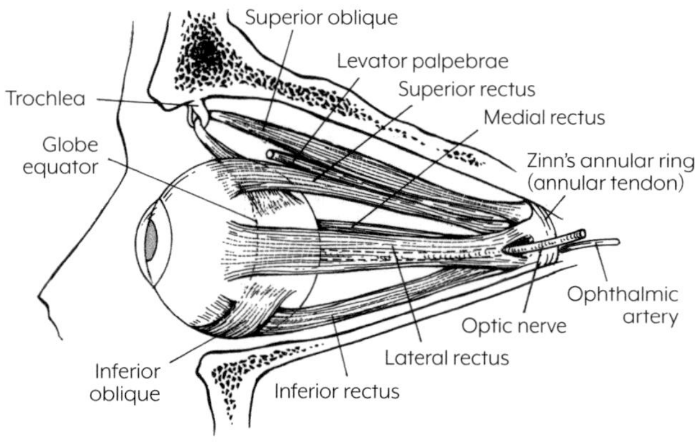

Figure 3.16

Extrinsic eye muscles. Semi-realistic view of the left eye after removal of the lateral wall of the orbit. The levator palpebrae muscle has been severed

3.4.2 Extrinsic ocular motility

The eyeball is moved by six muscles within the orbit: four rectus muscles (superior, medial, inferior, and lateral) and two oblique muscles (superior and inferior). These muscles are innervated by three cranial nerves (oculomotor, trochlear, and abducens) (Figure 3.16). They are activated by supranuclear motor systems originating from the cortex and vestibular nuclei and are coordinated by the brainstem reticular formation, superior colliculi, cerebellum, and basal ganglia. Another orbital muscle, the levator palpebrae superioris, is responsible solely for lifting the eyelid.

Extrinsic eye muscles

The *four rectus muscles attach* posteriorly to the annulus of Zinn, a tendinous structure that adheres to the apex of the orbit, and anteriorly to the globe in front of the equator. *Superior oblique muscle* travels from the annulus of Zinn to the medial wall of the orbit, where it reflects over a cartilaginous pulley called the trochlea, reversing its course and inserting onto the globe behind the equator. The inferior oblique muscle originates from the medial wall of the orbit and runs beneath the globe, also inserting behind the equator. The globe is surrounded by the *Tenon's capsule*.

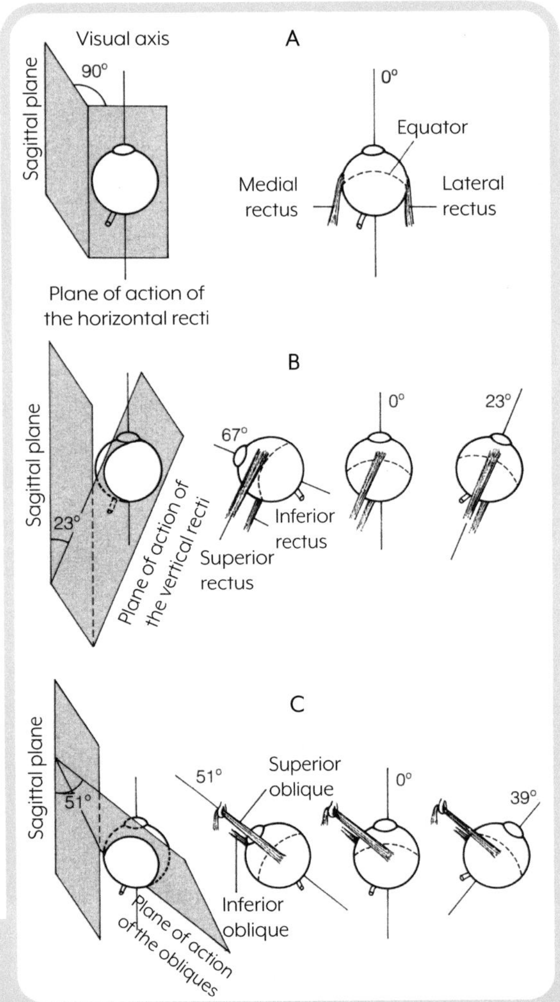

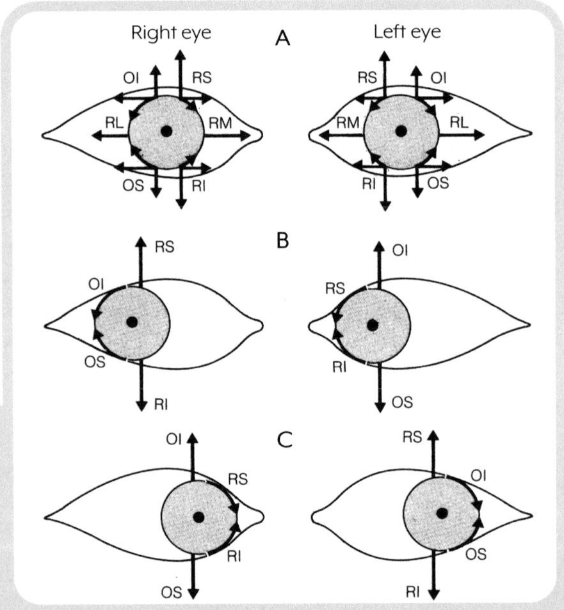

Figure 3.18

Combined action of the extrinsic ocular muscles. A) Global actions of the six ocular muscles. B, C) Lateral rotation of the eyes; the vertical rectus muscles act purely as elevators-depressors in the abducted eye and as pure rotators in the adducted eye. The opposite occurs for the oblique muscles (note that the lines of force of the oblique muscles are mirror images with respect to the insertion points). MR = medial rectus; LR = lateral rectus; SR = superior rectus; IR = inferior rectus; SO = superior oblique; IO = inferior oblique.

Figure 3.17

Action plan of the extrinsic eye muscles. Right eye seen from above. A) Plane of horizontal recti; the action of the muscles is exclusively exerted on this plane. B) Plane of vertical recti; the action of the muscles is purely elevating (superior rectus) and depressing (inferior rectus) when the eye is abducted by 23°; it is purely rotational when the eye is adducted by 67°; it appears combined in intermediate degrees. C) Plane of obliques; the action of the muscles is purely elevating (inferior oblique) and depressing (superior oblique) when the eye is adducted by 51°; it is purely rotational when the eye is abducted by 39°; it is combined in intermediate degrees. The primary position of the eyes coincides with oo (Modified from Cogan, 1966).

The muscles can be grouped into three pairs: the horizontal recti (medial and lateral), the vertical recti (superior and inferior), and the oblique muscles (superior and inferior). When the eyes are looking straight ahead (*primary position*) the visual axis, which is the path of a ray reaching the fovea, aligns with the sagittal and axial planes of the head (Figure 3.17). The action of the horizontal recti muscles is confined to the horizontal plane, which coincides with the axial plane of the head (Figure 3.17A): the medial rectus rotates the eye inward (adduction), and the lateral rectus rotates the eye outward (abduction).

The *action of the vertical recti muscles* occurs in a vertical plane that diverges from the sagittal plane by 23° (Figure 3.17B). Therefore, the action of the vertical recti muscles becomes purely vertical when the visual axis aligns with the plane of action of these two muscles, which occurs when the eye is abducted by 23°. In this position, the superior rectus muscle elevates the eye (elevation), and the inferior rectus muscle depresses the eye (depression). In the primary position, the combined action of the two vertical recti muscles causes adduction, while the action of a single muscle causes torsion of the eye around its axis, inward for the superior rectus muscle (internal torsion), and outward for the inferior rectus muscle (external torsion).

The *action of the oblique muscles* also occurs in a vertical plane that diverges from the sagittal plane by 51° (Figure 3.17C) and becomes purely vertical when the eyeball is adducted by 51°. The superior oblique muscle rotates the eye downward, and the inferior oblique muscle rotates the eye upward. In the primary position, the combined action of the two oblique muscles, inserted behind the equator, causes abduction, while the action of a single muscle causes torsion, inward for the superior oblique muscle and outward for the inferior oblique muscle.

The actions of the six muscles are summarized in Figure 3.18. Together, the rectus muscles pull the globe backward, and the oblique muscles pull it forward. Coordinated movements of the two eyes, or gaze movements, require the action of complementary pairs of muscles. For example, during rightward gaze, the right lateral rectus muscle and the left medial rectus muscle become agonists.

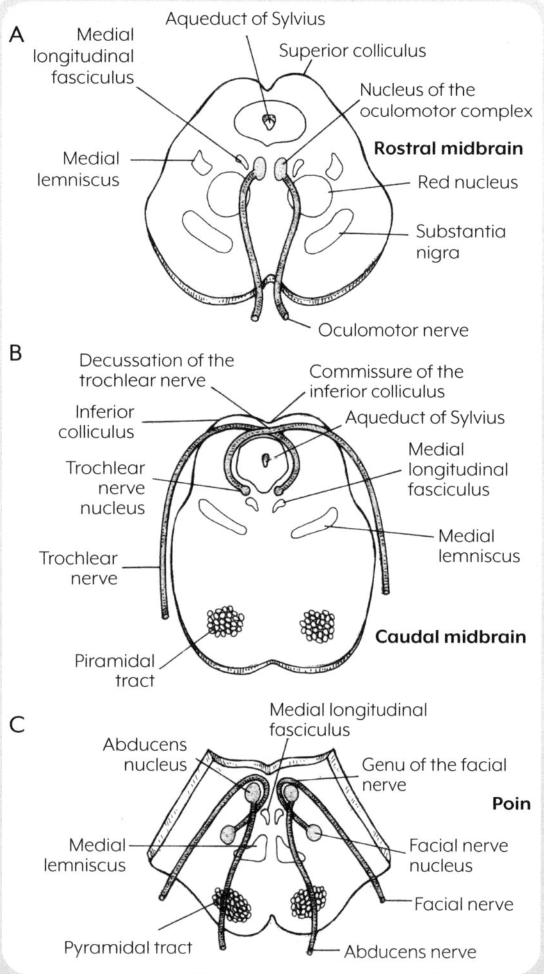

Figure 3.19

Oculomotor nerves: oculomotor (3rd), trochlear (4th), abducens (6th). A) Axial section of the midbrain at the level of the superior colliculi to show the origin of the oculomotor nerve. B) Axial section of the midbrain at the level of the inferior colliculi to show the origin of the trochlear nerve (note that this is the only nerve that crosses). C) Axial section of the pons to show the origin of the abducens and facial nerves.

Nuclei and Oculomotor Nerves

The *oculomotor nerve* (3rd cranial nerve) originates from a cluster of nuclei located in the paramedian region of the midbrain tegmentum, ventral to the Sylvian aqueduct. The fibers traverse the red nucleus, substantia nigra, and the medial portion of the cerebral peduncle, compacting together to emerge from the interpeduncular fossa (Figure 3.19A). It courses through the subarachnoid space at the base, passing between the superior cerebellar artery and posterior cerebral artery. It then traverses the entire lateral wall of the cavernous sinus and enters the orbit through the superior orbital fissure along with the 4th and 6th cranial nerves, as well as the 1st branch (ophthalmic) of the trigeminal nerve. The oculomotor nerve innervates the levator palpebrae, superior rectus, medial rectus, inferior rectus, and inferior oblique muscles. The fibers for the levator palpebrae and superior rectus muscles originate from the oculomotor nuclei on both sides. A group of medial and posterior

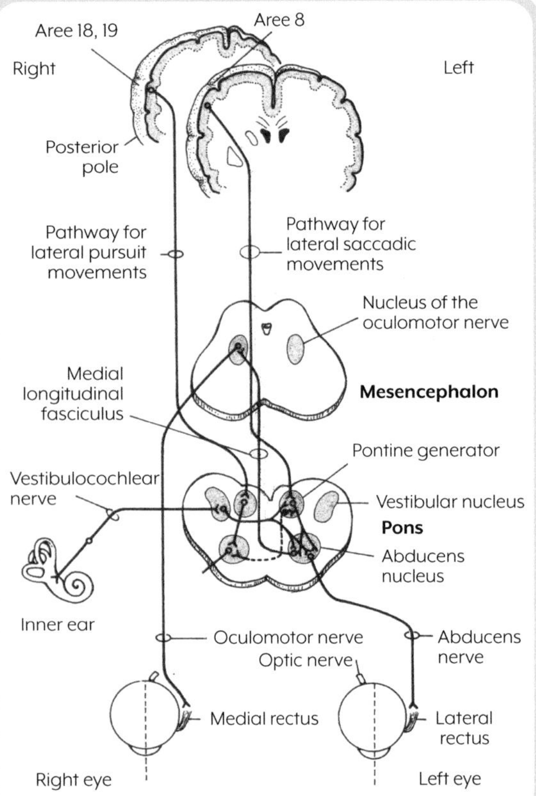

Figure 3.20

Pathways for lateral eye movements. The pathway for voluntary saccadic movements originates from the frontal cortex (area 8); the pathway for pursuit movements (reflexive responses to visual stimuli) originates from the parieto-occipital cortex (areas 18 and 19); the pathway for vestibular movements (reflexive responses to labyrinthine stimuli) originates from the vestibular nuclei. The "pontine generator" organizes the activity of the ipsilateral abducens nucleus and, through the medial longitudinal fasciculus, the contralateral oculomotor nucleus. An inhibitory connection (represented by a black neuron with dashed axon) inhibits the antagonistic muscles (not marked in the diagram). The abducens nucleus has been arbitrarily depicted in a more ventral position than in reality.

cells behind the oculomotor nuclei (Edinger-Westphal nucleus) gives rise to preganglionic parasympathetic fibers that travel through the nerve to reach the ciliary ganglion, which innervates the intrinsic muscles of the globe (iris sphincter and ciliary muscle).

The *trochlear nerve* (4th cranial nerve) also originates from the midbrain, from a nucleus located caudally to the nucleus of the 3rd nerve. It ascends superiorly, encircling the central gray matter, and decussates in the roof of the midbrain, emerging behind the inferior colliculi (Figure 3.19B). It then proceeds forward, encircling the midbrain, traverses the subarachnoid space at the base, crosses the entire wall of the cavernous sinus inferiorly to the 3rd nerve and superiorly to the ophthalmic branch of the 5th nerve, and enters the orbit through the superior orbital fissure. The trochlear nerve innervates the superior oblique muscle of the opposite side.

The abducens nerve (6th cranial nerve) originates from the paramedian region of the pons. The abducens nucleus contains not only the motoneurons for the lateral rectus muscle but also interneurons whose fibers cross over, ascend in the medial longitudinal fasciculus, and reach the nucleus of the 3rd cranial nerve for the medial rectus muscle of the opposite side, for lateral gaze movements. The 6th nerve runs laterally to the pyramidal tract and emerges between the pons and medulla (Figure 3.19C). It passes in front of the pons, traverses the apex of the petrous pyramid, crosses the wall, and enters the cavernous sinus laterally to the internal carotid artery (Figure 3.8). It then enters the orbit through the superior orbital fissure.

Supranuclear Oculomotor Systems

These systems aim to keep the object of interest projected onto the fovea of both eyes. These functions are carried out by four systems: the saccadic system, which locates the target; the pursuit system, which tracks its movements; the vestibular/optic-kinetic system, which compensates for head oscillations; and the vergence system, which adjusts for distance. These systems converge on common effectors that give peculiar characteristics to the discharge of oculomotor motoneurons and ensure reciprocal innervation of agonist and antagonist muscles. The common effectors consist of neuronal circuits ("integrators") located in the pontine and mesencephalic reticular formations, respectively, for horizontal and vertical-torsional gaze movements.

The *pontine integrator* is bilateral and occupies the paramedian pontine reticular formation, at the lateral and medial margins of the 6th nerve nucleus. It projects to the ipsilateral 6th nerve nucleus, both to the motoneurons for the ipsilateral lateral rectus and to the interneurons for the contralateral medial rectus (Figure 3.20). Horizontal movements are disconjugate between the two eyes: when one eye rotates outward, the other rotates inward.

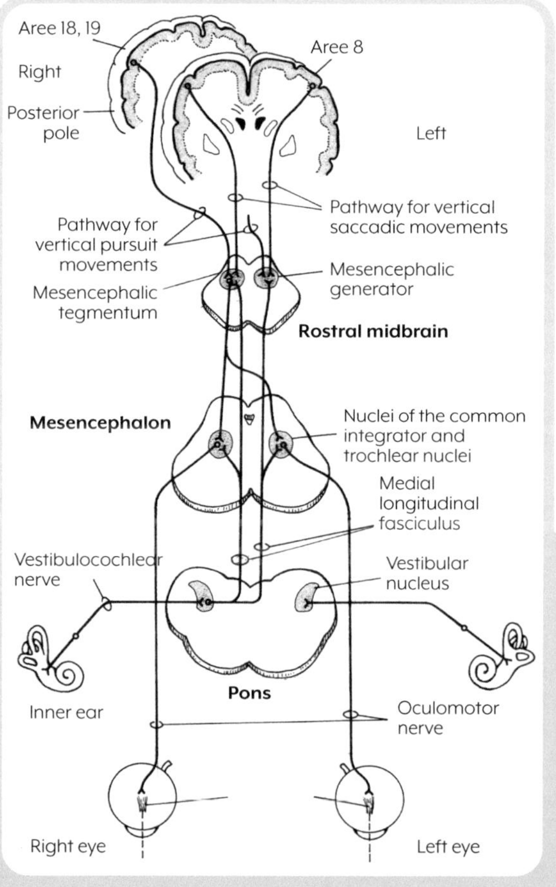

Figure 3.21

Paths for vertical eye movements. Similar to lateral movements, the pathway for saccadic eye movements originates from the frontal cortex, the pathway for pursuit movements originates from the parieto-occipital cortex, and the pathway for vestibular movements originates from the vestibular nuclei. The 'mesencephalic generator' organizes the activity of the oculomotor and trochlear nuclei on both sides.

The *mesencephalic integrator*, which is also bilateral, is strongly interconnected through the posterior commissure and occupies the midbrain tegmentum. It projects to the motoneurons of the 3rd and 4th nerve nuclei for the elevator muscles (superior rectus and inferior oblique) and the depressor muscles (inferior rectus and superior oblique). These muscles also allow torsion of the eye along the anteroposterior axis. The connections are bilateral because vertical-torsional movements are symmetric and complementary in both eyes, which rise, fall, and twist together (Figure 3.21).

Function of the integrator circuits is to activate agonist muscles while inhibiting antagonists, allowing the rotation of the eyeball against the viscoelastic resistance of orbital tissues and maintaining the eyeball in the reached position, preventing viscoelastic forces from bringing it back to the center of the orbit.

The *superior colliculus* contributes to target selection by integrating visual, acoustic, and somatic information, coordinates eye-head movements, and provides the start signal by blocking omnipause neurons. The cerebellum receives vestibular, reticular, and olivary nucleus information. The flocculonodular lobe and ventral portion of the vermis (vestibulocerebellum) stabilize the eyes during fixation and regulate the speed of pursuit movements, while the dorsal vermis regulates the speed, accuracy, and coordination of all movements, including eye-head coordination. The *basal ganglia* are traversed by a projection from the oculomotor fields, through the caudate, subthalamus, and substantia nigra, reaching the superior colliculus and facilitating the initiation and execution of saccadic movements, particularly in learned behaviors.

Saccadic System | Generates voluntary, spontaneous, and visually triggered movements that bring a selected target or a target appearing in the visual field onto the fovea. The pathway originates from the cortex, with the frontal oculomotor fields (area 6, 4) contributing more to internally generated movements and the parieto-occipital fields (areas 19, 37, 39) to reflexive movements. Descending pathways reach neurons in the interstitial nucleus of the medial longitudinal fasciculus, the ventral pontine reticular formation, and from there, the cerebellum and superior colliculus. Saccadic movements are rapid (200°-400° per second) and ballistic, meaning they cannot be corrected during execution phase: if the target is moved after the movement has started, the eyes reach the original position and then reacquire the target with a new saccade.

Tracking System | Generates movements that keep a target on the fovea (fixation reflex). If the target is moving, the eyes track it in space, potentially anticipating its trajectory; if the target is stationary, the gaze is held fixed by suppressing outward saccades. Tracking movements are slow (30°-50° per second) and produced reflexively, based on foveal information and through a long pathway: retina, lateral geniculate nucleus, striate and extrastriate areas, frontal and posterior oculomotor cortex, dorsolateral pontine reticular formation, cerebellum, and integrator and oculomotor nuclei of the brainstem. The pathway crosses twice, in the midbrain and pons, and the system appears to be more competent for tracking movements to the same side. The length of the pathway accounts for the fragility of tracking movements, which are compromised in many pathological conditions and by certain drugs.

Vestibular/Opticokinetic System | The vestibular system generates eye movements that compensate for head rotation and translation. The movement is reflexive and originates from the receptors of the labyrinth, consisting of the ampullae of the semicircular canals for rotation and the maculae of the utricle and saccule for translation. The maculae also provide information about the absolute position of the head in space. The information, collected by bipolar cells of the Scarpa's ganglion, converges on the vestibular nuclei and is then transmitted (directly or through the medial longitudinal fasciculus) to the motoneurons of the three oculomotor nuclei, spinal motoneurons, and the cerebellar vermis (see Figures 3.20 and 3.21).

Vergence System | Adapts the convergence of the eyes to the distance of the target. The movement, generated reflexively by the disparity of images on the two retinas, is very slow (approximately 10° per second) and can also be performed voluntarily. The pathway originates from the visual cortex and oculomotor fields, reaches the reticular formation of the mesencephalic tegmentum, and projects to the motoneurons of the medial rectus muscles (third nerve nuclei) and lateral rectus muscles (sixth nerve nuclei). Convergence is accompanied by accommodation and miosis (*accommodative triad*).

Coordinated action of supranuclear systems | The integration between the vestibular and saccadic systems occurs when the subject is placed on a rotating chair and the fixation reflex is prevented by Frenzel goggles (convex lenses of 20 diopters that make clear vision impossible). The eyes perform a compensatory movement of vestibular origin in the opposite direction of head rotation, maintaining the original direction; when the position becomes too eccentric, a cortical saccade brings them back to the primary position. The repetition of this sequence generates *vestibular nystagmus*. The integration between the optokinetic and saccadic systems emerges when clear vision is allowed. On a rotating chair or other moving device, the eyes instinctively fixate on a particular point in the visual field, and visual information suppresses the vestibular reflex. This phenomenon is evident in a subject looking out of the window of a moving train and can be reproduced in a stationary subject by rotating a cylinder with vertical stripes in front of their eyes. The eyes slowly track a target until a compensatory head movement is necessary. At this point, a saccade brings the gaze back, and the tracking resumes on another target. This is known as *optokinetic nystagmus*.

Examination of eye motility

It is used to assess the functioning of individual muscles and supranuclear motor systems.

The individual muscles are examined by moving the patient's eyes in the direction of action of each muscle. There are no doubts for horizontal movements and for the action of the medial and lateral rectus muscles. Vertical movements are explored with the eyes rotated laterally, first to one side and then to the other:

in this position, the superior and inferior rectus muscles act as elevator and depressor in the abducted eye, while the oblique muscles act as elevator and depressor in the adducted eye (note: the inferior oblique acts as an elevator and the superior oblique as a depressor). If a muscle is paretic, the visual axes of the two eyes are misaligned (*strabismus*); the projections of a target fall on non-corresponding points on the two retinas, and the subject perceives two images, one "true" from the healthy eye and one "false" from the paretic eye (*diplopia*). There are some rules to identify the affected muscle:

1) When looking in the direction of action of the paretic muscle, strabismus and the distance between the true and false images increase.
2) The false image is shifted in the direction of action of the paretic muscle.
3) The false image is eccentric compared to the true image.
4) To reduce diplopia, the subject deviates their head in the direction of action of the paretic muscle.

Let's suppose there is a deficit in the right lateral rectus muscle (Figure 3.22A). In the primary position, the two eyes may appear aligned, but when the patient looks to the right, the left eye rotates while the right eye remains immobile, increasing the strabismus. The target is projected onto the fovea of the left eye but falls on the nasal retina of the right eye. Since the brain locates the images of the right nasal retina to the right, the false image is seen to the right of the true image, i.e., in the direction of action of the right lateral rectus muscle, and it is eccentric compared to the true image. To reduce diplopia, instead of rotating the eyes, the subject tends to rotate the head to the right, in the direction of action of the paretic muscle.

If the deficit affects the right medial rectus muscle (Figure 3.22B), when the subject looks to the left, the left eye rotates while the right eye remains immobile. The target is projected onto the temporal retina of the right eye, and the false image is located to the left of the true image, again in the direction of action of the paretic muscle and eccentric compared to the true image. The patient tends to keep the head rotated to the left. To separate the images of the two eyes, one eye is occluded with the hand, and the patient is asked to indicate which image disappears. Placing a red lens in front of the right eye facilitates the examination.

Saccadic movements are evaluated by observing spontaneous movements continuously produced during conversation, asking the subject to look horizontally and vertically, to look at the examiner's hand as it moves, and to alternate between looking at the examiner's two hands. The following aspects should be assessed: numerosity, latency, speed, accuracy, and the ability to move the eyes while keeping the head still. For pursuit movements, a target is moved in

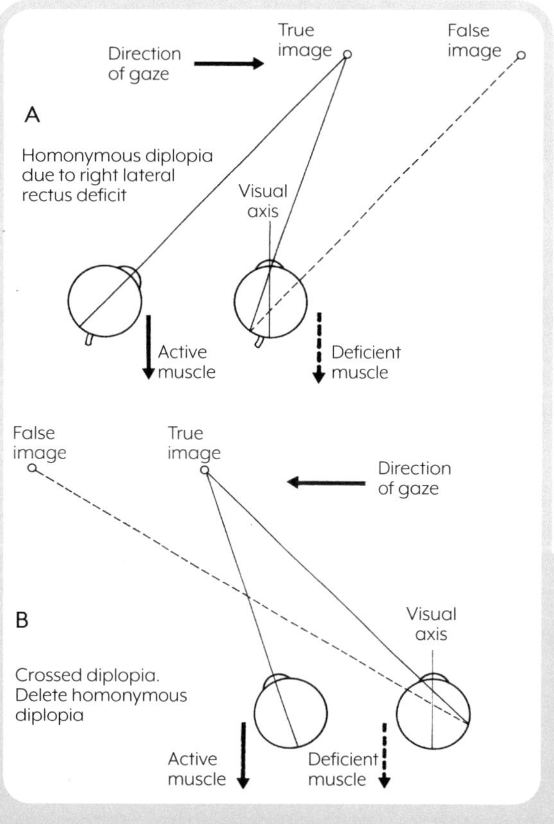

Figure 3.22

Diplopia in horizontal rectus muscle deficits. The eyes are seen from above, and the deficit affects the right eye. A) Lateral rectus muscle deficit; the false image is positioned in the direction of the deficient muscle's action and is eccentric to the true image; the diplopia is homonymous (deficient muscle on the right, false image to the right of the true image). B) Medial rectus muscle deficit; in this case as well, the false image is positioned in the direction of the deficient muscle's action and is eccentric to the true image, but the diplopia is crossed (deficient muscle on the right, false image to the left of the true image).

front of the patient's eyes at various speeds and in horizontal and vertical directions. It is observed whether the movement is smooth or fragmented by saccades to recapture the target.

To examine *vestibular movements*, the subject is asked to fixate on the examiner's nose. A sudden passive rotation of the head (approximately 15°) is applied, and if the vestibular system is functioning properly, the eyes maintain fixation. If there is a deficit, the subject must make an adjustment saccade. An ophthalmoscope can be used: the optic disc is observed at close range from the subject's face, and the subject is asked to make alternating rotational movements of the head (15°, twice per second). If the system is working, the optic disc remains still (even during head tremors, the optic disc appears still). In a comatose subject, a passive rotation of the head or irrigation of the ear with cold water is performed (see 8th cranial nerve). For optokinetic movements, a common tailor's measuring tape (preferably with alternating colors) is passed in front of the patient's eyes, and they are instructed to fixate on it. *Convergence movements* are assessed by having the patient alternately focus on a nearby target (examiner's finger) and a distant one.

Eye movement disorders

They depend on three conditions:

a) Altered balance of the eye muscles (non-paralytic strabismus).
b) Paralysis of the eye muscles (paralytic strabismus).
c) Lesions of the supranuclear oculomotor systems (gaze palsy).

Non-paralytic strabismus | The balance of eye muscles appears congenitally imperfectly regulated. This condition can remain latent (*heterophoria*) or become manifest (*heterotropia or strabismus*). In the latent form, the imbalance between the eye muscles is actively compensated by the supranuclear motor systems. The alignment effort may become insufficient when the individual is fatigued or in old age, leading to the appearance of fluctuating strabismus and diplopia. It also becomes decompensated when there is a visual deficit in one eye or paralysis of an eye muscle, further complicating the characteristics of diplopia.

In the manifest form, strabismus (either *divergent/exotropia* or *convergent/esotropia*) is present from birth or develops in early childhood, sometimes in association with an intercurrent illness, which is mistakenly attributed as the cause. The deviation angle of the eye axes remains constant in all gaze directions (*concomitant strabismus*); and there is no diplopia because the conflict between the two images is resolved at the cortical level through functional exclusion of one eye. If the condition is not treated early with alternate occlusion of the two eyes, the loss of visual acuity becomes permanent (*amblyopia ex anopsia*). The excluded eye (referred to as "lazy") exhibits a normal retina, optic disc, and pupillary reflexes but perceives only light.

Paralytic strabismus | It is caused by the deficit of one or more eye muscles and results in diplopia. The lesion can be localized in the brainstem, nerve, neuromuscular junction, or eye muscles.

Brainstem lesions are usually lateralized and cause an alternate syndrome with deficits of one or more oculomotor nerves and other structures on the side of the lesion, along with long tract signs and contralateral neurological signs. Eponymous syndromes have lost much of their localizing value with the advent of magnetic resonance imaging. The most classic ones include:

- Benedikt's syndrome: paramedian tegmental lesion of the midbrain (involving the fibers of the 3rd nerve, red nucleus, pyramidal tract, superior cerebellar peduncle; resulting in 3rd nerve palsy and contralateral hemiparesis, chorea, ataxia). In Claude's syndrome, which is also paramedian tegmental, the pyramidal tract is spared.
- Weber's syndrome: ventral tegmental lesion of the midbrain (involving the fibers of the 3rd nerve and pyramidal tract, causing 3rd nerve palsy and contralateral facio-brachio-crural hemiplegia).
- Foville-Millard-Gubler syndrome: pontine tegmental lesion (involving the nuclei of the 6th and 7th nerves and the pontine integrator, medial lemniscus, spinotalamic tract, pyramidal tract; resulting in ipsilateral gaze palsy and contralateral tactile and

thermosensory anesthesia, facio-brachio-crural hemiplegia).

Causes can include ischemic foci, cavernous angiomas with hemorrhagic foci, infiltrating gliomas, demyelinating plaques, other autoimmune pathologies, Wernicke's disease, and tuberculomas.

Sometimes, the oculomotor nuclei are congenitally hypoplastic. The most common condition is hypoplasia of the 3rd nuclei, which causes congenital eyelid ptosis, usually on one side only. Hypoplasia of the 6th nucleus leads to fibrosis of the lateral rectus muscle and hypertrophy of the medial rectus muscle, resulting in congenital abduction deficit of one eye and retraction of the eyeball during adduction (Duane syndrome)

Nerve injuries. They can affect the ocular nerves individually or in combination. *Paralysis* of the 3rd nerve results in a deficit of all the ocular muscles on one side, except for the superior oblique and lateral rectus muscles. The eye is closed due to the deficit of the levator palpebrae; the globe tends to rotate outward, and the head turns in the opposite direction of the paralysis side; the pupil is dilated due to involvement of the pupilloconstrictor parasympathetic fibers. The nerve can be compressed by aneurysms of the posterior communicating artery, basilar artery, and supraclinoid segment of the internal carotid artery, parasellar meningiomas, pituitary adenomas, tumors of the base, and granulomatous meningitis. It is frequently compromised in diabetes due to a central infarct that typically spares the pupillary fibers running in the upper portion of the nerve. Conversely, mydriasis is the initial sign in uncal herniation of the hippocampus during expansive supratentorial lesions.

Isolated 4th nerve lesions are usually caused by closed head trauma and sometimes by increased intracranial pressure. The eye tends to elevate and rotate outward, and diplopia worsens when looking downward and inward.

6th nerve palsy is common. The globe tends to rotate inward, and the head turns towards the side of the paralysis. It occurs in cases of increased intracranial pressure, subarachnoid hemorrhages, meningitis, following head trauma, and is not uncommonly bilateral. It is also observed in diabetes, osteitis of the apex of the petrous pyramid together with Gasser ganglion lesion (Gradenigo's syndrome).

Tolosa-Hunt syndrome is a granulomatous inflammation of the cavernous sinus region on one side, responsive to corticosteroid treatment. It causes paralysis of the three ocular nerves and orbital pain in the territory of the 1st branch of the 5th nerve. It can also be caused by meningiomas, cavernous sinus thrombosis, and carotid-cavernous fistulas. The three ocular nerves and the 1st branch of the 5th nerve have a common blood supply and are affected together in occlusion of the inferolateral branch of the internal carotid artery.

The three ocular nerves are typically affected bilaterally, often at different times, in tumors of the cranial base and granulomatous or carcinomatous meningitis. The impairment is bilateral and acute in cranial inflammatory polyneuropathies (Fisher syndrome).

Junctional and ocular muscle injuries. The former develop in myasthenia and myasthenia-like syndromes and begin with levator palpebrae deficit and ptosis; the latter in ocular myopathies. They are part of muscular diseases.

Gaze palsy Laterality paralysis | *Laterality paralysis.* Frontal or capsular lesions interrupt the pathway of saccadic movements, making it difficult to direct or maintain gaze towards the opposite side. Contralateral hemiparesis is often present, and therefore, the eyes have difficulty looking towards the side of paresis. The deficit appears in the acute phase of an ischemic or hemorrhagic stroke; in a depressed state of consciousness, the eyes (and to a lesser extent, the head) tend to rotate towards the non-paretic side. The disturbance tends to resolve in the days following the episode and with the recovery of vigilance. Pursuit movements are preserved.

Parieto-occipital lesions affect pursuit movements, which tend to fragment. Due to the double decussation of the pathway, pursuit is more compromised when the target moves towards the non-paretic side but can be disturbed in both directions.

Lesions in the paramedian region of the pons involve the pontine integrator of lateral movements and cause paralysis of lateral gaze towards the side of the lesion. The pyramidal tract is usually involved, and contralateral hemiparesis occurs. In pontine lesions, there is a dissociation between the eyes, which cannot gaze towards one side, and the limbs that are paretic on the opposite side (Foville's syndrome). Oculomotion deficit from a pontine lesion is much more severe and persistent than in hemisphere damage; due to the unopposed action of the intact pontine structures on the healthy side, the eyes are forcibly rotated towards the side of hemiparesis and do not cross the midline voluntarily or with pursuit movements. Vestibular movements may be spared, but this depends on the extent of the lesion.

Internuclear paralysis. The lesion is located in the medial longitudinal fasciculus, interrupting the crossed pathway that connects the nucleus of the 6th nerve with the nucleus of the 3rd nerve and activates the contralateral medial rectus muscle during lateral gaze (Figure 3.20). Let's assume that the lesion affects the left medial longitudinal fasciculus: during rightward lateral gaze, the right lateral rectus muscle is normally innervated and rotates the eye outward, while the left medial rectus muscle is disconnected and the eye does not move; however, the left eye, which appeared incapable of adduction, easily crosses the midline during convergence, as the pathway reaches the nucleus of the 3rd nerve from above and bypasses the lesion. The abducted eye (the right eye in our example) exhibits nystagmus, which is actually the most frequent sign of internuclear lesion. Due to the paramedian course of the medial longitudinal fasciculus, a single lesion can interrupt the pathway from both sides: in this case, both eyes show nystagmus during abduction, adduction paralysis, and normal convergence. Internuclear paralysis is characteristic of multiple sclerosis but is also observed in infiltrating gliomas, pontine infarctions, and Arnold-Chiari malformation.

"One-and-a-half syndrome". It is the combination of lateral gaze paralysis and internuclear paralysis due to a unilateral pontine lesion affecting the integrator and the medial longitudinal fasciculus. The affected eye does not perform horizontal movements: it does not abduct due to the pontine integrator lesion and does not adduct due to the medial longitudinal fasciculus lesion ("one"); the contralateral eye does not adduct due to the pontine integrator lesion ("and-a-half"); both eyes can converge.

Vertical paralysis. It results from lesions in the dorsal midbrain, affecting the pretectal region and the posterior commissure, and compromising the mesencephalic integrator on both sides and their reciprocal connections. The deficit can involve all vertical movements but more frequently affects upward movements, including both saccadic and pursuit movements, while vestibular movements, controlled by pathways ascending from the pons, may be spared. Convergence paralysis, upper eyelid retraction, midriasis, and reduced pupillary light reflex (Parinaud syndrome) are also observed. It can result from thalamic and mesencephalic hemorrhages and infarctions, hydrocephalus, pineal tumors, and encephalitis. Vertical movements are compromised in some degenerative parkinsonism disorders.

3.4.3 Intrinsic Ocular Motility

There are four smooth muscles in the eye with vegetative functions:

- The *iris sphincter*, which constricts the pupil (miosis), and the *ciliary muscle*, which adjusts the focal length of the lens (accommodation), both innervated by the parasympathetic nervous system.
- The *iris dilator*, which dilates the pupil (mydriasis), and *the Müller's tarsal muscle*, which assists in lifting the upper eyelid, both innervated by the sympathetic nervous system.

Functional Organization of the Pupils

The size of the pupils depends on the balance between parasympathetic and sympathetic innervation and is regulated reflexively (Figure 3.23). The afferent pathway of the reflex originates from retinal receptors, especially macular receptors. The fibers cross over at the optic chiasm following the general distribution of optic fibers, travel through the optic tract, and near the geniculate body, they diverge from the visual pathway and enter the superior colliculus arm, terminating in the pretectal region of the mesencephalon. From

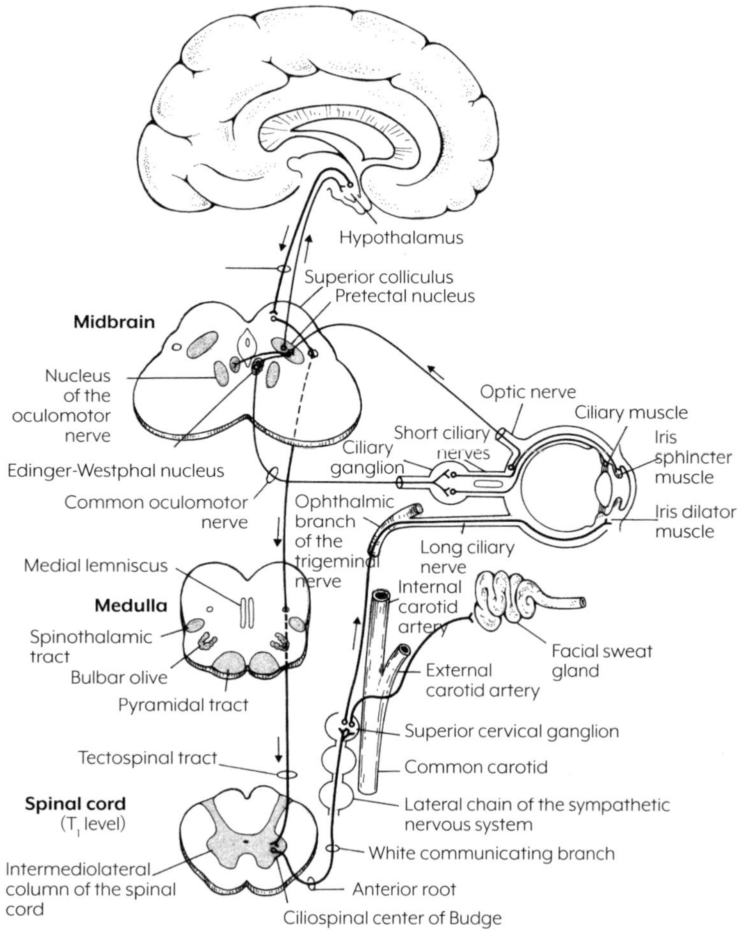

Figure 3.23

Pupillary pathways. The parasympathetic pathway starts from the Edinger-Westphal nucleus and travels through the oculomotor nerve, the ciliary ganglion (where it synapses), and the short ciliary nerves to reach the sphincter muscles of the iris and ciliary body. The sympathetic pathway starts from the ciliospinal center of Budge and travels through the sympathetic chain, the superior cervical ganglion (where it synapses), the pericarotid sympathetic plexus, the ophthalmic branch of the trigeminal nerve, and the long ciliary nerve to reach the dilator muscle of the iris. It is initiated by the hypothalamus through the dorsal longitudinal fasciculus and tectospinal pathway.

there, interneurons project to the Edinger-Westphal nucleus on both sides.

The *parasympathetic pathway*, which is cholinergic, originates from the Edinger-Westphal nucleus located in the mesencephalic tegmentum, dorsally and medially to the oculomotor nucleus. The axons run in the upper quadrant of the oculomotor nerve, a position that makes them susceptible to extrinsic compression. Upon reaching the orbit, they travel through the inferior division of the oculomotor nerve, detach via the short ciliary root, and reach the ciliary ganglion located at the orbital apex, where they make contact with the second neuron. The postganglionic fibers reach the eyeball via the short ciliary nerves, pierce the sclera at the posterior pole, and terminate on the sphincter and ciliary muscles.

The *sympathetic pathway*, which is adrenergic, originates from the hypothalamus and descends without crossing over in the lateral tegmentum of the brainstem and spinal cord, terminating in the intermediolateral column at the C8-T1-T2 levels (Budge's ciliospinal center). The preganglionic fibers leave the spinal cord through the T1-T2 anterior roots, reach the sympathetic chain via the white communicating ramus, which runs in the thoracic cavity behind the pleura of the apical lung, cross the inferior cervical ganglion (stellate ganglion) and middle cervical ganglion, and terminate at the superior cervical ganglion located above the carotid bifurcation, between the internal carotid artery and internal jugular vein, where they make contact with the ganglionic neurons.

The postganglionic fibers follow the internal carotid artery and, in the middle cranial fossa, leave the artery by accompanying the first branch of the trigeminal nerve, entering the orbit through the superior sphenoidal fissure. They detach from the branch as long ciliary nerves, reach the posterior pole of the eyeball, and ultimately innervate the dilator of the iris and tarsal muscles. Some fibers follow the ophthalmic artery, a branch of the internal carotid artery, to reach the eyeball. The sudomotor and vasomotor sympathetic fibers, which supply the sweat glands and vascular branches of the face, follow the external carotid artery.

Examination of the pupils

Under normal conditions, the diameter of the pupils ranges from 5 to 2 mm and tends to decrease with advancing age. The pupils are circular (isocyclic) and equal in size (isocoric). They become irregular (anisocyclic) due to pathologies of the anterior chamber of the eye. In 10% of individuals, there may be minimal differences in size (anisocoria), but occasionally larger differences can be observed due to the occasional use of eye drops in the hours preceding the examination.

The *light reflex* occurs following the sudden illumination of one eye and results in miosis by activating the Edinger-Westphal nucleus on the same side (direct pupillary reflex) and the opposite side (consensual or crossed reflex). It is advisable to have the subject look into the distance and project the light obliquely to avoid accommodation. The extent and duration of miosis should be evaluated.

The *accommodation reflex* occurs during fixation on a near target. The response is activated by visual afferents to the striate and peristriate areas, from where a projection reaches the pretectal region and causes accommodation, convergence of the ocular axes, and miosis.

The *ciliospinal reflex* is elicited by painful stimuli in the cervical region and results in weak mydriasis due to activation of Budge's ciliospinal center.

Pharmacological reactivity is helpful in assessing the functionality of the autonomic innervation. Cholinergic agents such as methacholine and pilocarpine induce miosis by stimulating cholinergic receptors, and the response increases if the parasympathetic pathway is compromised and the pupil has developed denervation hypersensitivity. Hydroxyamphetamine releases adrenaline from sympathetic nerve endings and causes mydriasis if the postganglionic fibers are intact. On the other hand, apraclonidine causes mydriasis when the adrenergic fibers are degenerated, and the pupil has developed denervation hypersensitivity.

Pupillary Syndromes

The pupillary pathways follow a long central and peripheral course, adjacent to the structures that regulate wakefulness, and are highly resistant to metabolic damage. In disorders of consciousness, but not limited to them, pupillary alterations are a significant indicator of structural lesions. Moreover, they exhibit specific modifications during certain intoxications.

Bilateral Miosis | It is observed in bilateral lesions of the pons, which interrupt the central sympathetic pathway, and in opiate intoxication and generally in narcotic intoxication, which exert a central effect. The pupils can reach sizes smaller than a millimeter (pinpoint pupils), and further constriction to light may only be observed with magnification.

Bilateral Mydriasis | This results from lesions of the mesencephalic tegmentum, which centrally interrupt the parasympathetic pathway, and from bilateral lesions of the 3rd cranial nerve that interrupt the pathway to the periphery. It is also observed in cocaine and amphetamine intoxication, which inhibit the reuptake of norepinephrine by adrenergic terminals, and in atropine and scopolamine intoxication, which block cholinergic receptors. Tricyclic and serotonergic antidepressants also cause mydriasis due to cholinergic inhibition. In brain death, the pupils tend to dilate due to elastic effects.

Unilateral Miosis | Associated with narrowing of the palpebral fissure due to paralysis of the tarsal muscle, it is observed in unilateral lesions of the sympathetic pathway (Bernard-Horner syndrome). The enophthalmos, the third classic element of the syndrome, is apparent and depends on the palpebral narrowing. Other associated symptoms may include loss of sweating (anhidrosis) and vasodilation on the ipsilateral half of the face. The syndrome can occur due to:

a) Central lesions in the hypothalamus, lateral tegmentum of the medulla, and cervical spinal cord;
b) Preganglionic peripheral lesions, from the central root T1-2 to the superior cervical ganglion;
c) Postganglionic peripheral lesions, at the level of the internal carotid artery, cavernous sinus region, and superior orbital fissure.

The most frequent causes include bulbar strokes, syringomyelia, tumors of the lung apex, carotid dissection, trigeminal autonomic cephalalgias, and cavernous sinus syndromes. Central lesions are accompanied by signs of damage to long pathways and cranial nerves. In lesions involving the common carotid artery, there is a loss of sweating on the ipsilateral half of the face. Pharmacological reactivity aids in localizing the damage. Hydroxyamphetamine causes dilation in central or preganglionic peripheral forms but is absent in postganglionic peripheral damage. The response to apraclonidine in inducing mydriasis is strong, but over time, it also appears in central and preganglionic lesions due to depletion of adrenergic synaptic terminals and subsequent hypersensitivity.

Unilateral Mydriasis | It occurs in lesions of the 3rd cranial nerve. Pupillary fibers are particularly sensitive to compressive damage at the exit of the nerve from the midbrain. The causes have been reported in lesions of the 3rd cranial nerve.

Loss of Light Reflex | It can result from lesions of the afferent or efferent branch. Lesions of the optic nerve interrupt the afferent branch, and illumination of the affected eye does not elicit a response in either eye, while the response is bilaterally normal when illuminating the healthy eye. Loss of the reflex, as well as its reduction or comparatively rapid exhaustion of the response, are highly sensitive indicators of damage to the maculopapillary bundle. On the other hand, lesions of the 3rd cranial nerve interrupt the efferent branch of the reflex and abolish the pupillary response on the affected side, whether illuminating either eye.

Argyll Robertson Pupil | It is almost pathognomonic of late-stage syphilis of the nervous system, but it can also be observed in compressive lesions of the pretectal region. The pupils are miotic and sometimes anisocoric and anisocyclic; they do not react to light but respond normally to accommodation, which should be observed carefully or with a lens. The lesion is located in the pretectal region and bilaterally interrupts the afferent pathway of the light reflex. However, it spares the descending cortical pathways responsible for accommodation.

Adie's Tonic Pupil | It occurs in young age, usually in females, and almost always affects only one side. The lesion consists of an acute injury to the ciliary ganglion, followed by incomplete reinnervation of the iris sphincter muscle by fibers destined for the ciliary muscle. The unreinnervated muscle fibers develop denervation hypersensitivity. The pupil appears midriatic under normal illumination and does not respond to light. After prolonged exposure to bright light, it may show a slight reduction in size, but usually the variations are minimal. However, it responds to accommodation with intense, but slow, tonic and persistent miosis. In approximately half of the cases, the Achilles and patellar reflexes are absent. Denervation hypersensitivity is demonstrated by 0.1% pilocarpine eye drops, which induce a prompt miosis, while being ineffective on a normal pupil. The cause is unknown, but the condition is benign.

3.5 Neurotology

Neurotology studies the neurological aspects of balance and hearing function. The receptors are located in the membranous labyrinth of the inner ear, which is contained within the bony labyrinth inside the petrous pyramid of the temporal bone. The two systems transmit information to the central nervous system through two separate branches: the vestibular nerve (for balance), originating from Scarpa's vestibular ganglion, and the cochlear nerve (for hearing), originating from Corti's spiral ganglion. The two ganglia possess bipolar neurons connected peripherally to the receptors and centrally to the nuclei of the brainstem. They are located at the beginning of the auditory canal and in the axis of the cochlea, giving rise to the vestibulocochlear nerve (8th cranial nerve), which travels through the auditory canal and exits through the internal acoustic meatus on the wall of the temporal pyramid, laterally to the 7th nerve. It crosses the region of the cerebellopontine angle and enters the lateral surface of the brainstem at the caudal border of the pons.

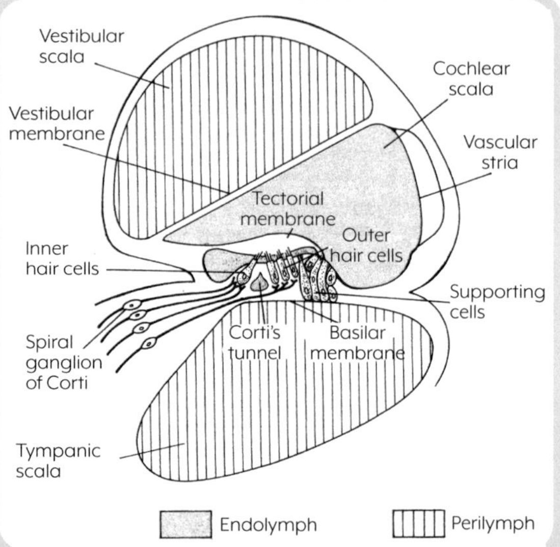

Figure 3.25

Cross-section of the cochlea. The scala media (or cochlear duct), bounded by the basilar and vestibular membranes and the vascular stripe, separates the vestibular scala from the tympanic scala. The basilar membrane supports the inner row and the three outer rows of receptor cells, covered by the tectorial membrane. The vascular stripe provides energy to the organ of Corti and regulates the composition of the endolymph in the scala media. The cochlea is housed within the temporal pyramid.

3.5.1 Vestibular System

Functional organization

The *membranous labyrinth*, the peripheral organ of the vestibular system, consists of a series of interconnected cavities, including the cochlear duct (leading to the cochlea), containing *endolymph* (Figure 3.24).

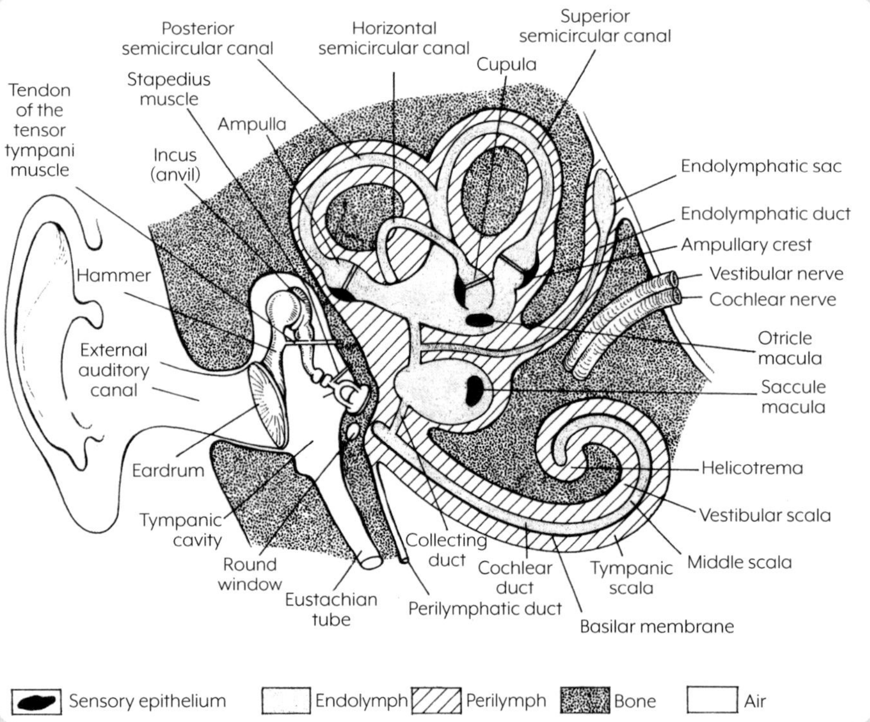

Figure 3.24

Schematic representation of the vestibular and auditory organs. The membranous labyrinth (vestibular) and the cochlear duct (auditory) communicate through the vestibular duct. Vestibular receptors are located in the maculae of the saccule and utricle, as well as in the ampullary crests of the semicircular canals; auditory receptors are located in the cochlear duct.

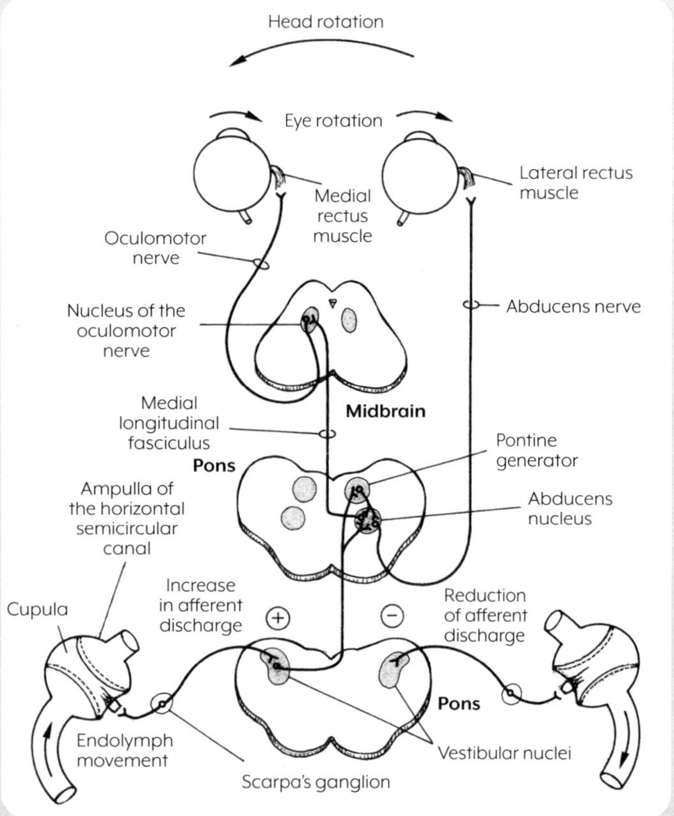

Figure 3.26

Functioning of the horizontal semicircular canals. The head is seen from above. When the head rotates to the left (arrow pointing up), in the left semicircular canal, the endolymph moves forward by inertia (ampullopetal movement), activating the receptor cells, while in the right semicircular canal, it moves backward (ampullofugal movement), inhibiting them. The afferent discharge activates the left vestibular nucleus and the right lateral rectus muscle and the left medial rectus muscle, which deviate the eyes to the right and maintain the gaze in the original direction. This reflex is the basis of the "doll's eye phenomenon".

Endolymph is produced by the vascular stria of the cochlear duct (Figure 3.25) and drained into the venous sinuses of the dura mater by the endolymphatic duct. It is surrounded by *perilymph*, which separates it from the walls of the bony labyrinth, produced by the arterioles of the labyrinthine periosteum and drained into the subarachnoid space by the perilymphatic duct.

It is divided into two subunits: the *otolithic organs* (utricle and saccule) and the semicircular canals, which have the same type of receptor cells.

Receptor Cells | These cells are located in specialized areas of the walls, known as the *maculae* of the utricle and saccule, and the *ampullary* crests of the canals. The ampullary crests are situated in a dilated portion of the canal adjacent to the utricle, called the ampulla. They are innervated at one end by the peripheral extensions of Scarpa's ganglion neurons (Figure 3.26). At their free ends, they expand into a series of aligned microvilli called *stereocilia*, one of which, the *kinocilium*, is situated on one side and is more prominent. The cilia protrude into the cavities of the labyrinth and insert into the *gelatinous membrane*, mainly composed of mucopolysaccharides. Like a compass, the labyrinthine receptor has a morphological axis of orientation and exhibits tonic resting activity modulated by the position of the cilia. Displacement of the stereocilia towards the kinocilium depolarizes the cell and increases afferent discharge, while displacement in the opposite direction inhibits it.

Otolithic Organs | The receptor cells of the maculae have morphological axes oriented in the four directions around the *striola*. The gelatinous membrane (otolithic membrane) contains calcium carbonate crystals (otoliths) that make it heavier than the endolymph. The utricular macula is horizontally positioned on the floor of the cavity: when the head is upright,

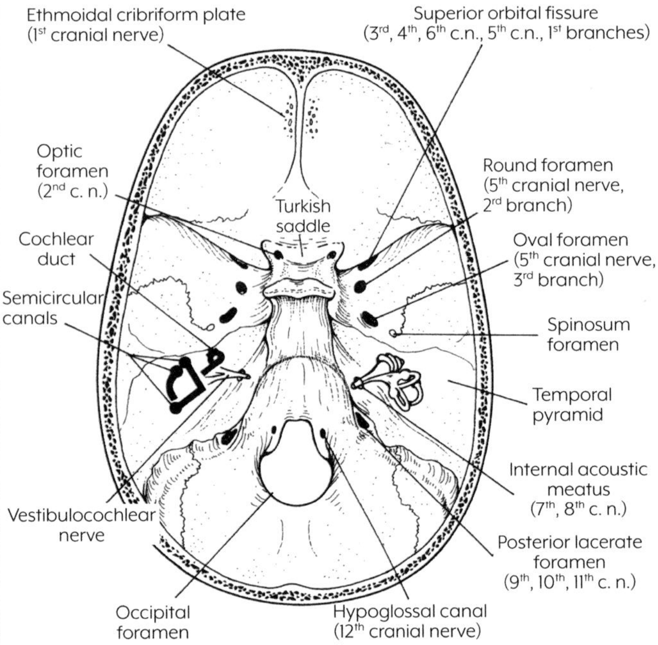

Figure 3.27

Arrangement of the vestibular and auditory organs in the temporal pyramid. View from above of the cranial base. On the left, schematic representation; on the right, semi-realistic representation. On the right, the exit holes of the other cranial nerves are also indicated.

the cilia do not undergo deformation, but when it is tilted, the membrane slides, bending the cilia and modifying the afferent discharge depending on the direction of inclination. When the head undergoes acceleration or deceleration, the membrane moves by inertia, similar to a free object in a car that starts or stops. The situation is similar in the macula of the saccule, which is positioned upright in a vertical orientation. In this way, the central nervous system is informed about the position and *linear accelerations* of the head.

Semicircular Canals | These canals are oriented in the three planes of space and converge in the utricle with the terminal dilation of the ampulla (Figure 3.27). The horizontal canal is inclined 30 degrees upward, while the vertical canals are arranged at right angles to each other. The morphological axes of the receptor cells of the crests all have the same orientation: in the horizontal canals, the kinocilium is directed towards the junction with the utricle, and in the vertical canals, it is arranged in the opposite direction. The gelatinous membrane or cupula, devoid of otoliths and with the same weight as the endolymph, extends from the crest to the roof of the ampulla and faithfully follows the movements of the endolymph. Due to the position of the kinocilium, in the horizontal canals, the displacement of the endolymph towards the ampulla (*ampullopetal*) is excitatory, while the opposite direction (*ampullofugal*) is inhibitory.

The canals on both sides work in pairs. The two horizontal canals lie on the same plane and function together; the anterior canal on one side lies on the same plane and pairs with the posterior canal on the opposite side. The nervous system derives information about *angular accelerations* of the head from the discharge of the six canals.

Vestibular Reflexes

The *vestibular nuclei* form a neuronal cluster beneath the floor of the 4th ventricle, in a lateral position at the border between the pons and medulla. They serve as the destination station for the axons of Scarpa's ganglion (Figures 3.26 e 3.28). They receive proprioceptive information about the posture and movements of the head and body,

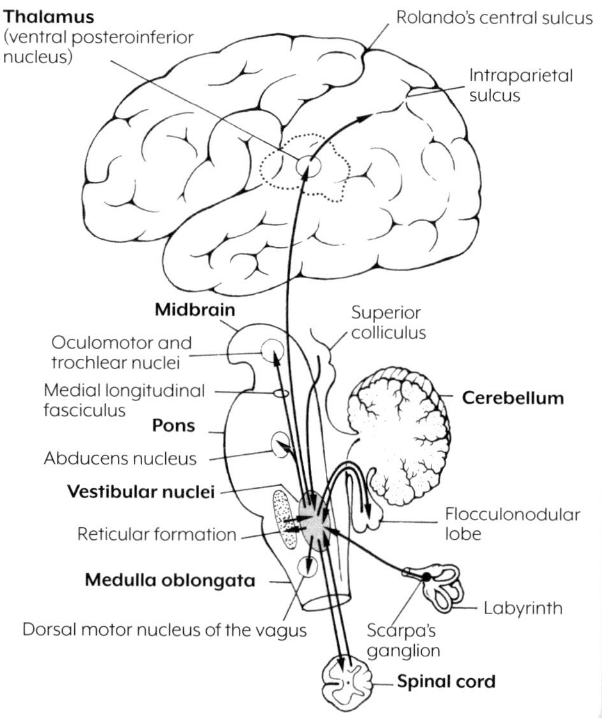

Figure 3.28

Connections of the vestibular nuclei. They receive information from the labyrinth, the cerebellum, the reticular formation, the superior colliculi, and the spinal cord; they project to the cortex (intraparietal sulcus) through the ventral posteroinferior nucleus of the thalamus, to the oculomotor nuclei through the medial longitudinal fasciculus, to the flocculonodular lobe of the cerebellum, to the reticular formation, the dorsal motor nucleus of the vagus, and the spinal cord.

cutaneous information about body support from the colliculus and reticular formation, and visual and auditory information. They have a powerful two-way connection with the *flocculonodular lobe* and the *vermis of the cerebellum*, which act as regulating organs.

In addition to the cerebellum, the efferent projections are directed to the parietal cortex for the physiological sensation of balance and spatial perception (body-environment relationships). In pathological conditions, this sensation becomes vertigo. They also project to the autonomic nuclei of the brainstem and spinal cord, responsible for the autonomic accompaniments of vertigo, and to the spinal motor systems (*lateral and medial vestibulospinal tracts*) for posture regulation. An important crossed and direct projection reaches the nuclei of the eye and neck muscles through the *medial longitudinal fasciculus*. The fasciculus, located beneath the floor of the 4th ventricle on both sides of the midline, continues into the *medial vestibulospinal tract* and extends from the midbrain to the cervical spinal cord. It plays a fundamental role in coordinating the eye muscles and the interaction between the eyes and the head.

There are four vestibular nuclei with specific functions: the superior nucleus of Bechterew and the medial nucleus of Schwalbe (vestibuloocular reflexes), the lateral nucleus of Deiters (postural control), and the inferior nucleus of Roller (vestibulo-cerebellar coordination). Overall, they serve as integrative stations for balance, posture, and the position of the eyes and head during body movements.

Reflexes of the otolithic organs are difficult to study because they require horizontal or vertical translation of the head. The effects of *rotation on the horizontal plane* (Figure 3.26) are easier to study. If the head rotates on its vertical axis to the left, the endolymph, due to inertia, moves forward in the left horizontal canal, dragging the cupula and cilia (ampullopetal movement, excitatory), and backward in the right canal (ampullofugal movement, inhibitory). Activation of the left horizontal canal triggers the contralateral lateral rectus muscle and, through the interneurons that cross and ascend again in the medial longitudinal fasciculus, the ipsilateral medial rectus muscle. Inhibition of the right horizontal canal deactivates the two antagonistic muscles: the ipsilateral lateral rectus and the contralateral medial rectus. As previously mentioned regarding supranuclear oculomotor systems, with inhibited fixation reflex, the eyes slowly move in the opposite direction of the rotation due to the vestibular action and are brought back by a rapid cortical-originated jerk (*rotatory vestibular nystagmus*). If the rotation speed is constant, after 30-45 seconds, the endolymph rebalances, and the two ampullary crests return to a resting state. The sudden stop of rotation displaces the endolymph backward in the left canal, which becomes inhibited, and forward in the right canal, which becomes activated. This generates *post-rotatory nystagmus*, with a slow deviation in the direction of the just-completed rotary movement and a rapid jerk in the opposite direction. This is easy to observe and is used in the diagnosis of vertigo. Equivalent reflexes are generated by the other canals for anteroposterior and lateral angular movements. *Flourens' law* states that each semicircular canal gives rise to a movement on the same plane as the canal.

Other vestibular reflexes can be activated by proprioceptors in the neck and changes in posture, which are normally immersed in the general plane of movement. They remain recognizable in newborns and reemerge in coma and after diffuse cortical or corticofugal pathway injuries. When labyrinthine afferents are disturbed or vestibular pathways are damaged, the reflex distribution of tone becomes unbalanced, affecting balance, posture, and eye position. These disturbances are usually transient because the vestibular system possesses remarkable plasticity and quickly adapts to the new condition.

Examination of the Vestibular System

The sensations reported by the patient are not always clear, but it is usually easy to distinguish between vertigo and *pseudovertigo*. Vertigo is characterized by a sensation of body rotation or displacement or a shifting of the environment around the body. It is accompanied by autonomic phenomena (nausea, vomiting, sweating, pallor) and a strong urge to minimize head movements. It is similar to motion sickness and can sometimes be reproduced by rapid and repeated head rotations. Pseudovertigo, on the other hand, is a sensation of instability and insecurity that often accompanies anxious and depressive states, along with other cenesthetic disturbances. It can also occur with postural hypotension, anemia, or hypoglycemia and is comparable to the sensations caused by 2-3 minutes of forced ventilation. In English-speaking neurology, pseudovertigo is referred to as *dizziness*, contrasting it with *vertigo*.

Postural Asymmetries | The patient is seated or standing with their eyes closed, arms outstretched, and index fingers facing those of the examiner. It is observed whether there is a slow and reproducible deviation of one or both index fingers. The test can be sensitized by asking the patient to touch the examiner's finger with their eyes closed after taking aim: the finger misses the target, passing beyond it in the direction of the spontaneous deviation ("past pointing"). In the upright position with eyes closed (Romberg's test), the deviation of the body axis is highlighted. In the step test (stepping in place with eyes closed) and the star gait test (three steps forward and three steps backward with eyes closed), the tendency to rotate oneself is observed. Walking (especially tandem walking, with the heel touching the toe step by step or a few steps with eyes closed) shows deviation in one direction (lateropulsion).

Nystagmus | It should be examined with the eyes in the primary position and in various gaze directions, observing both distant targets and the examiner's finger. Labyrinthine-origin nystagmus is enhanced by suppressing visual inputs. If Frenzel glasses are not available, the patient can be asked to look at a white surface of a paper placed 20-30 centimeters from the eyes, or the optic disc in the fundus can be examined with an ophthalmoscope while keeping the other eye closed (due to the crossing of light rays, the direction of optic disc movement, but not the torsion, is opposite to that of the anterior segment). Central nystagmus, on the other hand, is enhanced by fixation and can be observed by having the patient follow the examiner's finger in various gaze directions.

The *direction* of nystagmus is usually defined based on the fast phase (nystagmus beating to the left, i.e., with a fast phase to the left). However, this complicates interpretation

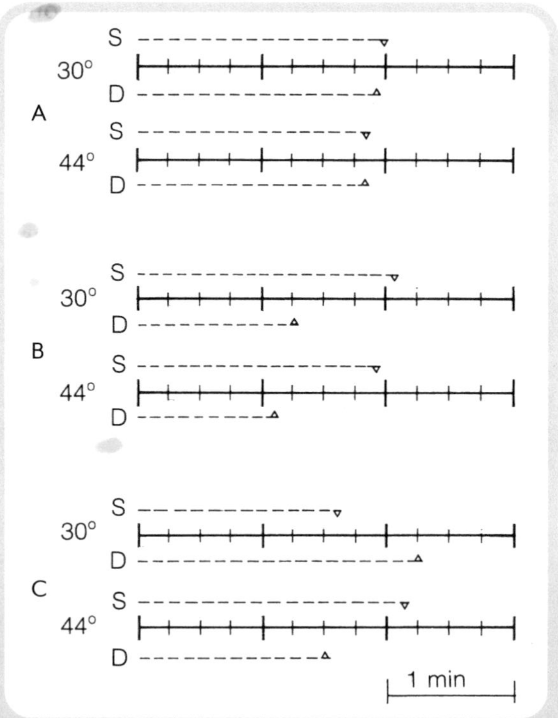

Figure 3.29

Caloric labyrinthine test. The auditory canals are irrigated with cold water (30°C) or hot water (44°C), alternating between left (L) and right (R), while measuring the duration of nystagmus. A) Normal subject; the response is symmetrical. B) Right canal paresis; both cold and hot water elicit a shorter duration response on the right side. C) Tonic directional preponderance to the right; the eyes tend to spontaneously deviate to the right, and cold stimulation of the right ear or hot stimulation of the left ear, which reinforce this tendency, generate longer duration responses.

since the essential component is the slow deviation, not the compensatory fast phase of cortical origin. Therefore, it is useful to explicitly add "nystagmus with a slow phase to the right.

Instrumental Tests | *Rotational Test.* The rotational test involves the patient sitting on a rotating chair with their head tilted forward by 30 degrees to match the inclination of the horizontal canal. This is done in a dark room or with Frenzel goggles. The chair completes ten revolutions in 20 seconds and then abruptly stops. The post-rotatory nystagmus is observed, which appears after 10-15 seconds and lasts for 20-50 seconds, with the slow phase in the direction of rotation. After a few minutes, the test is repeated by rotating the chair in the opposite direction. By bending the head 90 degrees (shoulder direction), the vertical canals are evaluated. The rotational test does not allow for separate examination of the two labyrinths because it activates one side's canal and inhibits the other side's canal.

Caloric Test (Figure 3.29). After ensuring in the patient's medical history that there are no infectious conditions or perforation of the eardrum, the patient is seated with the head tilted back by 60 degrees or lying down with the head tilted forward by 30 degrees to vertically align the horizontal canal with the ampulla positioned upwards. The external auditory canal is irrigated with 50 ml of cold water. This generates a slow eye rotation toward the irrigated side (ampullofugal) in the horizontal canal adjacent to the external auditory canal. In conscious individuals, nystagmus occurs, while in comatose patients, only tonic deviation toward the irrigated side is observed (remember "FROM" - cold on the same side). In the laboratory, hot and cold water can be used, allowing for separate examination of the labyrinths on both sides. Caloric stimulation can reveal the following in the acute phases of labyrinthine disorders: an exaggerated response of one labyrinth with significant subjective symptoms (labyrinthine hyperexcitability), a reduced response (canal paresis) typically seen in stabilized pathologies of the inner ear or the acoustic nerve, and a predominance of nystagmus in one direction (directional preponderance) observed in both peripheral and central impairments.

Vestibular Syndromes

The characteristics of the disturbances resulting from labyrinth and central pathway lesions typically allow for localization of the damage.

Peripheral Vestibular Syndrome | In labyrinthine lesions, the information is imbalanced from the start, and the imbalance is reflected harmonically in all the functions coordinated by the system. The slow phase of nystagmus, the indices, the body axis, and gait deviate in the same direction and are proportionate in magnitude. Vertigo can be accompanied by hearing disturbances and is significantly influenced by medical therapy.

Central Vestibular Syndrome | In central lesions, labyrinthine afferents are normal, but the circulation of information is imbalanced at the level of distributive circuits. Not all structures are equally affected by the disorder, and nystagmus, index deviation, body axis deviation, and gait are not proportional and congruent; in other words, the symptoms are *disharmonious*. For example, marked lateropulsion can be observed without index deviation. Auditory signs are absent, while other neurological signs are often present. Vertigo is less responsive to therapy.

Pathology of the Vestibular System

Nystagmus | Nystagmus is a conjugate, repetitive, and asymmetric eye movement characterized by a slow deviation in one direction followed by a rapid jerk in the opposite direction. The direction, plane of movement, amplitude, velocity, and symmetry in both eyes should be observed. Nystagmus varies depending on the site of the lesion.

Labyrinthine Nystagmus. Acute lesions of one labyrinth suddenly disrupt vestibular afferents. Nystagmus is very evident initially but tends to subside within days or weeks. Typically, it is horizontal with a rotary component, and its direction remains constant, reflecting the predominance of the healthy labyrinth. Therefore, the slow phase is directed toward the affected labyrinth, and the amplitude increases when the eyes are rotated in the opposite direction (tonic asymmetry, which tends to deviate the eyes to the right, is more pronounced when the patient looks to the left). The amplitude increases when fixation is suppressed, with Frenzel goggles, and when the other eye is closed while examining the fundus oculi. Nystagmus changes with head position and increases after head shaking (which may be poorly tolerated and requires the subject's consent). It is accompanied by vertigo, nausea, and sometimes hypoacusis and paracusis. Saccadic and pursuit movements are preserved. Caloric tests show canal paresis. The most frequent causes are Meniere's disease, positional vertigo, and inflammatory, traumatic, or toxic labyrinthopathies.

Nystagmus from Acoustic Nerve. It occurs in one-fourth of cases of acoustic nerve neurinoma and is usually horizontal, occasionally with a rotary component, and the slow phase is directed toward the side of the lesion. . It is accompanied by unilateral hypoacusis and canal paresis. In advanced stages, central signs can occur when the tumor compresses the brainstem.

Central Nystagmus. It appears in lesions of the vestibular pathways. It persists much longer than labyrinthine nystagmus and can become permanent, but it is highly polymorphic. It is mostly pure, either horizontal, vertical, or rarely rotary. Its direction can change depending on the direction of gaze, worsens with fixation, and becomes more apparent when examining the fundus oculi while keeping the other eye open. It is not accompanied by hypoacusis, while other signs of central damage are often present. Saccadic and pursuit movements may be affected. Instrumental tests show directional preponderance or mixed patterns. The characteristics vary with the site of the lesion.

In *bulbar lesions* (lateral ischemic lesions, cerebellar and posterior fossa malformations, syringobulbia), a vertical nystagmus can be observed with slow phase directed upward and rapid jerk downward (*downbeat nystagmus*), which is more evident in downward gaze. It has also been described in cases of lithium intoxication. In bulbar lesions (lateral ischemic lesions, cerebellar and posterior fossa malformations, syringobulbia), a vertical nystagmus can be observed with slow phase directed upward and rapid jerk downward (downbeat nystagmus), which is more evident in downward gaze. It has also been described in cases of lithium intoxication. In *lateral pontine lesions*, along with difficulty in rotating the eyes to the side of the lesion, horizontal nystagmus with slow phase directed toward the center (*gaze-paretic nystagmus*) occurs. In paramedian pontine lesions affecting the medial longitudinal fasciculus, nystagmus appears in the abducted eye, which is the first symptom of internuclear ophthalmoplegia. In lesions of the *midbrain tegmentum*, vertical nystagmus can be observed, more pronounced in upward gaze, with rapid phase downward (*upbeat nystagmus*), sometimes accompanied by retraction and convergence of the eyeballs (*retraction nystagmus*).

Cerebellar pathologies present a variety of types of nystagmus: it can appear in all gaze directions, change direction depending on the gaze direction, sometimes occur in the primary position, and be mixed with saccadic intrusions. In lateralized lesions, it may indicate hyperactivity of the ipsilateral vestibular nuclei with slow phase directed toward the opposite side of the lesion.

Saccadic Intrusions and Nystagmoid Movements | Injuries to the brainstem and cerebellum, particularly in multiple sclerosis, can lead to movements that do not fall under the definition of nystagmus. The most common ones are:

a) *Ocular dysmetria*: excessive saccadic eye movements beyond the target (overshoots), followed by progressively smaller corrective adjustments. They are common in multiple sclerosis and result from cerebellar damage.
b) *Square wave jerks*: involuntary, sudden, horizontal saccadic movements of a few degrees, causing the eyes to deviate from the target. After a brief period of fixation, the eyes return to their original position. They are also present in normal individuals but increase in cases of cerebellar lesions.
c) *Macrosquare wave jerks*: similar to the previous type, but larger in amplitude and occur in bursts. They are observed in cerebellar lesions;
d) *Ocular bobbing*: rapid downward jerks followed by slow return upward. They appear in comatose states due to acute pontine lesions and have an unfavorable prognosis.
e) *Opsoclonus*: continuous saccadic eye movements in all directions, interrupted by periods of quiescence. They are observed in brainstem encephalitis.
f) *See-saw nystagmus*: rapid, dissociated eye movements, with one eye moving upward and the other moving downward. When this pattern is tonically maintained, it is referred to as *skew deviation*. It is observed in acute cerebellar lesions.

Pendular nystagmus | Pendular nystagmus is a repetitive eye movement characterized by symmetrical oscillations in both directions, with the same speed and amplitude. However, in extreme lateral gaze, the return movements may become faster. It can be congenital (with or without visual acuity deficits), acquired, or part of an infantile syndrome known as spasmus nutans.

Congenital Pendular Nystagmus. It usually appears in the first months or years of life, is horizontal, and remains consistent in all gaze directions. It is conjugate and increases with visual attention but decreases with convergence (which allows for good near vision) and eye closure. The presence of a neutral zone in certain eye positions, where the amplitude is reduced, leads to deviations and sometimes head oscillations. In most cases, it does not show visual deficits. In a quarter of cases, it is associated with strabismus, and in 10% of cases, it is associated with visual acuity deficits, usually due to ocular pathologies (albinism with macular degeneration, retinopathies, high myopia, congenital cataracts, corneal opacities). It can be familial.

Acquired Pendular Nystagmus. It can be horizontal, vertical, or torsional, and may change direction, be disconjugate, and show differences in amplitude between the two eyes. It can occur after acquired visual deficits, in multiple sclerosis, metabolic myelin disorders, oculopalatal myoclonus syndrome, and focal brainstem lesions.

Spasmus Nutans. It is a rare infantile syndrome that appears around the 4th to 12th month of life and spontaneously resolves by the age of 3. It is characterized by irregular head tremors, spastic torticollis, and intermittent, high-frequency, disconjugate nystagmus, which can be horizontal or vertical and is more pronounced in the abducted eye. The cause is unknown. It is necessary to rule out tumors of the third ventricle that can cause similar disturbances.

Vertigo | Vertigo, one of the most common neurological symptoms, is a hallucinatory sensation of movement or altered body orientation in space, usually accompanied by nystagmus, ataxia, and nausea. The sensation originates from cortical disarray of sensory information from the two vestibules. Nystagmus and ataxia reflect the alteration of vestibular reflexes, while nausea and other vegetative symptoms (vomiting, sweating, pallor, bradycardia, hypotension) indicate involvement of autonomic structures.

Objective vertigo (where the space appears to move relative to the body) is distinguished from *subjective vertigo* (where the body feels like it is moving in space), but there is no real difference as the movement is always a relative phenomenon. However, it is important to differentiate vertigo from *pseudovertigo* (as mentioned above).

Labyrinthine vertigo is by far the most common condition, and the three recurring forms (benign paroxysmal positional vertigo, Meniere's disease, recurrent benign vertigo) account for 90% of vertigo syndromes. In general, vertigo lasting seconds or tens of seconds is positional, those lasting minutes are circulatory, those lasting hours are associated with Meniere's disease, and those lasting days are related to labyrinthitis or toxic labyrinthopathies.

Motion sickness. It is a discomfort experienced in cars or boats due to the discrepancy between the vestibular input, activated by repetitive motion, somatic input, which does not signal any motor activity, and especially visual input, which indicates a stationary environment (such as the enclosed cabin, a page being read, or even the rear seats of a car). It can be prevented by anticipating motion, as in driving, and improves with a panoramic view of the moving environment, such as on the deck of a ship or in the front seats of a car. The symptoms are vegetative (nausea, vomiting, sweating), and psychological conditioning and gastric content play a decisive role (liquid foods should be avoided). The medical prophylaxis follows that of labyrinthine vertigo.

Benign positional vertigo. It is the most frequently observed vertigo syndrome. It is characterized by brief vertiginous attacks (10 seconds to one minute) triggered by positional changes such as lying down, getting up, extending the head, and especially turning in bed. The attacks recur for days or weeks, and the specific movement is usually unique to each patient; they may recur periodically. It is caused by the detachment of otoliths from the utricular macula, which enter the posterior semicircular canal (*cupulolithiasis*), transforming the cupula into a static position receptor. During the active phase, it can be reproduced with the *Dix-Hallpike positional test* (which can be disturbing and should be authorized): with the patient seated, their head in the examiner's hands, the torso is suddenly tilted backward, with the head hyperextended and rotated 45° towards the examiner. After a latency period of 4-20 seconds, intense and disturbing vertigo and vertical and rotatory nystagmus with a slow phase downward occur, which subsides in a few tens of seconds. If the maneuver is ineffective, it should be performed after a few minutes by rotating the head to the other side (the compromised labyrinth is the one facing downward). If the patient can be convinced, repeating the maneuver 3-4 times will reduce and eliminate the vertigo and nystagmus. Involvement of the horizontal canal, which requires a different maneuver (torso tilted backward and head held horizontally), is rarer. The condition can occur in idiopathic form in adulthood or old age, more commonly in females, or it can occur after head trauma. Vertigo can cause nocturnal awakenings due to involuntary sleep movements. Vestibular or audiometric tests are normal for the patient's age.

The positional test can also be positive in acute vascular lesions of the brainstem, but the vertigo and nystagmus are immediate and lack the characteristic latency and exhaustibility of the positional form.

Meniere's disease. It occurs in adulthood and is due to labyrinth hydrops with rupture of the membranous labyrinth. It is characterized by sudden, violent vertigo attacks lasting for hours, which require almost complete immobility, recurring with free intervals of months or years. They are accompanied by low-pitched tinnitus, a sense of "ear fullness," and unilateral or, more rarely, bilateral sensorineural hearing loss, which worsens during the attacks and over the years, while the vertigo episodes become less frequent. Nystagmus usually shows a slow phase toward the affected labyrinth, but the direction depends on the position of the rupture relative to the ampulla. Vestibular tests show canal paresis, while audiometric tests show sensorineural hearing loss that starts with intermediate frequencies and progresses to higher frequencies.

Vestibular neuritis (labyrinthitis). It consists of an inflammatory affection of the labyrinth, which occurs in young individuals, possibly caused by viral infections. Bacterial forms can complicate otomastoiditis. It presents with an intense vertiginous episode lasting a few days, usually a single occurrence, accompanied by nausea, vomiting, and the need for immobility, without cochlear symptoms. Vertigo may indicate damage to the semicircular canals and be rotatory, or it may indicate damage to the otoliths and cause a sense of levitation, displacement, or an unstable floor sensation. There is deviation of indices, lateropulsion, and nystagmus with a slow phase toward the affected side. Caloric tests show canal paresis. The disorder regresses without residual effects.

Recurrent benign vertigo. It is also called "recurrent acute labyrinthitis" or "paroxysmal vertigo of childhood." It is characterized by recurrent disabling vertigo attacks lasting 1-24 hours, with variable frequency (from once a week to less than once a year), without tinnitus or hearing loss, and with normal vestibular and auditory function tests. It occurs in childhood or adulthood and is interspersed with episodes of torticollis and migraine headaches. It is often familial. The differential diagnosis from Meniere's disease is based on the early onset, longer duration of vertigo, and lack of auditory disturbances.

Labyrinthine apoplexy. It is an acute vascular syndrome caused by occlusion of the anterior inferior cerebellar artery or its branch, the internal auditory artery, which leads to prolonged vertigo, ataxia, hypoacusis, tinnitus, and leaves a stable vestibular and auditory deficit. Transient ischemic attacks can occur in the same territory.

Toxic labyrinthopathics. They occur after prolonged therapy with aminoglycoside antibiotics (streptomycin, gentamicin, amikacin) and manifest as prolonged or recurrent vertigo triggered by movement, with bilateral canal paresis in caloric tests. Hearing is also compromised. The condition persists for days or weeks and leaves stable sequelae.

The therapy for labyrinthine vertigo is symptomatic. The most useful medications are: scopolamine (0.5 mg transdermally), antihistamines (diphenhydramine 50 mg, dimenhydrinate 100 mg, cyclizine 50 mg, buclizine 50 mg, meclizine 25 mg), phenothiazines (promethazine 25 mg, prochlorperazine 10 mg; thiethylperazine 12 mg, which can cause neuroleptic malignant syndrome), vasodilators (betahistine 16-24 mg). In positional vertigo, there are specific maneuvers to remove the otoliths from the canal. The most commonly used one is the Dix-Hallpike maneuver: when the vertigo has subsided, the head is rotated to the other side while keeping the neck down, then the patient rotates in a prone position with the head down, and finally sits up; all done very slowly with pauses of 10-15 seconds between positions. It is also helpful to habituate the labyrinth with the following maneuver (to be repeated, sitting on the bed, 10-20 times, several times a day): lie on one side, sit up, lie on the other side, waiting in each position for the vertigo to extinguish.

Acoustic nerve neurinoma. Vertigo is recurrent but of low intensity because the slow progression allows compensation of vestibular asymmetry. Symptoms consist of a sense of instability, which can be mistaken for a neurotic symptom and occurs during vigorous movements or in conditions of difficult balance (e.g., on buses).

Troncoencephalic and cerebellar vertigo. They occur in acute lesions of the vestibular nuclei and their connections and in cerebellar lesions. Vertigo can be intense and prolonged and manifests as a disordered vestibular syndrome. It can recur and leave residual effects that are slowly compensated. It is not accompanied by hearing disturbances since the vestibular and auditory pathways follow different routes. Instead, other signs of focal damage are present, and caution should be exercised when vertigo appears in isolation. Stimulation tests show a directional preponderance or mixed patterns. The most common conditions are lateral bulbar infarctions, which cause Wallenberg's syndrome (see vascular pathologies), cerebellar hematomas, and demyelinating plaques.

Epileptic vertigo. Epileptogenic foci in the parietal and temporal cortex can manifest as rotational or linear vertiginous seizures lasting seconds or minutes, accompanied by head and eye rotation usually contralateral to the focus. They exhibit the unpredictable course of epilepsy.

3.5.2 Acoustic System

Functional organization

The *cochlea*, the peripheral organ of hearing, is composed of three parallel and spiral-shaped channels (Figure 3.25). The upper channel (*scala vestibuli*), closed by the oval window, and the lower channel (*scala tympani*), closed by the *round window*, contain perilymph and communicate at the top of the spiral through an opening called the *helicotrema*. The middle channel (*scala media or cochlear duct*) contains endolymph and communicates with the membranous labyrinth. It has a triangular cross-section and is enclosed by the basilar membrane, vestibular membrane, and vascular stria, which form its floor, roof, and lateral wall, respectively. It separates the scala vestibuli from the scala tympani and ends blindly. The *receptor cells* are arranged in parallel rows on the *basilar membrane*, vestibular membrane, and vascular stria, which form its floor, roof, and lateral wall, respectively. It separates the scala vestibuli from the scala tympani and ends blindly. The receptor cells are arranged in parallel rows on the basilar membrane, with one row on the inside and three rows on the outside. They are equipped with cilia at their free end, which come into contact with the *tectorial membrane*, a gelatinous mass anchored to the inner corner of the scala media. At their other end, they are innervated by the peripheral extensions of the spiral ganglion neurons of Corti, located at the center of the cochlea, whose central extensions form the *cochlear nerve*.

Sounds, conducted through the external auditory canal, are collected by the tympanic membrane and transmitted to the oval window through the chain of ossicles (*malleus, incus, and stapes*) in the middle ear (*air conduction*). Two synergistic muscles (the tensor tympani, 5th nerve, attached to the malleus, and the stapedius, 7th nerve, attached to the stapes) reflexively reduce the vibration of the ossicular chain and protect against sounds that are too intense and prolonged (but not against sudden sounds). Sounds are also transmitted through the temporal bone (*bone conduction*), causing the ossicular chain and the bony labyrinth to vibrate, bypassing the tympanic membrane.

The oscillation of the oval window is transmitted to the perilymph and travels as a mechanical wave towards the helicotrema, causing the basilar membrane of the scala media to oscillate. The mechanical properties of the basilar membrane, which widens and becomes less rigid from the oval window to the helicotrema, and the physical structure of the receptor cells, which have longer and more flexible cilia as one progresses from the oval window to the helicotrema, give the basilar membrane a specific resonance to different frequencies, with a very narrow oscillation peak located at the beginning of the scale for high-pitched sounds and at the terminal part for low-pitched sounds. The basilar membrane

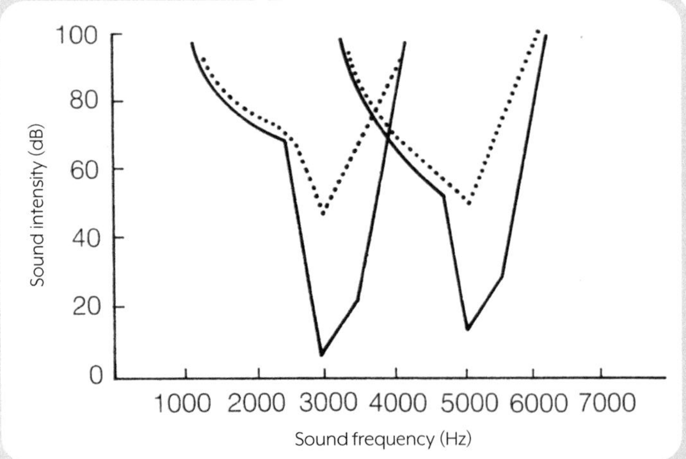

Figure 3.30

Response curve of the auditory nerve fibers. In normal subjects, individual cells exhibit a characteristic response frequency (solid lines). In lesions of the organ of Corti, the curve flattens (dashed lines), and small increases in sound intensity recruit a greater number of receptor cells than usual. This behavior forms the basis of supraliminal audimetry. (Modified from Schmidt and Thews, 1983).

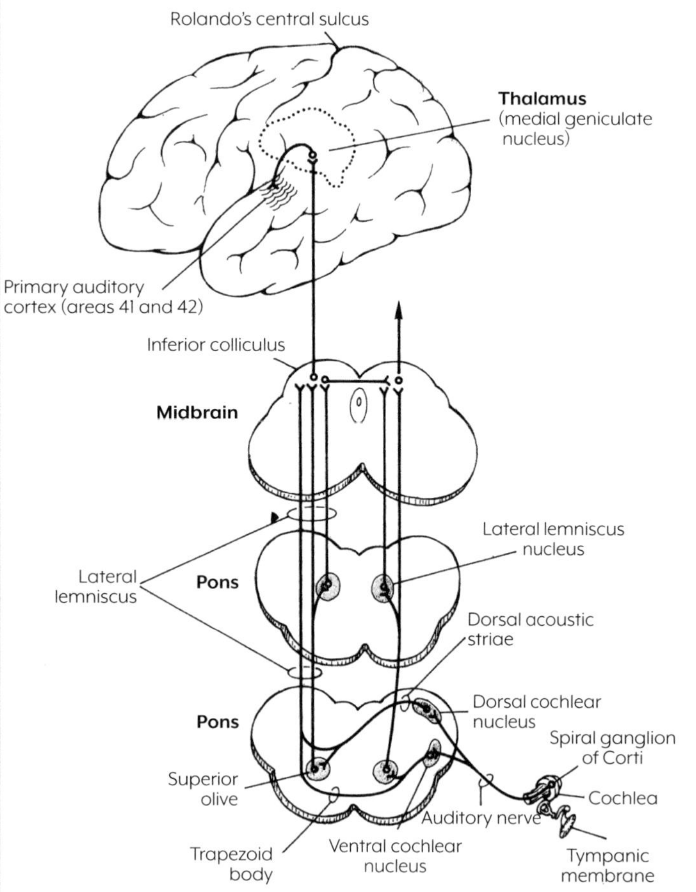

Figure 3.31

Auditory pathways. The central projections of the cochlear nuclei are bilateral, although predominantly contralateral. The intermediate stations include the superior olive, the lateral lemniscus nucleus, the inferior colliculi, and the medial geniculate body. The primary auditory cortex is located in the superior temporal gyrus, corresponding to Brodmann areas 41 and 42.

and the tectorial membrane oscillate with a different angle of insertion, displacing the cilia of the receptor cells. As the sound intensity increases, neighboring cells are progressively recruited (Figure 3.30). Therefore, the cochlea encodes frequencies in terms of activated cell series and intensities in terms *of activity and the number* of recruited cells. Upon entering the brainstem, the fibers of the cochlear nerve split into two contingents, which terminate in the *ventral and dorsal cochlear nuclei* (Figure 3.31), located laterally at the borders between the medulla and the pons. From the ventral cochlear nucleus, the *trapezoid body originates*, reaching the ipsilateral and contralateral superior olivary nucleus, from where the pathway continues in the *lateral lemniscus* on both sides. From the dorsal cochlear nucleus, the *acoustic striae originate*, reaching the contralateral lateral lemniscus. The lemnisci ascend in the lateral portion of the pons and midbrain, encounter the nucleus of the lateral lemniscus, and terminate in the inferior colliculus. The pathway continues through the brachium of the *inferior colliculus* to the *medial geniculate nucleus* of the thalamus, from where the acoustic radiations originate. Through the posterior part of the internal capsule, they terminate in the superior temporal gyrus, in the primary auditory area (areas 41 and 42). The main characteristic of the auditory pathway is the bilateral projection; consequently, unilateral lesions of the central auditory pathways do not alter the hearing threshold. Therefore, hearing impairments are almost always of peripheral origin, caused by lesions in the middle or inner ear or the auditory nerve.

The bilaterality of the pathway is also the basis for sound localization. A sound coming from a lateral source reaches the opposite ear with a slight delay and, due to the head's screening effect, also has slightly lower intensity. In the superior olive, there are neurons that selectively respond to sounds presented with latency or intensity gradients between the two ears. This type of analysis is further refined in the auditory cortex, where cortical areas are organized in an orderly manner based on frequency (tonotopic distribution) and also based on interaural latency and intensity differences. There are cellular columns that receive information from one or both ears and allow for the analysis of sound origin. The decomposition of the auditory reality in terms of frequency, volume, rhythm, timbre, and origin enables sophisticated analysis required for language comprehension and music listening. In general, the contralateral ear is dominant, and cortical lesions leave the hearing threshold intact but impair the ability to localize the source of sounds, especially from the contralateral space.

There is also an important *centrifugal projection* that descends from the auditory cortex to the cochlear nuclei and terminates on the receptor cells of the cochlea through the *olivocochlear bundle*. It is possible that this projection plays a role in selective attention to certain sounds.

Pathophysiology of hearing disorders

The loss of auditory sensitivity is called hearing loss or *hypoacusis*, and in severe degrees, deafness. There are four types of hearing loss.

In *conductive hypoacusis* (also known as *transmission hypoacusis*) the disorder affects the transmission of sound energy from the tympanic membrane to the oval window. Sounds conducted through the air are attenuated, while sounds conducted through bone are heard better than in the healthy ear because there is no interference from environmental sounds, and the cochlea has adapted to low sound volume, enhancing the sensitivity of the receptor cells.

In *sensorineural* or *cochlear hypoacusis*, the disorder affects the receptor cells, which become less sensitive to low sound intensities. Sounds are heard less both through the air and through bone, with the air pathway remaining advantageous. Additionally, by increasing the sound intensity, the damaged ear recovers because the receptor cells, which are not activated by specific frequencies at low intensities, are recruited in large numbers as soon as the sound exceeds a certain threshold (Figure 3.30). This phenomenon is the basis of "recruitment," which improves performance at high sound intensities and tends to reduce the difference between the two ears. However, the diseased ear loses selectivity for nearby frequencies, compromising language comprehension.

In *neural* or *retrocochlear hypoacusis*, the disorder affects the nerve fibers, and the hearing loss involves both air-conducted and bone-conducted sounds, similar to sensorineural hearing loss. However, unlike cochlear lesions, there is no recovery of sensation by increasing sound intensity, and the sensitivity difference between the affected ear and the healthy ear remains the same at all sound intensities.

In *central hypoacusis*, the disorder affects the transmission of information within the nervous system. In this case, all acoustic sources are cut off, but this condition is very rare because the auditory pathways become bilateral as soon as they enter the brainstem, and bilateral interruption in the brainstem, radiations, or at the level of the primary auditory areas is infrequent and often accompanied by other serious complications.

Sensorineural and neural hearing loss are combined under the term *sensorineural hypoacusis* and contrasted with the conductive form. In general, conductive hypoacusis affects low-pitched sounds more, while sensorineural hypoacusis affects high-pitched sounds more.

Examination of auditory function

Sounds have two qualities: *frequency*, measured in cycles per second or Hertz (Hz), and *intensity*, measured on an arbitrary logarithmic scale in decibels (dB) relative to a reference sound of 3,000 Hz that is just audible to the human ear. The human ear is sensitive to a limited range of frequencies (approximately 20 to 20,000 Hz), while it distinguishes a wide range of intensities. The loudest sound perceived without discomfort is nearly a million times greater than the threshold. The noise level in a soundproof room is below 18 dB, ambient noise is around 35 dB, conversation is around 65 dB, and the threshold for annoying noises is around 100 dB.

Clinical examination | In a low ambient noise room with one ear manually occluded, a normal individual can hear a whispered voice at a distance of 6 meters. *Hypoacusis* (*hearing loss*) is mild if the whispered voice is heard between 1 and 6 meters, moderate if heard at less than 1 meter, and severe if the full voice is not heard even at a distance of 1 meter. The ticking of a clock can also be used, slowly approaching the patient's ear and comparing it to the examiner's ear, or rubbing a piece of paper near the patient's ear.

Tuning fork tests | A tuning fork at 512 Hz allows separate examination of air conduction and bone conduction, distinguishing between transmission defects and sensorineural defects. When the prongs of the tuning fork are placed in front of the external auditory meatus, the sound is conducted through the air, while when the base of the tuning fork is placed on the mastoid, the sound is predominantly conducted through bone. In the *Rinne test*, the tuning fork is held on the mastoid until the subject reports no longer hearing the sound, and then it is brought close to the ear. A normal individual and a patient with sensorineural hearing loss still perceive the sound because air conduction is more efficient than bone conduction (normal or positive Rinne test), while a patient with conductive hearing loss continues to hear nothing (abnormal or negative Rinne test). In the *Weber test*, the tuning fork is placed on the vertex of the head, and a normal individual localizes the sound in the center. In cases of conductive hearing loss, the sound is lateralized to the affected ear, while in cases of sensorineural hearing loss, it is lateralized to the healthy ear. The *Schwabach test* compares the patient's bone conduction with that of the examiner, and in cases of conductive hearing loss, the patient has an advantage.

Audiometric threshold testing | This is performed in a soundproof booth in an audiology laboratory and is the fundamental technique

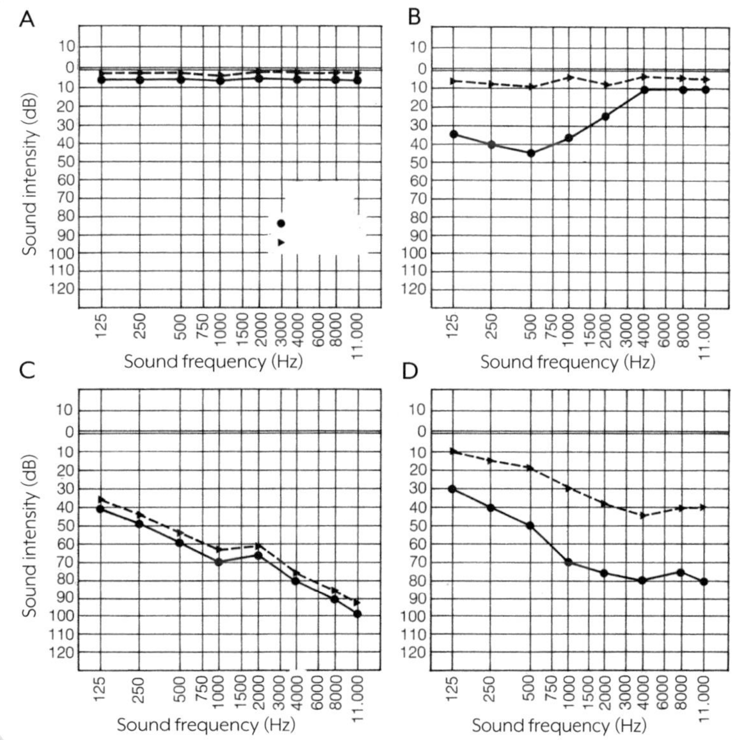

Figure 3.32

Audiogram of threshold tonal in normal and pathological conditions. A) Normal subject; B) Conductive hearing loss (middle ear lesion); C) Sensorineural hearing loss (acoustic nerve lesion); D) Mixed hearing loss (advanced otosclerosis).

for evaluating hearing defects. Pure tones of different frequencies are delivered through headphones or via a vibrator in contact with the mastoid. The tone intensity is progressively increased until it is detected, and the threshold intensity is plotted on a graph (audiogram) with frequency in Hz on the horizontal axis and intensity in dB on the vertical axis (Figure 3.32). In *conductive hearing loss* (Figure 3.32B), the drop occurs in air conduction, while bone conduction is normal. All tones are affected, but low-frequency tones to a greater extent. In *sensorineural hearing* loss (Figure 3.32C), the drop occurs in both air conduction and bone conduction, predominantly affecting high-frequency tones. In *otosclerosis* (Figure 3.32D) mixed-type curves are observed.

Pure-tone audiometry | It allows differentiation between sensorineural hearing loss, which can be improved by increasing the intensity of sounds, and neural hearing loss, which does not improve. In sensorineural defects, as the intensity of sounds increases, the difference between the two ears (one healthy and one affected, or one more impaired than the other) tends to disappear (*positive recruitment*), while in neural hearing loss, it remains unchanged (*negative recruitment*). Additionally, the ear with sensorineural defects can better discriminate differences in intensity compared to neural defects and normal ears, and in tests involving increasing or decreasing sounds, it can recognize a higher percentage of variations.

Evoked auditory potentials | They are generated by the repetition of a "click" sound and consist of a series of waves with known latency. The first wave is unilateral and generated by the distal portion of the cochlear nerve, while the subsequent waves are bilateral and generated in the brainstem. They help identify compression of the auditory nerve, where the first wave is preserved, but the subsequent waves are delayed and distorted. They are not helpful in the differential diagnosis of hearing loss (see Chapter 8 Electroneurography, electromyography, and evoked potentials).

Tympanometry | It is an otologic test that measures the impedance of the tympanic membrane to airborne sounds, which is altered in middle ear lesions. By delivering an intense sound, the *stapedial reflex* can be evaluated, which involves an increase in impedance due to contraction of the small muscles of the ossicular chain.

Pathology of the auditory system

Conductive hearing loss | It is caused by occlusion of the external auditory canal due to earwax blockage, canal atresia, traumatic rupture of the eardrum, acute otitis media, chronic otitis media with cholesteatoma , and fractures of the petrous bone with damage to the ossicles. The reduction in hearing primarily affects the air conduction pathway and predominantly involves low-frequency sounds. The most common cause of hearing loss in adults is *otosclerosis*, which shows an autosomal dominant pattern of incomplete penetrance. It is usually bilateral and characterized by excessive bone production around the oval window, leading to progressive immobilization of the stapes; as the disease progresses, signs of sensorineural hearing loss appear, resulting in a mixed-type deficit. Reconstructive microsurgery allows significant improvements.

Sensorineural hearing loss | It can be congenital, resulting from cochlear aplasia in an autosomal dominant form or intrauterine cochlear damage due to rubella. In childhood, it can be a consequence of extension of middle ear infection to the inner ear due to measles or vaccination. In adults, it can result from acoustic trauma (industrial environments, discos, rock music, shooting) with initial loss limited to a specific frequency range. The most common causes are age-related degeneration of the cochlea, Meniere's disease, toxic iatrogenic damage from salicylates, quinine, loop diuretics (ethacrynic acid), aminoglycoside antibiotics (streptomycin, gentamicin, etc.), which block the ion pumps that regulate the composition of the endolymph, and chronic meningitis. The hearing loss affects both air conduction and bone conduction, with a predominant impact on high-frequency sounds, and recruitment is positive. It impairs speech comprehension by hindering consonant discrimination.

Neural hearing loss | It can result from congenital conditions and progressive hereditary neuropathies, often associated with degeneration of other neural systems, chronic basal meningitis, or demyelinating plaques affecting the cochlear nerve at its entry into the brainstem. It primarily affects high-frequency sounds and interferes with speech comprehension; the recruitment phenomenon is negative. The most common cause of unilateral hearing loss is *acoustic neurinoma* (*Schwannoma*) of the auditory nerve, accounting for nearly 10% of primary intracranial tumors and can develop at any age, with a median onset in the 5th decade. As the tumor progresses, balance disorders, facial paresthesia due to involvement of the trigeminal nerve, peripheral facial weakness, and headaches may occur. Audiometry shows unilateral neural hearing loss, and auditory evoked potentials are altered in 95% of cases. Bilateral acoustic neuromas can occur in the context of neurofibromatosis type II. Early tumor removal (when the size is less than 2 cm) is low-risk and does not result in permanent deficits.

Central deafness | These are very rare and observed in cases of bilateral interruption of the auditory pathways in the brainstem (infiltrating tumors), bilateral lesions of the acoustic radiations (multiple subcortical infarctions), or bilateral destruction of the temporal cortex (multiple cortical infarctions of embolic origin).

Tinnitus | In many patients, the main symptom is a hallucinatory sensation of noise, *called tinnitus*, which usually accompanies the initial phase of hearing loss but can persist for a long time independently. It is likely due to irritation of the receptors and neural structures. The noise is predominantly heard in silent environments and causes a lot of discomfort, especially in emotionally susceptible individuals. In pathologies of the middle ear, it usually has a low pitch, while in inner ear and nerve disorders, it has a high pitch. In Meniere's disease, a characteristic low-frequency roaring sound (a "roaring" tinnitus) is present. As the functional loss worsens, tinnitus tends to decrease.

The patient may also report a pulsating noise synchronous with the pulse, caused by blood flow in an intracranial arteriovenous malformation, which can be heard by the examiner by placing the stethoscope on the mastoid. This should not be confused with the simple pulsation that many normal individuals hear when resting their ear on a pillow.

The therapy for tinnitus is often disappointing. Medications such as carbamazepine, betahistine, amitriptyline, and benzodiazepines can be tried, and it is useful to avoid excessive silence by maintaining a low-volume sound source (e.g., a turned-on radio).

3.6 Cranial bulbar nerves

Of the four nerves that originate from the medulla, the glossopharyngeal, vagus, and cranial root of the accessory nerve have largely common motor, sensory, and autonomic functions. The spinal root of the accessory nerve (true accessory nerve) is the motor nerve of the trapezius and sternocleidomastoid muscles, while the hypoglossal nerve is the motor nerve of the tongue.

3.6.1 Glossopharyngeal (9th), Vagus (10th) and cranial root of the accessory (11th)

The three nerves exit the lateral surface of the medulla with a series of rootlets (Figure 3.33) and leave the skull through the *jugular foramen*.

The *glossopharyngeal nerve* presents the superior (somatic afferents) and petrous (visceral afferents) ganglia at the level of the foramen. It descends on the lateral aspect of the pharynx, laterally to the internal carotid artery, and branches into terminal branches at the base of the tongue.

The *vagus nerve* presents the jugular (somatic afferents) and nodose (visceral afferents) ganglia at the level of the foramen and gives off the auricular and meningeal branches. It descends in the neck within a common sheath with the carotid artery and internal jugular vein and gives off the pharyngeal branches and the superior laryngeal nerve.

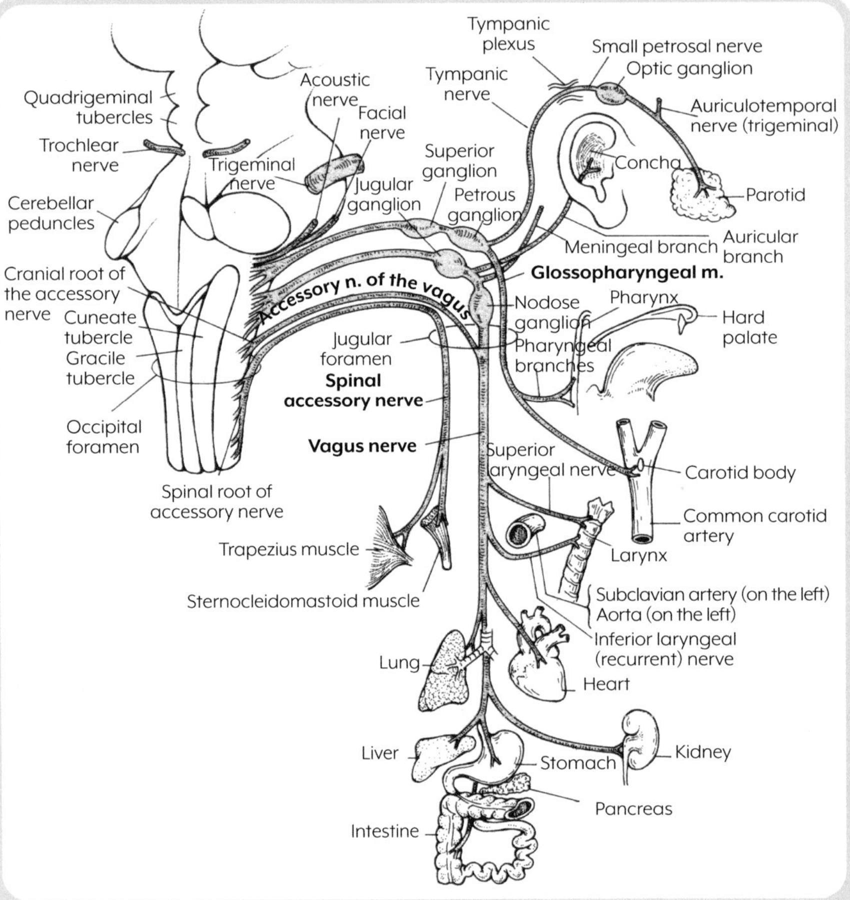

Figure 3.33

Bulbar Nerves: Glossopharyngeal (9th), Vagus (10th), and Accessory (11th). They are shown originating from the brainstem (viewed posteriorly and from the right) and their main branches (the fibers of the vagus nerve directed towards the viscera make contact with the post-ganglionic neurons located in the walls of the viscera, not labeled in the figure).

It passes to the right in front of the subclavian artery and to the left in front of the aortic arch, emitting the recurrent laryngeal nerve, which ascends posteriorly surrounding the subclavian artery and aortic arch. Finally, it attaches to the esophagus and penetrates the abdomen through the esophageal hiatus of the diaphragm.

The c*ranial root* (*internal branch*) of the *accessory nerve* is an aberrant bundle of the vagus nerve, originating from the nucleus ambiguus and rejoining it immediately after the jugular foramen.

The *motor contingent* of the three nerves, of the special visceral type, originates from the nucleus ambiguus, located deep in the lateral bulbars region. A group of fibers takes the route of the glossopharyngeal nerve, while the majority follow the vagus nerve, directly or through the cranial root of the accessory nerve. The distribution of fibers between the two nerves is somewhat individual. The glossopharyngeal nerve carries fibers for the stylopharyngeus muscle (elevator of the pharynx and larynx) and possibly some fibers for the pharynx. The vagus nerve carries almost all motor fibers for the palate, pharynx, and larynx; the latter reach the nerve through the cranial root of the accessory nerve.

The *sensory contingent* consists of three groups of fibers:

a) *General somatic* afferent fibers originate from the superior (glossopharyngeal) and jugular (vagus) ganglia and terminate in the trigeminal nuclei. They carry painful, thermal, and tactile information. They innervate the concha of the auricle (vagus and partly glossopharyngeal), the dura of the posterior cranial fossa (vagus, along with cervical spinal branches), and the mucosa of the posterior part of the tongue, tonsils, soft palate, pharynx, Eustachian tube, and middle ear (glossopharyngeal).

They also innervate the mucosa of the larynx (vagus).

b) *General visceral* afferent fibers originate from the petrous (glossopharyngeal) and nodose (vagus) ganglia and terminate in the solitary nucleus. Some sensations, such as hunger, satiety, and nausea, reach consciousness, while most regulate reflex visceral activities. Notable are the afferents from the baroreceptors of the carotid sinus (glossopharyngeal), which regulate heart rate and blood pressure, as well as those from the tracheobronchial mucosa, stomach, and abdominal viscera (vagus) involved in cough reflex, glandular secretion, and visceral motility (vomiting reflex, etc.). Painful afferents from the thoracic and abdominal viscera largely travel with the spinal nerves.

c) *Special visceral* afferent fibers originate from the petrous (glossopharyngeal) and nodose (vagus) ganglia, terminate in the solitary nucleus, and carry taste information, as described previously.

The *autonomic contingent* consists of efferent fibers of general visceral parasympathetic nature, secretory and motor, originating from the *inferior salivatory nucleus* located at the border of the pons and medulla, and the *dorsal motor nucleus* located in the medulla, below the floor of the fourth ventricle. The fibers of the inferior salivatory nucleus take the route of the glossopharyngeal nerve and, following a tortuous course reach the otic ganglion. They synapse there and, as postganglionic fibers, join the third branch of the trigeminal nerve to reach the parotid gland through the auriculotemporal branch. The fibers of the dorsal motor nucleus continue in the vagus nerve and reach the ganglia plexuses of the viscera for secretory and visceral motility in the thoracic and abdominal regions.

During the *clinical examination*, the first thing to evaluate in the patient is the voice, whether it is loud, hypophonic, or biphonic, as occurs in the paralysis of a vocal cord. Additionally, nasal tone should be assessed, as seen in palatal paralysis. *Swallowing* should be investigated by having the patient take a sip of water. In the *examination of the palate and pharynx*, the glossopharyngeal nerve should be considered the sensory nerve, while the vagus-accessory nerve is the motor nerve. The most indicative afferent deficit is the loss of sensitivity in the pharynx, tonsils, and soft palate (as well as the loss of taste in the posterior third of the tongue). Mechanical stimulation of the lower edge of the palate and the posterolateral wall of the pharynx (palatal and *pharyngeal reflexes*) does not elicit responses. Unilateral motor deficits manifest as drooping of the soft palate. When pronouncing the letter "A," the palate does not elevate, while the uvula and the posterior wall of the pharynx are pulled toward the healthy side due to the unopposed action of the contralateral superior pharyngeal constrictor muscle. Dysphagia, usually not severe, becomes disabling in bilateral lesions since the bolus, propelled by the tongue into the pharynx, does not progress due to the deficit of the pharyngeal constrictor muscles, while paralysis of the palate leaves the nasal cavities open, causing food to reflux into the nose. The voice acquires a nasal tone.

Examination of the *larynx* requires laryngoscopy since unilateral lesions are often paucisymptomatic. The involved branches depend on the vagus nerve and are the superior laryngeal nerve, which provides sensation to the larynx and innervates only the cricothyroid muscle (tensor of the vocal cord), and the recurrent laryngeal nerve (terminating as the inferior laryngeal branch), the motor branch for all other laryngeal muscles.

In *unilateral vagus nerve* lesions, before the detachment of the superior laryngeal nerve, the vocal cord is immobile and assumes an intermediate position between abduction and adduction (*cadaveric position*).The voice becomes biphonic, but vocal disturbances are transient since the cord of the healthy side crosses the midline, compensating for the deficit. Concurrently, the ipsilateral *palatopharyngeal paralysis* described earlier occurs. In *bilateral lesions*, the cords are immobile in an intermediate position, resulting in complete aphonia, ineffective coughing, severe dysphagia, and a high risk of food reflux into the trachea. However, there are no obstacles to airflow and breathing.

Unilateral *recurrent laryngeal nerve injuryè* is a frequent event, especially on the left side, due to the nerve's long course. It can be caused by pathologies of the cervical lymph nodes, thyroid and mediastinal tumors, and neck surgeries. Additionally, on the left side, it can be injured by aortic aneurysms and left atrium enlargement, while on the right side, it can be affected by subclavian aneurysms. Often, no demonstrable causes are found, and the injury presents in an idiopathic form. The cricothyroid muscle and the cord on the affected side are spared, lying close to the midline with minimal residual motility. The voice is usually biphonic but transiently. There may be swallowing difficulties due to incomplete closure of the cricopharyngeal sphincter, but the palate and pharynx move normally, and breathing is normal.

Bilateral lesions of the recurrent laryngeal nerve, especially if acute, such as after thyroidectomy, allow for a reasonable phonation, but the abducted position of the vocal cords obstructs the passage of air and causes serious dyspnea. Dyspnea is even greater in incomplete bilateral lesions, as the abductor muscles of the cords are compromised first (Semon's law).

The autonomic functions of both the glossopharyngeal and vagus nerves are of clinical relevance in diagnosing *neurogenic syncope*. *Glossopharyngeal neuralgia* manifests with acute paroxysms of pain, localized in the tonsillar region, base of the tongue, external auditory canal, and with specific "triggers" (swallowing, chewing, speaking, coughing). They can be associated with *syncope* due *to cardioinhibition*, from direct or reflex activation of afferents from carotid baroreceptors. *Hyperreflexia of the carotid sinus* can develop in elderly individuals due to carotid atheromas and can cause syncope upon mechanical stimulation of the lateral neck region, even sudden rotation. Under normal conditions, *cardioinhibitory* and *vasodilatory reflexes* mediated by the vagus nerve are responsible for orthostatic vasovagal syncope, common and benign events occurring during blood draws, wounds, upon seeing blood, emotions, indigestion, vomiting, exposure to hot environments, or prolonged upright posture. Cold-water baths after meals and syncope occurring within the context of neurodegenerative autonomic insufficiency are risky events.

The three nerves are typically affected together, in association with the accessory spinal nerve (Vernet's syndrome), with the hypoglossal nerve (Sicard-Collet syndrome), and with the addition of the pericarotid sympathetic plexus (Villaret's syndrome), in pathologies of the cranial base, the region of the jugular foramen, and the space below the lateral condyle and retro-parotid (meningitis, epidural abscesses, tumors of the jugular glomus, metastases, neurinomas of the three nerves, chondromas, cholesteatomas, meningiomas, nasopharyngeal tumors, leukemic infiltrates, vertebral artery aneurysms, bone remodeling in Paget's disease, platybasia, Arnold-Chiari malformation, skull fractures), as well as in the *occlusion of the ascending pharyngeal artery*, a branch of the external carotid artery. Moreover, the glossopharyngeal and vagus nerves are acutely affected in the posterior fossa due to vertebral dissection and upon exiting the skull due to carotid dissection. Bilateral lesions are observed in the extensive form of Guillain-Barré acute inflammatory polyneuropathy and in diphtheric neuropathy.

At the bulb level, the fibers of the ambiguous nucleus are easily involved in lateral softening (Wallenberg's syndrome, already discussed with the trigeminal nerve). In motor neuron disease, the motor neurons of the ambiguous nucleus degenerate along with spinal motor neurons and the motor nuclei of the trigeminal, spinal accessory, and hypoglossal nerves.

Due to the bilateral pyramidal innervation of the ambiguous nucleus, unilateral pyramidal lesions practically do not give symptoms; however, bilateral lesions (pseudobulbar syndrome) become highly debilitating, manifesting with spastic dysarthria, dysphagia for liquids, spastic laughter and crying, urinary urgency, and pyramidal signs in all four limbs with a small-step gait.

3.6.2 Spinal accessory nerve (11th cranial nerve)

It is a motor branch composed of special visceral fibers, originating from the accessory nucleus, a gray column that extends from C2 to C5, in line with the ambiguous nucleus. It emerges between the anterior and posterior spinal roots, ascends through the occipital foramen as the spinal root (Figure 3.33), joins the cranial root, and exits the skull again

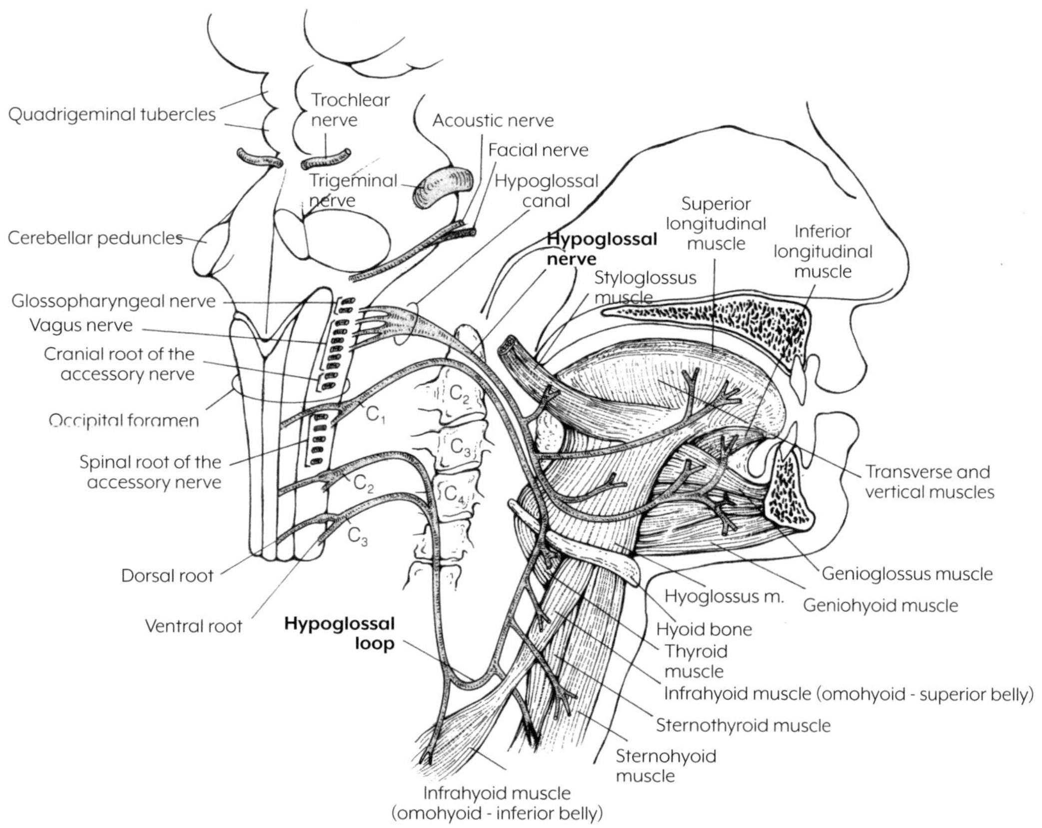

Figure 3.34

Bulbar Nerves: Hypoglossal (12th). The origin of the trunk (seen posteriorly and from the right), the branches to the muscles of the tongue, and the anastomosis with the first three cervical roots (hypoglossal loop) for innervation of the infrahyoid muscles are shown. Cl, C2, C3, C4: cervical roots and vertebrae.

through the jugular foramen. The cranial root returns to the vagus nerve; the spinal root descends in the neck along with the internal jugular vein, penetrates the *sternocleidomastoid muscle* where it gives branches, exits to the posterior direction between cervical lymph nodes, and reaches the *trapezius muscle*, where it branches with terminal fibers (the lower portion of the trapezius is innervated by the 3rd and 4th spinal root). Pyramidal projections for the sternocleidomastoid muscle are predominantly crossed, while those for the trapezius are exclusively crossed.

Isolated injuries occur in surgery of the posterior triangle of the neck or in cervical lymph node pathology. It is usually damaged together with other bulbar nerves (Vernet and Sicard-Collet syndromes). The sternocleidomastoid muscle rotates the head towards the opposite side, and the deficit is noticeable during rotation or when lifting the head from the bed in a supine position. The trapezius muscle elevates the scapulae and raises the upper limb beyond 90° with the upper fibers, while the lower fibers adduct the scapula; its paralysis limits the elevation of the upper limb and causes the detachment of the scapula from the chest wall (winged scapula); the sign appears when extending the arm anteriorly below the horizontal line and is less pronounced than in the deficit of the serratus anterior muscle (long thoracic nerve), where the sign appears when extending the arm anteriorly above the horizontal line. The lower bundles of the trapezius muscle, innervated by spinal roots, are spared in accessory nerve injuries.

3.6.3 Hypoglossal nerve (12th cranial nerve)

It is composed of general somatic efferent fibers from the homonymous nucleus, a bulbar continuation of the anterior horn of the spinal cord, located near the midline, below the floor of the 4th ventricle. It exits the medulla with a series of rootlets located between the pyramid and the olive, aligned with the anterior spinal roots, and leaves the skull through the *hypoglossal canal* or *condylar canal* (Figure 3.34).

It passes laterally to the internal and external carotid arteries and reaches the base of the tongue, distributing to the intrinsic and extrinsic muscles of the tongue, as well as the geniohyoid. After the canal, fibers from the first cervical root join the nerve and, together with fibers from the second and third roots, form the *hypoglossal loop* for the infrahyoid muscles.

The most important muscles in the clinical examination are the *genioglossus* and the styloglossus. The genioglossus, attached to the inner arch of the mandible and the base of the tongue, protrudes the base of the tongue forward, deviating the tip towards the opposite side. In unilateral nerve injuries, the patient is unable to press the tip of the tongue against the cheek on the affected side, and during protrusion, the tip deviates towards the affected side due to the unopposed action of the genioglossus on the unaffected side. The *styloglossus*, attached to the styloid process and the base of the tongue, retracts and elevates the tongue. In unilateral injuries, with the tongue at rest in the oral cavity, the tip deviates slightly towards the unaffected side due to the unopposed action of the styloglossus on that side. Atrophy of the intrinsic muscles becomes evident with a reduction in tongue volume. In bilateral injuries, the tongue lies in the oral cavity, and food cannot be pushed under the teeth or collected for swallowing; speech is also significantly impaired. Fasciculations and fibrillations are clearly observed.

Isolated injuries are rare and occur as a result of fractures of the cranial base, wounds or surgery in the retromandibular region, pathologies of the retromandibular lymph nodes, tortuosity, aneurysms, or dissection of the internal carotid artery before entering the skull, or arachnoid cysts of the posterior fossa. More often, the nerve is injured along with other nerves in the region in base pathologies Within the medulla, it generally escapes vascular injuries; sometimes it is injured along with the pyramidal fibers before the decussation, resulting in a rare alternate syndrome with ipsilateral paralysis of the tongue and contralateral paralysis of the limbs. Unilateral pyramidal lesions only transiently cause paresis of the opposite half of the tongue, while bilateral lesions significantly impair tongue motility.

Finally, the tongue is frequently involved in spontaneous and *pharmacological tardive* dyskinesias.

Bibliography

Abbruzzese G. et al., Hemifacial spasm, Handb Clin Neurol 100:675, 2011.

Adour K.K., Diagnosis and management of facial paralysis, N. Engl J Med 307, 348,1982.

Berardelli A. et al., Corticobulbar and corticospinal projections to neck muscle motoneurons in man. A functional study with magnetic and electric transcranial brain stimulation, Exp Brain Res 87:402, 1991.

Brodal A., The cranial nerves. Anatomy and anatomico-clinical correlations, Blackwell Scientific Publications, Oxford, 1972.

Cruccu G. et al., Trigeminal neuralgia: New classification and diagnostic grading for practice and research, Neurology 87:220, 2016.

Sonne J., Lopez-Ojeda W., Neuroanatomy, Cranial Nerve (StatPearls, Internet, November 19, 2020, prelevato dicembre 2021).

4 ANATOMICAL BASES OF COGNITIVE PROCESSES

Marco Canevelli, Fabrizia D'Antonio,
Alessandro Trebbastoni, Giuseppe Bruno

Understanding the mechanisms underlying cognitive processes and theories of mind presupposes knowledge of the anatomical bases associated with them. The cerebral cortex and subcortical structures, which are anatomically and functionally interconnected, are the elective sites of such processes. Different regions can be distinguished, which are variably named and classified based on cytoarchitectural characteristics, topographic localization, and functional specificity.

Primary Cortices

Distinguished into sensory and motor cortices, they represent the initial stations for analyzing the most elementary components of sensory experiences (such as somatosensory, visual, auditory, gustatory, etc.) and the final site for motor response planning, respectively. These are modality-specific areas that exclusively respond to specific stimuli within a given sensory or motor modality. They can, therefore, be considered as the sites of primary input for stimuli from the external environment and output for movement execution. Lesions in these areas result in "elementary" deficits (motor, sensory, olfactory, visual disturbances, etc.).

Unimodal Associative Areas

Also divided into sensory and motor areas, they integrate different and specific information for a single modality, performing much more sophisticated processing of various stimuli compared to primary cortices. Taking visual function as an example, the unimodal associative areas integrate information related to different aspects of visual experience (such as shape, color, size, and movement of objects), which have already been individually analyzed in the primary visual cortex. Regarding motor activity, on the other hand, the primary motor cortex exclusively encodes the force and degree of contraction of different muscle groups, while the associative motor areas carry out more complex processes such as movement planning and the learning of new motor sequences. Lesions in associative areas result in complex clinical symptoms and signs (agnosias, disturbances of body schema, exploration of extrapersonal space).

Heteromodal associative areas

They integrate information from multiple sensory modalities and are closely interconnected with motor areas. Therefore, they represent the anatomical substrate of the most complex cerebral and cognitive activities such as perception, language, memory, consciousness, thought, and behavior. Heteromodal associative areas are represented by the prefrontal regions, the limbic lobe, and the parietal-temporal cortex.

It is possible to hypothesize that environmental stimuli reach the primary sensory cortices, where they are decomposed into different sensory components that are processed in parallel. The information then reaches the unimodal associative areas, where all the individual components related to a single sensory modality are integrated, and

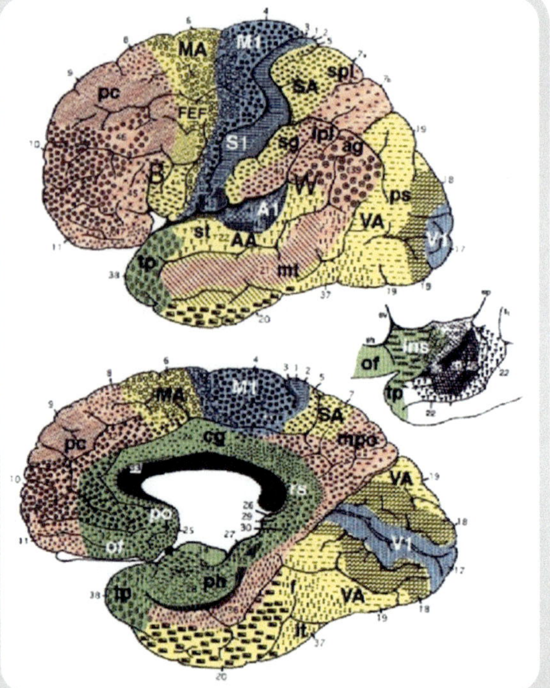

Figure 4.1

In blue, primary cortices; in yellow, unimodal association areas; in red and in green heteromodal and limbic association areas. (Brain area map according to Brodmann, modified).

Table 4.1 CORTICAL AREAS AND THEIR FUNCTIONS

CEREBRAL AREAS	LOCALIZATION
Primary cortices	
Somatosensory	Postcentral gyrus, parietal
Visual	Calcarine sulcus, occipital lobe
Auditory	Heschl's gyrus, temporal lobe
Olfactory	Junction between insular, orbitofrontal, and temporopolar areas
Vestibular	Posterior part of Sylvian fissure
Motor	Precentral gyrus, frontal lobe
Unimodal associative areas	
Somatosensory	Posterior parietal cortex
Visual	Occipito-temporal and occipito-parietal junction
Auditory	Superior temporal gyrus.
Motor	Premotor and supplementary motor areas, frontal lobe.
Heteromodal associative areas	
Limbic lobe	Medial surface of the cerebral hemispheres
Prefrontal cortex	Dorso-lateral surface of the frontal lobe located in front of the motor areas.
Posterior area	Temporo-parietal junction

finally reaches the heteromodal areas that integrate different modalities, giving rise to conscious perception. In these regions, sensory information is transformed into a motor/behavioral response that is transferred to the motor associative areas and from there to the motor cortex in the form of movement and/or language.

Figure 4.1 and Table 4.1 represent and list the different cortical regions.

4.1 Memory

The term "memory" refers to the ability to acquire, store, and use knowledge and new information. It can be classified based on temporal characteristics and the nature of the information (Figure 4.2).

In terms of temporal dimension, there are the following distinctions:

- *Immediate or sensory memory:* primarily concerns auditory (echoic) and visual (iconic) stimuli and is characterized by extremely rapid and transient (milliseconds) processing of information. Depending on their cognitive salience, i.e., their relevance to the individual, the information is further elaborated and converted into short-term memory.
- *Short-term memory:* allows for the storage of a limited amount of information for a short period (a few seconds). It is also referred to as "working memory" as it serves as a system for the temporary maintenance and manipulation of information during the execution of various cognitive tasks such as comprehension, learning, and reasoning.
- *Long-term memory:* enables the permanent storage of an unlimited amount of information.

In terms of information characteristics, long-term memory can be further divided into:

- *Explicit or declarative memory*: so named because the information can be volun-

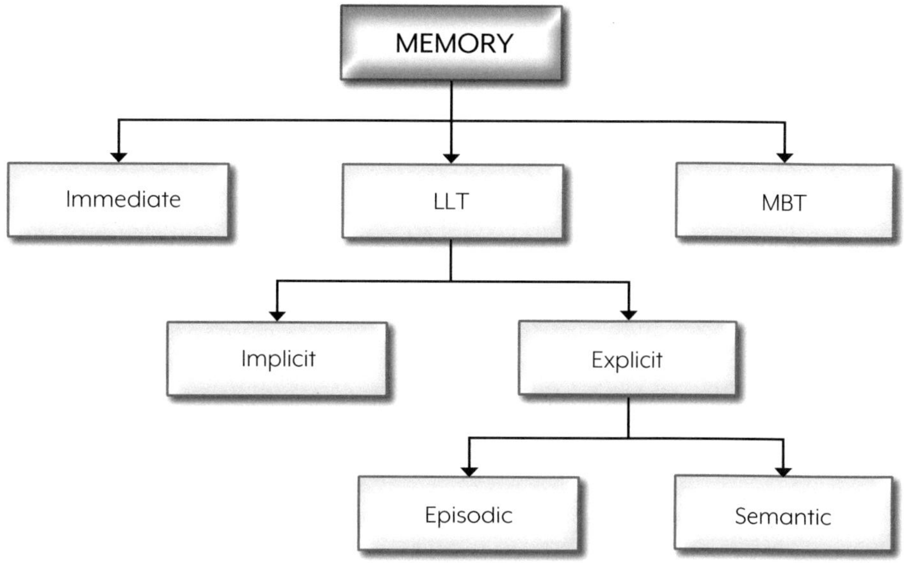

Figure 4.2

Memory classification. LLT: long-term memory; MBT: short-term memory.

tarily recalled and verbalized. It includes knowledge of facts, concepts, and meanings. It is further distinguished as:
- *Episodic: pertaining to personal events and experiences.*
- *Semantic:* relating to knowledge of concepts, words, and meanings.

– *Implicit or procedural memory*: concerns perceptual experiences and motor actions that cannot be verbally expressed and often translate, after numerous attempts, into the execution of motor tasks and behaviors that do not require conscious intervention. Examples of implicit memory include learning procedures, rules, and motor skills.

The processes leading to the creation of different forms of memory take place in distinct brain areas. The structures of the temporal lobe, particularly the hippocampus, are essential for the formation of explicit memories, which are then stored in the unimodal and heteromodal associative areas. Traces of semantic memory are widely distributed and stored in the cortical areas. On the other hand, the cerebellum, striatum, amygdala, motor systems, and sensory systems are involved in the formation of implicit memories derived from different learning processes. The prefrontal cortex plays a central role in working memory formation. Therefore, there are no exclusive locations for memory localization, rather, memory is a widely distributed function across various cortical areas.

From a neurobiological perspective, the storage of information as short-term and long-term memory depends on synaptic transmission modifications (presynaptic facilitation and inhibition), gene expression, as well as long-term synaptic potentiation processes.

Neurological pathologies of any nature (degenerative, tumorous, infectious, etc.) can be associated with long-term memory disorders, forming an amnesic syndrome that can be defined as:

– *Anterograde:* characterized by the inability to learn new information.
– *Retrograde:* characterized by prominent difficulty in recalling events or episodes that occurred before the pathological event (both immediately preceding the event and related to recent or remote periods of the patient's life).
– *Anteroretrograde:* with mixed characteristics.

4.2 Executive functions

Executive functions can be defined as the abilities that allow an individual to make choices, make decisions, implement strategies aimed at achieving a goal, and perform goal-directed behaviors. They consist of activities such as planning, programming, inhibition, critical thinking, judgment, and abstract reasoning, and they are intimately connected to the mechanisms that regulate behavior, affectivity, and personality.

Executive functions are primarily regulated by the prefrontal areas, particularly the connections of these cortical regions with subcortical structures such as the basal ganglia and the thalamus. There are three main frontal-subcortical circuits or loops that originate from three distinct portions of the prefrontal cortex, which are:

- The dorsolateral area, located anteriorly to the premotor region.
- The orbitofrontal area, located at the level of the basal region.
- The frontomedial area, which occupies the medial region and including the anterior cingulate gyrus.

These cortical regions are connected to specific portions of the basal ganglia and thalamus and form circuits (Figure 4.3) that terminate in the same cortical areas of origin, exerting distinct functions.

The *dorsolateral prefrontal circuit* primarily governs executive functions. Its alterations lead to the onset of a dysexecutive syndrome characterized, from a clinical perspective, by difficulties in programming, planning, abstract reasoning, and inhibiting interfering stimuli, as well as the presence of perseveration and deficits in working memory.

The dorsolateral prefrontal dysexecutive syndrome can be recognized in neurodegenerative diseases, depressive disorders, and psychotic disorders.

The *lateral orbitofrontal circuit* primarily integrates emotional states, thoughts, and memories into appropriate behavioral responses to different contexts. Lesions affecting the different components of this circuit can therefore cause profound changes in personality, alterations in social behaviors, depressive symptoms, obsessive-compulsive disorders, and affective blunting.

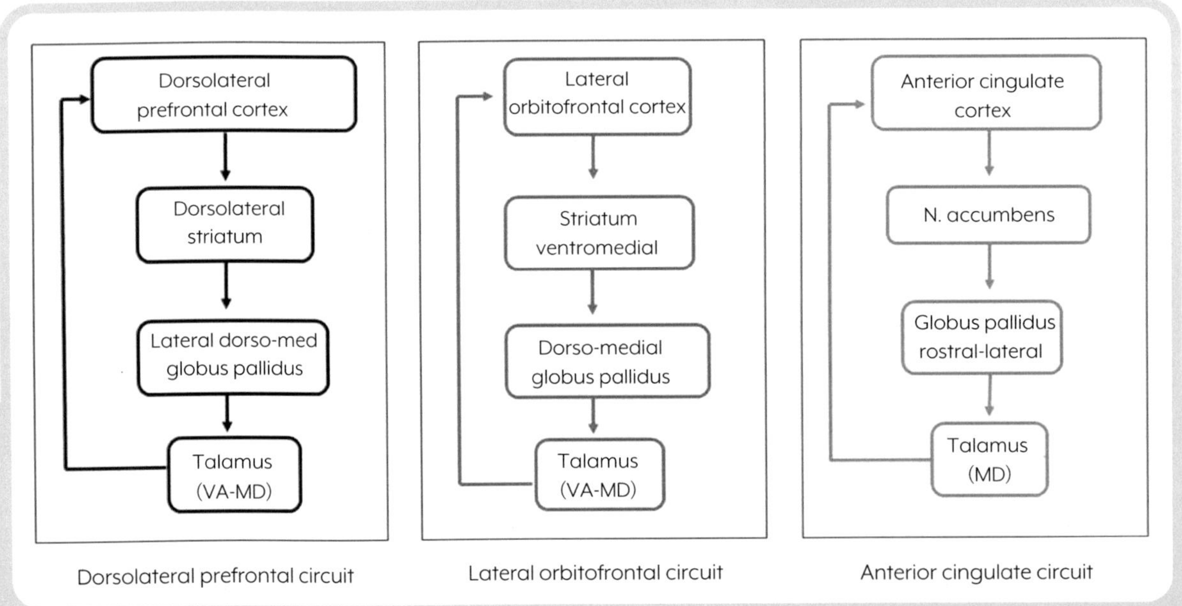

Figure 4.3

Representation of the frontal-subcortical circuits. VA: ventral anterior nucleus; MD: mid-dorsal nucleus.

The orbitofrontal syndrome is typically recognizable in obsessive-compulsive disorder, apathetic syndrome, and frontotemporal dementia.

The *anterior cingulate circuit* is closely interconnected with the orbitofrontal regions and limbic areas, integrating cognitive and emotional aspects to modulate motivated behaviors. Symptoms and clinical signs resulting from alterations in this loop include apathy, abulia, loss of interest, and motivation towards the surrounding environment. The anterior cingulate gyrus syndrome is involved in a broad spectrum of clinical conditions characterized by the presence of apathy: Alzheimer's disease, Parkinson's disease, frontotemporal dementia, ischemic strokes, and traumatic brain injuries.

4.3 Attention

The term "attention" refers to the ability to maintain focused awareness of relevant information while excluding irrelevant or interfering stimuli from both the external and internal environment (such as emotions, thoughts, and perceptions). There are two important categories of attention:

- *Sustained attention:* This enables the maintenance of cognitive performance over an extended period. It includes a prolonged tonic component, which corresponds to the state of vigilance, and a phasic component (arousal), which relates to the physiological reactivity to external stimuli.
- *Selective attention:* This allows filtering and countering of stimuli that act as "distractors," enabling the focus of cognitive resources on relevant information and selecting only some of the multiple solicitations from the external environment.

The state of vigilance and arousal are controlled by the brainstem reticular formation, interlaminar thalamic nuclei (with diffuse projections), and monoaminergic transmission nuclei. Prefrontal areas are crucial for the selection, inhibition, and control of stimuli. Posterior-inferior parietal regions (especially in the right hemisphere), the superior colliculus, and the thalamus are involved in stimulus orientation and spatial attention. Lesions in these regions result in spatial exploration disorders and hemi-inattention (neglect). Attention disorders manifest as distractibility, inattentiveness, forgetfulness, and even confusion.

4.4 Language

Language can be understood as the ability to transform thoughts and ideas into symbolic communication. It consists of a purely motor-articulatory component, which includes the muscular and nervous structures involved in producing sounds, and a symbolic component that relies on syntactic, grammatical, and phonological conventions to enable communicative use. The left hemisphere plays a central role in language processing and regulation, except in a small percentage of left-handed individuals where right hemisphere dominance occurs.

The study of patients with aphasic disorders has identified two critical cortical regions for language: Broca's area, located at the base of the third frontal convolution, responsible for language production; and Wernicke's area, situated in the posterior portion of the superior temporal gyrus, primarily responsible for language comprehension. These two areas are interconnected by a bidirectional system of fibers known as the arcuate fasciculus. These "primary" areas are surrounded and supported, in language perception and production, by other associative areas located in the temporal pole, prefrontal, temporal, and inferior parietal cortices. The right hemisphere, on the other hand, plays an essential role in language expressiveness and prosody, which involves attributing different meanings to language through pauses, changes in intonation, and syntactic structures.

The clinical evaluation of language is based on the analysis of the following elements:

- *Spontaneous speech:* verbal fluency, the content of information, syntactic structure characterized by either poverty or excess of grammatical elements (referred to as agrammatism and paragrammatism, respectively), presence of phonemic substitutions or paraphasias (substituting a syllable or sound within a word) and semantic substitutions (replacing a word with another correctly pronounced but inappropriate word), repetitions, and neologisms; non-verbal aspects of language such as intonation and melody.

- *Repetition.* Generally, test phrases are used, mostly devoid of meaning.
- *Naming.* The patient is asked to name some visually presented objects.
- *Auditory comprehension.* The patient's ability to follow simple and complex commands.
- *Writing.*
- *Reading.*

The term "*dysarthria*" refers exclusively to a motor disorder characterized by articulation impairments in speech. Although the speech may be difficult to understand, it is correctly processed and, therefore, communicative. The patient's speech may appear "slurred," "stuttered," "staccato," or "explosive," but it is not associated with impairments in comprehension, writing, or reading. Dysarthria represents the clinical expression of lesions in the neural structures that control the speech articulatory system (cranial nerve nuclei, particularly the trigeminal, facial, glossopharyngeal, and hypoglossal nerves; corticobulbar pathways; basal ganglia; cerebellum).

On the other hand, the term "*aphasia*" defines a clinical disorder characterized by an acquired impairment, more or less severe, in the symbolic use of language, resulting from cortical lesions in the dominant hemisphere. Table 4.2 summarizes the clinical characteristics of the main aphasic syndromes.

In clinical practice, it is difficult to observe aphasic syndromes that fully satisfy the criteria listed in the table, as well as brain lesions confined to specific language areas. In most cases, clinical presentations with mixed characteristics are observed. However, in general, in non-fluent aphasias, the patient tends to be aware of their expressive difficulties, leading to "catastrophic" and depressive reactions. In fluent aphasias, on the other hand, individuals tend to ignore their deficits. In transcortical aphasias, repetition is

Table 4.2 THE MAIN APHASIA SYNDROMES

TYPE OF APHASIA	SPONTANEOUS SPEECH	COMPREHENSION	REPETITION	SITE OF LESION
Non-fluent aphasias				
Broca's aphasia	Non-fluent speech, produced with difficulty; phonemic paraphasias; agrammatism	Preserved	Altered	Left posterior frontal cortex (Broca's area)
Transcortical Motor Aphasia	Reduced verbal fluency, explosive language	Preserved	Preserved	Regions surrounding Broca's area (mostly located anteriorly and superiorly)
Global aphasia	Limited, non-fluent, and minimally informative language	Altered	Altered	Extensive left hemisphere lesions
Fluent aphasias				
Wernicke's aphasia	Fluent, verbose, sometimes verbose but poorly informative speech; semantic paraphasias; paragrammatism.	Altered	Altered	Left superior temporal cortex (Wernicke's area)
Transcortical Sensory Aphasia	Fluent, paraphasic	Altered	Preserved	Regions surrounding Wernicke's area (mostly located posteriorly and inferiorly)
Conduction aphasia	Fuent, phonemic and semantic paraphasias	Preserved	Altered	Angular gyrus, supermarginal gyrus, insular cortex (involvement of the arcuate fasciculus)

typically preserved because it is believed that information from Wernicke's area can directly reach the motor areas. Aphasic syndromes are frequently associated with other focal neurological symptoms and signs, such as right hemiparesis/plegia, right hemianesthesia/hypoesthesia, homonymous hemianopsia, and impairments in other symbolic functions such as praxis and gnosis.

4.5 Praxic functions

Praxis refers to the abilities that enable the execution of "refined" movements and sequences of movements. Therefore, apraxia is defined as the impairment of intentional gestural activity, which occurs in the absence of motor, sensory, perceptual, and cognitive deficits that could affect the capacity to execute and understand the task at hand. It can involve both transitive gestures, characterized by intentionality and purpose (such as using an object), and meaningless motor acts.

The distinctive feature is represented by "automatic-voluntary dissociation": the gesture is spontaneously produced in response to internal instructions or environmental stimuli but becomes altered or compromised when performed upon external request.

The critical brain areas for praxis functions are the heteromodal associative parietal and prefrontal cortices of the dominant hemisphere. The parietal areas receive input from visual, auditory, and somatosensory areas and send information to the prefrontal cortex, premotor areas, and orbitofrontal areas. The prefrontal areas receive input from the parietal cortex and send information to the premotor areas and primary motor cortex, which are responsible for movement planning and execution. These two extensive brain regions are connected to the homologous areas of the contralateral hemisphere through the commissural fibers of the corpus callosum. Generally, lesions in the left frontal and parietal regions (dominant hemisphere) tend to cause bilateral apraxic impairments, while lesions in the non-dominant hemisphere can result in unilateral left-sided apraxias.

In clinical practice, the presence of apraxic impairment is evaluated by asking the patient to perform specific movements:

- *Buccofacial movements:* blowing a kiss, clicking the tongue, whistling, etc.
- *Transitive gestures:* mimicking the use of an object (a toothbrush, nail, hammer, comb, etc.).
- *Intransitive gestures:* generally conventional gestures (military salute, sign of the cross, etc.).
- *Sequential gestures:* non-purposeful motor sequences.
- *Goal-directed actions:* lighting a candle, opening and closing a padlock, etc.

Different forms of apraxia can be distinguished:

- *Ideational apraxia*: the inability to perform complex sequences of movements due to difficulties in the mental representation of the gesture. Patients can recognize and correctly name common objects but do not know how to use them, making gross errors (altered or reversed movement sequence, incorrect use of the object, omissions). The patient, therefore, "does not know what to do." Movement execution tends to improve with imitation. This form of apraxia is generally associated with lesions in the posterior regions of the left hemisphere (temporo-parieto-occipital junction). Before accepting these behaviors as evidence of an autonomous disorder, it is necessary to exclude the presence of other pathologies that could cause motor impairments as a consequence of different functional alterations. The main alternatives are:
  1) *Dementia or confusion.*
  2) *Agnosia*. The possibility that the patient cannot use the object because they do not recognize it can be easily excluded both by its correct naming - which often occurs - and by the fact that the object is also held in hand. Therefore, the deficit is not confined to a single sensory channel as in agnosia.
  3) *Presence of a severe form of ideomotor apraxia*. In principle, errors in ideomotor apraxia should be easily distinguishable because the general idea of the gesture is still maintained, thanks to proprioceptive information that comes from manipulating the object. In

practice, however, in very severe forms of ideomotor apraxia, it can be difficult to determine whether the incorrect use of an object is due to a defect in ideation or execution because the patient ends up using objects incorrectly.

- *Ideomotor Apraxia*: it is the inability to translate the motor sequence into the executive program. The patient "knows what to do, but doesn't know how to do it." Unlike ideational apraxia, movement execution does not improve after imitation. It is mainly manifested following parietal lesions and tends to predominate in the right limb.
- *Gait Apraxia*: it is the partial or total inability to walk, even in the absence of motor deficits. The patient may have difficulties in standing up/sitting down, maintaining balance, initiating walking, and changing direction during walking.
- *Dressing Apraxia:* it is the selective inability to perform and coordinate the trunk and limb movements necessary to dress oneself. It is mostly associated with dysfunction in the right parietal regions.
- *Constructional Apraxia*: it is a clinical condition, not detectable in an ecological context, characterized by difficulty in reproducing a visual stimulus (drawing, puzzle, etc.). It can have different clinical features depending on the lesion location: in left-sided lesions, the copy tends to correspond to the model but is highly simplified; in right-sided lesions, on the other hand, spatial property alterations prevail, and the copy tends to deviate from the model in terms of overall characteristics and proportions.

4.6 Gnostic functions

Gnostic functions constitute the set of capacities that enable the recognition of a sensory stimulus and its meaning. Agnosia is defined as a perceptual disorder characterized by the inability to recognize and interpret a sensory experience in the absence of alterations in the organs and sensory pathways.

To understand the complexity of gnostic functions, it is necessary to briefly recall the mechanisms of visual perception. The information that reaches the brain does not have stable characteristics but continuously varies depending on light, motion, and depth. An object in motion sends a series of different retinal images, yet it is perceived as the same object. Therefore, the brain must extract the salient and invariant characteristics of objects from the multitude of information it receives. To recognize the surrounding reality, it cannot solely analyze the images presented to the retina but must construct a visual world.

The visual cortical system, like other sensory systems, is hierarchically organized into primary, secondary, and associative areas. The primary or striate visual cortex is located in the posterior part of the occipital lobe (areas V1 and V2). In this projection area, the fibers from the retina terminate after following a path that passes through the optic nerve, optic chiasm, optic tract, and lateral geniculate body, before fanning out in the optic radiation. The primary visual cortex is in turn connected to the secondary visual cortex, consisting of the prestriate cortex and the inferotemporal cortex. The prestriate cortex comprises many highly specialized cortical areas for different tasks: some cells (V3) respond to shape, others (V4) are sensitive to light wavelengths and line orientations, and still others (V5) respond to motion. There are two functional systems originating from the primary visual cortex: a) the ventral pathway, which passes through the prestriate cortex and reaches the inferior temporal cortex, and b) the dorsal pathway, which passes through the prestriate areas and terminates in the posterior parietal cortex. The ventral stream seems to be involved in the recognition of visual stimuli ("what"), while the dorsal stream is responsible for the spatial analysis of the stimulus ("where").

Agnosias can be confined to a single sensory modality (tactile, visual, auditory, etc.) or manifest in a complex form. They can be distinguished as follows:

- *Apperceptive forms*: represent a disorder of the early stages of the perceptual process. They are characterized by the inability to integrate the individual components of a stimulus into a structured perception. The patient may have difficulty recognizing the shapes of objects correctly when they are rotated, inverted, resized, or viewed from a different angle; they may perceive different details of a stimulus without deriving an integrated image from it.

- *Associative forms*: are characterized by difficulty in assigning meaning to correctly processed and perceived stimuli. The patient can perceive a stimulus, but not to attribute meaning to it, resulting in deficits in naming, finding associative links between different stimuli, and using objects (this cannot be referred to as apraxia in this case because perception is compromised).

Agnosias are conventionally classified according to the affected sensory modalities (visual, auditory, tactile). The following are the most common forms of agnosia.

4.6.1 Visual Agnosias

These are the result of lesions in the occipital and inferior temporal cortex (in most cases due to posterior circulation ischemia).

Object Agnosia | The patient has difficulty in recognizing (and consequently naming) visually presented objects. However, their ability to describe the characteristics of the same object when verbally evoked remains intact.

Pure Alexia | Also known as "alexia without agraphia." It consists of a selective inability to recognize words and write, but not to read. The patient can copy and write dictated text but is unable to reread what they have written.

Color Agnosia | It involves a selective difficulty in recognizing colors. The patient is unable to name colors or color black and white figures representing common objects with the appropriate colors.

Prosopagnosia | It is a selective agnosic disorder for faces. It consists of the inability to recognize familiar people (family members, acquaintances, famous individuals). Recognition becomes possible through cues such as voice, surrounding environment, clothing, walking style, etc.

4.6.2 Auditory Agnosias

These are disorders of recognition of auditory stimuli.

Non-verbal auditory agnosia | is the difficulty in understanding and recognizing non-verbal sounds (e.g., bells, animal noises, etc.). It is supported by lesions involving the right temporoparietal cortex.

Pure word deafness | is the selective impairment of comprehension of verbal sounds (spoken language), in the absence of aphasia and hearing disorders. The patient can write spontaneously or copy, understand written commands, but is unable to write under dictation or comprehend verbal commands. It can be the clinical expression of lesions surrounding the Wernicke's area and disconnecting it from auditory areas.

Amusia | is the selective inability to perceive, comprehend, and produce musical sounds.

4.6.3 Tactile Agnosia

Tactile agnosia is characterized by the inability to recognize objects through touch in the absence of somatosensory perception disorders. The patient can discriminate some details of the object through touch, but not recognize it. These are often unilateral disorders that depend on lesions affecting the contralateral inferior parietal cortex.

4.7 Body Schema

The *body schema* refers to the spatial image that each person has of their own body. The concept refers to a complex synthesis function that allows recognizing one's body as a unit, to identify its morphology, the relationships between its various segments, and the changing position in space.

Recent observations suggest that the construction of the body schema uses not only sensory information (such as vision and hearing) but also mnemonic and emotional components. It is supported by the activity of a genetically determined, spatially distributed neural network that is also subject to epigenetic influences.

Disorders of the body schema can be bilateral or unilateral and are categorized as positive or negative. Positive disorders include phantom limb, which is the illusion of the existence of body parts that the patient has lost due to surgical removal or an accident. Negative disorders indicate the neglect of a part of one's own body, usually involving one side of the body (hemineglect).

Bilateral disorders of the body schema are rare and include symptoms such as autotopagnosia, which affects the entire body, as well as digital agnosia and Gerstmann syndrome. Autotopagnosia is a disorder that involves the patient's inability to localize a body part, with the lesion typically located in the left parietal lobe. Digital agnosia was described by the Austrian neurologist J. Gerstmann, who studied an ambidextrous patient with a right parietal tumor. This patient was unable to distinguish, name, or select, upon command, the individual fingers of their own hands or someone else's hands, or fingers depicted in a drawing. Gerstmann later observed that digital agnosia was frequently associated with right-left disorientation, acalculia, and agraphia. Taken together, these different symptoms constitute a condition known as Gerstmann syndrome. The presence of at least three signs of this syndrome in a patient indicates the presence of a lesion in the dominant hemisphere's parietal lobe.

Unilateral body schema disorders | These disorders are included within the broader scope of the so-called "neglect" disorders. The term refers to patients who do not respond to stimuli or are unable to receive information from the contralateral side of the damaged cerebral hemisphere. This is commonly referred to as hemineglect.

Neglect can be referred to as external space neglect (extrapersonal neglect) or bodily space neglect (personal or extrapersonal neglect). Extrapersonal neglect can pertain to information obtained through visual, auditory, somesthetic pathways, as well as mental images or topographic memory functions. In many situations, patients are unable to reproduce, for example, the left half of an original drawing or construction with cubes, or they may fail to read the first words of each line.

Alterations of neglect in intrapersonal space are most frequently represented by hemisomatagnosia and anosognosia.

Hemisomatognosia is characterized by a deficit in synthesizing sensory inputs from different channels, leading to a lack of awareness of the contralateral half of the body to the lesion or a deficit in attention for half of the space, including the hemibody. It is found in approximately one-third of individuals with retro-rolandic right hemisphere lesions, while only a small percentage of cases are attributed to lesions of the left hemisphere. The individual does not perceive the left half of their body as their own and, therefore, may only shave or apply makeup to the right half of the face, for example. The retro-rolandic location of the lesion involves the parietal lobe, including the subcortical part of the right hemisphere, and less frequently the left hemisphere.

Anosognosia, or Anton-Babinski syndrome, is characterized by denial or lack of recognition of a motor, sensory, or other type of deficit and typically occurs in the presence of hemiplegia. The patient ignores the paralysis and claims that the paralyzed limb shown to them by the examiner is not theirs.

4.8 Neuropsychological Assessment

Neuropsychological assessment allows for the evaluation of normal cognitive functioning and, in cases of brain damage, enables the identification of the affected cognitive processes, the areas involved, and the severity of the pathology with a high degree of reliability. Any lesion, even if localized, commonly produces inevitable repercussions on the surrounding interconnected areas. On the other hand, it rarely destroys all the nerve elements in that area; those that remain continue to function under pathologically different conditions.

The assessment can be an integral part of a diagnostic process or provide support for patient management and care planning. It allows for evaluating the effectiveness of a treatment, providing medicolegal information, or it can be targeted toward research. In many cases, multiple objectives can coexist, but the examiner must always bear in mind the reasons why the patient is undergoing the examination and select the most suitable tools, adapting them to the patient's conditions. From a certain perspective, this type of assessment can be considered a series of experiments that generate explanatory hypotheses in the clinical setting.

The investigative methodology consists of neuropsychological tests, which record cognitive functions in standardized and replicable situations, including learning and memory, language, praxis and visuospatial abilities, abstract conceptual thinking, attention, and cognitive flexibility. For this purpose, the test provides quantitative data that can be compared with values obtained from a control population of the same sex, age, and education level.

Table 4.3 presents the main tests used for a basic cognitive evaluation.

Table 4.3 MAIN TESTS USED FOR BASIC COGNITIVE EVALUATION

Verbal short-term and long-term memory
Rey's 15-Word Test Digit-span Brief narrative Buschke-Fuld Supra-Span Verbal Learning Serial position curve
Visuo-spatial short-term and long-term memory
Rey Complex Figure (recall) Corsi Block-Tapping Test Benton Visual Retention Test
Praxis functions
Rey Complex Figure Copy Drawing Copy with and without programming elements Orofacial Apraxia Test Ideomotor Apraxia Test
Visuo-spatial functions
Line Orientation Test Overlapping Figures Test (Poppelreuter-Ghent)
Attention
Attentive Matrices Stroop Test Trail Making Test Digit Symbol Line Cancelation Test
Executive Functions
Modified Card Sorting Test Frontal Assessment Battery Tower of London Cognitive Estimation Test
Language
Phonemic Verbal Fluency Test Semantic Verbal Fluency Test Naming Token Test

4.8.1 Diagnostic question

The primary and most important purpose of neuropsychological assessment is to reach a diagnosis with a high degree of accuracy. In daily clinical practice, errors such as false positives or negatives can have significant psychological and therapeutic implications for both patients and their families. Especially in elderly patients, it is crucial to distinguish cognitive changes related to physiological aging processes from alterations characteristic of an early stage of dementia. Hence the importance of a "tailored" evaluation for the patient, taking into account parameters such as fatigue and reduced motivation to perform long and mentally demanding tasks.

A second purpose is related to differential diagnosis. The etiological characterization of a neurological pathology leads to entirely different prognostic and therapeutic approaches, ranging from a judgment of irreversibility of the process, as in the case of degenerative dementias, to a benign prognosis in focal forms, to the possibility of therapeutic interventions in cases of depressive pseudo-dementias or subcortical degenerative pathologies. The methodological approach consists of a basic screening to differentiate the "organic" nature from the "non-organic" nature of a cognitive disorder or pathologies that involve different levels of cognitive organization (e.g., cortical degenerations vs. subcortical degenerations).

The final purpose of the assessment is to determine the severity of the disorder and, concurrently, the remaining capabilities upon which rehabilitative interventions can be based. Hence the need to determine not only the extent of the disorder itself, which is useful primarily for care-related decisions (e.g., disability recognition) or research, but also the intact cognitive functions. In other words, the presence or absence of compensatory strategies and motivation to undertake rehabilitative pathways. Describing a cognitive profile with generic definitions is of no practical utility to the patient or their family members, who won't know which capabilities to leverage in managing everyday practical problems.

The levels of investigation that make up the examination are essentially three:

1) Descriptive diagnosis, which illustrates the complex of symptoms and cognitive signs;
2) Functional diagnosis, which identifies the impaired cognitive processes;
3) Localization diagnosis, which defines the brain area associated with the symptoms.

The numerical data provided by the test constitutes the quantitative dimension of the neuropsychological examination, but a quantitative deficit does not necessarily imply the existence of an organic pathology: tests that obtain similar scores can provide completely different indications regarding the patient's actual difficulties, and direct towards one diagnostic hypothesis rather than another. Therefore, it is necessary to obtain additional elements of judgment.

The qualitative dimension - the observation of how the patient thinks and acts in front of the tests - is essential for a correct evaluation and allows for the interpretation of test results from a broader perspective: many conditions can contaminate cognitive performance or overestimate a symptom that may instead be attributable to anxiety, depression, or lack of confidence with intellectual tools. Therefore, the examination also encompasses the patient's reactions to the test demands, which activate emotional and motivational functions. For example, when a personality disorder is present within the symptomatology, this type of observation becomes essential in the overall evaluation of the patient. In the diagnosis of certain forms of dementia, behavioral disturbances largely prevail even in the early stages of the disease and represent an important element for differential diagnosis. In depressive states, reduced performance may be erroneously attributed to primary cognitive decline.

The interpretation of the data is therefore based on both primary cognitive symptoms - which most reveal the nature and degree of deficits - and secondary symptoms in the form of adaptive strategies.

4.8.2 Procedural Aspects

An accurate neuropsychological examination requires, first and foremost, the examiner's familiarity with neuroanatomy and neurophysiology, knowledge of clinical and cognitive psychology, and an understanding of brain functions and their respective neuroanatomical correlates.

The score assigned in a test also assumes diagnostic relevance only when evaluated in light of the patient's background, allowing for the delineation of a pre-illness level of performance, which can vary from relatively high to relatively low. The most appropriate context for interpreting test data can only be obtained by considering the patient's clinical and occupational history, lifestyle, social status, and the circumstances underlying the request for examination—all elements that should be gathered during an interview with the patient or their family members. The so-called "blind analysis," where the examiner evaluates test results without reviewing clinical documentation, is a harmful practice for making clinical decisions. On the contrary, active listening to the patient and the way they describe their condition is essential, as it offers important insights into the true nature of the deficit.

Once the preliminary clinical interview is conducted, the examiner assesses all hypotheses and selects the most appropriate techniques for a proper evaluation. They determine the functions to investigate and the level of complexity of the tools, adapting them to the patient's sociocultural factors and any physical limitations.

During the examination, observing the patient's behavior will be a key element in interpreting test performance, including work style, language content and context, self-care, excessive familiarity, and emotional lability. All these so-called "informal" elements provide valuable information about how the patient approaches new and relatively stressful situations. When combined, qualitative and quantitative data ultimately create the reference context for understanding the patient's behavior and the functioning of their cognitive processes.

Finally, it should be emphasized that neuropsychological assessment must be carried out by specialized personnel with adequate clinical training. In clinical practice, both specialist and non-specialist physicians can rely on rapid cognitive and functional screening tests for initial identification of any critical issues, such as the Mini-Mental State Examination (MMSE), Activities of Daily Living (ADL), and Instrumental Activities of Daily Living (IADL). For calculating ADL and IADL scores, a simplified scale is used, which assigns one point for each independent function, resulting in a score ranging from 0 (complete dependence) to 6 (ADL) and 8 (IADL) (independence in all functions) (see sheets on the following page).

Bibliography

Blundo C., Neuroscienze Cliniche del Comportamento. Elsevier, 2011.

Boller F., Grafman J., Handbook of Neuropsychology. Elsevier, Amsterdam, 2000.

Kandel E.R., Schwartz J.H., Jessell T.M., Principi di Neuroscienze, Casa Editrice Ambrosiana, 2003.

Lezak, M. Neuropsychological Assessment. Oxford University Press, 2012.

Luria A.R., Come lavora il cervello. Il Mulino, Bologna, 1977.

Mesulam M.M., Principles of Behavioral Neurology. Oxford University Press, 2000.

Tulving E., Craik F., The Oxford Handbook of Memory. Oxford University Press, 2000.

Mini-Mental State Examination (MMSE)
(Folstein, 1975)

Patient: ____________________ date: ____________________

1. Temporo-spatial orientation

The patient must report the day of the month, the year, the month, the day of the week, and the season 0 1 2 3 4 5

The patient must report the location where they are, the floor, the city, region, and state 0 1 2 3 4 5

2. Memory

The doctor pronounces out loud the names of three objects (house, bread, cat).
The patient must repeat them until they have learned them (maximum 6 repetitions).... 0 1 2 3
Attempt n°.........

3.Attention and calculation

Subtract 7 units, starting from 100, five times 0 1 2 3 4 5
If the patient has difficulty with calculation, have them spell the word 'mondo' backwards, letter by letter.

4. Recall of the three objects

Report the three objects previously learned 0 1 2 3

5. Language

The patient must recognize an object:
What is this called? (pointing to a pencil);
What is this called? (pointing to a clock). 0 1 2

"The patient must repeat "no if, or, but"........ 0 1

The patient must perform a task on command:
a)Take a sheet of paper with your right hand;
b) fold the sheet of paper in half;
c) place the paper on the table........ 0 1 2 3

The patient is presented with a sheet of paper with the following inscription:
"Close your eyes". The patient must obey the order........ 0 1

Have the patient write a sentence consisting of at least a subject and a verb........ 0 1

Have the patient copy the indicated drawing 0 1

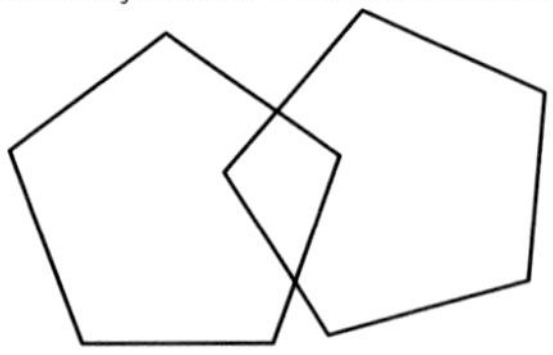

Overall score .... /30

0-10: severe deficit
11-20: moderate deficit
21-23: mild deficit
24-30: normal

	Age range				
Years of scooling	65-69	70-74	75-79	80-84	85-89
0-4 years	+0,4	+0,7	+1,0	+1,5	+2,2
5-7 years	-1,1	-0,7	-0,3	+0,4	+1,4
8-12 years	-2,0	-1,6	-1,0	-0,3	+0,8
13-17 years	-2,8	-2,3	-1,7	-0,9	+0,3

The coefficient is added (or subtracted) to the raw score of the MMSE to obtain the adjusted score.

FUNCTIONAL EVALUATION

Activities of Daily Living Autonomy Scale

A) BATHING (bathtub, shower, sponge bath)

1 Bathes independently (enters and exits the bathtub alone)
1 Requires assistance only with cleaning a specific body part (e.g., back)
0 Requires assistance with multiple body parts

B) DRESSING (getting clothes from the wardrobe and/or drawers, including underwear, clothes, use of fasteners and suspenders if used)

1 Takes clothes and dresses completely without assistance
1 Takes clothes and dresses without assistance except for tying shoelaces
0 Requires assistance in getting clothes or dressing or remains partially or completely undressed.

C) TOILETING

1 Uses the bathroom, cleans themselves, and dresses without assistance (may use supportive aids such as a cane, walker, or wheelchair; may use a bedpan at night and empty it in the morning)
0 Requires assistance in using the bathroom, cleaning themselves, dressing, and using a bedpan
0 Does not use the bathroom for elimination

D) TRANSFERRING

1 Transfers in and out of bed and chair without assistance (may use canes or a walker if needed)
0 Requires assistance for these transfers
0 Bedridden, does not leave the bed

E) CONTINENCE CONTROL

1 Completely controls bowel and bladder functions
0 Occasional "accidents"
0 Requires supervision for bowel and bladder control, uses a catheter, or is incontinent

F) FEEDING

1 Independent in feeding without assistance
1 Assistance only needed for cutting meat or spreading butter on bread
0 Requires assistance in bringing food to the mouth or is partially or completely fed through parenteral means

TOTAL SCORE

FUNCTIONAL EVALUATION

IADL - Instrumental Activities of Daily Living Autonomy Scale

A) ABILITY TO USE THE TELEPHONE
- 1 Uses the telephone independently: looks up phone numbers and dials
- 1 Dials only a few well-known numbers
- 1 Answers the phone but cannot dial a number
- 0 Unable to use the telephone

B) SHOPPING
- 1 Takes care of shopping independently
- 0 Able to make only small purchases
- 0 Needs to be accompanied for any type of purchase
- 0 Completely unable to do shopping

C) MEAL PREPARATION
- 1 Plans meals, prepares them properly, and serves them independently
- 0 Prepares adequate meals only if provided with all the ingredients
- 0 Can only heat up pre-prepared meals or prepares meals inconsistently, resulting in inadequate nutrition
- 0 Needs pre-prepared meals and to be served

D) HOUSEHOLD CARE
- 1 Manages household chores independently or with occasional assistance for heavy work
- 1 Performs light household chores such as washing dishes, making the bed, etc.
- 1 Performs light household chores but cannot maintain an adequate level of cleanliness
- 0 Needs help with all household cleaning
- 0 Completely disinterested in any household matters

E) LAUNDRY
- 1 Washes all their own laundry
- 1 Washes all their own laundry
- 0 All laundry needs to be done by others

F) OUTDOOR MOBILITY
- 1 Travels independently, using public transportation or their own car
- 1 Uses taxis but cannot use public transportation
- 1 Uses public transportation only when assisted or accompanied
- 0 Travels by car or taxi when assisted or accompanied by others
- 0 Unable to travel

G) MEDICATION MANAGEMENT
- 1 Is capable of taking medication correctly
- 0 Is capable of taking medication only if prepared and separated in advance
- 0 Is unable to take medication on their own

H) MONEY MANAGEMENT
- 1 Manages personal finances independently (accounts, checks, rent, and other expenses, banking); monitors income
- 1 Handles daily expenses and bills but needs assistance for major operations (going to the bank, writing checks or large expenses, etc.)
- 0 Is unable to handle money independently

TOTAL SCORE

5 NEURORADIOLOGY DIAGNOSTICS AND THERAPEUTICS

Patrizia Pantano, Costanza Gianni, Claudio Colonnese, Marco Fiorelli

5.1 Computed Tomography

Computed Tomography (CT) is a radiological technique that uses ionizing radiation to evaluate the density (ability to retain radiation) of the analyzed tissues.

The equipment consists of a radiographic tube that emits ionizing radiation and a system of detectors, placed diametrically opposite to the tube, which detects the radiation not absorbed by the patient. The tube-detector system rotates around the patient, and each individual layer is traversed by radiation at a different angle of incidence. Therefore, the layer is divided, like a grid, into many small parts called pixels, where the absorption of radiation can be evaluated. Density is measured in Hounsfield units (HU), named after G. Hounsfield, the creator of CT. Tissues denser than water (which is arbitrarily assigned a value of 0) will have a positive value, while less dense tissues will have a negative value. The density values of each pixel can be represented either as numerical values or as grayscale images, creating an image of the examined section of the human body. CT is usually performed with axial scans of varying thickness, depending on the organs being examined and the diagnostic question related to the patient. Images on planes other than the axial plane are obtained through subsequent reconstructions starting from the axial images. Technological advancements have increased the rotation speed of the tube-detector system, allowing for scans of 320/640 slices per second.

With CT, sequential images can be obtained by examining one complete layer at a time, in succession. Alternatively, with the spiral volumetric technique, images can be acquired during the continuous movement of the table on which the patient lies. The spiral volumetric technique provides information about volumes of matter that can be subsequently reconstructed on the three planes of space.

Regarding the nervous system, CT examines the morphology and density alterations (Figure 5.1). The ventricular system may be compressed and/or deformed due to the presence of various types of cerebral space-occupying processes, or it may appear larger in the presence of cerebral atrophy or secondary to obstruction of cerebrospinal fluid outflow. The subarachnoid spaces may be dilated in atrophic processes or compressed by space-occupying lesions. The density of cerebral tissues may be reduced (hypodensity)

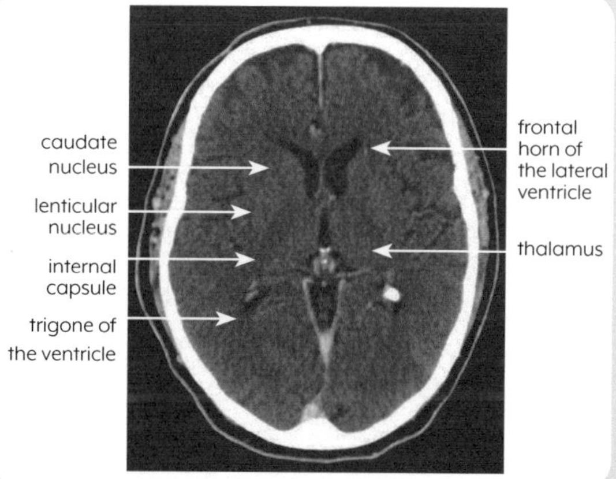

Figure 5.1

Cerebral CT from a healthy subject.

or increased (hyperdensity) depending on the nature of any cerebral pathological processes.

Iodine-based contrast agents, administered intravenously, increase the density of cerebral tissue only in the presence of an alteration of the blood-brain barrier. Blood-brain barrier disruption can occur as a result of acute ischemic injury, inflammatory processes, or neoangiogenesis, as seen in neoplasms or post-ischemic and post-inflammatory reparative processes.

CT is used for the study of spinal cord and vertebral pathology when there is an indication for a detailed examination of bony structures or in cases of degenerative lumbar disc arthropathy. For such indications, reconstructions on the three planes of space are useful.

5.1.1 Angio-TC

Angio-CT involves acquiring radiological images during the controlled administration of contrast medium. The contrast medium, within the vascular compartment, is denser than blood, resulting in the arterial and venous vessels appearing denser than the surrounding tissues. The acquired volume can be reconstructed in three dimensions on different planes of space using a technique capable of detecting areas with an identical increase in density.

Angio-CT allows for the assessment of the caliber of intra- and extracranial vessels and the quantification of any channeling defects, providing information about stenotic or occlusive pathologies or potential alterations of the arterial vessel wall (Figure 5.2). Angio-CT enables accurate diagnosis of intracranial vascular aneurysms and arteriovenous malformations (AVMs). Lastly, with current dual-energy equipment, it is also possible to subtract bone density and study vascular regions that are not easily visible due to being intraosseous (for example, the intrapetrous segment of the internal carotid artery).

5.1.2 Cerebral Perfusion

Cerebral perfusion with CT allows the assessment of cerebral blood volume (CBV), expressed in ml per 100 grams of tissue, cerebral blood flow (CBF), expressed in ml per 100 grams of tissue per minute, and mean transit time (MTT). The technique involves the intravenous injection of iodinated contrast medium at a quantity of 60-80 ml at a constant rate of 4-5 ml/sec. The density variation of each individual pixel associated with the passage of the contrast medium is calculated, and transit

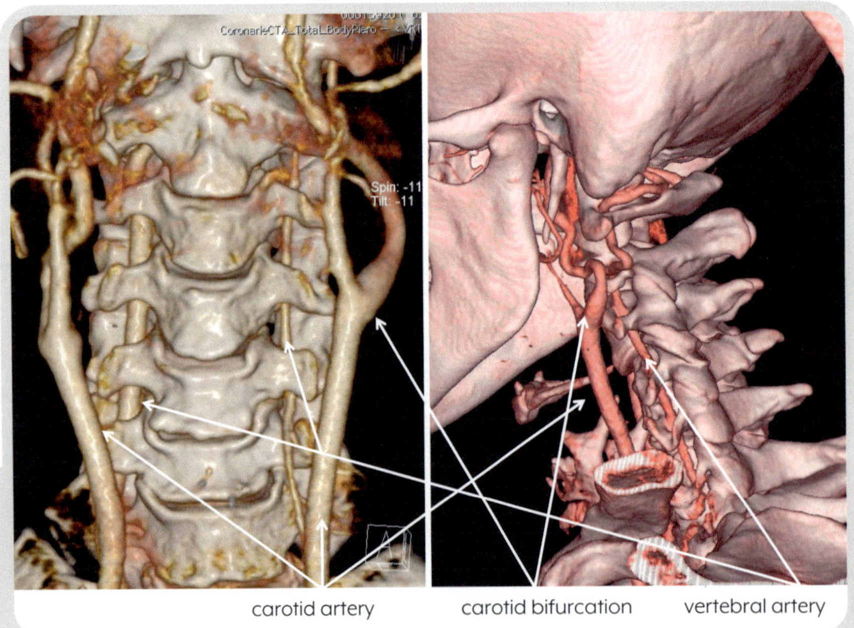

Figure 5.2.

Epiaortic vessels Angio-CT from a healthy subject (volumetric reconstruction).

curves of density variations of individual pixels in different sections are generated. Hemodynamic parameters can be derived from these obtained curves.

5.2 Magnetic Resonance Imaging

For an understanding of the physical phenomena underlying Magnetic Resonance Imaging (MRI), please refer to more specific texts. MRI allows obtaining images of body regions in three spatial planes. The necessary technical information is as follows: all atoms with an odd atomic number behave as an electric dipole due to the elliptical shape of the electron rotation movement around the nucleus. The electric dipole acts as a small magnet sensitive to high magnetic fields. MRI examines the modifications induced by the magnetic field (of the MRI itself) on the hydrogen atom of the subject under examination. Research-focused MRI equipment can study modifications induced in other atoms as well. When all hydrogen atoms in the patient's body are immersed in the stable magnetic field of the MRI equipment, the hydrogen atoms align themselves parallel to the magnetic field, mostly in the same direction and with the same polarity. Consequently, the patient's body undergoes longitudinal magnetization with the same direction and polarity as the equipment's magnetic field (behaving like a magnet). At this point, to obtain images, the patient's magnetization is interfered with by stimulating the patient with electromagnetic waves that depend on both the stable magnetic field of the equipment and a constant specific to each atom (in this case, the hydrogen atom). In this way, the state of equilibrium reached in the stable magnetic field is disturbed (the resonance of an atom is the result of this stimulation mode). The modifications obtained with the magnetic coils (which are necessary to induce interference) on the patient's magnetization involve the loss of longitudinal magnetization and the acquisition of transverse magnetization. When the coils of the MRI equipment stop transmitting energy, the system returns to the equilibrium state; the patient's body loses transverse magnetization and regains longitudinal magnetization. These phenomena occur within two characteristic time constants for each tissue. This time, called "relaxation time," is T2 (for the loss of transverse magnetization) and T1 (for the recovery of longitudinal magnetization). By modifying the magnetic stimulation parameters, it is possible to obtain images that are weighted or dependent on either T1 or T2 time. By adjusting the equipment parameters, it is also possible to obtain different sequences. Among the most common are the so-called FLAIR T2 (Fluid Attenuated Inversion Recovery) sequences, capable of suppressing the signal from the cerebrospinal fluid (Figure 5.3), or other image sequences that subtract the signal from fat, which is known to be a major component of myelin. Finally, it is also possible to obtain Gradient Echo images, which are highly sensitive to the presence of haemoglobin degradation products and calcium, known as T2* images.

For the study of the cerebral cortex, a strongly T1-weighted gradient inversion (IR) sequence can be used. For the evaluation of nerve roots, a myelographic sequence can be used, which allows for optimal visualization of the perimedullary and periradicular liquor spaces. In T1-weighted images, the cerebrospinal fluid appears hypointense compared to the parenchyma, and gray matter appears hypointense compared to white matter. In T2-weighted images, cerebrospinal fluid appears hyperintense compared to the parenchyma, and white matter appears hypointense compared to gray matter. In general, most central nervous system lesions have a reduced T1 and increased T2 compared to healthy tissue, but depending on the pathological alterations, the modifications of T1 and T2 can also be reversed. In general, T2-weighted images provide better contrast between pathological tissue and normal tissue, while T1-weighted images provide better anatomical detail. It is worth noting that in conventional images, vascular structures are highlighted due to the so-called "flow void."

In MRI studies, the contrast agent administered intravenously is gadolinium, which has the characteristic of significantly reducing the T1 relaxation time. Gadolinium remains localized in the blood vessels if the

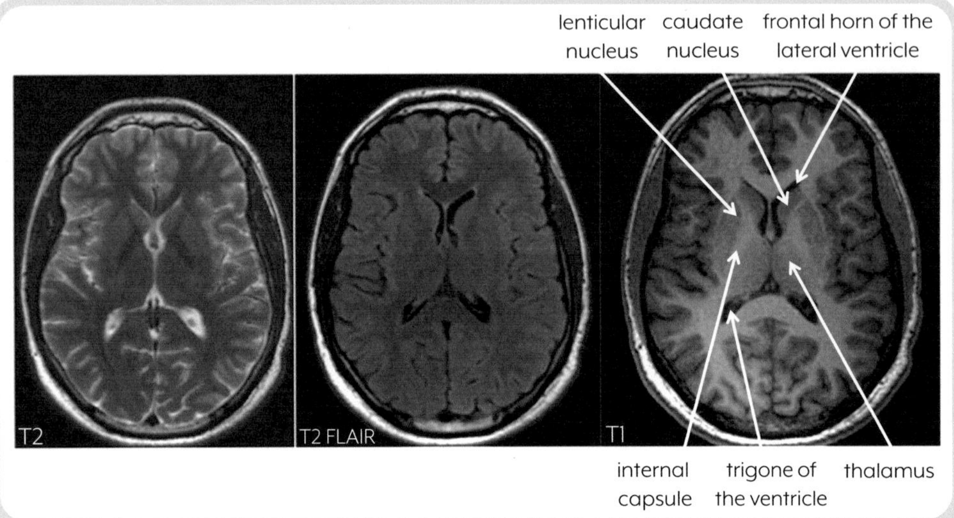

Figure 5.3

Brain MRI from a healthy subject (same sections as Figure 5.1).

blood-brain barrier is intact; otherwise, it accumulates in the tissue. Side effects (allergic reactions) related to the use of contrast agents are very rare; however, recently, the possibility of systemic fibrosis has been reported in patients with severe renal insufficiency. There has been growing concern about the accumulation of gadolinium in the basal ganglia and dentate nuclei.

5.2.1 Angio-RM

The most commonly used techniques are time-of-flight (TOF), phase contrast (PC), and contrast-enhanced (CE) techniques.

The TOF technique is routinely used for the study of the intracranial arterial circulation (Figure 5.4). For the study of intracranial venous vessels, phase-contrast Angio-MRI (PC) is preferred. Unlike TOF, this technique allows activation of the gradient based on the flow velocity being investigated. Angiographic images can then be acquired during the administration of a bolus of contrast agent (contrast-enhanced technique). This technique is used for the study of epiaortic vessel structures (Figure 5.5). Finally, it is possible to perform sequential angiographic studies of cerebral vessels, separately documenting the arterial and venous phases, using ultra-fast sequences acquired during contrast administration (CEMRA or 4D). This technique is particularly useful for the study of arteriovenous malformations (AVMs).

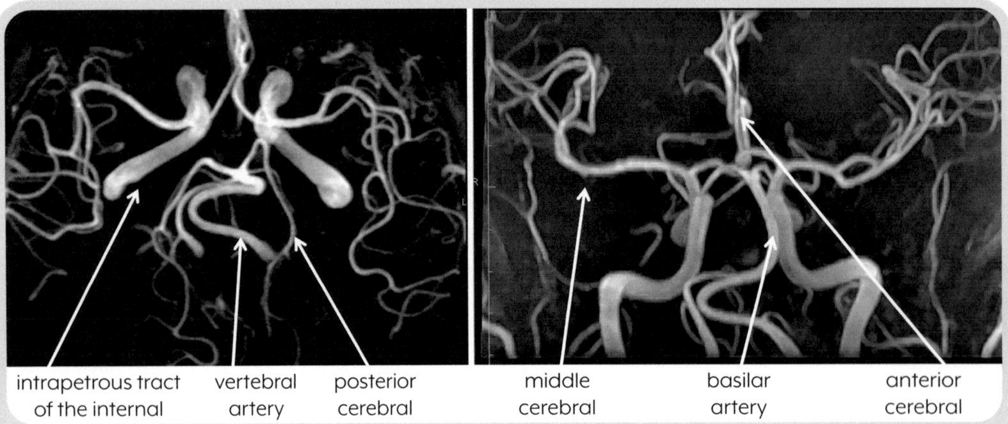

Figure 5.4

Intracranial angio-MRI from a healthy subject

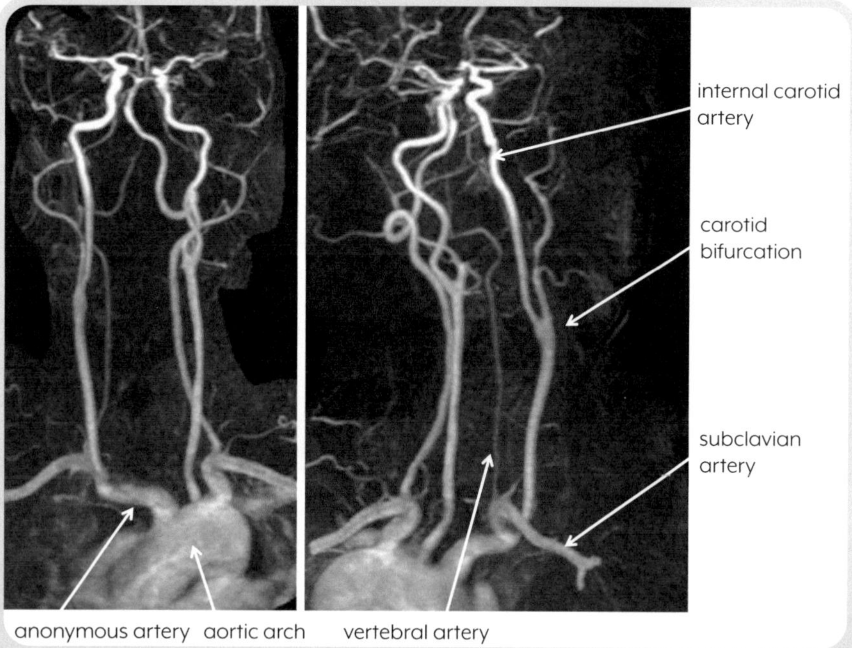

Figure 5.5

Epiaortic vessels Angio-MRI from a healthy subject.

5.2.2 Diffusion MRI

Diffusion MRI is a technique in which the signal depends on the diffusion coefficient, which is related to the Brownian motion of water molecules (diffusion), measured in mm^2/s. In diffusion images, tissues with high water molecule movement appear hypointense, while those with slowed movement appear hyperintense. Diffusion images are also influenced by the T2 relaxation time of brain tissue. To obtain images solely conditioned by diffusion, one can calculate maps of the apparent diffusion coefficient (ADC) (Figure 5.6). In these maps, areas with slowed movement exhibit low values. The movement of free water in the interstitial space occurs in all directions (isotropic movement). Depending on the tissue organization, the movement of water molecules is more restricted, such as in white matter where the movement of water molecules is constrained by the direction of fiber bundles and occurs parallel to the fibers themselves (anisotropic movement). Therefore, techniques that exploit the anisotropy of diffusion, such as diffusion tensor imaging (DTI), provide information about the orientation of nerve fiber bundles.

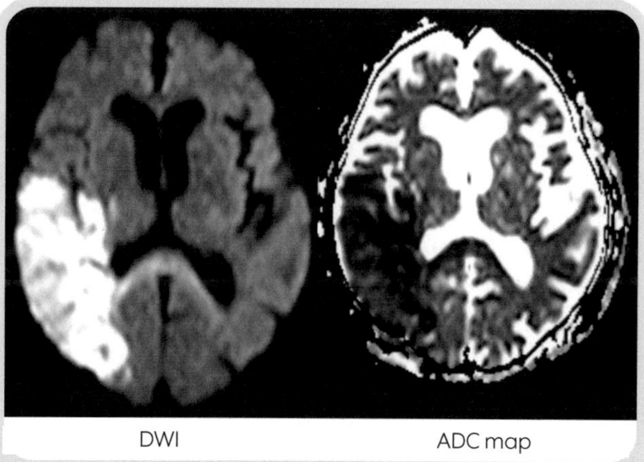

Figure 5.6

Brain MRI, DWI sequence and ADC map. Cerebral ischemia in the territory of the right middle cerebral artery.

Tractography represents a reprocessing of such information. Basic parameters studied with this technique allow the measurement of mean diffusivity (MD) and fractional anisotropy (FA). MD indicates tissue integrity and organization, measured in absolute terms (mm^2/s), while FA represents the alignment of cellular structures within white matter and is measured on a scale from 0 to 1.

5.2.3 Perfusion MRI

Perfusion MRI involves acquiring ultra-fast sequences with T2*-weighted sequences during the injection of contrast agent. Perfusion sequences can study sections of the entire brain with a thickness of a few millimeters every 1.5-2 seconds. From these images, the variations in signal intensity, proportional to the changes in tissue concentration of the contrast agent, can be calculated pixel by pixel, resulting in intensity/time curves. From these curves, several hemodynamic parameters can be calculated, such as cerebral blood volume (CBV), mean transit time (MTT), and cerebral blood flow (CBF), similar to perfusion studies with CT. The data obtained are particularly relevant in the study of acute ischemia and brain tumors. There are perfusion techniques that do not require exogenous contrast agents, such as the technique called Arterial Spin Labeling (ASL), which allows for regional quantitative assessment of CBF.

5.2.4 RM in Spectroscopy

Magnetic Resonance in Spectroscopy (MRS) is a technique that allows the detection of certain chemical components in tissues, based on the analysis of resonance frequencies of different components. MRS is commonly presented in the form of two-dimensional graphs, where the x-axis represents the frequency position that characterizes the nature of the component, and the y-axis represents the intensity of the associated signal, which is closely related to its quantity. The investigation is performed using two types of spectroscopic techniques: single-voxel spectroscopy and multivoxel spectroscopy. The former allows the acquisition of signals from a region of interest; it is more spatially limited but more precise. The latter is capable of providing information about larger brain areas and can be displayed as a color map or presented in the form of multiple graphs; it is generally less precise but provides information about both the region of interest and the surrounding tissue.

The studied metabolites are: myoinositol (mI), choline (Cho), creatine (Cr), N-acetyl-aspartate (NAA), lactate (Lac), and lipids.

Myo-inositol (mI) is a glial marker, and its peak increases in conditions of gliosis, as can occur in the temporal lobe or cingulate gyrus in patients with Alzheimer's disease, or in low-grade glial tumors. Choline (Cho) is a marker of membrane turnover and increases where there is destruction of cellular membranes and active proliferation, such as in tumors (Figure 5.7). The increase is proportional to the degree of malignancy. Creatine (Cr) is an energy marker as it is involved in ATP metabolism and used as a reference index (the heights of other peaks are compared to the height of the creatine peak). N-acetylaspartate (NAA) is a neuronal marker, and its peak decreases in all conditions where there is neuronal loss or replacement by pathological tissue (tumors, inflammation, ischemia, etc.). Lactate (Lac), an expression of anaerobic glycolysis, is absent in normal tissue and appears in conditions of ischemia, necrosis, or a mismatch between vascularization and cellular activity (seizure crisis or rapidly growing tumor). Lipids, absent in healthy tissue and an expression of the destruction of cellular membranes, are present in some tumors with necrosis.

5.2.5 Functional Magnetic Resonance Imaging (fMRI)

fMRI allows the assessment of the functional activity of certain brain areas based on local modifications of the oxygen/deoxyhemoglobin ratio. fMRI is associated with the development of so-called "ultrafast" sequences, such as single-shot echo-planar imaging. The technique known as Blood Oxygenation Level Dependent (BOLD) is the most commonly

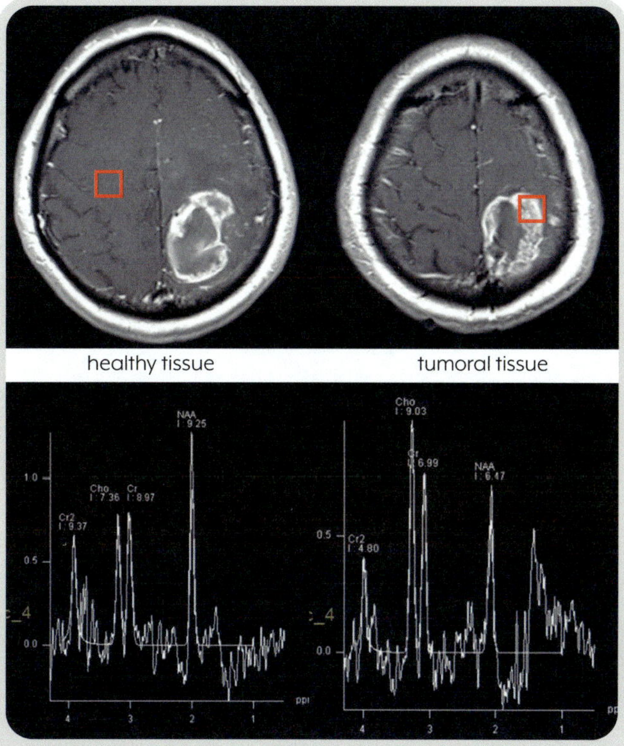

Figure 5.7

MR spectroscopy: glial tumor.

used. In the brain, the activation of brain structures leads to an increase in local blood flow that exceeds the increase in oxygen consumption. This results in a reduction in the concentration of deoxyhemoglobin in capillaries and veins, which, in turn, causes a modification of the magnetic properties (oxyhemoglobin is diamagnetic, while deoxyhemoglobin is paramagnetic), so that deoxyhemoglobin acts as an endogenous contrast agent. The BOLD technique is based on variations in the content of oxyhemoglobin and deoxyhemoglobin in the microcirculation, with corresponding changes in signal intensity. During the execution of a task (motor, visual, verbal, etc.), it is possible to visualize the brain areas connected to that specific function and evaluate their involvement in the case of tumors or vascular malformations. In pre-surgical or pre-endovascular intervention studies, such acquisitions are now considered indispensable (Figure 5.8).

The BOLD technique can also be applied under resting conditions, where the subject does not perform any specific task. Analysis techniques developed for this purpose are capable of assessing the functional connections between different brain areas. Two analysis methods are possible: the first involves defining a specific brain area and calculating the areas that exhibit synchronous signals with the selected area. Alternatively, independent component analysis (ICA) can be applied, which allows for the identification of the so-called resting-state networks (RSNs). An RSN is a set of brain areas, even topographically distant, that exhibit synchronous signals and are therefore considered to belong to the same network, such as the Default Mode Network (DMN).

5.3 Cerebral Angiography

Cerebral angiography is an invasive diagnostic technique that involves the intra-arterial administration of a water-soluble iodinated contrast agent and the subsequent acquisition of radiographs. This technique allows visualization of both the arterial and venous phases of cerebral circulation, as well as the capillary phase. The procedure is typically performed using transfemoral catheterization. After local anesthesia at the

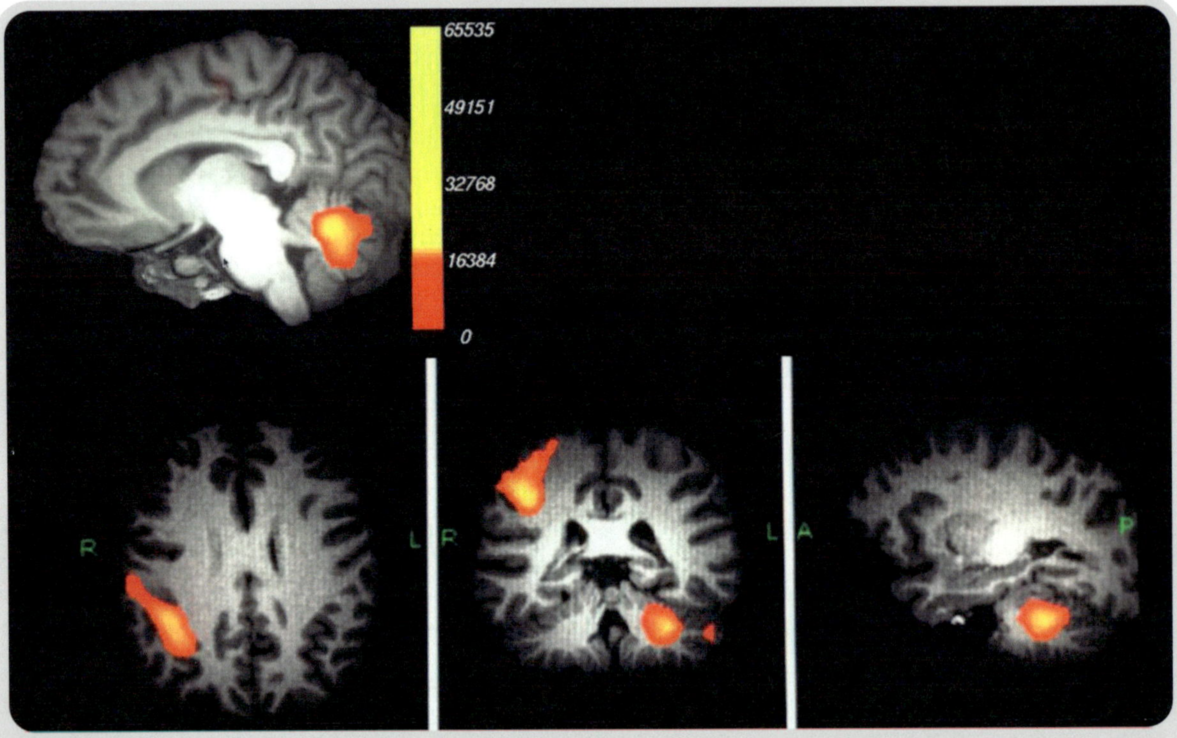

Figure 5.8

Functional MRI. It is evident the activation of the motor cortex and the contralateral cerebellar emisphere.

groin level, the femoral artery is cannulated with a needle and introducer sheath, and a flexible radiopaque guide wire is inserted through the needle. Once the guide wire is in place and the needle is removed, an introducer sheath is placed over the guide wire to separate the tissues from the guide wire. The size of the introducer sheath may vary depending on whether the examination is purely diagnostic or has interventional purposes as well. After the catheter is positioned, selective catheterization of individual arterial branches is performed, allowing the injection of contrast medium to visualize specific vessels. With specially designed microcatheters, it is now possible to achieve highly selective catheterization, even reaching the terminal branches of different cerebral arteries. Catheter angiography is the only technique capable of providing comprehensive information on the quantity, velocity, and direction of blood flow. Among the interventional applications, we can mention intra-arterial fibrinolysis and mechanical thrombectomy.

Using equipment with a dual radiographic tube (biplane angiography system), images can be obtained in two orthogonal planes with a single contrast medium injection. This allows diagnostic imaging with low contrast doses and the use of small-caliber catheters. Three-dimensional angiography, which involves rotating the radiographic tube around the patient during the contrast medium injection, allows the operator to obtain three-dimensional reconstructions of the cerebral vessels, enabling comprehensive visualization. This equipment is ideal for endovascular therapy of vascular malformations and aneurysms.

There are no absolute contraindications to angiographic examination. Complications can be local, such as hematomas, femoral artery lacerations, vessel dissection with subintimal contrast injection, formation of pseudoaneurysms, and arteriovenous fistulas. Approximately 0.51% of patients may experience focal neurological complications, which are more common in patients with arteriosclerotic disease. The main causes of central neurological complications are embolus detachment or clot formation at the catheter tip. Systemic reactions are related to potential allergic reactions to the contrast medium.

5.4 Spinal Angiography

Spinal angiography is performed by administering iodinated contrast medium directly into the radiculomedullary arteries via femoral catheterization and utilizing the digital subtraction technique for various angiographic phases. The spinal cord is supplied by three arteries: the anterior spinal artery and the two posterior spinal arteries. These arteries arise from the vertebral arteries. The radiculomedullary arteries, numbering 6-8, divide into anterior and posterior branches, which along with comb-like branches vascularize the spinal cord. The great radicular artery, originating from a radiculomedullary artery, mostly between D6 and D10, has only an anterior branch. The spinal arteries terminate at the level of the conus by anastomosing with each other.

With spinal angiography, it is necessary to perform a comprehensive study that also investigates the vertebral arteries, the thyrocervical trunk, and all intercostal and lumbar arteries. This study is essential in vascular malformations of the spinal cord, allowing for accurate localization of any fistulas and their afferent and efferent vessels. This methodology is indispensable for the planning and execution of endovascular treatment.

5.5 Interventional Neuroradiology

Interventional radiology is used for the treatment of intracranial, extracranial, and spinal pathologies. In cranial cases, endovascular treatments are performed using microcatheters, usually with an arterial approach, and less commonly with a venous approach. Depending on the patient's specific pathology, the technique allows for the delivery of coils, glues, particles to occlude abnormal cerebral vessels or those with malformations, tubular metallic endoprostheses (stents), and fibrinolytic drugs. Mechanical procedures can also be performed to remove any vascular obstructions. General anaesthesia is generally preferred to ensure the patient's complete immobility.

The main pathologies that can be treated via endovascular approaches are:

- Cerebral and spinal vascular malformations
- Cerebral aneurysms
- Stenosis of cerebral vessels at the extracranial and intracranial levels
- Arterial occlusions of embolic nature

Furthermore, at the vertebral level, pathological vertebral body fractures can be treated using vertebroplasty and kyphoplasty to alleviate pain.

5.5.1 Carotid Stenting

Carotid stenting involves the placement of a tubular metallic endoprosthesis at the site of a vascular stenosis, resulting in the restoration of vascular lumen and mechanical protection against potential embolus detachment. It is currently widely used due to the low incidence of complications attributed to the improved quality of the products used. Compared to carotid endarterectomy, carotid stenting has the same incidence of focal neurological complications but eliminates the risk of potential cranial nerve injuries in the vascular-nerve tree of the neck.

5.5.2 Endovascular Treatment of Aneurysms

The goal of aneurysm treatment is to exclude them from the cerebral circulation to prevent rupture or rebleeding after rupture. Endovascular treatment involves filling the aneurysm with thin platinum wires, resulting in the exclusion of the aneurysm from the circulation. The choice of endovascular treatment, as an alternative to the more traditional neurosurgical approach, is based on the characteristics of the aneurysm, its location, and the patient's clinical features. Reduced mortality and morbidity have been demonstrated in patients treated with endovascular methods compared to those treated surgically. The endovascular technique achieves complete occlusion in less than 60%

of cases. Furthermore, follow-up examinations have shown an increase in the residual aneurysm volume without an increased risk of bleeding. For these reasons, neurosurgical intervention is considered the treatment of choice in young patients, intact anterior circulation aneurysms, Sylvian aneurysms, and all low-risk patients. Current technology also allows the use of stents suitable for large-sized aneurysms.

5.5.3 Treatment of Arteriovenous Malformations (AVMs)

The treatment of AVMs includes neurosurgical intervention, endovascular embolization, radiosurgery, or increasingly, a combination of these treatments. The choice of treatment is based on the patient's clinical characteristics, age, location, and size of the AVM. Endovascular embolization employs glues (such as isobutyl cyanoacrylate) or more recently, Onyx.

5.5.4 Endovascular Treatment of Ischemic Stroke

Endovascular treatment of ischemic stroke has become an essential technique in the management of patients with acute cerebrovascular ischemic events. This method, which can be applied alone or in combination with systemic thrombolysis, allows the treatment of patients with certain contraindications to systemic thrombolytic therapy and extends the intervention time beyond the onset of the pathology. Different treatment systems exist, such as the use of stents that capture and mechanically remove the thrombus, or thromboaspiration, which allows for aspiration and removal of the thrombus from the vessel.

5.5.5 Treatment of painful vertebral fractures through vertebroplasty

Pathological vertebral fractures are caused by osteoporosis, neoplastic pathology, and angiomas. Vertebroplasty involves injecting radiopaque cement (PMMA - Polymethylmethacrylate) into the fractured vertebral body, allowing for rapid fracture consolidation and significant reduction in pain. The cement is introduced through the vertebral pedicle under fluoroscopic or CT guidance.

5.6 Main clinical indications

5.6.1 Brain tumors

The preferred technique for brain tumors is Magnetic Resonance Imaging (MRI). Even in cases where the diagnosis is made using CT, integration with MRI is essential.

With MRI, brain neoplasms generally appear hypointense in T1 and hyperintense in T2. It is essential to complete the study with intravenous administration of contrast medium to evaluate whether the tumor exhibits neo-angiogenesis or alteration of the blood-brain barrier. MRI is particularly useful in highlighting indirect signs of neoplasms and in the differential diagnosis between extraparenchymal and intraparenchymal lesions. Spectroscopy and perfusion studies are particularly useful for studying the concentration of cerebral metabolites and neoangiogenesis within the tumor context. Specifically, spectroscopy allows for staging of the tumor, potential changes in tumor malignancy, and differentiation between radionecrosis and tumor recurrence. In selected cases, integrating the study with tractography and functional MRI (fMRI) is valuable to assess the relationships between the surgically resectable lesion, eloquent areas, and major white matter tracts.

The most common extraparenchymal neoplasms are meningiomas, which appear isointense or hypointense in T1 and hyperintense in T2, with homogeneous enhancement after contrast medium administration (Figure 5.9). Meningiomas can rarely present necrosis or calcifications, and in some cases, perilesional edema can affect the adjacent brain parenchyma, especially if the tumor reaches large dimensions. Other tumors located extraparenchymally include neurinomas, which primarily affect the

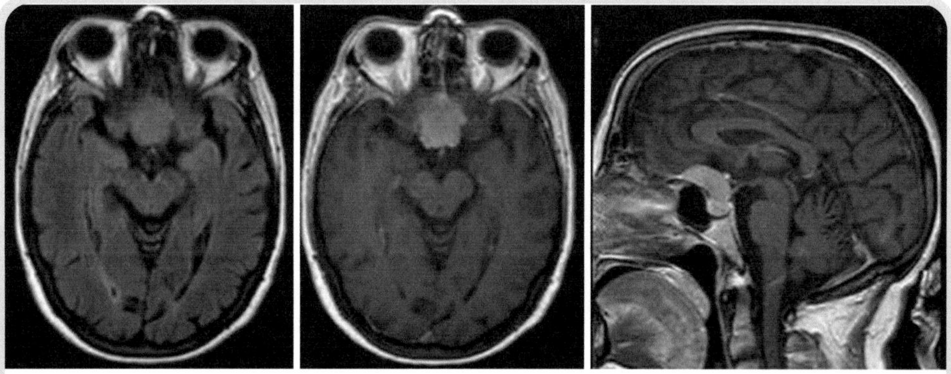

Figure 5.9

Brain MRI. Meningioma of the olfactory groove.

cerebellopontine angle as they predominantly involve the cranial nerve VIII. Other cranial nerves, mainly the V and VII, and spinal nerves can also be affected. Neurinomas have similar characteristics to meningiomas, but the presence of contrast enhancement within the internal auditory canal is typical in the case of cranial nerve VIII neurinomas.

The most common intraparenchymal tumors are glial tumors, classified into 4 grades based on histopathological classification (WHO - World Health Organization). More recently, molecular medicine has revolutionized the classification of brain tumors, making it more correlated with patient prognosis and improving differentiation between histotypes. The most relevant molecular profiles included in the latest WHO classification are IDH mutation, which correlates with increased survival, 1p19q codeletion, which typifies oligodendrogliomas and correlates with better prognosis, and MGMT methylation, which affects chemotherapy response.

Except for Grade I gliomas, which are circumscribed, all others have the characteristic of infiltrating the surrounding parenchyma, making it challenging to distinguish the tumor boundaries from healthy tissue. Gliomas appear hypointense in T1 and hyperintense in T2; depending on the histopathological grade, they may exhibit contrast enhancement. Spectroscopy and perfusion provide information about malignancy grade and neoangiogenesis (in Figures 5.7, 5.10, 5.11, and 5.12).

A particular form of astrocytoma, typical in pediatric age, is pilocytic astrocytoma (Grade I), which presents cystic components, pseudocystic components with walls, and solid components that enhance after contrast medium administration.

Oligodendroglioma (Grade II), a well-differentiated slow-growing tumor, is more frequently localized in the frontal region and often presents internal calcifications; Gradient Echo MRI (FFE or T2*) sequences or alternatively a CT are useful for highlighting the calcifications.

The most aggressive glioma is glioblastoma (Grade IV), which exhibits a heterogeneous appearance, even after contrast medium administration, due to the coexistence of necrotic/hemorrhagic areas and neoangiogenesis.

Medulloblastomas, typical in pediatric age, originate from embryonic cells and are mostly located in the posterior cranial fossa, specifically in the cerebellar vermis. They

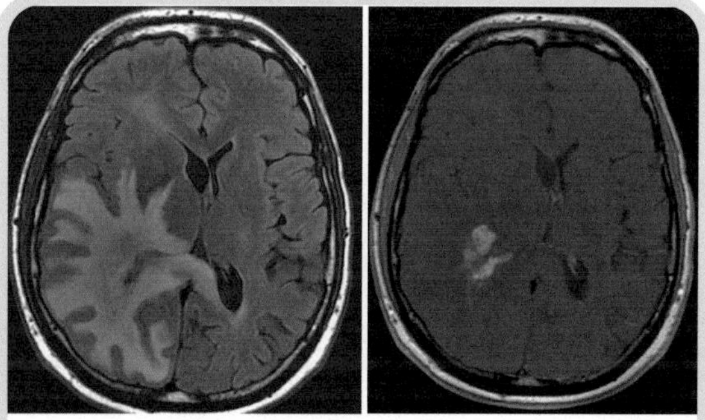

Figure 5.10

Brain MRI. Anaplastic astrocytoma, grade III-IV WHO.

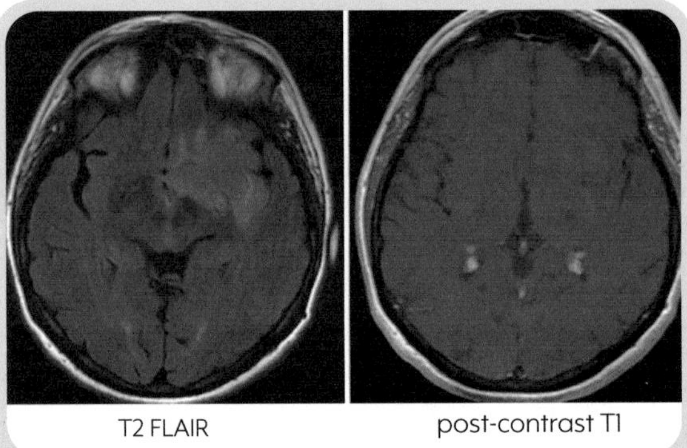

Figure 5.11

Brain MRI. Astrocytoma, grade II WHO.

appear hyperintense in T2, with enhancement after contrast medium administration. They are aggressive neoplasms (Grade IV) with a tendency for cerebrospinal fluid dissemination to the spinal cord.

Given the significant vascularity of the brain, metastatic brain tumors resulting from hematogenous spread of primary tumors outside the central nervous system are among the most frequent neoplasms. They appear as generally multiple lesions, hyperintense in T2, iso- to hypointense in T1, with irregular enhancement, often peripheral, and accompanied by abundant perilesional edema.

The sellar region is affected by craniopharyngiomas, more typical in pediatric and young adult age, which present both cystic and solid components, often with calcifications, and enhance in intensity after contrast medium administration. Craniopharyngiomas can reach large dimensions and are usually located at the suprasellar level, with endosellar extension, and more rarely exclusively intrasellar. There are also forms that are localized within the third ventricle. The most frequent tumors in the pituitary region are adenomas, which are classified as macroadenomas (size > 1 cm) and microadenomas. Macroadenomas are localized within the sella but can cause suprasellar expansion, resulting in structural changes in the surrounding bone. They appear hyperintense in T2 and enhance after contrast medium administration. Microadenomas, measuring up to 10 mm, are visualized as nodular intraglandular areas, mostly hyperintense in T2 and hypointense

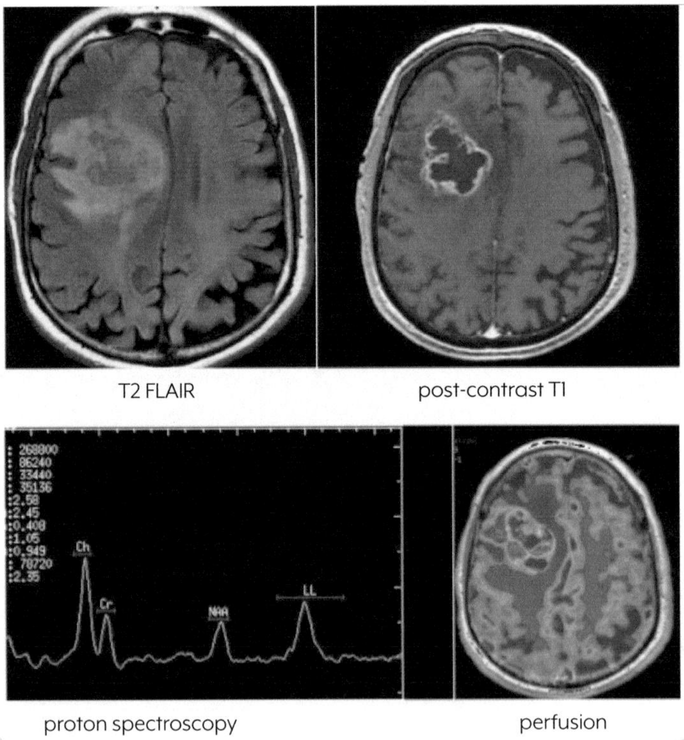

Figure 5.12

Glioblastoma. MRI without and with contrast agent, MR spectroscopy and MR perfusion.

in T1. After contrast administration, they exhibit reduced enhancement compared to healthy glandular tissue and often cause contralateral displacement of the pituitary stalk. Dynamic study during contrast medium administration is useful for identifying the lack of enhancement in early post-contrast sequences for microadenomas.

5.6.2 Cerebrovascular Diseases

Vascular-type brain injuries can be studied using CT scans. In the case of transient ischemic attack, the CT scan may yield negative results. In the case of ischemic injuries within the first few hours of the event, the CT scan can reveal early signs of this condition, characterized by a lack of density differentiation between white matter and gray matter, mild flattening of the sulci, and sometimes increased density in a cerebral vessel where the clot is located (see Figures 5.13 and 5.14a). It is important to assess the topographic extent of the early signs of damage (which is crucial for potential thrombolytic therapy). Quantification methods of early damage, such as the ASPECT study (refer to Chapter 13, Cerebrovascular Diseases), are currently used for this purpose.

A comprehensive CT study of a patient with an acute cerebrovascular event includes a parenchymal study, a triphasic CT angiography, with the arterial phase extending from the aortic arch to the vertex, and the venous and capillary phases throughout the brain. If available, integration with cerebral perfusion studies is essential, especially in the presence of a Stroke Unit.

In acute ischemic lesions, MRI is highly sensitive when weighted diffusion sequences (DWI) are used, and apparent diffusion coefficient (ADC) maps are calculated (see Figures 5.6 and 5.15).

Neuroradiological investigation of a patient with an acute cerebrovascular event also requires the study of the vascular system and cerebral perfusion, which can be easily obtained with both MRI and CT. The main indication for MRI in patients with acute ischemia is uncertain timing, such as when symptoms occur upon awakening. In such cases, images from DWI with corresponding apparent diffusion coefficient (ADC) maps, the mismatch between perfusion-weighted imaging (PWI) and DWI, and between DWI and fluid-attenuated inversion recovery (FLAIR) images strongly indicate the time of onset. A lesion visible in DWI but not yet in FLAIR is certainly recent.

A complication of ischemic pathology is haemorrhagic infarction (Figure 5.14b), characterized by hyperdensity in the hypodense lesion on CT and hyperintensity on T1-weighted and hypointensity on T2-weighted MRI, especially when using the T2 Echo Gradient sequence (T2*, FFE, or GRE). The prognosis for the patient will be worse if the haemorrhagic infarction is extensive.

After the acute phase, the ischemic lesion appears hypodense on CT due to vasogenic edema and more hyperintense on T2-weighted and hypointense on T1-weighted MRI.

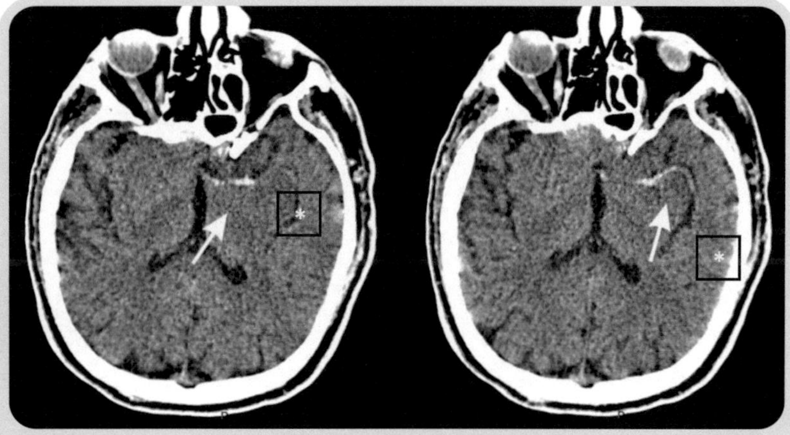

Figure 5.13

Cerebral CT: cerebral ischemia, middle cerebral artery hyperdensity (arrow) and flattening of cerebral sulci in the left temporal lobe (*).

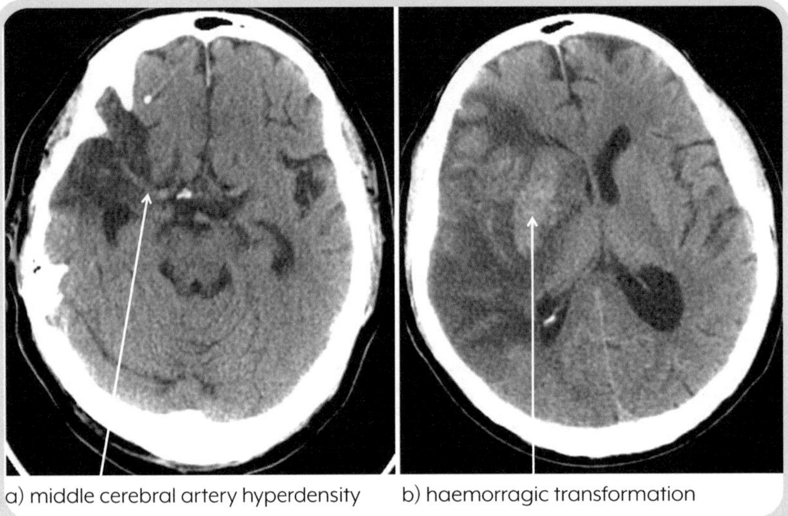

Figure 5.14

Cerebral CT: cerebral ischemia.
a) vessel occlusion, b) same patient after 5 days.

When the ischemic lesion becomes chronic, the images appear clearly hypodense on CT and hyperintense on T2-weighted and hypointense on T1-weighted MRI, but there is a marked reduction in the volume of the ischemic area, which no longer exerts a compressive effect (as in early lesions) on adjacent structures. Instead, there is a sectoral ex-vacuo dilatation of the ventricular system and subarachnoid spaces.

In the case of acute haemorrhagic lesions, the CT scan will immediately show an area significantly hyperdense compared to the brain parenchyma (Figure 5.16). If the examination is performed while the bleeding is still ongoing, a small enhancing intracranial nodule can be detected after contrast administration (spot sign). However, the CT examination should be repeated within 24 hours to assess whether the lesion tends to increase in volume. Radiological investigations with CT allow for the localization of the site of bleeding. Typical bleeding sites, such as the basal ganglia region (in hypertensive and elderly individuals, sometimes with amyloid angiopathy), can be distinguished from atypical sites, such as haemorrhages in different cerebral lobes, brainstem, or cerebellum (the haemorrhage in these cases is likely secondary to neoplastic lesions, vascular malformations, or other causes), which are better visualized with MRI.

With MRI, early changes due to bleeding are less evident compared to CT, although the

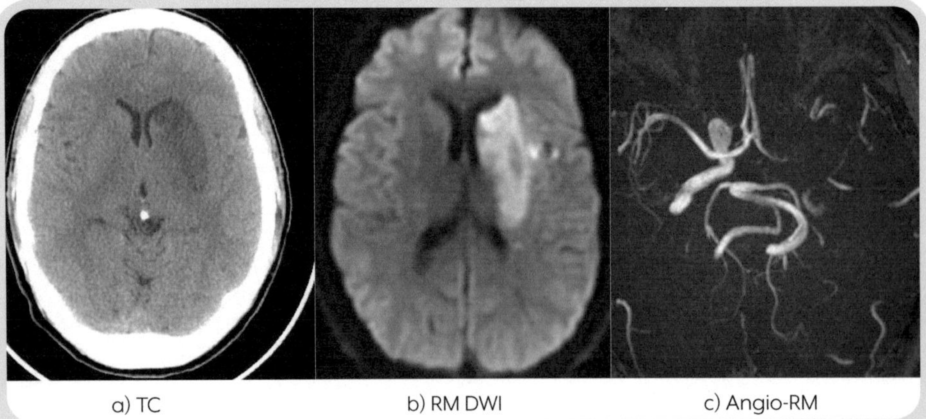

Figure 5.15

a) Cerebral CT, b) Brain diffusion MRI, c) Cerebral Angio-MR. Cerebral ischemia in the territory of left lenticulostriate arteries.

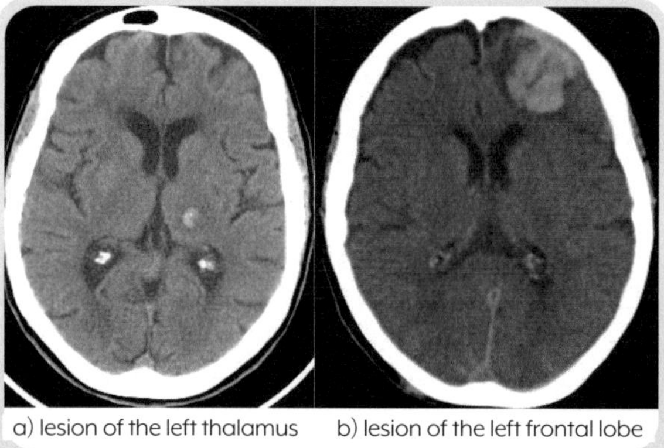

Figure 5.16

Cerebral CT. a) typical site haemorrage; b) atypical site haemorrage.

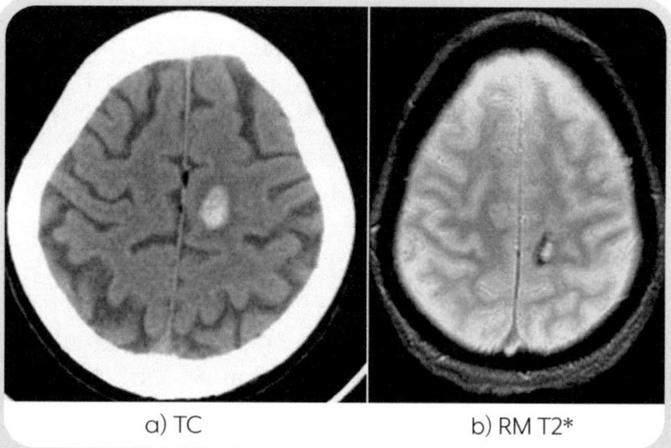

Figure 5.17

Cerebral haemorrage in a) cerebral TC and in b) brain MRI of the same patient.

identification of different signals resulting from the presence of oxyhemoglobin, deoxyhemoglobin, and methemoglobin allows for temporal evaluation of the bleeding. The use of T2 Echo Gradient sequences is still useful in early-phase haemorrhages (Figure 5.17). Atypical haemorrhagic events in cerebral cerebrovascular pathologies resulting from the rupture of vascular malformations can occur in mostly young patients without cerebrovascular risk factors. In these cases, it is essential to complete the study with CT angiography, contrast-enhanced MRI, and MR angiography.

Regarding cerebral vascular malformations, notable conditions include cavernomas, sometimes hereditary, with a tendency to cause haemorrhagic phenomena, particularly in the infratentorial regions (Figure 5.18), arteriovenous malformations, fistulas, and dural arteriovenous fistulas. Another important malformation type is cerebral aneurysms, which are often responsible for subarachnoid haemorrhage. For arteriovenous malformations, aneurysms, and dural arteriovenous fistulas, angiography is necessary to complete the study.

5.6.3 Cranial Trauma

Being an acute and urgent condition, the preferred technique is Computed Tomography (CT). This method is also useful for detecting any bone fragments and even small haemorrhagic collections.

Injuries resulting from cranial trauma can be extraparenchymal or intraparenchymal.

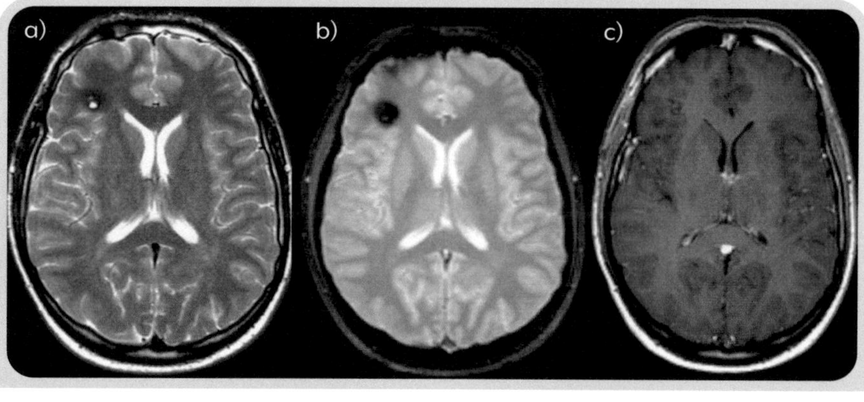

Figure 5.18

Brain MRI of a right frontal cavernoma in a) T2, b) T2* and c) T1.

Among the most common extraparenchymal injuries is epidural hematoma, which appears on CT as a hyperdense area with a biconvex lens-shaped morphology located between the cranial vault and brain parenchyma. Epidural hematoma is commonly associated with a fracture of the cranial vault, often involving the temporal bone, and is caused by injury to branches of the middle meningeal artery. Subdural hematoma has the same density and appears as a crescent-shaped collection with a medial concavity. In this case, bleeding is caused by the rupture of bridging veins between the meninges and the dural sinuses. In elderly individuals, the presence of concomitant cerebral atrophy increases the frequency of bleeding. Chronic subdural hematoma, especially in the elderly, gradually decreases in density and appears hypodense. Cranial trauma can also result in subarachnoid haemorrhage.

Intraparenchymal injuries consist of hematomas within the cerebral cortex, parenchymal hematomas (involving both white and gray matter), contusions, and diffuse axonal injury. Post-traumatic haemorrhagic lesions may not be immediately evident after the traumatic event but can be detected in subsequent examinations, after 12 or 18 hours. Diffuse axonal injury is an extremely serious condition from a clinical perspective but is relatively poor in characteristic signs, at least in the immediate aftermath of the trauma. Easily detectable changes include small haemorrhagic petechiae, mostly in the corticosubcortical junction or in the vicinity of the basal ganglia. Only at a later stage can secondary cerebral atrophy resulting from deafferentation be observed.

5.6.4 Infectious Pathologies

Alterations due to infectious causes can affect the meninges, parenchyma, ependyma, or all of these structures. In herpes encephalitis, inflammatory alterations are characteristically localized in the temporal lobes. The lesions are easily visualized with magnetic resonance imaging (MRI) as hyperintense areas in T2, often with a haemorrhagic component and slight restriction of diffusion. Abscesses initially appear as a heterogeneous region of parenchymal damage (cerebritis), hypodense on CT and mildly hyperintense on T2-weighted MRI. Subsequently, within the abscess, a liquefied area and a peripheral capsule form. On CT, the abscess appears hypodense centrally with enhancement of the capsule after contrast administration. On MRI, the abscess shows central hyperintensity on T2 and hypointensity on T1, with enhancement of the capsule after contrast administration. The necrotic tissue appears markedly hyperintense on diffusion-weighted images (Figure 5.19). Inflammation affecting the meninges is characterized, in FLAIR sequences, by a faint hyperintensity of cerebrospinal fluid in the cisterns, with diffuse

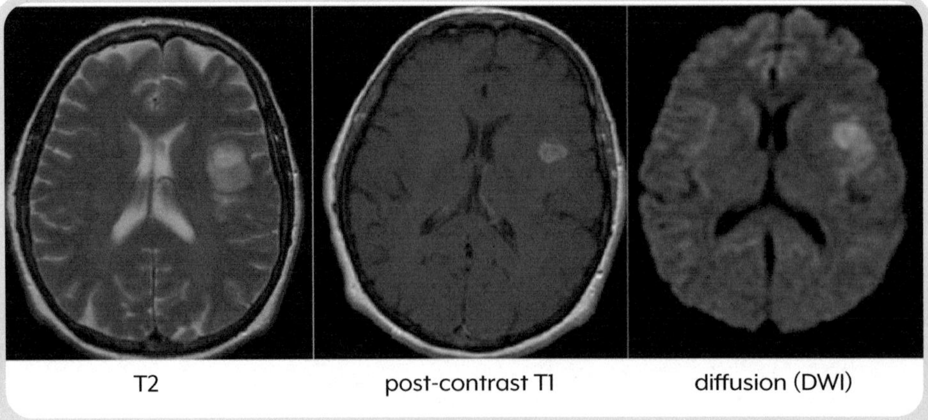

Figure 5.19

Brain MRI. Cerebral abscess in early phase.

enhancement after contrast administration (in bacterial meningitis) or localized enhancement mainly affecting the basal cisterns (as seen in tuberculous meningitis).

5.6.5 Multiple Sclerosis

MRI is the preferred method and should investigate both the brain and the spinal cord. Generally, it is also performed after the administration of a contrast agent. Useful sequences are considered T2 FLAIR, which suppress the hyperintense signal of cerebrospinal fluid, allowing for a better evaluation of the lesions (which are also hyperintense), especially if they are located in the periventricular area. Multiple sclerosis lesions appear hyperintense in T2, small, oval-shaped, with a longer axis perpendicular to the ventricles. In the brain, they are primarily located in the white matter, with a particular predilection for the periventricular zone and the corpus callosum. Active lesions enhance after the administration of a contrast agent, either peripherally or involving the entire plaque (Figure 5.20). Some lesions appear markedly hypointense in T1 and indicate tissue loss since axonal damage can be associated with demyelination.

MRI is crucial for the diagnosis of multiple sclerosis, especially in the early stages of the disease, and is based on the criteria of spatial and temporal dissemination of the lesions. Spatial dissemination of the disease involves demonstrating multiple lesions located in five specific regions (cortical, juxtacortical, periventricular, subtentorial, and spinal). Temporal dissemination involves demonstrating lesions in different stages on the initial MRI examination, such as a single lesion with enhancement after the administration of a contrast agent, or, in the absence of this, showing the appearance of a new lesion on subsequent MRI examinations that was not present on the previous examination.

MRI is particularly useful in evaluating the presence of Progressive Multifocal Leukoencephalopathy (PML), a feared complication of some immunomodulatory therapies (such as Natalizumab) used for multiple sclerosis. The appearance on T2, more widespread lesions, peripheral hyperintensity on DWI, heterogeneous enhancement after contrast administration, and a punctate appearance ("Milky Way") may raise suspicion of this complication in at-risk patients.

The differential diagnosis includes all multifocal white matter pathologies. In particular, Acute Disseminated Encephalomyelitis (ADEM) presents the greatest challenges in differential diagnosis. In ADEM, the lesions are generally larger than those of multiple sclerosis, often showing enhancement after contrast administration, and subsequent follow-up examinations demonstrate the monophasic nature of the disease.

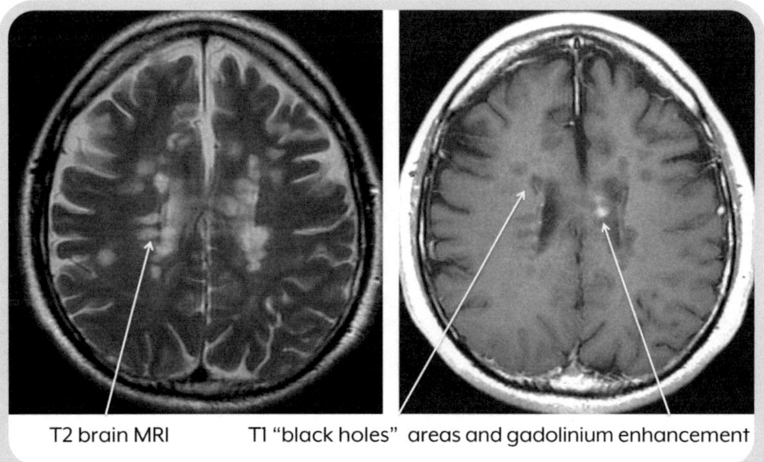

Figure 5.20

Brain MRI. T2 sequence and T1 sequence after contrast agent injection in a patient with multiple sclerosis.

5.6.6 Degenerative Diseases

In degenerative pathology of the central nervous system, both specific and nonspecific alterations indicating neural damage can be observed.

In dementia, nonspecific signs include ventricular enlargement and subarachnoid space dilation (cerebral atrophy), and sometimes the accumulation of ferromagnetic substances in deep gray matter nuclei. More specific signs include hippocampal atrophy in Alzheimer's dementia, predominantly affecting the temporal horns with dilatation of the dentate gyrus. Spectroscopy may show increased myo-inositol in the cingulate gyrus (Figure 5.21). Frontotemporal dementia often presents with hyperintensity in T2-weighted images of the cerebral white matter, accompanied by predominant frontal or temporal atrophy. Asymmetric temporal atrophy between the right and left temporal lobes is not uncommon (Figure 5.22). Multi-infarct dementia is characterized by numerous ischemic vascular lesions and diffuse T2 hyperintensity in the cerebral white matter. Typical signs of normal-pressure hydrocephalus include ventricular dilatation with relative preservation of the subarachnoid spaces and signs of cerebrospinal fluid resorption through the ependyma, represented by T2 hyperintensity and hypodensity on CT scans.

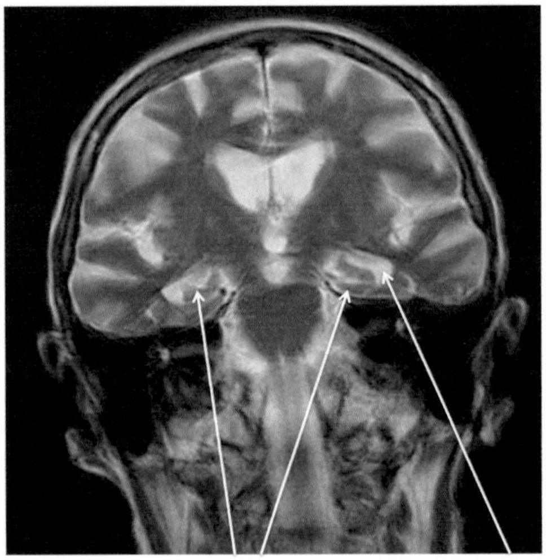

Figure 5.21

Brain MRI. T2 sequence on coronal plane in a patient with Alzheimer dementia.

In prion encephalopathy, MRI reveals altered signal intensity, appearing increased in diffusion-weighted sequences, primarily localized in the basal ganglia and later in cortical areas, often asymmetrically. Only at a

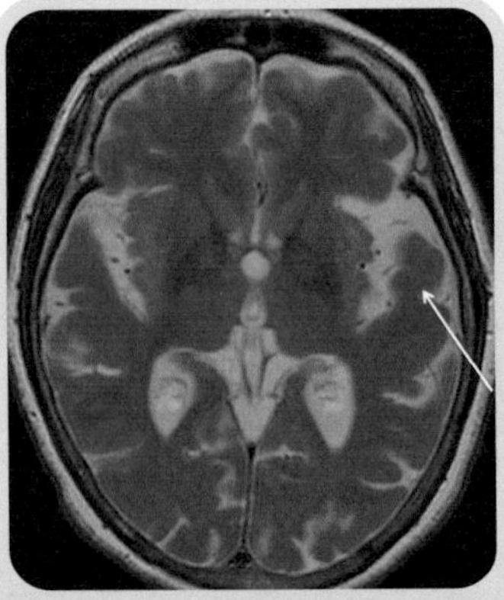

Figure 5.22

Brain MRI. Fronto-temporal dementia (temporal atrophy).

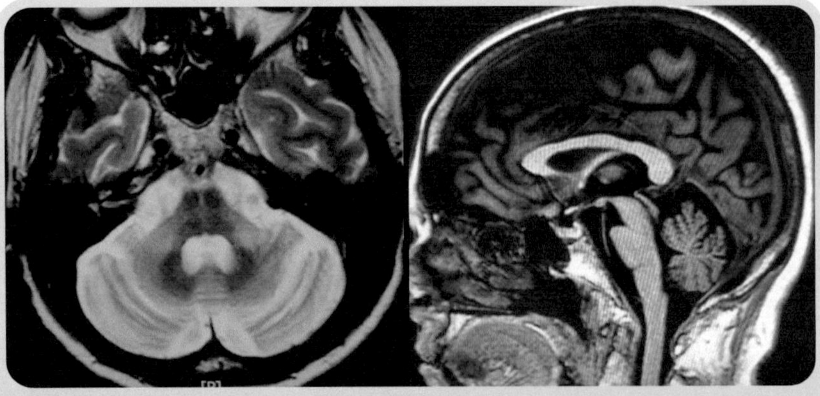

Figure 5.23

Brain MRI. Patient with MSA-C.

later stage does the signal become hyperintense in T2 FLAIR sequences. In limbic encephalitis, T2 hyperintensity is characteristic in the hippocampal regions, sometimes bilaterally. Hyperintensity is also present in diffusion-weighted images, but sparing of the basal ganglia allows for differential diagnosis from prion encephalopathy.

MRI is useful in Parkinson's disease for excluding other pathologies and certain secondary forms of parkinsonism (e.g., vascular). The use of high-field (3T) and ultra-high-field (7T) magnets can reveal morphostructural alterations affecting the compact part of the substantia nigra. Atypical parkinsonism (multiple system atrophy - MSA, progressive supranuclear palsy - PSP, corticobasal degeneration - CBD) can show morphovolumetric changes in the basal ganglia and brainstem. Accumulation of ferromagnetic substances in the putamen is often observed in parkinsonism. A characteristic feature of PSP is the "hummingbird sign," where the midbrain profile on the sagittal plane resembles the shape of a hummingbird due to selective atrophy of the mesencephalon. In MSA, a "cross" appearance of the pons can be seen on axial T2 images, resulting from the contrast between persistent longitudinal fibers and the loss of axial fibers (Figure 5.23).

Furthermore, nuclear medicine, particularly with DaTSCAN, plays an important role in the diagnosis. DaTSCAN is a technique that studies dopamine receptors in the basal ganglia using 123-iodineioflupane as a tracer. It allows for the detection of altered dopaminergic uptake in the putamen in Parkinson's disease and demonstrates normal uptake in essential tremor.

In advanced stages of motor neuron disease, T2-weighted images may reveal hyperintensity in the pyramidal tracts due to axonal degeneration (Figure 5.24).

5.6.7 Epilepsy

In patients with epilepsy, it is essential to perform a neuroradiological study, particularly in late-onset epilepsy and focal forms. The most commonly found lesions in patients with epilepsy are brain neoplasms, alterations in cortical organization, dysplasias, vascular malformations, sequelae of previous conditions (traumatic, vascular, or infectious), and mesial temporal sclerosis. Mesial temporal sclerosis is characterized by the presence of scar tissue in the hippocampal region, visible as hyperintensity in T2, with volumetric reduction of the hippocampus and dilation of the temporal horn (Figure 5.25). Focal cortical dysplasia appears as a hyperintense area in T2, even more evident in T2 FLAIR, with reduced signal differentiation between the underlying gray and white matter (blurring).

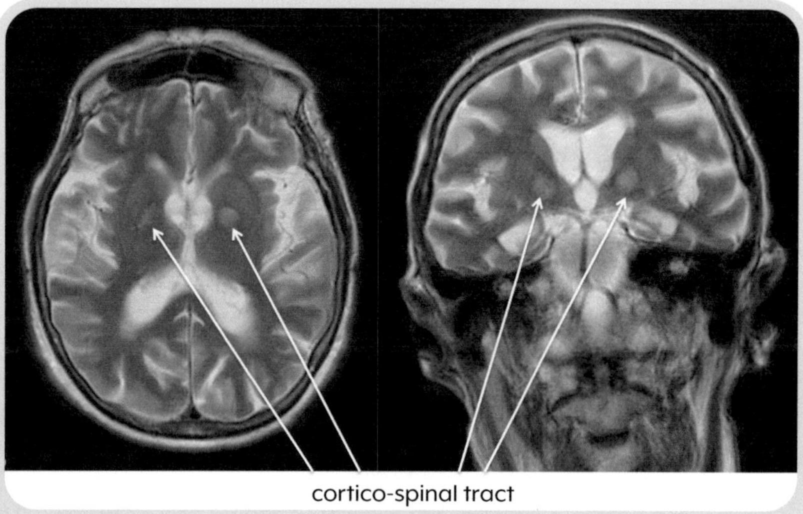

Figure 5.24

Brain MRI. Patient with SLA with loss of fibes in the cortico-spinal tract.

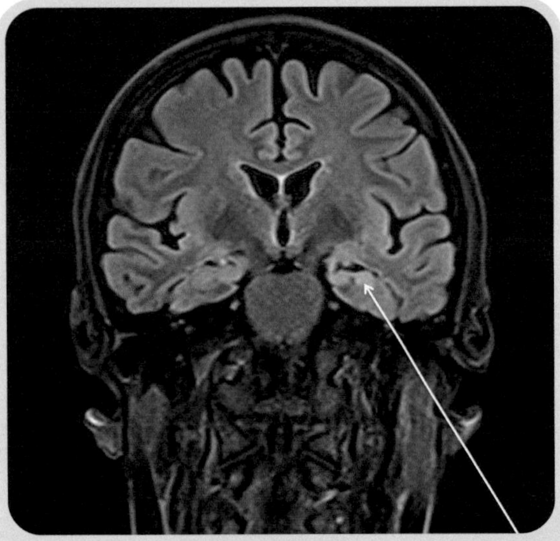

Figure 5.25

Brain MRI. T2 sequence on the coronal plane. Mesial temporal sclerosis.

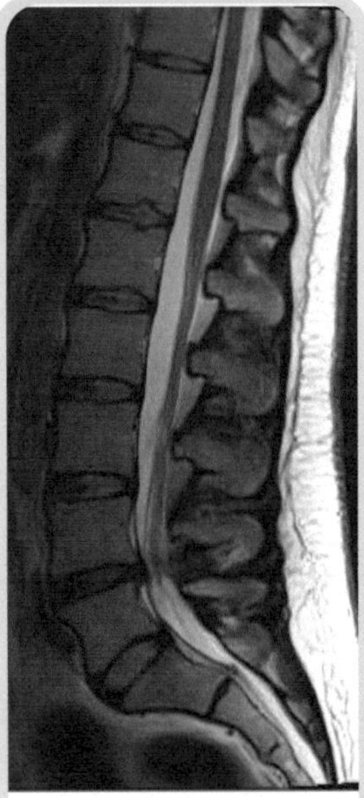

Figure 5.26

Lumbosacral segment MRI from a healthy subject.

5.6.8 Study of the Spinal Column

Regarding the spinal column, it is important to remember that CT is mainly indicated for the study of bony components, while MRI is indispensable for the study of the spinal cord, nerve roots, and ligaments. In the case of traumatic pathology, it is particularly useful to complement traditional radiographic studies with computed tomography, especially with the extended multi-segment spiral acquisition technique in cases of severe trauma. Several studies have shown that CT can detect up to 20% of vertebral fractures not visible on conventional radiographs. MRI is beneficial for patients with neurological deficits.

Neoplastic pathology is examined in detail using MRI, which allows distinguishing neoplasms as extradural and extraparenchymal (such as bone metastases), extraspinal intradural (such as meningiomas and neurinomas), and intramedullary neoplasms (such as astrocytomas, ependymomas, and hemangioblastomas).

Regarding degenerative pathology of the cervical and thoracic spine, MRI is preferred as the only modality capable of providing information about the state of the spinal parenchyma. Additionally, sagittal plane imaging enables the examination of multiple spinal cord segments (Figure 5.26). In the cervical segment, degenerative disc disease often leads to compression of the spinal arterioles, resulting in ischemic damage to the spinal cord (spondylotic myelopathy). Degenerative pathology in the lumbosacral segment can be studied using both CT and MRI to visualize osteophytosis, disc herniation, canal stenosis, intervertebral foramen stenosis, and hypertrophy of the facet joints. Conventional radiography is still useful in the study of spondylodegenerative alterations that cause spinal instability, especially when dynamic testing (flexion-extension of the spine) is also employed.

For a more comprehensive discussion of individual neuroradiological techniques, their respective indications, and characteristic aspects in different neurological pathologies, please refer to the following reference: Colonnese Bozzao A., C., Pantano P. Lezioni di Neuroradiologia (Società editrice Esculapio, September 2014).

Bibliography

2016 Updates to the WHO Brain Tumor Classification System: What the Radiologist Needs to Know. Johnson DR, Guerin JB, Giannini C, Morris JM, Eckel LJ, Kaufmann TJ. Radiographics. 2017 Nov-Dec;37(7):2164-2180. doi: 10.1148/rg.2017170037. Epub 2017 Oct 13. PMID: 29028423 Review.

Stroke Imaging. Kamalian S, Lev MH. Radiol Clin North Am. 2019 Jul;57(4):717-732. doi: 10.1016/j.rcl.2019.02.001. Epub 2019 Apr 8. PMID: 31076028 Review.

Mechanical Thrombectomy in Acute Ischemic Stroke: A Systematic Review. Lambrinos A, Schaink AK, Dhalla I, Krings T, Casaubon LK, Sikich N, Lum C, Bharatha A, Pereira VM, Stotts G, Saposnik G, Kelloway L, Xie X, Hill MD. Can J Neurol Sci. 2016 Jul;43(4):455-60. doi: 10.1017/cjn.2016.30. Epub 2016 Apr 13. PMID: 27071728 Free PMC article. Review.

Epilepsy imaging in adults: getting it right. Friedman E. AJR Am J Roentgenol. 2014 Nov;203(5):1093-103. doi: 10.2214/AJR.13.12035. PMID: 25341150 Review.

Traumatic Brain Injury: Imaging Patterns and Complications. Schweitzer AD, Niogi SN, Whitlow CT, Tsiouris AJ. Radiographics. 2019 Oct;39(6):1571-1595. doi: 10.1148/rg.2019190076. PMID: 31589576 Review.

Diagnosis and Treatment of Multiple Sclerosis: A Review. McGinley MP, Goldschmidt CH, Rae-Grant AD. JAMA. 2021 Feb 23;325(8):765-779. doi: 10.1001/jama.2020.26858. PMID: 33620411 Review.

Imaging of cerebritis, encephalitis, and brain abscess. Rath TJ, Hughes M, Arabi M, Shah GV. Neuroimaging Clin N Am. 2012 Nov;22(4):585-607. doi: 10.1016/j.nic.2012.04.002. Epub 2012 Sep 28. PMID: 23122258 Review.

The Role of Magnetic Resonance Imaging for the Diagnosis of Atypical Parkinsonism. Chougar L, Pyatigorskaya N, Degos B, Grabli D, Lehéricy S. Front Neurol. 2020 Jul 17;11:665. doi: 10.3389/fneur.2020.00665. eCollection 2020. PMID: 327.

The following authors are thanked for their contribution: Francesca Caramia, Giulio Guidetti, Stefano Martini, Emanuela Rastelli, Francesco Biraschi, Valentina Martines.

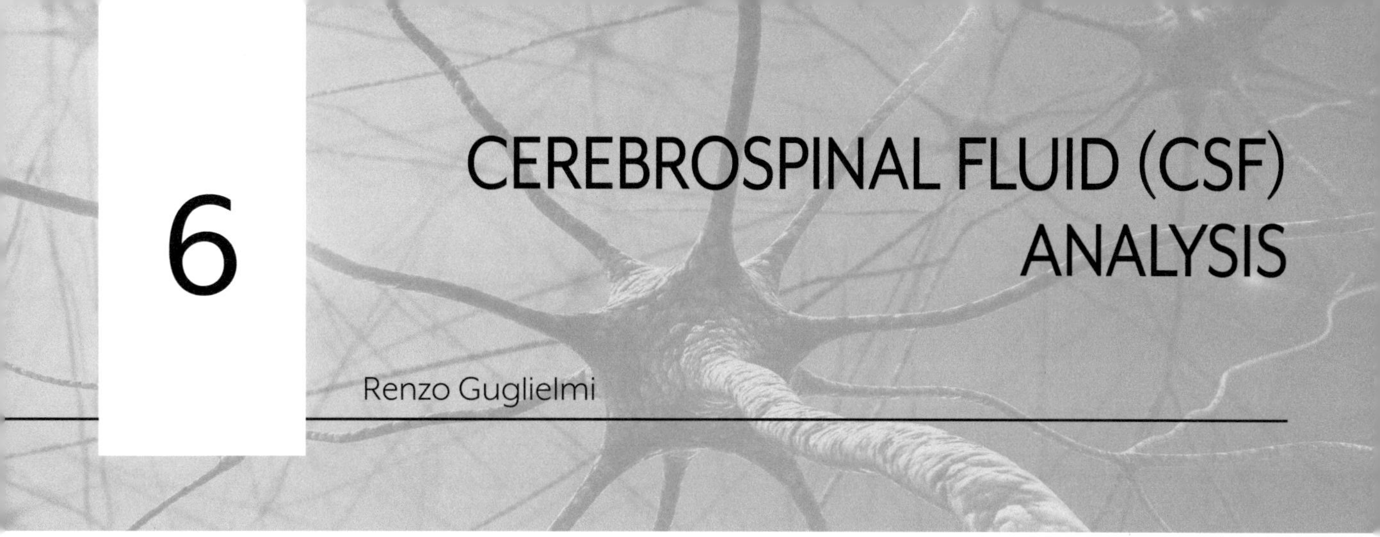

6 CEREBROSPINAL FLUID (CSF) ANALYSIS

Renzo Guglielmi

6.1 Cerebrospinal Fluid

Cerebrospinal fluid (CSF) is a liquid contained in the cerebral ventricles and the subarachnoid space, which normally appears as a clear and colorless fluid. CSF is an important tool for understanding and diagnosing numerous neurological diseases. Unlike internal diseases, most neurological diseases do not cause significant changes in the blood due to the presence of the blood-brain barrier. The total volume of CSF is 90-150 ml, with variability related to age: 60-100 ml in children, 100-160 ml in adults, with an average of 135 ml. The production rate is 0.35 ml/minute, equivalent to about 500-600 ml/day, which means that CSF is renewed by the body 4-5 times a day. The distribution in adults is as follows: 35 ml in the ventricles, 25 ml in the subarachnoid space, and 75 ml in the spinal canal.

Among the main functions of CSF is the maintenance of homeostasis in the central nervous system (CNS). Its constituent elements are in balance with the extracellular fluid of the brain, thus maintaining a constant external environment for the cells of the nervous system. The homeostatic function is also expressed through an excretory function, removing metabolic products such as lactate, CO_2, H^+, pharmacological substances, and neurotransmitter metabolites. CSF provides support and mechanical protection to the nervous system. The liquid layer between the nervous system and the bony structures allows the brain to float, attenuates shocks and stresses, and reduces the actual weight of the brain from 1,500 grams to a relative weight of 50 grams. The volumes of CSF, blood content, and intracranial parenchyma are interrelated, providing a compensatory margin in conditions of intracranial hypertension.

6.1.1 Physiology and Pathophysiology

CSF is mainly produced by the choroid plexus in the lateral ventricles (70%), the brain parenchyma, ventricular ependyma, and the leptomeninges (pia mater and arachnoid). The choroid plexus consists of capillary networks surrounded by cuboidal or columnar epithelium projecting into the ventricles. The small plexuses, located in the roof of the third and fourth ventricles, join the two large plexuses located in the floor of each lateral ventricle. The structure of the villi that compose the plexus is illustrated in Figures 6.1 and 6.2. CSF production is quite complex, and there are multiple mechanisms regulating it, as illustrated in Figure 6.3. The definition of CSF as a “active secretion” appears to be the most appropriate. After being produced in the lateral ventricles, CSF flows through the Monro foramina into the third ventricle, and then through the Sylvian aqueduct into the fourth ventricle. From here, through three openings in the roof, represented by the median Magendie foramen and the two lateral Luschka foramina, it reaches the subarachnoid spaces between the dura mater and the pia mater. At the folds of the tissue at the base of the skull, the subarachnoid spaces expand, forming cisterns. CSF flows into the cisternal spaces at the base and then ascends into the subarachnoid spaces of the convexity (Figure 6.4). Another portion of CSF spreads caudally into the spinal subarachnoid

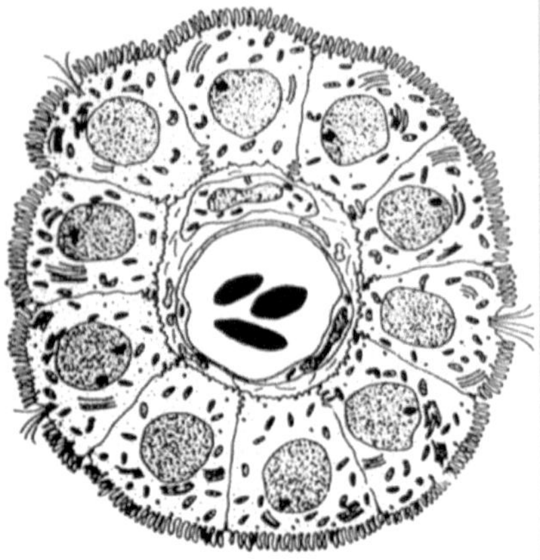

Figure 6.1

Structure of a choroid plexus villus. The central capillary (vascular pole) is delimited by a thin and fenestrated endothelium, surrounded by an interstitial layer of pial cells and collagen fibers on which the lining of cuboidal epithelial cells rests. These cells have the following characteristics: the basal cell membrane is folded; the apical surface, facing the liquor side, presents microvilli and sporadically tufts of 2-8 cilia; the cytoplasm contains numerous mitochondria, indicating high metabolic activity, as well as numerous pinocytic vesicles, expressing substance transport. The morphology of the villus suggests that the choroid plexus has a prominent active and selective secretory capacity.

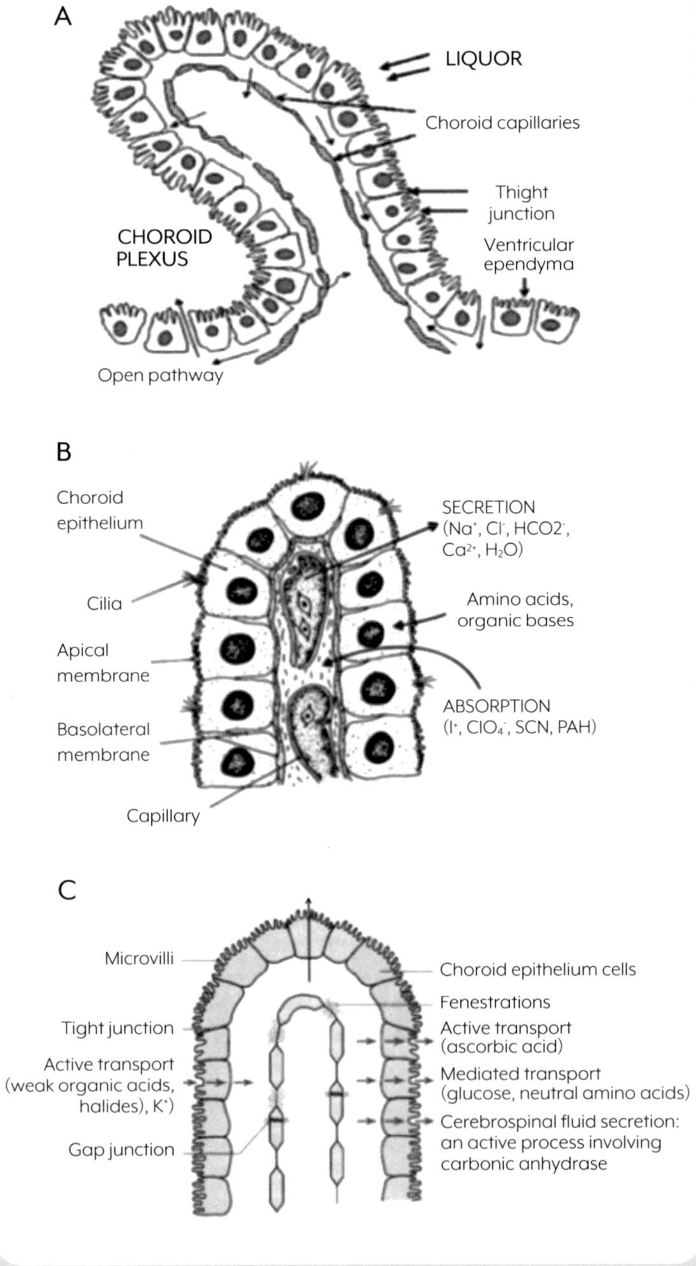

Figure 6.2

A) The *blood-brain barrier* is located at the level of the choroid plexus and, therefore, anatomically consists of the wall of the choroid capillaries and the cells of the choroid epithelium.
B) The *choroid plexus* is composed of choroid villi, each of which consists of a vascular axis, the choroid capillary, originating from the terminal branches of the choroid arteries, and a monolayer of cylindrical cells, the choroid epithelium, derived from the ependyma lining the ventricular walls.
C) While the capillaries are fenestrated, at the level of the choroid epithelium, there are tight junctions that restrict the free diffusion of solutes from the blood to the cerebrospinal fluid, thereby maintaining the chemical-physical homeostasis of the cerebrospinal fluid.

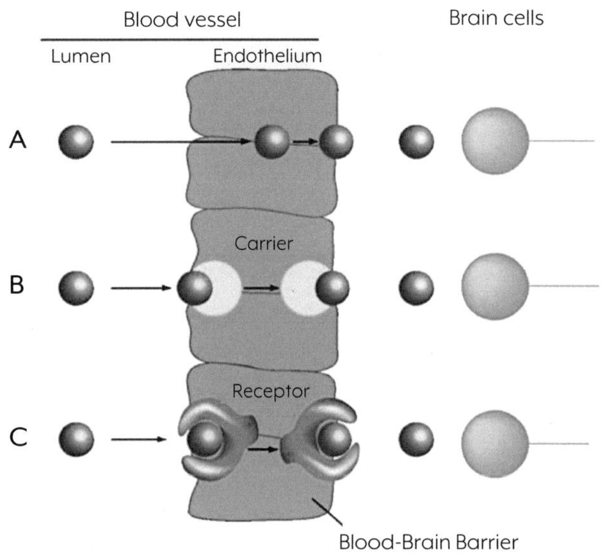

Figure 6.3

The transmembrane transport can be classified as follows: (A) Passive diffusion: lipophilic substances (alcohol, nicotine, and caffeine) pass through the membrane freely; (B) Active transport: substances that the central nervous system (CNS) requires (glucose, amino acids) are transported using carrier proteins; C)Receptor-mediated transport: a molecule binds to a receptor on the surface and is released on the opposite side (proteins, insulin).

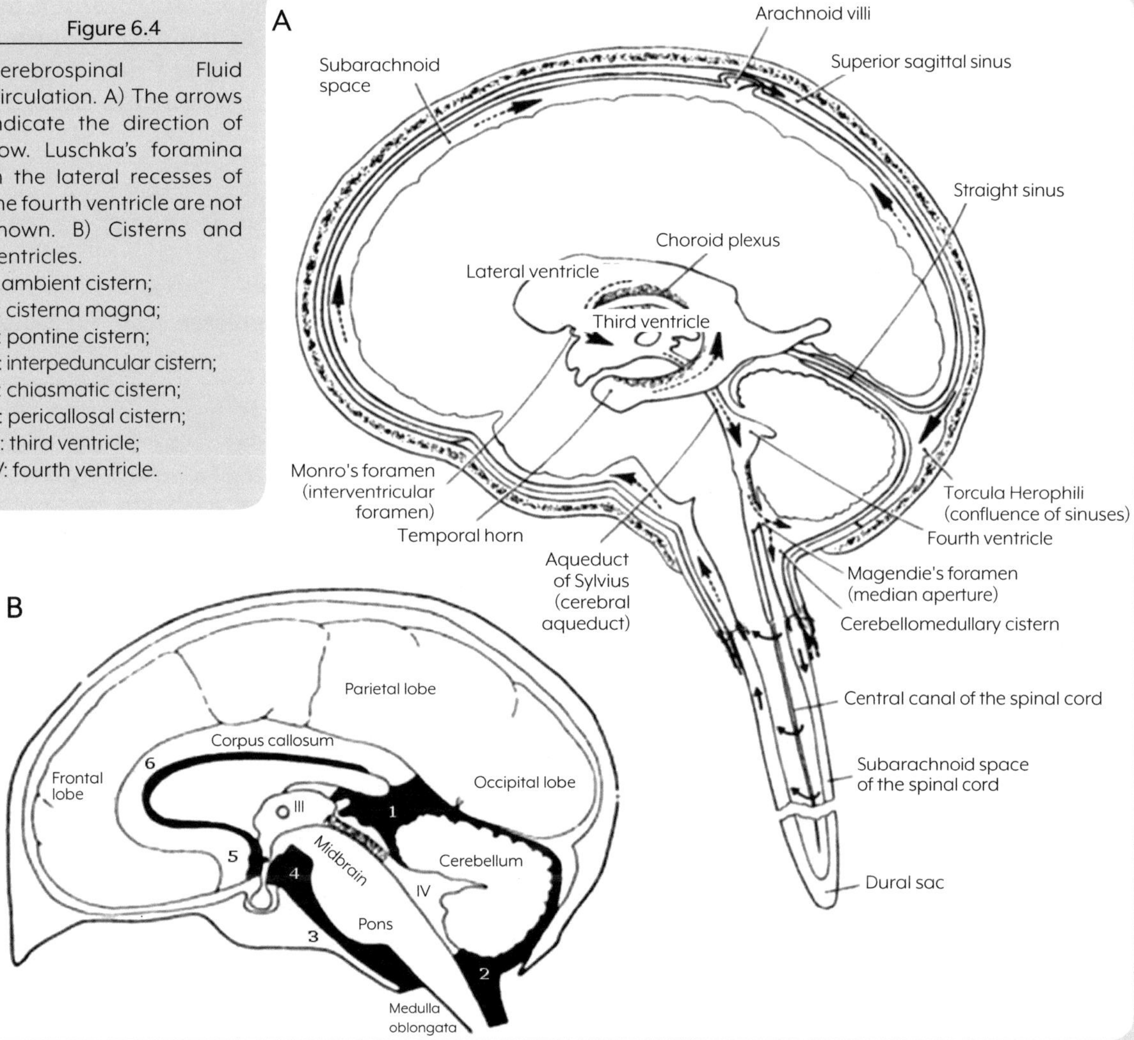

Figure 6.4

Cerebrospinal Fluid Circulation. A) The arrows indicate the direction of flow. Luschka's foramina in the lateral recesses of the fourth ventricle are not shown. B) Cisterns and ventricles.
1: ambient cistern;
2: cisterna magna;
3: pontine cistern;
4: interpeduncular cistern;
5: chiasmatic cistern;
6: pericallosal cistern;
III: third ventricle;
IV: fourth ventricle.

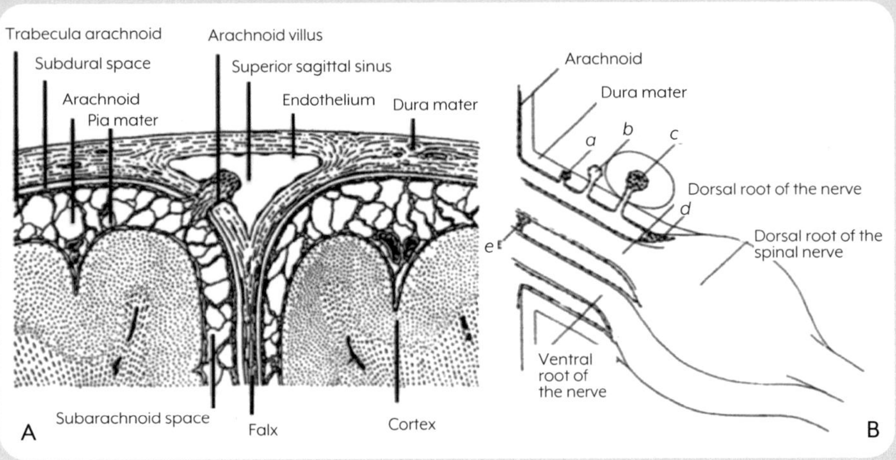

Figure 6.5

A) Structure of arachnoid villi projecting into the superior sagittal sinus in a coronal section of the brain.
B) Distribution of arachnoid villi along the spinal roots (from Pollay, 1972). a. villus terminating within the dura mater; b. villus traversing the dura mater; c. villus protruding into a spinal vein; d, e. arachnoid proliferations within the subarachnoid space.

spaces, while a minimal amount reaches the ependymal canal. This way, CSF fills the tubular expansion of the subarachnoid space, forming a sheath around the spinal cord. The lower limit of this space is variable but generally located at the level of the second sacral vertebra, below the lower end of the spinal cord.

At the level of the superior sagittal sinus, absorption occurs through arachnoid herniations into the dura mater (arachnoid villi projecting into the lumen of the sinus) (Figure 6.5). By crossing these villi, CSF enters the venous blood circulation of the sinus. CSF is absorbed, primarily in the superior sagittal sinus and to a lesser extent in the small arachnoid villi projecting into the spinal radicular veins. Interstitial fluid is reabsorbed into the blood within the brain parenchyma through the blood-brain barrier.

6.1.2 Cerebrospinal Fluid Pressure

The measurement of cerebrospinal fluid (CSF) pressure is performed before and after CSF extraction using simple graduated column manometers inserted on the needle through specific connectors. CSF pressure is an index of the real intracranial pressure, but only when measured at the intraventricular or subarachnoid level of the brain. Since CSF pressure is usually measured at the lumbar level, only these values are taken into consideration. In an adult patient in the lateral decubitus position, CSF pressure ranges between 10 and 15 mm/Hg, equivalent to 7-20 cm of H_2O, which decreases by 4-5 cm after CSF subtraction. Significantly lower values are observed in children. Conversely, in a patient in the sitting position, it is 20-40 cm of H_2O. Arterial pressure has little effect on CSF pressure, while venous pressure is determinant.

Valsalva Maneuver | It consists of manual compression of the abdomen, which causes intra-abdominal and intraspinal venous hypertension and increases CSF pressure by 5-15 cm of H_2O.

Queckenstedt Maneuver | It consists of compressing the jugular veins in the neck for 10-15 seconds, resulting in an increase in CSF pressure, recorded with a needle inserted into the subarachnoid space at the lumbar level.

6.1.3 Barriers between blood, brain, and cerebrospinal fluid and their functions

The central nervous system (CNS) and the cerebrospinal fluid surrounding it are isolated from the blood circulation by two active barriers: the blood-brain barrier and the blood-cerebrospinal fluid barrier. These barriers prevent the free diffusion of solutes from the blood to the brain and, through controlled production of CSF, maintain a necessary physical and biological homeostasis for the proper functioning of the CNS.

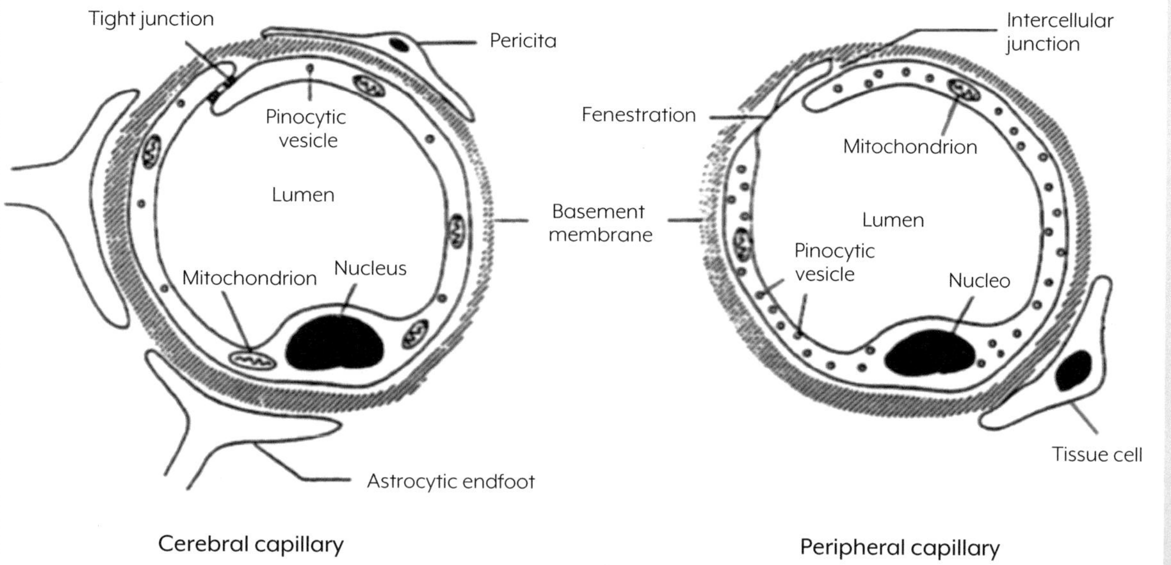

Figure 6.6

The cerebral capillaries differ anatomically from the peripheral systemic ones because they are composed of capillary endothelial cells equipped with tight junctions that prevent the free diffusion of solutes and an underlying basement membrane, and by pericytes, contractile cells separated from the basement membrane by an extracellular matrix of collagen.

Blood-Brain Barrier | It is the barrier effect due to the unique properties of the endothelium of cerebral capillaries. The anatomical-functional structure is represented by the luminal surface of the cerebral capillary endothelium, which differs from that of other tissues due to the presence of adjacent tight junctions and a basement membrane, upon which astrocytic pericytes rest, covering almost the entire extraluminal surface of the endothelium (Figure 6.6).

Blood-Cerebrospinal Fluid Barrier | It is the barrier between blood and CSF and is formed by the choroid plexus. The fundamental element of the plexus, the choroidal epithelium, consists of cylindrical cells derived from ependymal cells that rest on the capillary and are interconnected by tight junctions at the lateral surfaces. The apical surface, which produces CSF, is equipped with a brush border (Figures 6.1, 6.2). These cells, rich in mitochondria and with high metabolic activity, have numerous pinocytic vesicles that transport substances of high molecular weight. The barrier is responsible for the equilibrium between CSF and plasma, with a dynamic exchange occurring at all levels of the neuroaxis, depending on the size and solubility of the molecules (Figure 6.3).

The issue of the origin of lymphocytes present in CSF, ranging in number from 0 to 5 mm^3 under physiological conditions and originating from the blood, remains unresolved to this day.

6.1.4 Cerebrospinal Fluid Withdrawal

The method primarily used for cerebrospinal fluid (CSF) withdrawal is lumbar puncture (*spinal tap*). The lumbar puncture should be performed on a fasting patient for at least six hours and in a seated position, even when measuring CSF pressure. However, it would be more appropriate to place the patient in a supine position on the right lateral decubitus, with the back parallel to the bed and in a knee-chest position to maximize the interapophyseal distance, with arms around the legs and the head as close as possible to the knees. The puncture is generally performed between the L3-L4 spinous processes, but also between L4-L5 (the spinal cord ends at the upper margin of L2) (Figure 6.7). The lumbar puncture needle is 8 cm long, with a gauge of 18-22 and equipped with a stylet and an obliquely sharp tip. The patient should remain in the prone position for at least one hour to facilitate closure of the dural puncture hole. In the case of intracranial hypertension due to a space-occupying lesion in the cerebral hemisphere or a tumor mass in the posterior cranial fossa, lumbar puncture is not recommended because rapid removal of CSF at the lumbar level can cause herniation of the brain through the large occipital foramen. Generally, lumbar puncture is not very painful, but in the subsequent phase, one-third of patients experience headaches that last a few days, which are due to stretching of the meningeal attachments of the brain or leakage of CSF from the puncture site. Immediately after CSF withdrawal, it is helpful to administer fluids to the patient to promote CSF formation. The CSF withdrawal technique is used both to measure CSF pressure and to collect a sample for cytochemical examination, which is necessary for the diagnosis of many neurological diseases. For the analytical examination, it is sufficient to collect a total of 5-10 ml of CSF in three sequential aliquots, collected in sterile, transparent, and sequentially numbered vials. CSF withdrawal should be accompanied by a venous blood draw (Figure 6.8).

6.1.5 Cerebrospinal Fluid Examination

The basic examination of cerebrospinal fluid (CSF) involves evaluating its physical, biochemical, and cytological parameters. Under normal conditions, CSF is clear and

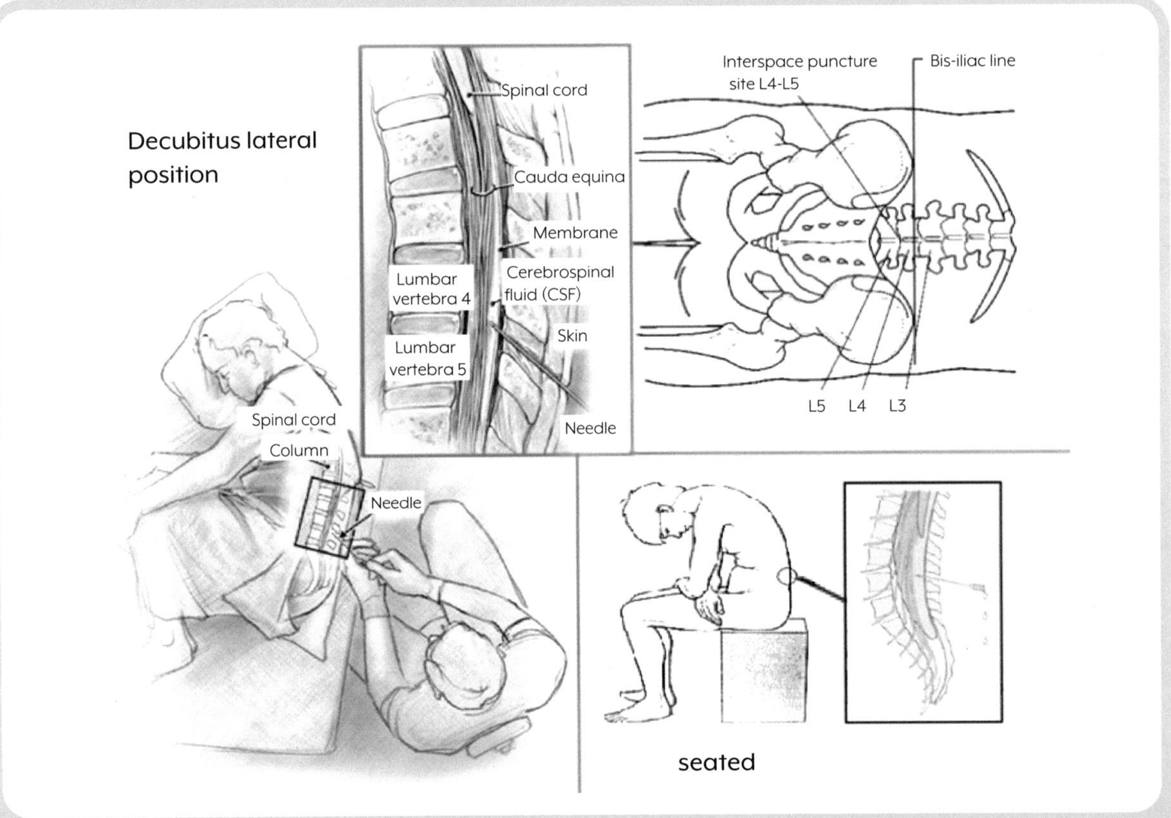

Figure 6.7

Spinal tap in both positions.

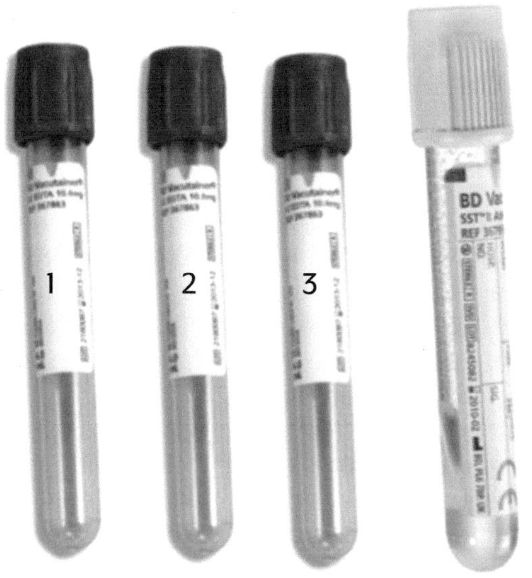

Figure 6.8

Tubes for collecting cerebrospinal fluid and blood samples.

colorless (like water). Any changes in the color of the CSF, excluding blood contamination, should be considered pathological. Clear CSF generally indicates physiological cellularity (up to 5 cells/mm^3), except in cases of "clear CSF encephalitis," where the CSF is clear despite presenting lymphocytic pleocytosis (increased cellular content). Opalescent appearance is observed in lymphocytic and tuberculous meningitis and is characterized by pleocytosis of mononuclear cells (glassy appearance of CSF). It can be turbid or purulent in pyogenic meningitis with pleocytosis of neutrophil polymorphonuclear cells. The color of the CSF generally indicates the presence of red blood cells, blood pigments, bacterial contamination, or increased protein levels. A reddish color, more or less intense, is caused by red blood cell contamination. The presence of blood in the CSF may be related to subarachnoid hemorrhage (SAH) or vessel injury caused by lumbar puncture needle insertion. The color becomes xanthochromic (brown) due to hemocatheresis. Red blood cells disappear from the CSF within 3-7 days, while xanthochromia starts to appear a few hours after hemorrhage, peaks after a week, and disappears in 2-4 weeks. Xanthochromic color, even if intense, can be produced by a massive entry of plasma proteins (albumin, bilirubin) into the CSF, as well as free bilirubin in severely jaundiced individuals. A straw-yellow color (yellow, more or less intense) always indicates increased CSF proteins.

Hemorrhagic CSF and Bilirubin | The classical collection of CSF in three tubes (in this case, containing blood) can differentiate subarachnoid bleeding from local blood contamination due to puncture. In the latter case, progressive reduction in blood coloration is observed from the first to the third tube and disappears after centrifugation. Spectrophotometry of CSF is the reference test for diagnosing SAH. In the first few hours after bleeding, the presence of hemoglobin with a peak at 415 nm is sought, and after 12 hours, bilirubin is determined with peaks at 440-460 nm. Bilirubin measurement is useful not only in cases where imaging diagnostics are inconclusive but also to establish the time elapsed since the presumed hemorrhagic event. While hemoglobin and its degradation products can be measured for up to 4-8 days, bilirubin remains in the CSF for 15-20 days at concentrations higher than physiological levels ($\leq$ 0.01 mg/dl).

In certain syndromes, CSF is characterized by increased viscosity due to the presence of specific and excessive solutes, which decrease its fluidity. The passage of fibrinogen and albumin into the CSF, caused by barrier damage, can be relatively modest and generate thin fibrin networks, resembling a spider web-shaped inverted funnel (*Mya's reticulum*), especially when CSF is left undisturbed in the tube for a few hours. This can be observed in brucellar or tuberculous meningitis. In *Froin's syndrome*, the high concentrations of fibrinogen and albumin in the CSF lead to massive spontaneous coagulation, resulting in xanthochromic-colored CSF. This occurs in occlusions of spinal subarachnoid spaces during intradural and medullary expansive processes.

Cells | Normally, in adults, CSF contains no more than 5 cells/mm3, which are mononuclear elements represented by B and T lymphocytes (60-70%) and monocytes (30-40%) derived from the blood. These cells pass through the endothelial cells of cerebral capillaries via a transcellular migration process of leukocytes into giant vacuoles. More than 10 cells/mm^3 indicate pathology. Pleocytosis always has a pathological significance and usually indicates meningeal irritation. Neutrophilic pleocytosis generally indicates an acute inflammatory process, while mononuclear pleocytosis is observed during viral or fungal infections. Mixed cell types, characterized by the presence of both mononuclear and polymorphonuclear cells, can be observed in all conditions of exacerbation of chronic infections (tuberculosis, syphilis, etc.). Eosinophils are present in variable percentages in all infectious conditions, often in parasitic infections. In addition to blood-derived cells, microorganisms (bacteria or fungi) responsible for infections can be found in the CSF. In such cases, it is important to proceed with bacteriological and cultural examinations or virological tests. The biochemical parameters considered clinically relevant include glucose, proteins, and certain electrolytes (Table 6.1).

Glucose | The concentration of glucose in the cerebrospinal fluid (CSF) depends solely on the blood glucose level and the metabolism of the nervous tissue, thus being functionally related to blood sugar levels. Under normal physiological conditions, the CSF/blood glucose ratio ranges from 0.6 to 0.7. Hypoglycorrhachia occurs in the presence of widespread neoplastic manifestations of the meninges (carcinomatosis and meningeal leukemia) as well as due to increased glucose consumption by nervous tissue, which enhances its anaerobic glycolysis (resulting in increased lactic acid in the CSF). It can also be caused by blood-brain barrier

Table 6.1 COMPOSITION OF NORMAL CEREBROSPINAL FLUID (CSF) COMPARED TO SERUM
(for comparative purposes, average serum values provided by Fishman, 1980 are reported)

Parameters	Cerebrospinal fluid	Serum
Erythrocytes/mm^3	Absent	3.5-5.9 milion (whole blood)
Leukocytes/mm^3	0-5	4500- 11000 (whole blood)
Leukocyte Types/mm^3	5 linfo-monocytes	7000
pH	7.33	7.41 (arterial)
Osmolarity	295 mOsm/l	295mOsm/l
CO_2 Pressure	47.0 mmHg	41.0 mmHg (arterial)
Total Liquids	1.5 mg/100 ml	750.0 mg/100 ml
Glucose	45-80 mg/100 ml	60-100 mg/100 ml
Lactate	1.6 mEq/l	1.0 mEq/l
Total Proteins	35 mg/100 ml	7 g/100 ml
Prealbumin	4%	Tracce
Albumin	65%	60%
Alpha 1	4%	5%
Alpha 2	8%	9%
Beta	12%	12%
Gamma	7%	14%
Urea	4.7 mmol/100 ml	5.4 m mol/100 ml
Creatinine	1.2 mg/100 ml	1.8 mg/100 ml
Chlorides	119 mEq/l	102 mEq/l
Sodium	138 mEq/l	138 mEq/l
Potassium	2.8 mEq/l	4.5 mEq/l
Calcium	2.1 mEq/l	4.8 mEq/l
Magnesium	2.3 mEq/l	1.7 mEq/l
Phosphorus	1.6 mg/100 ml	4.0 mg/100 ml
Bicarbonate	22.0 mEq/l	24.0 mEq/l (arterial)

damage, which reduces glucose passage from the blood due to altered membrane transport.

Proteins | The concentration of proteins in the cerebrospinal fluid of adults under normal conditions ranges from 15 to 50 mg/100 ml. The most commonly used method for measuring protein concentration is the colorimetric biuret method. The majority of CSF proteins originate from plasma. Other proteins, such as myelin basic protein, acidic gliofibrillary protein, S-100, and partially beta3 and beta2-microglobulin, come from the central nervous system (CNS). Some proteins, like transferrin, undergo modifications during the transition from the serum compartment to the CSF compartment. Additionally, immunoglobulins, particularly IgG class, can be synthesized by lymphocytes in the CNS in certain inflammatory diseases (intrathecal production). Prealbumin is synthesized by both the liver and the choroid plexus, so its CSF concentration is proportionally higher than its serum concentration.

Increased protein levels can be caused by:

1) serum-related abnormalities (alteration of plasma proteins);
2) intrathecal production;
3) barrier damage. Hyperproteinorrhea resulting from barrier damage can slow down protein reabsorption and establish a vicious cycle that worsens the barrier damage. Mild to moderate hyperproteinorrhea (50-100 mg%) is observed in lymphocytic meningitis, encephalitis, peripheral neuropathies, brain tumors, cerebrovascular lesions, and multiple sclerosis. Severe hyperproteinorrhea is detected in purulent and tuberculous meningitis, spinal cord tumors, spinal arachnoiditis with dynamic CSF block, acoustic neurinomas, neurofibromatosis of the cauda equina, and especially in acute or chronic idiopathic polyradiculoneuropathy (Guillain-Barré syndrome).

Barrier Index | It is calculated as (CSF albumin/serum albumin $\times 10^{-3}$) and indicates the integrity of the barrier in relation to age. The albumin was chosen as a marker to assess the overall permeability of the blood-CSF interfaces. Albumin was selected because it is exclusively produced by the liver, outside the CNS, and is well represented in both serum and CSF. (Table 6.2).

Pathological CSF Patterns | In certain neurological diseases, the physiological ratio between protein levels and cell count in the CSF is altered. Two distinct CSF patterns can be identified:

1) Albuminocytological dissociation, characterized by increased protein levels without a concomitant increase in cell count. This pattern is present in various conditions, notably in Guillain-Barré syndrome and spinal cord compression.
2) Cytological dissociation, characterized by increased cell count with normal protein levels. This pattern is observed in many inflammatory reactions of the CNS and meninges, particularly in aseptic meningitis and meningeal reactions.

Immunoglobulin Dosage | Determination of total protein levels in the cerebrospinal fluid (CSF) is essential but provides nonspecific and partial diagnostic information. It is useful to determine the total protein levels in the CSF using technologies that allow

Table 6.2 REFERENCE VALUES BASED ON AGE GROUPS

Age (years)	Albumin Range (mg/dl)	Range (mg/dl)	CSF Albumin/CSF Serum Albumin$_{Ratio}$
17 - 30	12.4 - 21.6	1.3 - 2.1	$< 5.7 \times 10^{-3}$
31 - 40	12.9 - 22.9	1.4 - 2.8	$< 6.2 \times 10^{-3}$
41 - 50	14.7 - 26.1	1.6 - 3.2	$< 7.2 \times 10^{-3}$
51 - 60	16.6 - 31.8	1.8 - 3.6	$< 8.9 \times 10^{-3}$
61 and beyond	16.3 - 31.1	1.7 - 3.5	$< 9.0 \times 10^{-3}$

for their fractionation and identification. The determination of intrathecal production proteins, particularly immunoglobulins, is particularly useful for diagnostic purposes as they indicate a local immune reaction. In many inflammatory conditions such as viral infections, multiple sclerosis, and others, immunoglobulins of the IgA, IgM, and especially IgG classes are found in the CSF, which are indicative of "intrathecal synthesis" universally recognized as a marker for many pathological conditions. The concentration of various classes of immunoglobulins in the CSF, as well as that of albumin, is approximately one hundred times lower than in the blood and varies depending on age (Table 6.2). For a rapid diagnosis of inflammatory diseases of the central nervous system (CNS), it is important to identify, as early as possible and with maximum sensitivity, a local immune response in the CSF, which means discriminating between IgG derived from blood and/or IgG intrathecal synthesis. For this purpose, mathematical formulas have been developed to calculate the intrathecal synthesis of IgG, taking into account both the CSF and blood concentrations of IgG and albumin. These formulas can be classified into two groups:

I. Linear Functions:

a) Link Index

$$\text{Link Index} = \frac{\text{IgG cerebrospinal fluid (CSF)}}{\text{IgG serum x Albumin serum}}$$

Normal values are considered to be <0.65; any value above this indicates intrathecal synthesis of IgG. Similar indices can also be calculated for IgA and IgM (Link, 1977).

b) Tourtellotte Index or IgG Synthesis Rate (mg/day)

II. Non-linear or Hyperbolic Functions: In all cases where there is a disruption of the blood-brain barrier, the intrathecal production of IgG is calculated using a non-linear function based on the Reiber and Felgenhauer formula (Figure 6.9).

6.1.6 Oligoclonal Band Search

To determine if the intrathecal synthesis of IgG (suggested by an increase in CSF IgG and a Link index value > 0.65) is oligoclonal

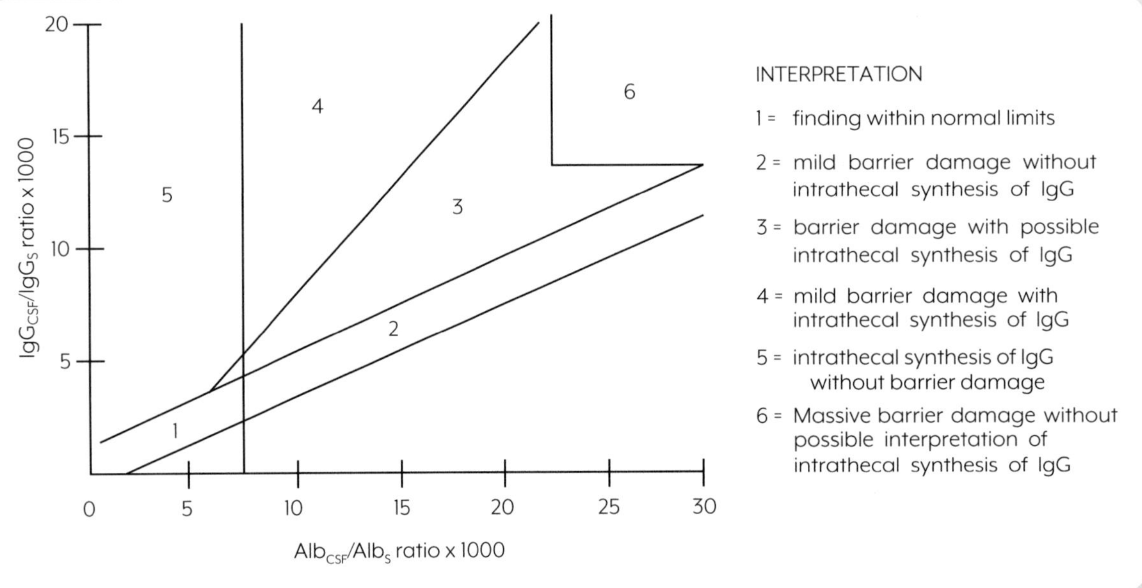

Figure 6.9

Interpretation of the Reiber chart: graphical evolution for different dysfunctions of the blood-brain barrier. On the x-axis: values of the ratio between the concentration of Albumin in the cerebrospinal fluid (CSF) and that in the serum; on the y-axis: values of the ratio between the concentration of IgG in the CSF and that in the serum. The numbers indicate the possible patterns.

in nature (resulting from the activation of individual B cell clones), it is necessary to search for oligoclonal IgG bands (OCBs). The most commonly used method involves isoelectric focusing of the CSF and serum proteins of each patient, followed by immunoblotting.

Isoelectric Focusing | Samples of CSF and serum from each patient, diluted in physiological solution to achieve the same IgG concentrations, are deposited into wells on an agarose gel with a pH gradient (3.5-9) and subjected to electrophoretic migration. Under these conditions, the proteins migrate on the gel until they reach their corresponding isoelectric point (zero charge).

Immunoblotting | After electrophoretic migration, the proteins are transferred (blotted) from the agarose gel to a nitrocellulose membrane by placing the gel in contact with the membrane, and the protein transfer onto the membrane occurs through capillarity. The membrane is incubated with a peroxidase-conjugated anti-IgG antibody and subsequently incubated with a substrate / chromogen solution. After the reaction development, the presence of IgG is detected as colored bands on the membrane corresponding to the alkaline pH region of the isoelectric focusing gel. IgG oligoclonal pattern refers to the presence of two or more bands in the CSF that are not present in the corresponding serum. The European Consensus identifies five distinct patterns (Figure 6.10). In multiple sclerosis, it is believed that the oligoclonal bands are mostly composed of complete IgG, while the detection of IgA and IgM is very rare. One characteristic of multiple sclerosis is that oligoclonal bands remain as an immunological "scar." In other diseases, however, the oligoclonal bands can change or disappear completely during the course of the disease. The increased synthesis of light and free chains accompanies the conditions of increased IgG production, both systemically and within the blood-brain barrier. In multiple sclerosis, an increased synthesis of K-type light chains has been documented in 90-95% of cases, with a higher specificity for the oligoclonal IgG fractions.

Oligoclonal bands are observed in meningoencephalitis, cerebral vasculitis, lupus, paraneoplastic neurological syndromes, and even in conditions that do not seem to have an immune-mediated component, such as Alzheimer's disease, motor neuron disease, primary metastatic brain tumors, and even cerebrovascular diseases such as subarachnoid hemorrhage. Therefore, despite their high sensitivity, the presence of oligoclonal bands is not specific to any CNS disease.

Figure 6.10

Immunoblot for the detection of IgG in cerebrospinal fluid (CSF) compared to serum (S) from the same subject in the 5 typical patterns identified by the European Consensus. 1. Normal pattern, characterized by a diffuse background of polyclonal IgG identical in CSF and serum; 2. Intrathecal synthesis pattern (oligoclonal IgG) characterized by the presence of at least two oligoclonal bands in CSF and absent in the corresponding serum; 3. "Mixed" pattern characterized by the simultaneous presence of patterns 2 and 5; 4. "Paraproteinemia" or paraproteinemic pattern, similar to the previous one but characterized by regularly spaced oligoclonal IgG bands in a pH gradient range, present in myeloma or benign paraproteins; 5. "Mirror" pattern characterized by the presence of oligoclonal bands in the serum and CSF at the same isoelectric point, indicative of systemic immune activation (gammopathy) with passive transudation of oligoclonal IgG from serum to CSF through an intact or altered barrier.

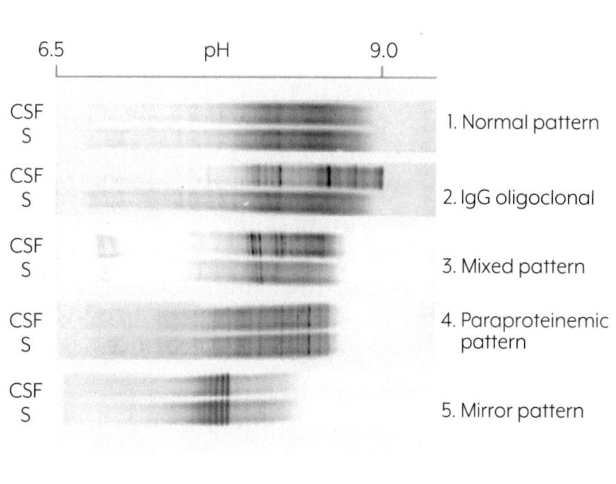

6.1.7 Quantification of specific antiviral antibody synthesis in cerebrospinal fluid

Immunoenzymatic methods (ELISA, etc.) allow for the evaluation of the concentration of pathogen-specific antibodies in cerebrospinal fluid (CSF) and serum. Their presence is diagnostically relevant in both acute infections, characterized by a monospecific immune reaction of the causative agent (such as herpes simplex, herpes zoster, HIV, toxoplasma, cytomegalovirus, measles, and Borrelia), and chronic inflammatory conditions (such as multiple sclerosis, chronic neuroborreliosis, and neurolupus) where virus-specific antibodies are produced as part of a polyspecific immune response.

Demonstration of the pathogen | Early diagnosis of the etiology of many inflammatory diseases of the central nervous system (CNS) is now possible through the application of PCR analysis of cerebrospinal fluid. PCR is a highly sensitive and specific method for rapid identification of genomic DNA from pathogenic microorganisms or viral particles in biological fluids and tissues.

6.2 Autoimmune diseases of the nervous system

An antibody response can occur as an expression of immune system activation against neuronal components in both the central nervous system (CNS) and the peripheral nervous system (PNS). This pathological immune system activation can involve:

a) The CNS (demyelinating diseases and encephalitis, paraneoplastic and non-paraneoplastic cerebellar syndromes, stiff person syndrome, and encephalomyelopathies) (Table 6.3a);
b) The peripheral nervous system (acute, subacute, and chronic radiculopleuropathies, paraneoplastic neuropathies) (Table 6.3b);
c) The neuromuscular junction (Table 6.3c);
d) The visual optic system (Table 6.3d).

The search for autoantibodies can be performed in the serum, cerebrospinal fluid, or other biological samples. In fact, antibodies

Table 6.3a CENTRAL NERVOUS SYSTEM

Demyelinating diseases and focal encephalitis
Type II histopathological multiple sclerosis
Hyperacute MS
Neuromyelitis optica (Devic's syndrome)
Rasmussen's encephalitis
Bickerstaff's brainstem encephalitis
Paraneoplastic syndromes
Limbic encephalitis
Cerebellar degeneration
Opsoclonus-myoclonus
Paraneoplastic Stiff-person syndrome
Necrotizing myelopathy
Morvan's chorea
Non-paraneoplastic cerebellar ataxias
GAD ataxia
Gluten ataxia (gliadin)
Stiff-person syndrome and encephalomyelopathic variants
Stiff-person syndrome
Progressive encephalomyelitis with rigidity (PEMR)
Stiff-limb syndrome
Jerking SMS

Table 6.3b PERIPHERAL NERVOUS SYSTEM

Acute/subacute and chronic radiculopathy(poly) neuropathies
Guillain-Barré syndrome and variants
Chronic inflammatory demyelinating polyneuropathy (CIDP)
Motor neuropathy with conduction blocks (MMNP)
Lewis-Sumner syndrome
Monoclonal gammopathy-associated neuropathies
Paraneoplastic neuronopathies
Sensory neuropathies
Subacute sensory-motor neuropathy
Peripheral nerve vasculitis
Peripheral nerve hyperexcitability syndrome
Autonomic neuropathy
Motor neuron disease

Table 6.3c NEUROMUSCULAR JUNCTION

Lambert-Eaton myasthenic syndrome
Myasthenia gravis
Polymyositis/dermatomyositis
Acute necrotizing myopathy
Carcinoid myopathy
Cachectic myopathy
Myotonia

Table 6.3d OPTIC-VISUAL SYSTEM

Autoimmune (Optic neuritis, CRION)
Paraneoplastic
Retinopathy (CAR, MAR)
Uveitis (typically associated with encephalomyelitis)

directed against antigens expressed by nerve cells, which are useful in the diagnosis of paraneoplastic diseases such as cerebellar degeneration and limbic encephalitis, are commonly found in the serum. The clinical situation will guide the research and, therefore, the measurement of antibodies directed against specific neuronal antigens (Tables 6.4 and 6.5). Two techniques can be used for the identification of these antibodies:

1) *Indirect immunofluorescence* on sections of brain tissue or peripheral nerve (Figure 6.11);
2) *Immunoblot*, where the presence of autoantibodies is tested by incubating the biological sample with specific antigens (Figure 6.12).

Among the autoantibodies of particular diagnostic importance, a recent discovery has identified an autoantibody in the serum

Table 6.4 ANTIBODIES IN PARANEOPLASTIC NERVOUS SYSTEM DISORDERS

Antigen	Paraneoplastic disorder	Associated tumor
Recoverin	Retinopathy	SCLC
Yo (PCA-1)	PCD	SCLC
Ma (Ma-1)	PCD, BE	Various
Ta (Ma-2)	BE, LE	Testicle
Hu (ANNA1)	PCD, PEM, BE	SCLS
Ri (ANNA2)	OM, PCD, BE	Breast, SCLC, Gynecological tumors
GAD	SMS	Breast, colon, SCLC
CV2 / CRMP4	PEN, SN	Thymoma, SCLC
Amphiphysin	SMS, SN	Breast, SCLC
mGluR1	PCD	Hodgkin's lymphoma
ANNA3	PCD, SN, PEM	SCLC
PCA-2	PEM, PCD, LEMS	SCLC
AGNA	PND	SCLC
Tr	PCD	Hodgkin's lymphoma

PCD, Paraneoplastic Cerebellar Degeneration; BE, Brainstem Encephalitis; LEM, Limbic Encephalitis; PEM, Paraneoplastic Encephalomyelitis; OM, Opsoclonus/Myoclonus; SMS, Stiff-Person Syndrome; SN, Sensory Neuropathy; LEMS, Lambert-Eaton Myasthenic Syndrome; PNS, Paraneoplastic Myasthenic Syndrome; PND, Paraneoplastic Neurological Disorders; SCLC, Small Cell Lung Carcinoma

Table 6.5 ANTI-NERVE ANTIBODIES IN IMMUNE-MEDIATED NEUROPATHIES

Antigen	Antibody isotype	Associated clinical form	Frequency of antibody	Type of clinical involvement	Nerve pathology
MAG/SGP/PO	IgM	PN+IgM	50%	S>>M	Demyelinating
Chondroitin sulfate C	IgM	PN+IgM	1%	SM	Axonal
Sulfatides	IgM	PN axonal PN+IgM	? 5%	S, S>M, SM SM	Axonal Demyelinating
Trisulfated heparin disaccharide	IgM	PN+IgM	8%	S>>M	Axonal
β-tubulina	IgM	CIDP	57%	M>>S	Demyelinating
GM1	IgM IgG	MMN±IgM GBS	20-80% 20-30%	M M>>S	Focal demyelination Axonal?
GM2	IgM IgG+IgM	PN+IgM GBS	? 6%	M>S SM	Demyelinating
GD1a	IgM IgG	PN+IgM GBS	2% >5%	M M>>S	demyelination Axonal?
Diasialo gangliosides (GD1b/GD1q)	IgM	PN+IgM	2%	S>>M	Demyelinating
GQ1b	IgG	MFS	>90%	MFS	Axonal

PN, Polyneuropathy; SM, S>>M, M>>S, M, S, Sensory Motor Neuropathy, predominantly sensory or motor, motor or sensory; PN+IgM, Neuropathy associated with IgM monoclonal gammopathy; CDIP, Chronic inflammatory demyelinating polyneuropathy; GBS, Guillain-Barré syndrome; MFS, Miller Fisher syndrome; MMN, Multifocal motor neuropathy

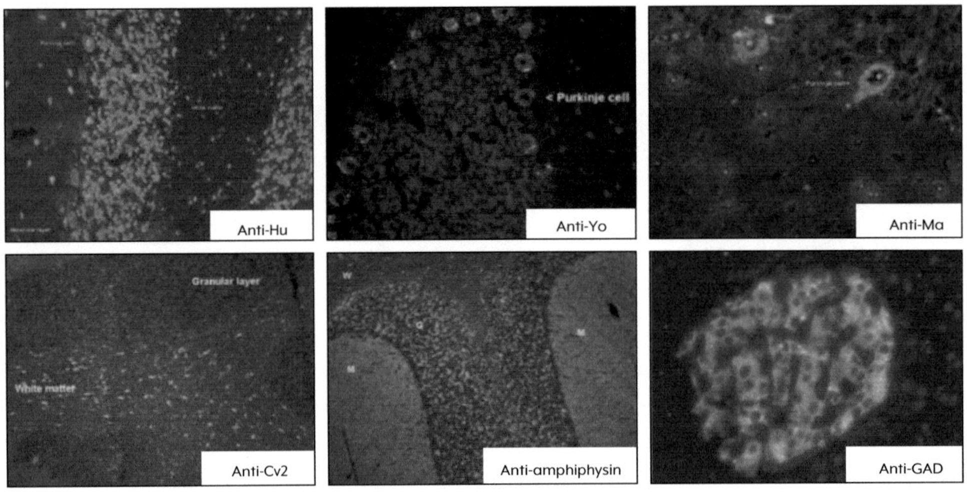

Figure 6.11

Indirect immunofluorescence on sections of brain or pancreatic tissue (for anti-GAD).

of patients with neuromyelitis optica (NMO) (absent in the serum of patients with multiple sclerosis or other inflammatory pathologies characterized by optic neuropathies or myelopathies). This autoantibody targets aquaporin-4 (AQP-4), the most abundant water-channel protein in the CNS. This discovery has made NMO the first demyelinating inflammatory pathology of the CNS to have a known autoantigen (Lennon et al., 2005). In 20% of NMO patients negative for anti-AQP-4 IgG, there are anti-myelin oligodendrocyte glycoprotein (MOG) antibodies. The combination of these two highly specific serological markers (anti-AQP-4 and anti-MOG) allows differentiation between NMO and multiple sclerosis.

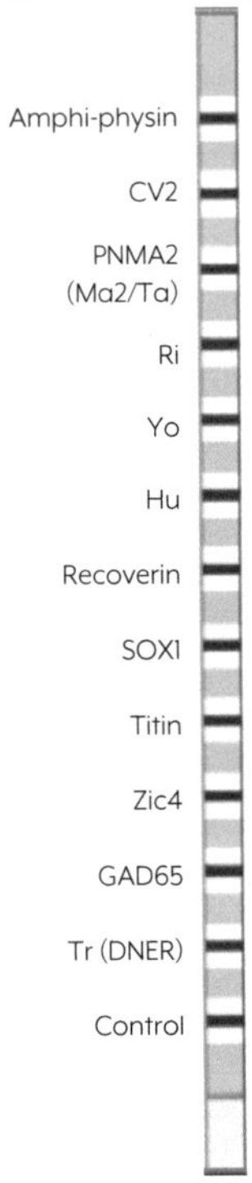

Figure 6.12

In immunoblot, the presence of autoantibodies is tested by incubating the biological sample with specific antigens.

In the autoimmune diagnosis of certain encephalopathies, the demonstration of the presence of antibodies against neuronal cell surface antigens is decisive. The antibodies are directed against glutamate receptors (NMDA or AMPA type), GABA B receptors, DPPX, voltage-gated potassium channels (anti-VGKC), or associated proteins (LGI1, CASPR2, TAG-1/contactin-2). Since these antigens play a direct or indirect role in synaptic signal transduction, associated autoimmune pathologies are typically characterized by epileptic seizures and neuropsychiatric symptoms. The resulting conditions include specific forms of autoimmune limbic encephalitis, neuromyotonia, or Morvan syndrome. These severe and potentially life-threatening syndromes can have a non-paraneoplastic etiology. The frequency of underlying tumors varies from 10 to 70% depending on the antibody type. The antibodies most likely play a causal role in the pathogenesis. Appropriate therapy (immunomodulatory intervention, tumor resection) leads to significant symptom regression in most patients, and early diagnosis is important for a favorable prognosis.

In Hashimoto's encephalitis, elevated serum and cerebrospinal fluid concentrations of thyroid autoantibodies have been reported: anti-thyroid peroxidase antibodies (AbTPO) and anti-thyroglobulin antibodies (AbTg), along with increased intrathecal production of oligoclonal IgG, detectable only in the cerebrospinal fluid. The diagnosis of Hashimoto's encephalopathy is mainly based on demonstrating high titers of thyroid antibodies during encephalitis and the effective response to corticosteroid therapy. Pathogenetic mechanisms include the possibility of vasculitis due to deposition of circulating immune complexes or, alternatively, an autoimmune reaction involving a common antigen between the thyroid and the brain (Table 6.6).

Table 6.6 OTHER IMPORTANT ANTIBODIES FOR DIAGNOSTIC PURPOSES

Antigen	Disease	Possible associated tumor
AQP-4, MOG	Neuromyelitis optica	
NMDA	Limbic encephalitis (psychiatric and behavioral abnormalities, memory impairment, movement disorders, seizures)	
AMPA	Encephalitis (hippocampus, cortex, basal ganglia, spinal cord)	Lung, thymus
GABA A	Acute encephalitis with status epilepticus	
GABA B	Typical limbic encephalitis (memory loss, seizures, behavioral changes)	Small cell lung carcinoma 50%
DPPX	Limbic Encephalitis (diarrhea, predominant hyperexcitability, memory loss)	
VGKC	Neuromyotonia	Lung, thymus, hodgkin
LGI 1	Limbic Encephalitis (medial temporal lobe)	
CASPR2	Morvan's syndrome	
TAG-1/contactin-2	Encephalitis (variable clinical manifestations)	
TPO, TG	Hashimoto's Encephalitis	

6.2.1 Research and demonstration of specific proteins

The search for certain proteins in the cerebrospinal fluid (CSF) can be of great importance for diagnosis.

This is the case with *beta2-transferrin* , an 827-amino acid glycoprotein involved in iron transport, which constitutes 10% of the CSF proteins compared to 4% of total serum proteins. Its serum electrophoretic mobility is in the beta1 region and shows 2 bands (Figure 6.13). Simply measuring glucose is not sufficient to use it as a marker for the sample.

In addition to these 2 bands in the beta1 region, transferrin in the CSF presents 2 other bands in the beta2 region, which constitute the "tau fraction" of CSF. Tau-transferrin accounts for 15% of the total concentration of transferrin in the CSF and is immunologically similar to the main fraction. *Clinical application:* The demonstration that beta2-transferrin is the product of a CSF fistula (e.g., rhinorrhea, otorrhea, etc.) is a fundamental diagnostic criterion and an integral part of the protocol for closing the fistula. The presence or absence of the tau-transferrin bands provides indications about the nature of the sample.

Beta-trace | Beta-Trace protein (betaTP), named for its position in electrophoretic migration, is a recently identified single-chain glycoprotein. It has prostaglandin D-synthetase7 enzymatic activity and is produced by the ependymal cells of the choroid plexus and secreted into the CSF. Its concentration in the CSF is approximately 35 times higher than in serum. BetaTP is a quantitative marker in nasal secretions strongly indicative of CSF fistula. A concentration of betaTP greater than 1.5 mg/L alone provides a definite diagnosis.

Prion Protein or Prion | It is believed that the pathogenic mechanism of transmissible spongiform encephalopathies is related to the presence of the protein called "prion," responsible for neuronal degeneration. The sporadic variant of spongiform encephalopathy, known as Creutzfeldt-Jakob disease, recognizes the protein 14-3-3 as a biological marker,

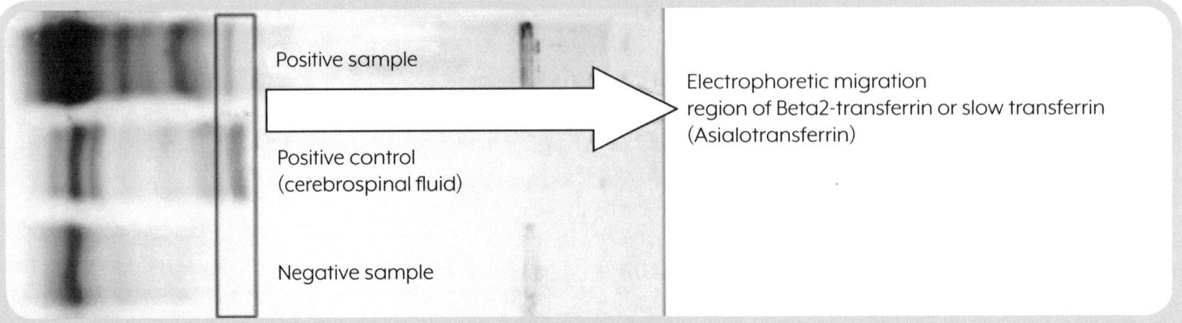

Figure 6.13

Beta2-transferrin (asialotransferrin). The presence or absence of the Beta2-transferrin band provides indications about the nature of the sample (cerebrospinal fluid). Beta2-transferrin is normally present in the cerebrospinal fluid (used as a positive control), but not in nasal mucus (negative control). Being the isoform of transferrin devoid of sialic acid groups, it separates easily with the isoelectric focusing (IEF) method. Beta2-transferrin is also present in the serum, accounting for approximately 4% of the total transferrin; therefore, the optimal sample to undergo IEF is the one free from blood contamination.

expressed by both neurons and glial cells and released into the CSF, where it can be detected by a specific antibody in an immunoblot. The test, with a predictive value of 92%, has a diagnostic sensitivity of 94% and specificity of 90%, values that can be further increased (98% and 100%, respectively) if tau proteins and A 1-42 are also measured.

Beta2-microglobulin | It is a potential prognostic marker in patients with HIV-1 infection. In fact, in HIV-1-seropositive individuals, CSF concentrations of beta2-microglobulin > 5mg/L increase the risk of developing HIV-related neurological disease by 17 times.

Proteins in Neurodegenerative Diseases (Dementia) | An increasing number of studies, thanks to expanding knowledge about CSF composition and its alterations in various pathologies, have proposed a series of proteins as biological markers for different diseases and, therefore, as tools for early diagnosis.

Firstly, it has been found that patients with Alzheimer's disease have elevated concentrations of beta-amyloid and phosphorylated tau protein (P-tau) in the CSF compared to age-matched individuals without the disease.

Beta-amyloid | is the main component of amyloid (or senile) plaques and originates from the *Amyloid Precursor Protein* (APP) in a two-step process. APP is a membrane protein encoded by a gene located on chromosome 21, and its function is to promote cell growth. Specifically, it is a transmembrane protein expressed in various types of cells, particularly in the brain, heart, spleen, and kidneys. At least 10 isoforms have been identified so far, derived from alternative splicing. The three most common isoforms are called C (predominantly present in neurons), B (common in T lymphocytes), and A, consisting of 695, 751, and 770 amino acids, respectively.

Tau | It is a phosphoprotein associated with microtubules located mainly in neuronal axons. It exists in six isoforms with variable molecular weights ranging from 50 to 65 kDa, characterized by 30 potential phosphorylation sites. Its function is to promote microtubule assembly and stability, allowing for transport along the axon. The neurofibrillary tangles found in individuals with Alzheimer's disease consist of hyperphosphorylated Tau protein. In this state, the molecule has reduced binding capacity to microtubules and decreases their stability, hindering their function. Tau levels in the CSF reflect the extent of neuronal damage. Elevated levels of Tau have been observed in individuals with cerebral infarction, Creutzfeldt-Jakob disease, and Alzheimer's disease, while normal levels of this marker have been found in individuals with depression, alcoholic dementia, and Parkinson's disease.

P-Tau | It is the hyperphosphorylated form of Tau protein, not only a marker of neuronal damage but also providing information about the phosphorylation status of Tau in individuals with Alzheimer's disease. It reflects the progression of neurofibrillary degeneration. Normal or slightly increased levels have been found in individuals with Creutzfeldt-Jakob disease, while a marked increase has been observed in individuals with Alzheimer's disease (Table 6.7).

Phosphorylation of P-Tau is an essential condition for its subsequent deposition in neurofibrillary tangles, which in turn are the cause of neuronal degeneration. P-tau is, therefore, a reliable and specific indicator of the degenerative process that underlies Alzheimer's disease.

The combined determination of three protein markers in cerebrospinal fluid can increase the sensitivity and specificity of the diagnosis, providing a laboratory data that, when associated with the patient's clinical condition, can help the clinician identify which individuals with cognitive deficits and neurological alterations will progress toward Alzheimer's disease or other forms of dementia. Therefore, currently, the primary indication for these three markers is the differential diagnosis among different types of dementia (Alzheimer's, frontotemporal, Lewy body, vascular). From a practical perspective, due to the markers' limited stability, especially beta-amyloid, the following pre-analytical procedures are recommended:

- sterile polypropylene collection tubes;
- exclusion of blood samples;
- centrifugation at 2000 rpm for 10 minutes at 4°C;
- storage at –80°C in sterile polypropylene tubes, avoiding repeated freeze-thaw cycles.

Table 6.7 INCREASE IN TOTAL TAU PROTEIN, PHOSPHORYLATED AND NON-PHOSPHORYLATED (T-TAU) IN CEREBROSPINAL FLUID OF ALZHEIMER'S DISEASE PATIENTS

Around 300% compared to healthy controls and other dementias	
Age-related:	
21-50 years	< 300 pg/ml
51-70 years	< 450 pg/ml
70-93 years	< 500 pg/ml
Specificity	65 – 85%
Sensitivity	40 – 86%

Lactate and Pyruvate | Investigations into cerebral metabolism, mentioned in relation to CSF glucose levels, are further explored by measuring lactate and pyruvate in the CSF (using spectrophotometry). The lactate/pyruvate ratio reflects the state of cerebral energy metabolism. Under physiological conditions, the concentration of lactate in the CSF is 9.90-21.90 mg/dl and is independent of serum levels because the molecule is ionized and therefore poorly crosses the blood-brain barrier. An increase in CSF lactate is found in inflammatory processes, particularly those of bacterial or fungal etiology (where CSF glucose decreases), providing greater indications of glycorrachia in the differential diagnosis compared to viral meningitis (where lactate levels remain within the physiological range). Lactate production is due to glucose consumption through anaerobic pathways, and its levels correlate with the severity of prognosis. Any cause of cerebral hypoxia (CNS hemorrhage, abscess, trauma, seizures, cerebral arteriosclerosis, hypotension) is responsible for elevated CSF lactate. It remains elevated after the start of therapy, so it is not a good marker of therapeutic response, but it does indicate the presence of infection even in patients undergoing antibiotic treatment.

The measurement of lactate in the CSF is diagnostically useful in support of a mitochondrial encephalopathy hypothesis.

6.2.2 Bacteriology and Virology

Direct research of microorganisms

Neurosyphilis | The extreme difficulty in isolating the etiological agent (*Treponema pallidum*) in cerebrospinal fluid and cultivating it in vivo has led researchers to develop highly sensitive and reliable specific tests. The first screening test is VDRL (Veneral Disease Research Laboratory), which involves a rapid flocculation test. Although it is a fairly sensitive examination, it is poorly specific. It can yield positive results even in the absence of syphilis, such as during pregnancy, autoimmune diseases (lupus, rheumatoid arthritis), acute viral infections (hepatitis, chickenpox, measles, mononucleosis), or chronic or bacterial infections (leprosy, tuberculosis, malaria). The TPHA test, or agglutination test (Treponema Pallidum Hemoagglutination Test), on the other hand, has greater specificity as it tends to remain positive for a long time regardless of therapy. Therefore, in the presence of a positive VDRL result, a confirmatory TPHA test should be performed. Microorganisms are directly sought by collecting fresh cerebrospinal fluid in sterile tubes, prior to initiating any therapy. Gram staining is used for bacterial flora, while Ziehl-Neelsen staining is used for fungi. Subsequently, cultivation is performed on specific media to promote the growth of fungi and aerobic and anaerobic germs. Cryptococci are directly identified using the India ink test.

Virus research | Utilizing techniques such as ELISA, RIA, and Western blot, viral antigens can be searched for in cerebrospinal fluid. However, currently, an early etiological diagnosis of many viral diseases, and not only, is possible with the DNA amplification technique using PCR (Polymerase Chain Reaction), a highly sensitive, specific, and rapid method: within a few hours, genomic DNA of pathogenic microorganisms or viruses in tissues and biological fluids such as cerebrospinal fluid can be identified. On the other hand, the isolation of viral particles requires several weeks and is carried out on cell cultures, chicken embryos, and laboratory animals.

Research of anti-viral antibodies | The most frequently employed techniques for serological diagnosis are ELISA, RIA, and Western blot, which allow for the identification of specific anti-viral antibodies, as well as their quantitative determination in the form of a titer (i.e., the highest dilution of the sample at which the test still yields positive results). Mathematical formulas, both linear

Table 6.8 ANALYTICAL PARAMETERS IN CEREBROSPINAL FLUID FOR NERVOUS SYSTEM DISORDERS

Pathological condition	Appearance, pressure (P), particular findings	Leukocytes/μl	Prevalent leukocytes	Proteins mg/100ml	Blood-brain barrier	Glucose
Cerebral abscess	Clear, Increased P	5-100	Granulocytes	50-100	Normal or altered	Decreased in 98% of cases
CNS parasitic infections		< 30	Eosinophils		Normal or altered	
Tabes dorsalis and progressive paralysis	Clear, Normal P, increased globulins, positive specific reactions	15-150	Lymphocytes	45-100	Altered	Normal
Brain tumors	Clear, Normal or increased P, tumor cells in 20%	5-20	Lymphocytes	75-100	Altered	Normal
Meningeal carcinomatosis	Clear or turbid, Normal or increased P, tumor cells in 80%	5-500	Lymphocytes	45-1000	Altered	Diminuito
Spinal tumors	Clear or xanthochromic, Normal or decreased P, massive reticulation or coagulation	5-100	Lymphocytes	50-3000	Altered	Normal
Subarachnoid hemorrhage	Bloody or xanthochromic, Increased P, erythrocytes	up to 2000	Same as in blood	50-1000	Altered	Normal or decreased
Cerebral hemorrhage	Bloody or xanthochromic clear in 20%, increased P, erythrocytes	up to 2000; normal in 20% of cases	Same as in blood	15-1000	Altered	Normal or decreased
Cerebral infarction	Clear, Normal or increased P	0-50	Lymphocytes, granulocytes	15-100	Altered	Normal
Guillain-Barré syndrome	Clear or xanthochromic, Normal P, protein-cell dissociation, oligoclonal bands in 30%	0-15	Lymphocytes	15-600	Altered	Normal
Diabetic neuropathy	Clear, Normal P, protein-cell dissociation	0-5	Lymphocytes		Normal	60-80% of the value in blood

Table 6.9 ANALYTICAL PARAMETERS IN CEREBROSPINAL FLUID INFLAMMATORY DISEASES

Clinical picture	Appearance, Pressure (P), Specific findings	Leukocytes/µl	Prevalent leukocytes	Activated B lymphocytes	Proteins (mg/100ml)	Blood-brain barrier	Intrathecal synthesis of antibodies, (*) predominant class, (■) detected since the onset or during the course of the disease (Δ)			Glucose (% case)
							Oligoclonal IgG	IgM	IgA	
Acute bacterial meningitis	Turbid, increased P, bacteria, positive culture tests	< 30 – < 300 (reparative phase) > 300 (proliferative exudative phase)	Granulocytes	Present	50-1500	Altered	Δ (40% of cases)		Δ*	Decreased (98%)
Viral Meningitis	Clear, normal or Increased P	< 300 - > 300	Lymphocytes	Present	50-100	Normal or altered				Decreased (20%)
Herpes Simplex Encephalitis	Clear, normal or increased P	< 30; < 300; > 300	Lymphocytes	Absent	15-400	Normal or altered	Δ (98% of cases)	Δ	Δ*	Decreased (20%)
Herpes Zoster Meningitis	Clear, normal or increased P	< 30 - <300	Lymphocytes	Present		Normal or altered	Δ (40% of cases)			Normal
HIV	Clear, normal or increased P	< 30	Lymphocytes	Present		Normal or altered	Δ (40% of cases)	Δ*		Normal
Mumps	Clear or opalescent, normal orincreased P	< 30; < 300; > 300	Lymphocytes, granulocytes	Absent		Normal	Δ (40% of cases)	Δ	Δ	Decreased (30%)
Posterior Encephalomyelitis	Clear, normal P	< 30	Lymphocytes	Presenti	15-80	Normal	Δ (40% of cases)	Δ		Decreased (50%?)
Fungal Meningitis	Clear, opalescent or turbid, Normal or Increased P, viscous, fungi, positive culture: specific antigens and antibodies	< 30 - < 300	Initially granulocytes, later iymphocytes	Absent	50-500	Normal or altered	Δ (50% of cases)			Decreased (90%)
Tuberculous Meningitis	Clear, opalescent or turbid, Increased P, Koch's bacillus in 20%, positive culture in 80%, Mya's reticulum not constant	< 30 (adhesive arachnoiditis) < 300 (granulomatous phase) > 300 (recurrent invasive phase)	Lymphocytes, monocytes, granulocytes	Present	50-500	Altered	■ (50% of cases)		■*	Decreased (90%)
Neurosyphilis	Clear or opalescent, normal P, VDRL and TPHA positive	0 - < 300	Lymphocytes granulocytes	Present	45-100	Normal or altered	■ (80% of cases)	■*		Decreased (50%)
Acute neuroborreliosis	Clear or opalescent, normal P	< 300	Lymphocytes, monocytes	Present		Altered	■* (50% of cases)	■*	■	Normal
Chronic Neuroborreliosis	Clear, normal P	0 - 5	Lymphocytes, monocytes	Absent		Normal or altered	■ (40%of cases)	■		Normal
Multiple Sclerosis	Clear, normal P	0 - 5 < 30 (in 61% of case)	Lymphocytes, plasma cells	Present (91% of case)	50-100	Normal (20% of case)	■ (98% of cases)	■	■	Normal
Opportunistic toxoplasmosis	Clear, normal P	0 - 5	Lymphocytes, eosinophils	Absent		Normal or altered	■ (40% of cases)	■	■	Decreased (70%)
CMV Opportunistic Infection	Clear, normal P	0 - 5	Lymphocytes	Absent		Normal or altered	■ (40% of cases)	■	■	Decreased (30%)
Neurolupus	Clear, normal P	< 30	Lymphocytes, monocytes	Absent		Normal	■ (40% of cases)			Normal
Neurobrucellosis	Clear, normal P	< 30	Lymphocytes	Absent		Normal	■ (40% of cases)			Decreased (90%)

and nonlinear, can be applied to assess the intrathecal synthesis of specific antibodies across various classes of immunoglobulins. Acute neurosyphilis and neuroborreliosis exhibit a predominance of intra-blood-brain-barrier synthesis of IgM. Neurotuberculosis, bacterial meningoencephalitis, and Herpes simplex have a higher frequency of IgA synthesis, in contrast to multiple sclerosis and HIV infection. The main cerebrospinal fluid patterns of the nervous system are summarized in Tables 6.8 e 6.9.

Bibliography

Avasarala J.R., Cross A., Trotter J.L., Oligoclonal band number as a marker for prognosis in Multiple Sclerosis. Arch Neurol; 58:20442045, 2001.

Cruickshank A.M, Revision of national guidelines for cerebrospinal fluid analysis in suspected subarachnoid haemorrage. Ann Cli Biochem; 45:236-238, 2008.

Lennon V.A. et al., A serum autoantibody marker of neuromyelitis optica: distinction from multiple sclerosis. Lancet; 364:21062112, 2004.

Probstel A.K. et al., Anti-MOG antibodies are present in a subgroup of patients with a neuromyelitis optica phenotype. J Neuroinflammation; 12:46-52, 2015.

Reiber H., Felgenhauer K., Protein transfer at the blood-cerebrospinal fluid barrier and the quantification of the humoral immune response in the central nervous system. Clin Chim Acta; 163:319-328, 1987.

Reske D., Petereit H.F., Heiss W.D., Difficulties in the differentiation of chronic inflammatory diseases of the central nervous system value of cerebrospinal fluid analysis and immunological abnormalities in the diagnosis. Acta Neurol Scand; 112(4): 207-213, 2005.

Tourtellotte W.W., Potviv A.R., Fleming J.O. et al., Multiple sclerosis: measurement and validation of central nervous system IgG synthesis rate. Neurology; 30:240-244, 1980.

7

ELECTROENCEPHALOGRAPHY AND RELATED TECHNIQUES

Oriano Mecarelli, Patrizia Pulitano, Edoardo Vicenzini

The electroencephalogram (EEG) is an instrumental investigation that allows the recording, from the scalp, of the brain's bioelectric activity. The extracellular currents, recordable as an EEG signal, originate from the pyramidal cortical neurons and the topographic organization of their dendrites, which are parallel to each other and perpendicular to the cortical surface. The synchronized activity of large cellular aggregates can be detected by extracellular recordings, and in these cases, the recorded signals are called *field potentials*.

Surface EEG can therefore be considered as the result of *field potentials* produced by fluctuations in the electrical activity of large populations of cortical neurons. These extracellular current flows are generated by the spatial summation of postsynaptic potentials of activated cells. The synchronous activation of over 100 cortical neurons in an area of at least 6 cm^2 is necessary to produce an EEG signal, whose amplitude depends mainly on the synchronization of the activated cells.

To understand the importance of cortical cell synchronization in the generation of the EEG, it is necessary to keep in mind that the electrical contribution of each cortical neuron is minimal and that the signal must pass through various "non-neuronal" layers of tissue, including the meninges, cerebrospinal fluid, cranial bones, and the scalp. Each layer has different conductivity and susceptibility properties that attenuate the electrical signal before it reaches the electrodes placed on the scalp. Consequently, thousands of simultaneously activated neurons are required to generate an EEG signal large enough to be detected on the scalp surface.

The EEG is the graphical representation of the electrical potential difference between an "active" electrode, placed above the site where neuronal activity takes place, and a theoretically "indifferent" electrode located at a certain distance from the first one. It is a dynamic measure since the potential difference is represented as a function of time. Therefore, surface EEG measures the electrical potential difference between different areas of the scalp and reflects the current flowing in the cerebral cortex during the synaptic activation of the dendrites of many pyramidal neurons.

However, considering the EEG solely as the result of cortical electrical activity is limiting. Although subcortical structures produce potentials that are not directly detectable on the scalp due to the decrease in the electric field intensity with the square of the distance from its source, they can still be indirectly recorded by the EEG. EEG rhythms depend on the synchronization of waves derived from the summation of synaptic potentials generated by the activity of thalamo-cortical neurons. The precise role of specific thalamic structures and details about their "pacemaker" activity in the generation of the EEG signal are still being studied.

In light of the extensive neurophysiological basis on which it is founded and the various anatomical structures directly and indirectly explored, electroencephalography, nearly a century after its first use, finds increasing clinical indications. These include the identification of epileptiform activity, differential diagnosis between epileptic and non-epileptic episodes (syncope, psychogenic seizures, cardiac rhythm disorders, etc.), monitoring of antiepileptic therapy, sleep architecture analysis, assessment of consciousness level, monitoring of bioelectrical activity in intensive care and during surgical procedures, and confirmation of its cessation. In brain death diagnosis these are just some of the possible uses of electroencephalography in clinical practice. These indications are further satisfied and expanded by polysomnography, which allows simultaneous recording of muscle activity (using electrodes placed on the muscles under investigation), cardiac activity (ECG), and respiratory activity. For example, the quantitative study of the relationship between the EEG signal and muscle activity (back-averaging) is important for establishing any correlation between involuntary muscle activity and brain activity and for classifying a motor phenomenon as epileptic or non-epileptic (differential diagnosis between cortical and subcortical myoclonus). The simultaneous ECG monitoring can clarify the presence of cardiac rhythm abnormalities, responsible for episodes of loss of consciousness mistakenly interpreted as epileptic seizures.

7.1 EEG Execution Techniques

Electrodes, derivations, and montages

Electrodes serve as the connection system between the brain tissues where the bioelectric activity is generated or conducted and the inputs of the amplifiers. They can come in various types and shapes and constitute an interface between the patient and the recording apparatus. For EEG recordings from the scalp at laboratory, electrodes used are bridge or cup electrodes, held in place on the scalp with elastic or pre-wired headsets or various adhesives. In comatose patients, intradermal needle electrodes are used instead. For studying brain regions that are difficult to investigate using conventional surface electrodes, special invasive or semi-invasive electrodes can be used (sphenoidal, ethmoidal, nasopharyngeal, zygomatic, supraorbital, and tympanic electrodes). In pre-surgical studies of patients with drug-resistant epilepsy, special electrodes such as subdural electrodes (electrocorticography) or depth electrodes (stereoelectroencephalography) are used. Surface electrodes are positioned on the scalp according to the International 10-20 System, a naming convention derived from the percentage calculation of the distance between electrodes along ideal longitudinal and transverse lines drawn from specific anatomical landmarks (nasion, inion, preauricular points). The traditional standard numbering of the International 10-20 System involves placing even-numbered electrodes on the right side of the skull and odd-numbered electrodes on the left side, identifying them with letters that indicate the cranial zone where they are located: Fp2, F4, F8, C4, P4, T4, T6, and O2 for the right hemisphere, and Fp1, F3, F7, C3, P3, T3, T5, and O1 for the left hemisphere. This measurement system, therefore, involves identifying 21 standard electrode positions, including midline electrodes (Fz, Cz, and Pz) and two reference earlobe electrodes (A2 and A1). The development of digital EEG and the advent of advanced techniques (High-Density EEG) have necessitated an increased number of electrodes (> 70), with modifications to their nomenclature as well (10-10 and 10-5 systems). Therefore, the electrodes T4, T3, T6, and T5 are currently referred to as T8, T7, P8, and P7, respectively. Even in routine recordings, it is preferable to apply 25 electrodes on the scalp, adding 2 additional temporal chains to the ones already planned.

In electroencephalography, in addition to electrode placement on the scalp, the combination and connection mode to the amplifiers (montages and derivations) are essential. According to international guidelines, it is necessary to: record at least 16 EEG channels; at least 21 electrodes according to the 10-20 system; use bipolar and referential montages; specify the electrode connections for each channel at the beginning of each montage; maintain continuous lines for electrode connections in bipolar derivations, with equal inter-electrode distances; channels in an anteroposterior direction; add at least 2 polygraphic parameters (e.g., ECG, EMG) to the EEG channels. The choice of montage type depends closely on the type of EEG activity/pattern being studied and its localization (Figure 7.1).

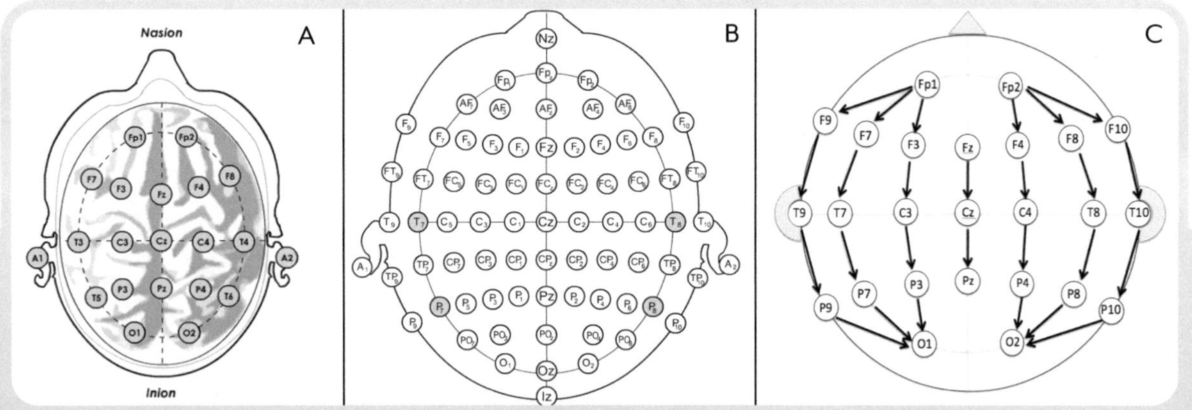

Figure 7.1

A: standard positions of 19 scalp electrodes according to traditional 10-20 system; B: modified 10-10 system, with 73 electrode positions on the scalp; C: new standard montage with 25 electrodes according to the recommendations of International Federation of Clinical Neurophysiology (2017). Note that the electrodes T8, P8, T7, and P7 replace the electrodes formerly named T4, T6, T3, and T5.

7.2 General characteristics of physiological EEG signals and patterns

Rhythms and physiological EEG graphoelements during wakefulness | The brain's bioelectrical activity is represented by EEG in the form of graphoelements, and to distinguish between physiological and pathological patterns, it is necessary to analyze their fundamental characteristics of morphology, localization, appearance mode, and repetitiveness.

Morphology identifies the graphoelement as a whole, that is, it expresses how it appears. This concept includes other aspects such as duration, which refers to the time interval between the beginning and end of a single wave or complex, expressed in milliseconds (ms). The waveform shape (rounded, pointed) is directly correlated to the duration (pointed graphoelements generally have a shorter duration compared to rounded ones). Phase refers to the point at which the signal leaves the isoelectric line, distinguishing between mono- and polyphasic signals. If a signal appears in different channels of bipolar derivations with common electrodes, the phenomenon of phase opposition (phase reversal) may occur: the graphoelement in the upper channel will have a different phase from the one below, with the two pointed peaks tending to coincide.

The amplitude of a graphoelement, that is, its height, depends on its voltage and is expressed in mV. It is measured "peak-to-peak," and the voltage value of the signal (mV/mm) is given by the product of the "peak-to-peak" wave height in mm and the sensitivity of the amplifier.

In the case of regular signals (or graphoelements) that repeat within a unit of time, the fundamental parameter to evaluate is the frequency, which refers to the number of complete cycles of repetitive waves or complexes occurring in one second. This parameter is expressed in Hertz (Hz), not cycles per second.

Since EEG is the graphical representation of the bioelectrical activity of different brain regions, the evaluation of the topographic localization of graphoelements based on electrode placement on the scalp is essential. Thus, a graphoelement can be focal when it is represented only in a specific brain region, multifocal if present in different regions of a single hemisphere or both hemispheres, or diffuse or generalized if uniformly or synchronously present in both hemispheres. Additionally, the comparison between signals recorded from multiple channels in both hemispheres must always be performed to

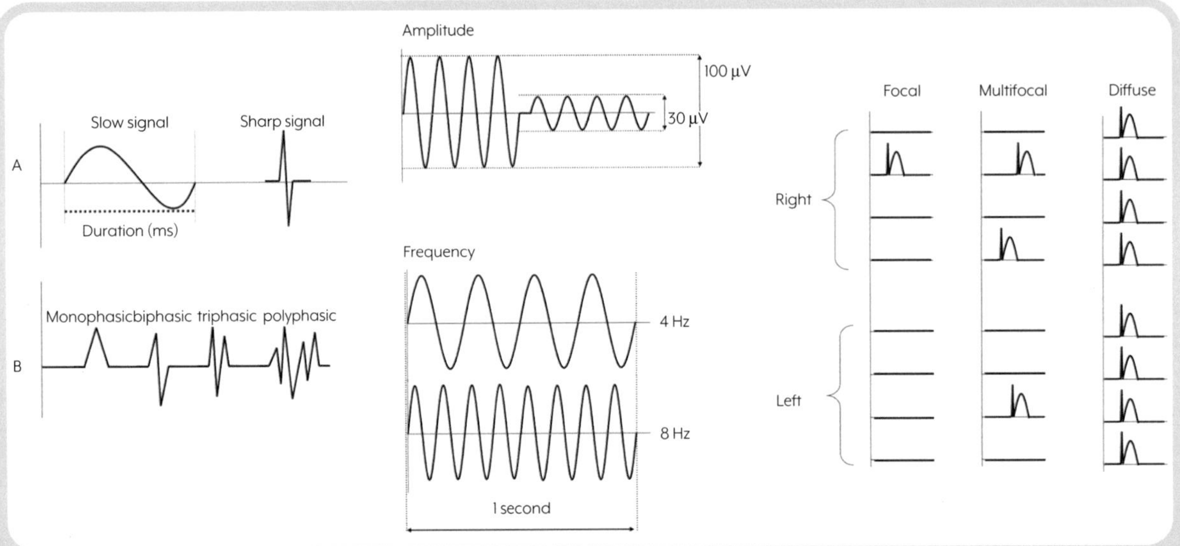

Figure 7.2

Characteristics of morphology, amplitude, frequency and localization of EEG signals.

determine the symmetry/asymmetry of the EEG signal.

The characteristics of morphology, amplitude, frequency, and localization are schematically shown in Figure 7.2.

The evaluation of an EEG tracing generally begins with the identification and description of the background activity, which can be characterized by various frequency bands, assessable either qualitatively (visual analysis of the tracing) or through dedicated software (quantitative analysis). The frequency bands that are more easily recognizable through visual analysis are: the delta band (0.1 to < 4 Hz), the theta band (4 to < 8 Hz), the alpha band (8 to 13 Hz), and the beta band (> 13 to 30 Hz). Within each frequency band, there are slower and faster variants that characterize interindividual variability. The EEG signal also includes ultraslow (0 to 0.3 Hz) and ultrafast (30 to 1000 Hz) frequency bands, which are not appreciable in traditional EEG recordings but are of great scientific interest.

Each frequency band can appear in well-defined physiological and pathological situations, which is why it should always be evaluated considering the entire trace and the recording circumstances, in terms of localization and reproducibility. For example, delta activity, considered pathological in wakefulness EEG, represents part of the physiological pattern of NREM sleep EEG, while beta activity, fast in nature, is related to various mental processes (concentration, calculation, etc.), but also to anxiety states or the use of psychoactive substances (e.g., benzodiazepines). Even the alpha activity, described below, typically characteristic of quiet wakefulness, can be present during the early stages of propofol sedation, although typically anteriorized.

Based on the most represented frequency bands over time, it is possible to describe proper rhythms.

The alpha rhythm constitutes the fundamental characteristic of the awake EEG of an adult subject in a state of psychosensory relaxation with closed eyes. It typically presents in the temporo-parieto-occipital region, although a tendency toward anterior transmission is frequently observed. The alpha rhythm has a frequency within the alpha band range (8-13 Hz), is well-synchronized with closed eyes and relaxed wakefulness, and promptly blocks upon eye opening and/or during mental activity and sensory stimuli (arrest reaction) (Figure 7.3A-B). It is presumed that this hypersynchronous activity is the result of complex interactions between cortico-cortical and thalamo-cortical systems.

The mu rhythm is characterized by rhythmic sequences of potentials with the same frequency as alpha (at 8-13 Hz, typically 9-10

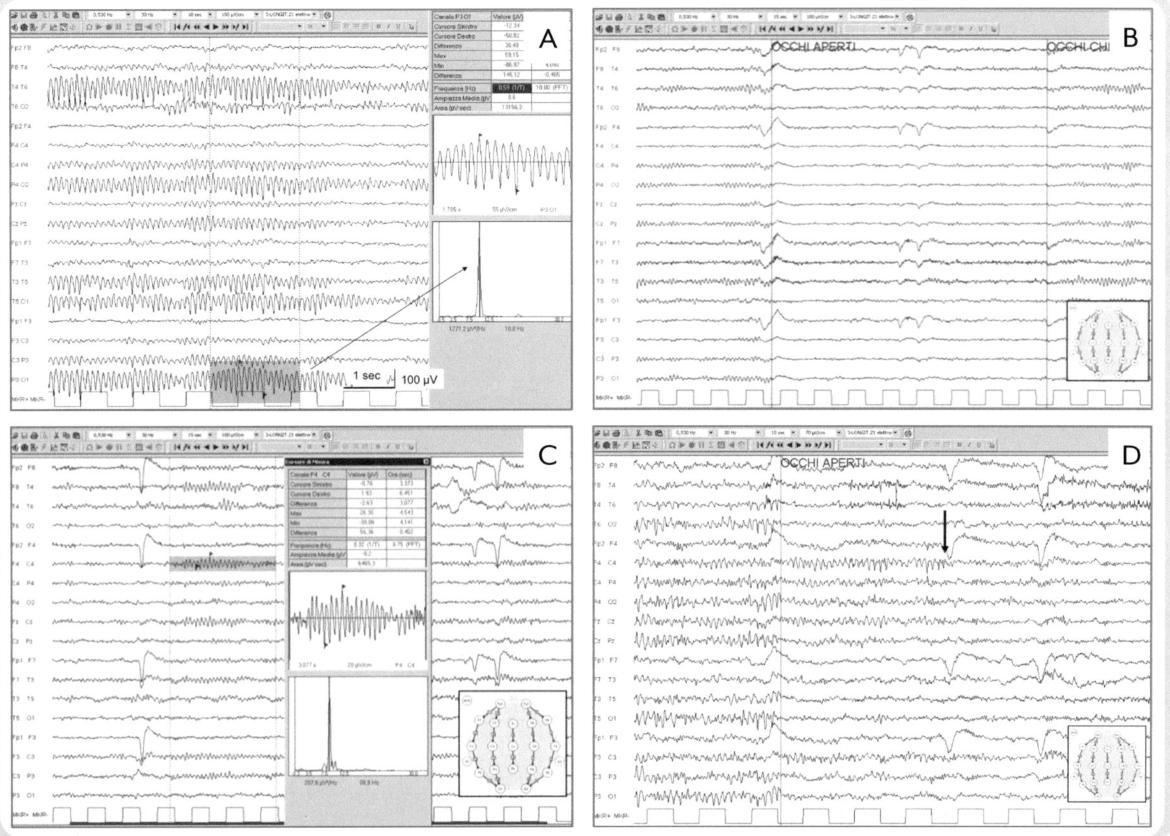

Figure 7.3

A. Alpha rhythm in an awake adult subject with eyes closed. B. Normal reactivity of alpha rhythm with eyes opening. C. Sequences of mu rhythms, more evident in right central region, blocked by asking the subject to tighten the contralateral hand (D, at arrow).

Hz), but with maximum spatial representation in central or rolandic regions (below electrodes C4, C3, Cz). Unlike alpha, it can be appreciated with both eyes open and closed, and it is blocked by movements (active, passive, or reflex) or tactile stimulation of the contralateral limb, as well as by the mere mental planning of movement (Figure 7.3C-D). It is also a physiological rhythm of wakefulness, whose neurophysiological basis is not well understood.

Lambda waves are sharp, low-amplitude graphoelements recorded in the majority of

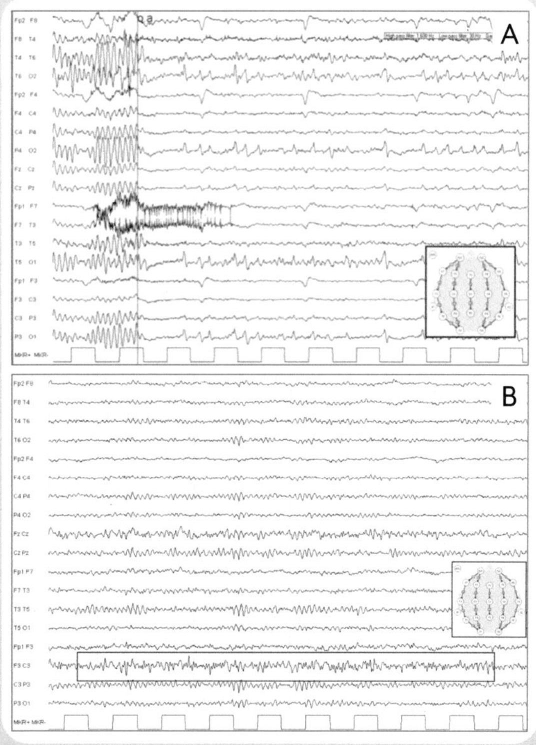

Figure 7.4

In A, posterior open-eye lambda waves. In B, an example of a left fronto-central breach rhythm.

young-adult subjects with eyes open (during visual exploration) in the parieto-occipital region. Lambda waves appear when the subject views text or a complex image and are closely related to saccadic eye movements. Therefore, they are primarily of interest for the study of the visual system and should not be confused, due to their sharp morphology, with epileptiform graphoelements (Figure 7.4A).

The Breach (breach rhythm) refers to a unilateral subcontinuous activity of mixed frequency (beta, alpha, and theta) with occasional superimposed sharp graphoelements, observable in scalp regions (> central-temporo-parietal) where there are disruptions of cranial continuity (sequelae of cranial trauma, neurosurgical interventions, etc.). It fundamentally depends on impedance variations, thus it does not react to various stimuli, and it is present both in wakefulness and sleep (Figure 7.4B). To correctly interpret it, knowledge of the patient's clinical history, particularly regarding the cranial situation, is indispensable to avoid mistakenly confusing it with epileptiform activity.

Characteristic EEG patterns of sleep | The EEG during sleep is profoundly different from that during wakefulness (Figure 7.5). During prolonged sleep, the EEG activity exhibits

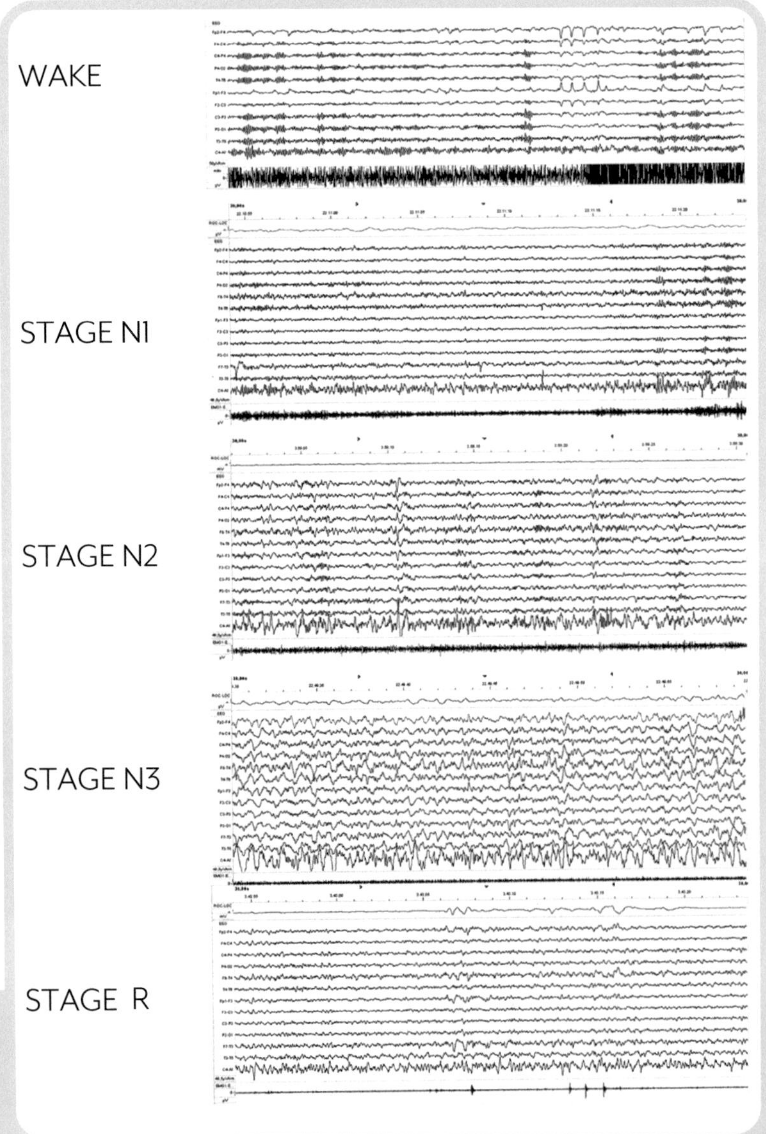

Figure 7.5

Modifications of the EEG pattern from wakefulness to the progression of various stages of spontaneous sleep.

different morphologies and organizations, allowing for the classification of sleep into various stages (macrostructure). The traditional classification divides the cyclic modifications of sleep EEG into Stages 1-2-3-4 NREM and REM stage (REM: Rapid Eye Movements). The new scoring rules developed by the American Academy of Sleep Medicine (2007) include the following stages: N1 (NREM 1), N2 (NREM 2), N3 (NREM 3+4), R (REM). The transition from wakefulness EEG (W, wake) to sleep involves a more or less rapid desynchronization of the physiological alpha rhythm, progressively replaced by slow activity, first theta and then delta, which is diffuse, increasingly persistent, and of high amplitude (NREM Stages 1-4). In Stages 1-3 NREM, physiological graphoelements such as vertex sharp waves, K-complexes, and sleep spindles are observed. The identification of REM stage is based on three basic characteristics: desynchronized background activity, mixed-frequency, and low-voltage activity; presence of rapid eye movements, which occur only during a portion of the stage and are generally absent at the beginning and end; drastic reduction in muscle tone. REM sleep in adults begins approximately 70-90 minutes after the onset of sleep, and REM periods are shorter and less frequent in the first part of the night compared to the second. To identify the cyclicality of sleep stages in a nocturnal EEG recording, it is necessary to correlate the EEG pattern with polygraphic parameters, especially electrooculography (EOG) and electromyography (EMG). A complete polysomnography includes, in addition to EEG, EOG, and EMG, a nasal, thoracic, and abdominal pneumogram, video recording of body movements, snoring recording, measurement of O2/CO2 saturation, pH and intraesophageal pressure evaluation, and monitoring of penile erection. During sleep, it is also possible to study a microstructure using EEG, characterized by the presence within each NREM stage of periods characterized by an alternation between monotonous and phasic activity (Cyclic Alternating Pattern - CAP).

7.3 Pathological EEG Patterns

Although the correct evaluation of an EEG, like any other instrumental examination,

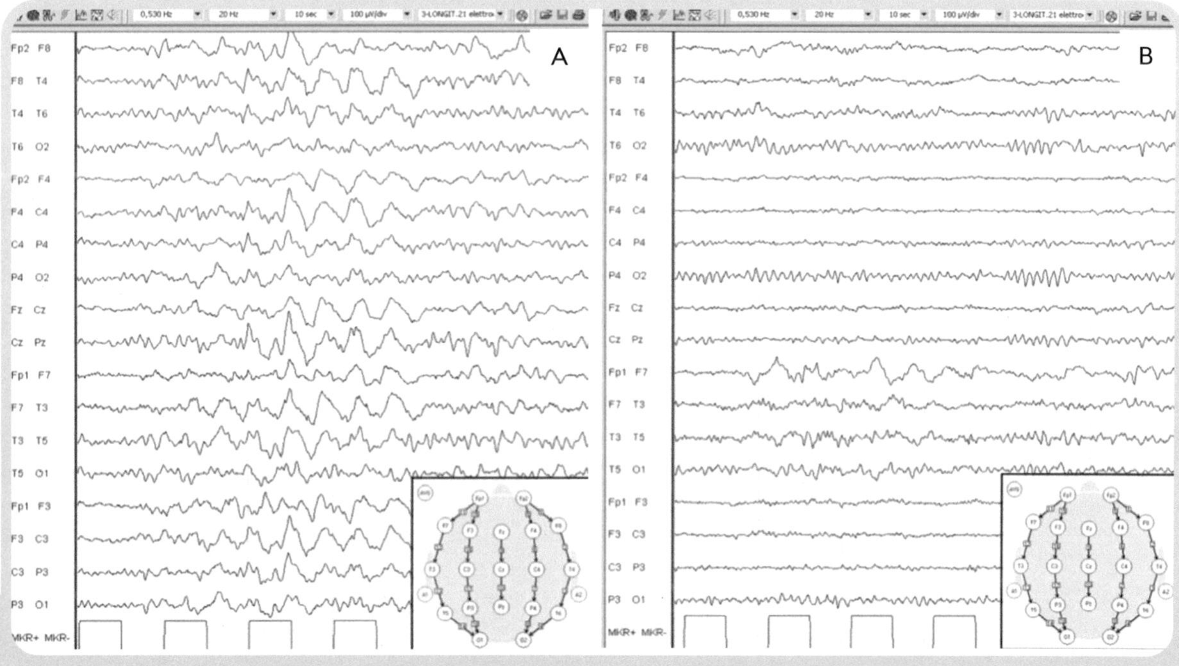

Figure 7.6

Examples of diffuse (A) and focal (B) EEG slowings.

cannot be separated from the knowledge of the patient's clinical history, some graphoelements and EEG rhythms are considered typically pathological.

Slowings | An important initial distinction should be made based on the topography between diffuse and focal slowings (Figure 7.6). While the former are an expression of a pathological process involving the entire brain (of disendocrine-dismetabolic, inflammatory-infectious, degenerative, toxic, or post-critical nature), the latter address towards a focal pathology affecting a specific brain area (ischemia, hemorrhage, abscess, neoplasm).

In specific circumstances, slowings, mostly represented by delta graphoelements with high voltage, can be diffuse, monomorphic, and show a repetitive pattern. In this case, it is called Rhythmic Delta Activity (RDA), with variable distribution (frontal, temporal, occipital) but symmetrical between the two hemispheres. This activity is generally indicative of brain damage involving subcortical structures, particularly the thalamus.

Epileptiform Graphoelements | They are represented by spikes and sharp waves, spike and slow wave complexes (Figure 7.7). Epileptiform graphoelements can be single, well distinguished from the background activity, or organized into critical discharges, focal or diffuse, associated or not with a clinical component. The latter aspect generally depends on the duration of the discharge.

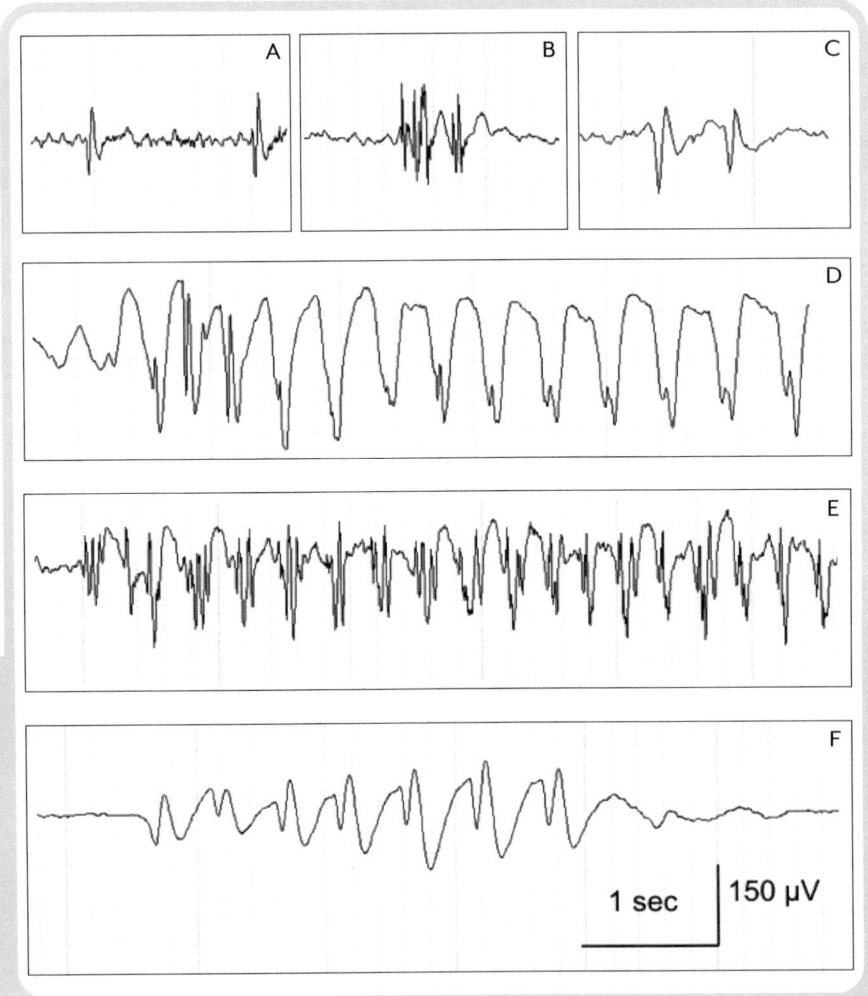

Figure 7.7

Examples of epileptiform abnormalities:
A) spikes;
B) sharp waves;
C) spike waves;
D) spike-and-wave complexes;
E) polyspike-and-wave complexes;
F) sharp and slow wave complexes.

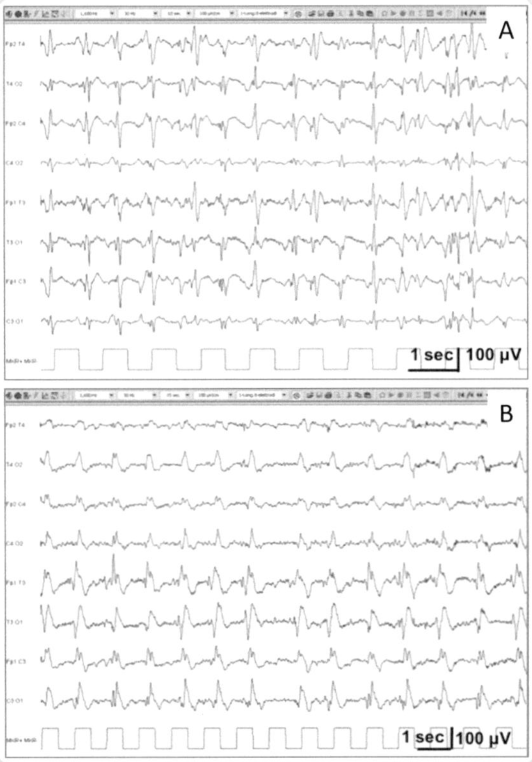

Figure 7.8

In (A) EEG pattern with diffuse periodic abnormalities at short intervals; in (B) periodic lateralized pattern in the left hemisphere, with a tendency for contralateral transmission.

Periodic EEG Patterns | The term periodic or quasi-periodic refers to a graphoelement that tends to repeat in sequence at regular intervals. Periodic patterns can be diffuse, with short or long intervals, or lateralized. The characteristics of periodicity in terms of frequency, topographic distribution, wave morphology, and temporal behavior are important to recognize because they sometimes have a precise pathognomonic significance. An example is the triphasic wave pattern, characteristic of Creutzfeldt-Jakob disease, caused by diffuse periodicities at short intervals (0.5-4 sec.) which, in the advanced stages of the disease, evolve into an alpha coma pattern and subsequently electrocortical depression. The presence of focal periodic patterns indicates focal pathologies, mostly of hemorrhagic and/or inflammatory-infectious nature (Figure 7.8).

Attenuation/Suppression and Electrocerebral Inactivity | Severe dysfunctional and/or lesioned conditions of brain structures can lead to a depression of electroencephalographic activity of variable degree and duration (attenuation or suppression), up to the so-called electrical silence, more accurately defined as electrocerebral inactivity, which is typical of brain death. A marked alternation of periods of flattened tracing and bursts of EEG activity with various morphologies (delta/theta waves mixed with rapid potentials) and amplitude characterizes the pattern known as burst-suppression. This electrical pattern is observed in severe brain pathologies but can also be iatrogenic in origin (excessive sedative/anesthetic level).

7.4 Activation tests

Approximately 50-80% of patients with epilepsy show EEG tracings without interictal epileptic abnormalities under basal conditions. Therefore, in routine laboratory practice, activation tests of the tracing are performed, which are techniques that facilitate the emergence of EEG alterations that are absent in the resting tracing. In routine recordings, it is necessary to regularly perform both hyperventilation (HV) (or hyperpnea) and intermittent photic stimulation (IPS) in all laboratories. For specific clinical questions, recordings during sleep or after sleep deprivation may also be required.

Hyperventilation (HV) | Involves faster and deeper breathing than normal, performed rhythmically while sitting or lying down, for a variable period of 3 to 5 minutes. In young normal subjects, HV can lead to a physiological slowing of background activity and the appearance of diffuse theta/delta slowing, dominant posteriorly in children and anteriorly in adolescents and young adults. EEG abnormalities unmasked or accentuated by HV can manifest as pathological slowing (focal and/or diffuse) or clear epileptic-type abnormalities (Figure 7.9). The precise pathophysiological mechanism by which hyperventilation causes slowing of EEG activity or the appearance of epileptiform abnormalities is not yet fully understood, but hypocapnia and consequent

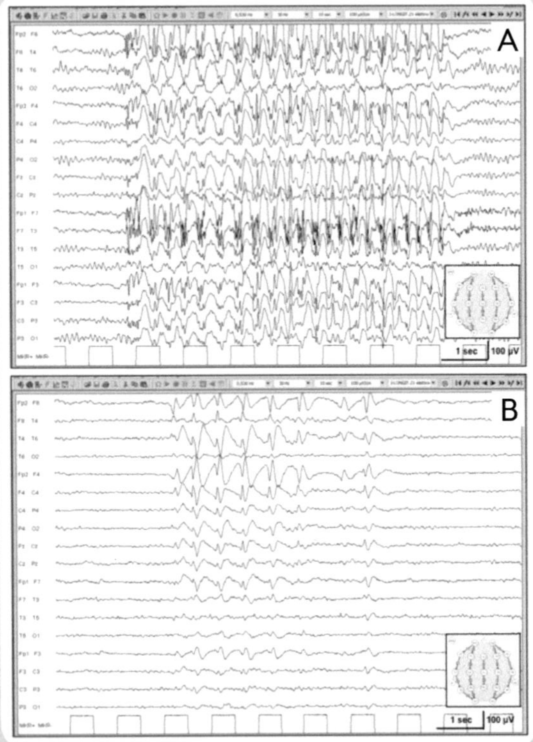

Figure 7.9

Examples of a generalized (A) and focal (B) epileptic discharge induced by hyperventilation.

alkalosis, due to hyperventilation, play a crucial role. These changes induce cerebral vasoconstriction and hypoxia; it has also been hypothesized that there is disinhibition of the synchronizing structures of the midbrain reticular formation, primarily responsible for the genesis of slow waves.

Intermittent photic stimulation (IPS) | or photic stimulation is used as an activation test to highlight EEG abnormalities, with or without clinical correlation (Figure 7.10). The equipment required to perform IPS consists of a stroboscope, which should be positioned frontally, approximately 30 cm from the patient's nasion and at an angle of 13°. Generally, IPS is performed under reduced lighting conditions (dim light) and is typically done with both eyes open and closed, without neglecting the opening-closing phase.

7.5 Poligraphy and Special EEG Recordings

Poligraphy | is an electrophysiological investigation method that allows the acquisition and simultaneous recording of

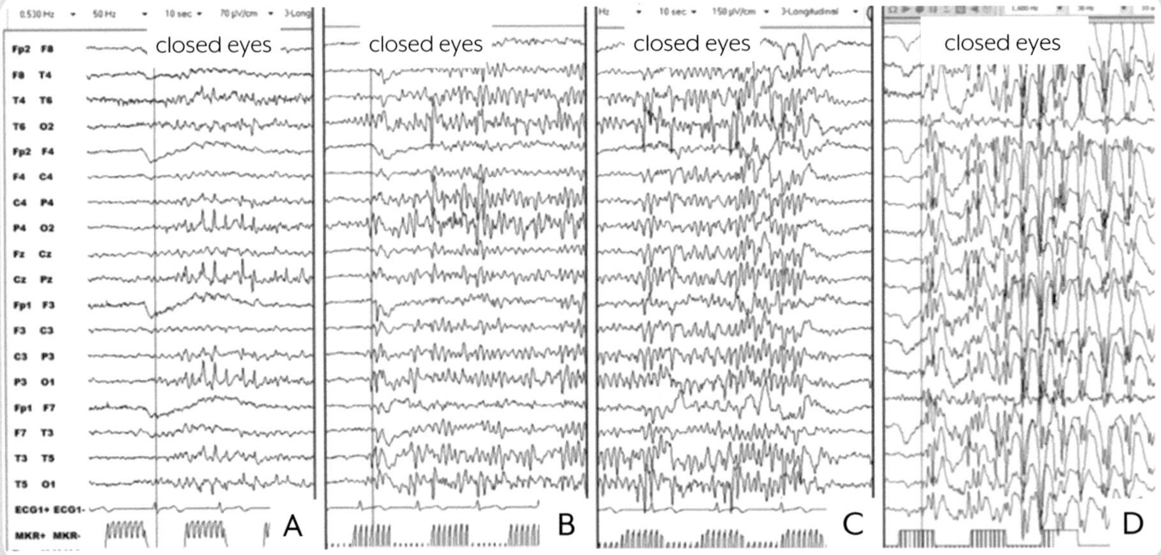

Figure 7.10

Increasingly severe examples of epileptic-like anomalies induced by intermittent light stimulation, varying in intensity and distribution, from A to D.

multiple biological signals, even for long periods. In poligraphy, in addition to EEG, parameters of bioelectric nature such as EOG (Electrooculogram), EMG (Electromyogram), ECG (Electrocardiogram), and SSR (Sympathetic Skin Response) can be recorded.

Ambulatory EEG (A-EEG) | refers to the prolonged monitoring (12 or 24 hours) of EEG under dynamic conditions: the patient is not required to stay in a confined environment but is free to engage in common daily activities. The main clinical application of ambulatory EEG is in epilepsy, from diagnostic assessment to therapy effectiveness evaluation. A-EEG allows demonstrating the possible correlation between events described by the patient and epileptiform activity, as well as evaluating sleep architecture and the presence of critical or intercritical epileptiform activity during sleep. To perform dynamic EEG on the patient, electrodes are applied to the scalp in a laboratory setting, connected to a small, portable signal acquisition unit worn on the shoulder. In this way, the EEG is continuously recorded in wakefulness and sleep in a comfortable environment, which is particularly helpful for patients with behavioral disorders that result in poor cooperation. In case of critical events, a home video recorded by caregivers can also enable electroclinical correlation.

However, precise electroclinical correlation is only possible with *Video-Electroencephalography (V-EEG).* | The essential purpose of Video-EEG monitoring is to analyze in detail the behavioral manifestations, documented by video recordings, along with concomitant modifications in EEG activity. The main clinical application of Video-EEG is therefore the study of critical epileptic manifestations and the differential diagnosis between epileptic and non-epileptic seizures. It should be noted that modern digital technology allows Video-EEG to be performed in any laboratory or even at the patient's bedside using portable devices. There are specialized centers for Long Term Monitoring (LTM) where Video-EEG is performed for several days, with patients confined to bed or free to move within the department, using surface or deep electrodes. This type of video-EEG monitoring is required for pre-surgical epilepsy evaluation. Magnetoencephalography (MEG) is a technique that allows the recording of extremely low-intensity magnetic fields generated by neuronal currents in the human brain. While EEG measures potential differences between two electrodes, MEG detects the absolute magnetic field value at the recording point. MEG provides useful information in various neurological and psychiatric fields, allowing a better understanding of the pathophysiological mechanisms underlying various diseases or the possibility of refining therapeutic-rehabilitative intervention techniques. In epileptology, MEG, currently performed in very few centers, mainly due to its cost and the need for highly specialized personnel, is useful for identifying the deep sources of epileptic activity with greater precision. Techniques correlating high-density EEG (involving the application of 256 electrodes to the scalp) with functional neuroimaging are also interesting for the same purpose.

Bibliography

AASM Manual for the Scoring of Sleep and Associate Events. Rules, terminology and technical specifications. Westchester, American Academy of Sleep Medicine, 2007.

Acharya J.N., Hani A., Cheek J., Thirumala P., Tsuchida T.N. American Clinical Neurophysiology Society Guideline 2: Guidelines for Standard Electrode Position Nomenclature. J Clin Neurophysiol. 2016; 33: 308-311.

Acharya J.N., Hani A.J., Thirumala P.D., Tsuchida T.N. American Clinical Neurophysiology Society Guideline 3: A proposal for standard montages to be used in clinical EEG. J Clin Neurophysiol. 2016; 33: 312-316.

Amzica F., Lopes Da Silva F.H. Cellular substrates of brain rhythms. In: Niedermeyer's Electroencephalography. Basic principles, clinical applications and related fields. DL Schomer & FH Lopes da Silva Eds, 7th edition, 2018; Oxford University Press.

Hirsch L.J., La Roche S.M., Gaspard N., et al. American Clinical Neurophysiology Society's

Standardized Critical Care EEG Terminology: 2012 version. J Clin Neurophysiol 2013; 30:1-27.

Hirsch LJ et al. American Clinical Neurophysiology Society's Standardized Critical Care EEG Terminology: 2021 version. J Clin Neurophysiol 2021; 38:1-29.

Kane N., Acharya J., Benickzy S. et al. A revised glossary of terms most commonly used by clinical electroencephalographers and updated proposal for the report format of the EEG findings. Revision 2017. Clinical Neurophysiology Practice 2017; 2: 170-185.

Krishnan V., Chang B.S., Schomer D.L. Normal EEG in wakefulness and sleep: adults. and elderly. In: Neidermeyer's Electroencephalography. Basic Principles, Clinical Applications, and Related Fields. D.L. Schomer & F.H. Lopes da Silva Eds, 7th edition, 2018, pp 202-228. Oxford University Press.

Mecarelli O. Manuale teorico-pratico di Elettroencefalografia clinica. Springer Healthcare Communications, 2009, pp 1-649.

Mecarelli O. Clinical Electroencephalography. Springer Nature Switzerland 2019, pp 1-822.

Morgenthaler TI, Deriy L, Heald JL, Thomas SM. The evolution of the AASM Clinical Practice Guideline: another step forward. J Clin Sleep Med 2016; 12:129-135.

Seeck M., Koessler L., Bast T., et al. The standardized EEG electrode array of the IFCN. Clin Neurophysiol. 2017; 128: 2070-2077.

Strigaro G, Bisulli F, Assenza G, Mecarelli O et al. Translation and adaptation into the Italian language of the glossary of terms most commonly used by clinical electroencephalographers and proposal for the format of the EEG report (IFCN 2017 Revision). . Clin Neurophysiol Pract 2022; 7: 325-365.

8 ELECTRONEUROGRAPHY, ELECTROMYOGRAPHY AND EVOKED POTENTIALS

Antonella Conte, Andrea Truini, Maurizio Inghilleri, Alfredo Berardelli

8.1 Electroneurography and electromyography

The study of nerve conduction velocity, known as Electroneurography (ENG), and the study of muscle activity, known as Electromyography (EMG), allow for the assessment of the anatomical and functional integrity of the peripheral nervous system, neuromuscular junction, and muscles. ENG-EMG examination helps localize the site of peripheral nervous system impairment, determine whether the alterations affect motor or sensory nerve fibers, identify involvement of the axon, myelin, or both, assess whether the alterations are acute, subacute, or chronic, and, when performed regularly over time, track the progression of the pathology, prognosis, and response to pharmacological treatments. EMG examination is also crucial in diagnosing myopathy. However, it is essential to interpret the electrophysiological results in light of clinical alterations.

The necessary equipment for performing ENG/EMG consists of an amplification and filtering apparatus, as well as analog-to-digital signal conversion, for the analysis and computer recording of the bioelectrical signal.

8.1.1 Electroneurography

Motor Conduction Velocity (MCV) and Sensory Conduction Velocity (SCV) | The study of motor and sensory conduction velocities (MCV, SCV) allows for the assessment of the functional integrity of motor and sensory nerve fibers in the peripheral nerves. It is performed using surface electrodes.

For accurate recording of motor conduction velocities, a recording electrode with an active electrode function is necessary. It is placed on the muscle belly near the neuromuscular junction, while a reference electrode is placed in an inactive region close to the muscle being recorded (usually on the tendon).

Stimulation is carried out using two stimulation electrodes with the cathode or negative pole placed above the nerve near the recording electrodes. With stimulation, nerve depolarization occurs beneath the cathode.

The parameters to consider in the study of MCV and SCV are as follows:

- Amplitude of the potential: conventionally measured from the isoelectric line to the negative peak (which is the deflection above the isoelectric line) for motor potentials and from the negative peak to the positive peak for sensory potentials (Figure 8.1);

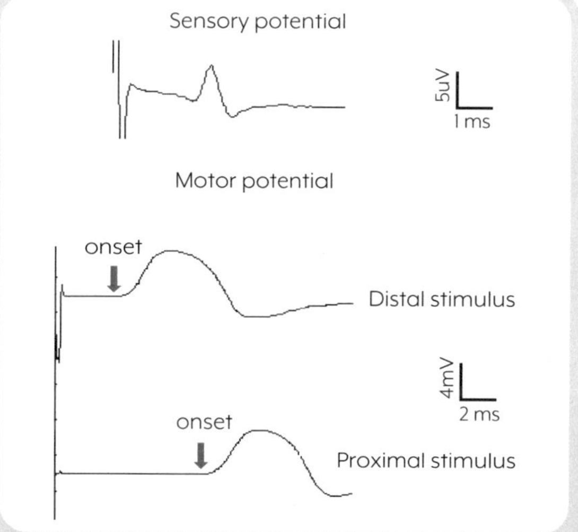

Figure 8.1

- Area of the potential: a function of the amplitude and duration of the potential, it represents a measure of the number of activated fibers.
- Latency of the potential: the time interval between the stimulus and the appearance of the response. In the case of motor response (*Compound Motor Action Potential* CMAP), the latency of the motor potential from distal stimulation reflects the conduction time between the site of stimulation and the neuromuscular junction, the time for crossing the neuromuscular junction, and the time for muscle fiber depolarization.
- Duration of the potential: the time between the onset of the negative deflection and the point at which the negative phase crosses the isoelectric line again. This parameter represents the synchronization of activated fibers and increases under conditions of conduction slowing. Variations in potential duration are also referred to as "dispersion".
- Conduction velocity (CV): the maximum conduction velocity, expressed in meters per second (m/s), obtained by measuring the conduction velocity of the fastest motor fibers (MCV) in the nerve trunk. This is achieved by stimulating the nerve trunk at a distal and proximal point and recording the response from a muscle innervated by the stimulated nerve trunk. MCV is calculated by dividing the distance between the two stimulation points by the difference in latency between the distal and proximal responses. The sensory conduction velocity (SCV) of the nerve trunk is obtained by calculating the maximum conduction velocity of sensory fibers (in m/s) using the ratio of the distance between the stimulation point and recording point to the latency of the potential. Conduction velocity reflects the integrity of myelin and normally has a value of 50-60 m/s.
- The factors that influence electroneurographic parameters are age (with a decrease in potential amplitude and conduction velocity as age increases) and ambient temperature (low temperature increases distal latency and reduces conduction velocity).

In the case of peripheral nerve damage, ENG examination can determine whether there is primary involvement of the axons or myelin. In the presence of axonal damage, reduced amplitude sensory and motor potentials are recorded, but conduction velocity is preserved. In the case of myelin alterations, there is a reduction in both sensory and motor conduction velocity with normal amplitude action potentials, although sometimes with increased duration. In the specific case of compressive-based peripheral nerve damage, such as carpal tunnel syndrome affecting the median nerve, ENG examination will show reduced amplitude of the sensory potential (and in severe cases, also the motor action potential) and a slowing of distal conduction velocity. In general, the reduction in amplitude of sensory and motor potentials recorded during ENG can be caused by a reduction in the contingent of nerve axons, blockage of conduction in a fiber contingent, or an uneven reduction in conduction velocity resulting in temporal dispersion of the signal along the fiber, associated with slowed conduction. In the latter case, the potential will have low amplitude but increased duration. Significant slowing of conduction velocity can occur due to loss of fibers with higher conduction velocities or pathologies involving demyelination of the peripheral nerve (segmental demyelination). ENG is also an essential electrophysiological test for defining the topographic distribution of peripheral nerve damage: mononeuropathy, mononeuritis multiplex, or polyneuropathy. This is of great importance in the clinical management of patients because the diagnosis of various forms of neuropathy requires different diagnostic and therapeutic approaches. Examples of polyneuropathies with predominant axonal damage include diabetic neuropathy, alcoholic neuropathy, uremic neuropathy, toxic and deficiency-related neuropathies, paraneoplastic neuropathies, and amyloidosis-associated neuropathies. Polyneuropathies with predominant demyelinating damage include acute inflammatory demyelinating polyradiculoneuropathy (Guillain-Barré syndrome), chronic inflammatory demyelinating polyradiculoneuropathy (CIDP), certain forms of diabetic neuropathy, and type II Charcot-Marie-Tooth neuropathy (see Chapter 20 - Diseases of the Peripheral Nervous System). Multifocal neuropathies are generally of the axonal type (due to vasculitis and consequent alterations in nerve vascularization).

In the case of mononeuropathy, ENG is able to classify nerve damage into three types: neuropraxia (preserved nerve continuity but demyelination of larger caliber/faster conducting fibers), axonotmesis (disruption of axonal continuity but preservation of connective tissue sheath structures), and neurotmesis (complete nerve interruption). The accurate characterization of the type of focal nerve lesion is crucial for formulating a prognosis because neuropraxia offers the potential for complete functional recovery within 2-3 weeks. In the case of axonotmesis, functional recovery will not be complete and may take several months, while neurotmesis typically does not show significant improvement.

ENG also allows for the study of electrophysiological responses that reflect the functionality of spinal roots (H-reflex and F-wave) (Figure 8.2).

H Reflex | The H reflex, also known as the Hoffmann reflex, is a *late muscle response* that serves as an electrophysiological equivalent to the monosynaptic stretch reflex. The H reflex is a muscle response evoked by low-intensity and long-duration electrical stimuli. Its afferent branch consists of intrafusal fibers (Ia fibers) from a mixed nerve, while the efferent branch involves alpha motor neurons.

The latency of the H reflex reflects the conduction velocity of Ia afferent fibers, motor fibers, and synaptic time at the spinal level. An increased latency of the H reflex or the absence of the response in the presence of a normal distal motor response suggests a proximal damage in the peripheral nervous system (root). In clinical practice, the most commonly studied H reflex in the lower limb is the H reflex recorded from the soleus muscle after stimulating the tibial nerve at the popliteal fossa, which assesses S1 radiculopathy.

F Wave | The F wave is a *late muscle response* evoked by supra-maximal electrical stimuli (i.e., above the threshold for producing further amplitude increase of the Compound Muscle Action Potential derived from the stimulated nerve). Supra-maximal electrical stimulation activates nerve fibers orthodromically, directly activating the muscle to produce the Compound Muscle Action Potential (CMAP). It also depolarizes the nerve fibers along the proximal segments of the

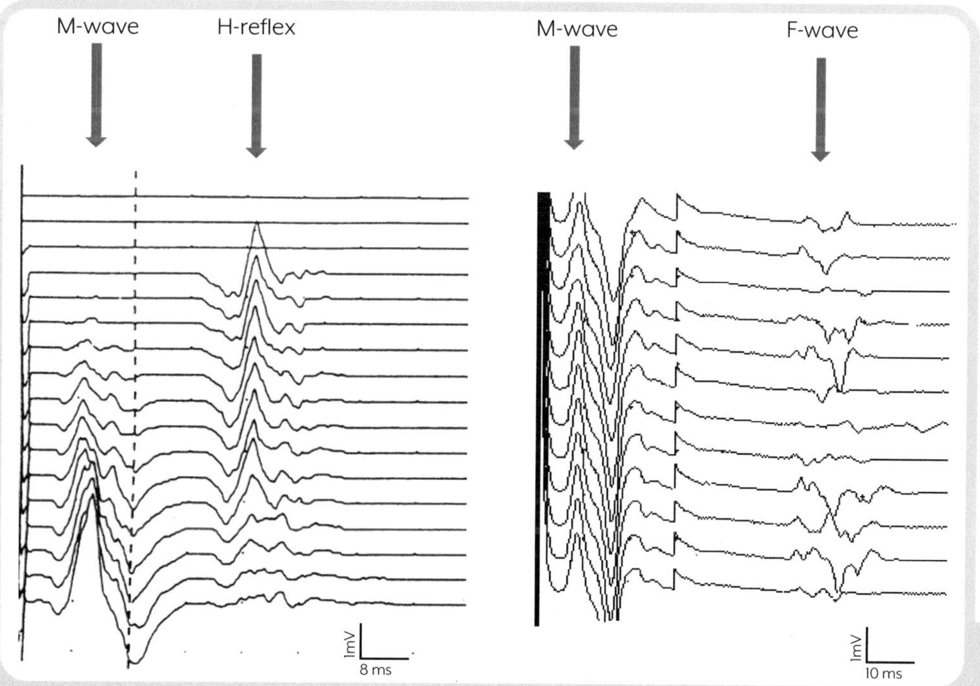

Figure 8.2

nerve in an antidromic fashion, exciting the cell body of motor neurons at the anterior horns of the spinal cord. In some of these motor neurons, reactivation of the motor axon occurs, which conducts the efferent impulse to the muscle, leading to its reactivation and the appearance of the F wave. The parameters commonly used to evaluate the F wave are the minimum latency, persistence, and chrono-dispersion (difference between the minimum and maximum latency of the F wave, indicative of fibers with different conduction velocities in the nerve). The appearance and minimum latency of the F wave reflect the excitability of spinal motor neurons, axonal integrity, and the degree of myelination along the entire course of the nerve trunk. The study of the F wave is particularly useful in assessing the functionality of nerve roots and in cases of diffuse involvement of the peripheral nervous system, with a specific involvement of the proximal nerve tracts (Guillain-Barré syndrome, chronic inflammatory demyelinating polyradiculoneuropathy - CIDP).

8.1.2 Study of repetitive nerve stimulation

It is the most commonly used method in clinical practice, although less sensitive than single-fiber EMG, to study the functionality of the neuromuscular junction. Under normal conditions, the end-plate potential always generates a muscle action potential. The amplitude of the end-plate potential sufficient to generate muscle contraction is defined as the "safety factor of the neuromuscular junction" (see Chapter 1 - Motor System). In normal conditions, the end-plate potential has a significantly larger amplitude than the minimum amplitude required to induce a muscle potential. The ratio between the amplitude of the end-plate potential and the threshold amplitude for generating a muscle potential expresses the so-called safety factor of the neuromuscular junction. During prolonged (or repetitive) stimulation at low frequency (3Hz), the available ACh for release in the synaptic cleft decreases. Consequently, the number of bonds between ACh and postsynaptic receptors and the amplitude of the end-plate potential decrease (synaptic fatigue). Conversely, during prolonged stimulation at high frequency (>10Hz), Ca++ accumulates in the presynaptic terminal, increasing the mobilization of ACh from storage reserves and the immediately available quantity of ACh, thus increasing the amount of ACh released in the synaptic cleft. This results in an increase in the amplitude of the end-plate potential. After 10 seconds of sustained muscle contraction, calcium accumulates in the presynaptic terminal, leading to increased mobilization of synaptic vesicles and ACh exocytosis, producing end-plate potentials of increasing amplitude. This phenomenon, known as "post-exercise facilitation," in normal conditions results in an increase in the amplitude of the CMAP that does not exceed 140% of the CMAP before physical exertion (incremental response). The repetitive nerve stimulation test is performed by stimulating motor fibers with supra-maximal intensity and recording the CMAP derived from the muscle innervated by the stimulated nerve. Typically, the ulnar nerve is studied with recording from the abductor digiti minimi muscle, the circumflex nerve with recording from the deltoid muscle, and the facial nerve with recording from the orbicularis oculi muscle. Repetitive stimulation simulates a sort of neuromuscular junction fatigue similar to the phenomenon of fatigability typical of myasthenia. In patients with myasthenia, low-frequency repetitive stimulation results in a decremental response, with a reduction in the amplitude of the evoked muscle potential starting from the 3rd or 4th stimulus. In cases of presynaptic muscular junction alteration (Lambert-Eaton syndrome), the repetitive stimulation test shows a reduced resting CMAP amplitude, a decremental response at 3Hz, but an abnormal facilitation of the response after voluntary muscle exertion or high-frequency repetitive stimulation (>20 Hz).

8.1.3 Electromyography

Electromyography (EMG) involves the recording of muscle electrical activity using a needle electrode inserted into the muscle. The recording of a motor unit potential through the extracellular space is represented by a waveform with a triphasic morphology (positive-negative-positive). The first positive deflection represents the propagation of the depolarization wave toward the recording electrode, the second negative deflection represents the propagation of the wave beneath the electrode, and the third positive deflection represents the departure of the depolarization wave from the electrode (Figure 8.3). EMG involves inserting the needle electrode into the resting muscle to evaluate the presence of insertion activity or any potential spontaneous pathological activity. Subsequently, the amplitude, duration, and morphology of motor unit potentials are evaluated during voluntary muscle contraction at low effort. Finally, the recruitment of motor units is evaluated during increasing efforts and maximal muscle exertion.

Resting activity | Under normal conditions with the muscle at rest, the insertion and movement of the needle electrode cause mechanical excitation of the adjacent muscle fibers, resulting in short-duration and low-amplitude potentials. The absence of normal insertion activity indicates muscle necrosis, reduced insertion activity indicates muscle atrophy with replacement of muscle tissue by connective or fatty tissue, while increased insertion activity (pathological spontaneous activity) indicates muscle membrane instability, as seen in the acute phase of a neurogenic injury, myositis, or myotonia. When recording near the neuromuscular junction in a healthy muscle, a specific electrical activity called "end-plate activity" is recorded.

Pathological spontaneous activity at rest is represented by fibrillation potentials, positive sharp waves, fasciculation potentials, myotonic discharges, and complex repetitive discharges (Figure 8.3). Fibrillation potentials are characterized by a biphasic shape, low amplitude (100-200 µV), and short duration (1-3 ms), with a variable appearance frequency between 1 and 30 Hz. Positive sharp waves represent the action potential of the individual damaged muscle fiber and are characterized by an initial positivity followed by a prolonged, low-amplitude negative wave that gives it a "sawtooth" appearance. Both fibrillation potentials and positive waves indicate a muscle fiber lacking its innervation and are present in neurogenic lesions and inflammatory myopathies, appearing 2-3 weeks after the onset of the lesion. Fasciculation potentials are the electrophysiological correlate of fasciculations

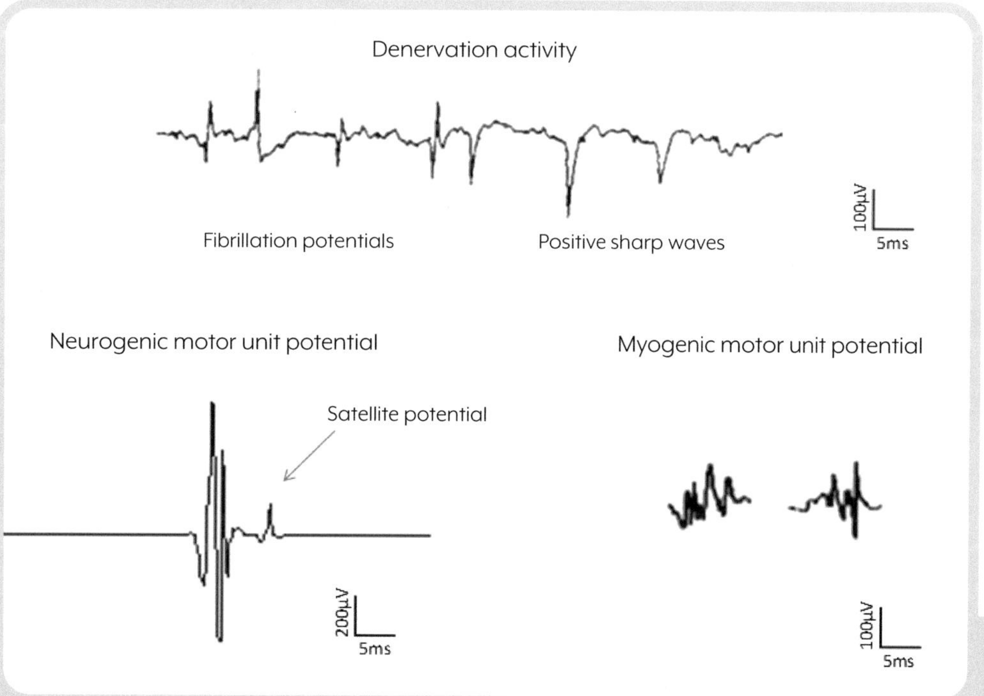

Figure 8.3

and originate from the spontaneous discharge of a group of muscle fibers innervated by the same motor neuron. They have an irregular discharge frequency and can be frequent or sporadic. They are commonly found in healthy individuals, with or without associated cramps (benign fasciculations), but in this case, they have a higher discharge frequency compared to pathological fasciculations. Pathological fasciculations are common in motor neuron disease affecting the second motor neuron, polyneuropathies, radicular compressions, and thyrotoxicosis. Myotonic discharges are potential discharges similar to fibrillation potentials but with a characteristic increasing-decreasing discharge frequency pattern, which gives the characteristic "dive-bomber" sound. Myotonic discharges are characteristic of congenital myotonia (Thomsen's disease), myotonic dystrophy (Steinert's disease), and paramyotonia congenita. Complex repetitive discharges consist of synchronous discharges of a group of presumably denervated muscle fibers, activated by ephaptic transmission from a fibrillating fiber acting as a pacemaker. They appear and disappear abruptly and have a constant discharge frequency. Complex repetitive discharges can be recorded both in neurogenic lesions (motor neuron disease, radiculopathies, neuropathies) and myogenic lesions (polymyositis, muscular dystrophies, endocrine myopathies), therefore, they have limited diagnostic significance due to their non-specificity.

Motor unit potentials | The motor unit potential is generated by the temporal and spatial summation of the potentials from muscle fibers of the individual motor unit during voluntary muscle contraction. The motor unit consists of an alpha motor neuron and the muscle fibers connected to it (typically around 20 in normal conditions). The analyzed parameters are the amplitude, duration, and morphology of the motor unit potential. The amplitude of the motor unit potential, expressed as peak-to-peak amplitude, varies in individual muscles, and the variability depends on fiber density, fiber diameter, synchrony of fiber discharge within the motor unit, and distance of the fibers from the needle electrode. In general, the motor unit potential recruited during mild muscle contraction does not exceed 2 mV in amplitude (Figure 8.4). The duration of the potential reflects the synchrony of discharge among the muscle fibers comprising the motor unit and normally ranges from 5 to 15 ms. The morphology of the motor unit potential is considered normal if triphasic or biphasic, while it is considered pathological if the number of phases exceeds 4 (in this case, the motor unit potential is defined as polyphasic). Under normal conditions, each muscle is characterized by a certain percentage of polyphasic potentials, typically not exceeding 10%. The presence of short-duration and low-amplitude polyphasic potentials suggests myogenic damage, but polyphasic motor unit potentials with short duration and reduced amplitude can also be recorded in cases of recent reinnervation (referred to as "nascent potentials") in neurogenic conditions (Figure 8.3). In myopathies, EMG examination shows reduced amplitude and duration of motor unit potentials due to the reduction in muscle fibers. In contrast, in neurogenic lesions, EMG examination reveals polyphasic potentials with increased amplitude and duration. The polyphasic morphology, increased amplitude, and duration of the motor unit potential are determined by the increased number of muscle fibers connected to the motor neuron of the individual motor unit through reinnervation processes by residual axons (Figure 8.4). In general, variations in morphology, duration, and amplitude reflect the "size" of the motor unit. Neurogenic potentials with significantly increased amplitude (up to 10 mV), relatively simple morphology (giant potentials), are indicative of a previous and stable motor neuron disease (e.g., poliomyelitis) or a chronic course (e.g., spinal muscular atrophy).

Recruitment of motor units | An evaluation of the recruitment pattern of motor units is performed for progressively increasing intensity of effort. Under normal conditions, for mild muscle exertion, motor units are activated at a frequency of approximately 5-10 per second. The progressive increase in effort intensity initially results in an increase in the discharge frequency of already active fibers and then the recruitment of higher threshold fibers. The EMG trace during "single oscillations,"

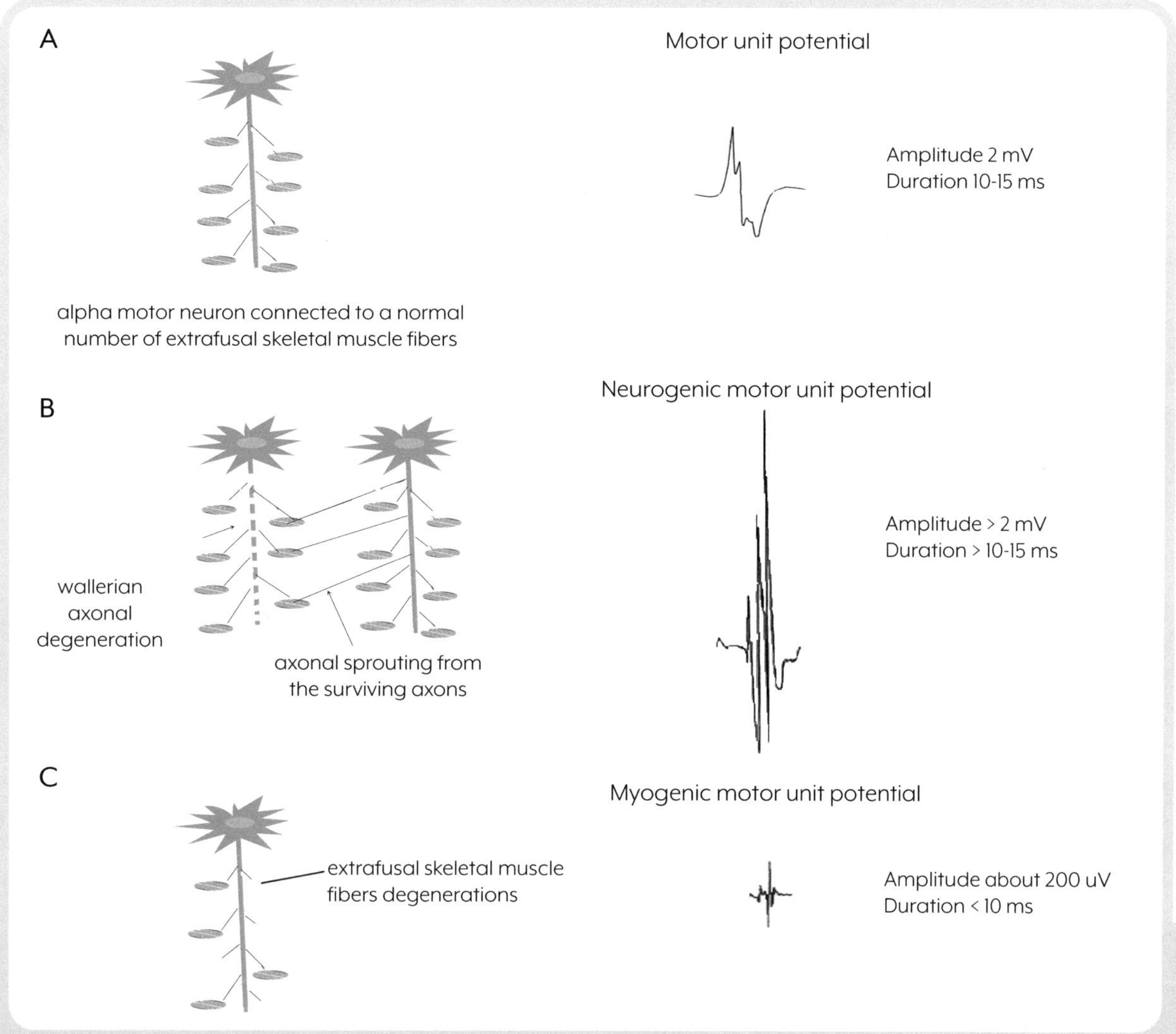

Figure 8.4

A) Motor unit under normal conditions and the motor unit potential (MUP) generated by it during muscle contraction, recorded by electromyographic examination. The MUP has a biphasic morphology, an amplitude of less than 2 mV, and a duration of less than 10 ms. These parameters are determined by the fact that the motor unit is typically composed of one axon and approximately 20 muscle fibers connected to it. B) Case of axonal injury and degeneration due to peripheral nerve lesion. Adjacent axons, through collateral reinnervation, will innervate the muscle fibers orphaned by the degenerated axon. As a result, the number of muscle fibers connected to the surviving axon will be higher than normal. The motor unit activated during muscle contraction will generate a potential with increased amplitude and duration, exhibiting a polyphasic morphology (neurogenic MUP) due to the heterogeneous synaptic transmission times in the reinnervated fibers. C) Case of primary myogenic damage. In this situation, due to myopathy-related necrosis of muscle fibers, the number of muscle fibers connected to the axon will decrease. During muscle contraction, the motor unit will generate a MUP with reduced amplitude and duration, exhibiting a polyphasic morphology.

which is characteristic of mild exertion, becomes richer in potentials, and in moderate exertion, it is referred to as "intermediate," where only potentials with greater amplitude are distinguishable. At maximum effort, motor units are indistinguishable from each other, and the trace is referred to as "interference pattern" (Figure 8.5). Neurogenic lesions are characterized by a reduction in the recruitment of motor units at maximum effort and an increase in the discharge frequency of fibers that can still be activated by contraction.

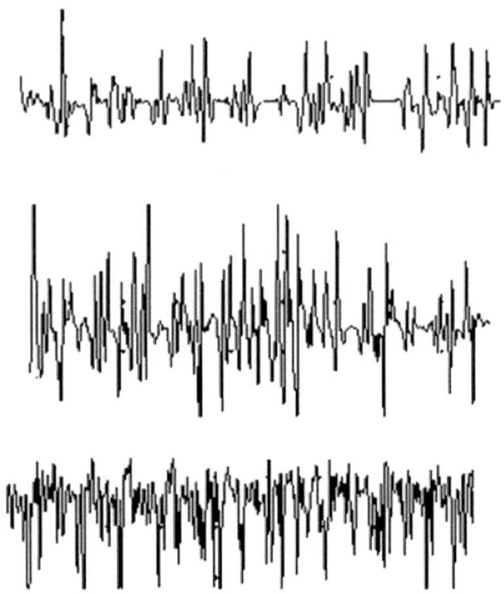

Figure 8.5

In the case of loss of muscle fibers in myogenic pathology, motor units, characterized by a lower number of intact muscle fibers, develop less force. Therefore, to perform an effort, even a mild one, it is necessary to recruit a greater number of motor units, which results in a disproportionate recruitment compared to the actual force generated. The EMG trace in myopathies is, therefore, of the "interference pattern" type for non-maximal muscle exertion and is referred to as "early interference pattern." A characteristic recruitment pattern also occurs in cases of first motor neuron injury. In these circumstances, however, there is a reduction in recruitment, but the activated motor units do not increase the discharge frequency (temporal recruitment deficit).

In summary, the combination of parameters considered during the execution of an EMG examination (resting activity, morphology of motor unit potentials, and recruitment for maximal efforts) allows differentiation between neurogenic and myogenic pathologies. Regarding neurogenic EMG alterations secondary to nerve trunk damage, initially, there will be an increase in insertion activity or a reduction in the number of recruited potentials (Table 8.1). After approximately 2-3 weeks from the onset, denervation activity appears (fibrillation potentials, positive sharp waves, complex

Table 8.1 ELECTROPHYSIOLOGICAL FINDINGS OBSERVABLE IN CASE OF PERIPHERAL NERVE LESION IN RELATION TO THE ACUTE/SUBACUTE AND CHRONIC PHASES OF THE CONDITION

Electrophysiological techniques	Acute/subacute phase (0-20 days)	Chronic phase (>1 month)
ENG	· Reduction in amplitude of sensory and motor potentials · Motor conduction block · Absence/reduction in the frequency of late responses	· Partial recovery of sensory and motor potential amplitudes · Reappearance/improvement in the frequency of late responses
EMG	· Presence of resting denervation potentials at approximately 15-20 days from the onset of symptoms	· Disappearance of denervation activity · Appearance of reinnervation potentials (neurogenic motor unit potentials) · Improvement in recruitment grade at maximum effort

repetitive discharges), along with a reduction in recruitment during maximum effort (variable in severity depending on the lesion, but with an increase in the discharge frequency of remaining fibers). The process of reinnervation is initially manifested by the appearance of short-duration polyphasic potentials (incipient potentials). As reinnervation progresses, motor unit restructuring occurs (Table 8.1 and Figure 8.4). The number of muscle fibers per motor unit increases, and the motor unit potential increases in amplitude and duration (due to increased fiber density). In the course of motor neuron disease, there will be signs of neurogenic involvement with denervation activity in multiple non-contiguous body regions and reduced recruitment during maximum effort due to motor neuron loss if exclusive involvement of the second motor neuron is present. Alternatively, there may be a temporal recruitment deficit if there is concurrent involvement of the first motor neuron. EMG examination in demyelinating peripheral nervous system pathologies has limited indicative value. The only electrophysiological element is a reduction in recruitment during maximum effort due to conduction blocks.

Myogenic EMG alterations, resulting from muscle damage, are generally characterized by spontaneous activity at rest (fibrillation potentials, positive sharp waves, complex repetitive discharges) in the case of inflammatory myopathies such as polymyositis or myotonic discharges in myotonic dystrophy. Motor unit potentials are characterized by low amplitude, reduced duration, and polyphasic morphology due to a reduction in the number of muscle fibers comprising the motor unit and variation in fiber caliber (Figure 8.4). The recruitment of motor units is of an early interference pattern type.

Single-fiber electromyography | Single-fiber electromyography is an EMG technique performed using a specialized needle electrode with a small recording surface, high impedance, and reduced capacitance, allowing for the decomposition of the motor unit potential into individual potentials from the muscle fibers comprising it. Single-fiber EMG involves the extracellular recording of individual muscle fibers activated with minimal contraction. The analyzed parameters are *"jitter"* and fiber density. If the electrode is positioned to record the activity of two muscle fibers belonging to the same motor unit, the temporal interval between the potentials generated by the activation of the two fibers can be calculated. The temporal interval between the potentials of two individual muscle fibers belonging to the same motor unit varies and is related to the stability of the motor endplate. This variability, called *"jitter,"* increases in neuromuscular junction disorders (myasthenia gravis and Lambert-Eaton syndrome). Fiber density is an indicative parameter of the number of fibers simultaneously discharging within the area explored by the electrode and is increased in cases of reinnervation processes.

8.1.4 Trigeminal reflexes

Trigeminal reflexes assess the integrity of the trigeminal system, including its peripheral and brainstem components. They involve a series of reflex responses mediated by large-caliber myelinated fibers (A-beta fibers). The trigeminal reflexes commonly used in clinical practice are the *blink reflex* and the masseter inhibitory reflex. The *blink reflex* is a trigeminal-facial reflex, with the first division of the trigeminal nerve as the afferent branch and the facial nerve as the efferent branch. It is elicited by surface electrode stimulation of the supraorbital nerve and the recording of two muscle responses in the orbicularis oculi muscle. The first response, R1, is an early unilateral response on the stimulated side, mediated by a paucisynaptic pontine circuit. The second response, R2, is bilateral and corresponds to the blink, mediated by a polysynaptic bulbopontine circuit (Figure 8.6). The masseter inhibitory reflex is a trigeminal-trigeminal reflex, with the second or third division of the trigeminal nerve as the afferent branch and the efferent branch corresponding to the inhibition (mediated by a pontine inhibitory interneuron) of the trigeminal motoneurons. The masseter inhibitory reflex is elicited during voluntary contraction of the masticatory muscles by surface electrode stimulation of the infraorbital or mental nerve and the recording of two distinct reflex inhibitory responses in the masticatory

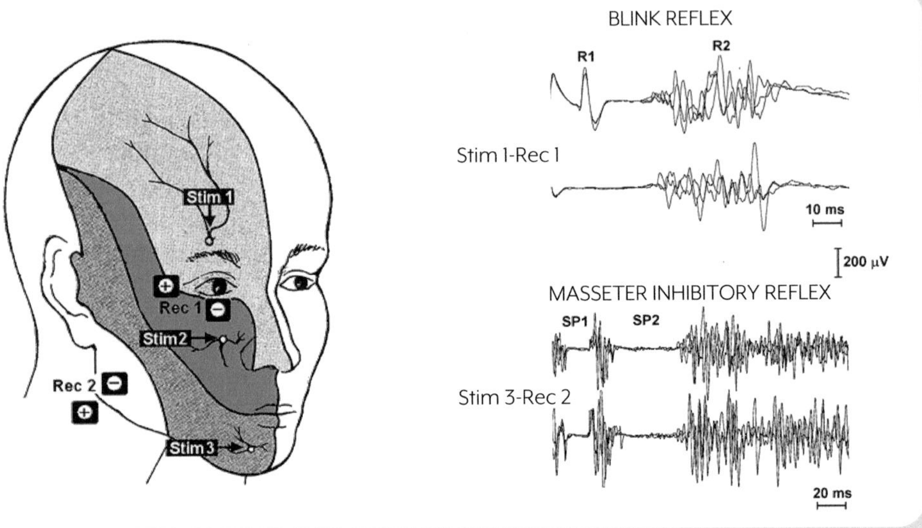

Figure 8.6

muscles. The first response (SP1), with a short latency, is mediated by a paucisynaptic pontine circuit, while the second response (SP2), with a longer latency, is mediated by the polysynaptic bulbo-pontine circuit. Trigeminal reflexes are a simple and reliable tool in the evaluation of facial pain because they accurately differentiate pain secondary to structural damage to the trigeminal system, such as tumors in the posterior cranial fossa, skull base, or brainstem plaques in multiple sclerosis. Trigeminal reflexes also have high sensitivity and specificity (around 90%) in the differential diagnosis between the classic (idiopathic) and secondary forms of trigeminal neuralgia: they are normal in the former condition and altered in the latter.

8.2 Evoked Potentials

Evoked potentials are bioelectrical signals generated in the central nervous system following sensory stimulation and, at the muscular level, after stimulation of the motor cortex. Evoked potentials allow investigation of the central nervous system circuits but do not provide information on the etiology of any abnormalities. They are a useful diagnostic tool for the anatomical and functional correlation of central nervous system alterations. The results obtained with evoked potentials should always be interpreted in relation to the patient's clinical presentation.

8.2.1 Visual Evoked Potentials (VEPs)

They explore the functionality of the visual pathways. They are performed by recording bioelectrical signals generated by the primary visual cortex in the occipital region in response to visual stimuli characterized by luminance variations (flash VEPs) or contrast variations (pattern VEPs). The most commonly used test in clinical practice is the pattern VEP (Figure 8.7). The visual stimulus consists of a checkerboard pattern in which white squares alternate with black squares in a rhythmic sequence. Each eye is stimulated individually for hemifields or in full-field. The visual evoked potential is generated by averaging 250-500 visual stimuli and consists of three components: the first component has a negative polarity and an average latency of about 75 ms (N75); the second component has a positive polarity and an average latency of 100 ms (P100); the last component has a negative polarity and an average latency of 145 ms (N145). The neurophysiological parameter useful for clinical interpretation is the absolute latency of P100 and the latency difference between the two sides. An unilateral increase in P100 latency, with full-field monocular stimulation, suggests pathology of the ipsilateral optic nerve, while a bilateral increase in P100 latency with monocular full-field stimulation suggests involvement of the retrochiasmatic pathways. Full-field VEPs are normal for

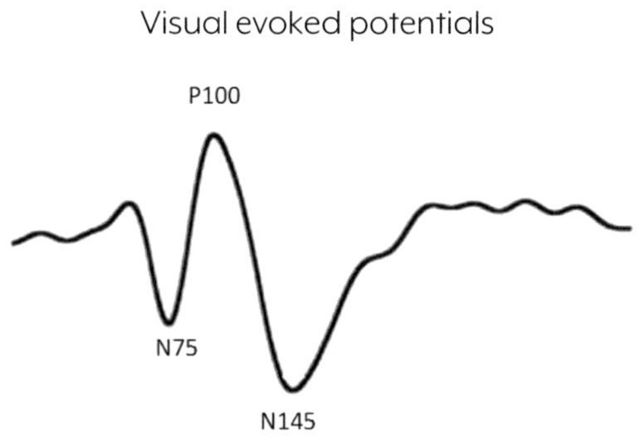

Figure 8.7

unilateral hemispheric lesions. In such cases, hemifield VEPs are necessary to obtain pathological responses. The clinical indication for VEP testing aims to demonstrate optic nerve alterations in the retrobulbar segment in patients with demyelinating diseases of the central nervous system, nutritional and toxic optic neuropathies, Leber's optic atrophy, extrinsic or intrinsic compressive optic nerve lesions, and in general, visual pathway impairments.

8.2.2 Auditory evoked potentials

Clinically relevant auditory evoked potentials refer to bioelectrical signals generated in the brainstem and recorded from the cranial vault (an electrode on the vertex and another on the earlobe or mastoid) in response to repetitive acoustic stimuli, such as 100 ms clicks delivered at a frequency of 20-30 Hz and intensity of 70-80 dB. Auditory evoked potentials are visualized as a sequence of seven positive waves at the vertex with an amplitude of less than 1 μV (Figure 8.8). The I wave is generated in the distal portion of the VIII cranial nerve; the II wave is generated by the proximal portions of the VIII cranial nerve and in the cochlear nucleus; the III wave is generated in the pontine region between the cochlear nucleus and the superior olivary nucleus by the fibers of the trapezoid body; the IV and V waves are generated in the upper pons by the lateral lemniscus and inferior colliculus; the VI and VII waves are less easily recorded and are believed to be generated in the medial geniculate body and temporal radiations, respectively. In clinical practice, due to considerable interindividual variability in responses, the latency difference between the I and III waves and between the III and V waves is used as a reference. An increase in the latency difference between the I and III waves indicates an alteration in the proximal portion of the VIII cranial nerve and the caudal pontine region. An increase in the latency difference between the III and V waves indicates an alteration in the rostral pontine region and the mesencephalon. The clinical indication for studying brainstem auditory evoked potentials is currently limited to evaluating patients with demyelinating diseases of the central nervous system, acoustic neuromas, and in the diagnosis of coma or brain death.

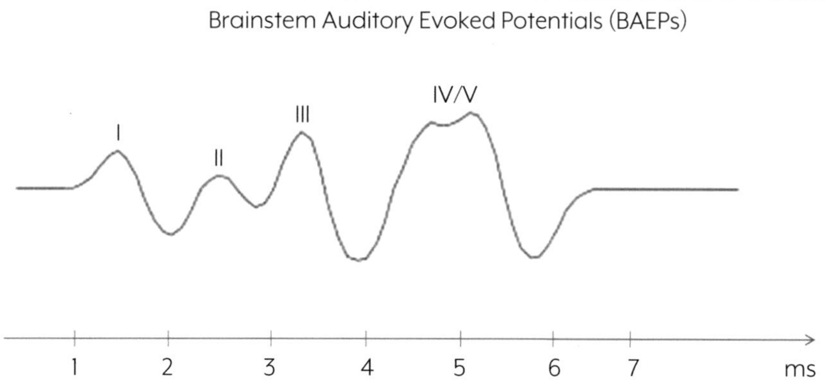

Figure 8.8

8.2.3 Somatosensory evoked potentials (SEP)

They are represented by bioelectrical signals generated by the electrical stimulation of a mixed or sensory peripheral nerve (usually the median nerve for the upper limb and the tibial nerve for the lower limb). For the study of upper limb SEPs, recording electrodes are placed 1) at the supraclavicular level (Erb's point) to record the propagation of the stimulus along the structures of the brachial plexus (N9); 2) at the spinous process of the fifth cervical vertebra to record the components generated at the spinal cord level (N13); 3) at the post-rolandic parietal cortical region. This last recording line identifies a succession of components that correspond to the activation of structures in the cervicobulbar region (caudal portion of the medial lemniscus) (P14), the superior colliculus and thalamic nuclei (P18), and the post-rolandic cortex (N20, P27, N35). In clinical practice, an increased signal latency at Erb's point indicates peripheral pathology, an increased N9-N13 interval indicates radiculospinal pathology, while an increased latency difference between N13 and N20 represents an alteration in the central conduction of the lemniscal pathway. In the case of SEPs from tibial nerve stimulation, the N22 component is recorded, which is comparable to the N13 component from the median nerve and represents the activation of neurons in the posterior horns. The arrival of the afferent signal in the cortex is represented by the P38 component, recorded at the vertex of the skull (Figure 8.9). As in all electrophysiological investigations, the negative polarity is conventionally represented above the isoelectric line in SEPs. The absolute latencies of N22 and P38, as well as the N22-P38 interval representing the central conduction of the lemniscal pathway, are considered. The clinical indication for SEPs is found in patients with demyelinating diseases of the central nervous system, Friedreich's ataxia, subacute combined sclerosis, vitamin E deficiency, coma, and brain death. In particular, the cortical components of SEPs are commonly used to obtain, albeit rough, information about the prognosis of coma patients. The absence of cortical components, in fact, indicates with good approximation an unfavorable prognosis for the functional recovery of the comatose patient.

Somatosensory Evoked Potential (SSEP) from the lower limb

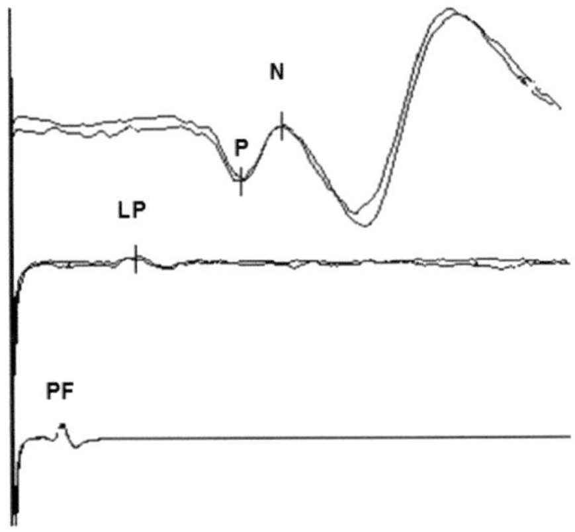

Figure 8.9

8.2.4 Motor evoked potentials (MEP)

The study of MEPs is the functional study of the corticospinal pathways using transcranial magnetic stimulation. The magnetic stimulator delivers magnetic stimuli through a coil placed on the scalp, inducing an electric current in the brain parenchyma and activating the neurons of the primary motor cortex via transsynaptic pathways. Transcranial activation of the descending motor pathways evokes short-latency muscle responses that can be recorded using surface electrodes. The required magnetic field intensity to activate the corticospinal pathway and evoke MEPs is reduced with a slight contraction of the target muscle. The parameters considered are the absolute latency of the MEP and the central conduction time. The central conduction time is defined as the difference between the latencies of the MEPs from cortical stimulation and the latency of the MEPs from radicular stimulation performed by placing the coil at the cervical region for upper

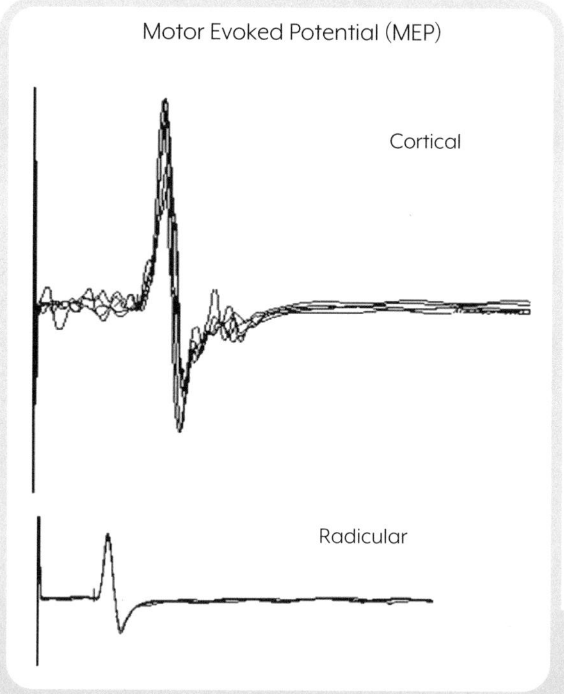

Figure 8.10

limb MEPs and at the lumbosacral region for lower limb MEPs (Figure 8.10).

In clinical practice, the main abnormalities of MEPs include the absence of the cortical MEP, increased MEP latency, and increased central conduction time. These alterations occur in cases of conduction block or slowing of the corticospinal fibers. The study of MEPs is indicated in patients with demyelinating diseases of the central nervous system, such as multiple sclerosis, amyotrophic lateral sclerosis, traumatic or spondylogenic myelopathy, and cerebrovascular lesions.

8.2.5 Laser Evoked Potentials (LEP)

Laser evoked potentials investigate the pain pathway. The stimulus consists of a brief laser radiation that causes a sudden increase in the temperature of the irradiated cutaneous region. This temperature increase activates the mechano-thermal nociceptors associated with Aδ and C fibers, generating an afferent input conducted along the spinothalamic system. Laser evoked potentials consist of two main components: N1, generated by the secondary somatosensory area (S2), and the biphasic complex N2-P2, generated by the insular cortex and cingulate gyrus. The recording for clinical-diagnostic purposes is performed with an electrode in the temporal region to study the N1 component and one at the vertex to study the N2-P2 complex. The main clinical application of laser evoked potentials is the study of peripheral and central nervous system pathologies involving the pain system. Therefore, they represent the elective method in diseases such as syringomyelia or small fiber neuropathy, characterized by selective damage to the pain afferents.

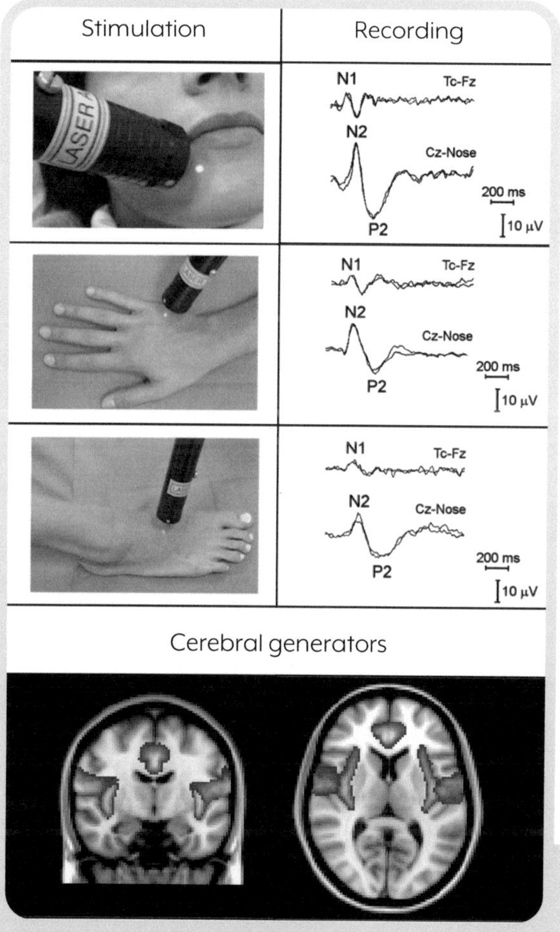

Figure 8.11

Bibliography

Currà A., Modugno N., Inghilleri M., Manfredi M., Hallett M., Berardelli A., Transcranial magnetic stimulation techniques in clinical investigation. Neurology; 59(12):1851-9, 2002.

Deuschl G., Eisen A., Reccomendations for the practice of clinical Neurophysiology: guidelines of the international Federation of clinical Neurophysiology. Elsevier, 1999.

Kimura J., Electrodiagnosis in diseases of nerve and muscle: principles and practice. Oxford University Press, 2001.

Lenman J.A.R., Ritchie A.E., Elettromiografia Clinica. Raffaello Cortina Editore, Milano.

Ludin H.P., Electromyography in Practice. New York: Thieme-Stratton, 1980.

Ubiali E., Elettroneurografia-Testo Atlante. Scienza Medica.

Preston D.C., Shapiro. B.E. Electromyography and Neuromuscular Disorders: Clinical-Electrophysiologic Correlations. Elsevier Inc. 2013.

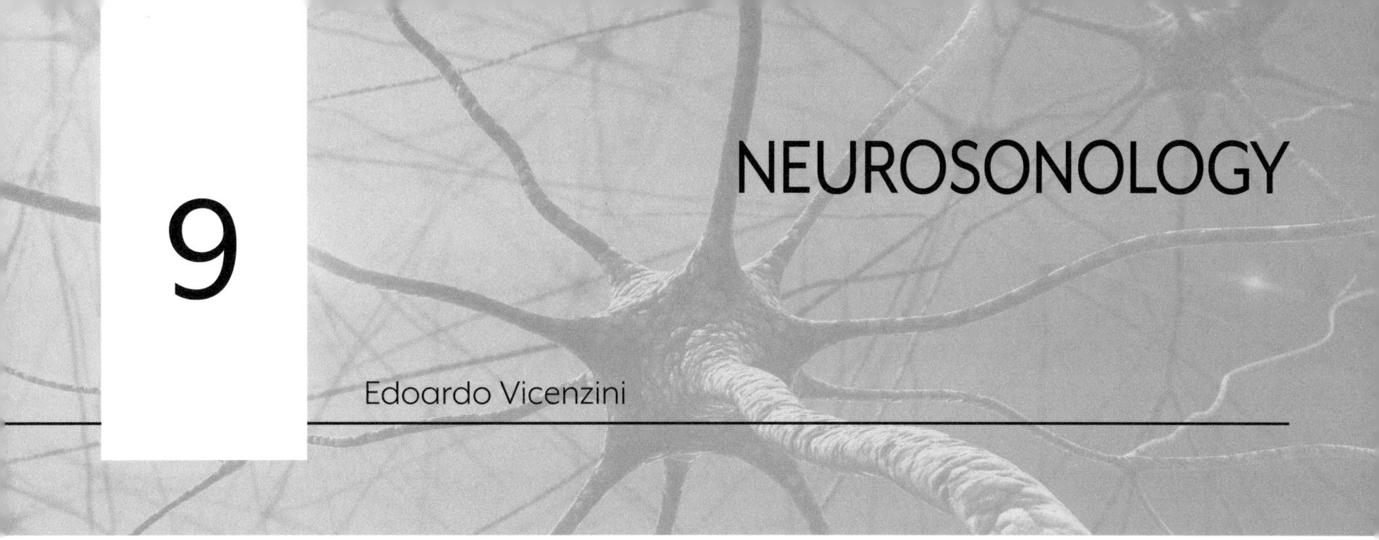

9 NEUROSONOLOGY

Edoardo Vicenzini

Neurosonology is part of the non-invasive vascular diagnostics in Neurology. It includes eco-color Doppler of the supra-aortic vessels and transcranial Doppler/color Doppler studies. The specific applications of transcranial studies include evaluating the diagnosis of paradoxical shunt (right → left) in the case of *patent foramen ovale*, diagnosing cerebral circulatory arrest in cases of brain death, and assessing the echogenicity of the substantia nigra and basal ganglia in movement disorders. Other recent applications of neurosonology involve studying the orbit to evaluate the diameter of the optic nerve sheath and performing ultrasound imaging of muscles and peripheral nerves.

9.1 Principles of ultrasound imaging

Ultrasound imaging is a technique based on ultrasound, which are sound waves with frequencies higher than 20.000 Hz, not audible to the human ear. A piezoelectric crystal, housed in a probe, is stimulated by electrical pulses and vibrates, producing ultrasound waves. The "targeted" tissues, which are insonated by the ultrasound waves, generate a reflected acoustic signal called "echo." The characteristics of the returning echo signal depend on the *impedance, acoustic attenuation* of the tissue, and the *intensity of the emitted* ultrasound. To obtain a visually interpretable two-dimensional representation of the returning echo, the most commonly used *imaging system* involves transforming the echo intensities into a grayscale scale (Brightness, B-Mode), in a bidimensional image. With this system, lipid-rich structures and fibrous tissue, which are partially penetrated by ultrasound waves, generate a low-intensity echo, resulting in "dark" hypoechoic images. Bones and air induce complete reflection of the sound waves, resulting in high-intensity echoes and a "bright" hyperechoic appearance. Muscular and fibrous structures, which are only partially penetrated by ultrasound waves, generate echoes of medium intensity and an appearance that is intermediate between the previous two, referred to as isoechoic. Additionally, calcified structures are not penetrated by ultrasound waves, generating highly hyperechoic images with a characteristic "acoustic " beneath, which means a lack of acoustic signal below them.

9.2 Doppler effect and velocimetry

The basis of ultrasonographic vascular diagnostics lies in the physical principle of the "Doppler effect," which refers to the frequency variation of sound waves reflected from a moving object. The equation described by the Austrian physicist Christian Doppler takes into account the emitted frequency (*f*0), the received frequency (*f*D), the angle of insonation (q), and the speed of sound propagation in tissue (c).

$$v = fD\frac{c}{2f0\cos\vartheta}$$

By knowing the frequency of the emitted ultrasound waves at start and the angle of insonation, it is then possible to calculate the direction and velocity of a moving structure being examined. In other words, structures approaching the probe produce a response echo with a higher frequency than the emitted one, while structures moving away from the probe generate an echo with a lower frequency.

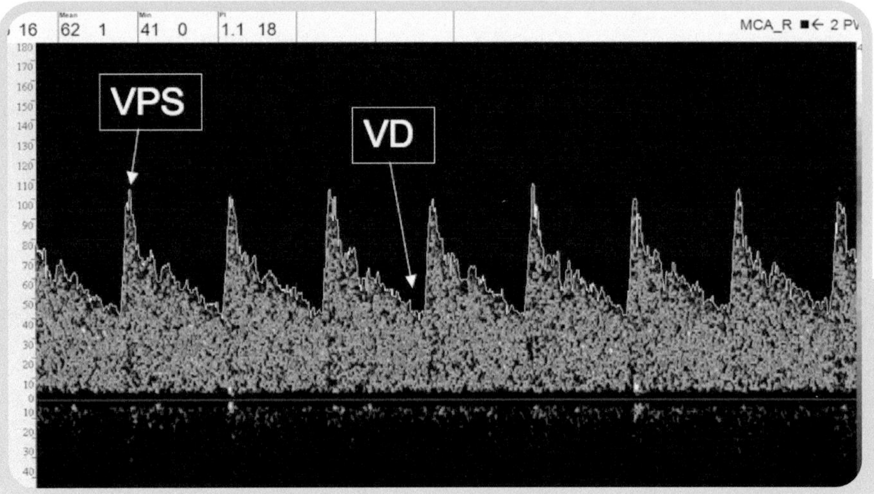

Figure 9.1

Typical Spectrogram of the Middle Cerebral Artery with Peak Systolic Velocity (VPS), Mean Velocity, and Diastolic Velocity (Min), VD.

An illustrative example of this effect in daily common experience is the different perception of the siren of an approaching or receding ambulance by our ears.

The Doppler effect is employed in medicine for "velocimetry," which is the study of blood velocity and direction within vessels. The movement of blood within arteries is represented by a typical "spectrum" that identifies the Peak Systolic Velocity (PSV), the Diastolic Velocity (DV), and the Mean Velocity (MV) (Figure 9.1).

By combining these three velocities, it is possible to obtain indices that reflect the elasticity of the examined vessel and the "resistance" of the downstream circulation to which they contribute: the Pulsatility Index (PSV-DV/MV) and the Resistance Index (PSV-DV/PSV). The intracranial circulation is typically a territory of "low resistance," and the arterial vessels that supply it (internal carotid arteries and vertebral arteries) have high DV. Conversely, the tributary arteries of the muscular districts (external carotid arteries, subclavian arteries, peripheral vessels) exhibit high PSV and low DV, indicating that blood flows predominantly during systole and tends to stagnate during diastole, resulting in "high resistance".

9.3 Eco-color-Doppler

Velocimetry alone is a "blind" investigative technique, as it relies solely on the examiner's experience to assess the vessels without any visual relief, based on predetermined points above the skin. For this reason, during the development of the method, B-Mode ultrasound was associated with velocimetry, giving rise to the "duplex-scan," which is a two-dimensional ultrasound that securely identifies the vessel to be explored with velocimetry. Subsequently, through further application of the Doppler effect, color coding (color Doppler) of blood direction and velocity was added to B-Mode ultrasound. These three techniques gave rise to the "triplex-scan," the eco-color Doppler (Figure 9.2 A), which allows for: the ultrasound study of vessel morphology in B-Mode, color coding of blood flow, and analysis of velocity parameters. Another development in color coding is represented by power Doppler, which visualizes blood flow not based on velocity and direction but on the amplitude of reflected Doppler frequencies. This technique allows for the visualization of slower flows and more tortuous vessels without dependence on the angle of insonation (Figures 9.2 B e C).

9.3.1 Eco-color-Doppler of the supra-aortic vessels

Eco-color Doppler of the supra-aortic vessels include the evaluation of the carotid district (common carotid, internal carotid, and external carotid), the subclavian-vertebral district, the brachiocephalic trunk, and the internal and external jugular veins. From a

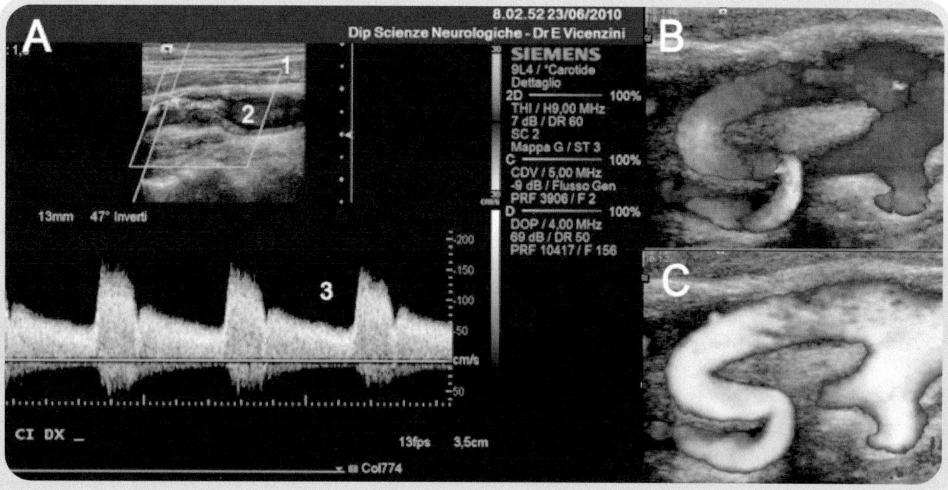

Figure 9.2

Triplex scan:
A) echo (1) color (2) Doppler (3) of a hemodynamic stenosis of the internal carotid artery.
B) color Doppler;
C) power Doppler.

technical point of view, it is performed with linear probes anteriorly and posteriorly to the sternocleidomastoid muscle, using longitudinal and transverse scanning planes.

Caliber and course of the vessels | Among the most frequently encountered caliber abnormalities affecting the carotid bifurcation, the dilation of the carotid bulb, known as carotid bulb ectasia, should be mentioned. It is typically a fusiform dilation with a diameter of approximately 1-1.5 cm anteroposteriorly, involving the distal segment of the common carotid artery and the origin of the internal carotid artery. It is often found in hypertensive patients and fibromuscular dysplasia. The diameters of the dilation can be easily measured using B-mode images, while color Doppler can visualize the turbulence associated with consequent hemodynamic alterations (Figure 9.3 A).

Asymptomatic course abnormalities can be classified as "tortuosity," "coiling," and "kinking." The latter (Figure 9.3 B, C), is frequently encountered and refers to an angulation of the vessel course in the longitudinal plane exceeding 90°, while below this value, it is referred to as a "tortuosity".

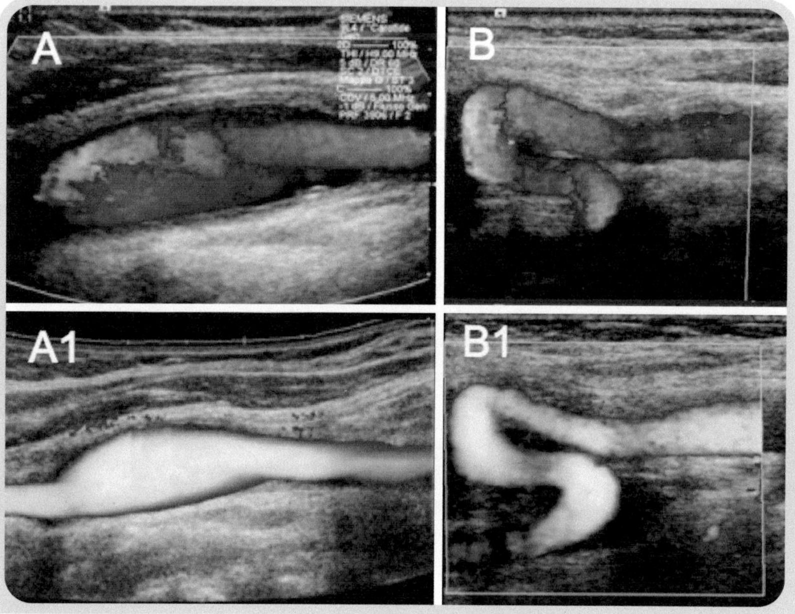

Figure 9.3

A-A1) Color and power Doppler of a case of carotid bulb ectasia. Note the flow turbulences in the color Doppler images. B-B1) Color and power Doppler of distal kinking of the internal carotid. In the power Doppler images (B1), the course of the vessel is visible with improved definition.

Coiling, on the other hand, involves angulation in both the longitudinal and transverse planes. Course tortuosities are typically found along the common carotid artery and the internal carotid artery, most commonly in the distal segment. These alterations are more prevalent in females and can be congenital or secondary to arteriosclerosis and fibromuscular dysplasia. When encountered in the vertebral arteries in the extracranial and intervertebral segment, they may be indicative of significant arthritic changes in the cervical spine. Kinking is asymptomatic and it does not have clinical relevance in a healthy individual but can be of fundamental importance in evaluating a surgical approach. The tortuous course of the vessel can hinder, for example, the endovascular positioning of a stent or make endarterectomy procedures more challenging. Tortuosities are visualized on eco-color Doppler as curvatures in the vessel course, accompanied by changes in the flow direction. Power Doppler, in general, can provide a more comprehensive visualization as the tortuous segments are more prone to color signal artifacts (Figure 9.3B e 9.3B1), related to flow direction changes.

Intima-media thickness of the common carotid artery | In B-Mode ultrasound images of the common carotid artery, a "double-line pattern" appearance of the vessel wall has been described, characterized by alternating hyperechoic layers (adventitia and intima) with a hypoechoic layer (media). Intima-media thickness (IMT) is measured in the distal pre-bifurcation centimeter of the common carotid artery on the posterior wall, which is usually more clearly visualized. The thickness is calculated using single, multiple, or computerized measurements, from the outermost sub-adventitial hypoechoic point to the innermost hyperechoic point of the vascular lumen (Figure 9.4). Pathological intimal thickening, correlated with chronological age, is considered > 1.0 mm and is typically observed in patients with arterial hypertension or vascular dysplasia. It is an indicator of atherosclerotic disease and is related to the condition of the coronary arteries. Therefore, systematic measurement of IMT as screening in young individuals is essential to identify general atherosclerotic changes and to potentially subject the patient to other cardiovascular investigations aimed at identifying coronary pathology, such as stress EKG.

Morphology and quantification of carotid stenosis | Color Doppler ultrasound allows for the characterization of carotid stenosis by visualizing the vessel wall, plaque appearance, and hemodynamic variations through the stenosis. The fundamental advantage of this technique is its real-time nature, allowing not only the evaluation of moving structures but also the adjustment of visualization during the examination by the operator, to obtain the "best view". When assessing carotid stenosis to evaluate the risk of stroke, the quantification of the degree of stenosis and the morphological characteristics of the plaque should always be considered. The following characteristics should be examined for plaque morphology characterization:

1) Structure: homogeneous or heterogeneous;
2) Echogenicity: hyperechoic with acoustic shadow (calcified), hyper- and isoechoic (fibrous), hypoechoic (hemorrhagic or lipid-rich);
3) Surface appearance: regular, irregular, or ulcerated;

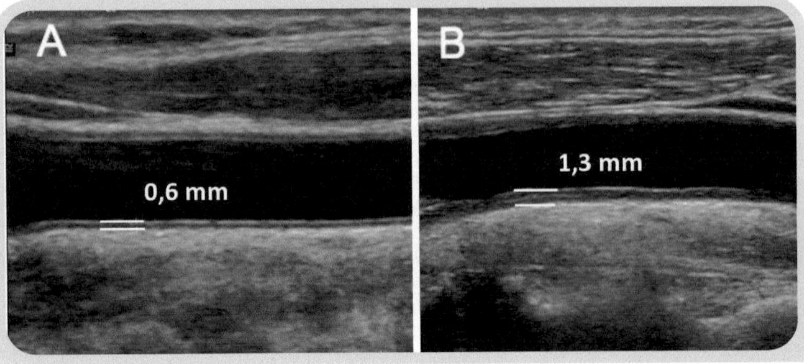

Figure 9.4

High-resolution B-Mode images of the intimal thickness of the common carotid artery, normal (A) and increased (B).

4) Percentage of stenosis: based on both visual and velocity criteria;
5) Location and extent of the lesion.

Accurate quantification of the degree of stenosis is of fundamental importance. As a matter of fact, according to the literature, stenoses greater than 70% have a specific indication for endarterectomy, even in primary prevention, as the surgical risk, with a qualified team, is lower than the risk of stroke when a medical and conservative approach is chosen. The degree of stenosis should be evaluated: a) based on visual criteria, by calculating the area and/or diameter of the stenosis, and b) based on velocity criteria, which rely on the fluidodynamic principle that blood velocity values increase proportionally with the degree of stenosis through the stenotic segment.

Visual and velocity criteria should be closely integrated to obtain precise quantification of the degree of stenosis. It should be noted that, although "numerical" and precise, the evaluation of the degree of stenosis is of a "semi-quantitative" nature, and decimal values (e.g., stenosis of 37.2%) derived solely from mathematical calculations based on the evaluation of stenosis areas should be avoided as they are strictly "operator-dependent." For stenosis less than 70%, surgical intervention is considered in cases of symptomatic stenosis in secondary prevention and the presence of unstable plaques. Plaques with a heterogeneous structure, iso- or hypoechoic, irregular or ulcerated surface with moderate-to-severe stenosis are considered more "unstable" and at risk of embolization (Figure 9.5A). The latest generation ultrasound devices allow for better spatial resolution and enable the evaluation of additional features of plaque "instability," such as thinning of the fibrous cap, plaque movement within the vessel, and the presence of fissures with adherent thrombi on its surface. The use of ultrasound contrast agents and "contrast-specific" imaging, which detects and visualizes the distribution of the contrast agent at the capillary level, has also increased the diagnostic sensitivity in the morphological evaluation of the plaque (e.g., detecting surface fissures) and, above all, in assessing plaques neovascularization, which reflects the inflammatory state of the lesion and, therefore, "plaque activity." Therefore, with these recent advancements, color Doppler ultrasound evaluation transforms from a

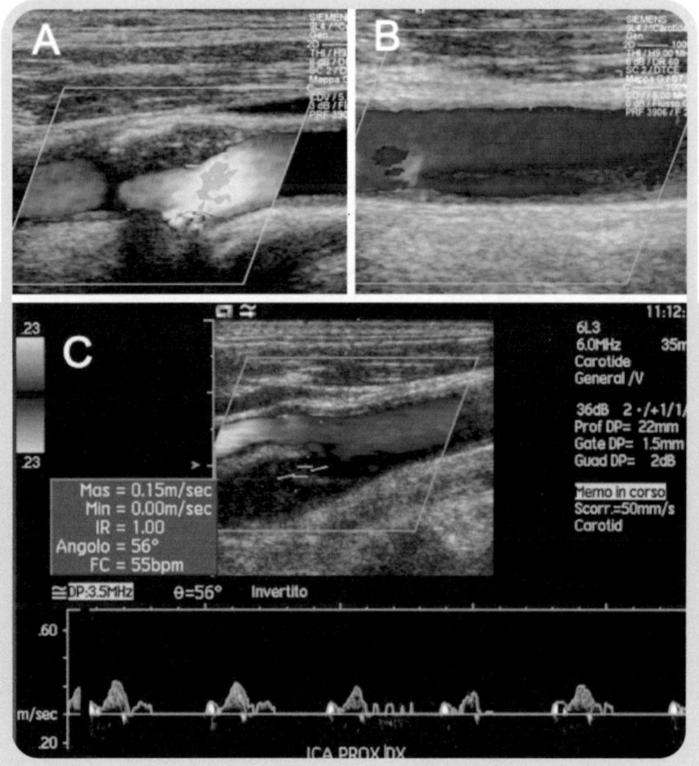

Figure 9.5

A) Eco-color Doppler of a moderately severe stenosis of the internal carotid artery due to an uneven plaque, with hyperechoic calcific heterogeneous components, acoustic shadowing, and areas of lower echogenicity. The surface shows a small ulceration in the proximal part, visible as a color signal alteration. B) Eco-color Doppler of a common carotid dissection: the double lumen is clearly visible, with reversed flow direction in the false lumen. C) Eco-color Doppler of an occlusion of the internal carotid artery: the color signal is not visible within the vessel, and no flow is detected by pulsed Doppler velocimetry.

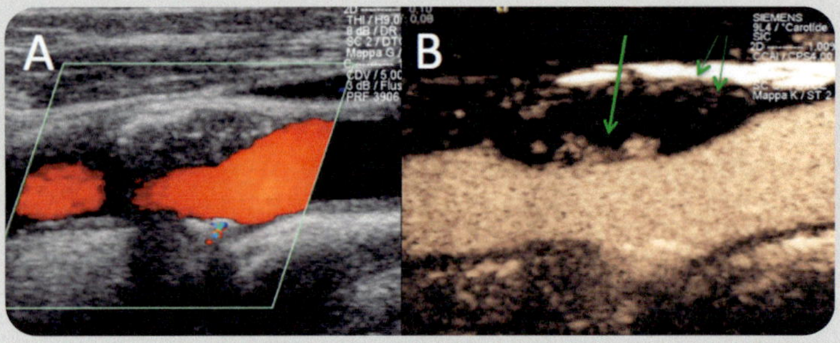

Figure 9.6

A) Eco-color-Doppler of a carotid artery stenosis caused by a heterogeneous plaque, seemingly with a smooth surface; B) Evaluation of the same lesion using contrast-enhanced ultrasound: the large arrow identifies the rupture of the plaque surface, while the small arrows show the diffusion of the contrast into the tissue of the plaque, indicating neoangiogenesis.

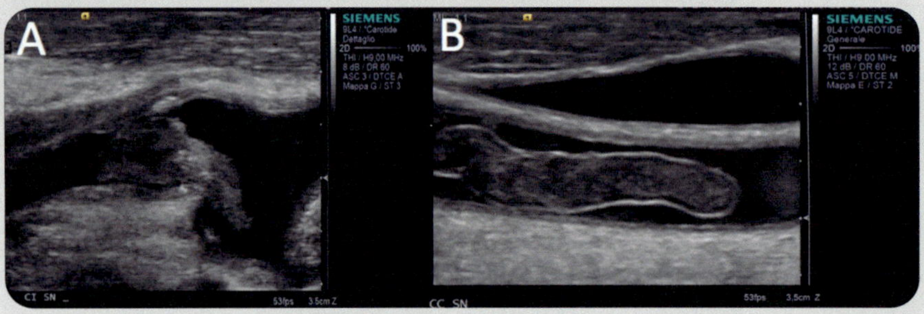

Figure 9.7

B-Mode evaluation of two cases of carotid occlusion due to a cardiac-origin embolus, localized 'opposite the bifurcation of the internal and external carotid arteries (A)' and 'in the middle segment of the common carotid artery (B).

"morphological" imaging to a true "functional" imaging, with undeniable value in the study of vascular pathology (Figurc 9.6 A, B).

Occlusion and dissection | The occlusion of the internal carotid artery is characterized by the absence of flow signal, both on color Doppler ultrasound and pulsed Doppler (Figure 9.5 C). In cases of distal intracranial occlusion of the internal carotid artery, vessel patency is observed at the carotid bifurcation level, but with increased resistance indices and a typically "basculating to-and-fro" flow that is zero or reversed in diastole. A particular clinical condition that can lead to internal carotid artery occlusion is the dissection (Figure 9.5 B). The separation of the intima from the outer layers at the bifurcation forms a "false lumen" below the dissection, accompanied by wall hemorrhage. This, combined with the underlying systolic wave, can result in vessel occlusion. Using color Doppler ultrasound, it is possible to detect the absence of signal in both color Doppler and pulsed Doppler in cases of occlusion due to dissection. A typical feature of dissection is the presence of a "double lumen" with the "intimal flap" of the dissected and mobile intima within the vessel, and a hypoechoic appearance in B-Mode images corresponding to the intraparietal hematoma that occludes the artery. Furthermore, it should be noted that occlusion of the internal carotid artery does not exclusively occur due to the degeneration of atherosclerotic carotid stenosis but can also result from the presence of cardiac emboli. With the high spatial resolution of ultrasound imaging and its real-time capabilities, these emboli can be more easily identified compared to conventional static radiological imaging (Figure 9.7 A, B).

Vertebral Pathology and "Subclavian Steal Syndrome" | An often-observed aspect related to the vertebral arteries is asymmetry in caliber typically with dominance on the left side. When the vessel caliber is less than 2 mm, it is referred to as hypoplasia, and an increase in resistance indices with a reduction in systolic and diastolic velocities is observed. Correlating the velocity findings with the vessel caliber is crucial for the differential diagnosis of a distal intracranial occlusion, where reduced velocity values and increased resistance indices occur in a vessel with a normal caliber. Simultaneous performance of transcranial Doppler is essential in these cases to identify the distal intracranial pathology. A specific condition in the subclavian-vertebral district is "subclavian steal syndrome." Severe stenosis or occlusion of the subclavian artery before the origin of the vertebral artery leads to a compensatory circulation aimed at maintaining blood supply to the upper limb ipsilateral to the occlusion. Blood from the contralateral subclavian artery reaches the basilar artery and reverses the flow direction in the vertebral artery, which becomes the vessel supplying the upper limb irrigated by the occluded subclavian artery, resulting in a true "stealing" of blood from the brain.

9.3.2 Transcranial Doppler and Transcranial Color-Doppler

The ultrasonographic study of intracranial vessels represents, in selected patients, the "completion" of the study of epiaortic vessels. It can be performed using two different and complementary techniques: Transcranial Doppler (TCD) and Transcranial Color Doppler (TCCD). TCD involves the application of Doppler velocimetry to measure velocity values in the major intracranial arteries (middle cerebral arteries, anterior cerebral arteries, posterior cerebral arteries, vertebral arteries, and basilar artery) (Figure 9.1). It is performed using a relatively simple device called a "transcranial Doppler system" with 2 MHz probes, through the temporal, suboccipital, and transorbital "acoustic windows". In the temporal region, the cranial bone is thinner, allowing the passage of ultrasound waves for the evaluation of intracranial structures, while in the suboccipital region, the bone is absent. On the other hand, TCCD is performed using dedicated ultrasound devices with sector probes of 2-3 MHz, similar to those used in cardiology, but with different presets. The flow results are encoded in a color image, allowing for visual identification of the Willis polygon (Figure 9.8). However, it should be noted that this is a "duplex" method: the visualization of the vessel is a result of detecting the movement of blood flow inside it, while the arterial wall is not visualized. For both techniques, the main limitation for performing the examination is the inadequacy of the temporal "acoustic window," which does not provide good visualization of intracranial structures in approximately 5% of subjects (usually older individuals and females).

TCD and TCCD find application in the following fields:

1) In primary and secondary prevention of cerebral ischemia and in patients with vascular risk factors, for the identification of hemodynamic intracranial stenosis, which can be detected through increased velocity findings in TCD and alterations in color signal encoding in CDTC;
2) In the acute phase of cerebral ischemia, for the identification of arterial occlusion, which can be detected by the absence of signal or significant changes in symmetry indices, and for subsequent monitoring of potential recanalization processes;
3) In the evaluation of the functionality of intracranial compensatory circuits, such as the activation capacity of communicating arteries following common carotid compression manoeuvers, which simulate intraoperative clamping, or in the case of carotid occlusion and vasomotor reserve, which measures the vasodilation/

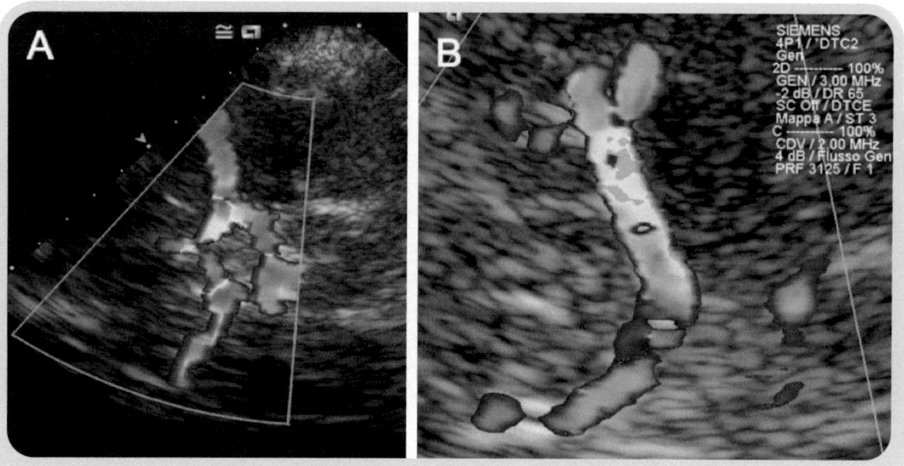

Figure 9.8

Transcranial Color Doppler: Overview of the Willis polygon (A) and detailed view of the middle and anterior cerebral arteries (B), showing the visualization of the distal branches of the middle cerebral artery and trifurcation.

vasoconstriction capacity in response to hypo/hypercapnia stimuli. This evaluation is performed in patients undergoing carotid endarterectomy;

4) In subarachnoid hemorrhage, for the assessment and monitoring of vasospasm, a frequent cause of neurological symptom worsening in the days following the acute event;
5) In the determination of brain death, for evaluating the cessation of circulation at the level of intracranial vessels.

Cerebral circulatory arrest in the case of brain death | The law provides that, in specific cases (children under one year old, presence of central nervous system depressant drugs that interfere with instrumental clinical assessment, clinical situations that do not allow for a certain etiopathogenetic diagnosis or the execution of brainstem reflexes, apnea test and EEG recording), the initiation of brain death diagnosis procedure should be preceded by the evaluation of cerebral blood flow, typically using traditional angiography or Transcranial Doppler. Diffuse cerebral edema and intracranial hypertension result in the progressive transformation of the cerebral vascular territory from low resistance to high resistance, with a gradual reduction, reversal of direction, and disappearance of the diastolic component of the flow. These patterns, known as "reverberant flow" and "systolic spikes", are pathognomonic of circulatory arrest and brain death. Transcranial Doppler for the diagnosis of cerebral circulatory arrest has a diagnostic sensitivity of 97% (with false positives in patients with decompressive craniectomy or external ventricular drains) and a specificity of 100%, and it offers the clear advantage of being a non-invasive technique that can be performed at the patient's bedside in critical cases (Figure 9.9 A, B, C, D).

Right-to-left circulatory shunt and patent foramen ovale (PFO) | In healthy individuals, peripheral venous blood reaches the right heart chambers, and the pulmonary filter allows for oxygenation and 'filtration.' In the presence of abnormal communications between the right and left cardiac chambers, such as in the case of atrial septal defects, patent foramen ovale (PFO), or pulmonary arteriovenous malformations, peripheral venous blood can bypass the pulmonary filter and directly reach the systemic arterial circulation. PFO can be found in up to 30% of healthy and asymptomatic individuals in the general population. Under certain conditions, if associated with atrial septal aneurysm or coagulopathies, including those iatrogenic due to hormone replacement therapy or contraceptive use, PFO can become an embolic source. When combined with deep venous thrombosis, the detachment of embolic material can lead to a so-called "paradoxical embolism", where the embolus bypasses the pulmonary filter and directly enters the systemic arterial circulation through the right-to-left shunt. The presence of PFO may represent a risk factor for paradoxical embolism, even in scuba divers and high-altitude pilots who are more prone to gas embolism formation during

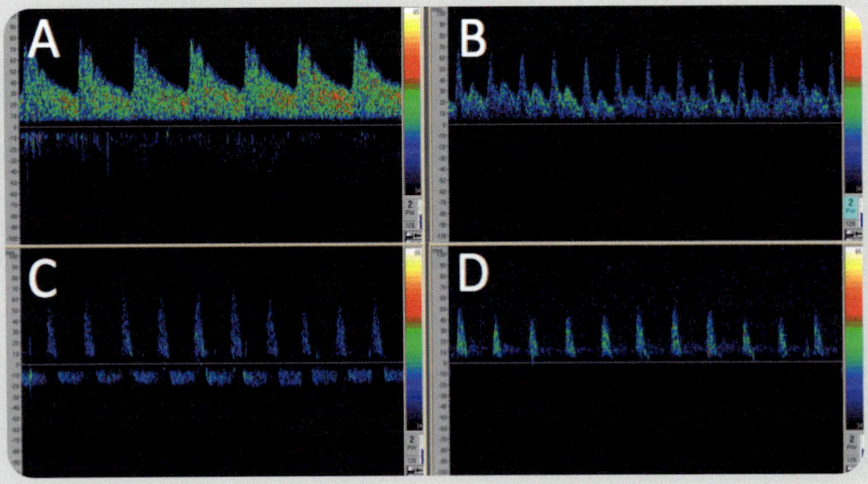

Figure 9.9

Evolution of the spectrogram of the middle cerebral artery with increasing intracranial pressure until circulatory arrest. A) Normal; B) Increase in resistance indices due to intracranial hypertension; C) Reversal of the direction of diastolic flow - "reversed flow"; D) Disappearance of the diastolic component "systolic spikes". Frames C and D are pathognomonic of intracranial circulatory arrest.

decompression phases. Furthermore, there is a non-causal association between PFO and patients with migraine with aura.

The morphological characterization of PFO is performed by transthoracic echocardiography with saline contrast and transesophageal echocardiography, which is an invasive technique reserved for selected patients. On the other hand, transcranial Doppler with saline contrast is a less invasive method for diagnosing right-to-left circulatory shunt. The technique is simple and carries no risks for the patient. Middle cerebral arteries are monitored using an externally applied fixation device resembling a "helmet" (Figure 9.10), and a "saline contrast" mixture, consisting of 9 cc of saline solution and 1 cc of air, is injected through a peripheral vein and rapidly mixed using a three-way stopcock. The "intact" pulmonary circulation normally arrests the microbubbles of the saline contrast, whereas they are observed in the intracranial circulation in the case of a right→left shunt, such as in the presence of PFO (Figure 9.9). In selected cases, the possibility of surgical closure of PFO using an endovascular technique may be considered.

However, the performance of transcranial Doppler examination for the detection of right→left shunt should be limited to selected cases and should always be pursued in cases of "cryptogenic" stroke, i.e., without an evident cause, especially in young patients.

Other applications of neurosonology | The development of more recent technologies involves the use of ultrasound contrast agents for the *semi-quantitative evaluation of cerebral perfusion* and for "*sonothrombolysis*", which is the combined use of ultrasound and contrast agents as adjuvants in the recanalization process during acute phase of cerebral stroke, in case of intracranial arterial occlusion. In patients with adequate acoustic windows, it is also possible to study certain areas of the brain parenchyma. A relatively recent introduction is the possibility of evaluating, through high-resolution transcranial B-mode ultrasound, the modifications of the *Substantia Nigra* (SN) and the *basal ganglia* in patients with movement disorders. An increase in the echogenicity of the SN, attributable to an increase in iron deposits at that level, has been observed in over 90% of patients with Parkinson's disease, without significant correlations with the severity of the clinical picture and without substantial changes in echogenicity during the course of the disease. The hyperechogenicity of the SN and alterations in other basal ganglia can be helpful in the differential diagnosis between Parkinson's disease, essential tremor, and other parkinsonian syndromes (Figure 9.11). The recognition of the triad consisting of a) hyperechogenicity of the SN, b) anosmia, and c) motor disturbances can be considered a marker of Parkinson's disease, even in its early stages. To obtain increasingly detailed and reliable evaluations, the recently introduced "fusion" technology allows for the integration and overlaying of previously acquired Magnetic Resonance Imaging images on the ultrasound machine screen, enabling true "real-time" ultrasound navigation. Furthermore, the use of ultrasound is finding increasing applications

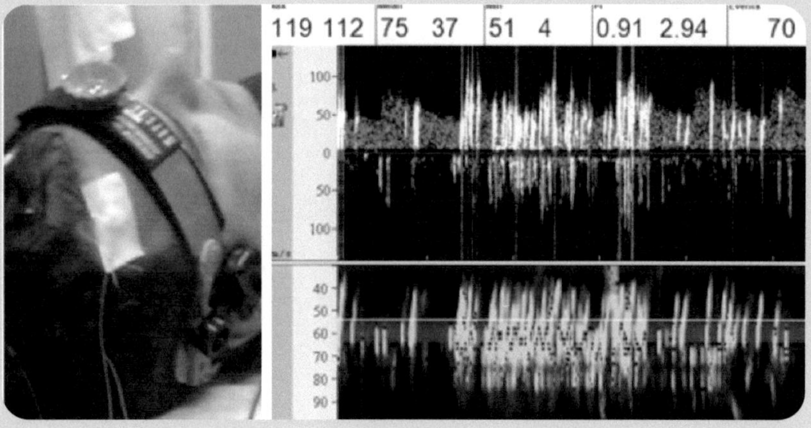

Figure 9.10

Transcranial Doppler with a test for the diagnosis of right-to-left shunt. By applying a bilateral monitoring 'helmet,' the gaseous microbubbles of the agitated saline solution that pass through the interatrial septal foramen ovale can be easily identified in the Doppler spectrogram of the middle cerebral artery as short-duration, high-intensity signals (High Intensity Transient Signals - HITS or Micro Embolic Signals - MES).

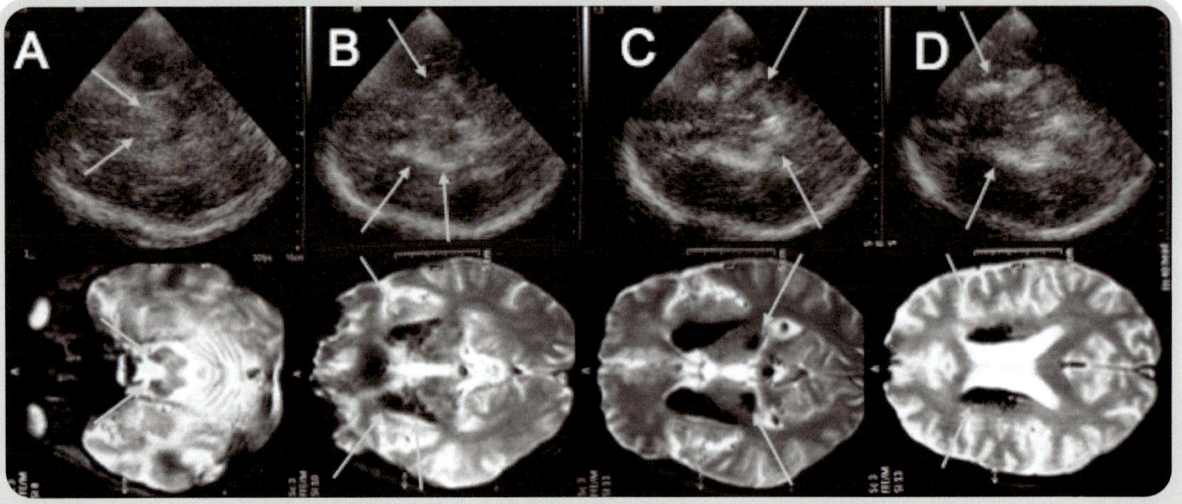

Figure 9.11

B-Mode ultrasound (top) and corresponding Magnetic Resonance Imaging (bottom) images documenting (arrows) the altered echogenicity of the substantia nigra and calcifications in the basal nuclei in a patient with Fahr's disease.

in neurology, such as in the study of the optic nerve sheath and peripheral nerves. The optic nerve sheath is an outpouching of the meninges, in direct communication with the subarachnoid spaces, and its "swelling" is universally recognized as a sign of increased intracranial pressure; therefore, measuring the thickness of the optic nerve sheath provides a rapid and non-invasive tool for neuromonitoring critically ill neurological patients in intensive care (Figure 9.12). Peripheral nerve ultrasound also offers the possibility of non-invasively evaluating the microstructure of peripheral nerves along their entire course in the limbs - with a higher spatial resolution than magnetic resonance imaging - and, in association with classical neurophysiological studies, provides early data on the morphology and topography of nerve lesions that are difficult to visualize, such as cysts, transection injuries, tumors, and signs of degeneration, which are essential in the diagnostic and therapeutic work-up process.

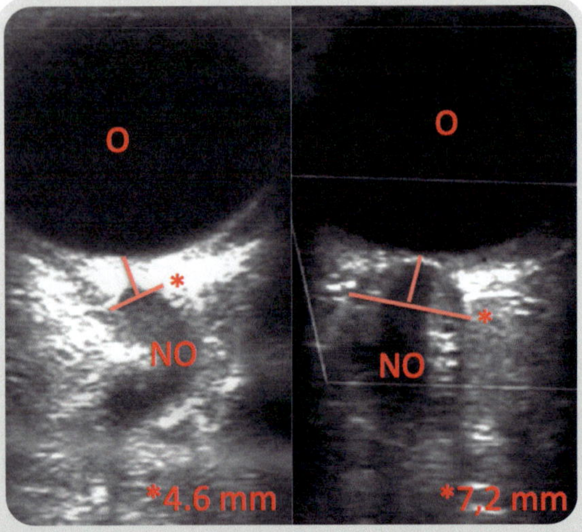

Figure 9.12

B-Mode Imaging of the Eye and Optic Nerve in a Healthy Patient (left) and in a Patient with Intracranial Hypertension (right). The significant increase in optic nerve sheath thickness (horizontal line, 7.2 mm), conventionally measured 3 mm from the optic disc, is documented in cases of malignant intracranial hypertension. O: eye; NO: optic nerve.

Bibliography

Bartels E., Color-Coded Duplex Ultrasound of the cerebral vessels. Atlas and Manual. Ed Schattauer, 1999.

Berardelli A., Wenning G.K., Antonini A., Berg D., Bloem B.R., Bonifati V., Brooks D., Burn D.J., Colosimo C., Fanciulli A., Ferreira J., Gasser T., Grandas F., Kanovsky P., Kostic V., Kulisevsky J., Oertel W., Poewe W., Reese J.P., Relja M., Ruzicka E., Schrag A., Seppi K., Taba P., Vidailhet

M., EFNS/MDS-ES/ENS recommendations for the diagnosis of Parkinson's disease. Eur J Neurol; 20(1):16-34, 2013.

Baumgartner R.W., Transcranial color-coded duplex sonography. J Neurol; 246: 637-647, 1999.

Csiba L., Baracchini C., Manual of Neurosonology. Cambridge University Press, 2016.

Hennerici M.G., The unstable plaque. Cerebrovasc Dis; 17(Suppl 3):17-22, 2004.

Gasparotti R., Padua L., Briani C., Lauria G., New technologies for the assessment of neuropathies. Nat Rev Neurol; 13(4): 203-216, 2017.

Toscano M., Spadetta G., Pulitano P., Rocco M., Di Piero V., Mecarelli O., Vicenzini E.,Optic Nerve Sheath Diameter Ultrasound Evaluation in Intensive Care Unit: Possible Role and Clinical Aspects in Neurological Critical Patients' Daily Monitoring. Biomed Res Int. :1621428, 2017.

Vicenzini E., Ricciardi M.C., Puccinelli F., Altieri M., Vanacore N., Di Piero V., Lenzi G.L., Common carotid artery intima-media thickness determinants in a population study. J Ultrasound Med; 26: 427-432, 2007.

Valdueza J.M., Schreiber S., Roherl J.E., Klingebiel R., Neurosonology and Neuroimaging of Stroke. Ed Thieme, 2008.

Vicenzini E., Giannoni M.F., Puccinelli F., Ricciardi M.C., Altieri M. Di Piero V., Gossetti B., Benedetti-Valentini F., Lenzi G.L., Detection of carotid adventitial vasa vasorum and plaque vascularization with ultrasound cadence contrast pulse sequencing technique and echocontrast agent. Stroke; 38: 2841-2843, 2007.

Vicenzini E., Ricciardi M.C., Sirimarco G., Di Piero V., Lenzi G.L., Extracranial and intracranial sonographic findings in vertebral artery diseases. J Ultrasound Med; 29: 1811-1823, 2010.

Vicenzini E., Pro S., Pulitano P., Rocco M., Spadetta G., Zarabla A., Di Piero V., Mecarelli O., Current practice of brain death determination and use of confirmatory tests in an Italian University hospital: a report of 66 cases. Minerva Anestesiol.;79(5):485-91, 2013.

10 CONSCIOUSNESS AND ITS DISORDERS

Francesco Orzi, Michele Cavallari, Marco Salvetti

The meaning of the word "consciousness" varies depending on the context. In the medical field, it refers to the awareness of one's self and the surrounding environment. *Consciousness* remains challenging to describe. Current definitions are essentially tautologies, and an operational definition is lacking. It also remains unclear why the brain is conscious and what the evolutionary advantage of consciousness may be. Neuroscience seeks to address questions that are inherently linked to ancient philosophical quests regarding the relationship between the physical and phenomenal world, whether the world we perceive is real or a construct of experience, and the biological and psychological mechanisms that mediate the interpretation of sensory stimuli reaching the brain.

The neurological approach to consciousness is reductionist and less sophisticated. The main objective of a neurologist is to identify the underlying cause of an altered state of consciousness. However, the assessment of consciousness can pose a challenge due to the elusive nature of its definition. As a subjective experience, consciousness is difficult to subject to empirical investigation. One indirect approach to accessing consciousness is through the examination of its expressions. A conscious individual has facial expressions and gaze that vary in response to stimuli. If the "internal" perspective of consciousness is entirely private and ungraspable from the outside, the "external" perspective relies on language, motor function (eye movements in particular), muscle tone, and posture. These expressions involve the functioning of the motor systems that mediate them. Therefore, there is a phenomenology of consciousness, but its expression implies the function of anatomical and functional structures independent from consciousness. Making inferences about the state of consciousness in the presence of severe motor impairment can be challenging. The neurologist must distinguish altered states of consciousness from conditions in which consciousness is intact, but its phenomenology is absent or reduced due to severe sensory, motor, or psychiatric disturbances that prevent its externalization (e.g., the locked-in syndrome). Some patients may no longer be able to respond to stimuli, even though they have a conscious experience of the stimuli themselves. This condition may arise from sensory disconnection, motor dysfunction, or severe impairment of executive functions, for instance during sleep, under anesthesia, or as a result of brain injuries.

Ongoing research aims to discover investigative tools that may reflect the state of consciousness and serve as surrogates when the "traditional" phenomenological aspects of consciousness are compromised. These tools include the assessment of changes in functional brain parameters following stimulation (e.g., auditory, visual, or transcranial magnetic stimulations), using functional neuroimaging or electroencephalography.

With a reductionistic but practical approach, from a medical standpoint consciousness can be categorized into two aspects: vigilance and content. Vigilance (*wakefulness*) can be evaluated from the individual's ability to respond to stimuli. Content (*awareness*) is represented by the individual's collective emotional, cognitive,

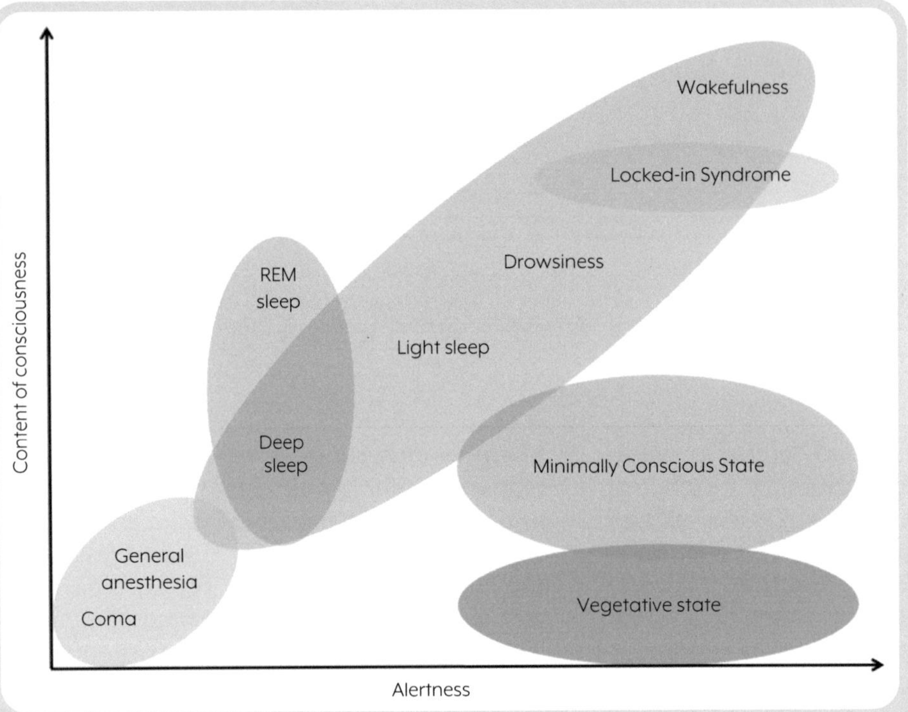

Figure 10.1

Consciousness and vigilance contribute to characterizing various physiological and pathological conditions (Laureys, 2007).

and behavioral expressions, which can be evaluated through verbal and non-verbal language. These two phenomenological aspects have their own identity, to the extent that they can be present or absent in an individual in a dissociated manner. From a clinical perspective, the level of consciousness of a patient can be represented by a diagram in which *vigilance* and *content* are plotted on the x and y axis, respectively (Figure 10.1). Dreaming can be considered a condition of reduced vigilance with unchanged content of consciousness. Except for this specific physiological condition, states of altered vigilance always entail an altered content of consciousness. Conversely, vigilance can be present under conditions of severe impairment of consciousness.

10.1 Anatomical bases of consciousness

10.1.1 Vigilance

Observations in subjects with Wernicke's encephalopathy or lethargic encephalitis, conducted during an epidemic that affected Europe between 1915 and 1920, as well as later pivotal studies of experimental neurophysiology by Moruzzi and Magoun, have pointed to the role of the brainstem reticular formation in mediating cortical *arousal* functions. More recently, it has been established that the ascending activation system includes several circuits that extend from the brainstem to the hypothalamus. They include diffuse ascending projections from the reticular substance and neurons located in the locus coeruleus, hypothalamic nuclei, dorsal raphe nucleus, mesencephalic tegmentum, and Meynert's basal nucleus, which are active during wakefulness. Several neurotransmitters are implicated in the function of those systems, including adrenaline and noradrenaline (locus coeruleus), acetylcholine (Meynert's nucleus), glutamate (reticular substance), and serotonin (raphe nucleus and tegmental area). Orexins, discovered in 1998 and produced by neurons in the lateral posterior hypothalamus, regulate wakefulness and sleep, among other functions. Orexins and their receptors are also present outside the nervous system, particularly in organs involved in nutrition and energy metabolism, such as the gastrointestinal tract and pancreas. These networks, either collectively or independently, modulate cortical functions and are responsible for maintaining vigilance. From a clinical perspective, the presence of vigilance necessarily implies the functional activity of the brainstem.

10.1.2 Consciousness content

Clinical conditions in which vigilance is preserved while the content of consciousness is altered include the *vegetative state*, *minimally conscious state*, *akinetic mutism*, and certain types of epileptic seizures. These areas are extensive and bilateral, in line with the concept of cognition as an "emerging" function. This term is central to complex systems theories and reflects the notion that consciousness is a distributed function that arises from the integration of multiple neural systems (with their respective functions), each of which is relatively simple compared to the function that emerges from their integration. Electrophysiological tools demonstrate that during a conscious experience, cortical areas exhibit high connectivity. The thalamus serves as the functional hub of this diffuse neural network and is itself targeted by major activating systems from the brainstem and hypothalamus. This implies that a disorder of consciousness is generally the expression of a widespread, bilateral brain dysfunction. The dysfunction can result from structural damage to cortical areas or areas projecting to the cortices (e.g., the brainstem or thalamus), or metabolic abnormalities (e.g., endocrine disturbances, electrolyte imbalances, or other internal medicine conditions). From a practical standpoint and with some approximation, an alteration of consciousness often implies extensive, bilateral cortical dysfunction. Table 10.1 lists the most common pathological alterations of consciousness. In this chapter, we will discuss coma, *vegetative state*, and *locked-in syndrome*. Although locked-in syndrome is not characterized by any alteration of consciousness, it can present differential diagnosis challenges with respect to coma. From a clinical perspective, a loss of consciousness content implies brainstem dysfunction or widespread bihemispheric dysfunction.

Table 10.1 PATHOLOGICAL ALTERATIONS OF CONSCIOUSNESS

Transient	Coma Acute Confusional Episode Concussion Narcolepsy Syncope Epilepsy
Prolonged	Minimally Conscious State Unresponsive Wakefulness Syndrome (Vegetative State)

10.2 Coma

Coma is a transient condition of altered vigilance, with the potential for recovery of consciousness, regression to a vegetative state, or death. The duration varies but is typically less than 30 days. A comatose patient lies with closed eyes and does not respond (or responds only partially) to stimuli. Impaired vigilance is often accompanied by vegetative dysfunctions that lead to disturbances in heart rhythm, blood pressure, and breathing.

10.2.1 Causes

The causes of coma can be divided into two groups: brain injuries, and systemic or metabolic abnormalities.

Figure 10.2, outlines the leading causes of coma due to brain injuries and metabolic causes. Coma caused by brain injuries is typically associated with focal neurological signs and positive findings on neuroimaging, such as brain computed tomography (CT) or magnetic resonance imaging (MRI). The injuries can be supratentorial or infratentorial. In order to cause coma, supratentorial injuries must be extensive and bilateral. Alternatively, they may result from secondary damage to the brainstem through the "mass effect" of a brain lesion, leading to brain herniation through the tentorium of the cerebellum. Transtentorial herniations can involve: a) downward wedging of brain structures, which compress the diencephalon and then the brainstem structures, leading to progressive dysfunction in a rostrocaudal direction (rostrocaudal deterioration); b) displacement of the medial portion of the temporal lobe (uncus),

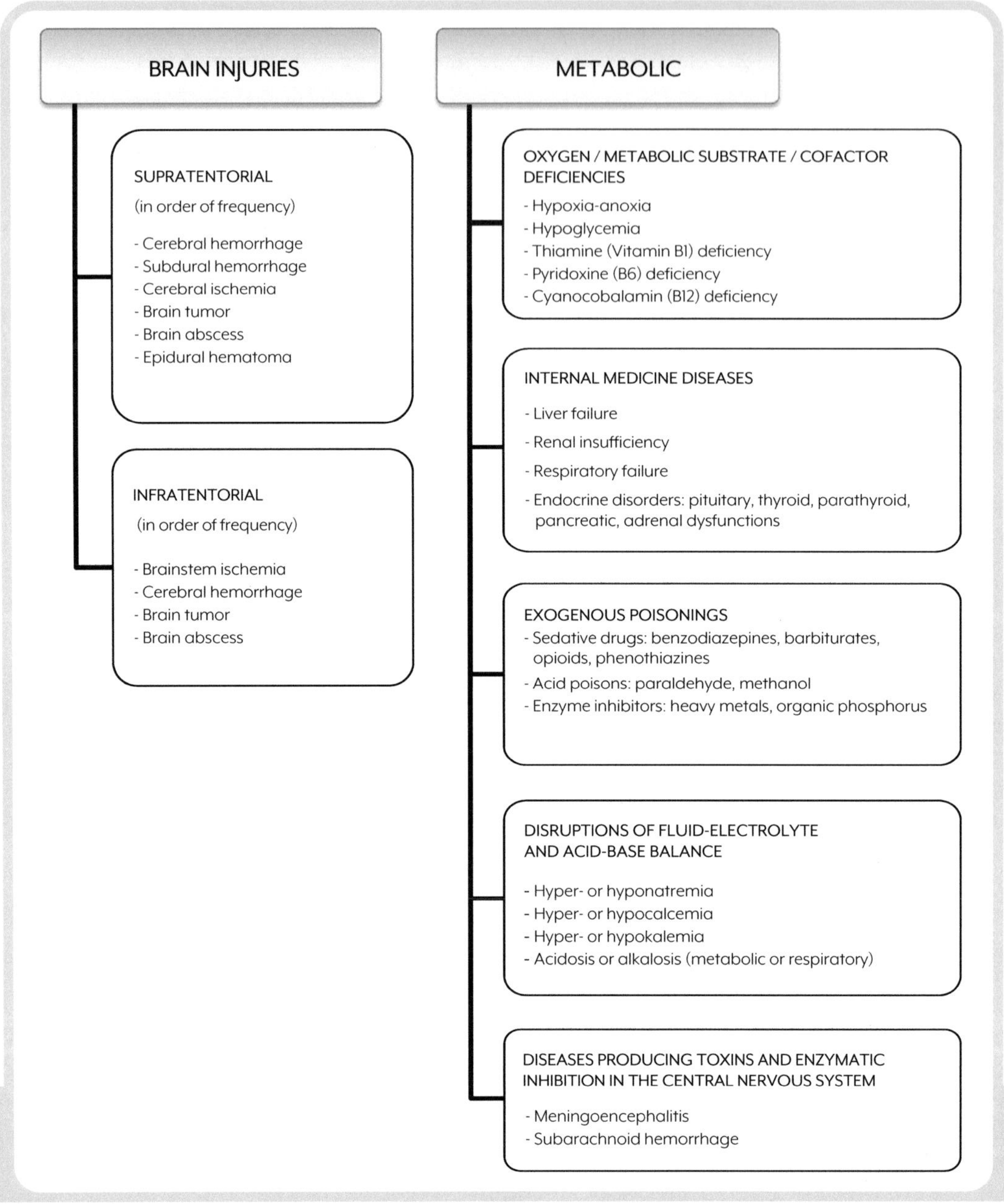

Figure 10.2 Causes of coma.

resulting in compression of the mesencephalic structures. In this case, the third cranial nerve compression causes fixed ipsilateral mydriasis. Increased intracranial pressure is another mechanism implicated in coma from supratentorial brain lesions, although its role is still debated. In contrast, infratentorial lesions cause coma through direct involvement of the ascending activating system. Metabolic coma is usually not accompanied by focal neurological signs, except when hypoglycemia is the cause. Metabolic causes lead to coma through diffuse brain dysfunction. Iatrogenic forms and substance abuse, such as sedative medications, alcohol, drugs, and toxins, are among the most common causes of metabolic coma. Other possible causes include nutritional deficiencies, metabolic substrate disorders (hypoxia and hypoglycemia), and electrolyte or acid-base imbalances.

10.2.2 Diagnosis

The diagnostic workflow starts with the medical history. It is important to assess:

1) *The onset of coma*. Sudden onset may suggest subarachnoid or intraparenchymal hemorrhage, head trauma, or cardiac dysfunction. A sudden coma without apparent signs of focal brain damage suggests severe cerebral hypoperfusion, often due to cardiac causes. Gradual onset may indicate a non-traumatic brain lesion or metabolic causes.
2) *Symptoms immediately preceding the alteration of consciousness*. Headache or focal neurological signs and symptoms (e.g., limb weakness, focal sensory deficits, diplopia) may indicate a compressive brain lesion.
3) *History of recent traumas.*
4) *Any pre-existing conditions that may lead to coma*, with particular attention to diabetes, renal insufficiency, heart disease, and psychiatric disorders.
5) *Use of sedative medications* (benzodiazepines, barbiturates, neuroleptics) or substance abuse.

The neurological examination of a comatose patient differs from the "standard" examination. A simple inspection can help understand the etiology of coma. It is important to look for the following:

- Direct or indirect signs of head trauma, including periorbital or periauricular ecchymosis (Battle's sign) suggestive of basal skull fracture.
- Pupillary anisocoria with mydriasis, indicative of compression of the third cranial nerve due to ipsilateral herniation of the uncus, suggestive of increased intracranial pressure and/or other serious pathology (e.g., aneurysmal dilation).
- Tongue biting or sphincter release, suggestive of an epileptic seizure.
- Petechiae, potential expression of meningitis or disseminated intravascular coagulation.
- Signs of substance abuse, such as alcoholic breath or injection marks.
- Clues to metabolic causes such as ketosis breath, asterixis, or multifocal myoclonus.
- Hypothermia, potentially suggestive of sedative intoxication, severe hypothyroidism, sepsis in older adults, or drowning.
- Hyperthermia, indicating central nervous system infection, sepsis, or neuroleptic malignant syndrome.

The neurological examination proceeds with the assessment of ocular motility, motor response to painful stimulation, brainstem reflexes, breathing, and nuchal rigidity. These parameters can be coded within scales (Table 10.2) that provide a numerical value of the depth of the coma. Scales can provide a rapid and standardized assessment of the comatose patient. However, a description of the patient's neurological status is often preferred in clinical practice.

Levels of impaired consciousness | The intensity of the stimulus required to elicit a response and the quality of the response define the level of impaired consciousness. The following clinical scenarios can be outlined:

1) *Obtundation*. The patient shows present but delayed response to low-intensity stimuli.
2) *Stupor*, The patient can only be awakened with vigorous (e.g., nociceptive) or prolonged stimulation.
3) *Coma*, The patient lies with eyes closed and does not respond appropriately to stimuli, even if it is of high intensity (i.e., unarousable unresponsiveness). Incongruous or stereotyped motor responses to nociceptive stimulation may be present. The examiner should always administer the stimuli bilaterally to ensure that the possible lack of response is not due to sensory or motor deficits that may be associated with the cause of coma.

Postural responses | Postural responses are stereotyped trunk and limb responses evoked or exacerbated by nociceptive stimuli. They can be divided into two types:

1) Decerebrate posture, which is characterized by flexion of the upper limbs (finger flexion and limb adduction) and extension (with internal rotation and plantar flexion) of the lower limbs.
2) Decorticate posture, which is characterized by extension of the upper and lower limbs, and occasionally associated with opisthotonos.

Generally, decorticate response indicates a supratentorial brain lesion (approximately

Table 10.2 COMA RATING SCALES

Glasgow Coma Scale (GCS) (Teasdale e Jannett, 1976)		
Eye Opening	Spontaneous	4
	To verbal stimulus	3
	To painful stimulus	2
	Absent	1
Verbal Response	Oriented and appropriate	5
	Disoriented and confused	4
	Inappropriate words	3
	Incomprehensible sounds	2
	Absent	1
Motor Response	Follows simple commands	6
	Localizes painful stimulus	5
	Withdraws from painful stimulus	4
	Flexion response to painful stimulus	3
	Extension response to painful stimulus	2
	Absent	1
Total	3-15	

FOUR Score (Full Outline of UnResponsiveness) (Wijdicks et al, 2005)		
Eye Opening	Spontaneous, follows commands or winks on command	4
	Spontaneous, but not following commands	3
	To verbal stimulus	2
	To painful stimulus	1
	Absent	0
Motor Response	Follows simple commands	4
	Localizes painful stimulus	3
	Flexion response to painful stimulus	2
	Extension response to painful stimulus	1
	Absent	0
Brainstem Reflexes	Pupillary and corneal reflexes present	4
	Unilateral pupillary reflex	3
	Pupillary or corneal reflex absent	2
	Pupillary and corneal reflexes absent	1
	Pupillary, corneal, and cough reflexes Absent	0
Respiration	Non-intubated, normal respiratory pattern	4
	Non-intubated, Cheyne-Stokes breathing	3
	Non-intubated, irregular breathing	2
	Respiratory rate > mechanical ventilation	1
	Respiratory rate < ventilator or apnea	0
Total	0-16	

above the quadrigeminal tubercles) and represents a less severe condition compared to decerebrate response, which suggests a brainstem lesion. In patients with coma due to head trauma, decorticate posture recovers in approximately 1 out of 3 cases, while decerebrate posture recovers in 1 out of 10 cases. Decorticate and decerebrate posture can also be observed in metabolic coma.

Ocular reflexes | Assessing the brainstem function and reflexes provides valuable insights into the severity of coma and the localization of cerebral dysfunction (see Tables 10.3 and 10.4). In proceeding schematically in a rostrocaudal direction, the following features should be examined:

1) *Pupil diameter and pupillary light reflex.* The pupillary light reflex is mediated by the midbrain nucleus of the involuntary parasympathetic component of the oculomotor nerve (Edinger-Westphal nucleus). Light stimulation causes ipsilateral miosis (direct reflex) and contralateral miosis (consensual reflex). The afferent branch of the pupillary reflex is the optic nerve, while the efferent branch is the oculomotor nerve. Pupil diameter and pupillary light reflex vary depending on the location of the cerebral lesion responsible for the coma. A diencephalic lesion is characterized by miosis and preserved pupillary reflex. This pattern is also typical for metabolic coma. A midbrain lesion is associated with intermediate and non-reactive pupils. The ciliospinal reflex (i.e., mydriasis evoked by painful stimulus) is preserved. This is a fundamental sign for distinguishing midbrain lesion coma from brain death in the absence of other brainstem reflexes. Compression of the oculomotor nerve caused by herniation of the uncus of the temporal lobe through the tentorium of the cerebellum results in fixed ipsilateral mydriasis. Lesions of the pons lead to bilateral miosis (i.e., pinpoint pupils); intoxication with opioids (heroin or morphine overdose) should be considered for differential diagnosis.
2) *Corneal reflex.* The reflex is elicited by gently touching the surface of the cornea with a sterile gauze. The response consists of bilateral closure of the eyelids and upward eye deviation (Bell's phenomenon). The afferent branch of the reflex is the trigeminal nerve and the efferent branch is the facial nerve. The absence of response implies a brainstem lesion.

Table 10.3 PUPILS

	Diameter	Light reaction	Interpretation
Bilateral	+	–	Mesencephalic lesion
Bilateral	–	+	Metabolic encephalopathy, bilateral deep hemisphere lesions (hydrocephalus, thalamic hemorrhage), drugs, pontine lesion
Unilateral	+	–	Lesion of the III cranial nerve (uncal herniation)

Table 10.4 OCULAR MOTILITY

Phenomenon	Interpretation
Spontaneous erratic conjugate horizontal movements	Common in coma, excluding mesencephalic lesion
Conjugate horizontal deviation	Opposite-side pontine lesion or frontal lobe lesion on the same side
Ocular bobbing	Bilateral pontine lesion
Preserved oculomotor reflex	Intact brainstem function

3) *Ocular position, motility, and oculocephalic* (or "doll's eyes") *reflex*. Effective eye movements require intact consciousness and rely on the motility dysfunction. Analysis of gaze fixation, voluntary pursuit movements, and saccades are useful in defining the clinical and anatomical-functional aspects of altered consciousness states. Some involuntary eye movements are typically associated with alterations of consciousness and may help localize the brain structures involved (the patient "looks at" the lesion) and its location in the frontal eye fields (Brodmann area 8). Dysconjugate gaze deviation suggests a lesion or dysfunction involving one or more oculomotor cranial nerves (i.e., oculomotor, trochlear, and abducens nerves). It is important to note that increased intracranial pressure can also cause paralysis of ocular motility due to dysfunction of the abducens nerve (not the nucleus). While examining the position of the eyeballs, it is critical to evaluate the possible presence of spontaneous movements. Slow and random movements of the eyeballs are typically observed in metabolic coma. Rapid saccades that mimic nystagmus can be observed in altered states of consciousnesses due to epileptic seizures. Ocular bobbing is often observed in coma as well. It consists of intermittent ocular movements, often conjugate and vertical, typically with a rapid downward phase followed by a slow return to the primary position. This phenomenon likely reflects residual motor function in patients with severe impairment of conjugate eye motility. The oculocephalic reflex is examined by passively mobilizing the patient's head on the horizontal plane. Before proceeding with this maneuver, it is mandatory to ensure that there is no cervical trauma, which would potentially make the maneuver dangerous in the event of a cervical spine fracture. Head rotation causes vestibular stimulation that evokes a reflex response from the oculomotor system. This response consists of conjugate deviation of the eyeballs in the opposite direction to the head rotation ("doll's eyes"). The reflex serves to maintain gaze during head movement. In awake subjects, the cortical voluntary control predominates over the reflex, thus inhibiting the "doll's eyes" phenomenon. In comatose patients, voluntary control is lost, and the reflex is present unless the structures responsible for the reflex are damaged. Therefore, in comatose subjects, the presence of the

oculocephalic reflex implies the integrity of the vestibular pathways in the midbrain and pontine tegmentum; while the absence of the reflex indicates impairment of these structures.

4) *Oculo-vestibular reflex.* The oculo-vestibular reflex can be assessed by the so-called caloric test. With the patient in a supine position, the head is tilted approximately 30° on the plane of the bed (to place the horizontal semicircular canal of the inner ear in a vertical position and maximize the response to the stimulus). Cold water (15-20 °C) is injected into the ear canal using a syringe of approximately 50 ml. The response consists of a conjugate gaze deviation toward the irrigated ear. The afferent branch of the reflex is the vestibular pathway that projects to the pons, and the efferent pathway involves the oculomotor system in the pons and midbrain. Therefore, the presence of the reflex indicates the integrity of these structures, in the absence of vestibular dysfunction, which can be caused by neuroleptic drugs or tricyclic antidepressants (Table 10.5).

Nuchal Rigidity | Nuchal rigidity refers to the spontaneous resistance to flexion of the head. It is important to remember that the maneuver to assess nuchal rigidity can be dangerous in the case of cervical trauma because there is a risk of injuring the spinal cord. Brudzinski's sign (passive forward flexion of the head in a supine patient causes flexion of the lower limbs), Kernig's sign (inability to extend the leg on the thigh while keeping the thigh flexed at 90° on the pelvis), and Binda's sign (in supine position, passive rotation of the head causes elevation of the contralateral shoulder) have the same clinical significance in assessing nuchal rigidity. The presence of nuchal rigidity may indicate meningeal irritation caused by meningitis, neoplasia, or subarachnoid hemorrhage.

Table 10.5 ESSENTIAL DIFFERENTIAL DIAGNOSIS

Phenomenon	Interpretation
Reactive and equal-sized pupils, presence of vestibular reflex	Bilateral hemispheric lesion/dysfunction
Fixed pupils, absence of vestibular reflex	Mesencephalic lesion

Breathing | Alterations in respiratory rhythm are often associated with coma and allow for evaluating the degree of neurological impairment. The anatomical and physiological substrates of breathing are not entirely understood. For practical purposes, it is sufficient to know that the respiratory centers are located in the caudal portion of the brainstem and modulate the respiratory rhythm based on chemical stimuli, primarily the partial pressure of respiratory gases in the arterial circulation. Four characteristic respiratory patterns of coma of increasing severity can be distinguished:

1) *Cheyne-Stokes respiration,* is characterized by a periodic alternation of two cyclical phases. The first phase consists of increasing and decreasing amplitude of respiratory movements (i.e., the hyperpnea phase), followed by a brief phase of apnea. This respiratory pattern is attributed to the deafferentation of the brainstem respiratory centers from more superior brain structures, resulting in increased sensitivity of the respiratory centers to chemical stimuli, CO_2 in particular, which leads to increasing hyperventilation during the hyperpnea phase. Hyperventilation causes a decrease in CO_2 in the arterial blood below the threshold to stimulate the brainstem respiratory centers, resulting in a temporary cessation of breathing (i.e., the apnea phase).
2) *Central neurogenic hyperpnea* is characterized by increased frequency and amplitude of respiratory movements, leading to secondary respiratory alkalosis. Neurogenic hyperpnea is defined based on arterial blood gas analysis values (e.g., elevated pH and partial pressure of O_2, reduced partial pressure of CO_2). It should be distinguished from the hyperventilation associated with some instances of metabolic coma. From a pathophysiological perspective, neurogenic hyperpnea results from the deafferentation of groups of neurons located in the upper midbrain and characterized by a high frequency of intrinsic discharge. When released from reflex control by other structures, this discharge leads to an increased frequency of respiratory movements.

3) *Apneustic respiration*, is characterized by respiratory pauses lasting 2-3 seconds at the end of maximal inspiration.
4) *Ataxic or Biot's respiration* is characterized by a chaotic succession of respiratory movements in terms of frequency, depth, and duration. This respiratory pattern is considered secondary to damage affecting a population of neurons located in the most rostral part of the spinal cord, which generates the respiratory rhythm in physiological conditions.

The pathological respiratory patterns may help assess the depth and cause of the coma. In a coma caused by structural brain lesions, the clinical features, including pathological breathing patterns, depend on the rostrocaudal progression of cerebral dysfunction. Cheyne-Stokes respiration indicates impaired diencephalic brain function that does not involve the brainstem respiratory centers. Neurogenic hyperpnea has been rarely observed in certain mesencephalic tumors or primary central nervous system lymphomas, even without direct involvement of the brainstem. Apneustic respiration may indicate bilateral pontine lesions, typically caused by basilar artery occlusion. Ataxic respiration reflects a compromised pontomedullary junction. In metabolic coma, the initial alteration in breathing is often Cheyne-Stokes respiration. This may be followed by a prolonged phase of hyperventilation (distinct from central neurogenic hyperpnea), which represents compensation for metabolic alkalosis (e.g., in diabetic or uremic coma) or is sustained by direct stimulation of the respiratory centers (e.g., in hepatic coma or sepsis).

Syndromes | The combination of clinical features can help localize the lesion or dysfunction underlying the coma (Table 10.6). Three syndromes corresponding to three anatomical levels can be schematically outlined:
1) *The diencephalic syndrome* is characterized by Cheyne-Stokes respiration, pinpoint pupils, and "doll's eye" reflex.
2) *The mesencephalic syndrome* is characterized by central neurogenic hyperventilation, non-reactive intermediate pupils, and decerebrate motor response.
3) The *pontine-bulbar syndrome* is characterized by apneustic or ataxic breathing, non-reactive intermediate pupils, and absence of the oculocephalic reflex.

The rostrocaudal deterioration syndrome indicates worsening clinical conditions in a comatose patient, often secondary to cerebral herniation with downward displacement of axial structures and involving the progression from the diencephalic to the pontine-bulbar syndrome.

Biochemical and Instrumental Tests | Clinical examination is a fundamental step of the diagnostic workflow for coma. It requires a short time yet provides critical information for diagnosis and treatment. Findings from the clinical examination define the subsequent diagnostic workup, which includes the following biochemical and instrumental tests:
1) *Blood and urine tests*. Albeit rarely, focal neurological signs may be present in some cases of metabolic coma. Therefore, performing venous blood sampling for routine blood tests in all comatose patients is advised. It is important to include glucose levels (in urgent circumstances, a capillary blood glucose evaluation may suffice), electrolytes, and toxicological screening. In case of severe hypoglycemia requiring glucose infusion therapy, it is recommended to administer a 10% glucose solution, due to the potential risk of edema caused by the administration of a hypotonic solution

Table 10.6 LOCALIZATION

	Subcortical	Mesencephalon	Pons	Medulla
Breathing	Cheynes-Stokes	Central neurogenic hyperpnea	Apneustic or cluster	Ataxic
Pupils	Small and reactive	Intermediate or large and fixed	Small "pinpoint" and fixed	Intermediate or irregular and fixed
Oculocephalic reflex	Present	Absent or abnormal	Absent or abnormal	Absent

(e.g., 5% glucose solution). In cases of hyponatremia, sodium correction should be slow (i.e., < 10 mEq/L per day) to avoid iatrogenic central pontine myelinolysis due to osmotic demyelination. Arterial blood gas analysis should also be performed if signs of respiratory insufficiency or acid-base imbalances are present. In women, a pregnancy test (e.g., human chorionic gonadotropin) is advised to evaluate contraindications to radiological exams.

2) *Neuroimaging.* Brain CT should be performed in all patients with coma of uncertain etiology. Neuroimaging is not always indicated, for instance, in case of coma due to hypoglycemia that resolves after glucose administration. Contrast media should be used in case of a suspected brain tumor or steno-occlusion of cerebral vessels. Prior to contrast administration, renal function should be evaluated through blood tests. The main advantage of CT over MRI is the rapidity of the procedure, which not only speeds up the investigation process but also reduces the risk of artifacts caused by patient movements. A limitation of CT is its lower accuracy in detecting hyperacute ischemic lesions within 24 hours or hemorrhagic lesions in the third week after onset, which are both isodense to the brain parenchyma. Brain MRI is less commonly used in emergency settings. The advantages of MRI, which justify its use in selected cases, include increased sensitivity in detecting focal cerebral lesions, particularly acute ischemic lesions (e.g., using diffusion MRI). Furthermore, it enables the evaluation of intracranial arterial circulation without the need for contrast media and the assessment of venous circulation using MR angiography, which is more sensitive than CT in detecting cerebral venous thrombosis. Before performing an MRI exam, it is necessary to obtain relevant medical history to rule out contraindications, such as the presence of a pacemaker or metal implants.
3) *Lumbar puncture.* In cases of coma of uncertain etiology, a lumbar puncture may be considered. It is recommended to conduct this procedure after completing the neuroimaging evaluation. If there is evidence of brain displacement from neuroimaging, lumbar puncture should not be performed because it could facilitate cerebral herniation. Cerebrospinal fluid diagnostics include the examination of glucose, proteins, immunoelectrophoresis, bacterial and fungal cultures, detection of neurotropic viruses using polymerase chain reaction, and cytological examination to detect and characterize neoplastic or immune cells.

10.2.3 Evaluation and treatment of comatose patients

Coma is a medical emergency. Therefore, the clinical approach must prioritize providing adequate oxygen and glucose supply to the brain. The diagnostic process begins only after stabilizing vital parameters. The so-called "ABC" (Airways, Breathing, Circulation). protocol ensures adequate blood flow and oxygen supply to the brain tissue. A – Airways: Ensure airway patency by removing secretions, foreign bodies, or any other physical obstruction to air entry into the airways. B – Breathing: Ensure adequate ventilation, if necessary through endotracheal intubation. Generally, a subject is considered to have adequate ventilation if the respiratory rate is > 8 breaths/minute and the vesicular murmur is audible on auscultation of both lung bases. Arterial blood gas analysis is recommended. The target is to achieve pO_2 > 100 mmHg and pCO_2 = 35-40 mmHg; C – Circulation: Maintain adequate circulation in terms of heart rate and blood pressure. Electrocardiographic and blood pressure monitoring are necessary. The target mean arterial pressure (1/3 systolic blood pressure + 2/3 diastolic blood pressure) is 70-80 mmHg. In the acute setting, hypertension is treated only if the diastolic blood pressure is > 120 mmHg.

The brain tissue requires a continuous supply of glucose (in addition to oxygen). Blood glucose levels should be maintained between 80 and 110 mg/dL. Hypoglycemia or hyperglycemia should be treated by administering glucose or insulin. It should be noted that a glucose load can precipitate Wernicke's encephalopathy, a clinical condition characterized by ocular motor disturbances, imbalance, mental confusion, and coma due to thiamine (vitamin B1) deficiency resulting from alcohol abuse or malnutrition. Therefore, it is recommended to administer also thiamine when administering glucose to a comatose patient. In emergency situations, it is appropriate to infuse a glucose solution while awaiting the laboratory test results in cases of suspected hypoglycemia.

Body temperature is another parameter to consider in assisting a comatose patient. Hyperthermia can be caused by infections, brain injuries (central fever resulting from impaired thermoregulatory centers), or metabolic dysfunctions, all of which can lead to coma. Hyperthermia is potentially harmful because it increases the metabolic demand of the brain tissue, can promote detrimental inflammatory responses from the immune system, and worsen hypoxic or hypoglycemic damage. On the other hand, hypothermia can facilitate infectious complications, cardiac arrhythmias, electrolyte and acid-base imbalances, and coagulation dysfunction. If the temperature exceeds 38 °C, antipyretics should be administered after performing blood cultures. Body temperature below 35 °C should be treated using thermal blankets and may require respiratory support.

In the early phase of assisting a comatose patient, treatment of specific pathological features may be necessary before completing the diagnostic process. For instance, in case of a brain lesion causing mass effect with increased intracranial pressure and progressive clinical deterioration, it is recommended to administer osmotic agents (e.g., intravenous mannitol boluses). The use of corticosteroids should be limited to cases with evidence of a brain tumor since they can increase blood pressure, which in turn can exacerbate other pathological conditions (e.g., cerebral hemorrhage and ischemia). Seizures should be treated since repeated seizures can further damage the brain tissue. The drugs typically used are intravenous lorazepam or diazepam. For the treatment of status epilepticus, please refer to the corresponding chapter. If drug intoxication or substance abuse is suspected, specific antagonists should be administered, such as naloxone for opioid intoxication and flumazenil for benzodiazepine intoxication. It is important to note that these therapeutic procedures can cause withdrawal syndrome, especially in individuals with chronic substance use. Therefore, these antagonists should be reserved for selected cases and require patient monitoring.

Implementing strategies to prevent complications during the acute phase, such as infections and deep venous thrombosis, is also recommended. Inserting a urinary catheter is useful if urinary control is lacking. If there is a risk of aspiration pneumonia due to dysphagia, it is recommended to insert a nasogastric tube. To prevent stasis-related deep vein thrombosis, subcutaneous heparin or alternatively elastic stockings (e.g., in cases of bleeding) can be used. Adequate conjunctival lubrication and frequent oral cavity cleaning are essential to prevent infectious complications.

10.2.4 Prognosis

Coma is a transient condition. The patient may improve and regain consciousness or progress to a vegetative state, death, or rarely, locked-in syndrome. Prognostic studies mainly refer to two categories: post-traumatic coma and post-anoxic coma (e.g., secondary to cardiac arrest). Generally, post-traumatic coma has a better prognosis in terms of mortality: 40-50% in post-traumatic coma and 54-88% in post-anoxic coma.

In post-traumatic coma, the main adverse prognostic factors include low *Glasgow Coma Scale* score (Table 10.2), advanced age, long duration of coma (> 2 weeks), absence of pupillary reflex, presence of arterial hypotension, hypoxia or intracranial hypertension, and focal lesions or subarachnoid hemorrhage on neuroimaging.

In non-traumatic coma, prognosis is influenced by many factors, with the underlying cause being the primary factor. Regardless of the cause, three parameters affect the prognosis of non-traumatic coma: long duration of the coma, presence of neuro-ophthalmological signs, and absence of motor response to nociceptive stimuli. Scales such as the Glasgow Coma Scale and FOUR also hold prognostic value. The short-term mortality risk during coma and hospitalization is negligible for Glasgow Coma Scale scores> 8 and FOUR scores > 12.

10.3 Vegetative state and minimally conscious state

Vegetative State (VS) or *Unresponsive Wakefulness Syndrome* (UWS) corresponds to a condition in which the individual is awake and responds to simple stimuli but lacks awareness. Patients maintain an apparent sleep-wake cycle, with the eyes open when "awake" and closed when "asleep." They breathe spontaneously and have preserved autonomic functions, tendon reflexes, and intact cranial nerve function. Grimacing, eye movements, partial facial mimicry, limb spasticity, possible purposeless limb movements, and pseudobulbar paralysis may be present. However, to the extent this can be assessed, self-awareness and awareness of the environment are absent. Therefore, these patients cannot think, perceive, feel, or have any experience. The main objections to these diagnostic criteria arise from the difficulty in defining the absence of awareness operationally. Since there are no objective tools to assess *awareness*, it would be difficult to deny its presence confidently. This view does not exclude the possibility that a person in a vegetative state may have their own subjective experience and, potentially, experience suffering. Ongoing research is trying to assess functional brain activity instrumentally (e.g., using functional neuroimaging) in patients with VS. Research in this field is often not entirely independent from ideological positions. Based on currently available data from neuroimaging, evoked potentials, and neuropathological studies, it appears that individuals in a vegetative state lack *awareness*.

10.3.1 Diagnosis

The diagnosis of VS is based on a condition of *unawareness* of the self and the environment. Typical signs are: sleep-wake cycle with open and closed eyes; spontaneous breathing; aimless eye blinking and movement; nystagmus; emission of sounds, but not words; brief, non-purposeful gaze; facial expressions in response to pain; yawning, swallowing, and chewing movements; non-purposeful limb movements; decorticate posture; flexion withdrawal to painful stimuli; brief head movements and eye movements towards noises or motion in the environment; startle response to auditory stimuli.

The vegetative state can be a transient, chronic, or irreversible condition. It is defined as "persistent" after more than 1 month from the brain injury or in neurodegenerative disorders. A vegetative state that persists over 12 months after a brain injury or 3 months after anoxic brain injury is essentially considered "permanent." The probability of recovering *awareness* in these conditions is less than 1%.

However, it is difficult to be certain about the irreversibility of the condition. Anecdotal cases have reported "awakenings" after long periods of apparent vegetative state. They mainly consist of individual clinical case reports without neuroimaging and therefore raise legitimate concerns about the appropriateness of the diagnosis. Recent clinical studies, albeit often from individual cases, have reported the emergence of expressions of consciousness following brain stimulation (e.g., thalamocortical network stimulation through vagus nerve stimulation) in individuals in a vegetative state. These findings require caution in interpretation and may reflect an *overinterpretation* of motor responses. Nonetheless, they raise doubts about the irreversibility of VS and emphasize the inadequacy of current diagnostic criteria. Ideological positions also influence these issues. Many argue that considerations regarding civil rights, quality of life, the ability of self-determination, and communication with the environment should prevail over the attention to minimal brain functions. The issue is of enormous medical and ethical significance. The label "permanent" raises bioethical perspectives that authorize the discontinuation of therapy or the cessation of nutrition and hydration. The adjective "permanent" thus implies a diagnostic decision that can substantially affect medical management. Some patients with extensive brain damage show signs of awareness and cannot be diagnosed as VS. As previously mentioned, the problem lies in objectifying awareness or agreeing on its phenomenology. Some guidelines suggest rudimentary operational definitions of awareness that allow neurologists to make diagnostic assessments. The following behaviors, for example, are considered expressions of *awareness*:

1) Executing basic commands.
2) Responding with either a physical or verbal affirmation or negation to inquiries.
3) Verbalizing with meaning.
4) Showing intentional actions in response to intense stimuli, such as reaching for items in a way that aligns with their location and gesture direction, handling objects appropriately to their shape and size, maintaining gaze on a moving target, and responding appropriately to emotional stimuli (e.g., laughter or tears).

Similar conditions but with preserved *awareness* are defined as Minimally Conscious States (MCS) or Minimally Responsive States.

The diagnostic recognition of these conditions demonstrates that consciousness is not an all-or-nothing phenomenon. Rather, its clinical presentation is a continuum ranging from brain death to complete cognitive integrity. Due to the potential bioethical implications of the diagnosis of permanent VS, the diagnosis of MCS indicates a qualitatively different condition. However, the diagnostic criteria have limitations regarding a clear differentiation between VS and MCS, as well as in attributing the label "permanent" to VS. Future neuroimaging studies will likely lead to improved diagnostic criteria by incorporating instrumental exams to overcome limitations related to a diagnostic workflow that relies mainly on clinical assessment. Neuropathological observations consistently indicate that the vegetative state is associated with extensive cortical or thalamic lesions, often resulting from traumatic brain injury. The final stages of neurodegenerative diseases such as Alzheimer's, Parkinson's, or Huntington's disease may also lead to MCS.

10.3.2 Differential Diagnosis

The distinction between VS and MCS is not simple and not always possible. Clinical assessments should be repeated over time, and the examiner should allow time for delayed responses. The effect of sedative drugs should also be considered when evaluating the patient's response to stimuli. Nursing staff and family members should be consulted to verify if they have witnessed congruent behaviors.

The differential diagnosis also includes Locked-in Syndrome, which is typically caused by a pontine vascular lesion that affects all motor pathways except those controlling vertical eye movement. Locked-in Syndrome is not a disorder of consciousness. Both *wakefulness* and *awareness* are intact. In the differential diagnosis, conditions caused by advanced forms of Guillain-Barré Syndrome, myasthenia gravis, or other severe paralyzing diseases should also be considered. Furthermore, there are other states of profound apathy that in extreme cases can simulate VS or MCS, including akinetic mutism, abulia, or catatonia. These disorders share a dysfunction of the circuits involving the frontal lobes, diencephalon, and ascending dopaminergic projections, which are essential for motor and cognitive functioning. Akinetic mutism is an extreme form of abulia: the patient is seated or lying passively on the bed and responds to questions only occasionally or with a long delay. The disorder is considered to be motor in nature rather than cognitive. Non-convulsive status epilepticus is another condition to consider in the differential diagnosis.

10.3.3 Clinical case report

A 53-year-old man with a history of hypertension, diabetes mellitus, hyperlipidemia, and factor V deficiency is brought to the Emergency Room (ER) for headache, language alterations, weakness, and paresthesia in the left upper limb. All these symptoms have progressively worsened over the past 7-8 hours. The patient is taking warfarin for deep vein thrombosis prophylaxis following knee surgery. During the ER observation, the patient's level of consciousness deteriorates to a Glasgow Coma Scale score of 4. The patient is then intubated for assisted ventilation and transferred to the Intensive Care Unit (ICU). Neurological examination in the ICU shows no response to commands and absence of oculocephalic and corneal reflexes. The following day, the patient partially recovers, spontaneously opens the eyes but still does not respond to stimuli, and exhibits a decerebrate posture in response to painful stimuli. A brain CT scan shows bleeding extending from the ponto-bulbar junction to the upper pons, predominantly on the ventral side. Seven days later, the patient can move the eyes in response to commands. However, the association between command and seemingly voluntary movement is difficult to establish due to constant involuntary eye movements characterized by sudden and spontaneous downward deviations (i.e., ocular bobbing). Seven days after the onset, the patient remains tetraplegic and anarthric. At 10 days, upward eye mobility improves and becomes reproducible on command. Electroencephalography, auditory and visual evoked potentials performed 5 weeks later are normal.

These clinical features may suggest a diagnosis of Minimally Conscious State, but the electroencephalography and evoked potential results are unusual for this diagnosis. The correct diagnosis is Locked-in Syndrome. The hemorrhage occupies the ventral part of the pons, leaving the dorsal part that contains the ascending reticular formation relatively preserved. Tetraplegia, paralysis of lower cranial nerves, anarthria, and preserved consciousness (evidenced by response to commands) are consistent with the diagnosis of Locked-in Syndrome. The patient was initially comatose, possibly because the hemorrhagic lesion initially extended into the pontine tegmentum.

10.4 Delirium

Delirium is a syndrome characterized by an acute state of confusion. Confusion indicates cerebral insufficiency (or brain failure) and has two fundamental features. First, it lacks focal cerebral dysfunction (i.e., absence of focal neurological signs and symptoms). Second, it represents the clinical expression of a common final pathway for multiple pathogenetic mechanisms. Although delirium was traditionally classified among disorders of consciousness, it is currently considered primarily a cognitive-behavioral disorder, sometimes associated with signs of altered consciousness content (awareness) and reduced awareness of the surrounding environment.

10.4.1 Diagnosis

The clinical diagnosis is based on the acute onset of fluctuating mental dysfunction characterized by inattention, disorganized thinking, and psychomotor disturbances. Spatial and temporal disorientation, memory impairment, misperception (illusions or hallucinations), alterations in the sleep-wake cycle, and emotional disturbances (e.g., irritability, anxiety, paranoia, depressive mood tone, apathy, euphoria) may also be present. From a psychomotor standpoint, delirium can present in three clinical variants: hyperactive, hypoactive, or mixed. In hyperactive delirium, the patient appears uncooperative, agitated, and misperceptions are often present. Especially in older individuals, delirium is often hypoactive and manifests as lethargy and global bradykinesia. Hypoactive delirium is associated with a poor prognosis compared to hyperactive delirium, likely because it is more challenging to recognize. Mixed delirium can exhibit a combination of psychomotor agitation and lethargy.

Typically, delirium is episodic and lasts for hours or days if the underlying cause resolves. However, it can persist for a more extended period. Delirium in hospitalized patients persists until discharge in approximately 45% of cases and for at least one month in 33%. The temporal characteristics of the disorder, the acute onset in particular, facilitate the differential diagnosis from dementia (■ Table 10.7) or depression. The occurrence of delirium is associated with an increased risk of subsequent dementia. However, it remains unclear whether poor long-term cognitive outcomes in patients who experience delirium result from delirium and related factors or rather delirium indicates an underlying and progressively worsening cognitive disorder. Like the duration, the severity of delirium can vary considerably. In less severe cases, the diagnosis is facilitated by brief screening tests that can be performed at the patient's bedside. The diagnosis of delirium is based on: a) the presence of cognitive fluctuations following

Table 10.7 DIFFERENTIAL DIAGNOSIS

	Delirium	Dementia
Onset	Acute	Insidious and progressive
Duration	Hours or days (can be prolonged)	Years
Attention	Altered focus, shift, maintenance	Typically normal except in severe cases
Consciousness	Fluctuating and/or reduced	Intact
Language	Incoherent and distractible	Organized, anomia, or aphasia

the acute onset; b) impaired attention, which can be assessed by asking the patient to count backward in a sequence of 3-4 numbers or name the days or months of the year; c) disorientation and disorganized thinking, which can be assessed by asking about the current place and date, the name of the hospital, and by checking the consistency of thoughts; d) psychomotor disturbances (e.g., lethargy or hypervigilance) and altered level of consciousness. Severely hypoactive or hyperactive delirium may pose differential diagnosis challenges with psychiatric illnesses.

10.4.2 Causes

The leading causes of delirium are listed in Table 10.8. The etiology of delirium is often multifactorial and typically involves the exposure of a vulnerable individual (with predisposing factors) to one or more precipitating factors. Age and comorbidity of cognitive disorders or chronic conditions play a prominent role as predisposing factors. The most significant precipitating factors include surgery, anesthesia, sedative and narcotic medications, acute neurological diseases (such as stroke, cerebral hemorrhage, and meningoencephalitis), anemia, dehydration, infections, exacerbations of chronic illnesses, and sleep deprivation. Although the prevalence of delirium is relatively low in the general population (1-2%), it increases with age and reaches 14% in older adults over eighty-five. In about half of the cases, delirium occurs during hospitalization, often following surgical procedures. Delirium occurs in 10-15% of adults admitted to the emergency department. In hospitalized patients, the incidence varies from 6% to 56% in the general population.

The treatment of delirium primarily involves addressing its precipitating factors (Table 10.9). Often, discontinuation of sedative medications or hydration leads to improvement or resolution of delirium. In some cases, it is necessary to use medications to manage severe behavioral disturbances or hallucinations. Antipsychotics appear to offer the most favorable cost-benefit ratio. However, it is advised to limit their use to the minimum necessary, due to the potential risks associated with sedation and other complications. Benzodiazepines are only recommended for treating delirium caused by alcohol or benzodiazepine withdrawal.

Table 10.8 DELIRIUM: CAUSES

Causes	Examples
Toxic	Alcohol or substance abuse intoxication, or withdrawal syndrome
Metabolic	Hypoxemia/hypercapnia, hypo/hyperglycemia, hypo/hyperthermia, hypovitaminosis (e.g., Wernicke's syndrome)
Medications	Psychoactive medications, especially sedatives, hypnotics, narcotics, and anticholinergics
Electrolyte Disorders	Dehydration, hyponatremia
Infections	Urinary and pulmonary, most common ones
Systemic Diseases	Specifically, potential causes of cerebral hypo-perfusion (anemia, hypotension, cardiac dysfunctions)
Neurological Disorders	Space-occupying lesions, head trauma, stroke, cerebral hemorrhage, meningoencephalitis

Table 10.9 DELIRIUM: FREQUENT TRIGGERING FACTORS AND SUGGESTED INTERVENTIONS

Factors	Interventions
Medications	Consider the risk-to-benefit ratio of psychoactive medications. Verify if new medications have been taken or if dosages have been modified. Alcohol or opioids
Electrolytes	Assess hydration status, thyroid and renal function
Infections	Particularly urinary and pulmonary infections
Internal diseases	In particular, potential causes of cerebral hypoperfusion (anemia, hypotension, cardiac dysfunctions)
Reduced sensory input	Check vision, hearing. Facilitate contact with relatives
Sleep-wake cycle disturbances	Sleep hygiene, melatonin

Bibliography

Giacino J.T., Ashwal S., Childs N., Cranford R., Jennett B., Katz D.I., Kelly J.P. et al., The minimally conscious state: definition and diagnostic criteria. Neurology; 58(3):349-53, 2002.

Jaynes J. Il crollo della mente bicamerale e l'origine della coscienza. Adelphi Edizioni, 1984.

Kock C., Massimini M., Boly M., Tononi G. Neurla correlates of consciousness: progress and problems. Nature Rev Neurosci; 17:307-321, 2016.

Laureys S., Eyes open, brain shut. Scientific American; 96(5):84-9, 2007.

Plum F., Posner J.B., The diagnosis of stupor and coma. Contemporary neurology series; 10:1-286, 1972.

Teasdale G., Jennett B., Assessment and prognosis of coma after head injury. Acta neurochirurgica; 34(1):45-55, 1976.

Wijdicks E.F., Bamlet W.R., Maramattom B.V., Manno E.M., McClelland R.L., Validation of a new coma scale: The FOUR score. Annals of Neurology; 58(4):585-93, 2005.

We would like to thank Dr. Emanuela Onesti for her contribution to the chapter in the previous edition.

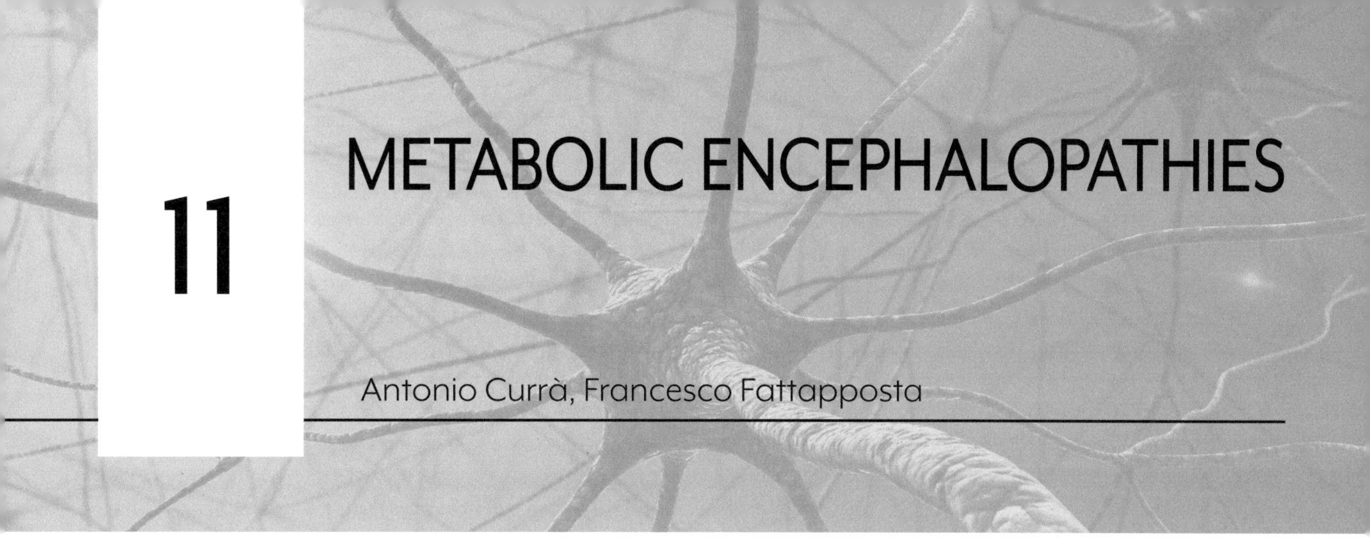

11 METABOLIC ENCEPHALOPATHIES

Antonio Currà, Francesco Fattapposta

The concept of "metabolic encephalopathy" was introduced in 1927 by Kinnier Wilson to describe a neurologic condition with heterogeneous etiology, characterized by an alteration of brain activity in the absence of parenchymal inflammation or gross structural abnormalities. Therefore, this concept does not possess a diagnostic value but rather a semiotic value, indicating a state of multifocal or diffuse cerebral dysfunction induced by a systemic disturbance, which can manifest with variable clinical intensity. The critical factor in encephalopathy is the alteration of consciousness, which presents as hyper-alertness and agitation, drowsiness, or psychomotor abnormalities (restlessness, alterations in the sleep-wake cycle).

The systemic disturbance is identified as the functional decompensation of an organ not belonging to the nervous system (heart-lungs, liver, kidney), generally responsible for regulating the otherwise toxic concentration of endogenous substances (carbon dioxide, ammonia, urea) or supplying critical substrates (oxygen, nutrients).

Despite being protected from the rest of the body by the blood-brain barrier (BBB), the central nervous system (CNS) proves vulnerable to the action of endogenous substances that can become toxic in high concentrations (glucose, peptides, electrolytes, water). In some cases, the medical history and clinical examination allow the identification of the dysfunctional organ or system, while in other cases, laboratory tests are necessary.

Metabolic encephalopathies usually develop acutely or sub-acutely and revert following the removal of the underlying internal cause. Therefore, at least in the initial stages, they represent functional alterations of the brain, devoid of neuropathological correlates. In cases where it is impossible to rapidly eliminate or correct the underlying cause, the "metabolic" brain damage can convert into secondary structural damage. This occurs, for example, in certain types of liver failure, where tissue hypoxia leads to edema and even necrosis.

11.1 Acute metabolic encephalopathy

Encephalopathy is the clinical expression of susceptibility to imbalances of various nature in the neural circuits distributed diffusely throughout the brain, responsible for functions such as the ability to focus on elements of interest (perception, attention, and directing capacity), the overall state of consciousness (vigilance), and self-memory (continuous comparison between current and past experiences, underlying the perception of identity). When one or more of these functions are compromised in rapid temporal progression, acute encephalopathy occurs; in cases due to metabolic imbalances, it is referred to as acute metabolic encephalopathy. Direct neuronal damage from trauma, vascular injury, or infection is therefore excluded. Instead, direct, or indirect damage resulting from systemic disorders such as hypoxemia, hepatic or renal failure, and endocrine dysfunction is taken into consideration. It is thus a syndrome with an acute onset and fluctuating course, which manifests in the context of an internal or systemic pathology. Typically transient and reversible, this syndrome can become chronic with permanent outcomes.

The clinical manifestations of encephalopathy present as signs of diffuse cerebral distress (global signs, predominantly indicating distress of the hemispheres or brainstem) or localized signs (focal signs, related to the specific compromised cerebral area), in varying combinations in terms of quality and quantity.

Observation of the global neurological signs of metabolic encephalopathy begins with the recognition of essential elements such as the alteration of the level of consciousness and the diffuse alteration of cognitive functions with an acute onset (confusional state), in the presence of an underlying metabolic process. The effects on consciousness result from the reduced integrative capacity of the neocortex. Cognitive impairment follows the alteration of consciousness and is expressed as attentional dysfunction (specifically selective or focused attention), which can range anywhere on the *continuum* between hyperactive agitation and coma. The inability to maintain coherent and organized flows of thoughts or actions makes patients distracted and hypersensitive to environmental stimuli, of which they fail to recognize the order of relevance. It is important to note the frequent dissociation between cognitive deficits (orientation, perception, language, memory, abstraction, introspection, and judgment) and the state of vigilance and awareness.

The confusional state clinically manifests in three behavioral or psychomotor modalities:

- Hyperactive psychomotor pattern: Patients exhibit restlessness, agitation, hyper-alertness, and often delusions or hallucinations.
- Hypoactive psychomotor pattern: Patients are sedated or lethargic, respond slowly to questions, and show a scarcity of spontaneous movements. They are often elderly individuals erroneously considered depressed or demented.
- Mixed psychomotor pattern: Patients exhibit characteristics of both hypo-activity and hyper-activity.

Other frequent global neurological signs include oral or facial automatisms, the presence of primitive reflexes (such as the grasp reflex, suckling reflex), the appearance of tremors, and alterations in muscle tone (ranging from paratonia to decerebrate posturing). Seizure episodes of varying clinical intensity, up to *status epilepticus*, can also occur in certain metabolic disorders, withdrawal syndromes, and forms of encephalopathy due to pharmacological toxicity. The clinical expression of reduced inhibitory control varies greatly among patients and characteristically within the clinical course of the same individual (fluctuations). Associated with the distinctive psychomotor expressions of global cortical and brainstem neurological signs (including coma) are autonomic symptoms originating from the diencephalon or brainstem: changes in respiration and heart rate, hypertension, hyperthermia, sweating, piloerection, dizziness, nausea, and vomiting.

Regarding focal signs, i.e., neurological manifestations resulting from the compromise of a specific cerebral area located in a particular hemisphere or the brainstem, they combine with varying clinical penetrance with global signs, making their definition sometimes difficult. Signs or symptoms that may have a hemispheric or brainstem localization value are considered semiotically "focal." Campimetric deficits, aphasia, apraxia, sensorimotor or ataxic disturbances with hemisomatic distribution have a hemispheric focal value. Brainstem focal value includes alterations in cranial nerves, nystagmus, other disorders of conjugate gaze, abnormalities of brainstem reflexes (blinking, sucking, swallowing, etc.), dysarthria, dysphagia, respiratory disturbances, sensorimotor or ataxic disturbances with congruous distribution (such as quadriparesis and corresponding alterations of tendon reflexes), and myoclonus.

11.1.1 Pathophysiology of encephalopathy

Direct neuronal damage induced by hypoxia, hypoglycemia, and other metabolic causes results in energy deprivation, leading to alterations in the synthesis and release of neurotransmitters and the propagation of impulses, particularly along the neural networks underlying attentive and cognitive functions.

Cerebral metabolism depends almost entirely on the metabolism of systemically derived substrates. Approximately three-quarters of hepatic glucose production is utilized by the brain, and 90% of the entire cerebral glucose metabolism follows the Krebs cycle and the butyrate (GABA *shunt*) pathway, which converts glutamate to succinate via gamma-aminobutyric acid (GABA). During high metabolic demand, in specific cerebral areas, the brain extracts amino-acids and ammonia from the bloodstream. The resulting neurological picture is a multifocal cortical and subcortical disorder affecting the frontal lobes, the right parietal lobe, the thalamus, the basal ganglia, and the brainstem, with variable involvement of these regions.

The described biochemical alterations lead to neurotransmitters imbalance involving acetylcholine, dopamine, serotonin, norepinephrine, GABA, and glutamate.

Cholinergic neurons are widely distributed in the central nervous system (CNS) and are involved in the control of wakefulness, attention, memory, and sleep. Reduction of cerebral cholinergic activity (due to hypoxia, carbohydrate supply restriction, or cofactor deficiency) is one of the basic changes in the confusional state, as exemplified by iatrogenic cases involving drugs with prominent anticholinergic action. These include first-generation antihistamines (e.g., diphenhydramine, meclizine), tricyclic antidepressants (e.g., imipramine, amitriptyline), and centrally acting antispasmodics used for the treatment of overactive bladder (e.g., oxybutynin, tolterodine).

The reduction of cerebral cholinergic activity parallels with increased dopaminergic activity, as evidenced by the beneficial effect of antidopaminergic drugs in calming hyperactivity and agitation in the confusional state. More than changes in primary mediators, imbalance in the acetylcholine/dopamine ratio contributes to the confusional disturbance, as these neurotransmitters act as modulators of inattention and disorientation.

Serotonergic neurons are also ubiquitous in the CNS and are involved in motor and mnemonic functions as well as sleep. High serotonergic activity is associated with psychosis and confusional states. Under certain conditions, patients taking selective serotonin reuptake inhibitors (SSRIs) can develop serotonin syndrome, a hypermetabolic emergency condition in which the confusional state is prominent.

The role of GABA and other neurotransmitters is not well-known. GABAergic activity is thought elevated in hepatic encephalopathy and reduced in alcohol withdrawal syndrome.

11.1.2 Clinical and instrumental semiotics

Since patients with metabolic encephalopathy may present semiological aspects potentially expressed by other clinical conditions, the clinical history must be collected with particular care. The anamnestic report should confirm the acute change in mental status and cognitive functions, rapid or sudden onset, concomitant pathology of other organs or systems, use or abuse of drugs, possible abrupt cessation of voluntary substance intake, or significant changes in the living environment.

The clinical examination should indicate specific changes in mental status in terms of activity (ranging from abulia and hypoactivity to agitation), vigilance (ranging from hypervigilance to *stupor*), involved cognitive domains (attention, memory, language, executive functions), and possible perceptual disturbances (visual and auditory illusions or hallucinations). Typically, milder alterations affect selective attention and manifest as ease of distractibility and prolonged reaction times. In the presence of attention disorders, other cognitive functions such as mental calculation, fixation memory, and orientation are impaired. In patients with markedly reduced levels of vigilance (*stupor*) and unassessable mental status, it is necessary to test sensory-motor functions and cranial nerves to confirm or exclude focal lesions underlying the disturbance of consciousness.

Assessment of motor function may reveal involuntary movements (positive or negative myoclonus, tremor, choreic movements) and changes in muscle tone (rigidity and paratonia).

From an instrumental perspective, neurological alterations are better detected and monitored by functional neurophysiological techniques rather than structural ones. Electroencephalography (EEG) shows a pattern of generalized reduction in brain electrical activity frequency with a predominance of theta (5-7 Hz) and delta (up to 4 Hz) rhythms. In cases of alcohol or benzodiazepine withdrawal, rapid low-voltage electrical activity may be observed. In some patients experiencing withdrawal from pharmacological substances, the EEG reveals whether changes in cognitive and consciousness alterations reflect non-convulsive epileptic activity. Non-convulsive status epilepticus is, in fact, an imperative differential diagnosis in all patients clinically diagnosed with encephalopathy.

Since, by definition, the clinical picture of metabolic encephalopathy manifests in the absence of intracranial structural lesions, theoretically neuroimaging would have the role of excluding lesions in case of negativity. In this sense, computed axial tomography retains its diagnostic value as an initial assessment due to its wide availability and short examination time, especially in emergency situations. Otherwise, magnetic resonance imaging, now capable of detecting changes in nervous tissue preceding structural alterations, has renewed utility in the diagnostic and prognostic evaluation of patients with specific metabolic encephalopathy presentations

11.2 Specific patterns of metabolic or toxic encephalopathy

11.2.1 Hypoglycemic encephalopathy

Hypoglycemic encephalopathy is a syndrome associated with blood glucose levels below 50 mg/dl. In patients with poorly controlled diabetes, the same clinical manifestations can occur even with normal or slightly elevated blood glucose levels. It is important to distinguish between fasting hypoglycemia and reactive or postprandial hypoglycemia.

Generally, hypoglycemia is iatrogenic, caused by inappropriate administration of insulin (type 1 and type 2 diabetes) or oral anti-diabetic drugs (type 2 diabetes). Risk factors include a long history of disease, insulin treatment, and a positive history of previous hypoglycemia. Less frequently, hypoglycemia is due to prolonged fasting, chronic alcohol abuse (which depletes hepatic glycogen stores), pancreatic insulinomas, and certain forms of glycogen storage disease.

In terms of frequency and severity of hypoglycemia, patients with type 2 diabetes are less at risk compared to those with type 1 diabetes, who have an annual mortality rate from hypoglycemia ranging from 2% to 4%.

The pathogenic mechanisms of hypoglycemic encephalopathy are still being defined. With the depletion of glycogen stores, neurons tend to utilize ketone acids and intermediate glucose metabolites. Prolonged hypoglycemia leads to cellular damage due to ATP depletion. Prolonged and severe glucose unavailability depletes acetate (the end-product of glycolysis), thus preventing citrate formation in the Krebs cycle. The accumulation of oxaloacetate has two consequences: on one hand, it drives the tricarboxylic acid cycle to feed on substrates derived from amino-acid catabolism (particularly from aspartate deamination); on the other hand, it derails the physiological GABA *shunt*. These conditions significantly increase aspartate concentrations, which, by acting on extracellular NMDA receptors, exert an excitotoxic effect. Another pathogenic mechanism of hypoglycemic encephalopathy is mitochondrial swelling with DNA fragmentation, which occurs through processes that are not yet fully understood. Neurons in the neocortex, hippocampus, and basal ganglia are most vulnerable to hypoglycemia, while cerebellar and brainstem neurons are less susceptible.

The syndrome of hypoglycemia begins with symptoms caused by the activation of counter-regulatory substances, mainly catecholamines (anxiety, tachycardia, headache, cold sweating, lightheadedness, and hunger) (Table 11.1). These symptoms, which are warning signs of imminent risk of encephalopathy, can be dampened or abolished in cases of central or peripheral autonomic complications, as seen in long-standing diabetic patients. They can "slide" into hypoglycemic encephalopathy and coma almost without warning: the encephalopathy starts with a confused state and progresses, with reduction of blood glucose, to stupor and coma. The lower the blood glucose

Table 11.1 SIGNS AND SYMPTOMS OF HYPOGLYCEMIA SYNDROME

Blood Glucose Level (mg/dl)	Clinical/Instrumental Signs	Symptoms
>70	Normal	Absent
55-65	Initial alterations in psychometric tests	Cold sweating
45-55	Generalized alterations in psychometric tests	Anxiety, tremor, palpitations, flushing
35-45	Increased amplitude and reduced frequency of EEG	Generalized weakness, hunger, visual disturbances; possible hyperactivity and restlessness
25-35	Decreased amplitude and frequency of EEG	Altered consciousness: drowsiness or *stupor*
<25	Isoelectric EEG	Coma

level, the more likely critical events, usually convulsions, become. Focal neurological signs, including involuntary choreiform movements, cranial nerve deficits, and interhemispheric disconnection syndromes, are rare.

During the catecholaminergic response phase, the EEG shows increased amplitude and reduced frequency. The deepening of the disturbance of consciousness is characterized by the appearance of delta waves and subsequent attenuation of the signal to an isoelectric pattern. Standard neuroimaging examinations often show signal alterations similar to those of hypoxic-ischemic encephalopathy, with the difference being that they are reversible in mild cases with prompt normalization of blood glucose levels. In other words, visible imaging alterations depend on both the intensity and duration of hypoglycemia. In magnetic resonance imaging, in the most severe forms of encephalopathy, signal alterations (increased signal on T2-weighted images) involve the cortex, hippocampus, and basal ganglia. In milder forms, the deep white matter is affected, particularly the *centrum semiovale*, internal capsule, and *splenium of the corpus callosum*. These alterations can coexist. The involvement of the cerebellum and thalamus is rare, which is another useful feature for differentiating hypoglycemic from hypoxic-ischemic damage. Diffusion-weighted sequences, capable of revealing the earliest alterations, demonstrate signal restriction with three possible patterns: selective involvement of white matter, gray matter, or a mixed pattern, which is the most common. These patterns do not correlate with the initial blood glucose level but are predictive of neurological outcomes, even severe ones, depending on the distribution, extent, and, above all, degree of regression. Spectroscopy sequences are useful because lactate accumulation is not expected in hypoglycemic encephalopathy due to substrate degradation.

The therapy for hypoglycemic encephalopathy is based on the treatment of hypoglycemia with early administration of intravenous glucose solutions. Despite the apparent simplicity of the treatment, it is crucial, in diabetic patients, to implement every strategy to prevent hypoglycemia by performing frequent blood glucose monitoring, keeping a diary, instructing the patient to recognize prodromal symptoms, and ensuring they have self-administrable glucagon injections. Regarding neurological damage, predictors of unfavorable outcomes include prolonged duration and severity of hypoglycemia, normal or elevated body temperature, and low plasma lactate levels. Age, sex, the presence of diabetes, or the triggering cause of hypoglycemia are not negative predictors. Since lowering body temperature reduces energy demand during the substrate-deficient phase, therapeutic use of hypothermia has been proposed based on some anecdotal positive reports. Additionally, due to observations that lactate produced by astrocytes can be utilized by neurons as an alternative energy substrate to glucose, lactic acid infusion has also been proposed for neuroprotective purposes. However, neither of these measures is yet part of routine clinical practice (Table 11.2).

Table 11.2 NEUROIMAGING FINDINGS IN HYPOGLYCEMIC SYNDROMES

Main neuroimaging features	Pathogenetic mechanisms	Essential to check
MRI: Signal restriction on DWI with corresponding low ADC values in the affected regions	Energetic insufficiency and tissue alkalosis with aspartate release Selective neuronal necrosis in the cortex, basal ganglia, and hippocampus	Cortical or subcortical areas with restricted diffusion values
MRI: Cortical or subcortical alterations with sparing of cerebellum, thalamus, and brainstem, hyperintense on T2, iso-intense on T1		
Thalamic, cerebellar, and brainstem sparing		Absence of lactate peak on MRS
MRS: Absence of lactate peak		

11.2.2 Hyperglycemic encephalopathy

Hyperglycemic encephalopathy is a complication of uncontrolled diabetes. "Hyperglycemia" refers to a plasma glucose concentration equal to or above 140 mg/dl. When it complicates type 1 diabetes, hyperglycemia is associated with ketoacidosis, while in type 2 diabetes, it is referred to as hyperosmolar hyperglycemia (non-ketotic). Encephalopathy (including coma d'*emblée*) manifests at blood glucose levels above 250 mg/dl in the case of ketoacidotic hyperglycemia and above 600 mg/dl in the case of hyperosmolar hyperglycemia. Ketoacidotic coma tends to predominate in the younger population, while hyperosmolar coma is more common in the elderly. However, the increasing incidence of type 2 diabetes in children and young people is changing this trend. Hyperglycemic encephalopathy is characterized by a deficit in insulin secretion or increased insulin resistance. Hyperglycemia can occur spontaneously or during metabolic stress caused by infections, trauma, etc. The ketoacidotic state constitutes the first clinical event leading to the diagnosis of diabetes mellitus in approximately 15% of cases.

The pathogenesis of the disturbance of consciousness is likely due to dehydration of the neuronal systems involved in the Ascending Reticular Activating System. However, alteration of neurotransmitter systems, particularly in determining the seizure correlate of the syndrome, is not excluded.

Non-neurological clinical manifestations vary depending on the type of hyperglycemia (Table 11.3). Patients with ketoacidotic hyperglycemia appear dehydrated, exhibit dry mucous membranes, tend to be hypotensive, asthenic, and generally have headaches. They have a characteristically fruity breath. The level of ketoacids increases in both urine and blood, leading to acidosis. The ketone bodies can produce such high acidity that they can affect the cerebrospinal fluid and interstitial pH, directly excite the pneumotaxic center in the brainstem, thus inducing a specific respiratory pattern. This pattern, known as "Kussmaul breathing," is characterized by increased respiratory rate and depth, similar to

Table 11.3 LABORATORY DATA IN HYPERGLYCEMIC SYNDROMES

	Diabetic ketoacidosis	Hyperosmolar hyperglycemic syndrome
Blood glucose level	>250 mg/dl	>600 mg/dl
Plasma osmolarity	<320 mOsm/kg	>320 mOsm/kg
Acid-base balance	pH <7.3 HCO3- <18 mEq/L Anion gap >10	pH >7.3 HCO3- >18 mEq/L Variable anion gap
Ketosis	Present	Rare

Table 11.4 NEUROIMAGING FINDINGS IN HYPEROSMOLAR HYPERGLYCEMIC SYNDROME (NON-KETOACIDOTIC)

Main neuroimaging features	Pathogenetic mechanisms	Essential to check
TC: Unilateral or bilateral hyperdensity of the putamen with or without involvement of the caudate nucleus	Uncertain pathogenesis of signal changes; diverse pathological mechanisms acting in parallel	CT hyperdensity or MRI T1 hyperintensity of the putamen in a clinically[1] and laboratory[2] consistent context
MRI: Putaminal signal alteration with T1 hyperintensity and variable T2 changes		[1] Acute onset of unilateral motor disorder with involuntary, arrhythmic movements of the hemichorea-hemiballismus type
Absence of surrounding edema or mass effect		[2] Hyperglycemia
MRS: Absence of lactate peak		

the central neurogenic hyperventilation seen in structural coma from ponto-mesencephalic damage (in this case, however, laboratory tests do not show acidosis or ketonuria).

Patients with hyperosmolar hyperglycemia have normal levels of ketoacids and, if conscious, may experience fatigue and polyuria.

Neurological manifestations, on the other hand, are less differentiating. In both conditions, they accompany systemic symptoms but are more prominent in hyperosmolar hyperglycemia. They are characterized by global signs (alterations in the level of consciousness, up to coma), sometimes associated with focal signs. In hyperosmolar hyperglycemia, focal signs can manifest as hemiplegia, aphasia, or motor seizures, and more rarely, but selectively, as hemichorea and hemiballismus. This motor disorder is known as diabetic striatopathy or hyperglycemic chorea and represents a neurologic condition that is increasingly recognized. In these patients, neuroimaging reveals typically unilateral involvement of the basal ganglia: putamen (79-94% based on CT or MRI), caudate (48-42%), globus pallidus (28%). The involvement of the subthalamic nucleus is less frequent than the striatum. Functional alterations in the same structures related to regional blood flow (reduced) and metabolism (reduced) have also been reported.

The treatment of hyperglycemic encephalopathy involves correcting hyperglycemia (administration of insulin) and restoring fluid and electrolyte balance (intravenous infusion of 0.9% NaCl saline solution, with potassium supplementation if necessary). The correction of metabolic abnormalities should not occur too rapidly to avoid the formation of cerebral edema. In the presence of diabetic striatopathy, correction of hyperglycemia rarely leads to partial or complete resolution of the motor symptoms or neuroimaging abnormalities. In such cases, therapeutic supplementation with anti-chorea medications is necessary (haloperidol in 40% of patients, tetrabenazine in 4%, risperidone in 2%, clonazepam in 2%) (Table 11.4).

11.2.3 Hepatic encephalopathy

It is a potentially reversible neuropsychiatric syndrome related to liver failure (dysfunction that prevents the liver from properly detoxifying the blood). This occurs due to the depletion of liver function or the presence of portosystemic *shunt* that divert blood flow from the portal circulation, leading to an increase in systemic blood concentration of neurotoxic substances.

Hepatic encephalopathy can be a direct consequence of acute or chronic liver failure. Acute liver failure occurs within 6 months of the liver disease that caused it. Triggering causes include hepatitis, medications, toxins, vascular anomalies, Wilson's disease, and Reye syndrome. Chronic liver failure, on the other hand, occurs more than 8 months after the disease that caused it. The main triggering causes include alcoholic and non-alcoholic liver cirrhosis and transjugular intrahepatic portosystemic shunts (TIPS).

The classification of hepatic encephalopathy is based on the underlying pathological process.

Type A encephalopathy follows acute liver failure. Type B is caused by portosystemic shunting without intrinsic impairment of hepatocellular function. Type C occurs with cirrhosis, portal hypertension, or portosystemic shunting. Clinically, Type C can be divided into episodic, minimal (when there are no objective clinical findings and the syndrome is detectable only through specific psychometric evaluation), and persistent encephalopathy. "Minimal hepatic encephalopathy" causes deficits in attention, vigilance, and general integrative functions.

The pathogenesis of hepatic encephalopathy is still under study. The main hypothesis focuses on the increase in ammonia levels, a catabolite of nitrogen-containing compounds (produced by enteric mucosal or saprophytic bacterial enzymes), which enters the portal circulation and is normally transformed into urea by hepatocytes for elimination through the renal filter. Excess ammonia crosses the blood-brain barrier and is transformed by astrocytes into glutamine from glutamate (which becomes depleted), resulting in an inhibitory imbalance of neurotransmission and cellular energy deficit due to ATP overconsumption. Astrocyte distress also induces the production of inflammatory cytokines, which can alter the permeability of the blood-brain barrier. In patients with acute liver failure, the intracellular increase in glutamine induces osmotic intracellular water influx and swelling of astrocytes, leading to cytotoxic edema, intracranial hypertension, and the risk of cerebral herniation. The risk of cerebral edema increases with arterial ammonia levels >200 micromol/L. In patients with chronic liver failure, compensatory mechanisms are activated, such as extracellular shifting of myo-inositol and taurine.

The lack of correlation between blood ammonia levels and the severity of encephalopathy suggests the presence of other mechanisms underlying the clinical manifestations. One of these mechanisms is the enhancement of GABAergic transmission induced by increased neurosteroids (particularly allopregnanolone), compounds produced by glial cells that act as positive modulators of GABA-A receptors, over-regulating benzodiazepine receptors. The role of these receptors has been confirmed by repeated observations in which flumazenil temporarily improves both EEG activity and the mental state of patients. Another mechanism is the increase in aromatic amino-acids (tryptophan, tyrosine, and phenylalanine, which the liver can no longer metabolize) compared to branched-chain amino-acids (leucine, isoleucine, and valine, which are not subject to hepatic transformation). The imbalance between these two types of amino-acids promotes the synthesis of octopamine and phenylethanolamine, substances that act as false neurotransmitters in noradrenergic and dopaminergic systems. Elevated plasma and cerebral levels of histamine found in autopsied samples of patients with hepatic encephalopathy, along with the up-regulation of cerebral H1 receptors, also indicate that altered amino-acid metabolism also impairs histaminergic transmission. The serotoninergic deficit induced by increased serotonin turnover (increased synthesis and metabolism) and rearrangement of receptor populations also contributes to the overall increase in inhibitory tone. Other mechanisms under study include the increase in cerebral lactate levels or manganese (particularly in the globus pallidus), which can cause neurotoxicity through oxidative damage to astrocytes.

From a clinical perspective, hepatic encephalopathy due to metabolic decompensation is characterized by a progressive alteration of consciousness (■ Table 11.5). It starts with subtle personality changes and cognitive deficits detectable only through specific psychometric evaluation and progresses to a comatose state. The clinical presentation evolves over days or weeks, without necessarily following a worsening course but rather a fluctuating one, even within the same day.

Based on the level of consciousness, intellectual function, degree of personality changes, behavior, and associated neuromuscular manifestations, four stages (I-IV) of hepatic encephalopathy are traditionally distinguished. These stages follow the one defined as minimal hepatic encephalopathy, in which cirrhotic patients present variable degrees of attention deficit, psychomotor slowing, and impaired

Table 11.5 STAGING OF HEPATIC ENCEPHALOPATHY

Minimal hepatic encephalopathy	Alterations in psychometric tests only
Stage I	Insomnia, fatigue, attention deficit, mild depression and irritability, tremor or incoordination
Stage II	Lethargy, disorientation, amnesia, confusion, behavioral changes, dysarthria, hyporeflexia, ataxia, *flapping tremor*
Stage III	Drowsiness/*stupor*, marked cognitive deficits, hallucinations and delusions, muscle weakness, hyperreflexia, nystagmus, Babinski sign, clonus
Stage IV	Coma, pathological postures

coordination. These impairments are induced by a combination of hyperammonemia and peripheral inflammation, triggered by specific alterations in immunophenotype, and occur even before the progression to cirrhosis. Supporting this, peripheral lymphocyte infiltration into the cerebellum has been observed in the early stages of liver disease, indicating that peripheral inflammation changes induce neuroinflammation, which in turn alters neurotransmission and leads to neurocognitive impairment. This outcome is also confirmed by observations made with functional magnetic resonance imaging techniques in patients with minimal hepatic encephalopathy, which show altered resting-state connectivity in various neural circuits. These are functional interconnections between cortical and subcortical regions that activate when the individual is awake and at rest. Interestingly, such connectivity is also altered in neurodegenerative diseases that cause cognitive impairment, including early-stage Alzheimer's disease. Recognizing minimal hepatic encephalopathy is particularly important because it has been established that it serves as a predictive factor for overt hepatic encephalopathy and unfavorable outcomes in patients with cirrhosis. Both progressions are promoted by zinc deficiency, a key element in ammonia detoxification.

In Stage I (mild), patients complain of insomnia and fatigue, reduced attention span, mild irritability and depression, minimal tremor, or incoordination. Stage II (moderate) is usually characterized by lethargy and disorientation, amnesia, confusion, evident personality changes, and behavioral disorders. There is dysarthria, hyporeflexia, and ataxia. In Stage III (severe), patients are drowsy or stuporous, exhibit marked cognitive impairments, paranoid ideation, and hallucinations. There is muscle weakness, hyperreflexia, nystagmus, extensor plantar reflexes, clonus, and in some cases, rigidity. Stage IV is characterized by coma, often associated with opisthotonus or other abnormal postures. Seizures are not characteristic manifestations.

Among the motor manifestations, *asterixis* - a *flapping tremor* for anglophiles or negative myoclonus for experts in motor disorders - deserves mention. It consists of brief and arrhythmic inhibitions of voluntary muscle contraction, resulting in simultaneous involuntary interruptions of posture maintenance. This phenomenon is prominent in Stage II but not in Stage I and it is never seen in Stage IV. It is typically identified in the upper limbs by asking the patient to extend the arms with the wrists dorsiflexed, but it can also be observed in the cranial region (tongue) and lower limbs. In Stage IV encephalopathy, characteristic grasp reflexes and extensor posturing (classically indicative of structural damage) are observed but are completely reversible with correction of hyperammonemia.

In patients with acute fulminant hepatic decompensation without chronic liver disease, the clinical development of encephalopathy is a more condensed process. Increased resistance to passive mobilization of the limbs and neck (oppositive paratonia, rapidly evolving into frank rigidity) accompanies the progression of mental confusion.

For completeness, it should be noted that patients with hepatic encephalopathy due to functional hepatic decompensation show clinical signs of liver disease such as ascites, jaundice, and spider angiomas. In these cases, the neurological picture leaves no diagnostic doubt, and the measurement of ammonia levels (usually $>200\,\mu g/dL$) confirms it.

Depending on the stage of encephalopathy, the EEG may show desynchronization of fast activity with diffuse slowing, increased dysrhythmia, random and arrhythmic appearance of asynchronous delta waves followed by mixed slow and fast activity. Triphasic waves (defined as generalized periodic discharges with an initial negative and brief deflection, a second positive and slightly longer deflection, and a third negative and slow deflection) appear in Stages II and III, in a periodic or pseudo-periodic pattern but disappear in the coma state. The practical significance of using EEG in the evaluation of patients with hepatic encephalopathy is to exclude non-convulsive status epilepticus.

The neuroimages show areas of cerebral edema, particularly in type A (acute) hepatic encephalopathy. Longitudinal examinations allow for monitoring the evolution of edematous state during the clinical course. In patients with fulminant hepatic decompensation, careful observation of CT scans enables early detection because of the disappearance of Sylvian fissures and sulci, followed by narrowing and eventual obliteration of the basal cisterns. In these patients, the extent of cerebral edema is sufficient to induce intracranial hypertension syndrome, an emergency condition that requires neurosurgical consultation for the placement of pressure monitoring devices. The hemorrhagic complications of such procedures are minimized by recent pre-implantation INR control protocols.

Bilateral signal intensity changes with restricted diffusion are observed in the insular cortex and cingulate gyrus and are associated with less specific, asymmetric cortical and subcortical changes, and variable in location (Table 11.6). T1-weighted images may show hyperintensity due to manganese accumulation in the globus pallidus and limbic system. However, it should be noted that these deposits are attributed to chronic hepatopathy rather than the specific encephalopathic condition. Spectroscopy sequences reveal increased levels of glutamine and glutamate, associated with reduced peaks of myo-inositol and choline, likely indicating the expression of compensatory cellular mechanisms in response to ammonia overload. The various signal changes are reversible with standardized treatment of hyperammonemia.

Since in many cases it is possible to identify a precipitating factor for the encephalopathic condition (such as sepsis, bleeding from esophageal varices, excessive protein intake, electrolyte abnormalities, surgical events, placement of TIPS), the primary goal of treatment for hepatic encephalopathy due to functional hepatic decompensation is the removal or correction of that factor. In patients with acute liver failure, it is essential to control intracranial hypertension through mannitol infusion or hypertonic saline solution. Recently, the beneficial effect of mild hypothermia in preventing cerebral damage from acute liver failure has been demonstrated. Hypothermia reduces intracranial hypertension, blood ammonia concentration and cerebral metabolism, cerebral blood flow, cytokine production, accumulation of glutamate and lactate in the extracellular spaces, and oxidative stress. In patients with chronic hepatic encephalopathy, liver transplantation is the definitive treatment. In the meantime, medical therapy should aim to improve clinical symptoms within 72 hours, beyond which alternative diagnostic hypotheses of

Table 11.6 NEUROIMAGING FINDINGS IN HEPATIC ENCEPHALOPATHY

Main neuroimaging features	Pathogenetic mechanisms	Essential to check
MRI T1: Bilateral and symmetric hyperintensity of the *globus pallidus* and *substantia nigra*	Manganese accumulation Mild or diffuse edema Intra-astrocytic accumulation of glutamine	Bilateral and symmetric T1 hyperintensity of the globus pallidus and substantia nigra Typical changes on MRS Reversibility of changes after transplantation
MRI T2-FLAIR: Hyperintensity of the hemisphere white matter along or surrounding the corticospinal tract		
MRS: Increased glutamine/glutamate signal, reduced myo-inositol/choline signal, normal N-acetyl-aspartate signal		

encephalopathy should be considered. The purpose of medical treatment is to reduce ammonia levels through two fundamental measures: non-absorbable disaccharides and intestinal antibiotics, administered alone or in combination. The most used products are lactulose (a disaccharide that acidifies the colonic lumen, reducing the activity of urease-producing bacteria) at a dose of 15-30 ml orally twice a day, and rifaximin at a dose of 1100 mg per day. The use of neomycin, on the other hand, is associated with frequent side effects. Protein restriction in the diet (previously considered beneficial) is now regarded as harmful.

In patients with minimal hepatic encephalopathy, chronic treatment with probiotics reduces ammonia levels, improves quality of life, and slows down the progression to overt encephalopathy. In the same category of patients, the use of 5-phosphodiesterase inhibitors has been proposed to enhance cognitive performance.

11.2.4 Renal functional failure encephalopathy

Renal functional failure encephalopathy can be classified as a condition induced by organ insufficiency *itself* or as a result of its treatment (dialysis). Renal functional failure can be caused by acute or chronic organ failure (the clinical course is worse in the former case in terms of severity and speed of progression) and manifests with signs and symptoms such as fluid retention, hypercreatininemia, hyperazotemia, metabolic acidosis, hyperkalemia, and anemia. The neurological picture induced by acute renal failure is defined as uremic myoclonic-convulsive syndrome. The term uremic encephalopathy (chronic) is instead used to refer to the neurological alterations associated with uremia, which is severe chronic renal failure. Uremia, in its complete clinical expression indicating multiorgan functional failure, is caused by the accumulation of protein catabolism products and the loss of the kidney's endocrine and homeostatic function.

In uremia, protein degradation products that are not effectively removed by the kidneys accumulate in the blood. For this reason, the clinical picture of uremic encephalopathy has long been attributed solely to increased blood urea concentration. Currently, urea is believed to be responsible for uremic myoclonic-convulsive syndrome (where it would act as a neurotoxin), while other mechanisms are also considered to explain the alterations in uremic encephalopathy, briefly described below.

An important role is attributed to guanidine compounds (guanidinosuccinic acid, guanidine, methylguanidine, and creatinine), waste products of protein catabolism that are present in elevated concentrations in the serum, cerebrospinal fluid, and brain tissue in the uremic state. Some of these compounds have markedly proconvulsant activity even at low doses, through their blocking action on GABA-A and glycine receptors and agonistic action on NMDA receptors; other compounds have been associated with depression and cognitive disorders in clinical studies.

Advanced glycation end-products are proteins or lipids that become glycated as a result of exposure to carbamyl groups of reducing sugars. Cortically, these products can dose-dependently induce neuronal death and contribute to the size of cerebral infarction; through interaction with specific receptors, they induce cognitive deficits.

Metabolites of tryptophan (indoxyl sulfate, indole-3-acetic acid, kynurenine, quinolinic acid), in addition to their pro-inflammatory, pro-thrombotic, and profibrotic actions, exert neurotoxic activity through various mechanisms, including the inhibition of removal of neurotransmitters, their metabolites, or other neurotoxins by organic acid transporters.

Parathyroid hormone (PTH) plays a central role in calcium and phosphorus homeostasis. The appearance of uremia-induced resistance to PTH, together with reduced levels of ionized calcium in the serum (hypocalcemia), leads to excessive secretion of PTH. The pathogenic role of PTH in uremic encephalopathy is supported by the positive correlation between the number and degree of EEG abnormalities and plasma PTH concentrations. In animal models, these abnormalities are abolished by preventive parathyroidectomy. It is reasonable to assume that calcium homeostasis alterations in the brain modify neuronal membrane properties and, with them, the release of neurotransmitters, thus favoring epileptogenesis.

Other substances thought to be involved in the pathogenesis of uremic encephalopathy include p-cresyl phosphate (for its pro-oxidative action), homocysteine (for its pro-neuroinflammatory action), and β_2-microglobulin (for its pro-aging action).

Acute uremic encephalopathy (Table 11.7) manifests with initially mild cognitive and consciousness alterations, variably characterized by apathy, flattened affect, irritability, impaired attention, personality changes, and sleep disturbances. In this phase, motor abnormalities are represented by reduced dexterity (clumsiness). As the disturbance of consciousness progresses to confusion, *stupor*, and coma, there is a transient increase in personality and behavioral disorders, while myoclonus, *asterixis*, and kinetic and postural tremor become characteristic motor manifestations. In acute uremic encephalopathy, myoclonus is predominant and is associated with generalized convulsive manifestations, especially in anuric patients. In this phase, neurological examination reveals hypertonia, hyperreflexia, clonus, extensor plantar responses, and limb weakness that, in possible asymmetric combinations, mimics the presence of focal deficits. The presence of meningeal signs can be misleading. Respiratory changes in acute uremic encephalopathy include compensatory hyperventilation in an acidotic state, Kussmaul's respiration, and Cheyne-Stokes respiration. Hypocalcemia, finally, promotes tetanic phenomena.

Chronic uremic encephalopathy has a more insidious clinical manifestation (Table 11.7). The symptomatology is similar to that of acute renal failure, but the severity of signs and symptoms is attenuated. Disturbances of consciousness are characteristically fluctuating and progress more slowly. Headache and sleep disorders are frequent, as well as the movement disorder known as "restless legs syndrome," often associated with myoclonus (positive and negative) and tremor. Seizures, on the other hand, are rare in chronic uremic encephalopathy and tend to occur only in the late or terminal stages. Cases of reversible posterior encephalopathy syndrome have been reported in patients with advanced kidney disease undergoing dialysis. This is a clinical-radiological entity traditionally associated with arterial hypertension, characterized by headache, alteration of mental status, seizures, visual disturbances, and possible focal neurological deficits. The magnetic resonance imaging (MRI) findings show hyperintensity on T2-weighted sequences in the posterior regions of the brain (occipital and parietal lobes), indicating vasogenic edema. The syndrome, if adequately recognized and treated, is - by definition - reversible. Dialysis-treated nephropathic patients represent a higher-risk category for developing this syndrome due to multiple factors of endothelial dysfunction (hypertension, uremia, and certain treatments such as erythropoietin) that compromise the efficiency of cerebral vascular autoregulation systems.

Generally, the clinical diagnosis of encephalopathy due to renal functional failure is straightforward. Organ failure is evident through routine blood chemistry tests, but it should be noted that neither the levels of urea or creatinine nor the reduced glomerular

Table 11.7 CLINICAL PICTURE OF ACUTE AND CHRONIC UREMIC ENCEPHALOPATHY

	Uremic myoclonic-convulsive syndrome	Uremic encephalopathy
Onset	Acute	Insidious
Pathogenesis	Uremia	Uremia, accumulation of guanidinic compounds, altered calcium homeostasis
Alterations in consciousness	From attention deficit to coma, with possible rapid progression	Drowsiness, confusion, mild and slowly developing alterations in consciousness, fluctuating course
Motor manifestations	Myoclonus (predominant), asterixis, tremor, hypertonia, tetany, weakness	Myoclonus, restless legs syndrome, tremor
Seizure events	Generalized seizures	Only in terminal stages

filtration rate correlate with the severity of the encephalopathic picture. On the other hand, in patients with chronic kidney disease or acute renal failure, the diagnosis can become difficult in the presence of potentially confounding neurological and/or internal comorbidities. In such cases, the diagnosis becomes one of exclusion, confirmed only by the improvement of symptoms and cognitive function with dialysis.

The most common EEG alteration is generalized slowing, predominantly frontal. In cases of acute progression, within 48 hours of the onset of renal failure, irregular reduction in voltage, slowing of the background rhythm, occasional theta wave discharges, and prolonged and bilateral sharp delta waves may be observed. Paroxysmal activity may accompany it, frequently associated with clinical seizure correlates. Triphasic waves with anterior predominance are common, while spike-and-wave complexes are less frequent. The degree of observed slowing is often consistent with the clinical course.

Cerebrospinal fluid examination does not show alterations (except for a modest increase in protein levels), or it may reveal nonspecific changes. The diagnostic objective of the procedure is to exclude alternative etiological hypotheses (infections).

Neuroimaging studies are usually normal. In addition to the described reversible posterior encephalopathy syndrome, other rare abnormalities are found affecting the basal ganglia either unilaterally or bilaterally and the internal and external capsules (e.g., the "fork sign," which can be observed in patients with metabolic acidosis from any cause) (Table 11.8).

The main treatment for encephalopathy due to renal functional failure is hemodialysis and, in chronic forms, kidney transplantation. It should be noted that the same dialysis treatment can sometimes be responsible for neurological manifestations, as it is directly or indirectly associated with dementia, disequilibrium syndrome (a reaction to rapid changes in solute concentration that occur during hemodialysis), worsening atherosclerosis, cerebrovascular events due to arterial hypotension from ultrafiltration, hypertensive encephalopathy, Wernicke's encephalopathy, cerebral hemorrhage, subdural hematoma, osmotic myelinolysis, and intracranial hypertension.

Myoclonus generally responds to treatment with clonazepam. Seizures should be treated with anticonvulsants, taking care to use low dosages (to avoid precipitating nephrotoxicity) to be administered at the end of the dialysis session. Similar precautions should be taken for the administration of other medications. Vitamin C-based treatments are useful for restless legs syndrome in dialysis patients. It should be noted that patients with chronic renal failure have a high risk of bleeding, hypertension, and infections; therefore, they need to be carefully monitored and treated as appropriate.

11.2.5 Pulmonary functional failure encephalopathies

These are encephalopathy conditions induced by various forms of respiratory failure characterized by either isolated hypoxia

Table 11.8 NEUROIMAGING FINDINGS IN UREMIC ENCEPHALOPATHY

Main neuroimaging features	Pathogenetic mechanisms	Essential to check
MRI T2: Bilateral hyperintensity of basal ganglia and cortical areas	Uncertain but complex Likely multifactorial	Fork sign (hyperintensity of external capsule, internal capsule, and corresponding medullary laminae of the putamen)
MRI T2-FLAIR: Possible presence of the "fork sign"		
Atypical changes may include diffusion signal restriction from cytotoxic edema in the basal ganglia, particularly in the pallidum		

or hypoxia with hypercapnia. This failure can be attributed to environmental causes, mechanical respiratory problems, and systemic diseases, primarily cardiopulmonary diseases. Conditions resulting from dysfunctions of the brainstem-muscle axis, which can cause acute respiratory mechanical failure, are not considered.

Hypoxic pulmonary encephalopathy | Hypoxic pulmonary encephalo-pathy presents in two forms: acute and chronic. The acute form, also known as "acute mountain sickness," is a reversible neurological condition characterized by headache, nausea, vomiting, generalized fatigue, and mild to moderate alterations in consciousness (Table 11.9). It can occur when rapidly reaching high altitudes (typically above 4,000 m, but also above 3,000 m with stays longer than 12 hours) where the partial pressure of oxygen in the air decreases. The relevant factor in assessing the risk during ascent is the altitude at which the individual sleeps at night, considering the relative nocturnal hypoxemia compared to wakefulness. Mathematical models have calculated that the likelihood for an unacclimatized young woman to develop severe acute mountain sickness during a rapid ascent (<2 hours) to an altitude of 3,000 meters is less than 2%.

Risk factors for the development of encephalopathy include prolonged stays at altitudes of at least 900 m, underlying cardiopulmonary diseases, the speed of ascent, and previous episodes of acute mountain sickness. At higher altitudes, the presence of cerebral edema (known as high-altitude cerebral edema or HACE) exacerbates the listed symptoms and leads to confusion, trunk ataxia, and rarely seizures. In these cases, magnetic resonance imaging (MRI) shows hyperintensity areas in the *corpus callosum* on T2-weighted images, likely due to vasogenic edema. The neurological picture is often complicated by high-altitude pulmonary edema. The pathogenesis of acute hypoxic pulmonary encephalopathy is attributed to an increased blood-brain barrier permeability (induced by cerebral vasodilation) and the formation of vasogenic edema.

The most effective treatment is, of course, descent to lower altitudes. Other forms of therapy, in addition to prevention, include controlled hyperventilation (which induces cerebral vasoconstriction and prevents vasogenic edema) and a combination of medications such as acetazolamide and prednisone.

The chronic form of hypoxic pulmonary encephalopathy (or chronic mountain sickness) is neurologically similar but clinically associated with systemic abnormalities such as secondary polycythemia, pulmonary hypertension, and chronic *cor pulmonale* (common in individuals who live at high altitudes for extended periods).

Table 11.9 CLINICAL CHARACTERISTICS OF HYPOXIC, HYPERCAPNIC, AND CARBON MONOXIDE ENCEPHALOPATHIES

	Hypoxic encephalopathy (acute mountain sickness)	Hypercapnic encephalopathy	Carbon monoxide encephalopathy
Pathogenesis	Reduced partial pressure of oxygen at high altitude Vasogenic cerebral edema	Increased partial pressure of CO_2 in the blood Acidosis of cerebrospinal fluid, extracellular fluids, and cerebral vasodilation	Higher affinity of CO for hemoglobin compared to oxygen Acidosis and cerebral edema
Symptoms	Mild: headache, nausea, vomiting, drowsiness Severe: confusion, ataxia, seizures	Headache, papilledema, drowsiness, confusion, generalized tremors, asterixis, myoclonus (predominantly in the upper limbs), *stupor*, coma	Nausea, vomiting, throbbing headache, dizziness, cherry-red coloration, memory deficits, hallucinations, visual field deficits, alterations in consciousness
Risk Factors	Prolonged stays at altitudes above 900 m, rapid ascent, pre-existing conditions	Lung diseases, neuromuscular abnormalities	Prolonged exposure to the toxin, poorly ventilated environments
Progression	Possible progression to coma	Rare prolonged coma and irreversible brain damage	Possible delayed encephalopathy
Treatment	Descent to lower altitudes, sedatives, corticosteroids	Positive pressure ventilation	Hyperbaric oxygen

Patients with chronic obstructive pulmonary disease (COPD) can also develop hypoxic pulmonary encephalopathy, which negatively affects cognitive functions, particularly attention, deductive reasoning, and motor learning.

Hypercapnic pulmonary encephalopathy When the partial pressure of CO_2 in arterial blood exceeds 60 mmHg, a condition of hypercapnia is established. This is the most common cause of metabolic pulmonary encephalopathy and occurs in patients where hypercapnia complicates hypoxia. These patients may have obstructive and restrictive lung diseases, disorders of the respiratory regulatory centers, lower motor neuron diseases, peripheral nerve disorders, neuromuscular junction disorders, and muscle disorders.

It is a syndrome characterized by alterations in consciousness and behavior, headache, and papilledema (with variable concurrent intracranial hypertension) that rarely progresses to coma. Generalized tremors, *asterixis* (correlating with the degree of hypercapnia and acidosis), and myoclonus, particularly in the upper limbs, are the typical motor expressions of chronic hypercapnia. Seizures rarely occur and only in the presence of *asterixis*. Symptoms tend to worsen in the morning due to nocturnal hypoventilation typical of sleep (Table 11.9).

The pathogenesis of metabolic pulmonary encephalopathy is not yet fully understood. The most plausible mechanism explaining the syndrome is cerebrospinal fluid and interstitial fluid acidosis. The increase in arterial PCO_2 results in an increase in CSF PCO_2, leading to a decrease in pH and cerebral vasodilation. Acute respiratory acidosis has a greater impact on CSF pH than metabolic acidosis because carbon dioxide, due to its high lipid solubility, rapidly crosses the blood-brain barrier, unlike hydrophilic bicarbonate ions. Consequently, the symptoms of hypercapnic encephalopathic syndrome correlate more closely with changes in CSF pH than with arterial blood or partial pressure of CO_2. Within the brain, the choroid plexus responds to changes in CSF acidity by increasing bicarbonate secretion, but the rate of production is insufficient to counterbalance the pH drop. Cerebral acidosis is therefore responsible for alterations in neuronal metabolism and excitability.

Additional exacerbating factors include concurrent cerebral hypoxemia reflecting systemic arterial hypoxemia, intracranial hypertension resulting from cerebral artery vasodilation, coexisting cardiac and renal dysfunctions, electrolyte imbalances, and factors related to treatment (high fraction of inspired oxygen, sedative medications). It should be noted that many lung and heart diseases can induce chronic hypoxic-hypercapnic states, leading to nonspecific neurological manifestations such as headache, mental dullness, and drowsiness. Subtle deviations from normal cognitive capacities, psychomotor activity, memory, and reasoning abilities may manifest as delayed reaction times and abnormalities in constructive skills. In other cases, neurophysiological alterations reflecting increased central cognitive processing time (latency of the P300 potential) precede or accompany clinical signs. Patients with COPD, in fact, exhibit below-average performance in various neuropsychological domains, particularly in tests requiring sustained attention. In such circumstances, arterial blood gas analysis is useful to confirm alterations in arterial oxygen and carbon dioxide partial pressures.

Carbon monoxide encephalopathy | Carbon monoxide (CO) is a gas normally present in the body that, along with hemoglobin, forms the complex called carboxyhemoglobin, which constitutes less than 1% of the total hemoglobin. CO competes with oxygen for the same binding sites but has an affinity over 200 times greater. In conditions of overexposure, it rapidly induces tissue hypoxia and shifts the hemoglobin dissociation curve to the left, resulting in a reduced release of oxygen and further aggravation of hypoxia. When hypoxia is accompanied by hypotension, the hypoxic-hypotensive process leads to damage in the border zones of arterial territories. Hypoxia increases the level of excitatory amino-acids, induces an increase in nitrite levels, and causes subsequent cortical damage. While hypoxia plays a leading role in the genesis of brain damage, it is not the only pathogenetic mechanism involved in oxidative stress, cellular necrosis, apoptosis, and neuroinflammation. CO directly binds to cytochromes A and A3, exerting a toxic effect, while the reduction in cytochrome C oxidase levels inhibits mitochondrial metabolism, resulting in cellular respiration inefficiency. This function is further compromised by peroxynitrite resulting from the excess of NO induced by CO binding to heme proteins in platelets. The interaction between CO and platelets promotes aggregation with neutrophils, leading to degranulation, which contributes to lipid peroxidation, apoptosis, and inflammation. This inflammation is further amplified by microglial activation triggered by the immunological response to lipid peroxidation products that damage myelin basic protein.

Immediate CO encephalopathy is characterized by nausea, vomiting, throbbing headache, dizziness, memory deficits, and mild alterations in consciousness (▪ Table 11.9). These symptoms occur when the concentration of carboxyhemoglobin reaches 20-30% of the total hemoglobin concentration. At this level, the patient may already exhibit a cherry-red skin color. With higher concentrations of carboxyhemoglobin, the patient experiences hallucinations, syncope, visual field disturbances, and further alterations in consciousness. These symptoms progressively worsen until, at concentrations equal to or exceeding 80%, cardiac arrest follows respiratory arrest, resulting in death.

Neuroimaging may reveal the presence of cerebral edema and lesions in the basal ganglia (particularly bilateral necrosis of the globus pallidus), due to the vulnerability of these structures to the specific hypoxic-ischemic process resulting from reduced anastomotic network and the affinity of CO for heme iron in the pallidum. The cerebral white matter is the second most affected area, typically showing signs of demyelination and necrosis that become apparent weeks after the initial insult. Other frequent sites of injury include the *hippocampus*, *cerebellum*, and *substantia nigra*.

The measurement of serum neurogranin has been proposed as a new diagnostic *biomarker* for patients presenting to the emergency department with CO poisoning. Elevated levels of this small neuronal protein reveal neurological damage at a stage when no restriction on diffusion signal in magnetic resonance imaging is detected. Neurogranin is located in the soma and apical and basal dendritic spines of pyramidal neurons. It is abundantly found in the cerebral cortex, hippocampus, amygdala, caudate nucleus, and putamen, but is sparsely represented in the *cerebellum*, brainstem, and spinal cord.

Delayed CO encephalopathy refers to the neurological complex that manifests approximately 2-3 weeks after CO poisoning in survivors (approximately two-thirds of total cases). The syndromic complex can vary in severity depending on the intensity of gas exposure (exposure exceeding 24 hours is a risk factor). Three clinical-behavioral variants can be outlined: approximately 70% of survivors will have transient symptoms only in the acute phase, around 20% will have persistent symptoms from the acute phase into the chronic phase, and the remaining 10% will experience delayed neuropsychiatric sequelae, a combination of neuropsychological and motor disorders that develop after the apparent disappearance of poisoning symptoms (known as the lucid interval or pseudo-recovery period of 22 days).

One of the proposed mechanisms to explain the delayed development is the progression beyond the acute phase of focal demyelination of the brain's white matter induced by CO, resulting in neuronal loss or axonal damage. From a clinical perspective, the picture resembles that of hypoxic-ischemic encephalopathy, with language disorders, memory impairments, urinary disturbances, disruptions in voluntary movement organization including parkinsonism, dystonia, athetosis, as well as tremors and ataxia. Currently, no reliable method can predict which individuals with acute CO encephalopathy will develop the delayed syndrome. However, a positive correlation has been identified between this occurrence and the severity of consciousness disturbance, positivity of neuroimaging, and increased blood levels of CK, CK-MB, and LDH, all of which are considered suggestive elements of intense or prolonged exposure to the toxic gas.

There is no specific treatment for patients with CO encephalopathy, but hyperbaric therapy is believed to reduce its incidence in the acute phase (when carboxyhemoglobin levels exceed 40%).

Bibliography

Adams and Victor's Principles of Neurology, 8th Ed. McGrawHill, 2005.

Bradley W.G., Daroff B., Fenichel G.M., Jankovic J., Neurology in Clinical Practice, 4th Ed. Butterworth Heinemann, 2004.

Flaherty A.W., Rost N.S., The Massachusetts General Hospital Handbook of Neurology. Lippincott, Williams and Wilkins, 2007.

Laureys S., Tononi G., The Neurology of Consciousness Cognitive Neuroscience and neuropathology. Elsevier, 2009.

Lewis S.L. Encephalopathy, in Roos K.L., "Emergency neurology", Springer, 2012.

Manji H., Willis A., Kitchen N., Dorward N., Connolly S., Mehta A., Oxford Handbook of neurology. Oxford University Press, 2006.

Young G.B. Handbook of Clinical Neurology, Disorders of Consciousness. Elsevier, 2008.

12 EPILEPSY

Carlo Di Bonaventura, Alessandra Morano,
Anna Teresa Giallonardo, Jinane Fattouch, Alfredo Berardelli

The term "epileptic seizure" refers to an episodic and transient alteration of neurological functions caused by the abnormal and excessive discharge of a group of neurons. "Epilepsy" refers to a chronic disease, secondary to various etiologies, characterized by the predisposition to have recurrent epileptic seizures. The recurrency of seizures over a period of more than 24 hours is a necessary condition for diagnosis. Therefore, an isolated seizure as well as two seizures within a 24-hour period do not constitute epilepsy. However, a single seizure, together with evidence of brain lesions (such as deficits on the neurological examination or structural lesions on neuroimages) or with the presence of epileptiform abnormalities on the electroencephalogram (EEG), may point towards a diagnosis of epilepsy. The term "epileptic syndrome" refers to a distinct nosographic entity consisting of specific characteristics that include the type of seizures, etiology, EEG alterations, findings on the neurological examination, prognosis, and, in some cases, response to specific antiepileptic medications.

12.1 Epidemiology

After headache, epilepsy represents the second most common chronic neurological condition. The prevalence of epilepsy (the number of cases in a given population at a defined point in time) is approximately 1% (varying worldwide between 0.5% and 0.8%). The prevalence is relatively uniform in countries with similar socioeconomic development. Incidence (the number of new cases appearing in a specific population within a well-defined time interval) varies, however, ranging from 40 to 70 new cases per 100,000 individuals per year in industrialized countries, and from 100 to 190 new cases per 100,000 individuals per year in developing countries. The age-specific incidence curve has a bimodal distribution, with a peak in the first year of life and a second peak in late age, above 75 years. Including isolated seizures, that can occur at any moment in life, cumulative incidence rates (measuring lifetime prevalence) are considerable, ranging from 2% to 6%. The probability of having at least one seizure during one's lifetime is approximately 8%. The mortality rate in patients with epilepsy is 2-3 times higher than that of the general population. Death can be directly related to the cause of epilepsy (tumors, degenerative diseases, etc.) or occur accidentally during a seizure (asphyxia, secondary head trauma, drowning, etc.). In recent years, many studies have focused on the increased risk of *Sudden Unexpected Death in Epilepsy* (SUDEP), which accounts for 10% of deaths in epilepsy patients and is likely supported by cardiogenic mechanisms. The risk of recurrence after a first spontaneous seizure is high, approaching 80% after 3 years. Generally, remission with treatment is observed in 70-80% of cases, which allows for the possibility of discontinuing therapy after a period of observation and careful evaluation. However, when discontinuation is performed, there is a relapse in 17-50% of cases. From a prognostic point of view, patients with newly diagnosed epilepsy can be divided into four main groups: *spontaneously benign epilepsies* (excellent prognosis, spontaneous remission, possibility of not prescribing therapy), *pharmacosensitive epilepsies* (good prognosis, remission with treatment, well-being after discontinuing medications), *pharmacodependent epilepsies* (more reserved prognosis, need to maintain therapy, unpredictability of possible remission, frequent relapse after discontinuing medications), *pharmacoresistant epilepsies* (20-30% of cases, unfavorable prognosis, persistence of seizures despite the use of multiple drugs, impaired quality of life).

12.2 Etiology

The etiological framework of epilepsy is based on the patient's anamnestic and clinical data (from the type of seizures to the neurological examination) and on investigations obtained through genetic testing and neuroimaging techniques (particularly brain MRI). Based on etiology, epilepsies have long been classified into three main groups: *idiopathic, symptomatic, and cryptogenic.* However, this classification has recently been surpassed by the new proposal for the classification of seizures and epilepsies. The new schema, in fact, distinguishes etiological causes based on their possible therapeutic implications. The etiological categories identified in the new schema include structural, genetic, infectious, metabolic, immune, and unknown causes. Etiologies are not exclusive, as some epilepsies may have multiple etiologies.

Structural etiology | This etiological category includes visible alterations of brain tissue in neuroimaging. Structural etiologies can be acquired, such as vascular lesions (stroke or hypoxic-ischemic encephalopathy), traumatic and infectious conditions (encephalitis, meningitis, brain abscesses, etc.), or genetic, such as certain cortical developmental malformations (e.g., polymicrogyria, heterotopias, lissencephalies, etc.) and neurocutaneous syndromes (tuberous sclerosis, Sturge-Weber syndrome, neurofibromatosis). The identification of small structural lesions requires appropriate MRI studies with specific protocols and high-field magnets (1.5 or 3 Tesla). It is also important to guide the MRI examination and its interpretation based on the defined localization hypothesis according to the symptoms and signs of the seizures. There are well-known associations between epilepsies and structural lesions. These include the association between temporal lobe seizures and hippocampal sclerosis, gelastic seizures with hypothalamic hamartoma, Rasmussen's syndrome with progressive hemispheric atrophy, and many other conditions with specific seizures and corresponding characteristic MRI patterns.

Among the structural lesions, whose recognition has been made possible by the progressive advancement of MRI techniques, particular attention should be paid to cortical developmental malformations and mesial temporal lobe sclerosis (or hippocampal sclerosis). Cortical developmental malformations represent the result of alterations in brain maturation during its different phases (proliferation, migration, and organization) that typically occur in fetal life (first 3 months). In these disorders, neurons, often immature and with altered morphology, become arrested in "heterotopic" positions and fail to reach the outermost zone of the brain. Alternatively, once they reach the surface, they position themselves abnormally, disrupting cortical architecture (Figure 12.1). Once arrested in abnormal positions, these neurons establish reciprocal connections with the normally organized brain cortex and any other heterotopic areas, forming highly excitable circuits. Mesial temporal lobe sclerosis is a condition that likely develops, possibly acquired, as atrophy of hippocampal structures (Figure 12.2) leading to the formation of altered circuits that predispose to the onset of epileptic seizures. Although a genetic contribution and individual predisposition cannot be excluded to determine mesial temporal lobe sclerosis, it is believed to be the result of vascular and metabolic damages, secondary to prolonged febrile seizures or to the repetition of seizures in childhood. Mesial temporal lobe sclerosis represents one of the most common causes of drug-resistant focal epilepsy.

The structural lesions underlying epilepsy can vary depending on age. In infancy, the most frequent causes include hypoxic-ischemic injury (pre-, peri-, and postnatal), infections, metabolic disorders, cortical developmental malformations, and neurocutaneous syndromes. In adolescence and young adulthood, "fixed" structural

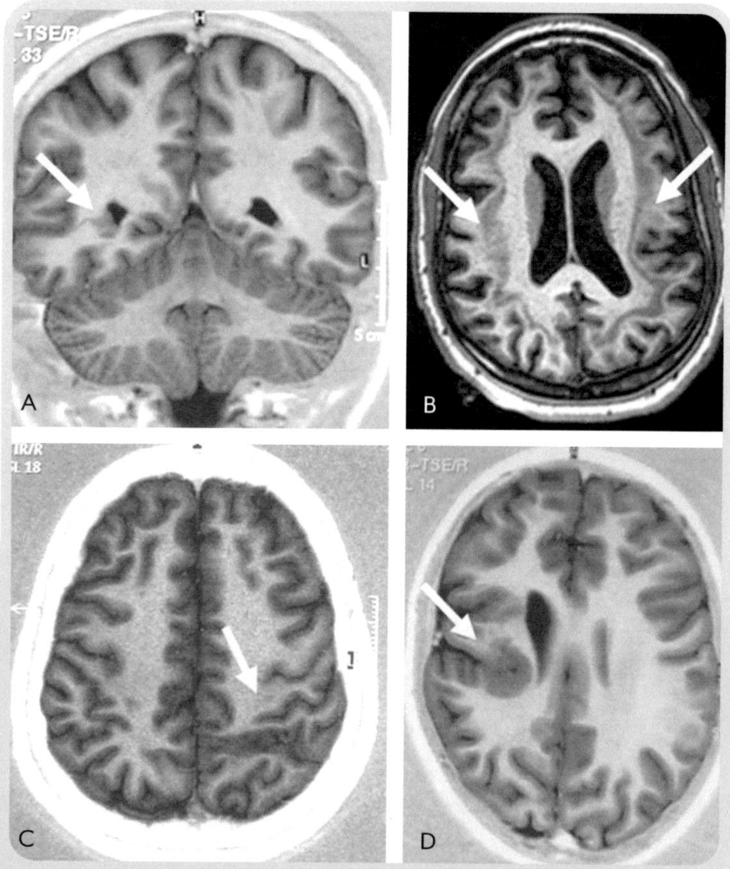

Figure 12.1

Different types of cortical development malformations are evident in the various MRI images (IR sequences). Specifically, a subependymal nodular heterotopia in the right hemisphere (A), a band or double cortex heterotopia (B), a complex left parietal heterotopia (C), and a heterotopia associated with right hemisphere schizencephaly (D) can be observed.

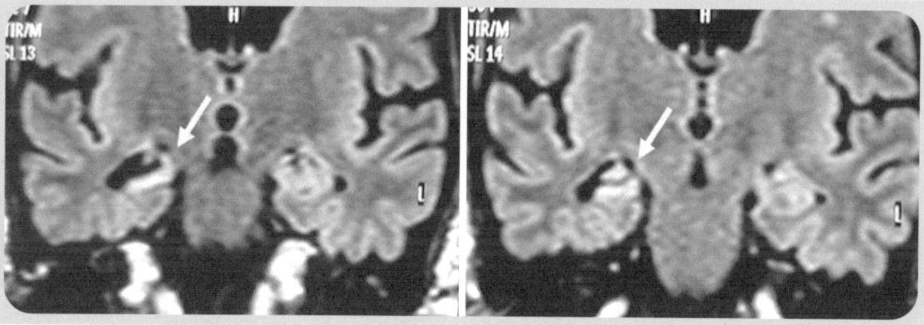

Figure 12.2

In the images on the coronal plane (FLAIR sequences), a typical picture of mesial temporal sclerosis can be observed, with evident hippocampal atrophy and the associated signal alteration (white arrow).

lesions, i.e., non-evolving lesions often present at birth or acquired in the early months of life, are often identifiable. In older age, the most frequent structural causes are represented by cerebrovascular diseases (cerebral hemorrhages or infarcts), tumors (including low-grade astrocytic tumors), and neurodegenerative diseases (such as Alzheimer's disease and other dementias).

Genetic etiology | This category includes forms of epilepsy that are the result of a known or presumed genetic mutation. There are various epileptic syndromes in which such etiology is involved, and in many cases, the underlying genes are still unknown. Genetic etiology can be hypothesized based on factors such as a family history of an autosomal dominant condition, clinical research in populations with the same epileptic syndrome (as seen, for example, in idiopathic generalized epilepsies), and the identification of causative gene mutations (molecular genetics has led to the identification of mutations in a large number of genes in up to 30-50% of cases of patients affected by epileptic encephalopathies). The main forms

Table 12.1 EXAMPLES OF GENETIC MUTATIONS ASSOCIATED WITH SOME EPILEPTIC SYNDROMES

Epileptic Syndrome	Transmission	Locus	Gene	Protein
Early-Onset Epileptic Encephalopathies				
Ohtahara Syndrome/ Early Infantile Epileptic Encephalopathy	AD	20q13.33	*KCNQ2*	Voltage-gated K channel, subfamily Q, member 2
	AD	2q24.3	*SCN2A*	Voltage-gated Na channel, subunit α2
	De novo (AD)	9q34.11	*STXBP1*	Syntaxin-1-binding protein
	XL	Xp22.1	*ARX*	Aristaless-related homeobox protein
	AR	11p15.5	*SCL25A22*	Glutamate carrier mitochondrial 2
	XL	Xp22.13	*CDKL5*	Cyclin-dependent kinase-like 5
	AR	17q21.32	*PNPO*	Pyridoxamine 5'-phosphate oxidase
	AR	7p22.3	*BRAT1*	ATM-activated BRCA1-associated protein
	XL	Xp11.4	*CASK*	Calcium/calmodulin-dependent serine kinase
	XL	Xp22.2	*PIGA*	Phosphatidylinositol glycan anchor biosynthesis, class A
Dravet Syndrome (and Dravet-like syndromes)	AD	2q24.3	*SCN1A*	α1 subunit of the voltage-gated Na channel
	XL (female)	Xq22.1	*PCDH19*	Protocadherin-19
	AD	19q13.11	*SCN1B*	β1 subunit of the voltage-gated Na channel
	De novo (AD)	9q34.11	*STXBP1*	Syntaxin-binding protein 1
	AD	5q34	*GABRA1*	α1 subunit of the $GABA_A$ receptor
	AD	15q26.1	*CHD2*	Chromodomain DNA helicase protein 2
	De novo (AD)	5p12	*HCN1*	Hyperpolarization-activated cyclic nucleotide-gated potassium channel 1
	AD	5q31	*GABRAG2*	γ2 subunit of the $GABA_A$ receptor
Childhood Epilepsy with Focal Migrating Seizures	AD	9q34.3	*KCNT1*	Sodium-activated potassium channel, subfamily T member 1
	AD	2q24.3	*SCN1A*	α1 subunit of the voltage-gated Na channel
	AR	11p15.5	*SLC25A22*	Mitochondrial carrier 2 of Glutamate
	AR	20p12.3	*PLCB1*	Phospholipase C β1
	AR	16p13.3	*TBC1D24*	TBC1-domain family member 24
	AD	2q24.3	*SCN2A*	α2 subunit of the voltage-gated Na channel
	AR	3p21.31	*QARS*	Glutaminyl-tRNA synthetase
	De novo, AD	12q13.13	*SCN8A*	α8 subunit of the voltage-gated Na channel
Infantile Spasms (other genes)	De novo (AD)	14q12	*FOXG1*	Forkhead box G1
	De novo (AD)	9q34.11	*SPTAN1*	Non-erythroid α spectrin 1
	De novo (AD)	9q34.11	*DNM1*	Dynamine 1
		Trisomy 21		
		Tetrasomy 12p		
Benign familial infantile/neonatal seizures				
Neonatal and infantile epilepsy Self-limiting familial	AD	20q13.33	*KCNQ2*	Voltage-gated potassium channel, subfamily Q member 2
		8q24.22	*KCNQ3*	Voltage-gated potassium channel, subfamily Q member 3
		2q24.3	*SCN2A*	α2 subunit of the voltage-gated Na channel
Familial infantile epilepsy Self-limiting	AD	16p11.2	*PRRT2*	Proline-rich transmembrane protein 2
		2q24.3	*SCN2A*	α2 subunit of the voltage-gated Na channel
		20q13.33	*KCNQ2*	Voltage-gated potassium channel, subfamily Q member 2
		8q24.22	*KCNQ3*	Voltage-gated potassium channel, subfamily Q member 3
Progressive myoclonic epilepsies				
Unverricht-Lundborg disease	AR	21q22.3	*CSTB*	Cystatin B
		4q21.1	*SCARB2*	Scavenger receptor class B, member 2
		17q21.32	*GOSR2*	Golgi SNAP receptor, member 2
Lafora disease	AR	6q24.3	*EPM2A*	Laforin
		6p22.3	*EPM2B*	Malin
Neuronal ceroid lipofuscinosis	AR	1p32	*CLN1*	Palmitoyl protein thioesterase
		11p15	*CLN2*	Tripeptidyl peptidase 1
		16p12	*CLN3*	Lysosomal transmembrane protein
		13q21–q32	*CLN5*	Lysosomal soluble protein
		15q23	*CLN6*	Reticular transmembrane protein
		4q28	*CLN7*	Lysosomal protein, MFS family
		8p23	*CLN8*	Reticular transmembrane protein
		11p15.5	*CN10*	Catepsin D
Myoclonus-dystonia syndrome with renal failure	AR	4q21.1	*SCARB2*	Scavenger receptor class B, member 2
Progressive myoclonic epilepsy-ataxia	AR	12q12	*PRICKLE-1*	Prickle homolog 1
Dentatorubral-pallidoluysian atrophy	AD	12p13.31	*ATN-1*	Atrophin-1
Myoclonic epilepsy with ragged red fibers (MERRF)	Diaginica	mtDNA (T8356C)	*MT-TK*	tRNA Lys
		mtDNA	*MT-TL1*	tRNA Leu1
		mtDNA (G12147A)	*MT-TH*	tRNA Hys
		mtDNA (T7512C)	*MT-TS1*	tRNA Ser1

Myoclonic epilepsy and ataxia due to potassium channel mutation (MEAK)	De novo, AD	11p15.1	*KCNC1*	Voltage-gated potassium channel, subfamily C, member 1
Genetic generalized epilepsies				
Juvenile Myoclonic Epilepsy	AD	6p 15q 5q34	*Unknown* *Unknown* *GABRA1*	Unknown Unknown $GABA_A$ receptor α1 subunit
Familial Benign Adult Myoclonic Epilepsy	AD	8q24 2p	*Unknown* *Unknown*	Unknown Unknown
GLUT-1 Deficiency Syndrome	De novo, AD	1p34.2	*SLC2A1*	Glucose Transporter 1 (GLUT1)
Genetic Epilepsies with Febrile Seizures Plus (GEFS+)				
GEFS+1	AD	19q13.11	*SCN1B*	β1 Subunit of the Voltage-gated Na Channel
GEFS+2	AD	2q24.3	*SCN1A*	α1 Subunit of the Voltage-gated Na Channel
GEFS+3	AD	5q31	*GABRG2*	γ2 Subunit of the $GABA_A$ Receptor
	AD	2q24.3	*SCN2A*	α2 Subunit of the Voltage-gated Na Channel
	XL (females)	Xq22.1	*PCDH19*	Protocadherin-19
Familial Focal Epilepsies				
Sleep-Related Hypermotor Epilepsy (SHE)	AD	20q13.2 1q21.3 8p21.2 9q34.3	*CHRNA4* *CHRNB2* *CHRNA2* *KCNT1*	α4 Subunit of the Nicotinic Acetylcholine Receptor β2 Subunit of the Nicotinic Acetylcholine Receptor α2 Subunit of the Nicotinic Acetylcholine Receptor K Na-dip Channel, T Subfamily, Member 1
Autosomal Dominant Epilepsy with Auditory Symptoms	AD AR AD	10q 7q22 22q12.2	*LGI-1* *RELN* *DEPDC5*	Epitempin Reelin Protein (DEP domain-containing 5) of the GATOR1 complex
Familial Epilepsy with Variable Foci	AD	22q12.2	*DEPDC5*	Protein (DEP domain-containing 5) of the GATOR1 complex
Epileptic Aphasias				
Landau-Kleffner Syndrome Continuous Spike-Wave during Slow Sleep Syndrome Atypical Rolandic Epilepsy (Centrotemporal Spikes)	AD	16p13.2	*GRIN2A*	NR2A Subunit of the NMDAR Receptor
Epilepsies associated with cortical developmental malformations				
Lissencephaly/Subcortical Band Heterotopia Spectrum (Double Cortex)	De novo (AD) AR AR XL De novo (AD) XL De novo (AD) De novo (AD) De novo (AD)	17p13.13 7q22.1 9p24.2 Xq22.3-q23 14q32.31 Xp22.1 12q13.12 6p25.2 17q21.2	*LIS1 (PAFAHIB1)* *RELN* *VLDLR* *DCX* *DYNC1H1* *ARX* *TUBA1A* *TUBB2B* *TUBG1*	β subunit of platelet-activating factor acetylhydrolase, isoform 1b Reelin Very Low-Density Lipoprotein Receptor Doublecortin Cytoplasmic Dynein 1 Heavy Chain 1 Aristaless-Related Homeobox Protein α-Tubulin 1A β-Tubulin 2B γ-Tubulin 1
Subependymal Nodular Heterotopia	XL AR De novo AD AR AR	Xq28 20p13 18q21 6q27 11p15.4 4q28.1 (1p, 4p, 5p, 5q, 6p, 9q)	*FLNA* *ARFGEF* *NEDD4L* *ERMARD* *DCHS1* *FAT4*	Filamin A BIG2 (Brefeldin A-inhibited guanine nucleotide exchange factor 1) NEDD4 family E3 ubiquitin ligase Membrane-associated RNA degradation protein Protocadherin-16 Atypical FAT Cadherin-4
Hemimegalencephaly (dysplastic megalencephaly)	AD	1q43-44	AKT3	Serine/Threonine Kinase 3
Focal Cortical Dysplasia	AD	10q23.31	PTEN	Phosphatase and Tensin Homolog
Polymicrogyria	AR AD De novo (AD) AD De novo (AD) AR De novo (AD) De novo (AD) De novo (AD)	16p13.11 8q12.2 14q32.31 2q23.1 12q13.12 22q11 6p25.2 16q24.3 6p21.33	NDE1 CHD7 DYNCHIH1 KIF5C TUBA1A TUBA8 TUBB2B TUBB3 TUBB	NudE-like nuclear distribution protein 1 ATP-dependent helicase CHD7 Cytoplasmic Dynein 1 Heavy Chain 1 Kinesin Family Member 5C α-Tubulin 1A α-Tubulin 8 β-Tubulin 2B β-Tubulin 3 β-Tubulin
Tuberous Sclerosis	AD AD	9q34.13 16p13.3	TSC1 TSC2	Hamartin Tuberin

of genetically determined epilepsy and their respective responsible genes are listed in Table 12.1. In general, many of the monogenic forms are associated with mutations in genes involved in the encoding of structural proteins of ion channels (e.g., sodium or potassium) or receptors for specific neurotransmitters (e.g., GABA), resulting in functional alterations of the implicated systems.

Infectious etiology | This category includes conditions in which seizures and epilepsy are directly correlated with an infection of the central nervous system (CNS), both in acute situations (e.g., meningitis, encephalitis) and chronic ones. Typical examples in certain regions of the world include pathologies such as neurocysticercosis, tuberculosis, HIV, cerebral malaria, subacute sclerosing panencephalitis, cerebral toxoplasmosis, and congenital infections from Zika virus and cytomegalovirus. These infections often lead to structural lesions.

Metabolic etiology | Many metabolic disorders are associated with epilepsy. This rapidly expanding field includes numerous conditions with partially characterized phenotypic spectra. This category encompasses disorders with well-defined metabolic defects characterized by correlated clinical manifestations and biochemical changes, such as porphyria, uremia, and aminoacidopathies. In many cases, the metabolic disorder is directly derived from a genetic defect, but in rare cases, it can be acquired (e.g., folate deficiency). The identification of specific metabolic causes is crucial for therapeutic implications and the prevention of potential intellectual disabilities.

Immune Etiology | This category includes immune-mediated conditions in which seizures represent a central symptomatic feature. Several autoimmune-based epilepsies with specific presentation characteristics have been recently identified in both children and adults. The spectrum of autoimmune encephalitis is rapidly expanding due to the identification of specific antibodies (the most representative examples being anti-LGI1 encephalitis and anti-NMDA encephalitis). Recognizing these forms is crucial for promptly guiding the choice of appropriate immunotherapy.

Unknown etiology | This category includes immune-mediated conditions in which seizures represent a central symptomatic feature. Several autoimmune-based epilepsies with specific presentation characteristics have been recently identified in both children and adults. The spectrum of autoimmune encephalitis is rapidly expanding due to the identification of specific antibodies (the most representative examples being anti-LGI1 encephalitis and anti-NMDA encephalitis). Recognizing these forms is crucial for promptly guiding the choice of appropriate immunotherapy.

12.3 Pathophysiology

Epilepsy and its clinical manifestations have always been considered as the expression of an alteration in the normal balance between excitatory and inhibitory processes that typically regulate brain functions. An epileptic condition occurs due to an abnormal recruitment of neurons secondary to:

1) Intrinsic modifications of neuronal properties,
2) Increased excitatory transmission,
3) Deficiency in inhibitory mechanisms,
4) Increased connectivity.

These factors contribute to the disruption of the excitation/inhibition balance, allowing neurons to become hyperexcitable and consequently discharge in a hypersynchronous manner. The electrical changes recorded during a seizure correspond to a depolarization of cortical pyramidal cells that is of greater magnitude and duration than normal (referred to as *paroxysmal depolarization shift*, PDS). The EEG correlate of the activity of a group of hyperexcitable neurons is characterized by the presence of distinct sharp potentials (referred to as *spike*), which are typically followed by slow potentials (*slow wave*), These slow waves represent the activation of inhibitory mechanisms, which are in turn triggered by the abnormal depolarization at the moment of its occurrence (this mechanism is implicated in explaining the self-limitation of the seizure).

Physiologically, the electrical charge at the level of the cell membrane is -70 mV (resting potential) and is determined by the distribution of ionic charges on both sides of the cell membrane (intracellular and extracellular). Excitatory and inhibitory synapses converge on the neuron. Inhibitory impulses hyperpolarize the membrane and depress its excitability, while excitatory impulses depolarize it, causing, when reaching -40 mV, the generation of the action potential. Normally, the activity of neurons relies on the function of sodium and potassium channels, which maintain a chemical and electrical gradient working as membrane pumps. Glial cells also play an important role in regulating the extracellular ionic concentration, thus influencing neuron activity. An alteration in the sodium/potassium balance (dysfunction of ion pumps or channels, or impairment of glial function) can lead to abnormal neuronal activity and determine seizures.

In maintaining an appropriate balance between excitation and inhibition, the action of various neurotransmitters, particularly gamma-aminobutyric acid (GABA) with its predominantly inhibitory action, and glutamate, which has a predominantly excitatory role, also contribute alongside neuronal membrane mechanisms. These neurotransmitters normally modulate brain activity.

In generating seizures, an important role is also played by the synchronization of neuronal circuits or *network*. A *network*, is a complex anatomofunctional entity in which neuronal aggregates are organized. It consists of anatomically and functionally interconnected cortical and subcortical brain structures. The clinical and EEG alterations typical of epilepsy manifest when the discharge involves a sufficiently structured *network*. The selective functional disorganization of a specific *network*, characteristic of epileptic seizures and varying across different forms of epilepsy, also accounts for the clinical and EEG stereotypy of ictal manifestations.

In genetically determined idiopathic generalized forms, seizures represent the expression of a reduced convulsive threshold. In absence seizures, the involvement of the thalamocortical network is presumed (Figure 12.3A). Numerous studies have demonstrated the crucial role of the circuit connecting the thalamus and cortex, which is necessary for the generation of generalized abnormalities (spike-wave discharges). Experimental studies using functional magnetic resonance imaging (fMRI) and co-registration with EEG (known as *EEG/fMRI*) of spike-wave discharges have documented activation of the bilateral thalamus, frontomesial cortex, insula, and cerebellum, as well as a deactivation (transient reduction of neural activity) in the bilateral frontal and parietal cortex, posterior cingulate gyrus, and left posterior temporal cortex. The deactivated structures are part of the *Default*

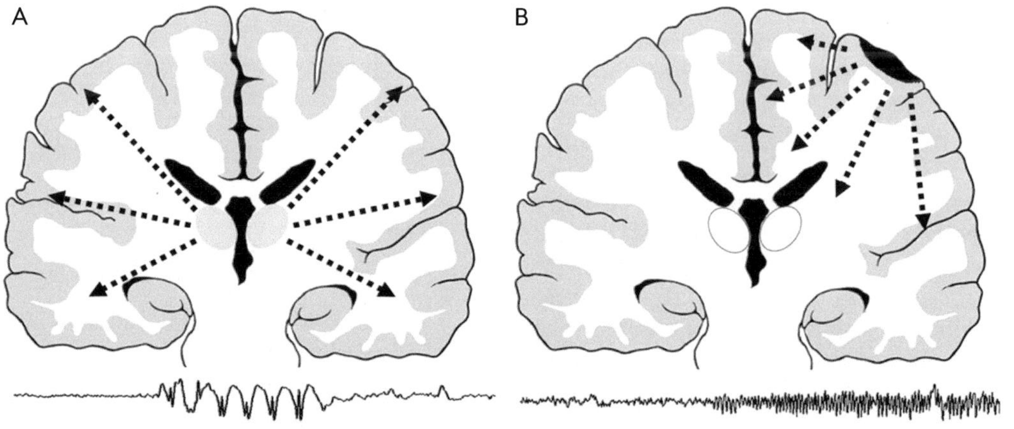

Figure 12.3

Simplified diagram of the networks underlying generalized seizures (A) and focal seizures (B). In generalized seizures, particularly absence seizures, the thalamo-cortical interaction is considered crucial in the generation of epileptic discharges. In focal seizures, the discharge originates from a very limited area of the cortex and then involves other cortico-subcortical structures during its propagation.

Mode Brain Network (DMN), a functional complex underlying consciousness and memory processes. During absence seizures, the deactivation of this network is now considered responsible for the state of reduced reactivity and consciousness alteration clinically characteristic of this type of seizure.

In focal forms, functional disorganization, often secondary to local pathological modifications in the brain (such as tumors or cortical malformations), leads to the appearance of focal seizures with possible recruitment of other neuronal structures (Figure 12.3B). The pathophysiological mechanisms of focal seizures also vary depending on different etiologies. Regarding symptomatic forms, animal models have been proposed in which the induction of tissue damage using chemicals (such as pilocarpine or kainic acid) or repeated electrical stimulation (known as *kindling*) results in closely spaced seizures and permanent modifications such as cell death, glial reaction, angiogenesis, tissue remodeling (e.g., formation of collateral axons from damaged neurons, known as *sprouting*), and altered synaptic reorganization. After a latency period following the induction of damage, spontaneous seizures occur. Recent studies on specific etiologies, such as temporal lobe or mesial-temporal sclerosis and malformations of cortical development, are providing important insights into the role of certain mechanisms (e.g., the role of glial cells, neuronal microenvironment, properties of complex *network*). Currently, there is a growing recognition of the role of *networks* in focal seizures. A paradigmatic example of focal epilepsies is the limbic/mesiotemporal *network*, which includes cortical structures (limbic structures, hippocampi, amygdalae, entorhinal cortex, insula, lateral temporal cortex) strongly interconnected with subcortical structures (thalamus and basal nuclei). The origin of seizures can occur in any part of the *network*, and the clinical manifestations reflect the involvement and disorganization of the entire system.

12.4 Clinical aspects and classification

Clinical manifestations and corresponding EEG characteristics are the foundation of epilepsy classification. The type of seizure, carefully evaluated in the overall context (which includes, for each individual patient, etiology, EEG data, neurological examination, response to therapy, and prognosis), allows for the classification of epileptic syndromes, which, in turn, is equivalent to recognizing specific nosological entities. In other words, defining an epileptic syndrome is comparable to a complex mosaic in which each element, starting from the type of seizure, becomes an irreplaceable tile. Similar to all other medical conditions, classifications of seizures and syndromes, essential for shared terminology and scientific schematization, are subject to continuous revision processes and therefore should be considered dynamic. In the case of epilepsy, the ongoing evolution of classifications is related to the acquisition of new information and knowledge offered primarily by neuroimaging and genetics.

The recent and new classification of epilepsies involves a multi-level organization that can be easily applied in various clinical contexts. The first level is dedicated to identifying the type of seizure, the second level to the type of epilepsy, and the third level to the type of syndrome.

12.5 Classification by type of seizure

According to the first level of classification, *seizures can be categorized as focal onset seizures, generalized onset seizures,* and *undetermined onset seizures* (Tables 12.2 and 12.3). Onset determination can be based on the reconstruction of clinical aspects or on the integration of clinical and EEG data.

12.5.1 Focal Onset Seizures

Focal seizures are characterized by a semiology that indicates the initial activation of a limited area in only one cerebral hemisphere (the so-called epileptogenic zone, which is the brain region where the epileptic discharge originates). The first symptoms/signs can be considered highly indicative of the location because they reflect the activation of the cortical area initially affected by the seizure. However, a focal seizure is usually not

Table 12.2 CLASSIFICATION OF EPILEPTIC SEIZURES

1. Focal seizures	2. Generalized seizures
1.1. With or without impaired consciousness A. With motor onset A.1. With automatisms A.2. Atonic A.3. Clonic A.4. Epileptic spasms A.5. Hyperkinetic A.6. Myoclonic A.7. Tonic B. With non-motor onset B.1. Autonomic B.2. With behavioral arrest B.3. Cognitive B.4. Emotional B.5. Somatosensory 1.2. From focal to bilateral tonic-clonic	2.1. Motor 2.1.1. Tonic-clonic 2.1.2. Clonic 2.1.3. Tonic 2.1.4. Myoclonic 2.1.5. Myoclonic-tonic-clonic 2.1.6. Myoclonic-atonic 2.1.7. Atonic 2.1.8. Epileptic spasms 2.2. Non-motor (absences) 2.2.1. Typical absences 2.2.2. Atypical absences 2.2.3. Myoclonic absences 2.2.4. Absences with eyelid myoclonia
	3. Seizures of unknown onset
Fisher RS, Cross JH, French JA, Higurashi N, Hirsch E, Jansen FE, Lagae L, Moshé SL, Peltola J, Roulet Perez E, Scheffer IE, Zuberi SM. Operational classification of seizure types by the International League Against Epilepsy: Position Paper of the ILAE Commission for Classification and Terminology. Epilepsia. 2017 Apr;58(4):522-530.	3.1. Motor 3.1.1. Tonic-clonic 3.1.2. Epileptic spasms 3.2. Non-motor 3.2.1. With behavioral arrest
	4. Unclassified seizures

constituted by a single clinical sign but by a variety of signs, often occurring in sequence, sometimes simultaneously, which are the expression of the anatomofunctional circuit involved in the seizure onset and spread. Since seizure onset and spread differ in different clinical conditions, the manifestations of seizures are extremely variable. Figure 12.4 schematically represents the theoretical organization of epileptic discharge during focal seizures. The EEG during a seizure typically shows the appearance of focal, unilateral anomalies at the onset of the seizure, which may be followed by propagation to homolateral and contralateral structures (Figure 12.5). According to the recent classification scheme for epileptic seizures, critical episodes are classified as either *focal seizures with preserved awareness or with consciousness impairment* (formerly known as complex partial seizures). During focal seizures, consciousness impairment is defined based on the response to environmental stimuli and on the individual's ability to retain

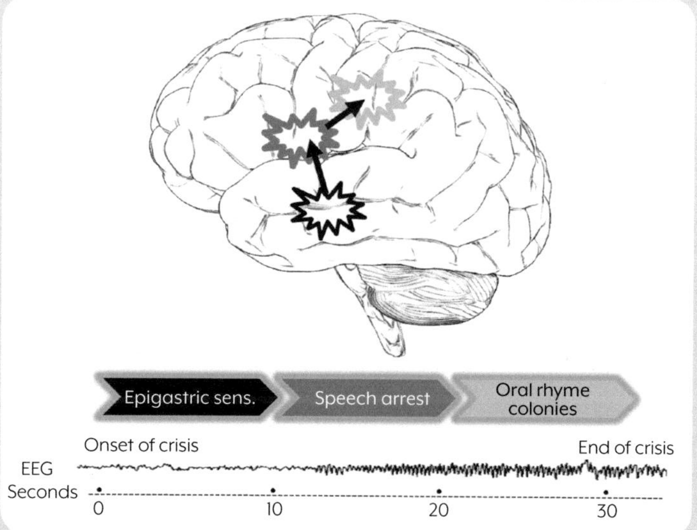

Figure 12.4

The dynamic evolution of focal seizures and their spatiotemporal organization is depicted. The critical discharge that originated in a brain area subsequently recruits other cortical areas, resulting in the progressive appearance of signs and symptoms characteristic of the various structures involved.

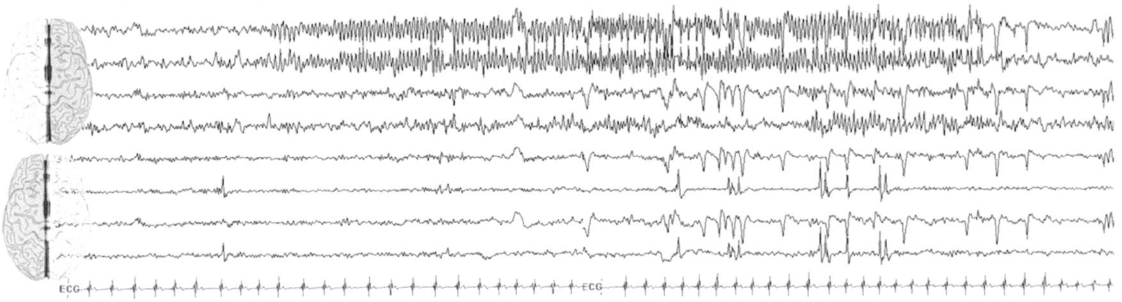

Figure 12.5

EEG Pattern of a Right Temporal Onset Focal Seizure with Subsequent Homolateral Hemisphere Propagation (recorded with 8 EEG channels + 1 ECG channel: the first 4 channels, in bipolar montage, record the brain activity of the right hemisphere, while the last 4 record the brain activity of the left hemisphere).

memory of the initial symptoms and stimuli or phenomena that occurred during the seizure. Clinically, it can manifest as cessation of ongoing activity, fixed gaze, unresponsiveness to stimuli, and a lack of appropriate response to simple commands; associated automatic activities (gestural, verbal, or oro-alimentary) are common. Such phenomenology often represents the expression of a partial impairment of consciousness. In general, it is believed that disturbances of consciousness are determined by the propagation of the critical discharge, which, starting from a highly delimited brain areas, progressively involves larger regions, particularly the associative cortical areas. In clinical practice, the disturbance of consciousness is considered significant because it indicates the lesser or greater intensity (and consequently the severity) of the critical event.

Once the degree of awareness involvement is defined, focal seizures are classified based on the predominant symptoms/signs at onset. These can primarily be motor in nature (motor onset focal seizures) or non-motor in nature (non-motor onset focal seizures).

Motor onset focal seizures

Motor onset seizures can be characterized by highly variable manifestations that include focal clonic movements, dystonic phenomena, tonic-postural changes, versive phenomena, incoordination, and dysarthria. The most characteristic motor signs (with significant localizing and lateralizing value) can manifest as isolated focal muscle contractions, limited to a single body part (e.g., the hand), or initially confined to one part of the body; there may be progressive involvement of different homolateral body parts (e.g., hand → face → tongue). Such progression, referred to as "Jacksonian march," documents the progression of the critical discharge that, during its propagation, involves different contiguous somatotopic regions of the Rolandic cortex. This type of motor manifestation has high localizing value, indicating the origin of the critical discharge at the contralateral primary motor area. Involvement of the premotor cortical areas results in seizures characterized by prolonged muscle contractions of the limbs and trunk. Versive seizures (lateral head and eye deviation) occur due to involvement of the lateral frontal cortex, phonatory and dysarthric seizures result from involvement of the opercular cortex, and motor seizures with inhibitory signs (motor inhibition, arrest of language, etc.) and specific postures (such as the fencer's position or the "figure of 4") are caused by involvement of certain frontal cortical areas (e.g., supplementary motor area).

In the recent seizure classification, importance is given to automatic activities, which include various manifestations: aggression, eyelid twitching, *head nodding*, manual automatisms (scratching, rubbing, manipulating objects, etc.), oro-facial automatisms (chewing, swallowing), sexual automatisms, pelvic thrusting, perseveration, ambulatory activities (walking, running), pedaling, vocalization, and verbal production. Some automatic activities, although common in temporal lobe seizures (with a clear predominance of oro-alimentary automatisms), do not have localizing value and are often interpreted as the expression of release activities originating from subcortical areas, especially during or at the onset of focal seizures with impaired awareness.

Focal seizures with non-motor onset

These seizures are characterized by extremely variable manifestations reflecting the involvement of different brain regions and *network*.

Focal seizures with autonomic manifestations | Autonomic alterations can occur as an initial symptom. The manifestations can be diverse and involve intrinsic ocular motility (mydriasis), thermoregulation (goosebumps, heat, sweating, chills, etc.), the cardiovascular system (pallor or flushing of the face, heart rhythm disturbances, general discomfort, etc.), the gastrointestinal system (abdominal sensations, nausea, belching, vomiting, etc.). Such manifestations, such as the classic ascending epigastric sensation, are particularly common in temporal lobe seizures. Their localizing value is not high since these manifestations occur in epileptic seizures originating from different cortical areas: a manifestation like "epigastric aura," often considered typical of mesial temporal lobe seizures, can accompany seizures originating from the operculoinsular or prefrontal regions.

Cognitive seizures | This group includes critical manifestations resulting from the involvement of brain areas associated with higher cognitive functions, symbolic functions. Among the most characteristic manifestations are dismnestic seizures, which are characterized by a sudden alteration of time cognition and memory: the patient has the impression of having already experienced or seen the present situation (*déjà vu e déjà vécu*) or experiences a sudden sense of unfamiliarity (*jamais vu*) or perceives a sensation of unreality, detachment, depersonalization with concurrent recall of past events (dreamy state). Cognitive epileptic phenomena also include aphasic disturbances, acalculia, amnesia, attentional disturbances, forced thinking, neglect.

Emotional or affective focal seizures | The most common clinical aspects are emotional and affective manifestations. Generally, the temporal lobe and frontal lobe are involved in their genesis. Affective seizures are characterized by the sudden appearance of an emotion (anxiety, anger, fear, joy, pleasure, etc.); their organization involves a circuit that includes numerous structures such as the temporo-mesial areas, the cingulate gyrus, and the temporo-frontal basal region. The recent new classification also includes laughter seizures (gelastic seizures) and crying seizures (dacrytic seizures) in this group.

Somatosensory focal seizures | This category includes phenomena characterized by perceptual experiences not caused by corresponding stimuli from the external world but by the critical involvement of specific brain areas. *Auditory focal seizures* are characterized by the emergence of noises, simple sounds and/or complex sounds (music, phrases, etc.) or illusional manifestations such as sound distortion. These manifestations suggest a localization of critical activity in a circuit involving auditory cortical areas (Heschl's gyrus, posterior portion of the superior temporal gyrus). *Olfactory* and *gustatory focal seizures*, also known as "uncinate seizures," are characterized by the presence of gustatory and/or olfactory illusions/hallucinations. Gustatory seizures likely involve the parietal operculum, while olfactory seizures are believed to involve the basal frontal cortex (straight gyrus and orbitofrontal cortex, areas involved in olfactory processing). Somatosensory *focal seizures* represent the expression of involvement of the primary sensory area (postcentral cortex): clinical manifestations can be characterized by sensory symptoms (tingling, numbness, electric shock sensation, pain, etc.) localized to the contralateral hemisoma. A sensory jacksonian march may also be present in this case. *Vestibular focal seizures*, which are rather rare and difficult to diagnose if clinically isolated, can manifest as "true" vertiginous seizures (impression of rotation of the external environment) or "pseudo-vertigo" (impression of body displacement relative to the external environment). In these cases, the cortex affected by the critical discharge is the posterior or temporo-occipital and inferior parietal cortex. *Visual focal seizures* are characterized by illusory manifestations (shape alteration) or simple or complex hallucinations (colored dots of light, flashes to the side, but also scenes, characters, etc.); negative symptoms such as scotomas, hemianopsia, etc., may also be present. In case of elementary hallucinations, either positive or negative, involvement of the contralateral pericalcarine occipital areas (areas 16 and 17) should be considered. Differently, in more complex visual manifestations, the origin of the seizure may be in the posterior temporal and parieto-occipital junction.

12.5.2 Generalized onset seizures

They are characterized by symptoms involving both cerebral hemispheres from the onset. Clinically, there are no apparent signs suggesting the involvement of a functional anatomical system localized in a single hemisphere; motor signs are bilateral from the beginning, and the EEG also shows bilateral interictal and ictal characteristics, classically synchronous and symmetrical in both hemispheres. There are different clinical expressions of generalized seizures.

Motor Generalized Seizures

Tonic-clonic seizures | They are usually characterized by three main phases: tonic, clonic, and postictal. Typically, the onset is characterized by a scream accompanied by an immediate loss of consciousness and sustained tonic contraction of all muscles (lasting 10-20 seconds). In this phase, significant autonomic disturbances occur (dilated pupils, changes in blood pressure, cardiac rhythm disturbances, excessive salivation, etc.). Lateral tongue biting and the appearance of apnea causing facial cyanosis are often observed. This is followed by the clonic phase (lasting about 30 seconds) with the appearance of synchronous bilateral muscle contractions that progressively decrease in frequency. The postictal phase can vary and last several minutes: the individual continues to have impaired consciousness (confusion may be apparent upon recovery), is hypotonic, and slowly resumes noisy respiration. Prolonged sleep is often present, sometimes accompanied by uncoordinated automatic activity. After the seizure, the patient may complain of diffuse muscle pain (often accompanied by elevated muscle enzymes), headache, and profound fatigue. The critical EEG shows the onset of low-voltage fast activity at the beginning of the seizure, followed by progressively decreasing spike and poly spike-wave anomalies during the clonic phase. This type of seizure can be observed in all generalized syndromes.

Clonic seizures | They are characterized by the presence of rhythmic clonic jerks, bilateral and involving the same muscle groups symmetrically, at a frequency of 2-3 Hz. Typically, there is a prolonged impairment of consciousness (critical and postcritical). They are typical of certain syndromes in children during early and late infancy. The EEG shows the presence of bilateral discharge of spike and polyspike-wave anomalies.

Tonic seizures | They are characterized by the onset of sustained and prolonged muscle contraction associated with a brief alteration of consciousness. They can affect the muscles of the neck and head (axial tonic seizures), the trunk (asso-rhizomelic tonic seizures), or the limbs (total tonic seizures). The sudden change in muscle tone can cause violent and often traumatic falls. They are frequent in non-benign evolving syndromes, such as epileptogenic encephalopathies. The critical EEG shows the presence of rapid rhythmic spike and/or diffuse poly spike anomalies.

Myoclonic seizures | Are characterized by the sudden, brief (<100 msec), involuntary contractions of variable intensity and location in a muscle or group of muscles with variable topography (axial, proximal, distal, mono or bilateral). They can be "positive" (muscle contraction with segmental movement) or "negative" (brief loss of postural tone due to transient interruption of muscle contraction). Typically, the jerks are bilateral and symmetric and occur without alterations in consciousness. They are accompanied by the presence of generalized abnormal discharges on the EEG, which are also very typical, defined as bilateral and synchronous poly-spike waves. They are frequent in idiopathic generalized syndromes in children/adolescents.

Myoclonic-atonic seizures | Are a type of generalized seizure characterized by myoclonic jerks that are accompanied by an atonic component (in the past, this type of seizure was referred to as myoclonic-astatic).

Myoclonic - tonic - clonic seizures | Are characterized by one or more myoclonic jerks in the limbs, followed bilaterally by a tonic-clonic seizure. Seizures with these characteristics are common in juvenile myoclonic epilepsy.

Atonic seizures | Are characterized by a sudden loss of postural tone that can affect only the neck, resulting in isolated involvement of the head. However, they typically also involve the trunk and limbs, causing sudden and traumatic falls. The EEG shows the appearance of rapid low-voltage activity with diffuse expression. These seizures are generally observed in epileptogenic encephalopathies.

Epileptic spasms | Are characterized by a sudden flexion or extension (or a combination of both) mainly affecting the trunk and proximal muscles. Typically, the motor phenomenon is more sustained than a myoclonic movement but not to the extent of a tonic seizure. Very limited phenomena such *grimacing, head nodding* (yes-yes movements of the head), and very discrete eye movements can occur. Epileptic spasms often occur in clusters, and infantile spasms are the most well-known form, but spasms can occur at any age.

Generalized non-motor seizures

Absences | Are characterized by brief and isolated alterations of consciousness. They have a sudden onset and termination. The individual abruptly interrupts ongoing activity, exhibits a fixed gaze, usually does not respond when called, and after a variable period of 5 to 40 seconds, resumes their activity as if nothing had happened. Absences can be accompanied by very discrete myoclonic motor phenomena (see below), reduction of postural tone (atonic absences), the presence of gestural automatisms or motor perseverations (absences with automatisms), and vegetative signs (absences with vegetative component). Generally, the semiological variants of absences only differ clinically and all are associated with a critical and absolutely typical EEG characterized by the presence of a bilateral, synchronous, and symmetrical discharge of generalized abnormalities (spike-wave complexes, usually at a frequency of 3 Hz) (Figure 12.6). These manifestations can be observed in idiopathic generalized syndromes in children and adolescents, less commonly in adults.

Atypical absences | Are longer in duration compared to typical absences and often accompanied by differential clinical elements such as motor components, often asymmetric, of tonic, atonic, and myoclonic types. The associated critical EEG shows a pattern of abnormalities similar to those accompanying typical absences but with a lower frequency (2-2.5 Hz) and associated with fast activity. This type of seizure is characteristic of epileptic syndromes with an unfavorable prognosis (such as epileptic encephalopathies), typically starting in childhood but persisting into adulthood.

Myoclonic absences | Are absences accompanied by imperceptible motor phenomena such as perioral and/or ocular clonic movements (myoclonic absences).

Eyelid myoclonus | Is characterized by eyelid movements at a frequency of at least 3 Hz, commonly associated with upward deviation of the eyes. They usually last less than 10 seconds and are often triggered by eye closure. They can be associated with a brief suspension of consciousness.

12.5.3 Unknown onset seizures

This category includes seizures for which it is not possible, based on clinical and EEG characteristics, to determine whether they have a focal or generalized onset. This group

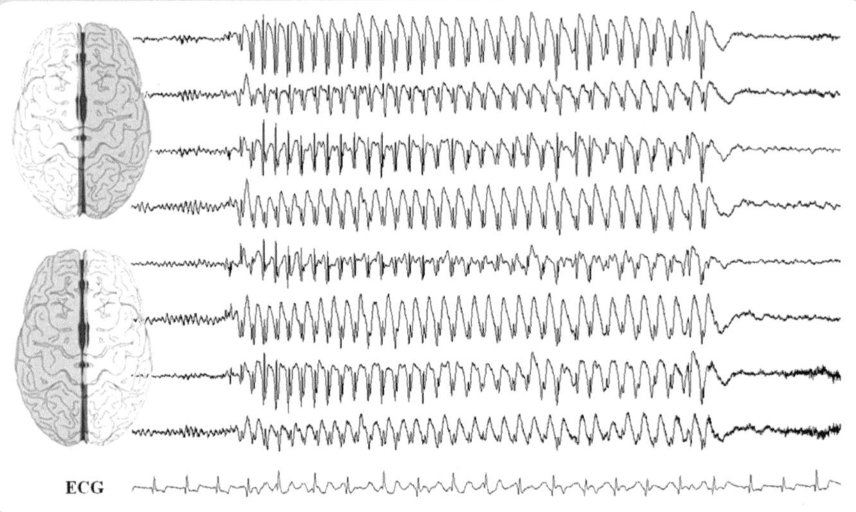

Figure 12.6

Tipycal EEG discharges of bilateral and synchronous 3 hz spike-and-wave complexes, corresponding clinically to an absence seizure (recorded with 8 EEG channels + 1 ECG channel: the first 4 channels, in bipolar montage, record the brain activity of the right hemisphere, and the last 4 channels record the brain activity of the left hemisphere).

includes motor seizures (further classified as tonic-clonic seizures and epileptic spasms) and non-motor seizures (essentially characterized by behavioral arrest).

12.5.4 Unclassified Seizures

This category includes seizures that cannot be classified due to incomplete information or the inability to place them in other categories.

12.6 Classification of epilepsy types and epileptic syndromes

The second level of the recent classification involves defining the type of epilepsy. According to the new terminology, there are *focal epilepsies*, *generalized epilepsies*, *combined focal and generalized epilepsies*, and *unknown epilepsies*.

Once the type of epilepsy is defined, it is possible to proceed with the third level, which involves *syndromic diagnosis*, i.e., the identification of specific epileptic syndromes. A specific syndrome is defined as the combination of certain clinical and instrumental aspects (seizure type, EEG, neuroradiological data) that tend to recur in a characteristic manner. Key syndromic aspects may include age dependency (onset and remission), precipitating factors, circadian rhythm relationship, prognosis, specific comorbidities such as intellectual and psychiatric disorders. The identification of specific syndromes has etiological, therapeutic, and prognostic implications.

Although the latest proposal for the classification of epilepsies (ILAE Commission, 2017) has outlined the main taxonomic aspects, an official classification of epileptic syndromes is not yet available. For this reason, this chapter presents a summary of the main aspects of the old classification (ILAE Commission 1989), which emphasized the role of etiology and epilepsy type (Table 12.3), as well as the new nosographic scheme that tends to categorize syndromes based on specific age of onset (Table 12.4).

12.6.1 Focal Epilepsies

These are conditions in which the clinical semiology and diagnostic data clearly define the focal origin of seizures and the type of epilepsy. Focal epilepsies can be further distinguished based on specific etiologies.

Structural, metabolic, infectious, and immune focal epilepsies

This group includes all focal epilepsies in which the presence of a brain lesion responsible for the seizures can be demonstrated. Based on the topographic origin of the seizures, epilepsies are distinguished into frontal lobe, temporal lobe, parietal lobe, and occipital lobe epilepsies. The clinical manifestations of seizures vary depending on the different lobes involved and, even more specifically, the different lobar structures affected by the critical discharge. The age of onset of symptoms and prognosis are variable, often related to the nature and type of underlying lesion and the associated epileptogenic *network*. A paradigmatic example of a symptomatic focal syndrome is temporal lobe epilepsy associated with hippocampal sclerosis. This is a syndrome, often drug-resistant, that is very common in young adults, although it can also begin in childhood. The clinical

Table 12.3 CLASSIFICATION OF EPILEPSIES AND EPILEPTIC SYNDROMES

1. Partial or focal epilepsies and syndromes

1.1 Idiopathic
- Benign childhood epilepsy with centrotemporal spikes
- Childhood epilepsy with occipital paroxysms
- Reading-induced reflex epilepsy

1.2 Symptomatic
- Continuous partial epilepsy of infancy (Kojewnikov syndrome)
- Syndromes with seizures triggered by specific precipitating factors (e.g., startle epilepsy)

1.3 Cryptogenic
- Probably symptomatic epilepsies with unknown etiology

2. Generalized epilepsies and syndromes

2.1 Idiopathic (in order of age)
- Benign familial neonatal seizures
- Benign neonatal seizures
- Benign myoclonic epilepsy of infancy
- Childhood absence epilepsy
- Juvenile absence epilepsy
- Juvenile myoclonic epilepsy
- Epilepsy with generalized tonic-clonic seizures on awakening
- Epilepsies with seizures triggered by specific precipitating factors

2.2 Cryptogenic or symptomatic
- West syndrome
- Lennox-Gastaut syndrome
- Myoclonic-astatic epilepsy
- Myoclonic absence epilepsy

2.3 Symptomatic
- Nonspecific etiologies
  - Early myoclonic encephalopathy
  - Early myoclonic encephalopathy with *suppression burst*
- Specific syndromes
  - Pathological conditions with epileptic seizures as the main manifestation

3. Indeterminate epilepsies and syndromes, whether focal or generalized

3.1 Indeterminate epilepsies and syndromes with focal and generalized seizures
- Neonatal seizures
- Severe myoclonic epilepsy of infancy
- Epilepsy with continuous spike-wave during sleep
- Acquired epileptic aphasia (Landau-Kleffner syndrome)
- Other indeterminate epilepsies not mentioned previously

3.2 Indeterminate epilepsies and syndromes without clear focal or generalized characteristics
- All cases in which electro-clinical features do not allow for a definitive classification

4. Special syndromes

4.1 Seizures related to specific situations
- Febrile seizures
- Isolated epileptic seizures or isolated status epilepticus
- Epileptic seizures in the course of acute alterations with toxic or metabolic basis

Table 12.4 EPILEPTIC SYNDROMES DEFINED ACCORDING TO AGE OF ONSET (classification proposal)

Neonatal/Infantile
- Self-limited neonatal seizures and self-limited neonatal epilepsy
- Familial infantile epilepsy
- Non-familial infantile epilepsy
- Early myoclonic encephalopathy
- Ohtahara syndrome
- West syndrome
- Dravet syndrome
- Childhood myoclonic epilepsy
- Childhood epilepsy with focal migratory seizures
- Myoclonic encephalopathy in non-progressive neurological disorders
- Febrile seizures plus, genetic epilepsy with febrile seizures plus

Childhood
- Epilepsy with myoclonic-astatic seizures
- Eyelid myoclonia epilepsy
- Lennox-Gastaut syndrome
- Childhood absence epilepsy
- Myoclonic absence epilepsy
- Panayiotopoulos syndrome
- Occipital epilepsy of childhood (Gastaut type)
- Photosensitive idiopathic occipital epilepsy of childhood
- Centrotemporal spikes epilepsy
- Atypical centrotemporal spikes epilepsy
- Epileptic encephalopathy with continuous spike-and-wave during sleep
- Landau-Kleffner syndrome
- Autosomal dominant nocturnal frontal lobe epilepsy

Adolescence/Adulthood
- Juvenile absence epilepsy
- Juvenile myoclonic epilepsy
- Epilepsy with generalized tonic-clonic seizures only
- Autosomal dominant epilepsy with auditory features
- Other familial temporal lobe epilepsies

Any Age
- Familial focal epilepsy with variable foci
- Reflex epilepsies
- Progressive myoclonic epilepsies

manifestations are characterized by typical signs of involvement of the mesial temporal structures and include autonomic, cognitive, and affective signs/symptoms (ascending epigastric sensation, déjà vu and déjà vécu, fear, etc.). Automatic gestural and oro-alimentary activities are frequent and appear early in the course of the seizure. MRI often shows the presence of focal atrophy in the hippocampus (hippocampal sclerosis). All these features constitute a defined syndromic condition, typical in individuals who have a history of prolonged and complex febrile seizures. The possible hemodynamic and metabolic damage to the hippocampal structures, mediated by intense convulsive activity in childhood, can predispose to the onset of epilepsy, often drug-resistant, in young adulthood.

Other focal syndromes should not be overlooked, as their prompt recognition allows for an appropriate choice of therapy and immediate prognosis definition. Among these syndromes are included some peculiar forms such as gelastic epilepsy, Kojewnikov syndrome, and Rasmussen syndrome. Gelastic epilepsy is characterized primarily by episodes of unprovoked and sudden laughter (so-called gelastic seizures); although very rarely, episodes of sudden crying (so-called dacrystic seizures) can also be observed. This epilepsy, sometimes having a negative outcome due to the occurrence of seizures with falls or the evolution into an encephalopathy, typically, though not exclusively, recognizes the presence of a hypothalamic hamartoma as its etiology. Kojewnikov syndrome, also known as *epilepsia partialis continua*, is characterized by prolonged critical episodes with motor semiology, structured as a persistent focal status epilepticus, expressing involvement of the Rolandic regions (frequent clinical manifestations are subcontinuous clonic movements affecting the contralateral hemisoma). From an etiological point of view, this form is usually secondary to lesions of various natures but often malformative (cortical dysplasias). Another well-defined nosographic entity, clinically resembling the previous one, is Rasmussen's encephalitis (or syndrome), an immunomediated pathology whose etiopathogenic aspects are not yet completely known (sometimes associated with the positivity of anti-Glu3 antibodies, directed against the glutamate receptor). The clinical picture is characterized by a typical combination of continuous focal epilepsy, deterioration of neurological functions (usually hemiparesis and cognitive impairments), and an MRI showing progressive cerebral hemiatrophy. More frequent in childhood, it requires, in addition to antiepileptic drugs, immunomodulating treatment (plasmapheresis, immunoglobulins, steroids), and in cases of drug-resistant and rapidly progressive epilepsy, surgical therapy (usually functional hemispherectomy).

Focal genetic epilepsies (or idiopathic)

They constitute a syndromic group that includes often age-dependent epilepsies, characterized by the absence of neurological and cognitive deficits and, in most cases, a good response to therapy. In some cases, responsible genes have been identified, often encoding for ion channel subunits, indicating that many of these forms belong to the group of channelopathies (with the exception of one syndromic form, autosomal dominant lateral temporal lobe epilepsy, which appears to be unrelated to channel alterations). The EEG shows a normal background rhythm and normal sleep organization; in some syndromes, there are evident anomalies with pathognomonic characteristics in terms of morphology, localization, and recurrence.

Among the focal genetic epilepsies, the following syndromes are notable:

Benign rolandic epilepsy (or rolandic spikes) | It is the prototype of focal genetic epilepsies. Seizures manifest with motor signs (localized clonic movements predominantly in the orofacial region, dysarthria, hypersalivation) occurring almost exclusively during sleep, with a possible tendency to generalize. The seizures originate from the opercular and perisylvian cortical structures, which are involved in motor function but are also connected to the insula.

Benign occipital epilepsy | (in its *variants of early onset* or *Panayiotopoulos syndrome* and *late onset* or *Gastaut syndrome*). In these conditions, similar to the previous one, the predominant clinical symptoms consist of vegetative, visual, and/or affective symptoms, typically reflecting involvement of the posterior temporal and parieto-occipital areas. Prolonged status epilepticus can be frequent (often manifesting only with vegetative signs such as nausea and vomiting).

Autosomal dominant nocturnal frontal lobe epilepsy | This form is characterized by brief clusters of motor seizures that occur at night, with dystonic/hyperkinetic manifestations. Mutations in the CHRNA4 and CHRNB2 genes (located on chromosomes 20 and 1, respectively) and loci on chromosome 15q have been identified. Neurological examination and neuroimaging are usually normal. The EEG, even when recorded during a seizure, may be negative due to the deep or mesial origin of the discharge, which is often difficult to explore with scalp EEG methods. These seizures need to be differentiated from psychogenic seizures and non-epileptic sleep-related events. These forms typically respond well to carbamazepine, depending on the specific gene mutation.

Autosomal dominant lateral temporal lobe epilepsy with auditory symptoms | This form is genetically determined by a mutation in the LGI1 gene (located on chromosome 10q24). Seizures are characterized by symptoms consistent with involvement of the lateral temporal cortex (auditory, vertiginous, visual, dysphasic, and less frequently, psychiatric and experiential manifestations). The EEG typically shows normal recordings or rare abnormalities, mostly slow waves localized in the posterior part of the temporal lobe. The response to therapy is generally good, although pharmacoresistant variants can be observed.

Autosomal dominant familial temporal lobe epilepsy | Is a form characterized by typical symptoms related to the involvement of the temporo-mesial structures, including vegetative, cognitive, experiential, and emotional manifestations. EEG and MRI are usually normal, with focal atrophy in the hippocampus rarely present. So far, no responsible gene has been identified.

12.6.2 Generalized epilepsies

Idiopathic and genetic generalized epilepsies

They constitute about one-third of all epilepsies. Genetic forms are generally benign conditions, as they are highly responsive to medical therapy, although they often require ongoing medication. Onset typically occurs in childhood and/or adolescence, but there are also cases that begin in adulthood and (more rarely) in the elderly. These forms are genetically determined, often having a family history, and are characterized by the presence of generalized seizures (absences, myoclonic jerks, generalized tonic-clonic seizures) occurring in patients without neurological abnormalities. EEG shows the presence of bilateral and synchronous critical and intercritical abnormalities (typically spike-wave, polyspike-wave, and polyspike discharges at a characteristic frequency of 3 Hz). The different syndromic forms, which probably represent a *continuum* of a single condition with different modes of expression, are distinguished by the type of seizures (prevalence of one type of seizure over the others, such as myoclonic jerks or absences), the age of onset of episodes, and the prognosis, which can vary from benign to more severe (while most cases respond well to medication). Some of the most representative idiopathic generalized syndromes are described below.

Childhood absence epilepsy (formerly known as "petit mal") | Typically has an onset between the ages of 4 and 8. It is characterized by absence seizures (brief but highly frequent) and rare generalized tonic-clonic seizures. EEG shows bilateral expression of typical spike-wave complexes at 3 Hz; intermittent photic stimulation is usually negative. A triggering condition easily demonstrated during EEG is hyperventilation. The response to therapy is usually excellent, and the prognosis is favorable (considered an age-dependent condition with complete resolution).

Juvenile absence epilepsy | This form has an onset between 10 and 17 years of age. It is characterized by absence seizures (less frequent but longer in duration compared to the childhood counterpart), rare myoclonic jerks, and generalized tonic-clonic seizures. The EEG shows diffuse spike-wave complexes at 3 Hz, and the photoparoxysmal response is negative. The response to therapy is excellent, but the prognosis is more uncertain compared to the infantile form.

Juvenile myoclonic epilepsy (Janz syndrome) | It has an onset between 12 and 18 years of age. It is characterized by myoclonic seizures, absence seizures (less frequent), and generalized tonic-clonic seizures. The EEG shows diffuse spike-wave and polyspike-wave discharges at 3.5-6 Hz (with variable frequency during the discharge). The presence of photosensitivity (photoparoxysmal response during the intermittent photic stimulation) is quite characteristic. Typically, seizures tend to occur within one hour from awakening, and conditions that facilitate them include sleep deprivation and alcohol use.

Epilepsy with generalized tonic-clonic seizures only | It has an onset between 6 and 35 years of age (peak at 18 years). It usually manifests with generalized tonic-clonic seizures (the so-called "grand mal" seizures) that predominantly occur upon awakening. These manifestations may sometimes be associated with "minor seizures." The EEG may be normal or show slow abnormalities or specific generalized spike-wave discharges, often associated with photosensitivity.

Within the realm of genetic generalized epilepsies, there are other nosological entities that are not clearly defined and not yet formally included in the classification: absence epilepsy with eyelid myoclonia, myoclonic-astatic epilepsy, epilepsy with myoclonic absences, and childhood myoclonic epilepsy. Each of these forms, characterized by specific electro-clinical patterns, can be distinguished by their possible association with varying degrees of intellectual disability. This last characteristic, in particular, and the possible presence of specific gene mutations, place these clinical entities at the boundaries with developmental encephalopathies or epileptic encephalopathies (their nosological placement is currently under discussion within the International League Against Epilepsy). One of the most representative forms in this group is undoubtedly absence epilepsy with eyelid myoclonia.

Absence epilepsy with eyelid myoclonia (Jeavons syndrome) | It has an onset between 2 and 14 years of age, with a higher prevalence in females. The seizures are characterized by eyelid myoclonia associated with eye deviation, and sometimes by absences (the alteration of consciousness can vary greatly) and rare generalized tonic-clonic seizures. Seizures with eyelid myoclonia are usually brief but can occasionally evolve into a status epilepticus. The EEG shows bilateral polyspike-wave complexes at 3-6 Hz (typically evoked by eye closure and suppressed by darkness) and a photoparoxysmal response. Conditions that facilitate seizures include photic stimulation, sleep deprivation, and alcohol use. The response to therapy is often inadequate.

There are numerous syndromic subgroups, and in addition to the listed forms, they also include *benign familial neonatal convulsions, benign infantile myoclonic epilepsy, and epilepsies characterized by specific provocation modalities*.

Focal and generalized combined epilepsies (or symptomatic generalized epilepsies)

They are composed of heterogeneous syndromes characterized by generalized seizures (myoclonus, often atypical absences, tonic seizures, atonic seizures, generalized tonic-clonic seizures) and focal seizures, variably associated with each other. Seizures are accompanied by neurological deficits (often intellectual delay) with or without the presence of anatomical abnormalities. This group includes phacomatoses (such as tuberous sclerosis, neurofibromatosis, etc.), aminoacidopathies, post-vaccination encephalitis, and some chromosomal abnormalities.

These are often epileptic encephalopathies and/or developmental conditions that represent conditions, often starting in childhood, in which severe epilepsy and epileptic activity contribute to impairment of cognitive and mental functions (intellectual delay or cognitive developmental regression, psychiatric disorders), sometimes progressive, more severe than expected based solely on the underlying pathology. The associated EEG often shows a disorganized background rhythm and the presence of generally multifocal, diffuse, or localized anomalies.

Among the most representative epileptic encephalopathies are West syndrome, Lennox-Gastaut syndrome, and Landau-Kleffner syndrome. West syndrome is a generally symptomatic epileptogenic encephalopathy with onset within the first year of life (peak between 4 and 7 months). Clinically, it is characterized by the appearance of spasms, mostly in flexion but also in extension and flexion-extension, affecting the neck and limbs, particularly the proximal districts, associated with severe regression of acquired psychomotor skills. The corresponding EEG is represented by hypsarrhythmia, a pattern of complete disorganization of the background activity, with the presence of slow waves and high-voltage irregular sharp elements, multifocal onset, and rapid spread throughout the entire brain. The prognosis is often unfavorable: the condition can lead to death or the development of Lennox-Gastaut syndrome, and only about 10% of patients experience recovery.

Lennox-Gastaut syndrome occurs in children between 1 and 7 years of age, in the presence of a concomitant organic condition (although the etiology remains unknown in at least 40% of cases). It is characterized by a typical triad of different types of epileptic seizures (atypical absences, tonic seizures, atonic seizures, myoclonic seizures, and tonic-clonic seizures), variable severity of intellectual disability, and a characteristic EEG pattern (slow spike-and-wave discharges at 2-2.5 Hz with diffuse expression).

Landau-Kleffner syndrome, also known as "acquired epileptic aphasia," is a rare condition with onset in childhood (peak between 4 and 7 years) characterized by a progressive, fluctuating phasic disorder inconsistently associated with learning difficulties and mental retardation. The EEG pattern shows continuous abnormalities localized in areas primarily responsible for language functions (the pathological activity can be structured during slow-wave sleep as status epilepticus).

Focal epilepsies of unknown etiology

This group includes all focal epilepsies in which the presence of a brain lesion responsible for the seizures cannot be demonstrated. In this case as well, the semiological characteristics of the seizures allow for distinguishing frontal, temporal, parietal, and occipital lobe epilepsies.

12.7 Diagnosis

In the presence of a paroxysmal event, it is important to determine whether the event is attributable to an epileptic seizure or another phenomenon. Regarding the differential diagnosis, there are numerous clinical conditions that can be similar to epileptic seizures. These include cerebrovascular disorders, syncope, migraine, psychogenic seizures, toxic-metabolic disorders, and movement disorders. The differential diagnosis can be challenging, especially in children and young adults, and diagnostic errors can have significant consequences for treatment, prognosis, and patients' quality of life. Table 12.5 summarizes the main conditions to consider in the differential diagnosis.

Once the epileptic nature of the event is confirmed, it is necessary to establish whether it is an acute symptomatic (or provoked) seizure, i.e., a phenomenon caused by a specific cause, or an "unprovoked" phenomenon indicative of epilepsy. The diagnostic algorithm includes a comprehensive synthesis of clinical data, neurophysiological findings (EEG and related techniques), neuroradiological investigations (particularly brain MRI), and laboratory tests aimed at defining the type of seizure and, once the diagnosis of epilepsy is established, the type of epileptic syndrome. The clinical element, which is primary and essential, is represented by a very detailed medical history, through which clinical information can be obtained from the patient and observers regarding the subjective and objective characteristics of the paroxysmal episodes. Occasionally, it may be useful to ask the patient and observers to capture amateur videos of the epileptic phenomena to directly observe the clinical signs, which are often described incompletely or not reported.

Table 12.5 DIFFERENTIAL DIAGNOSIS OF EPILEPTIC SEIZURES

	Epileptic seizure	Syncope	TIA	AGT	Metabolic	Psychiatric
Prodromal symptoms	None or "aura"	None or nausea, "discomfort"	None	None	None	None
Onset	Acute	Variable	Acute	Acute	Acute	Variable
Duration	1-2 minutes	Seconds - minutes	Minutes - hours	Hours	Minutes - hours	Minutes - hours
Motor pattern	Tonic-clonic movements	Trismus, myoclonus, loss of tone	Neurological deficits	None	Variable, myoclonus, tonic-clonic	Variable, sometimes with bizarre signs
Incontinence	Variable	None	None	None	None	None
Heart rate	Increased or decreased	Variable	Normal	Normal	Normal	Normal
EEG	Epileptiform pattern	Diffuse slow activity	Normal or focal slow activity	Slow activity (rare)	Diffuse slow activity	Normal
Trauma	Tongue biting or bruises	Bruises or fractures	None	None	Rare	None
Postictal phase	Confusion, drowsiness	Alert or mild confusion	Alert	Alert	Alert when treated	Alert

TIA: Transient Ischemic Attack; AGT: Transient Global Amnesia

Electroencephalography (EEG) | The recording of brain electrical activity through surface electrodes placed on the scalp, represents an indispensable technique. In general, the main pathological EEG activities can consist of slow waves in the theta and/or delta range and epileptiform abnormalities. Focal or generalized slow waves can represent indirect signs of brain injury, which may be limited to a specific region (e.g., in a tumor) or diffuse (e.g., in metabolic encephalopathies). More characteristic are the distinct epileptiform abnormalities, often classified based on their morphology, such as spikes, *sharp wave*, spike-wave complexes, poly-spikes, and poly-spike-wave complexes. From a topographic perspective, these abnormalities can have a focal or diffuse expression.

In the field of clinical epileptology, EEG can be used to: diagnose epilepsy, classify the type of seizure, localize the epileptogenic area (particularly in candidates for surgical intervention), quantify pathological activities (during seizures and interictal periods), support the decision regarding potential reduction/ discontinuation of therapy, and differentiate non-epileptic paroxysmal phenomena. Some considerations are crucial in the clinical interpretation of EEG results: it should be noted that a normal result, even in repeated recordings, can be found in 10-20% of patients with epilepsy, and conversely, a pathological result can be observed in 1-2% of individuals without a clinical history of epilepsy (this percentage increases up to 45% in first-degree relatives of patients with generalized epilepsy). EEG is particularly important as it can confirm the diagnostic hypothesis of epilepsy and guide to distinguish focal and generalized forms. *Intercritical abnormalities* (observed during periods between seizures) can be focal, mainly consisting of spikes, sharp waves, and spike-wave complexes localized in a specific region, or generalized, mainly consisting of spike-wave and poly-spike-wave complexes distributed bilaterally. In individuals with epilepsy, in addition to interictal abnormalities, *critical activities* corresponding to epileptic seizures can be recorded. In addition to standard EEG recordings, 24-hour EEG monitoring (dynamic EEG) and sleep-deprived or sleep EEG increase the possibility of demonstrating alterations in brain activity.

Morphological neuroimaging | Particularly brain MRI (with CT being less useful, except for specific conditions), is another essential element in the diagnostic approach to epilepsy. MRI usually allows the identification of any underlying pathologies associated with epilepsy, contributing to the etiological diagnosis. The sensitivity of MRI significantly increases when the examination is performed with high-field magnets (and specific parameters) and interpreted by expert neuroradiologists specializing in epilepsy based on clinical indications. As mentioned earlier, with the evolution of technical aspects (magnet strength, appropriate acquisition parameters, post-processing analysis capabilities), the proportion of epilepsies with unknown etiology has decreased.

Functional neuroimaging | Includes techniques such as SPECT, PET, fMRI, and MRS, which, in addition to providing information about brain structure, allow for valuable insights into brain function and, specifically, the evaluation of potential alterations in structures affected by epileptic processes. SPECT provides functional data through cerebral perfusion, PET through glucose metabolism, fMRI through the BOLD signal (based on increased cerebral blood flow and changes in the hemoglobin/oxyhemoglobin ratio in active areas), and MR spectroscopy through the modification of specific metabolites. These techniques are useful in clinical practice as complements to structural imaging in specific contexts and are essential for scientific research.

Other techniques and investigative methods | Are included in the diagnostic approach and can be planned according to different clinical contexts. In the case of newly diagnosed seizures, it is necessary to perform preliminary tests (including routine blood tests, ECG, etc.) or other investigations evaluated on a case-by-case basis, especially during the differential diagnosis phase. Once epilepsy is diagnosed, further diagnostic investigations may also involve more specific and advanced tests (e.g., genetic testing) for a better definition of the specific epileptic syndrome.

12.8 Therapy

Pharmacological therapy | Is the primary objective of epilepsy treatment, aiming to control seizures without significant side effects. The choice of medication(s) should be based on numerous factors, including the type of seizure and epileptic syndrome, age, sex, psychological profile, presence of comorbidities, socio-cultural conditions, and psychosocial aspects.

In general, antiseizure medications act through different mechanisms, resulting in increased inhibition, decreased excitation, or prevention of altered neuronal excitability. The mechanisms of action of antiepileptic drugs are not straightforward and, in some cases, not yet fully understood. Several drugs are characterized by multiple primary and secondary mechanisms of action. Some fundamental mechanisms of action can be recognized:

1) Stabilization effect on the cell membrane by blocking voltage-gated sodium and/or calcium channels (more recently also potassium channels). Drugs that exert their action through these effects include carbamazepine (CBZ), ethosuximide (ETS), eslicarbazepine (ESL), phenytoin (PHT), lacosamide (LCM), lamotrigine (LTG), oxcarbazepine (OXC), rufinamide (RFD), topiramate (TPM), and valproate (VPA).
2) Potentiation of GABA's inhibitory action through receptor stimulation, *reuptake* blockade, or inhibition of its degradation. Molecules capable of enhancing GABAergic transmission include benzodiazepines (BDZ), phenobarbital (PB), tiagabine (TGB), topiramate (TPM), vigabatrin (GVG), stiripentol (STP), and cenobamate (CNB).
3) Inhibition of excitatory mechanisms by acting on glutamate and aspartate through receptor blockade or inhibition of neurotransmitter release. Drugs with this activity include felbamate (FLB), lamotrigine (LTG), topiramate (TPM), and perampanel (PER).
4) Inhibition of neurotransmitter release at synaptic vesicles through binding to specific proteins (e.g., levetiracetam - LEV, brivaracetam - BRV). The main mechanisms of action of antiepileptic drugs are presented in Table 12.6.

To these fundamental mechanisms of action, additional mechanisms have recently been added, partially known, characterizing the therapeutic effects of cannabidiol (CBD).

Drug selection | Antiseizure medications, once initiated, are usually continued for several years or even for a lifetime. The essential prerequisite is a reasonable certainty, based on available data (clinical, neurophysiological, and neuroradiological), of the diagnosis of epilepsy. In the case of acute neurological conditions (e.g., ischemic or hemorrhagic brain injuries), the possible symptomatic seizures that occur in the very early stages (known as *early seizures*, i.e., within the first week of the acute event) are not necessarily a prelude to epilepsy. Therefore, in such cases, chronic therapy should not be recommended. In the case of isolated seizures, antiseizure medications should only be initiated in the presence of severe EEG abnormalities or demonstrable brain lesions on neuroimaging, or in the presence of "risky" professional activities. It is important to remember that antiseizure medications are a symptomatic therapy, capable of preventing the onset of seizures, but it does not have any properties to prevent epileptogenesis (the complex tissue changes that occur over time and lead to the susceptibility of the brain to develop unprovoked seizures).

Antiseizure medications should always be introduced cautiously, with slow titration, and gradually reduced or discontinued (abrupt

Table 12.6 MAIN MECHANISMS OF ACTION OF ANTIEPILEPTIC DRUGS

	Sodium channel blockade	Calcium channel blockade	Enhancement of GABA transmission	Binding to SV2A	AMPA receptor antagonism
First-generation drugs					
Acetazolamide*	-	-	+	-	-
Benzodiazepines	-	-	++	-	-
Carbamazepine	++	+	-	-	-
Ethosuximide	-	++	-	-	-
Phenobarbital	-	-	+	-	-
Phenytoin	++	?	-	-	-
Valproate	?	+	+	-	-
Second-generation drugs					
Eslicarbazepine	++	-	-	-	-
Felbamate	++	+	+	-	-
Gabapentin	?	++	?	-	-
Lacosamide	+	-	-	-	-
Lamotrigine	++	++	+	-	-
Levetiracetam	-	+	+	++	-
Oxcarbazepine	++	++	?	-	-
Pregabalin	-	++	-	-	-
Rufinamide	++	-	-	-	-
Tiagabine	-	-	++	-	-
Topiramate	++	+	+	-	+
Vigabatrin	-	-	++	-	-
Zonisamide	++	++	?	-	+
Third-generation drugs					
Brivaracetam	+	-	-	++	-
Cannabidiol**	-	++	-	-	-
Cenobamate	++	-	++	-	-
Perampanel	-	-	-	-	++
Stiripentol	-	-	++	?	-

++ Main mechanism of action; + Additional mechanism of action
* The main mechanism of action of acetazolamide is represented by the inhibition of Carbonic Anhydrase expressed in the central nervous system, which constitutes an additional target of Topiramate and Zonisamide.
** The main mechanisms of action are represented by the reduction of intracellular and extracellular calcium through the blocking of GPR55 receptors and the desensitization of TRPV1 channels, as well as the increase in adenosine levels through the inhibition of ENT1 pumps.

discontinuation being one of the most frequent causes of seizure recurrence or the onset of status epilepticus). The drug dosage should always be personalized and adjusted based on seizure control (in cases of persistent seizures, the recommendation is to increase the dosage to the maximum tolerated dose); in the case of toxic effects, the dosage should obviously be reduced. In theory, monotherapy is always preferable, as polytherapy increases the possibility of poor patient adherence, drug interactions, teratogenicity, and long-term toxic effects. However, for patients affected by pharmacoresistant epilepsy polytherapy cannot be avoided. In this context, the concept of "rational polytherapy" is emerging, meaning the use of combinations of molecules with different and complementary mechanisms of action that can act synergistically. Nevertheless, except for a few exceptions (such as the combination of valproate and lamotrigine), there is no evidence for specific synergistic combinations, and choices in clinical practice continue to remain heterogeneous and anchored to empirical procedures.

Regarding specific variables of the pathology, the choice of treatment is based on the type of seizures and epileptic syndrome. Focal seizures and focal epilepsies generally respond to all types of currently available drugs without clear specificity of action. Generalized seizures (particularly typical absences and myoclonic seizures) respond to more specific therapies. In some cases, the inappropriate use of drugs can worsen the frequency of seizures. In general, valproate is usually considered a very safe choice for generalized epilepsies, and carbamazepine for focal epilepsies. In a general and illustrative scheme, it is possible to remember some "classic" choices for specific types of seizures: for absences, valproate, ethosuximide, lamotrigine, levetiracetam, topiramate; for myoclonic seizures, valproate, phenobarbital, clonazepam, levetiracetam, perampanel, zonisamide; for tonic-clonic seizures (primary or secondary), valproate, phenobarbital, carbamazepine or phenytoin, and all the new generation drugs; for focal seizures, the sequence can be more variable and include carbamazepine, valproate, phenytoin, and all the new generation drugs; in specific syndromic contexts (e.g., West syndrome and Lennox-Gastaut syndrome), drugs considered as reference such as vigabatrin, clobazam, stiripentol, and rufinamide can be used, especially for the treatment of flexion spasms and tonic seizures. The general characteristics of the drugs and their respective indications for types of seizures and epileptic syndromes are reported in Table 12.7.

Adverse Effects | Numerous side effects can be observed, and their presence is now more carefully considered than in the past (it has been demonstrated that adverse effects have a greater impact on quality of life than the seizures themselves). Side effects can be either *idiosyncratic* or *non-idiosyncratic.* Idiosyncratic effects are often dose-independent, unpredictable, of acute onset, and often require a change in therapy. Thanks to the contribution of pharmacogenetics, the genetic basis of such conditions is increasingly being delineated. Almost all drugs are potentially responsible for idiosyncratic reactions (especially carbamazepine, phenytoin, and phenobarbital); among the newer drugs, lamotrigine can cause the development of Stevens-Johnson syndrome, a severe form of exfoliative dermatitis. Non-idiosyncratic effects can occur early, at the initiation of drug therapy, or later during prolonged treatment. The most frequent effects are related to cognitive dysfunction characterized primarily by a reduction in attention, concentration, and memory capacities. Some drugs can be responsible for specific side effects: phenytoin can cause cerebellar disorders and, in cases of prolonged overdose, cerebellar atrophy, while vigabatrin is often responsible for visual field disturbances (progressive narrowing) due to toxic effects on the retina. Psychological side effects should not be overlooked, as they often have a subtle onset, variable expression, and varying degrees of severity. These effects can include mild depressive symptoms and/or irritability, but also psychotic disorders and the emergence of suicidal ideation (increasingly reported, especially with the use of new drugs). The typical side effects of various drugs are reported in Table 12.7.

Table 12.7 METABOLISM, DOSAGES, ADVERSE EVENTS, AND CLINICAL INDICATIONS OF ANTIEPILEPTIC DRUGS

Drug	Indication	Metabolism/ elimination	Initial dose (mg)	Main. dose (mg)	Common adverse events	Severe adverse events
Acetazolamide	FE, GE	Renal metabolism, renal excretion	250	500-1000	Transient polyuria, hypokalemia, nephrolithiasis, asthenia, anorexia, drowsiness, paresthesia	Rash, rare Stevens-Johnson syndrome, aplastic anemia and thrombocytopenia (rare)
Brivaracetam	FE	Hepatic metabolism, renal excretion	50-100	50-200	Dizziness, drowsiness, influenza, dizziness, anorexia, insomnia, irritability, dyspepsia	Neutropenia, suicidal ideation/psychosis (rare)
Cannabidiol	LGS	Hepatic metabolism, fecal excretion	5/kg	10-20/kg	Drowsiness, anorexia, diarrhea, pyrexia, fatigue, vomiting	Marked sedation, worsening of seizures, suicidal ideation, weight loss
Carbamazepine	FE	Hepatic metabolism, urine >> fecal excretion	100-200	400-1800	Leukopenia, thrombocytopenia, dizziness, drowsiness, headache, impaired balance, rash, hyponatremia, nausea and vomiting, weight gain, fluid retention, asthenia, elevated liver enzymes, attention disturbance	Asterixis, dystonia, nystagmus (uncommon); Idiosyncratic reaction, hepatotoxicity, Stevens-Johnson syndrome, aplastic anemia, pancreatitis, arrhythmias (very rare)
Cenobamate	FE	Hepatic metabolism, urine >> fecal excretion	25	100-200	Drowsiness, dizziness, gait and coordination disturbances	Drug Reaction with Eosinophilia and Systemic Symptoms (DRESS)
Clobazam	FE, EG, cluster	Hepatic metabolism, renal excretion	10	10-30	Drowsiness, sedation, headache, concentration disturbances, anxiety, reduced l ibido, nystagmus, diplopia, tachycardia, nausea, vomiting, constipation, weight gain	Idiosyncratic rash, agitation and delirium (paradoxical reaction) (rare)
Clonazepam	FE, GE, cluster	Hepatic metabolism, renal excretion	1-2	1-6	Drowsiness, ataxia, dizziness, hypotonia, amnesia, tremor, behavior disturbances, nausea, sialorrhea/ dry mouth, nystagmus, palpitations	Idiosyncratic rash, thrombocytopenia, respiratory depression, heart failure, paradoxical reactions (rare)
Diazepam	FE, GE, cluster	Hepatic metabolism, renal excretion	5	10-30	Drowsiness, sedation, dizziness, ataxia, diplopia, asthenia, amnesia, nausea, constipation, sialorrhea/dry mouth	Respiratory and circulatory depression, paradoxical reactions (rare)
Eslicarbazepine	FE	Hepatic metabolism, renal excretion	400	800-1200	Dizziness, drowsiness, headache, tremor, dizziness, balance disturbances, diplopia, rash, nausea, anorexia	Hematologic disorder, acute cerebellar syndrome, psychotic disorder (rare)
Ethosuximide	GE, absence seizures	Hepatic metabolism, renal excretion	250	500-1500	Anorexia, headache, dizziness, drowsiness, ataxia, dyspepsia, abdominal pain	Rash, Stevens-Johnson syndrome, aplastic anemia (rare)
Felbamate	FE, LGS	Hepatic metabolism, renal excretion	400	1800-3600	Anorexia, insomnia/drowsiness, headache, dizziness, ataxia, asthenia, nausea, vomiting, diarrhea	Hepatic insufficiency, aplastic anemia
Phenytoin	FE, tonic-clonic seizures	Hepatic metabolism, renal excretion	200	200-400	Balance disturbances, diplopia, drowsiness, headache, nausea, vomiting, gingival hyperplasia, hematologic disorders, rash, osteopenia	Ataxia, tremor; Stevens-Johnson syndrome, ataxia, confusion (rare)
Phenobarbital	FE, GE, tonic-clonic seizures	Hepatic metabolism, 25% unchanged excreted	30-50	100-200	Drowsiness, sedation, ataxia, nystagmus, spindle-hand syndrome, osteopenia, megaloblastic anemia	Idiosyncratic reaction, hepatotoxicity, Stevens-Johnson syndrome, hematologic disorders (rare), osteomalacia, Dupuytren's

Gabapentin	FE	Unchanged excretion in urine	300	1800-3600	Drowsiness, dizziness, ataxia, leukopenia, infections, appetite changes, mood alterations, hypertension, edema, vasodilation, purpura, impotence	Increased seizures, hepatitis
Lacosamide	FE	Hepatic metabolism, renal excretion (40% unchanged)	50	300-400	Dizziness, headache, nausea, diplopia, balance disturbance, tremor, drowsiness, dysarthria, concentration impairment	Cardiac arrhythmia, psychotic disorder (rare)
Lamotrigine	FE, GE, LGS	Hepatic metabolism, renal excretion	25-50	100-400	Rash, headache, dizziness, tremor, drowsiness/insomnia, nausea, vomiting, diarrhea, dry mouth, asthenia, arthralgia	Idiosyncratic reaction, liver failure, rare Stevens-Johnson syndrome, severe hematological disorders, worsening of seizures, hepatopathy (rare)
Levetiracetam	FE, GE, myocl. seizures	Minimal metabolism (hydrolysis), renal excretion	250-500	750-3000	Drowsiness, headache, rhinopharyngitis, anxiety, depression, hostility/aggression, insomnia, nervousness, dizziness, tremor, balance disturbance, dyspepsia, diarrhea	Behavioral disorders, hematological disorder, hepatitis, Stevens-Johnson syndrome (rare)
Oxcarbazepine	FE	Hepatic metabolism, renal excretion	150-300	900-2400	Dizziness, drowsiness, headache, diplopia, vertigo, nausea and vomiting, hyponatremia, balance disturbance, diplopia, rash, depression, nervousness, diarrhea or constipation, asthenia, concentration impairment	Severe hyponatremia, arrhythmias, hematological disorder, pancreatitis, systemic lupus erythematosus (rare/very rare)
Perampanel	FE, tonic-clonic seizures	Hepatic metabolism, excretion in feces > urine	2	6-12	Dizziness, vertigo, drowsiness, balance disturbance, aggression, nausea, asthenia, back pain	Suicidal ideation, falls
Pregabalin	FE	Unchanged excretion in urine	50-75	100-600	Dizziness, drowsiness, headache, rhinopharyngitis, increased appetite, decreased libido, balance disturbance, euphoria, aggression, nausea, vomiting, diarrhea/constipation	Increased seizures, autonomic disorders, renal insufficiency (rare)
Rufinamide	LGS	Hepatic metabolism, renal excretion	200	1200-4800	Drowsiness, dizziness, headache, nausea, vomiting, infections, anorexia, asthenia, balance disturbance, anxiety	Rash, short QT interval, seizures (rare)
Stiripentol	SD	Hepatic metabolism, renal excretion	20 mg/kg	50 mg/kg	Decreased appetite, weight loss, insomnia/drowsiness, nausea, vomiting, irritability	Neutropenia, thrombocytopenia, hypotonia, dystonia
Tiagabine	FE	Hepatic metabolism, fecal excretion > urine	5	30-45	Dizziness, drowsiness, tremor, depression, nervousness, abdominal pain, bruising	Increased seizures, status epilepticus
Topiramate	FE, GE, LGS	Predominantly hepatic metabolism, renal excretion	25-50	75-200	Paresthesia, dizziness, drowsiness, anorexia, weight loss, nausea, vomiting, diarrhea, depression, tremor, anemia, language and attention disturbances, dysgeusia, balance disorders, diplopia	Renal calculi, cognitive impairment, hyperchloremic acidosis, hepatitis, visual disturbances (rare)
Valproate	FE, GE	Hepatic metabolism, renal excretion	200	4000-3000	Nausea, vomiting, transaminase elevation, tremor, weight gain, alopecia/hirsutism, paresthesia, gingival hyperplasia	Teratogenicity, acute pancreatitis, hepatotoxicity, thrombocytopenia, encephalopathy, polycystic ovary syndrome
Vigabatrin	FE, spasms in SW	85% unchanged excretion	500 mg	1000-2000	Drowsiness, asthenia, arthralgia, anemia, nausea, vomiting, weight gain, restlessness, headache, dizziness, attention/language/memory disturbances	Visual field defects (common), increased seizures, encephalopathy, suicide attempt (rare)
Zonisamide	FE	Hepatic metabolism, renal excretion	50-100 mg	200-600	Anorexia, weight loss, asthenia, dizziness, memory/attention disturbances, paresthesia, drowsiness, tremor	Rash, hematological disorder (very rare), cholelithiasis, liver abnormalities

FE = Focal Epilepsy; GE = Genralized Epilepsy; GTC: generalized tonic-clonic; LGS = Lennox-Gastaut Syndrome

Treatment management | Pharmacological therapy should be continued regularly. Clinical and laboratory monitoring, which is frequent at the beginning, will become less necessary with the passing of time, except in specific cases. Plasma monitoring serves to verify the correct intake and absorption of the drug but is less useful for determining the maintenance dose, which should be evaluated based on clinical response. Furthermore, plasma monitoring becomes important in the presence of an intercurrent illness requiring the use of other therapies, in the presence of gastrointestinal disorders (vomiting and diarrhea) that may affect drug absorption, if there are unexplained side effects, and when adding a second drug is necessary.

Discontinuation of therapy | Once initiated, treatment should be continued for a predetermined period based on the type of epilepsy. The drug can be safely discontinued when the epileptic form tends to spontaneously resolve. Paradigmatic examples are typical childhood absences, which tend to cease spontaneously with puberty, or benign childhood focal epilepsies (e.g., centrotemporal spikes), which tend to regress over the years. In all other cases, discontinuation of treatment increases the risk of relapse, even after seizure-free periods of 2-5 years (a seizure-free interval is necessary before considering treatment discontinuation). The relapse rate also depends on the type of epilepsy: in idiopathic generalized epilepsies with convulsive seizures and myoclonus, it is almost 90%, and in focal epilepsies, it ranges from 50% to 80%. The relapse rate is higher when epilepsy begins in childhood, when multiple drugs have been required to control seizures, or when a previous attempt to discontinue therapy has failed. Furthermore, it is higher when the EEG is still active at the time of treatment discontinuation and, especially, when the abnormalities worsen during the tapering of therapy. The use of 24-hour ambulatory EEG is much more useful than standard EEG, as it increases the observation time, allowing for an evaluation of the presence of abnormalities during sleep (including falling asleep and waking up). The relapse rate increases in symptomatic epilepsies.

Surgical therapy and other therapeutic strategies for drug-resistant forms | Approximately 20-30% of epilepsies are drug-resistant, meaning they do not adequately respond to pharmacological treatment. On average, the control of seizures is achieved in 70-80% of cases with the first drug used. In case of failure, a second drug is effective in only 10-20% of cases, and finally, the third drug is effective in only 3-5% of cases. Two main hypotheses have been proposed to explain the mechanisms underlying drug resistance. The first proposes an alteration of drug *targets* (e.g., conformational changes in neurotransmitter receptors), and the second suggests the central role played by drug-transporting proteins (excessive expression may reduce drug concentration around neurons in the epileptogenic area through active transport from brain tissue into capillaries). Surgical treatment is indicated for patients with drug-resistant focal epilepsy. After careful clinical, neurophysiological (crucially, seizure recording), neuroradiological, and neuropsychological evaluation, it is possible to select patients who are potential candidates for resection of the epileptogenic area. The necessary requirements are:

- A single and well-defined epileptogenic area
- Seizures without primary involvement of eloquent areas (to avoid permanent neurological outcomes)
- Correlation of anatomo-electro-clinical data.

The initial approach involves non-invasive study using video-EEG to analyze the electro-clinical aspects of seizures and adequately localize them. If video-EEG study is insufficient to define the onset area and seizure propagation, or if there is a discrepancy between clinical, EEG, and anatomical data, invasive study can be performed using specific EEG techniques (commonly *subdural grids* and *depth electrodes* through stereotactic approach). The most common procedure is temporal lobe resection (most implicated in resistant forms), where surgical intervention is often effective, resulting in complete seizure control in approximately 60-70% of cases. Surgical outcomes are less promising for extratemporal epilepsy forms, where the success rate tends to decrease, especially in cases where no clear anatomical lesion is evident. In some specific and highly selected cases, even if complete seizure control is unlikely, other types of surgical interventions can be proposed. If radical resection is not possible, alternative approaches such as callosotomy (section of the corpus callosum to control drop seizures), radiotherapy (using *gamma-knife* or *cyber-knife* for the treatment of specific conditions such as hypothalamic hamartoma), lvagus nerve stimulation, and more recently, *deep brain stimulation* can be considered. Among non-surgical approaches, for specific forms of epilepsy in childhood, a ketogenic diet (a special high-fat diet) can be used.

12.9 Epilepsy as a neurological emergency: status epilepticus

According to the latest definition (ILAE commission 2015), status epilepticus is a condition caused by the failure of mechanisms that inhibit seizures or, alternatively, the initiation of mechanisms that lead to an excessively prolonged seizure (this time limit is referred to as time 1 - t1). It is a condition that can result in long-term consequences after a prolonged interval of time (time limit referred to as time 2 - t2). Based on this new definition, the time limit for defining status epilepticus (previously indicated as a seizure lasting more than 30 minutes) has been reformulated. Currently, different time limits are considered depending on the type of status epilepticus: for convulsive status epilepticus, it is 5 minutes (t1) and 30 minutes (t2); for focal status epilepticus with impaired consciousness, it is 5 minutes (t1) and 60 minutes (t2); for absence status epilepticus, t1 is 10-15 minutes, whereas t2 is unknown. Currently, status epilepticus can be classified based on four main axes: semiology, etiology, EEG correlates, and age of onset (however, a comprehensive discussion of this topic is beyond the scope of this chapter).

Status epilepticus can complicate acute and chronic neurological disorders and febrile illnesses, often occurring in individuals without pre-existing epilepsy. However, in the majority of cases, it occurs due to the sudden or inappropriate discontinuation of therapies. Among *non-convulsive status epilepticus*, there are *absence status epilepticus* (repeated absences that generate a stable condition of mental confusion) and *focal status epilepticus with impaired awareness* (repeated focal seizures that cause fluctuating impaired consciousness and usually automatic motor manifestations). The most severe condition is represented by *convulsive status epilepticus*, in which motor manifestations of clonic or tonic-clonic type recur; the repetition of generalized seizures can be a life-threatening emergency due to intense cardiovascular and respiratory involvement. The incidence of status epilepticus is 40-60 cases per 100,000 population per year; it predominantly affects pediatric patients and, in one-third of cases, patients with a history of epilepsy. The overall mortality is estimated to be between 2.5% and 38%, with an increase correlated with both age and duration of status epilepticus.

Regarding treatment, it is necessary to initiate continuous monitoring of the patient to assess respiratory function (respiratory rate and oxygen saturation) and cardiovascular function (ECG and blood pressure), the main hematological and biochemical parameters, and brain electrical activity (EEG). The first pharmacological approach involves the administration of intravenous benzodiazepines, which, due to their liposolubility, ensure rapid and effective action in the brain. If status epilepticus persists, intravenous phenytoin should be used (with ECG and blood pressure monitoring) or other injectable antiepileptic drugs available (valproate, levetiracetam, lacosamide, brivaracetam). In case of failure, low-dose barbiturates can be attempted before the employment of anesthetics (propofol, midazolam, and finally thiopental) and subsequent management of status epilepticus in the intensive care unit.

Figure 12.7 shows the main therapeutic regimens used in the treatment of status epilepticus according to the most recent guidelines.

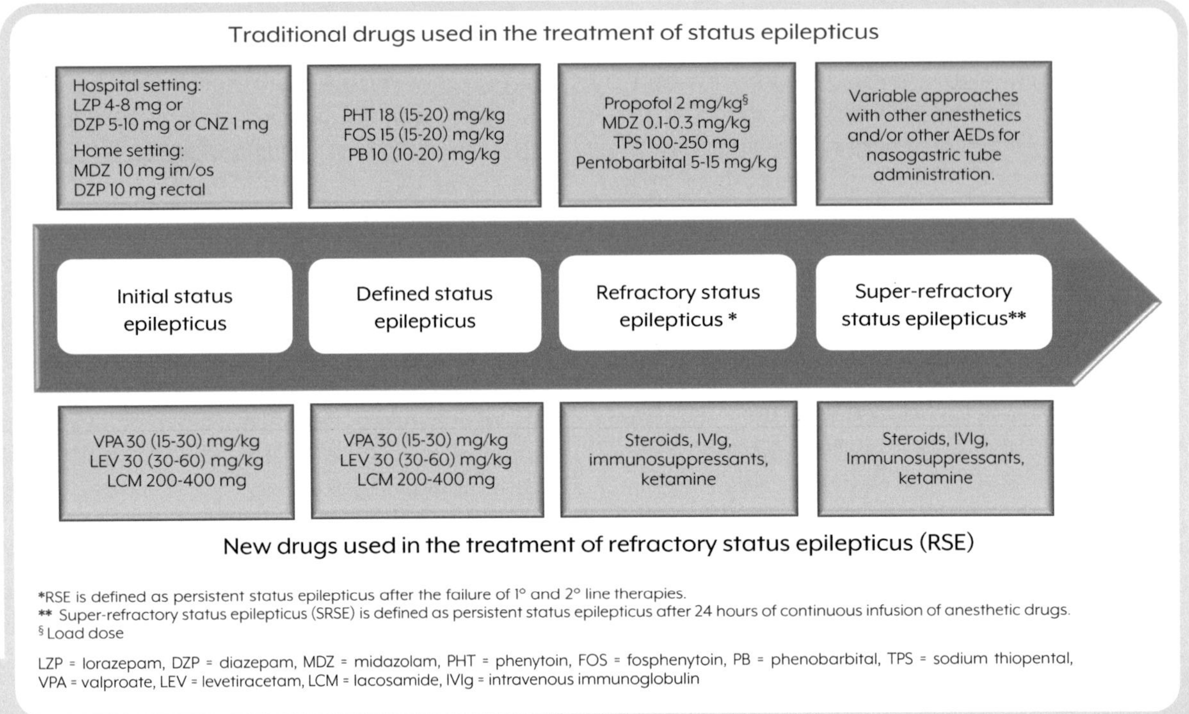

Figure 12.7

Therapeutic approach to status epilepticus.

Bibliography

Scheffer I.E., Berkovic S., Capovilla G. ILAE classification of the epilepsies: Position paper of the ILAE Commission for Classification and Terminology. Epilepsia, 58(4):512–521, 2017.

Fisher R.S., Cross J.H., D'Souza C, et al. on behalf of the ILAE Commission for Classification and Terminology. Instruction manual for the ILAE 2017 operational classification of seizure types. Epilepsia, 58(4):531–542, 2017.

Commission on Classification and Terminology of the International League Against Epilepsy. Proposal for revised classification of epilepsies and epileptic syndromes. Epilepsia; 30:389-99. 1989.

Duncan J.S., Sander J.W., Sisodiya S.M. et al. Adult epilepsy. Lancet; 367:1087-1, 2006.

Elger C.E., Schmidt D., Modern management of epilepsy: A practical approach. Epilepsy & Behavior; 12:501-539, 2008.

Kwan P., Sander J.W., The natural history of epilepsy: an epidemiological view. J Neurol Neurosurg Psychiatry; 75:1376-81, 2004.

Shorvon S., Handbook of epilepsy treatment. Oxford: Blackwell Science, 2000.

13 CEREBROVASCULAR DISEASES

Francesco Orzi, Danilo Toni

13.1 Vascular anatomy of the brain

From the aortic arch, the following arteries originate from right to left: the brachiocephalic trunk, the left common carotid artery, and the left subclavian artery (from which the left vertebral artery originates). The brachiocephalic trunk gives rise to the right common carotid artery and the right subclavian artery (from which the right vertebral artery originates). The common carotid arteries bifurcate into the external carotid artery and the internal carotid artery.

The internal carotid arteries do not have collateral branches outside the skull, which allows them to be distinguished from the external carotid arteries during angiographic or Doppler ultrasound examination of the supra-aortic trunks. The external carotid arteries emit branches for the neck, face, and scalp. Within the skull (Figure 13.1), the internal carotid

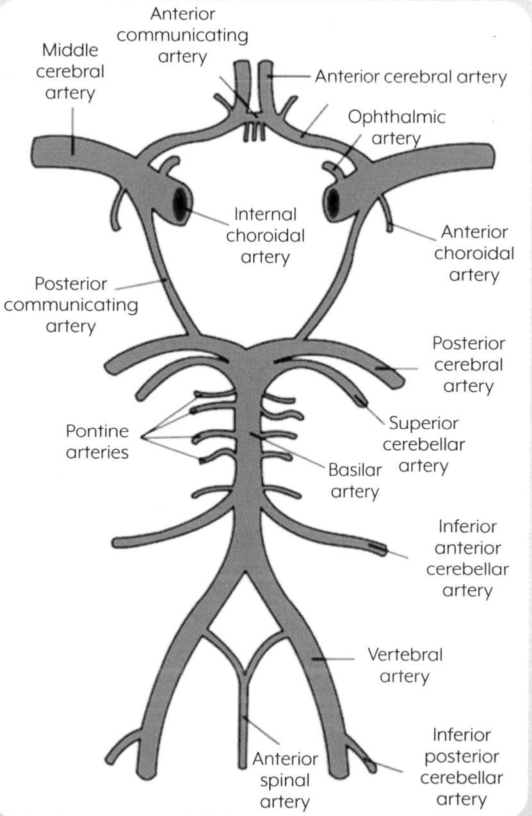

Figure 13.1

Schematic representation of the intracranial carotid and vertebrobasilar circulations and the Circle of Willis (formed by the posterior cerebral arteries, posterior communicating arteries, anterior cerebral arteries, and anterior communicating artery).

Box 13.1 ANATOMY AND CLINICAL FEATURES: KEY ASPECTS

- The *carotid artery*, in its course, comes into contact with the *sympathetic system of the carotid plexus*. Carotid artery injury (such as dissection) can cause *Horner's syndrome* (miosis, drooping eyelid).
- The carotid artery also comes into contact with the *hypoglossal nerve*; in case of nerve damage due to compression, tongue deviation is observed during protrusion towards the side of the lesion.
- The *ophthalmic artery* is the first intracranial branch of the carotid artery: amaurosis caused by artery obstruction suggests a carotid embolic pathogenesis.
- The *oculomotor nerve* emerges from the trunk, between the posterior cerebral artery and the superior cerebellar artery. The nerve is also in contact with the *Circle of Willis,* particularly with the posterior communicating artery. An aneurysm of this artery is a common cause of dysfunction or paralysis of the intrinsic cranial nerve III (mydriasis, loss of the pupillary light reflex), while diabetic mononeuritis affects the extrinsic cranial nerve III (drooping eyelid, paralysis of adduction and upward and downward rotation). However, in advanced stages, the aneurysm can cause complete paralysis of both the intrinsic and extrinsic cranial nerve III. An aneurysm of the posterior communicating artery can also compress the optic chiasm, resulting in a visual field defect.
- At the level of the cavernous sinus, the internal carotid artery comes into contact with *cranial nerves III, IV e VI* as well as the *maxillary branch of the trigeminal nerve* (see Cavernous Sinus Syndrome).

arteries pass through the cavernous sinus, from which the ophthalmic arteries originate (see Box 13.1). From the supraclinoid portion, the anterior choroidal arteries and posterior communicating arteries originate. The internal carotid arteries bifurcate into the middle cerebral arteries and anterior cerebral arteries. The anterior choroidal arteries have perforating branches to the globus pallidus, posterior limb of the internal capsule, temporal lobe, thalamus, and lateral geniculate body. The anterior cerebral arteries course along the corpus callosum and supply the anterior and medial areas of the hemispheres (where the lower limb of the motor and sensory homunculus is represented), the basal part of the frontal lobes, and the caudate nuclei. The two anterior cerebral arteries are usually connected by an anterior communicating artery, which allows compensatory circulation to the anterior cerebral artery and middle cerebral artery when the corresponding internal carotid artery is occluded. It is not uncommon for one anterior cerebral artery to be smaller (hypoplastic) than the other or for both anterior cerebral arteries to originate from the same internal carotid artery, resulting in a lack of compensation. The middle cerebral arteries course laterally and give rise, in their initial segment, to lenticulostriate arteries that supply the basal ganglia and internal capsule. At the Sylvian fissures, the middle cerebral arteries trifurcate into anterior temporal arteries, which supply the upper parts of the temporal lobes, and superior and inferior branches, which supply the lateral portions of the hemispheres above and below the Sylvian fissures. These areas correspond to the representation of the face and upper limb (motor and sensory homunculus).

The vertebral arteries, which originate from the subclavian arteries, ascend through the transverse foramina of the cervical vertebrae, enter the skull through the foramen magnum, and anastomose at the pontobulbar junction to give rise to the basilar artery. In the neck, the vertebral arteries supply spinal and muscular branches, and in the intracranial portion, they give rise to the anterior and posterior spinal arteries, penetrating branches to the medulla, and posterior inferior cerebellar arteries. The basilar artery ascends, giving rise to the anterior inferior cerebellar arteries, superior cerebellar arteries, and perforating branches to the brainstem, and terminates in the posterior cerebral arteries. The posterior cerebral arteries give rise to mesencephalic and thalamic penetrating branches and course posteriorly to the occipital and inferior temporal lobes (Figure 13.1). Anatomic variations of the posterior circulation are common, such as hypoplasia of a vertebral artery, the presence of a dominant vertebral artery that fully terminates in the basilar artery while the contralateral vertebral artery terminates in the posterior inferior cerebellar artery, or the so-called fetal origin of one or both posterior cerebral arteries from the internal carotid arteries.

Normally, the anterior, middle, and posterior cerebral arteries communicate with each other

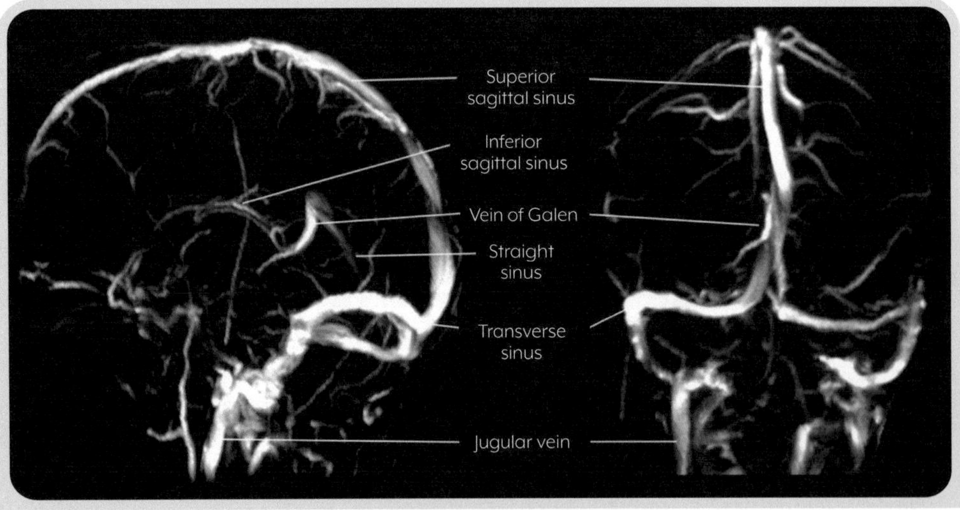

Figure 13.2

Brain Venous MR Angiography - Three-dimensional reconstruction in lateral-lateral and postero-anterior projection.

through the anterior communicating artery and two posterior communicating arteries, forming the circle of Willis, which allows for collateral flow in the event of occlusion of one of the major arteries (Figure 13.1). During acute arterial occlusions, leptomeningeal anastomoses also come into play, and their failure to activate can result in infarcts in borderzone vascular territories, which are sensitive to reduced territorial cerebral blood flow. Other collateral circulations are formed by the external carotid arteries, through the supraorbital artery connected to the ophthalmic artery, and by meningeal branches connected to the carotid siphon (in the petrous and cavernous segments), as well as by the vertebral arteries through the pharyngoccipital and cervical systems.

The anatomy of the venous system includes the dural venous sinuses and the superficial and deep veins. The longitudinal, sagittal, and transverse sinuses have walls formed by the dura mater. The superficial and deep veins drain into the dural sinuses, which in turn drain into the jugular veins (Figure 13.2).

13.2 Epidemiology

Stroke is the second leading cause of death (or third if neoplasms are considered as a whole) in industrialized countries. Over 2/3 (67-81%) of strokes are ischemic, 7-20% are intracerebral hemorrhages, 1-7% are subarachnoid hemorrhages, and 2-15% are strokes of undetermined cause. The incidence and prevalence (incident cases plus surviving cases from previous years) show national variations, with the highest incidence in Ukraine, Russia, and Japan, and the highest prevalence in the United Kingdom and Italy. The specific incidence increases for each decade of age. After the age of 55, the stroke rate doubles for each subsequent decade in both women and men, with 75-89% of strokes occurring in individuals over 65 years old. Stroke also occurs in young adults and children. The annual incidence is 2-3 new cases per 100,000 in the 20-24 age group, 5 new cases per 100,000 in the 30-34 age group, and over 30 new cases per 100,000 in individuals aged 45-49. Stroke is also one of the common causes of death in children, with an annual incidence of 2-13 per 100,000. Men have a higher incidence, with the exception of the 35-44 age group and those over 85 years old. Factors such as contraceptive use and pregnancy contribute to increased risk among women in the 35-44 age group, while early male mortality from heart disease contributes to the prevalence of stroke among older women. In general, 1/6 of women die from stroke, while in comparison, 1/25 die from breast cancer.

13.3 Ischemic stroke

13.3.1 Prognosis and risk factors

Ischemic stroke is associated with a mortality rate of 15-25%, and the majority of deaths occur within the first month. Among surviving patients, 20-30% show complete recovery within a month, 30-40% show nearly complete recovery, 20% require hospital assistance after 3 months, and 15-30% remain disabled. Approximately one year after the stroke, it can be estimated that 1/3 of individuals experience death, 1/3 significant disability, and 1/3 autonomy or complete functional recovery.

Despite significant advancements in therapy, prevention remains the best tool to reduce the medical, social, and human burden of stroke. A transient ischemic attack (TIA) or an episode of transient monocular blindness constitutes an immediate risk of stroke, which is around 1-5% within the first month and 10-20% within the subsequent 5 years. Primary prevention is important because individuals at risk can be identified and directed to specific treatments. The criteria for identification serve as a significant tool for medical intervention and consider various risk factors, generally categorized as: a) non-modifiable: age, sex, birth weight, ethnicity, and genetic predisposition; b) modifiable: hypertension, smoking, diabetes, atrial fibrillation and other cardiac conditions, dyslipidemia, carotid stenosis, postmenopausal hormone therapy, improper or poor diet, obesity, and body fat distribution; c) potentially modifiable: metabolic syndrome, excessive alcohol intake, drugs, oral contraceptives, breathing disorders during sleep, migraine, hyperhomocysteinemia, hyperlipoproteinemia, hypercoagulability, inflammation, and infection.

Familial predisposition for stroke is well-documented. A positive family history increases the risk of stroke by approximately 30%, and this can be attributed to heredity and susceptibility to risk factors, shared lifestyles and/or environmental factors, or the interaction between genetic and environmental factors. For instance, many known risk factors such as hypertension, diabetes, and dyslipidemia have both genetic and environmental components. Some coagulopathies associated with Factors V, VII, X, XI, and XIII are autosomal recessive. Chromosomal variants associated with stroke have been identified, including variants on chromosome 9p21 and chromosome 4q25. Some rare genetic diseases are associated with stroke, such as CADASIL, Marfan syndrome, Neurofibromatosis type I and II, Fabry disease, and sickle cell anemia. Intracranial aneurysms are also more common in individuals with a positive family history. Data on familial predisposition to stroke also open up possibilities for personalized medical care through the identification of genetic variability in cytochrome P450 2C9 (CYP2C9), vitamin K epoxide reductase complex 1 (VKORC1), or rare missense mutations in factor IX that determine the response to vitamin K antagonists. Hypertension remains one of the major risk factors. Even within the normal range, the higher the blood pressure, the greater the risk. For this reason, non-pharmacological blood pressure reduction is recommended even for individuals in the pre-hypertensive stage (systolic blood pressure of 120-139 mm Hg or diastolic blood pressure of 80-89 mm Hg). Antihypertensive treatment reduces the risk of stroke by 32%. Currently, there is no evidence that specific classes of antihypertensive drugs have a protective effect on stroke independent of their antihypertensive effect. Current guidelines recommend a blood pressure goal of <140/90 mm Hg (<130/80 mm Hg in individuals with diabetes).

Epidemiological data shows that smoking increases the risk of stroke, and quitting smoking reduces the heightened risk. Smoking can synergize with other risk factors, such as in young women using oral contraceptives or young adults carrying the ApoE4 allele.

Case-control studies and prospective epidemiological studies have confirmed that diabetes increases the risk of stroke from 1.8 to nearly 6 times. Glycemic control reduces microvascular complications but does not seem to negate the risk. Hence, in addition to glycemic control, individuals with diabetes also require blood pressure control with lower targets compared to the general population. In the presence of additional risk factors in individuals with diabetes, the use of statins should be considered even with normal cholesterol levels.

Many studies show an association between hypercholesterolemia and ischemic stroke and, although not consistently, between low cholesterol levels and hemorrhagic stroke. They also demonstrate an inverse relationship between HDL cholesterol and stroke. Reducing LDL cholesterol (with statins and lifestyle changes) is a form of primary prevention in individuals with coronary artery disease or high-risk conditions such as diabetes.

Atrial fibrillation, even in the absence of valvular disease, is associated with a 4-5 times increased risk of stroke. The risk is significantly reduced by oral anticoagulant therapy. Atrial fibrillation, therefore, represents a significant opportunity for primary prevention as it can be identified before a stroke. The stroke risk can be stratified based on the presence of other comorbidities using validated prediction tools.

Various other heart diseases can predispose to stroke, including sinoatrial node disease, primary cardiac tumors, valvular vegetations, prosthetic valves, dilated cardiomyopathy, coronary artery disease, valvular diseases, and endocarditis. The severity of the stroke is inversely proportional to the left ventricular ejection fraction. Congenital abnormalities such as a patent foramen ovale (PFO) and alterations or aneurysms of the interatrial septum can be associated with stroke.

Carotid plaques are also a risk factor, both for the first event and for recurrence if they result in 60%-70% stenosis.

Postmenopausal hormone replacement therapy is associated with an increased risk of stroke. A statistically weak but not negligible risk is also associated with the use of oral contraceptives, which should be discouraged in women with other risk factors. Physical inactivity, obesity, and metabolic syndrome are other conditions associated with stroke. In many observational studies, low alcohol consumption (<24 g per day) is associated with a reduced risk of stroke, while high consumption increases the risk.

Sleep apnea is a condition associated with a higher risk of stroke, regardless of age or the presence of other factors such as obesity, reduced left ventricular function, diabetes, sex, hypertension, atrial fibrillation, previous stroke, or smoking.

Elevated levels of homocysteine are associated with a 2-3 times increase in the risk of vascular diseases, including stroke.

States of hypercoagulability (thrombophilias), acquired or hereditary, are associated with an increased risk of venous thrombosis, while the relationship with arterial cerebral infarction is anecdotal or based on case-control studies. The association between elevated circulating levels of lipoprotein-associated phospholipase A2 (Lp-PLA2) and arterial thrombosis is documented; many studies also suggest an association between C-reactive protein (hs-CRP) and stroke. Currently, there is no indication for pharmacological treatment for primary prevention in individuals with elevated levels of Lp-PLA2.

Case-control and cohort studies suggest migraine as a risk factor for ischemic stroke. The risk would be higher for migraine with aura and in women using oral contraceptives. The correlation between migraine and stroke may be attributed to the coexistence, in these patients, of other potential risk conditions, such as mitral valve prolapse, atrial septal abnormalities, arterial dissection, antiphospholipid antibodies in the blood, and hyperhomocysteinemia.

13.3.2 Pathophysiology

The brain, weighing approximately 2% of body weight, consumes 20% of the oxygen and 25% of the glucose utilized by the entire body. In the absence of energy stores, the metabolic demands must be sustained by a continuous blood flow, approximately 57 ml/100 g of brain tissue/minute, equivalent to about 15% of resting cardiac output. Energy consumption and blood flow vary from cerebral area to area and also vary over time, depending on the functional activity of different brain areas. This marked heterogeneity of blood flow and energy consumption reflects the anatomical and functional heterogeneity of the organ.

Under normal levels of blood flow, the brain extracts about 50% of arterial oxygen and about 10% of arterial glucose. Oxygen passes from the blood to the tissue through diffusion, while glucose crosses the blood-brain barrier and enters neurons through a high-affinity protein carrier, and therefore, transport is passive (i.e., it does not require energy). Glucose is then metabolized through aerobic glycolysis with a net yield of 33 molecules of ATP per molecule of glucose. The energy derived from glucose oxidation is primarily used to reestablish the ionic membrane gradients. Glia cells utilize about 6% of the total energy.

If the blood flow were to stop, the brain would have enough energy to function for only a few minutes. This dependence of the brain on continuous energy support is supported by clinical experience. For example, after cardiac arrest, a person loses consciousness within a few seconds, and within a few minutes brain damage becomes irreversible. Within a few seconds, electrical activity ceases, primarily due to alterations in ion channels and membrane depolarization that cause significant changes in intra- and extracellular ion concentrations. Intracellular levels of sodium, calcium, and chloride increase, while potassium exits the cells. The efflux of K+ causes massive cellular depolarization, a condition known as "peri-infarct depolarization," similar to the "spreading depression" described by Leao. Membrane depolarization activates voltage-gated calcium channels and stimulates the release of neurotransmitters, including the excitatory amino acids glutamate and glycine. Glutamate binds to ionotropic (NMDA, AMPA, kainate) and metabotropic receptors. Activation of NMDA receptors, in particular, promotes calcium influx and the subsequent production of nitric oxide by nitric oxide synthase (NOS), along with the activation of intracellular enzymatic processes. During ischemia, especially during the early reperfusion period, increased production of free radicals exceeds the enzymatic capacities of superoxide dismutase and other defense mechanisms. Oxygen free radicals can oxidize proteins, lipids, and nucleosides (DNA, RNA). Alterations in ion channels lead to intracellular accumulation of Na+, water movement into the cell, passive cellular swelling, mitochondrial damage, and overall disruption of cellular homeostasis. The consequences include membrane lysis, release of intracellular constituents that evoke inflammation, cellular infiltration, and vascular damage. Edema typically encompasses two phases: cytotoxic and vasogenic. Cytotoxic edema begins within minutes of ischemia onset, at flow values around 20-30% of normal. After several hours of ischemia, the blood-brain barrier becomes disrupted, and vasogenic edema begins, peaking 1-2 days after onset.

The spatial and temporal distribution of the described events is not homogeneous. Following the occlusion of a blood vessel, a central zone of abolished or significantly reduced blood flow rapidly undergoes necrosis. The ischemic "core" is surrounded by an area where perfusion shows a gradient of values approaching normal. This peripheral area, subjected to incomplete ischemia, loses function but remains structurally intact. This perinecrotic zone, which has lost function but remains structurally intact, vital, and potentially recoverable, is defined as the "penumbra." Within the penumbra, the ischemic insult initiates a process of damage maturation, which has its inertia and proceeds even if blood flow returns to normal levels. This maturation process can lead to delayed death, healing, or recovery. Various forms of delayed or programmed cell death have been described in cerebral ischemia. Apoptosis is the most common and well-known morphological expression of programmed cell death. Other forms or mechanisms, including autophagy, seem to play a role. The process of damage maturation can last hours or days (and possibly even weeks) depending on the intensity of the insult and other local or systemic variables. The most important variables in determining the fate of the penumbra are the extent of residual blood flow, which depends on the amount of collateral circulation, and the duration of the insult before reperfusion (see ■ Box 13.2).

Within the context of post-ischemic damage maturation, significant attention has been given in the last decade to inflammation and the role of the neurovascular unit. There is growing awareness that blood vessels, particularly the endothelium, play much more significant roles than merely channeling blood flow. The slowing or cessation of blood flow within the vessel initially leads to endothelial alterations that trigger the coagulation cascade, further aggravating circulation. Adhesion molecules are translocated to the surface of endothelial cells and platelets, producing pro-inflammatory

Box 13.2 PATHOPHYSIOLOGY AND CLINICAL FEATURES: KEY ASPECTS

■ The *brain* has no energy reserves. Interruption of blood flow leads to necrosis within a few minutes. In cases where the flow is reduced, the tissue undergoes ***acute neurodegeneration***. This typically occurs in the ***perinecrotic zone*** (known as the "penumbra"), during a stroke. The ***penumbra*** is defined as an area of functional loss with preserved structure, offering potential for functional recovery. The penumbra is characterized spatially and temporally, with many local variables (primarily residual blood flow and duration of ischemic insult) and systemic factors (such as temperature, inflammation, and age) contributing to its definition. Spatially, the penumbra is a heterogeneous area with zones of varying degrees of damage within it. Temporally, the progression of damage is similarly heterogeneous, with some areas likely to undergo cell death and others expected to recover. ■ Clinicians cannot determine whether an ischemic injury is reversible or not, nor can they ascertain the "threshold" blood flow level below which the damage becomes irreversible. Consequently, there is no direct operational method for visualizing the penumbra. Clinicians must rely on indirect assessments or surrogates to infer the presence of the penumbra. In practical terms, it is assumed that there is a penumbra if the residual blood flow is 7-20 mL/100g/min (approximately two-thirds lower than normal) or if there is reduced perfusion without significant cytotoxic edema (known as PWI/DWI mismatch on MRI or hypoperfusion area on perfusion CT). ■ The penumbra provides the rationale for reperfusion and/or neuroprotective therapy. In the presence of necrosis, both interventions are either ineffective or harmful.

Box 13.3 A INFLAMMATION AND STROKE: KEY ASPECTS

Ischemic insult triggers an inflammatory response that involves both innate and adaptive immune response. Experimental data suggest that the ***early inflammatory response*** promotes cell death, but it is also clear that components of the immune response, especially the adaptive one, promote repair and recovery. Dissecting the two components of the inflammatory response (pro-death and pro-life, using extreme simplification) seems to be impossible. Contrary to what was believed a decade ago, the brain is far from being an "isolated" organ in terms of immunity. Lymphocytes enter and exit the tissue and communicate with the lymph nodes in the neck. Additionally, the brain interacts with systemic immunity. It is known, for example, that a systemic infection, trauma, or surgical intervention can activate microglia in cerebral areas. ***A neurologist must be aware that systemic infection or inflammation can increase susceptibility to stroke or worsen its prognosis.***

signals, including complement activation, disruption of the blood-brain barrier, and leukocyte passage (Box 13.3a). The phenomena initiated within the arterial vessel activate macrophages and microglia in the perivascular space. In the parenchyma, microglia are activated by nucleotides and cell degradation products (DAMP, "danger-associated molecular pattern"), leading to NF-kB activation and the production of hundreds of different cytokines. Activated microglia promote inflammation while also facilitating the production of trophic factors. It is known that activated microglia assume different morphological and functional states, along a spectrum ranging from the M1 (pro-inflammatory) phenotype to the M2 (neurotrophic) phenotype. Hours or days after ischemic insult, antigen-presenting cells (macrophages and dendritic cells) initiate adaptive immunity by transporting antigens to regional lymph nodes, where lymphocytes are sensitized or "primed".

Thus, ischemic insult activates both innate and adaptive immunity. While the role of early innate immunity appears to be predominantly detrimental, the role of late adaptive immunity remains uncertain and probably ambivalent, with aspects that are both detrimental and protective or neurotrophic. The entire phenomenon of ischemic damage maturation is characterized by the coexistence of mechanisms that promote cell death and endogenous protective mechanisms that promote survival by antagonizing damage mechanisms or facilitating recovery (Box 13.3b e c).

Box 13.3 B INFLAMMATION AND STROKE: KEY ASPECTS

Mechanisms	Damage mediators	Protective mediators
Hypoperfusion	Arterial occlusion, activation of the coagulation cascade, complement activation, and platelet activation	Production of vasoactive mediators, activation of eNOS. Expression of HIF1
Energetic defect	Malfunction of ion pumps, intracellular accumulation of Na+ and Ca2+, cytotoxic edema	Reduced protein synthesis, spike-arrest with closure of ion channels
Oxidative stress	Production of NO, free radicals, and arachidonic acid metabolites	Antioxidant response through Nrf2
Excitotoxicity	Excessive activation of NMDA receptors, intracellular accumulation of Ca2+, activation of intracellular enzymes	Release of inhibitory neurotransmitters
Programmed cell death	Activation of caspases, expression of pro-apoptotic factors	Expression of anti-apoptotic factors (Bcl2, IAP)
Inflammation	Complement activation, release of cytokines in the intravascular space, expression of adhesion molecules, disruption of the blood-brain barrier (BBB), leukocyte migration, activation of macrophages and microglia in the perivascular space and parenchyma, induction of adaptive immunity	Production of anti-inflammatory cytokines (IL-10, TGFβ), trophic factors, influx of anti-inflammatory lymphocytes (Treg, Breg)

Box 13.3 C INFLAMMATION AND STROKE: KEY ASPECTS

The phenomenon of ***damage maturation*** is complex, as many variables contribute to determining the outcome. The phenomenon is also redundant in the sense that the same result or biochemical process (e.g., cytokine production) can be achieved through different pathways. Mechanisms promoting cell death are accompanied by compensatory mechanisms. The distinction between ***damage and protection mechanisms*** is often ambiguous. In fact, the same phenomenon (e.g., glutamatergic stimulation of NMDA receptors or microglia activation) can induce biochemical processes that seemingly operate in opposite directions. A key point of endogenous neuroprotection concerns the role of ***peripheral organs***. Trophic factors such as EPO and IGF1 are produced by peripheral organs and reach the brain through residual circulation or reperfusion. Physical exercise stimulates the production of trophic factors (VEGF, BDNF) and promotes hippocampal neurogenesis. This endogenous neuroprotection can potentially be utilized for therapeutic or rehabilitative purposes. Mild ischemic stimuli induce ischemic tolerance. Tolerance can be early (minutes) or delayed (typically 12-72 hours) and can be produced by local stimuli (e.g., brief hypoxia or mild cerebral ischemia) or systemic stimuli (e.g., brief periods of mild ischemia to a limb). The stimulus is effective if applied before (pre-conditioning) or after (post-conditioning) the ischemic event. Much of the data on ischemic tolerance comes from laboratory animals. However, it is reasonable to assume that pre-conditioning could be used in individuals at high risk of stroke, while *post-conditioning* might (there are ongoing trials) be beneficial if applied during the acute phase of stroke.

13.3.3 Etiopathogenesis

There are three main etiopathogenetic subgroups of ischemic stroke: atherothrombotic (30-40% of cases), cardioembolic (30-40%), and lacunar (approximately 25%).

An ischemic stroke is classified as atherothrombotic when it is caused by atherosclerotic pathology affecting the arterial district, either carotid or vertebrobasilar, corresponding to the site of the stroke. Specifically, concerning the carotid district, a significant atheromatous plaque that reduces the lumen of the extracranial internal carotid artery by at least 50% up to occlusion is considered relevant. Plaques affecting the vertebral arteries are usually located at their origin from the subclavian arteries, and there is no specific critical stenosis value indicated. Atherothrombotic stroke originates from complications within the plaque (intraplaque hemorrhage with protrusion into the vessel lumen or ulceration of its surface) that occlude the vessel in the extracranial segment or embolize plaque fragments and platelet aggregates (arterioembolic stroke). Occlusion of the intracranial segment of the internal carotid artery and its branches is rarely caused by in situ thrombosis in Caucasian patients, less rarely in Asians or African Americans. Basilar artery occlusion due to in situ thrombosis is relatively frequent. Basilar artery thrombosis can involve its branches through either an ostial steno-occlusion or an artero-arterial embolism mechanism, similar to what has been described for the carotid district.

Cardioembolic stroke, as the term implies, results from the displacement of thrombotic material from the cardiac chambers into the intracerebral arteries, typically the left atrium in patients with atrial fibrillation. Less frequently, other mentioned pathological cardiac conditions are implicated as risk factors (see chapter on risk factors). Additionally, the role of plaques in the aortic arch is highlighted, particularly when they protrude into the vessel lumen by at least 4 mm and exhibit an irregular surface due to ulceration.

Lacunar stroke is caused by intrinsic pathology (lipohyalinosis or microatheroma) of the small intracerebral arteries, perforating branches originating from the middle cerebral artery or the basilar artery, often resulting from hypertension, diabetes, and/or hypercholesterolemia. These lesions have a diameter ranging from 1 to 15 mm and are generally located in the putamen, globus pallidus, thalamus, caudate nucleus, internal capsule, corona radiata, or pons. Larger lacunes may have a cardioembolic origin.

Rarely, the underlying pathogenic mechanism of stroke is hemodynamic in nature. In these cases, the lesions are located in the so-called "border zones," which are the border territories between the middle cerebral artery and the anterior cerebral artery or between the middle cerebral artery and the posterior cerebral artery, or between deep branches and deep branches of the superficial branches of the middle cerebral artery (internal "borderzone"). These areas receive reduced collateral flow. In the case of internal carotid artery stenosis/occlusion associated with a marked reduction in systemic blood pressure, these areas experience critical perfusion reduction and may sustain damage.

A minority of strokes are attributable to arterial dissection, prothrombotic mutations of coagulation factors, or other rare genetic disorders. Events that cannot be attributed to the described causes are classified as cryptogenic. Their incidence is higher in young patients and decreases in the elderly, accounting for up to 25-30% of cases.

13.3.4 Clinical aspects

Clinically, there is no way to distinguish an atherothrombotic stroke from a cardioembolic one. The more gradual onset of symptoms in the former case and a more rapid onset in the latter are not reliable indicators, considering that an arterioembolic mechanism can also underlie symptoms in the case of an atherothrombotic stroke.

Depending on the affected arterial district, different clinical pictures can be distinguished.

In the case of extracranial internal carotid artery occlusion, a clue is transient or permanent amaurosis (blindness of the eye corresponding to the occluded carotid, as the ophthalmic artery is the first branch originating from the internal carotid artery).

The clinical presentation of internal carotid artery occlusion is otherwise indistinguishable from that of middle cerebral artery occlusion unless good intracranial collateral circulation limits the damage to the "border zones" only.

Complete occlusion of the middle cerebral artery presents with conjugate gaze deviation towards the affected hemisphere, contralateral hemiplegia and hemianesthesia, homonymous hemianopsia on the side of hemiplegia, global aphasia if the dominant hemisphere is involved. Neglect, a tendency to ignore the hemiplegic side, can occur in the acute phase due to lesions in both the dominant and non-dominant hemispheres but tends to persist only in the latter case. Young patients with lesions encompassing the entire territory of the middle cerebral artery may undergo herniation of the affected hemisphere towards the brainstem with fatal consequences (malignant middle cerebral artery infarction) and may benefit from decompressive craniotomy. In the presence of good collateral circulation protecting the cortical structures, complete occlusion of the middle cerebral artery can lead to infarction of the basal ganglia alone, which can also result from embolic occlusion of the lenticulostriate arteries (striatocapsular infarction). The lesion manifests as a sensory-motor deficit, sometimes associated with cortical symptoms that tend to resolve in the following days. Occlusion of the main branches of the middle cerebral artery gives rise to partial clinical syndromes. Occlusion of the upper branches causes conjugate gaze deviation, hemiparesis, hemisensory syndrome, and, if the dominant hemisphere is involved, motor or expressive aphasia with preserved comprehension. Occlusion of the lower branches causes sensory-motor deficits, and in the case of dominant hemisphere involvement, fluent or receptive aphasia (the patient produces meaningless language without awareness or comprehension). Occlusion of the distal branches of the middle cerebral artery can lead to isolated motor or sensory deficits, which are difficult to distinguish from lacunar syndromes, or isolated cortical deficits.

The occlusion of the anterior cerebral artery is less common than that of the middle cerebral artery and presents with contralateral monoparesis of the lower limb. In some cases, there may be motor neglect, apraxia, and sometimes even transcortical motor aphasia characterized by limited verbal initiative.

The occlusion of the anterior choroidal artery results in faciobrachiocrural hemiparesis, hemi-hypoesthesia, and often reversible hemianopsia.

The occlusion of the posterior cerebral artery can lead to isolated hemianopsia. If the lesion is parieto-occipital, visual neglect may coexist. In the case of involvement of the thalamus or the posteromedial temporal regions, confusion, aphasia, mnemonic deficits, particularly affecting the processes of memorizing new traces, may be present. The two posterior cerebral arteries can be simultaneously affected

Table 13.1 ALTERNATING SYNDROMES

Anatomical site and name	Homolateral symptoms	Contralateral symptoms	Frequency
	BULBAR SYNDROMES		
Paramedian bulbar syndrome Dejerine syndrome	- Paralysis of the XII cranial nerve with lingual atrophy	- Hemiparesis or hemiplegia	Very rare
Lateral bulbar syndrome Wallenberg syndrome	- Thermopainful facial hemianesthesia - Bernard-Horner syndrome - Ataxia - Pharyngo-laryngo-palatal paralysis	- Thermopainful hemisomal anesthesia	Highly frequent
Extensive lateral bulbar syndrome Babinski-Nageotte syndrome	- Thermopainful facial hemianesthesia - Bernard-Horner syndrome - Ataxia - Pharyngo-laryngo-palatal paralysis associated with paralysis of the VI-VII, XI cranial nerves	- Thermopainful hemisomal anesthesia with hemiparesis	Highly frequent
Partial lateral bulbar syndrome Avellis syndrome	- Pharyngo-laryngo-palatal paralysis associated with sternocleidomastoid and trapezius paralysis - Thermopainful facial hemianesthesia - Ataxia	- Thermopainful anesthesia - Hemisomal anesthesia	Highly frequent
	PONTINE SYNDROMES		
Ventral pontine syndrome of the caudal third Millard-Gubler Syndrome	- Deficit of the VII and VI cranial nerves	Hemiparesis or hemiplegia	Frequent
Ventral pontine syndrome of the middle and rostral thirds Paramedian pontine syndrome	- Paraparesis or paraplegia - Tetraparesis or tetraplegia		Rare
Tegmental pontine syndrome of the caudal third Lower foville syndrome or Foville-Millard-Gubler syndrome	- Deficit of the VII and VI cranial nerves; lateral gaze palsy	Hemiparesis or hemiplegia	Frequent
Tegmental pontine syndrome of the middle third Alternate sensory syndrome or Grenet syndrome	- Global or thermopainful facial anesthesia - Occasionally paralysis of masticatory muscles	Hemisomal thermopainful anesthesia	Rare
Tegmental pontine syndrome of the rostral third: Superior foville syndrome or Raymond-Cestan syndrome	- Conjugate lateral gaze palsy - Hemiataxia, hemiasynergy - Choreoathetotic movements	Hypoesthesia (superficial and deep) hemisoma Ataxia	Frequent
Tegmental pontine syndrome of the rostral third: Superior cerebellar artery syndrome	- Ataxia - Bernard-Horner syndrome - Tremor or rhythmic myoclonus	Hypoesthesia (thermopainful or global), hypoacusia or deafness	Rare
Lateral pontine syndrome Marie-Foix syndrome	- Ataxia	Hemiparesis hypoesthesia (thermopainful) hemisoma	Very rare
	MESENCEPHALIC SYNDROMES		
Ventral mesencephalic syndrome Weber syndrome	- Paralysis of the III cranial nerve	Hemiparesis or hemiplegia	Frequent
Ventral tegmental syndrome Benedikt syndrome or inferior red nucleus syndrome	- Paralysis of the III cranial nerve	Hemiparesis, involuntary movements/ataxia	Rare
Inferior colliculus syndrome Superior cerebellar artery syndrome	- Ataxia - Bernard-Horner syndrome - Tremor or rhythmic myoclonus	Hypoesthesia (thermopainful or global), hypoacusia or deafness	Rare
Superior colliculus syndrome Parinaud syndrome	- Conjugate vertical ocular paralysis (upward or downward)		Frequent

in the occlusion of the apex of the basilar artery, causing cortical blindness.

In the case of occlusion of the vertebral artery, there is often an infarction affecting the lateral medullary fossa, supplied by the posterior inferior cerebellar artery originating from the vertebral artery. This results in the so-called Wallenberg syndrome, characterized in its complete form by miosis, enophthalmos, pseudo-ptosis of the eyelid, and anhidrosis of the half of the face (Bernard-Horner syndrome), nystagmus, limb ataxia, soft palate and vocal cord paralysis, and thermo-dolorific hypoesthesia of the ipsilateral face to the infarction, associated with thermo-dolorific hypoesthesia of the contralateral hemisoma (alternate syndrome, i.e., involvement of one side of the head and the opposite side of the rest of the body).

The occlusion of the posterior inferior cerebellar artery can spare the branches destined for the medulla and result in an infarction of the lower part of the cerebellum, manifesting as isolated vertigo.

The occlusion of a vertebral artery can also lead to more extensive infarctions affecting the brainstem or the cerebellum, giving rise to more complex syndromic pictures, such as those following steno-occlusive pathology of the basilar artery.

Complete occlusion of the basilar artery can manifest with dramatic acute-onset clinical pictures, such as a coma state (due to lesion of the ascending reticular formation) or tetraparesis or tetraplegia with preserved only ocular motility (locked-in syndrome). Occlusion of the apex of the artery, instead, determines often bilateral lesions in the territories of the superior cerebellar arteries, posterior cerebral arteries, and thalamoperforating arteries originating from them. Bilateral thalamic infarction causes a marked reduction in the level of consciousness. In these cases, a strong auditory or painful stimulus is necessary to obtain a short-lived purposeful response from the patient, with a return to a drowsy state as soon as the stimulus ends. Occlusion of the perforating branches of the basilar artery causes syndromic pictures involving cranial nerve nuclei and long motor, sensory, or spinocerebellar pathways, known as "alternate syndromes" (Table 13.1).

Lacunar stroke tends to manifest with stereotyped syndromic pictures. The most frequent syndromes are as follows: a) pure motor stroke (pure motor deficit, with faciobrachial or faciobrachiocrural distribution); b) pure sensory stroke; c) sensory-motor stroke; d) ataxic hemiparesis, which includes the clumsy hand-dysarthria syndrome; e) homolateral ataxia-crural paresis syndrome.

13.4 Transient ischemic attack

For a long time, TIA has been distinguished from stroke, but in recent years, a continuum between the two conditions has been recognized. The etiopathogenesis of TIA overlaps with that of stroke. The clinical presentations are also similar, with unilateral motor and/or sensory deficits with or without dysarthria and/or aphasia in a carotid territory TIA, and with diplopia, hemianopsia, balance disturbances, bilateral motor and/or sensory deficits with or without dysarthria in a vertebrobasilar territory TIA. Even transient monocular blindness (amaurosis fugax), often described as a "curtain" covering the eye for a few minutes, can be a TIA affecting the retinal vessels. What differentiates TIA from stroke is the duration of symptoms, which are transient in TIA and persistent in stroke. According to the definition given by the World Health Organization (WHO), a diagnosis of TIA can be made when the symptoms completely disappear within 24 hours of onset. However, clinical studies have shown that in over 60% of cases, the symptoms are completely resolved within 60 minutes of onset. In addition to the transient nature of the symptoms, the definition of TIA requires that no visible lesions be observed on neuroimaging. The increasingly frequent use of sophisticated neuroimaging techniques, such as Magnetic Resonance Imaging (MRI), has revealed that in 50-60% of clinically definable TIA cases (symptom regression within 24 hours), MRI identifies small infarcts consistent with the symptoms. This observation led the American Stroke Association to propose a new definition of TIA as a "transient episode of neurologic deficit caused by cerebral, spinal, or retinal ischemia without acute infarction".

Table 13.2 EARLY RECURRENT RISK SCORE IN PATIENTS WITH TIA – ABCD2

Variable	Value	Score
Age	≥ 60 years < 60 years	1 0
Blood pressure at admission	Systolic > 140 and/or diastolic > 90	1
Clinical presentation	Unilateral motor deficit Language disturbance with/without weakness Other	2 1 0
Duration of symptoms	≥ 60 min 10-59 min < 10 min	2 1 0
History of diabetes	Yes No	1 0

The total score ranges from 0 to 7. A score ≥ 4 indicates a moderate-high risk of TIA or stroke recurrence within 2-90 days.

The duration of symptoms is also an important prognostic indicator for the risk of early recurrence. In fact, a risk score called ABCD2 (Age, Blood Pressure, Clinical Picture, Diabetes, Duration of symptoms) (Table 13.2), has been developed, which allows for quantifying the risk of recurrence within the next 48 hours (up to 8%), 7 days (up to 12%), and the following month (up to 19%). This score can be used to decide whether or not to hospitalize a patient with TIA. The occurrence of multiple episodes within a few days should also prompt hospitalization and the search for a potential embolic arterial or cardiac source. Less frequently, hemodynamic mechanisms are involved, such as in the case of the so-called "subclavian steal syndrome," where stenosis of the subclavian artery before the origin of the vertebral artery diverts blood to the arm through the vertebral artery in an antidromic direction, "stealing" blood from the posterior circulation and causing vertebrobasilar TIA.

The diagnosis of TIA is certain when the physician has the opportunity to witness the disappearance of symptoms and neurological signs. Often, it is the patient or those around them who recount the event, so the diagnosis is based on the likelihood of reported symptoms. In this regard, a disturbance in strength and/or language is more indicative of a TIA diagnosis, while isolated sensory or visual disturbances may have a different nature. It is important to note that a diagnosis of TIA is not correct when the symptoms listed in Table 13.3 occur in isolation.

Table 13.3 SYMPTOMS THAT DO NOT ALLOW DIAGNOSIS OF TIA WHEN PRESENTED IN ISOLATION

- Loss of consciousness
- Feeling of instability
- Generalized fatigue
- Mental confusion
- Loss/decrease of vision associated with decreased level of consciousness
- Bowel and bladder incontinence
- Vertigo
- Diplopia
- Dysphagia
- Loss of balance
- Tinnitus
- Sensory symptoms confined to a part of a limb or the face
- Scintillating scotomas
- Amnesia
- Drop attack*

*Sudden falling to the ground, while maintaining an upright position or during walking, without loss or suspension of consciousness. The drop attack is a symptom, not a diagnosis, with an undefined cause in two-thirds of cases, while the remaining cases are of cardiogenic (a variant of syncope), critical, vestibular, or psychodynamic origin.

13.5 Transient global amnesia (TGA)

TGA is characterized by anterograde amnesia lasting several hours, during which the patient appears disoriented and confused, continuously asking "Where am I?" and "What is happening?" while maintaining awareness of self and identity. The pathophysiology of TGA is not clear, but it does not fall within the field of TIAs nor does it entail an increased risk of stroke. However, rare cases with ischemic lesions or transient epileptic amnesia have been observed. MRI studies in patients

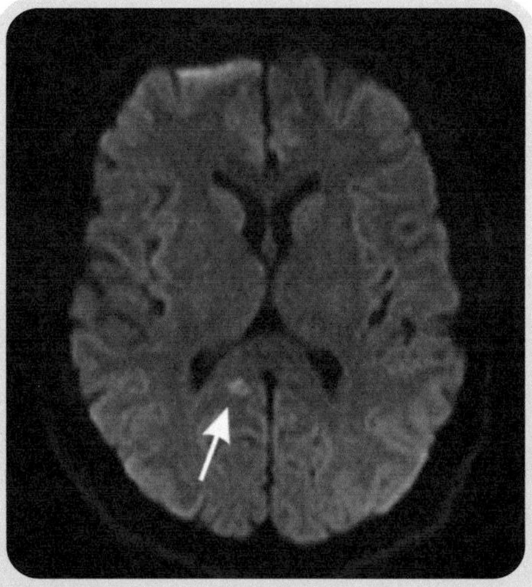

Figure 13.3

Episode of transient global amnesia with ictal etiology. A 53-year-old patient underwent angiography for stenosis of the left vertebral artery V2-V3 segment. Upon returning from the angiography room, the patient experienced confusion, temporal-spatial disorientation, and amnestic gaps related to the day, with complete recovery after a few hours. MRI reveals an acute ischemic lesion of approximately 6 mm in the right temporo-mesial region (arrow).

experiencing TGA have shown reversible signal hyperintensity in diffusion-weighted sequences in the temporomesial structures, suggesting a transient metabolic stress of the hippocampal neurons without structural sequelae. Nevertheless, it is still advisable to subject these patients to neuroimaging and screening for vascular risk factors (Figure 13.3).

13.5.1 Differential diagnosis

The sudden onset of symptoms and rapid attainment of maximal deficit strongly suggest a clinical suspicion of stroke. A more gradual onset and progressive worsening of symptoms over several days, on the other hand, favor alternative diagnoses such as neoplasm or chronic subdural hematoma, although a neoplasm, particularly a metastasis, can present with an acute focal deficit. The presence of fever may suggest an infectious pathology that has caused inflammation and destabilization of a carotid atherosclerotic plaque, endocarditis leading to septic embolic stroke, or simply reactive hyperthermia following the stroke, especially if the lesion is extensive. However, fever also requires differential diagnosis with viral encephalitis or cerebral abscess. The predominant presence of a confusional state or a clinical history of chronic infection, particularly involving the inner ear, can indicate encephalitis or abscess.

In young patients, an alternative hypothesis could be multiple sclerosis, which can be differentially diagnosed clinically if there is a history of monocular visual loss lasting a few days (retrobulbar optic neuritis) and/or if the neurological deficit simultaneously involves different parts of the central nervous system (spatial dissemination). The differential diagnosis is more challenging (and possible only with neuroimaging) when the deficit is isolated and of a sensory and/or motor nature, whether truncal or cerebellar. In young patients with stroke, intense headache, localized laterocervical/retro-orbital or retronuchal, should raise suspicion of arterial dissection, respectively carotid or vertebral. The presence of Horner's syndrome favors the diagnosis of extracranial carotid dissection. However, headache can be present in a variable percentage of cases (10-40% in carotid territory strokes, 20-70% in vertebrobasilar territory strokes), even in the absence of arterial dissection. Regarding TIA, the differential diagnosis should consider migraine attacks, especially when visual aura is not followed by headache, mimicking a retinal or vertebrobasilar TIA. Migraine is supported by the presence of an aura, often characterized by "positive" phenomena such as scintillating scotoma, photopsia, or paresthesia. Additionally, in migraine, symptoms evolve slowly, taking several minutes for visual disturbances to reach their maximum or for sensory disturbances to spread from the hand to the face. When a transient focal deficit tends to recur several times within a few days or within the same day, and in a stereotyped manner (i.e., always with the same clinical picture), an epileptic seizure should be considered. Epileptic seizures can manifest not only, as is frequently the case, with a paroxysmal increase in neurological function but also with a transient loss of function.

Another pathological condition that can cause stereotyped transient focal neurological deficits, known as "amyloid spells," is cerebral amyloid angiopathy with cortical siderosis, which involves the deposition of hemosiderin on the cerebral cortex, causing irritation.

Transient focal neurological deficits can also be caused by other central nervous system pathologies such as neoplasms or subdural hematomas, so it is always necessary to perform at least a brain CT when the possible conversion nature of the event has been ruled out. Occasionally, metabolic disorders can also give rise to transient focal deficits. This is the case with hypoglycemia and hyponatremia, the correction of which promptly normalizes the neurological picture.

13.5.2 Diagnostic-therapeutic pathway

The diagnostic-therapeutic pathway for patients with ischemic stroke consists of two phases:

a) Emergency phase: This phase includes the first 24 hours from symptom onset and aims to identify patients eligible for reperfusion therapies to salvage ischemic tissue that is not irreversibly damaged yet.
b) Urgency phase: This phase includes the following 48-72 hours from symptom onset and aims to identify the etiopathogenic mechanism underlying the stroke and the risk of recurrence in order to initiate targeted secondary prevention therapy.

Emergency phase | All patients should undergo an electrocardiogram (ECG), which can reveal atrial fibrillation or other arrhythmias, left ventricular hypertrophy due to hypertension, or acute myocardial infarction that may be concomitant with the stroke.

At the time of hospital admission, patients should also undergo standard blood tests, including:

a) Complete blood count, which can reveal leukocytosis (indicating an infectious condition or a stress response to the stroke), anemia (a potential marker of endocarditis), polycythemia, or thrombocytosis (known stroke risk factors), and thrombocytopenia (which could indicate a systemic disease or antiphospholipid antibody syndrome). Rarely, leukemias or lymphomas can cause a stroke.
b) Kidney function tests and electrolytes, which can indicate organ damage due to hypertension. Any electrolyte abnormalities that may cause focal or global neurological deficits should be promptly corrected.
c) Blood glucose levels, as hypoglycemia can mimic a stroke, while hyperglycemia can worsen its course and also serve as a risk factor for hemorrhagic transformation in patients undergoing thrombolytic therapy.
d) International Normalized Ratio (INR) and liver enzymes, which are indicators of normal liver function. For patients on prior oral anticoagulant therapy (OAT), it is necessary to know the INR value to assess whether the stroke is a result of inadequate OAT administration.

Neuroimaging can provide essential information on the extent of damage and the presence of salvageable ischemic tissue. Computed Tomography (CT) is the most commonly used neuroimaging modality in hospitals. It can easily differentiate between ischemic stroke, cerebral hemorrhage, subdural hematoma, or neoplasm. Furthermore, it can detect early signs of ischemia that result from cytotoxic edema present in the initial stages of stroke, and are more or less visible depending on the extent of ischemia and on time interval from stroke onset to imaging. These signs include the obscuration of the lentiform nucleus, loss of cortical definition in the insula, and compression of cortical sulci. Early signs involving more than one-third of the middle cerebral artery territory (Figure 13.4), or resulting in an Alberta Stroke Program Early CT Score (ASPECTS) score <7 (Figure 13.5), predict extensive infarction and a high risk of mortality, residual disability, and hemorrhagic transformation in case of intravenous thrombolysis. However, these signs are not contraindications to thrombolysis. Another early sign detectable on CT is hyperdensity of the middle cerebral

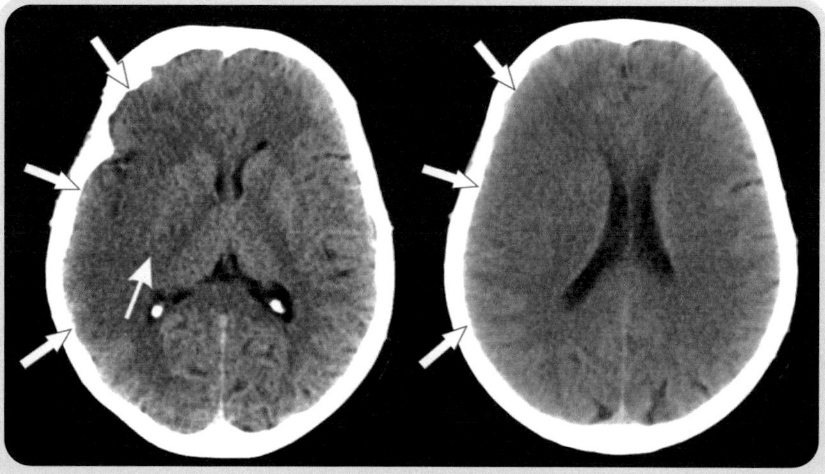

Figure 13.4

Early Signs of Cerebral Infarction. A 64-year-old patient with a sudden fall to the ground due to left hemiplegia with deviation of the head and gaze to the right. Brain CT scan shows flattening of cortical sulci in the right hemisphere and reduced representation of the right lentiform nucleus compared to the contralateral side (arrows).

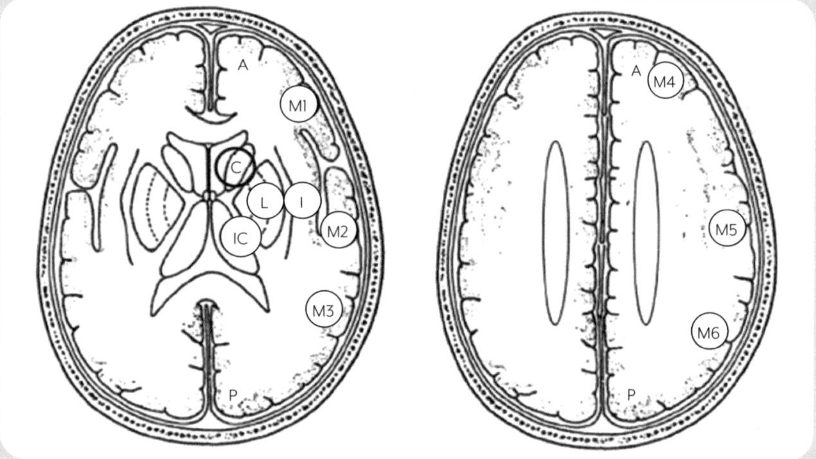

Figure 13.5

Schematic Representation of ASPECTS. C = caudate nucleus; IC = internal capsule; L = lentiform nucleus; I = insular cortex; M1-M6 = cortical sulci. Total absence of early signs = 10. Subtract 1 for each location of an early sign.
Score > 7 = non-extended early signs (<1/3 of ACM territory). Score ≤ 7 = extended early signs (>1/3 of ACM territory) with a high risk of death/disability at 3 months and of symptomatic hemorrhage.

artery, or of intracranial carotid bifurcation, or of basilar artery, indicative of an occlusive thrombus. CT can demonstrate already damaged brain tissue and quantify its extent, but it cannot visualize salvageable ischemic tissue. This information can be provided by Perfusion CT (CTp), which uses computer algorithms to differentiate between irreversibly damaged tissue (reduced flow and volume) and salvageable tissue (reduced flow but increased volume compensating for hypoperfusion). However, CTp is not yet standardized and widely available.

Conventional MRI with spin-echo sequences is no more sensitive than CT in identifying acute ischemic lesions. However, Diffusion-Weighted (DW) sequences are highly sensitive as they are based on the mobility of water molecules. In stroke, water mobility is reduced partly due to water displacement (resulting from alterations in the Na+/K+ pump) from the extracellular to the intracellular compartment where organelles and macromolecules restrict its movement, and partly due to neuronal swelling, which reduces interstitial space and hinders the movement of extracellular water. These factors lead to increased signal intensity, appearing white against the gray background of the surrounding parenchyma, and are visible within the first 15-30 minutes from symptom onset. The hyperintense area on DW is considered indicative of irreversible damage, although some studies have reported partial reductions in the final infarct area compared to the initially hyperintense area on DW. The hyperintensity on DW diminishes over time but remains visible up to two to four weeks after the ischemic event. Non-acute hyperintensities on DW can be differentiated from acute ones based on Apparent Diffusion

Coefficient (ADC) sequences (■ Figure 13.6 and 13.7). The reduction in ADC, present in the first few days after stroke onset, results in a hypointense signal appearing black against the gray background of the remaining parenchyma. Later, with the occurrence of massive necrosis leading to increased extracellular water, the ADC signal tends to increase and become higher than that of healthy tissue, resulting in hyperintensity. As time passes, the ischemic area tends to become hypointense on DW sequences while maintaining hyperintensity on ADC maps. Perfusion Weighted Imaging (PWI) sequences provide information on the regional reduction of cerebral blood flow secondary to arterial occlusion. The combination of DW and PWI sequences has led to the concept of a "mismatch," referring to the portion of brain tissue that appears non-hyperintense on DW but shows reduced blood flow on PWI, grossly corresponding to the ischemic penumbra (■ Figure 13.8).

For the selection of patients eligible for intravenous thrombolysis, knowledge of arterial occlusion and its location is not essential. However, it becomes crucial when considering intra-arterial revascularization interventions. CT angiography (CTA), with the possibility of 3D reconstruction, is a highly sensitive technique that uses contrast media to assess intra- and extracranial vascular patency. Triphasic CTA, with the first phase from the aortic arch to the vertex and the second and third phases from the base of the skull to the vertex, can reveal the presence of collateral circulation in the case of large vessel occlusion. Currently, CTA, preferably triphasic, is a standard examination for all patients with ischemic stroke identified by CT. Magnetic resonance angiography (MRA)

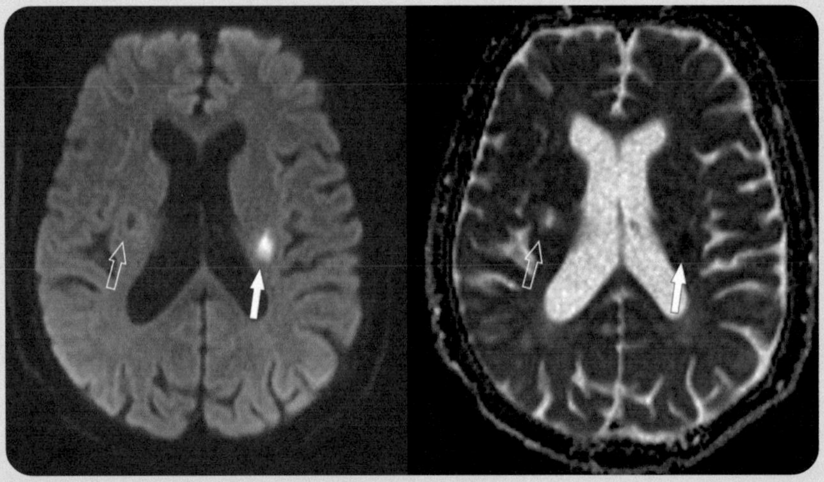

Figure 13.6

Acute ischemic injury and chronic injury on DWI and ADC MRI. 57-year-old patient with sudden onset of speech impairment and right hemisoma weakness. The MRI shows an acute ischemic lesion of approximately 1 cm in the white matter of the left-sided centrum semiovale, appearing hyperintense on DW sequences (left, white arrow) and hypointense on ADC maps (right, white arrow). In the contralateral white matter, a chronic ischemic lesion is evident, appearing hypointense on DW sequences (empty arrow) and hyperintense on ADC maps (empty arrow).

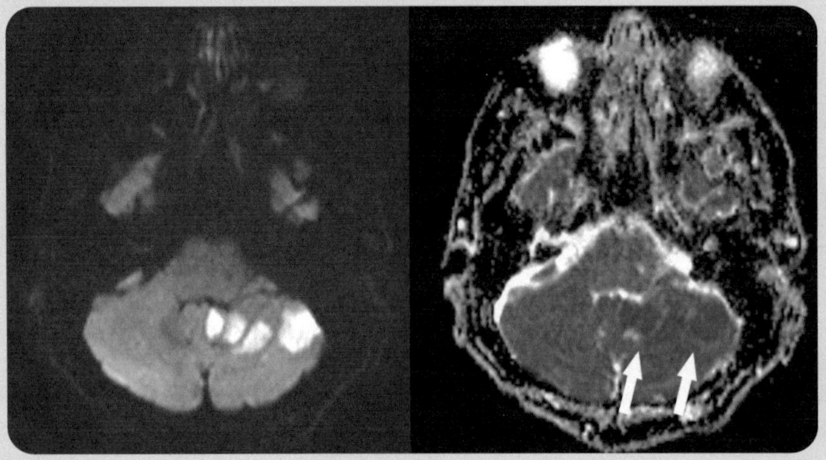

Figure 13.7

Subacute ischemic lesion on DW and ADC MRI. 61-year-old patient, smoker, hypertensive, with a history of myocardial infarction. Sudden onset of dizziness, vomiting, and ataxia. Brain MRI, performed one week after symptom onset, shows a subacute ischemic lesion, markedly hyperintense on DW sequences (left), weakly hypointense on ADC maps (right), involving the nodular flocculus and the basal corticosubcortical portion of the left cerebellar hemisphere.

Figure 13.8

DW/PW Mismatch. A 49-year-old patient, a smoker. Sudden onset of amaurosis in the right eye, followed by left-sided limb weakness, deviation of the head and gaze to the right, and a somnolent state. Brain MRI shows an acute ischemic lesion in the right frontobasal region in the DW sequences (on the left), and in the PW sequences (on the right) it shows an extensive area of hypoperfusion that extends beyond the boundaries of the lesion, defining a large PW/DW mismatch.

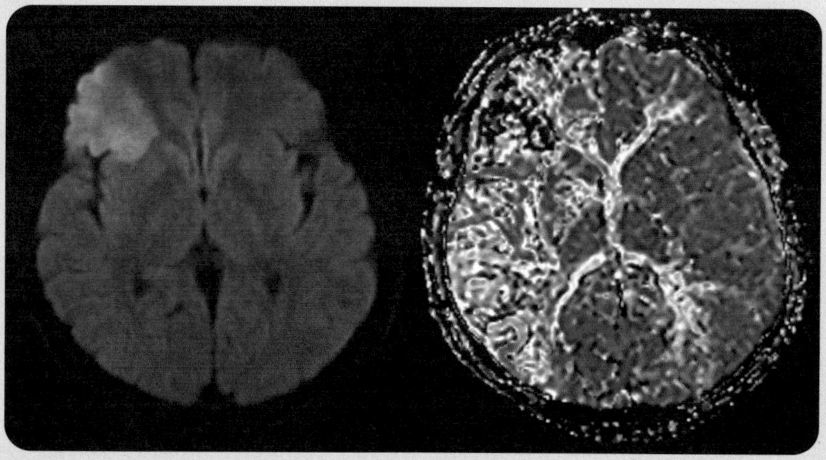

can be performed with or without contrast media, using *time-of-flight* (TOF) sequences. TOF-MRA is based on the magnitude of blood flow through the examined artery, and in the case of low flow due to significant stenosis, it may overestimate the clinical picture and give the appearance of occlusion (Figure 13.9). Other limitations of this technique include the time required (several minutes) for image acquisition, which requires patient cooperation and stillness, limited spatial resolution of peripheral branches of the middle cerebral artery, and suboptimal visualization of vascular branches in elderly patients. In some cases, catheter-based angiography, usually from the femoral artery, is necessary to clarify diagnostic uncertainties not resolved by CTA or MRA, and is essential for performing intra-arterial revascularization. However, since this approach carries risks (toxic effects of contrast media, possibility of thrombus fragmentation along the catheter path, risk of arterial dissection), the use of catheter-based angiography should be justified and not solely used for diagnostic purposes. Patients undergoing DWI and PWI MRI in the acute phase should also undergo MRA to identify possible large vessel occlusions.

Transcranial Doppler (TCD) is a non-invasive ultrasound technique that measures the velocity and direction of blood flow in the proximal portion of major intracranial arteries, allowing the detection of stenosis or occlusion in the carotid siphon, proximal middle cerebral artery (M1) segment, intracranial vertebral arteries, proximal basilar artery, and proximal posterior cerebral artery (P1) segment. Color Doppler TCD (Color DTC) also allows visualization of intracranial vessels and any stenosis or occlusions.

Figure 13.9

TOF MR Angiography and T1 Contrast-enhanced MR Imaging of MCA Stenosis. 36-year-old patient. Sudden onset of aphasia and right faciobrachial-crural hemiparesis. TOF MR angiography (left) reveals occlusion of the middle cerebral artery at the M2 segment with no visualization of distal branches (arrow). T1-weighted MR sequences with gadolinium (right) demonstrate non-occlusive stenosis of the MCA (arrow).

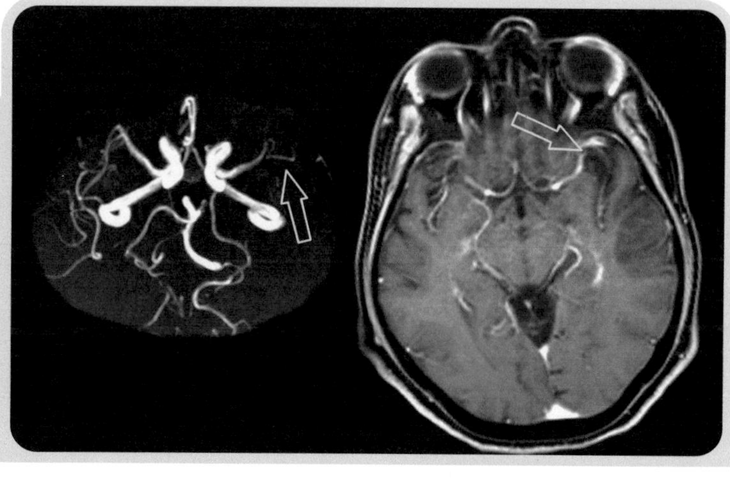

Urgency phase | In this phase, blood tests support etiopathogenetic hypotheses and help define the cardiovascular risk profile. The following tests are performed:

a) Erythrocyte sedimentation rate (ESR), C-reactive protein (CRP), and possible autoantibodies in the case of suspected vasculitis.
b) Blood cultures for suspected endocarditis or presence of infectious complications.
c) Cholesterol and triglyceride levels should be measured in all patients.
d) Thyroid hormone assays, particularly in patients with atrial fibrillation.
e) Toxicological investigations (blood and urine) if substance abuse is suspected.
f) Lumbar puncture when an infectious etiology is suspected.

Neuroimaging should determine the location and extent of the infarcted area and detect the presence of hemorrhagic transformation, which has significant prognostic implications. CT can show the lesion if it is larger than the resolution limit of the technique or if it is not within the context of marked leukoaraiosis. Conventional MRI reveals ischemic lesions as hyperintense areas on T2-weighted sequences. However, distinguishing them from pre-existing lesions, especially subcortical ones in the context of chronic vascular disease of the white matter, requires the use of DWI sequences. Secondary hemorrhagic transformation, characterized by variable amounts of blood ranging from petechiae to hematoma (spontaneous or resulting from thrombolytic or anticoagulant therapy), can be visualized on both CT and MRI (Figure 13.10). MRI, particularly with GRE sequences, can also detect micro hemorrhagic transformatuins that are not visible on CT. CT or MRI allows for morphological classification of infarcts as lacunar or non-lacunar, and in the latter case, it helps define the affected arterial territory and the extent of the damage, which has prognostic implications in terms of mortality and residual disability. The etiopathogenetic classification of non-lacunar infarcts as atherothrombotic/atheroembolic or cardioembolic requires further instrumental investigations.

Doppler, possibly combined with Color Doppler, allows the detection of steno-occlusive pathologies in extracranial arteries. The presence of a stenotic carotid atheromatous plaque narrowing the vascular lumen classifies the stroke as atherothrombotic/atheroembolic and indicates the need for endarterectomy or carotid stenting as secondary prevention. Similarly, vertebral artery steno-occlusion allows for the classification of an infarct in the vertebrobasilar territory as atherothrombotic or atheroembolic, but surgical indications are lacking, and stenting may be considered. Doppler and Color Doppler can suggest arterial dissection as the cause of the stroke, which then needs to be confirmed with neuroimaging.

The absence of carotid or vertebral pathology or the presence of minimal nonsignificant wall alterations necessitates further cardiac investigations to determine if the stroke can be classified as cardioembolic. The presence of a history of atrial fibrillation, whether permanent or paroxysmal, even if not present at the onset of the stroke, automatically leads to this

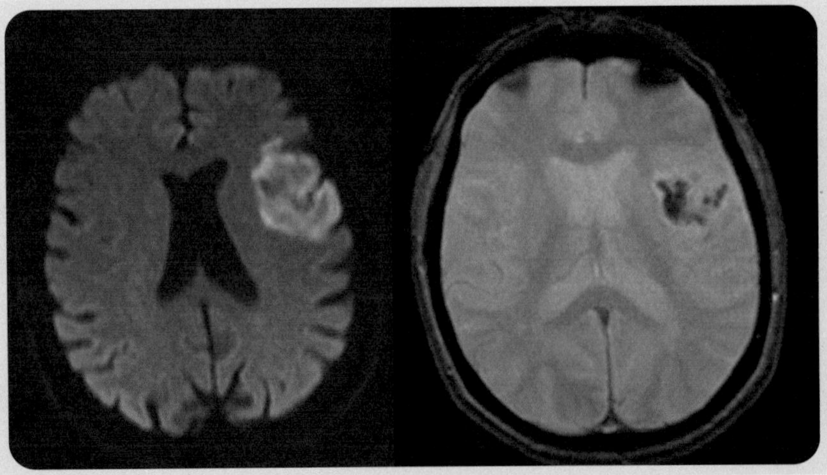

Figure 13.10

Hemorrhagic infarction due to ischemic lesion on MRI. A 74-year-old patient with arterial hypertension and atrial fibrillation. Sudden onset of hyposthenia in the right limbs and aphasia. Underwent thrombolytic treatment with improvement of symptoms. The MRI shows a hyperintense and heterogeneous area in the left fronto-insular cortical region on DW sequences (on the left), with a clearly visible hemorrhagic infarction on gradient echo sequences (on the right).

classification. In patients with a positive history of cardiac pathology (e.g., previous myocardial infarction), transthoracic echocardiography (TTE) is sufficient to detect potentially embolic conditions such as wall hypo-akinesia of the left ventricle and/or interventricular septum, significantly reduced ejection fraction, or the presence of intraventricular thrombi. Transesophageal echocardiography (TEE) is more sensitive than TTE in detecting potentially embolic conditions such as valvular vegetations, the presence of thrombi in the atrial or left atrium, or atheromatous plaques in the aortic arch. TEE is also essential for detecting the presence of a patent foramen ovale in young patients with cryptogenic stroke, possibly after screening with TCD, which accurately identifies patients with right-to-left shunts. Additional diagnostic investigations for cryptogenic cases are indicated as listed in Table 13.4.

13.5.3 Therapy

Therapies can be distinguished between those in the acute phase, aimed at preserving and potentially reperfusing the ischemic penumbra tissue, and those for secondary prevention, to be implemented in the immediate hours following the stroke.

Acute phase

Stroke Unit. Randomized clinical *trials* comparing the outcomes of stroke patients admitted to specialized units dedicated to cerebrovascular pathology (*stroke units*) versus those admitted to regular wards have unequivocally demonstrated the superior effectiveness of stroke units in reducing mortality and residual disability. The effectiveness of stroke units is not related to a specific therapy but to a care model, namely, admission to a dedicated area staffed by medical and nursing personnel exclusively devoted to stroke care, with the assistance of equipment for continuous monitoring of vital parameters such as blood pressure, heart rate and rhythm, oxygen saturation, and temperature. This allows for patient stabilization and timely prevention or treatment of complications that can negatively impact clinical outcomes.

Blood pressure. In the acute phase of ischemic stroke, particular attention should be given to blood pressure. Elevated blood pressure is observed in patients with and without a history of hypertension, due to a neurohumoral stress response or in the case of extensive lesions causing increased intracranial pressure. Since cerebral perfusion pressure is determined by the ratio of systemic pressure to intracranial pressure, if the latter increases, systemic pressure needs to increase to maintain a constant perfusion pressure. Generally, it is unnecessary and not recommended to treat arterial hypertension in the acute phase of ischemic stroke unless systolic blood pressure exceeds 200 mmHg and/or diastolic blood pressure exceeds 120 mmHg. However, arterial hypertension should be treated even if values are lower if the patient requires intravenous thrombolysis or if they present with concomitant heart failure, acute myocardial infarction, or a concurrent aortic dissection, which are hypertensive emergencies requiring treatment regardless of the presence of stroke. In any case, abrupt reductions in blood pressure should be avoided as they can critically reduce perfusion pressure in the ischemic penumbra, where autoregulatory mechanisms are impaired. Therefore, rapid-acting drugs such as sublingual calcium antagonists should be avoided, and intravenous administration of medications like labetalol or urapidil should be preferred. Spontaneous hypotension in the acute phase of stroke is a rare occurrence, mostly observed in cases of concurrent cardiac disease or dehydration. It should be

Table 13.4 ADDITIONAL DIAGNOSTIC INVESTIGATIONS TO BE PERFORMED ONLY IN CASES OF CRYPTOGENIC STROKE*

- Antiphospholipid antibody
- Autoantibody search in the hypothesis of vasculitis
- Screening for mitochondrial mutations
- NOTCH III gene (CADASIL)
- Leukocyte galactosidase A assay and search for related mutation (Fabry disease)
- Homocysteine assay and search for MTHFR mutation
- Syphilis serology
- HIV serology
- Potentially prothrombotic coagulation factor mutations: Factor V Leiden, Factor II
- Anticoagulant protein assay: antithrombin III, protein C, protein S

* For clinical/anamnestic data suggestive of the type of investigation to be performed, refer to the respective paragraphs.

Table 13.5 MOST COMMON COMPLICATIONS IN STROKE PATIENT

Complication (Harmful effect)	Causes	Interventions
Respiratory: Hypoxemia	- Chronic bronchopulmonary disease; - Aspiration pneumonia; - Hypoventilation due to extensive hemisphere lesions with secondary compression on the brainstem or primary lesions of the brainstem; - Cardiac decompensation; - Pulmonary embolism; - Status epilepticus	- SatO2 monitoring; - Administration of O2: indicated for SatO2 values < 92%; - Treatment of underlying causes
Cardiac: 15%-40% of cases Rhythm disturbances: - Atrial fibrillation - Ventricular arrhythmias - Sudden death Cardiac decompensation Acute myocardial infarction	- Pre-existing coronary artery disease, even if asymptomatic; - Electrolyte abnormalities: hypokalemia; - Medications that prolong the QT interval; - Ischemic injury involving the insula (particularly on the right side)	- Cardiac monitoring; - Correction of hypokalemia; - Careful dosing of medications that affect the QT interval (seek alternatives); - Coronary angiography for possible angioplasty in the presence of significant increase in cardiac enzymes and ECG signs of STEMI
Hydro-electrolytic:		
Dehydration	Patients rescued hours after the onset of symptoms who have lost urine and/or vomited, without the possibility of compensating for fluid losses	0.9% saline solution or 10% glucose solution (avoid hypotonic solutions, such as 0.45% saline or 5% glucose, due to the risk of reducing plasma osmolality that promotes cerebral edema)
Electrolyte imbalance at entry	Rare: Elderly patients with heart, renal, or hepatic failure. Use of diuretics or antidepressants (particularly SSRIs), especially in combination or with ACE inhibitors or angiotensin receptor antagonists.	
Electrolyte imbalances during hospitalization	Most common during the first few days, generally hyponatremia and/or hypokalemia, favored by osmotic diuretics used for anti-edema purposes, or hypernatremia usually resulting from dehydration or a renal conservation mechanism triggered by osmotic diuretics.	
Glycemic metabolism		
Hyperglycemia: 20%-50% of cases	Stress reaction from acute event in diabetics (known or newly diagnosed) or non-diabetics, especially in the case of more extensive lesions or lesions involving the insula. Previous nutritional deficiencies.	Correct if > 180-200 mg/dl with insulin at adjusted doses based on capillary blood glucose levels
Hypoglycemia: rare in acute phase		Correct with 33% dextrose boluses, with the addition of thiamine 100 mg in known alcoholics to prevent Wernicke-Korsakoff syndrome
Hyperthermia: 40%-50% of cases (aggravating effect due to increased release of neurotoxic amino acids and cerebral edema)	- Previous infectious pathology before stroke (consider endocarditis); - Secondary infectious complication (respiratory, urinary); - Stress reaction from acute event	Antipyretics to maintain body temperature ≤ 37°C; Investigate underlying infectious causes based on clinical suspicion: chest X-ray, urine culture, blood culture, echocardiography. Targeted antibiotic therapy
Dysphagia: 40%-50% of cases leading to: malnutrition, immune defense alteration, risk of aspiration pneumonia	- Bulbar lesion (Wallenberg syndrome); - Supratentorial lesion in patients with previous chronic vascular compromise	Enteral feeding with nasogastric tube. In patients with bulbar lesions, consider percutaneous endoscopic gastrostomy (PEG)
Pressure ulcers	- Diabetes with possible chronic microcirculation impairment - Malnutrition - Pressure on support points on the mattress (sacrum, heels)	Changes in position at predetermined hourly intervals, air mattresses, early mobilization, early sitting out of bed

Complication (Harmful effect)	Causes	Interventions
- Deep Vein Thrombosis (DVT) - Cause of pulmonary embolism in 15%-30% of cases	- Obesity; - History of previous DVT	- Low molecular weight heparin subcutaneously at prophylactic dose, from the first day of admission in case of ischemic stroke, after 48-72 hours in case of hemorrhagic stroke; - Elastic stockings not indicated - Intermittent pneumatic compression
Pain		
Shoulder pain		- Early mobilization - Proper positioning of the paralyzed limb (supported by a cushion to prevent shoulder subluxation)
Neuropathic pain	Generally, thalamic lesion	- Nonsteroidal anti-inflammatory drugs (NSAIDs) - Tricyclic antidepressants (amitriptyline); - GABAergic drugs: gabapentin, pregabalin
Depression	- Reactive; - Organic, due to brain lesion	- Antidepressants; - Psychological support
Seizures: 3%-43% of cases	- Acute phase: release of excitotoxic amino acids from the ischemic core	Treat individual seizures
Status epilepticus (SE): 4%-10% of cases	- Subacute/chronic phase: epileptogenic structural changes	SE therapy
Epilepsy: 3%-4% of cases	- More frequent lesions involving the cerebral cortex	- Antiepileptic therapy: preferred; - Levetiracetam, topiramate

promptly corrected with fluid administration, discontinuation of any antihypertensive drugs, and sometimes the use of inotropic agents. The main complications of the acute phase of stroke are listed in Table 13.5.

Thrombolysis. Intravenous thrombolysis with tissue plasminogen activator (tPA) has significantly contributed to the transformation of clinical management in ischemic stroke. tPA is one of the proteins involved in coagulation homeostasis, it is produced by the endothelium and it activates plasminogen to plasmin, which attacks and lyses fibrin attached to the clot. Intravenous thrombolysis is effective and safe within 4.5 hours of symptom onset, with the possibility of extending the time window up to 9 hours in selected cases using advanced neuroimaging techniques (DWI and PWI-MRI or CTp). Even very elderly patients (over 80 years old) and severe cases benefit from this treatment. Contraindications to intravenous thrombolysis are limited to a few specific clinically identifiable conditions and neuroimaging findings (Table 13.6a).

Pharmacological intra-arterial thrombolysis has the advantage of delivering the thrombolytic drug directly to the occluding thrombus, allowing for lower doses. However, the efficacy and safety of this approach have been demonstrated only in a small number of patients treated within 6 hours of middle cerebral artery occlusion, making it a non-standard treatment.

Mechanical Thrombectomy (MT). Patients with large intracranial vessel occlusion are candidates for MT in combination with intravenous thrombolysis or as a standalone treatment if intravenous thrombolysis is contraindicated, within the first 4.5 -9 hours from symptom onset. Beyond 9 hours and up to 24 hours from the last time patients were seen/heard to be in good health, MT can be performed in selected patients using advanced neuroimaging techniques (DWI and PWI-MRI or CTp) (Table 13.6b). The need for angiographic suites and expert interventional neuroradiologists limits intra-arterial approaches to more specialized hospitals with appropriate infrastructure and organization, to which patients with indications for mechanical thrombectomy should be referred.

Antithrombotic Therapies. Aspirin, administered within 48 hours of the onset of ischemic stroke symptoms, prevents death or disability in one out of every 100 patients without a significant risk of systemic or cerebral hemorrhagic complications. Although the effect is modest compared to intravenous thrombolysis, if aspirin were administered to 80% of all patients affected by a first ischemic stroke, approximately 1,000 patients per year in Italy would be saved from death or disability.

Unfractionated heparin and low molecular weight heparins are not effective in improving the clinical outcome of patients with acute stroke and carry an increased risk of bleeding complications. Therefore, anticoagulants are not indicated for the treatment of acute ischemic stroke, even in cases of worsening symptoms in the first few days after the event (progressing stroke), as the main cause of deterioration is not the extension of an occlusive thrombus but cerebral edema and enlargement of the ischemic penumbra area resulting from the release of excitotoxic amino acids. Hence, anticoagulants are not recommended for the prevention/therapy of progressing stroke, while it is recommended to prevent the extension of the penumbra area through early reperfusion with thrombolysis, treat cerebral edema, and manage homeostatic alterations.

Table 13.6a INDICATIONS AND CONTRAINDICATIONS FOR THE USE OF TPA IN PATIENTS WITH ACUTE ISCHEMIC STROKE

Indications

- Male and female patients aged ≥ 18 years
- Ischemic stroke resulting in measurable deficits in language, motor function, cognition, gaze, vision, and/or neglect
- Symptom onset within 4.5 hours (prior to rt-PA administration)
- Symptoms present for at least 30 minutes. Symptoms should be distinguished from those of a generalized ischemic episode (e.g., syncope), epileptic seizure, or migraine attack
- Patients (or a family member) must have received information about the treatment and given consent for the use of their data and follow-up procedures

Absolute contraindications	Relative contraindications**
- Stroke onset > 9 hours - Intracranial hemorrhage on brain CT scan - Clinical suspicion of early subarachnoid hemorrhage (SAH), even with normal CT scan - Intravenous heparin administration within the previous 48 hours and aPTT exceeding the upper limit of normal in the laboratory - Oral anticoagulant therapy with vitamin K antagonists and INR > 1.7 - Anticoagulant therapy with direct oral anticoagulants and unavailable specific tests - Platelet count < 100.000/mm^3 * - Known bleeding diathesis - Ongoing or recent severe bleeding - Suspicion of ongoing intracranial hemorrhage - Bacterial endocarditis, pericarditis - Acute pancreatitis - Neoplasm with increased bleeding risk - Severe hepatic impairment, including liver failure, cirrhosis, portal hypertension (esophageal varices), active hepatitis - Hemorrhagic retinopathy, e.g., visual disturbances in diabetic patients - Recent significant gastrointestinal or urinary bleeding - Active intracranial hemorrhage suspected - Major gastrointestinal ulceration (< 3 months) - Major surgery within the past 15 days - Myocardial infarction within the past 21 days - Previous/current aortic dissection - High bleeding risk due to comorbidities - Recent (< 10 days) traumatic external cardiac massage, childbirth, non-compressible vessel puncture (e.g., subclavian or jugular vein) - Lumbar puncture or non-compressible arterial puncture within the last 7 days	- Mild deficit or rapid symptom improvement (within 30 minutes) - Unknown time of symptom onset or stroke present upon awakening - Seizure at the onset of stroke - Patient with a history of stroke and concurrent diabetes - Glucose level < 50 or > 400 mg/dl - Previous stroke within the past 3 months - Uncontrolled severe hypertension - Clinically severe stroke (es. NIHSS >25) and/or based on appropriate neuroimaging techniques - Oral anticoagulant therapy with vitamin K antagonists and INR ≤ 1.7 - Anticoagulant therapy with direct oral anticoagulants and subtherapeutic anticoagulant activity, as measured by specific tests - History of CNS disorders: neoplasm, brain or spinal cord surgery, aneurysm - History of intracranial hemorrhage (parenchymal or subarachnoid) - Pregnancy - Major surgery or non-cranial major trauma (< 3 months)

* The current Actilyse prescribing information uses the term "very low platelet count." There are very limited data in the literature on patients treated with a platelet count <100,000, suggesting that alteplase treatment may be effective while maintaining safety. However, since the values at which treatment was performed are not explicitly stated, this option should be cautiously evaluated.

** Listed in the product summary of characteristics but no longer valid based on scientific literature.

Table 13.6b INDICATIONS FOR ENDOVASCULAR TREATMENTS

Patients with occlusion of intracranial artery (internal carotid artery, middle cerebral artery M1-M2 segments, anterior cerebral artery A1 segment, posterior cerebral artery P1 segment, basilar artery, dominant vertebral artery), with/without concomitant occlusion of extracranial artery (internal carotid or vertebral artery)*
Secondary treatments
After intravenous thrombolysis (bridging) when indicated. The endovascular intervention should not delay the initiation of intravenous thrombolysis, and intravenous thrombolysis should not delay the endovascular intervention.
Primary treatments
Onset of stroke > 9 hours and within 24 hours from the last time the patient was seen/heard in good health. Major surgery or severe recent trauma (< 3 months). Patient on oral anticoagulant therapy with vitamin K antagonist drugs and INR > 1.7. Patient on direct oral anticoagulant therapy with therapeutic anticoagulant activity, measured by specific tests, or with unmeasurable activity due to the absence of specific tests. Patient on anticoagulant therapy with low molecular weight heparins. Neoplasia with increased bleeding risk. History of cerebral or subarachnoid hemorrhage. Severe liver disease, including liver failure, cirrhosis, portal hypertension (esophageal varices), active hepatitis. Hemorrhagic retinopathy High bleeding risk due to comorbidities. Recent (< 10 days) traumatic external cardiac massage, childbirth, non-compressible blood vessel puncture (e.g., subclavian or jugular vein). Ulcerative disease of the gastrointestinal tract (< 3 months).
* Documented by Doppler ultrasound, CT angiography, or MR angiography.

Neuroprotection. Studies on animal models have suggested the potential efficacy of certain molecules classified based on their various mechanisms of action, but no clinical trials have confirmed their effectiveness in human pathology. In practice, a single molecule can block one mechanism but not the entire cascade of injury. Theoretically, hypothermia could have the ability to block the entire cascade, and pilot studies have shown its potential effectiveness in improving clinical outcomes. However, these preliminary data have not been confirmed by randomized trials, so hypothermia is not a therapeutic option for acute ischemic stroke. Recently, attention has shifted from the neurotoxic mechanisms of the acute phase to the progressive maturation of neuronal death through apoptosis triggered by the initial ischemic insult.

Treatment of Cerebral Edema. Impaired membrane pumps resulting from cerebral ischemia inevitably lead to cytotoxic edema. This causes swelling of the ischemic tissue, which, in more extensive infarcts, can be observed on neuroimaging as compression of cerebral sulci and ventricles. In the following days, alterations in the blood-brain barrier lead to water extravasation into intercellular spaces, resulting in vasogenic edema. Infarct swelling can last up to four weeks before edema completely resolves. As mentioned earlier, cerebral edema plays a key role in the early clinical deterioration of stroke patients, especially in cases of extensive infarction that can progress to uncal herniation and fatal compression of the brainstem (malignant middle cerebral artery infarction). Steroids do not have substantial efficacy and carry risks such as hyperglycemia and infectious complications. Mannitol is the most commonly used osmotic diuretic, but its efficacy is limited and temporary. In young patients with malignant middle cerebral artery infarction, regardless of the involved hemisphere, and in patients with infarction of a cerebellar hemisphere with secondary compression of the brainstem, decompressive craniotomy should be considered. This procedure involves the creation of a large craniotomy flap, which, in addition to saving lives, can lead to good functional recovery in approximately 30% of cases.

Secondary prevention

The patient with a transient ischemic attack (TIA) is at risk of a stroke, while the one with a stroke is at risk of recurrence, and both are at risk of myocardial infarction in the months and years following the initial event. The risk of stroke or recurrence is approximately 5% per year but can reach 30% in patients with significant carotid stenosis. Advanced age and the presence of multiple risk factors increase the danger of new events. For targeted secondary prevention, it is crucial to note that only 50% of recurrences recognize the same pathogenetic mechanism as the initial event, thus necessitating the assessment of the overall risk in individual patients.

Several interventions with proven efficacy from epidemiological studies and large *clinical trials* are currently available for secondary prevention.

Lifestyle. Quitting smoking reduces the risk by 50%. A healthy diet (Mediterranean diet), weight control, reduced alcohol consumption, and regular physical activity are the cornerstones of a lifestyle that helps control modifiable risk factors.

Hypertension. Hypertension is the primary risk factor not only for an initial stroke but also for a recurrence. It is recommended to maintain blood pressure below 140/90 mmHg in general and below 130/80 mmHg in diabetic individuals. In patients with significant carotid stenosis, hypotension should be avoided due to the risk of hypoperfusion. Apart from this limitation, blood pressure lowering poses no risks for stroke patients, and clinical trials show a beneficial effect of antihypertensive therapies in terms of secondary prevention, even in individuals who are normotensive.

Diabetes mellitus. Both type 1 and type 2 diabetes are well-known risk factors due to their association with atherosclerosis and hypertension. Glycated hemoglobin (HbA1c), an indicator of adequate medium-term glycemic control, should be maintained below 7% whenever possible. In diabetic patients, statins significantly reduce the risk of the first stroke and recurrence.

Hypercholesterolemia. While elevated cholesterol levels are a certain risk factor for coronary heart disease, they present a weak or uncertain risk for cerebral infarction. However, large clinical trials with lipid-lowering drugs, particularly statins and ezetimibe (which inhibits intestinal cholesterol reabsorption), and more recently, monoclonal antibodies inhibiting PCSK9 protein (responsible for LDL cholesterol receptor internalization and elimination in hepatocytes), have demonstrated the effectiveness of these therapies in reducing the risk of both the first stroke and recurrence. For every 1.0 mmol/L decrease in LDL cholesterol, there is an approximate 25% reduction in the risk of stroke or myocardial infarction (a greater effect than that of antiplatelet agents). Therefore, lipid-lowering therapy should be considered for all patients with TIA or stroke.

Anticoagulants. In patients with cardio-embolic stroke due to atrial fibrillation, oral anticoagulation is the preferred therapy. Its effectiveness is attributed to the primary role of the coagulation cascade in the formation of intracardiac thrombi, compared to the primary role of platelet aggregation in thrombus formation on an atherosclerotic plaque at the arterial level, which responds better to antiplatelet therapy. Despite the undeniable effectiveness, anticoagulant therapy in patients with atrial fibrillation is underused due to the fear of systemic or cerebral bleeding (which increases with patient age), the need for continuous INR monitoring, and the difficulty in maintaining it within the therapeutic range (between 2.0 and 3.0; optimal 2.5). The main challenges are interactions with vitamin K-containing foods and other medications. New oral anticoagulants, direct thrombin inhibitors (dabigatran) or activated factor X inhibitors (rivaroxaban, apixaban, edoxaban), have demonstrated similar, if not superior, efficacy compared to warfarin in reducing the risk of stroke or other embolic events in patients with atrial fibrillation, with a reduced risk of intracranial bleeding. Furthermore, these drugs have no interactions with food and minimal interactions with other medications. Currently, in patients with stroke and atrial fibrillation who cannot receive anticoagulant therapy, dual antiplatelet therapy with 75-100 mg/day aspirin plus 75 mg/day clopidogrel can be administered, unless there is a high risk of bleeding complications that dual antiplatelet therapy does not reduce. Alternatively, monotherapy with aspirin 75-100 mg/day has limited preventive efficacy. Percutaneous closure of the left atrial appendage can be a therapeutic alternative in these cases. Long-term oral anticoagulant therapy is also indicated in patients with mechanical valve prostheses, with or without atrial fibrillation, maintaining an INR between 3.0 and 4.0 (optimal 3.5), and in patients with dilated cardiomyopathy, primary or secondary to ischemic heart disease, with an ejection fraction < 40% and an optimal INR of 2.5. Short-term oral anticoagulant therapy is indicated in patients with stroke and concomitant acute myocardial infarction.

Antiplatelet agents. Acetylsalicylic acid (aspirin) is the most extensively studied antiplatelet agent in clinical trials. Meta-analyses demonstrate that in patients with TIA or stroke treated with aspirin, the relative reduction in the overall risk of stroke, myocardial infarction, or vascular death is 13%, representing modest yet significant epidemiological impact. Conversely, the risk of developing systemic bleeding is 2.7% per year, and the risk of intracranial bleeding is 0.5% per year. The most frequent systemic bleeding occurs in the gastrointestinal tract, while the most common side effect leading to therapy discontinuation (which can occur in up to 25% of cases) is dyspepsia. Adverse effects increase with higher doses, while the preventive effect does not substantially increase. Therefore, many guidelines recommend dosages between 75 and 100 mg/day for long-term therapy. Alternatively, clopidogrel 75 mg or the combination of extended-release dipyridamole 400 mg with 50 mg aspirin can be the first-line therapy instead of aspirin.

The combination of clopidogrel and aspirin, commonly used in cardiology, is no more effective than clopidogrel or aspirin alone, but it significantly increases the risk of hemorrhagic complications, especially cerebral, when administered long-term. However, dual antiplatelet therapy with clopidogrel and aspirin, initiated within the first 12-24 hours of a minor stroke (defined by an NIHSS score ≤ 3) or a high-risk TIA (defined by an ABCD2 score ≥ 4), and continued for 30-90 days, significantly reduces the risk of early recurrence with a tolerable risk of bleeding.

Surgery/Stenting. Patients with TIA or stroke due to carotid stenosis ≥ 70% (using the NASCET method: Figure 13.11) benefit from thromboendarterectomy (TEA), which reduces the risk of ipsilateral stroke recurrence from 12.5% at 2 years to 7.5% at 5 years. The advantage over medical therapy is greater in patients at higher risk of stroke (cerebral rather than ocular symptoms, ulcerated plaque, male sex, older age). Furthermore, the effectiveness is greater with earlier intervention, especially if TEA is performed within the first two weeks after the event. For patients with stenosis

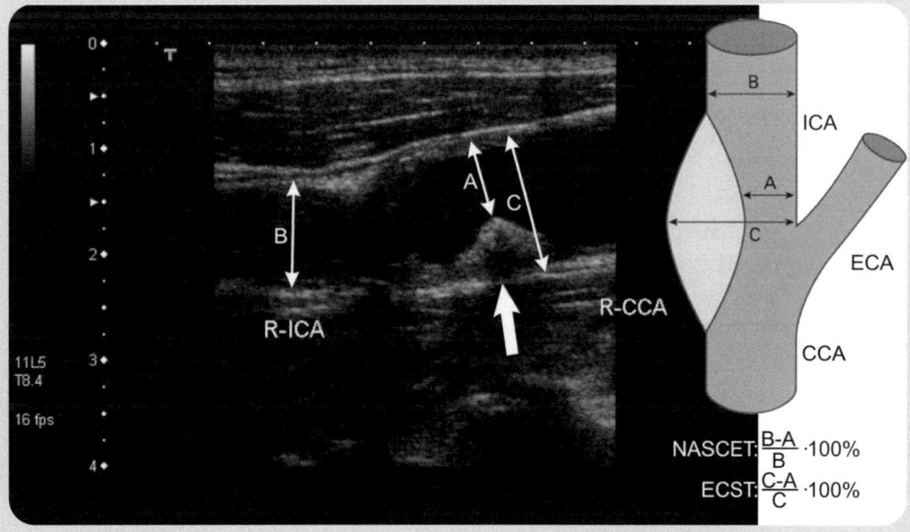

Figure 13.11

Schematic representation of NASCET and ECST methods for the measurement of carotid plaque stenosis (on the right; ICA, Internal Carotid Artery; ECA, External Carotid Artery; CCA, Common Carotid Artery). On the left, an ultrasound image of the common carotid artery and internal carotid artery showing an atherosclerotic plaque (arrow) located at the bulb.

between 50% and 69% (NASCET method), some degree of benefit has been demonstrated in subgroups at higher risk of stroke. Carotid stenosis can be detected without a history of ischemic cerebrovascular symptoms during screening in patients at risk or with a history of other vascular diseases (cardiac, peripheral arterial). In these asymptomatic individuals, TEA should be limited to cases at the highest risk of stroke, defined, for example, by considering the plaque morphology. As an alternative to TEA, carotid stenting has the theoretical advantage of being less invasive, not requiring surgical incisions, almost eliminating the risk of cranial neuropathies, and requiring shorter hospital stays. However, in all direct comparisons, TEA has consistently proven superior to stenting in reducing the risk of short-term stroke or death. Therefore, guidelines indicate TEA as the treatment of choice for patients with symptomatic carotid stenosis, reserving stenting for problematic situations for TEA (high surgical risk due to severe concomitant cardiac and/or pulmonary diseases, very high carotid bifurcation, restenosis following TEA, carotid stenosis due to radiation). No study has compared stenting with medical therapy in cases of symptomatic vertebral stenosis, for which TEA is not indicated due to surgical access difficulties. Therefore, in the case of recurrent stroke or TIA in the vertebrobasilar territory despite adequate pharmacological prevention, stenting may be considered.

13.6 Stroke from rare causes

Rare causes can be observed in young individuals aged between 15 and 49 years. In Western countries, the proportion of strokes occurring in individuals under 45 years of age is approximately 5.5% of all strokes, while it reaches 19% in developing countries. In young age, 30-day mortality is lower compared to older age, ranging from 10% to 34% (the latter figure in black patients), while approximately 16% of patients do not regain their functional autonomy. The average risk of recurrence is below 3% per year.

13.6.1 Arterial dissection

Arterial dissection accounts for 10-25% of cases of stroke in young individuals and globally represents 2% of all ischemic strokes. It can be spontaneous or associated with traumatic events (cervical whiplash, direct neck trauma), but often microtraumas during occupational or sporting activities or chiropractic maneuvers involving vigorous or repetitive head rotation and flexion-extension movements are implicated. Underlying connective tissue disorders such as Marfan syndrome, Ehlers-Danlos syndrome, cystic medial necrosis, polycystic kidney disease, osteogenesis imperfecta, or fibromuscular dysplasia may be present but are sometimes only presumed. Other genetically determined conditions related to dissection include α-1 antitrypsin deficiency and homozygous mutation-related hyperhomocysteinemia of the gene encoding methylenetetrahydrofolate reductase (MTHFR). Dissection is caused by blood penetrating between the intima and media, resulting in intimal detachment that can occlude the artery. The subintimal hematoma can become a source of emboli that cause stroke. It primarily affects the extracranial segments of the carotid or vertebral arteries, while multiple dissections of multiple cervicocerebral arteries occur in 15-20% of cases. A dissecting mechanism can also be involved in stenosis or occlusion of the supraclinoid segment of the intracranial internal carotid artery, where the artery passes over a bony prominence that can cause trauma following triggering events (e.g., carrying heavy objects on the shoulder with downward traction on the carotid arterial axis). The prognosis of stroke resulting from arterial dissection is primarily defined by the extent of damage. Mortality ranges from 4% to 5%, with 50% of survivors achieving complete recovery and 25% experiencing severe neurological sequelae. The average risk of recurrence is less than 1% per year and is higher in younger patients or those with a family history of arterial dissection-related stroke. Recurrence of dissection rarely affects the same artery as the initial event. However, the resolution of dissection, with reattachment of the intima, occurs more frequently, observed in 50-60% of cases.

Clinical presentations can include one of the syndromic patterns described earlier, and dissection is suspected in the presence of pain, typically lateral cervical or retro-orbital in carotid dissection and retro-nuchal in vertebral dissection. The pain may precede the onset of stroke by a few hours or days (less commonly weeks). Another sign is partial Horner's syndrome, characterized by pupillary miosis with pseudo-ptosis due to enophthalmos on the same side as the stroke location, without hemifacial anhidrosis, resulting from sympathetic fiber hypofunction originating from the ciliary ganglion and innervating the pupillary sphincter muscle, running along the outer wall of the internal carotid artery. Bernard-Horner syndrome can also occur due to infarction in the lateral medullary fossa (Wallenberg's syndrome) resulting from embolic occlusion of the posterior inferior cerebellar artery originating from a dissected vertebral artery. In cases of carotid dissection, the focal neurological deficit can also be transient, presenting as a TIA or transient amaurosis, and in 10% of cases, cranial nerve deficits such as IX, X, or XII can occur due to direct compression. In vertebral dissection, the infarct can involve the cervical spinal cord. Additionally, if the intracranial segment of the vertebral artery is involved, the clinical picture may include subarachnoid hemorrhage due to hematoma extension trough the adentitia layer.

The diagnostic suspicion is confirmed by ultrasound examinations, which can demonstrate narrowing of the lumen or sluggish flow distal to the carotid bifurcation and occasionally the pathognomonic double lumen. However, magnetic resonance imaging (MRI) and computed tomography (CT) are particularly useful, as axial scans can reveal the subintimal hematoma with a semilunar or double-target appearance if the vessel is not completely occluded (Figure 13.12). In cases of occlusion, CT angiography or MR angiography can demonstrate a typical "string sign" or "flute beak" appearance of the internal carotid artery immediately after the carotid bifurcation (Figure 13.13).

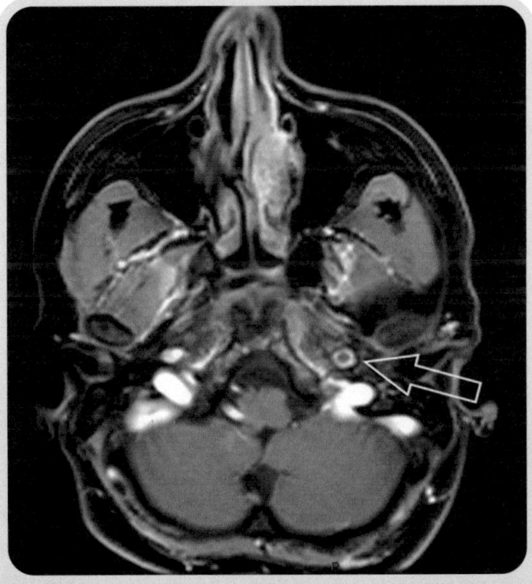

Figure 13.12

Intracranial internal carotid dissection. 'Double target' appearance on MRI. 35-year-old patient. Sudden onset of headache, dizziness, and paresthesia in the right hand, followed by right hemiplegia and aphasia. Post-contrast T1-weighted MRI sequences reveal the presence of a 'double target' appearance of the left internal carotid artery (arrow) within the intracranial segment.

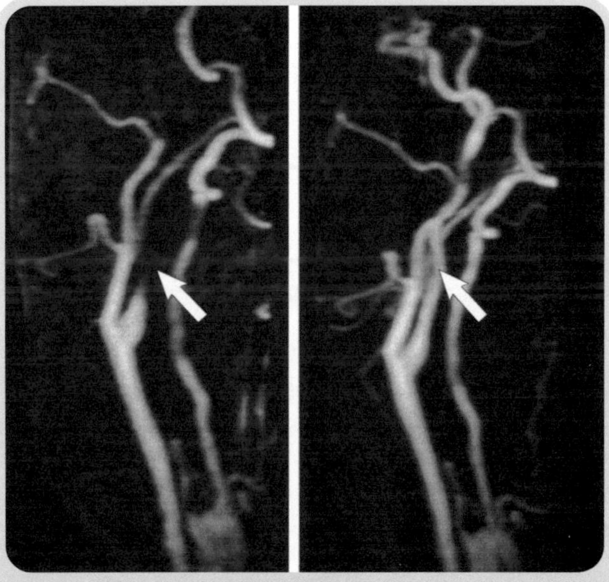

Figure 13.13

Dissection of the internal carotid artery detected by angio-MRI. 44-year-old patient. Transient episode of speech disturbance. TOF angio-MRI reveals progressive narrowing of the lumen of the internal carotid artery in a "flute beak" configuration, indicative of arterial dissection (arrow, left). On the right, complete recanalization of the vessel (arrow) is observed after 14 days of antiplatelet therapy.

The most frequently recommended treatment is currently antiplatelet therapy since a clinical trial has not shown the superiority of anticoagulant therapy over antiplatelet therapy in preventing recurrences. Antiplatelet therapy can be continued long-term, even to facilitate dissection resolution (Figure 13.13). Anticoagulant therapy should be avoided particularly in cases of intracranial dissection, due to the high risk of subarachnoid hemorrhage.

In cases of severe stenosis or complicated lesions with pseudoaneurysms, endovascular procedures have been used in some patients, but data from randomized studies are lacking to establish their safety and efficacy. Dissection is not a contraindication to intravenous thrombolysis in patients presenting within the appropriate time window for this therapy.

13.6.2 Vasculitis

Vasculitis accounts for 3-5% of cases of young stroke. Stroke occurs as a result of the inflammatory process affecting the blood vessel walls, leading to steno-occlusive processes and ischemic events. Less commonly, in advanced stages, vasculitis can cause aneurysm formation and intracerebral hemorrhage. Vasculitis can have infectious or autoimmune origins.

Infectious vasculitis can occur in the context of viral, bacterial, fungal, or tuberculous meningitis, with clinical prodromes typical of these meningoencephalitis conditions. Syphilis-related vasculitis tends to occur in the tertiary phase of the disease, several years after the initial infection.

HIV infection can also result in stroke as a complication of both HIV-related and non-HIV-related vasculitis, as well as due to endocarditis, immune responses, metabolic changes related to HIV, or iatrogenic causes. Specifically, metabolic alterations such as dyslipidemia, insulin resistance, and altered fat distribution have been reported due to chronic treatment with antiretroviral drugs, which can contribute as additional risk factors for cerebrovascular and cardiovascular diseases.

Viral vasculitis can also be caused by viral infections affecting other organs, such as hepatitis B and C.

Varicella-zoster virus (VZV) can cause necrotizing vasculitis of the central nervous system following primary infection, during chickenpox. However, the causal relationship between VZV and vasculitis during chickenpox is not proven. More typically, neurological deficits occur acutely 1-3 months after chickenpox, and unlike post-herpetic arteritis, there are no symptoms of diffuse encephalopathy. The role of VZV is more pronounced in vasculitis due to reactivation of herpetic infection, as the virus is present within the vascular wall, supporting the hypothesis of a direct pathogenic mechanism. In post-herpetic arteritis, stroke occurs weeks or months after trigeminal herpes zoster, affects immunocompetent individuals (usually over 60 years of age), is generally ipsilateral to the site of skin rash, is due to occlusion of a large intracranial vessel (carotid siphon or middle cerebral artery, less commonly posterior cerebral artery or basilar artery), and may not be associated with concomitant encephalitis. In 25% of cases, TIAs or symptoms indicative of diffuse encephalopathy are reported both before and after the stroke event. Cerebrospinal fluid analysis shows typical inflammatory findings. In immunocompromised individuals, both forms of VZV-related vasculitis preferentially involve small-caliber vessels, and the typical skin rash may be absent. In cases of clinical suspicion, specific DNA detection in the cerebrospinal fluid should be performed using PCR. The treatment involves administration of antiviral drugs (aciclovir 10-15 mg/kg three times a day for 7-10 days), with or without a short course of steroids (60-80 mg prednisone per day for 3-5 days). Among parasitic infections, cysticercosis can lead to ischemic stroke due to inflammation of the cerebral base arteries.

Autoimmune vasculitis can be associated with systemic collagen diseases, particularly systemic lupus erythematosus (SLE). In general, when stroke occurs, the disease is already established. However, there are cases where thrombocytopenia and positive VDRL (Venereal Disease Research Laboratory) test results, indicating cross-reactivity with antiphospholipid antibodies, raise diagnostic suspicion and warrant appropriate autoantibody testing. Furthermore, SLE can be complicated by non-infectious endocarditis (Libman-Sacks endocarditis), which can cause cardioembolic stroke, or by a prothrombotic state due to antiphospholipid antibodies. Cerebral vasculitis can also occur, albeit rarely, in the course of rheumatoid arthritis and systemic sclerosis; however, hypertension, which may have an etiological role, is often present in systemic sclerosis.

Autoimmune vasculitis can be primary, directly affecting the arteries independent of systemic diseases. In such cases, vasculitis can involve large, medium, or small vessels.

Among large-vessel vasculitis, Takayasu's disease and giant cell arteritis, also known as Horton's arteritis, should be mentioned.

Takayasu's disease, originally described in young Japanese women, involves progressive severe stenosis of the aortic arch and its branches, leading to the absence of carotid and radial pulses. Stroke is an infrequent complication. Anemia and elevated erythrocyte sedimentation rate (ESR) can support the diagnostic suspicion, and the diagnosis is confirmed by Doppler ultrasound and echocardiography, which reveal stenotic arteries with thickened or occluded walls.

Horton's arteritis affects the extracranial arteries, causing headache and visual disturbances, which can be accompanied by general malaise, muscle pain (polymyalgia rheumatica), weight loss, low-grade fever, marked increase in ESR (>50 mm in the first hour), elevated C-reactive protein, normochromic normocytic anemia, and increased platelet count. It predominantly affects medium to large-caliber arteries (carotid, vertebral, coronary, femoral, aorta) while sparing capillaries and veins. It most commonly involves branches of the external carotid artery (superficial temporal artery, facial artery, occipital artery) with symptoms such as headache, facial pain, scalp tenderness, and jaw claudication. On the occasion of painful accesses, the temporal artery appears swollen.

During painful episodes, the temporal artery may appear swollen.

The most frequent complication is anterior ischemic optic neuropathy, which can lead to blindness. Stroke is a rarer occurrence and manifests as a brainstem infarct resulting from involvement of the extradural vertebral artery.

A very high ESR supports the diagnostic suspicion, and confirmation is provided by temporal artery biopsy, which shows inflammatory cells in the internal elastic lamina. However, temporal artery ultrasound reveals an altered vessel profile and perivascular edema, allowing for diagnosis.

Prompt treatment with high-dose prednisone (40-80 mg/day in the first month) helps resolve general symptoms within a few days and normalizes the ESR in about a month. The dosage should then be gradually reduced while monitoring the ESR and clinical picture. In cases of poor response to steroid therapy, monoclonal antibodies can be considered.

Polyarteritis nodosa is the most important among the medium-sized vessel vasculitides, but it also affects smaller vessels. Stroke is a late complication, while peripheral complications are more frequent. Small-vessel arteritis, such as Wegener's granulomatosis and Churg-Strauss syndrome, often present with encephalopathy or peripheral symptoms, while stroke is a rare occurrence. Medium and small intracerebral arteries can be affected by primary central nervous system arteritis, which is a rather rare event. The clinical presentation often has a chronic course, with headaches and encephalopathy, but acute presentations with stroke are also possible. It can occur at any age, more frequently in males. Neuroimaging reveals multiple infarctions affecting small vessels, possibly associated with microhemorrhages. AngioCT or angioMRI may occasionally show segmental narrowing or appear normal. Cerebrospinal fluid may show pleocytosis and oligoclonal immunoglobulin bands.

With the exception of Takayasu's arteritis, Horton's arteritis, and primary central nervous system arteritis, central nervous system involvement in vasculitis is often late and constitutes a negative prognostic factor. Peripheral nervous system is instead more commonly affected with mono- or multi-neuropathies. Typically, there are significant systemic symptoms including fever, weight loss, generalized asthenia, anorexia, arthromyalgia, and signs of involvement of other organs such as the kidney or skin with petechiae, papules, and nodular erythema. These elements, along with elevated erythrocyte sedimentation rate (ESR) and C-reactive protein (CRP) values, should raise diagnostic suspicion and prompt specific immunological tests such as antinuclear antibody (ANA), anti-ENA antibodies, p-ANCA, and c-ANCA. Cerebrospinal fluid examination shows lymphocytic pleocytosis, increased protein levels, and elevated pressure in approximately 90% of cases. MRI can reveal multiple lesion areas, both lacunar and cortico-subcortical, often bilateral, enhancing with contrast medium, with frequent leptomeningeal involvement. Normal cerebrospinal fluid examination and MRI have important negative predictive value for the diagnosis of vasculitis. Confirmatory diagnosis is achieved through biopsy. In cases suspected of isolated granulomatous vasculitis of the central nervous system, diagnosis requires a biopsy to be performed on the temporal pole of the non-dominant hemisphere, associated with leptomeningeal sampling. In cases of systemic vasculitis, a skin, kidney, or other tissue biopsy can be performed based on the involvement of specific organs. False negatives in biopsies can occur, mainly due to the patchy distribution of vascular lesions. Biopsy should be complemented with culture of the sample to exclude an infectious etiology of granulomatous lesions.

There are no randomized studies on pharmacological interventions for the prevention of cerebrovascular complications in vasculitis. Similar to systemic vasculitis, immunosuppressive treatment with steroids is recommended for at least 6-12 months after clinical remission, monitoring the clinical picture and MRI. In severe cases, steroids may be combined with cyclophosphamide. Azathioprine and methotrexate are valid alternatives for long-term prevention of relapses if steroid therapy is contraindicated. In case of treatment failure, monoclonal antibodies, particularly rituximab, are a therapeutic option.

13.6.3 Hematological disorders

Sickle cell anemia (SCA) is the most common risk factor for stroke in children of African descent, with the highest prevalence in regions such as sub-Saharan Africa and India, where 10-40% of individuals are carriers. In Italy, the highest prevalence of heterozygous Hb-S carriers is found in Sicily (up to over 5% of the population). Approximately 10% of children with SCA experience a symptomatic stroke by the age of 20, with a recurrence risk of about 50% within 3 years. Additionally, 20% of SCA carriers develop clinically silent ischemic lesions. Stroke occurs due to steno-occlusive lesions in the proximal middle cerebral artery and distal internal carotid artery, with possible progression to a moya-moya-like pattern. There is also an increased risk of venous thrombosis and cerebral hemorrhage, especially in older individuals. The most effective intervention for preventing cerebrovascular events is regular blood transfusions (averaging 14 sessions per year) with the goal of reducing the percentage of Hb-S from a baseline value >90% to <30%. Transfusions should be repeated without a maximum time limit, considering potential long-term complications such as iron overload, infections, and alloimmunization. Acute-phase treatment requires exchange transfusion to reduce the percentage of Hb-S to less than 30%. For secondary prevention, transfusions targeting Hb-S levels between 30% and 60% are recommended. In patients who continue to have recurrent events despite transfusion therapy (or to reduce the risk of associated side effects), alternative treatments such as hydroxyurea or bone marrow transplantation may be considered. In adults with SCA who experience TIA or stroke, in addition to the therapeutic measures indicated for children, surgical bypass may be considered in cases with significant steno-occlusive alterations of cerebral vessels resembling moya-moya syndrome.

Antiphospholipid syndrome (APS) is an acquired coagulopathy that occurs as a result of systemic lupus erythematosus or as a primary condition. APS can cause TIA, stroke, cerebral venous thrombosis, and recurrent abortions. Cerebral infarctions are usually multiple, both lacunar and cortical, and generally not severe; however, a severe form with recurrent thromboembolic episodes has been described. Nevertheless, it is unclear whether antiphospholipid antibodies themselves are pathogenic or simply indicative of endothelial and platelet dysfunction predisposing to thrombosis. Another mechanism proposed is secondary cardioembolism due to nonbacterial thrombotic endocarditis. The presence of antiphospholipid antibodies can also be secondary to infectious diseases and the use of certain medications. For patients with arterial thrombotic events and isolated presence of antiphospholipid antibodies, secondary prevention is based on antiplatelet agents. In cases of stroke or TIA meeting the criteria for APS and associated with venous or arterial thrombotic events in various organs or recurrent abortions, long-term oral anticoagulant therapy with a target INR of 2.5 (range 2.0-3.0) is indicated. The INR may be increased to 3.5 (range 3.0-4.0) in cases of recurrent thrombotic events while on anticoagulation. Prophylactic anticoagulation for cerebral thromboembolic complications in asymptomatic patients with APS is not justified unless there is concurrent exposure to other risk factors. The use of oral contraceptives is not recommended.

The role of genetic polymorphisms is not yet well-defined. A meta-analysis of case-control studies analyzing 32 candidate genes identified a predictive role for cerebral stroke in only 4 genes: ACE I/D, factor V Leiden, prothrombin gene G20210A polymorphism, and MTHFR C677T. Factor V Leiden is associated with the risk of venous thrombosis, including cerebral thrombosis, and becomes a risk factor for stroke in young women who smoke and take oral contraceptives. Anticoagulant therapy is recommended to prevent venous thrombosis in cases of prolonged immobility of the lower limbs (e.g., immobilization in a cast after a fracture). The MTHFR polymorphism involves the enzyme methylenetetrahydrofolate reductase and homocysteine metabolism. Elevated homocysteine levels in the blood have an atherogenic and prothrombotic effect and exponentially increase the risk associated with other factors such as hypertension and smoking.

Thrombotic thrombocytopenic purpura (TTP) causes hemolytic anemia, thrombocytopenia, and multi-organ microinfarctions, including the brain, due to platelet-rich thrombi. TTP is related to a primitive or, more often, acquired deficiency of ADAMTS13 (A Disintegrin And Metalloprotease with ThromboSpondin type 1 repeats 13), the specific von-Willebrandt factor cleaving protease. The acquired form is caused by autoantibodies against ADAMTS13. Clinically, it presents with diffuse encephalopathy but can also include strokes, generally mild. Plasmapheresis is the treatment of choice, while the use of antithrombotic therapy should be evaluated based on the platelet count (avoid if < 60,000) and the potential risk of bleeding events.

T-cell angiocentric lymphoma, also known as granulomatous lymphomatosis or malignant angioendotheliomatosis, is an intravascular lymphomatous proliferation leading to arterial occlusion with multiple recurrent ischemic lesions, including severe infarctions. Diagnosis is typically made through biopsy or, more frequently, autopsy due to the unfavorable prognosis of the underlying disease.

13.6.4 Susac syndrome

Susac syndrome is a microangiopathy involving the retina, cochlea, and brain. It predominantly affects women, with a female-to-male ratio of 3:1, typically between the ages of 20 and 40. The etiology is not well-defined. The pathogenic mechanism appears to involve an autoimmune endotheliopathy characterized by arterial wall thickening without fibrinoid necrosis or amyloid deposits, resulting in microinfarctions in the white and gray matter of the brain, retina, and inner ear. Involvement of retinal arteries manifests as scotomas (sometimes scintillating) and decreased visual acuity; it is bilateral and clearly visible on fluorescein angiography. Involvement of cochlear arteries leads to noticeable hearing loss on audiometric examination, especially for mid-to-low frequencies. Symptoms such as dizziness, nausea, and ataxia may occur due to central and peripheral involvement of the vestibular pathways. Brain involvement presents with migraine-like headaches followed, even after months, by the appearance of psychiatric symptoms (character changes), cognitive deficits, and, more rarely, focal symptoms with ictal onset and cranial nerve deficits. Cerebrospinal fluid examination shows increased protein levels and mild pleocytosis. MRI reveals multiple signal abnormalities on T2-weighted sequences in both white matter, often involving the corpus callosum, and gray matter, with contrast enhancement of active lesions. Advanced stages show cortical atrophy. Due to clinical and MRI features, Susac syndrome should be considered in the differential diagnosis with multiple sclerosis, cerebral vasculitis, and acute disseminated encephalomyelitis. Immunosuppressive therapy based on steroids, cyclophosphamide, or intravenous immunoglobulins is recommended.

13.6.5 Sneddon's syndrome

Sneddon's syndrome is a non-inflammatory arteriopathy that involves small and medium-sized arteries and is characterized by livedo racemosa on the skin and recurrent cerebral infarctions. The literature reports an annual incidence of 4 cases per 100,000. In two-thirds of cases, it is a sporadic disease that predominantly affects females, with an average age of onset of 40 years (range 10-65 years). In the remaining cases, it has a familial distribution, and autosomal dominant transmission has been reported. The pathogenesis is uncertain because one-third of patients have anticardiolipin antibodies, lupus anticoagulant, and cardiac myxomas. Livedo racemosa appears as an erythematous-violaceous, irregular net-like pattern, primarily located on the lower trunk, buttocks, and thigh roots, but it can affect any part of the body. Livedo worsens with cold exposure, orthostatism, and sometimes during pregnancy. It can precede neurological symptoms by up to 10 years. Neurological symptoms manifest as migraine-like headaches, TIAs, and mild strokes with a tendency to recur in the following months or years. Hypertension, present in 60-80% of patients, can contribute to vascular damage. The disease's progression leads to a pseudobulbar syndrome and progressive cognitive decline. Peripheral venous thrombosis and ocular vascular abnormalities such as retinal thrombosis and microaneurysms have also been reported. Hematochemical and immunological investigations are generally normal, but as mentioned before, one-third of patients test positive for lupus anticoagulant and antiphospholipid antibodies. Carotid Doppler ultrasound is usually normal, while an echocardiogram should always be performed to rule out mitral valve myxomatous changes or atrial myxoma.

MRI reveals infarctions and areas of cortical atrophy and lacunar subcortical lesions. Cerebral angiography shows multiple occlusions and constrictions in the distal segments of small and medium-sized intracranial arteries and, in severe cases, fistulas and conditions resembling Moyamoya disease. The diagnosis is confirmed by a skin biopsy taken from the "pale" area within the livedo, which demonstrates arteriolar endothelitis with intimal hyperplasia and obliterative wall fibrosis without inflammatory infiltrates. There are no specific therapeutic interventions supported by studies; therefore, patients receive treatment with antiplatelet agents or, in the case of concurrent thrombophilia, oral anticoagulants.

13.6.6 Mitochondrial diseases

The disease known as "Mitochondrial Myopathy, Encephalopathy, Lactic Acidosis, and Stroke-like Episodes" (MELAS) can be considered in the diagnostic workup of juvenile stroke. It is caused by point mutations in mitochondrial DNA and has also been associated with microdeletions. MELAS presents with recurrent episodes of migraine with or without aura, partial or generalized epileptic seizures, vomiting, sensory hearing loss, somatic growth retardation and short stature, muscle abnormalities (asthenia, muscular atrophy, exercise intolerance with or without myalgia), endocrine disorders (hypogonadism, hypothyroidism, type I diabetes), cognitive deficits, psychiatric disturbances, ophthalmological abnormalities (cataracts, optic atrophy, retinitis pigmentosa, ptosis, and progressive ophthalmoplegia), cardiac abnormalities (conduction defects, hypertrophic or dilated cardiomyopathy), and polyneuropathy. TIAs or minor strokes can occur in early adolescence, presenting with clinical features such as hemianopsia, cortical blindness, ataxia, aphasia, or hemiparesis. They often have a subacute onset, can be associated with partial seizures or headache, and can be triggered by fever or infections.

Neuroimaging reveals lesions that do not correspond to the classic vascular territories, predominantly located in the cortex of the temporal-parietal and occipital lobes. Intracranial calcifications and areas of atrophy can also be observed. MR spectroscopy shows increased levels of lactic acid in the ischemic area. Increased levels of pyruvate and lactate can be detected in the blood and cerebrospinal fluid, which should be analyzed immediately after collection. Electromyography may reveal a myopathic pattern, while creatine phosphokinase (CPK) levels are often within the normal range. Muscle biopsy demonstrates “ragged red fibers” upon Gomori staining. The diagnosis is confirmed by analyzing mitochondrial DNA.

13.6.7 Fabry disease

Fabry disease is a lysosomal disorder caused by a deficiency of α-galactosidase A (α-Gal-A) enzyme, leading to the accumulation of globotriaosylceramide (GL3) in the nervous system, vascular endothelium, heart, kidneys, eyes, and gastrointestinal tract. The gene encoding the enzyme is located on the Xq22 chromosome, which is why the disease primarily affects males. However, females can also be affected, usually in milder form, likely due to the inactivation of one of the two X chromosomes. The typical course of the disease begins in childhood with polyneuropathy, characterized by recurrent episodes of painful acroparesthesia and debilitating pain in the extremities, accompanied by heat and cold intolerance and hypohidrosis. As patients age, these episodes tend to decrease. Gastrointestinal disturbances are common (typically starting in adolescence) and are characterized by abdominal pain, dyspepsia, bloating, postprandial swelling, and diarrhea.

Cutaneous angiokeratomas are present in 50% of males and approximately 11% of females. These are reddish-brown lesions, slightly raised due to vessel ectasia, typically found in the genital, gluteal, and peri-umbilical regions, but also in the oral epithelium or distal extremities. In the third to fourth decade of life, nephropathy develops, initially presenting with proteinuria and progressive renal insufficiency. Another characteristic feature is corneal opacities, particularly verticillate cornea, present in over 70% of cases but detectable only through slit lamp examination. Cardiac involvement manifests as hypertrophic or ischemic cardiomyopathy, arrhythmias, or valvular dysfunction. Neurosensorial hearing loss, the severity of which is correlated with the extent of white matter lesions in males, is also reported.

Stroke typically occurs in the fourth decade of life in hemizygous males and the fifth decade in heterozygous females, although earlier occurrences are possible. Stroke may also be the actual or apparent initial symptom, as prodromal manifestations have been so mild as to go unnoticed. An epidemiological study revealed Fabry disease as the cause of stroke in 4.9% of young men and 2.4% of young women with cryptogenic stroke, accounting for 1.2% of all strokes in individuals aged 18 to 55 years.

Stroke predominantly affects the posterior circulation, where megadolichoectasia of the basilar artery is often observed. Magnetic resonance imaging (MRI) also reveals alterations in the white matter, present as early as the age of 20 to 30 years and clinically asymptomatic for a long time. Bilateral calcifications of the pulvinar are also quite characteristic and may raise diagnostic suspicion.

In males, the diagnosis is based on the finding of reduced α-Gal-A leukocyte activity, which may be normal in heterozygous females. In both sexes, the diagnosis relies on identifying various mutations in the disease gene.

Enzyme replacement therapy through intravenous infusion of recombinant α-Gal-A has proven effective in slowing the progression of renal and cardiac damage and improving symptoms associated with peripheral and autonomic nervous system involvement. However, there is currently no available data on its efficacy in preventing new ischemic cerebral episodes.

In the presence of certain mutations known as susceptible, unstable and misfolded forms of α-Gal-A are produced. In these cases, migalastat can be administered, which is a chaperone molecule that establishes high-affinity, selective, and reversible bonds with the active sites of mutant forms of α-Gal-A. Binding with migalastat stabilizes these mutant forms of α-Gal-A in the endoplasmic reticulum and facilitates their proper trafficking to lysosomes. Once in the lysosomes, the dissociation of migalastat restores α-Gal-A inducing the catabolism of GL-3 and its related substrates.

13.6.8 CADASIL

Cerebral Autosomal Dominant Arteriopathy with *Subcortical Infarcts and Leukoencephalopathy* (CADASIL) is an autosomal dominant arteriopathy characterized by migraine, often with aura, multiple lacunar infarcts located in the basal ganglia, thalamus, or white matter, and progressive leukoencephalopathy that leads to subcortical vascular dementia. Some cases of CADASIL with severe cerebral hemorrhages have been reported, and there appears to be a high frequency of visible microbleeds on gradient-echo MRI sequences, although these alterations are not considered specific to this condition. The disease is caused by a mutation in the NOTCH3 gene, located on chromosome 19, which encodes for a transmembrane protein with an unknown specific function. The disease is characterized by a non-arteriosclerotic and non-amyloid microangiopathy with dense deposits on electron microscopy at the level of the basal membrane. The microangiopathy is widespread, so these alterations can also be found in peripheral nerves, muscles, and skin. Skin biopsy is a useful screening test. The presence of osmiophilic granulations in the skin biopsy has a specificity of 100%, but variable sensitivity ranging from a minimum of 50%. The diagnosis may require identification of the NOTCH3 gene mutation. The average age of onset of CADASIL is in the third to fourth decade of life (with headaches). The diagnostic suspicion is induced by cerebrovascular disorders that occur in the fifth to sixth decade of life and are followed by cognitive impairments. Some cases with few symptoms have also been described in the eldery.

MRI shows diffuse leukoencephalopathy involving the semioval centers and the external capsule. Fairly specific to CADASIL are the hyperintensity of the external capsule and, especially, the white matter alterations of the temporal pole.

13.6.9 Moya-moya disease

The term *Moya-moya* means "puff of smoke" and was coined to describe the network of fine collateral vessels that develop following the occlusion of both carotid arteries, either at their intra-cranial terminal segment or from their origin. The vertebrobasilar circulation is typically not involved. Although more commonly described in Japan, where the term was coined, it is also found in Western countries. The distribution has a bimodal peak, with the first peak in the first decade and the second peak in the third to fourth decade of life. In women, the incidence is almost double that of men. Familial cases account for 7-10% of the cases. Associations with chromosomes 3, 6, 8, and 17 have been reported.

Similar angiographic patterns are observed in other clinical conditions, such as secondary carotid occlusion due to radiation therapy or atherothrombosis, sickle cell anemia, fibromuscular dysplasia, neurofibromatosis, aortic coarctation, previous basal meningitis, polyarteritis nodosa, neonatal hypoxia, leptospirosis, tuberous sclerosis, Marfan syndrome, and Down syndrome. Clinically, it manifests in children with headache (a common initial symptom), epileptic seizures, TIAs, or minor ischemic strokes (typically presenting as mono-hemiparesis), possible choreiform movements, dystonia, and intellectual delay. In adults, it often presents with cerebral hemorrhage (isolated intraventricular or associated with parenchymal hematoma) resulting from rupture of the small collateral vessels subjected to significant circulatory overload. In ischemic forms, neuroimaging may reveal lesions in the basal ganglia or atypical infarcts, sometimes of the junctional type.

There is no proven effective therapy for preventing ischemic or hemorrhagic events. Surgical therapy with extra-intracranial bypass may be useful in delaying cognitive decline and improving performance in daily activities; however, it is unclear whether it has preventive efficacy against ischemic or hemorrhagic events.

13.6.10 Migrainous stroke

These are classified as strokes that occur at the peak of a migraine attack and for which no other etiological factors are identified. Typically, the symptoms resemble an aura that lasts longer than usual, and the infarction is usually located in the occipital region. This condition, although rare, should be distinguished from all cases of stroke that can be preceded or accompanied by migraines, such as in antiphospholipid antibody syndrome, CADASIL, MELAS, Susac syndrome, and all cases of stroke that can start with a headache but have a defined etiology.

Familial hemiplegic migraine should also be distinguished from migrainous stroke. It is a rare autosomal dominant channelopathy (with extremely rare sporadic forms) in which migraine is accompanied by focal neurological deficits lasting up to 24 hours without infarction.

In the differential diagnosis, consideration should also be given to the *Headache Neurological Disorder and Lymphocitosis* (HaNDL) syndrome, characterized not only by migraine and a neurological deficit that "mimics" a stroke, typically lasting no longer than 24 hours but also by an increase in lymphocytes in the cerebrospinal fluid in the absence of an infectious pathology.

13.6.11 Atrial septal abnormalities

In young patients with stroke of undetermined cause, the prevalence of a patent foramen ovale (PFO) and/or atrial septal aneurysm (ASA) can reach 50% of cases, compared to 15% in age-matched patients with stroke of determined causes. However, the role of these septal abnormalities in the pathogenesis of stroke is debated. It is unclear whether PFO has a pathogenic role and whether the stroke is attributable to paradoxical embolism from deep venous thrombosis and right-to-left atrial shunting, embolism originating within the PFO, or (especially in the presence of an atrial septal aneurysm) other mechanisms such as a high incidence of atrial fibrillation. Some studies have suggested that a PFO with massive passage of microbubbles, with shunting present at rest and not just after a Valsalva maneuver, and associated with a large atrial septal aneurysm, is the condition with the highest cardioembolic risk.

The preferred choice for secondary prevention therapy is percutaneous closure of the PFO using mechanical devices, which has been shown to be more effective than pharmacological therapy in clinical trials in patients up to 60 years of age. In particular, the efficacy has been demonstrated in patients with higher-risk PFO, as previously indicated. In cases where pharmacological therapy is chosen, anticoagulant therapy is superior to antiplatelet therapy.

13.6.12 Drug and substance abuse

Drug abuse may be implicated in approximately 2.5% of cases of young stroke. Heroin users are particularly at risk for endocarditis, primarily caused by *Staphylococcus aureus* and Candida, which can lead to cardioembolic ischemic events, typically TIAs or minor strokes. More rarely, embolization of foreign material and contaminants in the injected drugs, such as talc or cellulose, has been documented. Secondary vasculitis is also possible.

Neuroimaging reveals multifocal lesions. Antibiotic treatment reduces the risk of ischemic events due to endocarditis, except in cases of Candida. As in all cases of native valve endocarditis, anticoagulant therapy is contraindicated due to an increased risk of cerebral hemorrhagic complications. Septic emboli can also give rise to mycotic aneurysms that, when ruptured, cause cerebral hemorrhage, which can also occur as a rare manifestation of vasculitis. Lastly, overdose, leading to hypoventilation and hypotension, can cause bilateral ischemic injury to the globus pallidus, resulting in parkinsonism and behavioral changes.

Several sympathomimetic molecules (ephedrine, pseudoephedrine, dextroamphetamine, methamphetamine, methylphenidate, phenylpropanolamine, 3,4-methylenedioxymethamphetamine (MDMA) known as "ecstasy"), used as psychostimulants, nasal decongestants, and appetite suppressants, can cause acute confusional states, headache, hypertension, hypertensive and epileptic crises, hyperthermia, TIAs, stroke, and death in cases of overdose. Prolonged use can also cause cerebrovascular events, both ischemic and hemorrhagic, including subarachnoid hemorrhage. The mechanism is vasospasm, with angiographic patterns of multifocal vascular narrowing that often resolve spontaneously, typical of reversible segmental cerebral vasoconstriction syndrome.

Cocaine causes vasoconstriction by blocking the reuptake of norepinephrine from sympathetic nerve endings. The most common manifestations of acute and chronic cocaine toxicity are cardiovascular complications and psychiatric and neurological symptoms, such as epileptic seizures, movement disorders, and cerebrovascular complications. The latter include cerebral ischemia, intracerebral and subarachnoid hemorrhage. The pathogenic mechanism of cocaine-induced vasculopathy is likely multifactorial, involving not only vasoconstriction but also vasculitic-like changes, alterations in hemostasis and platelet function, and reduced cerebral blood flow.

Cerebrovascular complications can also arise from the use of LSD, marijuana, and phencyclidine.

13.6.13 Cerebral venous thrombosis

Thrombosis of the cerebral sinuses and veins, known as cerebral venous thrombosis, is a cause of venous infarction. It can be septic, secondary to facial cellulitis, middle ear infection, mastoiditis, or sinusitis, typically involving the cavernous sinus and transverse sinus. Bacterial meningitis can cause septic thrombosis of superficial veins. More commonly, venous thrombosis is non-septic and involves the dural sinuses, less frequently the cortical veins or deep veins. Elevated estrogen levels, such as during pregnancy, postpartum period, or in women taking combined hormonal contraceptives, are risk factors. The presence of factor V Leiden polymorphism is also a risk factor (detected in 10-21% of cases), especially when combined with concurrent oral contraceptive use. Mutations in factor II are also implicated, found in 6-50% of cases depending on the case series. Cerebral venous thrombosis can occur in individuals with sickle cell anemia. Severe dehydration can lead to thrombosis. Administration of high-dose steroids can be a potential cause of cerebral venous thrombosis. Behçet's disease, suspected in the presence of genital ulcers and uveitis, can cause thrombosis of the dural sinuses. An underlying malignancy can also result in a paraneoplastic prothrombotic syndrome. The cause remains undetermined in 20-35% of cases.

Clinical presentation includes focal neurological deficits that can mimic stroke, often accompanied by headache (which may precede the onset of symptoms by several days) or epileptic seizures. Severe cases may progress to coma. Thrombosis can also manifest with headache alone, without focal cerebral lesions, possibly associated with worsening signs of increased intracranial pressure (vomiting, papilledema, visual impairment) resembling pseudotumor cerebri. Subacute onset of focal neurological signs can also occur, mimicking an abscess or expansive process.

Isolated thrombosis of cortical veins is less frequent compared to extension of sinus thrombosis to these veins and is more challenging to diagnose; it may sometimes occur with subarachnoid hemorrhage. Deep vein thrombosis is rarer and can result in thalamic infarction, including bilateral involvement, with prolonged alteration of consciousness. Cavernous sinus thrombosis is also a rare event, usually of septic origin from facial cellulitis, characterized by pain, headache, fever, facial edema followed by proptosis and ophthalmoplegia. Non-septic cavernous sinus thrombosis can occur in the presence of carotid-cavernous fistula.

CT imaging reveals hypodensity of the white matter in 75% of cases, representing venous stasis ischemia with atypical, sometimes bilateral, localization, most commonly parasagittal or temporo-occipital, as the superior sagittal sinus and transverse sinus are primarily involved. In 10-50% of cases, the lesions may be hemorrhagic with significant perilesional vasogenic edema, and subarachnoid hemorrhages may coexist. Axial CT scans may show thrombus within the sagittal sinus, with the so-called "delta sign" appearing early but present in only 2%

of cases, or after contrast administration, the "empty delta sign", (Figure 13.14), which indicates central hypodensity surrounded by hyperdensity due to contrast enhancement. This latter sign is present in 35% of cases but is not visible in the first 3-4 days and may disappear after two to three months. Additionally, it is absent when the posterior third of the superior sagittal sinus is not thrombosed. MRI is more sensitive than CT in detecting parenchymal lesions, extent of edema, and hemorrhagic components. It can also visualize the absence of flow void normally seen in sagittal (superior sagittal sinus) or axial (transverse sinus) cuts due to thrombosis. Neuroimaging should be complemented with CT angiography or MR angiography with venous sequences (Figure 13.15). Hypoplasia of a transverse sinus may be misinterpreted as thrombosis by MR angiography; only comparison with axial MRI images, which demonstrate the normal "flow void" corresponding to the hypoplastic sinus, can resolve the diagnostic doubt.

The treatment for cerebral venous thrombosis is based on anticoagulation, even if the infarction is hemorrhagic. Treatment with unfractionated heparin or low-molecular-weight heparin aims to inhibit thrombus growth, promote spontaneous fibrinolysis, and improve venous outflow. Usually, it is sufficient to reduce intracranial pressure within a few days. Oral anticoagulation therapy should be added in the early days, to be continued for 3 months in cases secondary to a transient or modifiable risk factor (e.g., oral contraceptive use), 6-12 months in patients with idiopathic forms or mild hereditary thrombophilia (heterozygous factor V Leiden or G20210A prothrombin gene mutation), and indefinitely in patients with two or more episodes of idiopathic cerebral venous thrombosis or severe hereditary thrombophilia (antithrombin III deficiency, homozygous factor V Leiden or G20210A prothrombin gene mutation, or two or more associated thrombophilic conditions). In cases of septic origin thrombosis, broad-spectrum antibiotic therapy should be administered, even before obtaining the results of the antimicrobial susceptibility test, to be continued for at least two weeks after the resolution of local signs of infection.

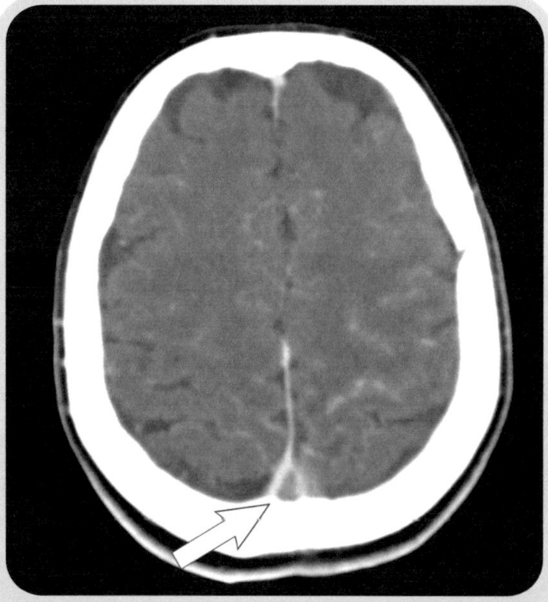

Figure 13.14

Venous Cerebral Thrombosis. A 64-year-old patient arrives at the Emergency Department due to persistent headache for several days. The CT angiography shows the presence of a signal void within the longitudinal sinus ("empty delta sign" - arrow), indicating venous thrombosis.

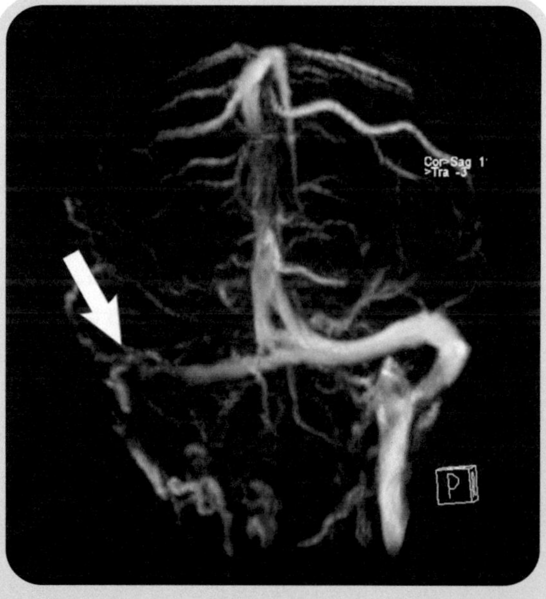

Figure 13.15

Cerebral venous thrombosis. 40-year-old patient, affected by poorly differentiated occult carcinoma in metastatic lymph node phase. Sudden onset of right homonymous lateral hemianopsia and headache. The MRI shows, in the venous angiographic sequences, the presence of thrombosis of the left transverse sinus and the left jugular vein (posterior projection).

In patients with isolated increased intracranial pressure and visual decline without venous infarction, therapeutic lumbar puncture is useful; in these cases, anticoagulant therapy should be initiated at least 24 hours after the last lumbar puncture. Administration of acetazolamide may be beneficial for patients with papilledema. If visual deterioration persists despite these therapies, invasive treatments such as ventriculoperitoneal shunting or optic nerve sheath fenestration should be considered. Additional measures can be implemented to manage increased intracranial pressure, such as elevating the head to approximately 30 degrees, hyperventilation (maintaining $PaCO_2$ at 30-35 mm Hg), infusion of osmotic diuretics, while avoiding hypovolemia and hypotension that can increase blood viscosity. Steroids should not be used due to the potential increased risk of venous thrombosis. For patients with massive cerebral edema at risk of herniation, decompressive craniotomy may be considered. Endovascular thrombolytic therapy or mechanical thrombectomy may be reserved for cases that do not respond to anticoagulant therapy.

The prognosis of cerebral venous thrombosis is generally favorable, with complete recovery in approximately 85% of patients and a mortality rate of around 12%, mainly associated with age, septic nature or underlying malignancy, deep sinus thrombosis, intracranial hemorrhage, male gender, and a Glasgow Coma Scale score <9. Clinical deterioration within the first few days of hospitalization occurs in about a quarter of patients, with the appearance of new lesions in one-third of cases, even in the presence of anticoagulant therapy, which may require several days of treatment before its effectiveness is evident. The risk of recurrence is approximately 10-12%, usually within the first year.

13.6.14 Posterior reversible encephalopathy syndrome (PRES)

In the differential diagnosis with cerebral venous thrombosis, as well as with a TIA or stroke, one should consider Posterior Reversible Encephalopathy Syndrome (PRES), which presents with headache, epileptic seizures, transient or persistent focal neurological deficits for several days, and altered consciousness. It occurs as a result of a sudden increase in systemic blood pressure that exceeds cerebral autoregulation limits, leading to the formation of vasogenic edema. The most common causes are eclampsia in pregnancy and a sudden increase in blood pressure due to renal pathology (e.g., unrecognized glomerulonephritis). It has also been described in cases of monoclonal antibody therapy and immunosuppressive therapy in transplant patients.

Diagnosis can be made using FLAIR MRI, which reveals predominantly posterior white matter involvement (hence the term), but in severe cases, other areas may also be affected (Figure 13.16). Aggressive management of hypertension typically results in complete regression of the leukoencephalopathy (Figure 13.16), although small infarct-like lesions or microhemorrhages may remain in more severe cases. An association with reversible cerebral vasoconstriction has also been described.

13.6.15 Marfan syndrome

Cohort studies report cerebrovascular complications in less than 4% of patients with Marfan syndrome, a condition that has a prevalence in the general population ranging from 1:10,000 to 1:20,000 and follows an autosomal dominant transmission, although approximately 1/4 of cases are sporadic. The classic diagnostic triad consists of skeletal abnormalities, such as long or disproportionate limbs in relation to the trunk, with or without tall stature, long and slender fingers, prognathism, joint hypermobility, pectus excavatum or carinatum, pes cavus, and a high-arched palate (*marfanoid habitus*); ectopia lentis, which is associated with myopia and predisposition to retinal detachment; and aortic aneurysm, which is associated with other cardiac abnormalities such as dilation of the aortic root with or without valve insufficiency, mitral valve prolapse, and the risk of aortic dissection. It should be emphasized that Marfan syndrome can also exist in oligosymptomatic forms with prominent vascular, ocular, or skeletal involvement. In the majority of cases, the underlying cause of this condition is a

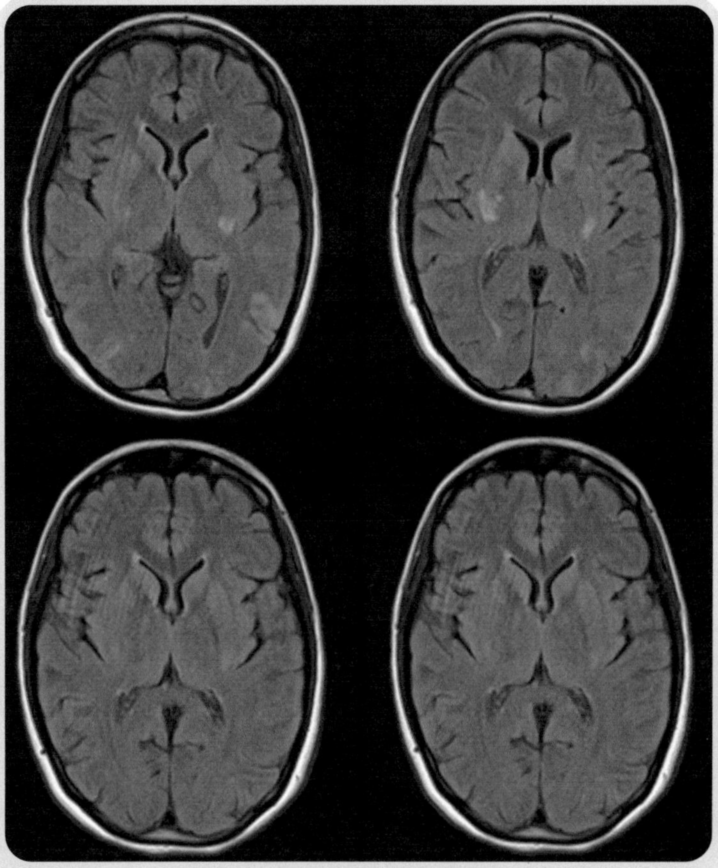

Figure 13.16

Reversible posterior encephalopathy syndrome - PRES. 20-year-old patient with preeclampsia, recent uncomplicated childbirth, and subsequent superior mesenteric vein thrombosis. Headache for a few days, followed by sudden onset of aphasia and weakness in the right upper limb. At the emergency department, epileptic seizure; blood pressure 160/120 mmHg. The MRI shows the presence of multiple hyperintense areas in T2 FLAIR in the temporo-parieto-occipital and bilateral lenticulocapsular regions (top image). The follow-up MRI performed after 4 days shows complete regression of the signal abnormalities in FLAIR (bottom image).

mutation in the fibrillin 1 gene (FBN-1), located on the long arm of chromosome 15, and less commonly in the fibrillin 2 gene (FNB-2) on chromosome 5. Fibrillin is a glycoprotein that is the main constituent of microfibrils found in various tissues, especially elastic tissue, and is particularly abundant in large-caliber blood vessels and the suspensory ligament of the lens. Alterations in fibrillin make elastic fibers more fragile, facilitating the formation of aneurysms and arterial dissections. Therefore, stroke results from dissection of the supra-aortic trunks, while the association with intracranial aneurysms remains controversial. Additionally, stroke can have a cardioembolic etiology due to rhythm disorders and valvular pathologies.

13.6.16 Ehlers-Danlos Syndrome

Ehlers-Danlos syndrome (EDS) presents cerebrovascular complications in approximately 2% of cases. EDS encompasses a group of hereditary collagen disorders characterized by skin hyperelasticity, joint hypermobility, and vascular lesions. There are various subtypes of EDS. Type IV is most predisposed to vascular complications and exhibits more pronounced cutaneous alterations compared to joint involvement: hyperextensible, thin, translucent skin with visible small vessels in the subcutaneous tissue, hyperpigmentation over bony prominences with venous ectasias, and a tendency to bruise easily. Patients look older for thei age. The prevalence of EDS type IV is estimated at approximately 1:50,000-1:500,000. The disease is caused by an autosomal dominant transmission of a mutation in the procollagen type III gene (COL3A1), resulting in the formation of abnormal pro $\alpha 1$(III) chains and increased vessel wall fragility. Cerebrovascular complications consist of dolichoectasia of the epiaortic vessels in young individuals, aneurysms of the internal carotid artery at the cavernous sinus or just distal to it, which can rupture and lead to carotid-cavernous fistula or subarachnoid hemorrhage (often the initial clinical manifestation of the disease), and spontaneous or minor trauma-induced dissection of the epiaortic vessels. The diagnostic suspicion of EDS type IV should be considered in all young patients who experience arterial ruptures or dissections unrelated to accidents, even minor ones, or surgical interventions. Diagnostic confirmation is obtained through histological and molecular investigations, which reveal the deficiency of type III procollagen. There is no medical therapy available for preventing vascular complications. Endovascular correction of fistulas or aneurysms is the treatment of choice, but it carries a higher risk of complications due to vessel fragility.

13.6.17 Loeys-Dietz syndrome

Loeys-Dietz syndrome (LDS) is a rare connective tissue disorder to consider in cases of arterial dissection-related stroke. It is transmitted as an autosomal dominant trait, and there are five types of LDS associated with mutations in the TGFBR1, TGFBR2, SMAD3, TGFB2, and TGFB3 genes. These genes encode for the Transforming Growth Factor-beta, which belongs to a family of multifunctional cytokines that control the proliferation, differentiation, migration, and death of many cell types, influencing various processes including the maintenance of the extracellular matrix and the morphogenesis of tissues such as cartilage, bone, and blood vessels.

There are two clinical phenotypes referred to as LDS 1 and LDS 2. LDS 1 phenotype presents with skeletal malformations (craniosynostosis, scoliosis, kyphosis, cleft palate), hypertelorism, pectus excavatum or carinatum, camptodactyly, ligamentous laxity with joint hypermobility, long fingers, cardiac anomalies (patent ductus arteriosus, atrial septal defects, bicuspid aortic valve), and tortuous blood vessels. LDS 2 phenotype presents with dystrophic scars, bifid uvula, hypertelorism, and joint hypermobility.

Patients with LDS are prone to aneurysm formation and dissections of large-caliber arteries, particularly the aorta and its branches, leading to cerebrovascular and cardiac ischemic events. Animal studies suggest that losartan or irbesartan (angiotensin II receptor antagonists) can block TGF-βactivity and slow the formation of aortic aneurysms, but there is no evidence of their efficacy in human pathology. Nonetheless, the use of antihypertensive medications to reduce vascular wall stress is recommended. In cases of aortic dissection, endovascular replacement of the aortic root with valve sparing is the preferred intervention.

13.6.18 Tortuous artery syndrome

Tortuous artery syndrome (ATS) is another rare connective tissue disorder to consider in cases of spontaneous arterial dissection. It affects medium to large-sized arteries that exhibit tortuosity and are prone to aneurysm formation, dissection, and stenosis of the pulmonary artery.

ATS is transmitted as an autosomal recessive trait and is caused by various mutations in the SLC2A10 gene, which encodes the glucose transporter 10 (GLUT10). Loss-of-function mutations in SLC2A10 affect proteoglycan biosynthesis, leading to disorganization of the extracellular matrix of connective tissue.

The syndrome typically manifests in neonatal or infantile age, although cases with onset in young adulthood have been described. Facial dysmorphisms (micrognathia, high-arched palate, beaked nose), lax and hyperextensible skin, inguinal, diaphragmatic, or hiatal hernias, joint hypermobility, and keratoconus may be present. In the most severe form, there is right ventricular hypertension, acute respiratory symptoms, and heart failure. Other serious clinical manifestations are associated with dissections causing cerebrovascular and cardiac ischemic events, as well as aneurysms with potential rupture and subarachnoid hemorrhage. The cardiovascular complications result in a mortality rate exceeding 12% of cases.

In cases of non-traumatic arterial dissection-related stroke, suspicion arises from evidence of tortuosity of the carotid arteries on CT angiography or Doppler ultrasound, and differential diagnosis includes Marfan syndrome, Ehlers-Danlos syndrome, and Loeys-Dietz syndrome. Total body angiography that demonstrates tortuosity of visceral arteries supports the diagnostic suspicion and warrants genetic mutation testing.

There is no preventive therapy available for the vascular complications associated with ATS, although endovascular treatments may be considered.

13.6.19 *Pseudoxanthoma elasticum*

Pseudoxanthoma elasticum (PXE) is a multisystem disorder of elastic tissue due to a point mutation in the *ATP-binding cassette transporter gene* (ABCC6) with autosomal recessive transmission, although rare cases with autosomal dominant inheritance have been reported, with a prevalence of approximately 1:100,000. It manifests with skin alterations, including laxity in the nape of the neck and other flexural areas such as armpits, elbow folds, and popliteal fossa, as well as areas with yellow-orange papules, similar to xanthomas, giving the skin an "orange peel" appearance. Ocular abnormalities may include unilateral or bilateral visual impairment, peripapillary neoangioid streaks, retinal hemorrhages, macular degeneration, and hyperpigmentation. Gastric abnormalities, such as gastritis, tortuous or occluded vessels, microaneurysms, and angiomata, can cause gastrointestinal bleeding. Cardiac complications may involve valvular and endocardial calcifications, mitral prolapse, restrictive cardiomyopathy, and coronary artery disease. Cerebrovascular complications include ischemic lesions in the white matter of the cerebral hemispheres, often multiple and asymptomatic; dolichoectasia of the epiaortic vessels; aneurysmal dilations that can cause both subarachnoid hemorrhage and cranial nerve deficits; epiaortic vessel dissection; moyamoya-like arteriopathy; and carotid-cavernous fistula. The cerebrovascular damage may also be partly mediated by the frequent occurrence of arterial hypertension in PXE. Skin biopsy demonstrates calcification and fragmentation of elastic fibers. Genetic analysis confirms the diagnosis.

13.6.20 Fibromuscular Dysplasia

Fibromuscular dysplasia (FMD) is a segmental angiopathy affecting large and medium-sized arteries with an unknown etiology. It predominantly affects young women, with an incidence ranging from 0.6% to 1%. FMD primarily involves the extracranial segment of the internal carotid artery, approximately 3-4 cm after the bifurcation, and less frequently the vertebral artery at the C2 level. It is bilateral in two-thirds of cases and is associated with intracranial aneurysms in 22-50% of cases, often multiple. FMD results in morphostructural alterations of the arterial wall, leading to stenosis, occlusion, or dissections. It can remain asymptomatic throughout life or manifest as TIAs or ischemic strokes, mainly in the carotid territory, due to thromboembolic events or as a result of dissections (25-30%) or subarachnoid hemorrhage from ruptured intracranial aneurysms. Hypertension, secondary to frequent renal involvement, may contribute to the development of cerebrovascular complications. The alterations of FMD can be visualized by CT angiography or MR angiography of the supra-aortic trunks, which can distinguish three types of FMD based on the pattern of stenosis: "string of beads" (Type 1, approximately 90% of cases) with multiple concentric constrictions alternating with normal or dilated arterial segments; tubular (Type 2, approximately 7% of cases) with concentric lesions and regular narrowing of the vessel lumen; focal segmental (Type 3), with a pouch-like appearance (carotid web). If FMD is identified before clinical manifestation, considering the risk of vessel dissection, it is advisable to avoid activities that involve cervical trauma or repeated microtrauma. In symptomatic patients, endovascular treatment may be considered in the presence of significant stenosis or aneurysms.

13.7 Intracerebral hemorrhage

13.7.1 Epidemiology and risk factors

Intracerebral hemorrhage accounts for 10-15% of all strokes, with an average incidence of 25 new cases per 100,000 person-year worldwide. The incidence increases with age, a major non-modifiable risk factor, ranging from approximately 2 new cases per 100,000 person-year under 44 years of age uo to about 200 in individuals aged over 85 years old. In African Americans and Japanese incidence is approximately twice that in Caucasians, suggesting a genetic predisposition, although the involvement of environmental and socioeconomic factors cannot be excluded.

One-month mortality varies from 13% to 61% in different case series and geographical areas, with an average of 40%, while one-year mortality ranges from 46% to 64%, with an average of 55%. One-third of surviving patients are functionally independent one year after the event. The main prognostic factors include age, baseline hematoma volume, supratentorial or infratentorial location of the hemorrhage, presence of intraventricular blood that may lead to secondary hydrocephalus, and the level of consciousness at onset. These features can be used to calculate a prognostic mortality score, known as the *Intracerebral Hemorrhage* (*ICH*) score (Table 13.7).

Similar to other types of stroke, both modifiable and non-modifiable risk factors are recognized for intracerebral hemorrhage. Among the non-modifiable factors, in addition to age, sex, and ethnicity, cerebral amyloid angiopathy (CAA) should be mentioned. CAA is characterized by the deposition of beta-amyloid protein, primarily in small- and medium-sized cortical arteries, which can be visualized histologically with Congo red staining. The amyloid is similar to that found in the plaques of Alzheimer's disease. CAA was initially observed in individuals with Alzheimer's dementia but it can also occur without clinical or histological evidence of Alzheimer's disease. While many cases are sporadic, hereditary forms also exist. Hemorrhages in CAA are almost exclusively lobar, often superficial or localized at the grey-white matter junction, and can be multiple. Approximately 10% of individuals over 70 years of age may have CAA, and this percentage rises to 60% in those aged over 90 years old. Therefore, the occurrence of a lobar hemorrhage in an elderly patient, especially if not affected bt arterial hypertension, highly suggests the diagnosis of CAA.

Cerebral hemorrhage associated with CAA is characterized by a high risk of recurrence, estimated at around 10% per year. In particular, individuals carrying the E4 and E2 alleles of the apolipoprotein E gene have a threefold higher risk of cerebral hemorrhage compared to with the carriers of the more common E3/E3 allele. Other non-modifiable risk factors include polymorphisms in coagulation factors, particularly factor XIII, which interfere with its normal role in thrombus consolidation by forming bridges between fibrin fibers.

Among the modifiable risk factors, hypertension is the most important, as there is a linear relationship between blood pressure values and the risk of cerebral hemorrhage, which can be significantly reduced by antihypertensive medications.

Alcohol consumption is the second most important modifiable risk factor, with a linear relationship existing between the amount of alcohol consumed and the risk of an event. This means that any amount of alcohol is associated with an increased risk compared to no consumption, and the risk increases with a "dose-response" effect. Smoking and diabetes are additional modifiable risk factors, while the role of cholesterol levels is controversial. Several studies have shown a correlation between low total and LDL cholesterol levels and the risk of cerebral hemorrhage.

Table 13.7 ICH SCORE*

Variables	
Glasgow Coma Scale	
3-4	2
5-12	1
13-15	0
Hematoma volume, cm^3	
≤30	
>30	
Intraventricular hemorrhage	
Yes	1
No	0
Infratentorial origin	
Yes	1
No	0
Age, years	
≤80	1
>80	0
Total	0-6

* The 30-day mortality rate is 13% for a score of 1, 26% for a score of 2, 72% for a score of 3, 97% for a score of 4, and 100% for a score of 5-6.

However, other studies have found that the increased risk is only present in patients with elevated blood transaminase levels, suggesting that hypocholesterolemia may be an epiphenomenon of poor dietary habits in low income social groups in which alcohol consumption is Higher.

13.7.2 Pathogenesis

Primary cerebral hemorrhage, which represents 80-85% of cases, should be distinguished from secondary hemorrhage, which accounts for the remaining 15-20%. In the first case, the hemorrhage is associated with one or more of the aforementioned risk factors, while in the second case, it can be associated with underlying conditions or iatrogenic causes. However, risk factors for "primary hemorrhage" may be present and play a contributing role in patients with other pathological conditions leading to "secondary hemorrhage".

Among the causes of secondary hemorrhage are aneurysms, which are generally sac-like dilations of medium or large arteries due to protrusions of the intima through a structural defect in the muscular layer of the vessel wall, and are typically located at bifurcations, especially in the circle of Willis. Aneurysms frequently cause subarachnoid hemorrhage (SAH) but can also lead to intracerebral hemorrhage, with or without SAH, in up to 20% of cases. The risk of rebleeding is 50% within the first 6 months, decreasing to 3% per year thereafter. Aneurysms develop in adulthood for reasons that are still unclear. Hypertension and smoking are risk factors. Mycotic aneurysms, which are secondary to septic emboli in the context of infective endocarditis, deserve mention as well. They are located in smaller cortical arteries and, if the infection is adequately treated, typically undergo a process of thrombization without consequences. Rarely, they may increase in size and rupture.

Tumors account for less than 10% of secondary intracerebral hemorrhages. Tumors that are more prone to bleed include metastases, especially from melanoma and renal carcinoma. Metastases from more common cancers (e.g., breast or lung) rarely cause intracerebral hemorrhage, but considering their high frequency, they should be considered in the differential diagnosis of atypical hemorrhages. In suspected cases, neuroimaging should be repeated a few weeks after the onset of cerebral hemorrhage to exclude the possibility of the bleeding obscuring the underlying neoplasm.

Arteriovenous malformations (AVMs) are a significant cause of cerebral hemorrhage in individuals under 40 years of age. Indeed, approximately 60% of individuals with AVMs experience hemorrhage, with a peak incidence between 25 and 40 years old. They have a prevalence in the general population of 0.1%-0.5%. In general, AVMs typically consist of a tangle of afferent arteries and veins without intermediate capillaries, communicating through one or more fistulas that form an arteriovenous shunt or through a mass of dysplastic vessels within the central part or nidus. AVMs are congenital and may increase in size with age. Hemorrhages can be intracerebral, subarachnoid, or intraventricular. Cerebral hemorrhages are typically lobar, but can also occur in the thalamus or basal ganglia. Risk factors for bleeding include advanced age, location in the deep regions of the brain (particularly basal ganglia and posterior fossa), small size, the presence of venous outflow stenosis, and the presence of associated aneurysms. After bleeding, the risk of recurrence is 18% per year. Mortality after a single hemorrhage is 10-13%, while residual disability is observed in 30% of cases.

Dural arteriovenous fistulas or malformations (dAVFs) are characterized by numerous arteries converging on a single venous structure. The arteries are typically dural, but in high-pressure fistulas, pial arteries may be involved. Venous drainage can occur into a sinus with/without stenosis or directly into cortical veins. These lesions are acquired, often as a result of minor trauma or asymptomatic cerebral venous thrombosis. They can be located anywhere within the dura mater, but they are frequently found near major sinuses, particularly the transverse sinus. Overall, the risk of hemorrhage is 2% per year, which increases to 4% per year for dAVFs that have previously bled and 7% if the dAVF is associated with an aneurysm.

Cavernous angiomas, also known as cavernomas or cavernous hemangiomas, have a prevalence of approximately 0.5% in the general population. Their etiology is unknown, but it has been suggested that they form in response to small hemorrhages in some cases. They can be familial and are often multiple. They have a peak incidence in the fourth and fifth decades of life and account for the 10% of all intracranial vascular abnormalities. Cavernous angiomas present as clusters of sinusoidal vascular channels, consisting of an endothelial layer and an inconstant fibrous adventitial layer. They can be associated with the development of microthrombi and microhemorrhages, are often asymptomatic and are occasionally discovered incidentally on neuroimaging performed for other reasons. However, they can also present with epileptic seizures or bleeding. The risk of bleeding from cavernous angiomas discovered incidentally or following an epileptic seizure is approximately 0.4-2% per year, while the risk of rebleeding from a cavernous angioma that has bled is approximately 4% in the first year. The risk of bleeding is higher for angiomas located in deep areas of the brain, such as those in the brainstem, thalamus, cerebellum, and basal ganglia.

Other causes of intracerebral hemorrhage include coagulation disorders. Hemophilia causes intracerebral hemorrhage or subdural hematoma in 2-5% of patients. Intracerebral hemorrhage is often associated with acute leukemia, thrombocytopenia, and disseminated intravascular coagulation.

Oral anticoagulants increase the risk of intracerebral hemorrhage by 8-10 times compared to that in patients not receiving anticoagulants, regardless of the presence other risk factors. However, in patients with a strong indication for anticoagulant therapy, the benefit outweighs the risk.

Antiplatelet therapy (aspirin) increases the risk of hemorrhage by 0.1% per year (higher percentage in elderly patients). The risk is largely offset by the benefit in secondary ischemic prevention. Cerebral hemorrhage can also occur in 2-4% of patients with ischemic stroke treated with intravenous thrombolysis, 9-10% of those treated with intra-arterial pharmacological thrombolysis, and 10-11% of those treated with mechanical revascularization techniques.

Finally, rare causes of secondary intracerebral hemorrhage include vasculitis, liver cirrhosis, Moyamoya disease, cerebral venous thrombosis, eclampsia, cerebral endometriosis, and traumatic brain injury.

13.7.3 Pathophysiology

Hypertension is responsible for the progressive hyaline degeneration of small lenticulostriate branches of the middle cerebral artery, small penetrating branches of the anterior cerebral artery and posterior cerebral artery, and paramedian penetrating branches of the basilar artery. The degenerative process leads to the weakening of arteriolar walls, eventually resulting in the formation of Charcot-Bouchard microaneurysms, the rupture of which causes hemorrhage. More recent observations identify these microaneurysms as subadventitial hemorrhages or extravascular clots resulting from endothelial damage caused by hypertension. Electron microscopy studies suggest that most hemorrhages occur at or near the bifurcation of the affected arteries, where arteriolar wall degeneration is most prominent. Neurons around the hematoma may die through necrosis or apoptosis related processes, or both. Additionally, in the peri-hematoma area edema develops which is initially cytotoxic, with onset a few hours after the initial event, and subsequently vasogenic, peaking at 10-20 days. The extent of cerebral edema is correlated with an unfavorable prognosis. Experimental data demonstrate that various mechanisms, in addition to the physical trauma caused by the blood itself and the mass effect, contribute to neurological damage in the regions surrounding the hematoma, indicating evolving damage mediated by hemodynamic and biochemical factors that could be targeted by therapeutic interventions. Many studies, for example, show reduced peri-hematoma blood flow, the pathogenetic significance of which remains unclear. In particular, it is uncertain whether the condition of these areas is comparable to ischemic penumbra. These findings would suggest caution in reducing systemic blood pressure in patients with intracerebral hemorrhage, as low pressure could worsen hypothetical hypoperfusion around the hematoma, favoring ischemic injury in still viable tissue. However, clinical trials have demonstrated partial efficacy of aggressive antihypertensive treatment, lowering systolic pressure to a target below 140 mmHg, in reducing the risk of hematoma enlargement without worsening clinical outcomes potentially due to blood pressure reduction, suggesting that the brain tissue surrounding the hematoma is not in a state of ischemic penumbra.

Thrombin, produced immediately after the hemorrhage, activates potentially harmful metabolic pathways, induces apoptosis, and activates microglia. Erythrocyte lysis, occurring several days after hemorrhage onset, appears to be associated with cellular damage, partly mediated by iron accumulation and oxidative stress.

Cerebral hematoma is a dynamic event. In approximately 40% of patients, it increases in volume, typically within the first hour in about two-thirds of patients and within the subsequent 24 hours in the remaining cases. The hematoma volume increase is an additional prognostic factor of unfavorable clinical outcomes. Furthermore, Hydrocephalus can develop, which is another important prognostic factor to consider, particularly in cases of cerebellar hematoma with compression of the third ventricle and Sylvian aqueduct, as well as in cases of hematomas that extend into the third ventricle, potentially obstructing the foramina of Monro.

13.7.4 Clinical aspects

Symptoms are related to the site of hemorrhage, which, in decreasing order of frequency, involve the striatum (34%), particularly the putamen, cerebral lobes (24%), especially the temporo-parieto-occipital zone, thalamus (20%), cerebellum (7%), pons (6%), and caudate nucleus (5%). In putaminal hemorrhage, the predominant manifestation is motor deficit, while in thalamic hemorrhage, contralateral sensory deficit prevails, sometimes accompanied by forced downward gaze, convergence paralysis, and miotic pupils unresponsive to light due to compression of the midbrain tectum. As the hematoma volume increases, the motor deficit worsens, and additional symptoms may appear, such as aphasia (if the hemorrhage is located in the dominant hemisphere), forced gaze deviation toward the lesion, and altered level of consciousness. Frontal lobe hemorrhages cause contralateral hemiparesis with forced gaze deviation toward the lesion. In posterior or frontoparietal lesions, sensory disturbances may also occur, and in the case of involvement of the dominant hemisphere, aphasia is present. A parietal hemorrhage results in sensory deficits accompanied by neglect/hemi-inattention. Hemorrhage in the dominant temporal lobe leads to fluent aphasia due to involvement of the Wernicke's area. In cases of excessive volume increase of supratentorial hematomas, the patient may progress into a coma due to increased intracranial pressure with subsequent herniation of the brain downward and compression of the brainstem. This typically occurs within the first 48-96 hours of the hematoma onset, although less frequently, the clinical course may be more rapid and tumultuous, with the patient entering a coma within a few hours or even minutes.

Regarding subtentorial hemorrhages, pontine hemorrhage presents with coma, pinpoint pupils, loss of oculomotor reflex, and tetraparesis. Hyperthermia and irregular respiratory rhythms may also follow. Extensive hematomas in this region are generally fatal.

Cerebellar hemorrhage, on the other hand, manifests with headache, vomiting, trunk or limb ataxia, nystagmus, gait disturbances, and possible subsequent coma due to brainstem involvement.

It should be noted that some of the pathological conditions causing secondary hemorrhage can present with signs or symptoms even before bleeding occurs. Specifically, AVMs can manifest with epileptic seizures, particularly if the lesion is large and involves the cerebral cortex. Focal symptoms such as hemiparesis, visual field deficits, or gradually worsening dementia can also occur in cases of large AVMs involving the basal ganglia. Motor or sensory deficits, with or without involvement of cranial nerves, can be seen in cases of brainstem AVMs. Recurrent microbleeds, multiple microinfarctions, reduced perfusion resulting from arterial stenosis, venous hypertension, and steal phenomena are all implicated mechanisms that could explain the progression of symptoms. Patients with AVMs may experience headache as an initial symptom (approximately 12% of cases). The pain is often unilateral and throbbing, making it difficult to distinguish from migraine. It is more common in case of dural or pial AVMs and tends to recur even after therapeutic treatment.

13.7.5 Diagnosis

A rapid alteration in the level of consciousness, along with the presence of headache and vomiting, are the three main variables to consider for the clinical differential diagnosis between cerebral hemorrhage and ischemic stroke. However, the alteration in the level of consciousness often develops gradually, and unlike bleeding in the subarachnoid spaces, bleeding in the brain parenchyma is typically painless since the brain lacks pain-related nociceptors and innervation. Therefore, patients with small deep hematomas do not experience headache, while headache is present in cases of very large hematomas or hematomas extending into the subarachnoid spaces. About half of the patients with supratentorial hemorrhage, more than half of those with subtentorial hemorrhage, and almost all those with cerebellar hemorrhage experience vomiting.

Overall, a clinical differential diagnosis between ischemic stroke and hemorrhagic stroke based on these variables is neither sensitive nor specific, and the use of neuroimaging is essential. Blood is immediately evident on CT scans as a distinct hyperdensity (Figure 13.17), which gradually decreases over the following days, becoming isodense with the brain parenchyma within 2 weeks and then hypodense. In patients with low hematocrit due to reduced hemoglobin concentration, the hemorrhage may be isodense since the acute phase. MRI can allow to approximately determine the age of the hemorrhage because the various phases of blood metabolic degradation correspond to specific MRI signal alterations.

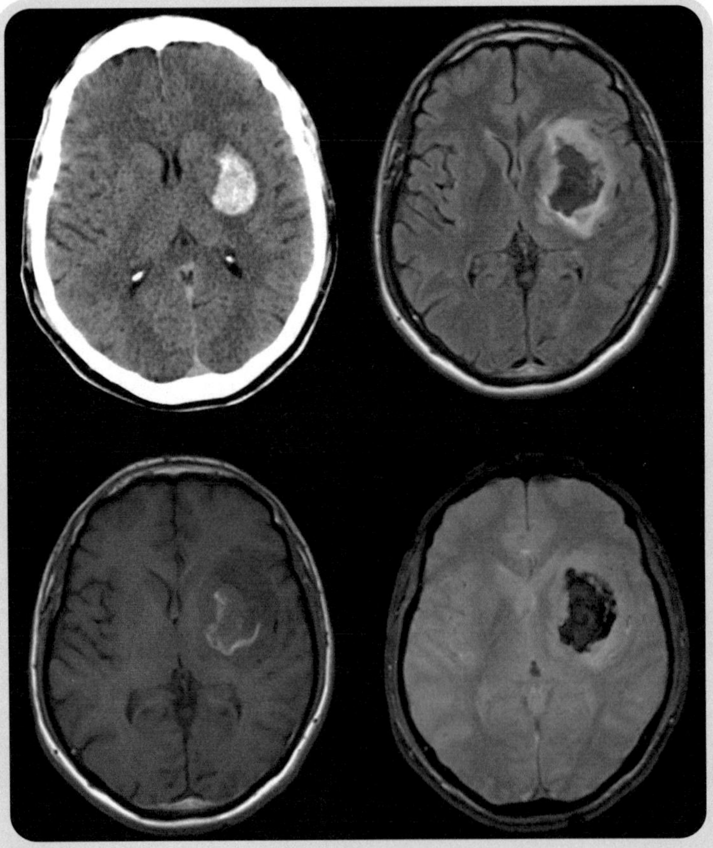

Figure 13.17

Intracerebral hemorrhage on CT and MRI. A 45-year-old patient with uncontrolled hypertension. Sudden onset of aphasia and weakness in the right upper limb. The urgent CT scan (top left) reveals a 3.2 cm diameter hemorrhage in the left lentiform nucleus. The MRI images, taken 4 days after the onset, show a 5 cm intraparenchymal hematoma in the left lentiform nucleus with perilesional edema. The T2-FLAIR sequence (top right), T1 sequence (bottom left), and GRE sequence (bottom right) are shown.

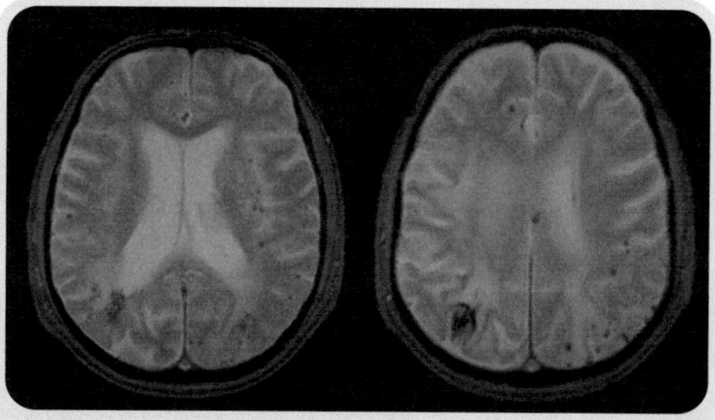

Figure 13.18

Amyloid angiopathy. A 70-year-old patient, heavy smoker, with multiple cerebral infarctions, right internal carotid artery occlusion, arterial hypertension, dyslipidemia, and impaired glucose tolerance. Admitted due to motor deficit in the right hemisoma caused by a left hemispheric cerebral infarction. MRI scans in GRE sequences show the presence of multiple hypointense bilateral lesions consistent with a diagnosis of amyloid angiopathy.

In the acute hematoma stage (hours to days), intracellular oxyhemoglobin transforms into deoxyhemoglobin (starting from the center of the hematoma). In this phase, the signal is iso- or slightly hyperintense on T1-weighted images and hypointense on T2-weighted images. The surrounding edema can cause a hyperintense T2-weighted halo peripherally (Figure 13.17). In the following weeks, intracellular deoxyhemoglobin evolves into intracellular methemoglobin (starting from the periphery), and the hematoma appears hyperintense on T1-weighted images. With cell lysis and the presence of extracellular methemoglobin, the signal becomes hyperintense on T2-weighted images as well. A hypointense ring due to hemosiderin remains for years, while the T1 and T2 hyperintensity gradually disappears. Gradient echo sequences (T2*) are highly sensitive to even small amounts of blood in all phases (Figure 13.17).

The analysis of the images and the location of the hematoma can provide clues regarding the possible etiology and the need for further investigations. Hemorrhage involving the basal ganglia, thalamus, internal capsule, periventricular white matter, pons, or cerebellum in patients with hypertension can be reasonably attributed to hypertensive arteriopathy, therefore additional diagnostic workup for etiological classification can be unnecessary. However, in the case of young patients or regardless of age in the absence of a history of hypertension, further diagnostic investigations such as CT angiography or MR angiography are indicated.

In cases of lobar hemorrhage in elderly patients where T2*-weighted MRI reveals multiple microhemorrhages, especially in the cortex, the diagnosis of CAA is almost certain (Figure 13.18). For prognostic evaluation, it is recommended to perform a follow-up neuroimaging study in the subsequent days to assess any hematoma enlargement or the presence of hydrocephalus in case of intraventricular bleeding.

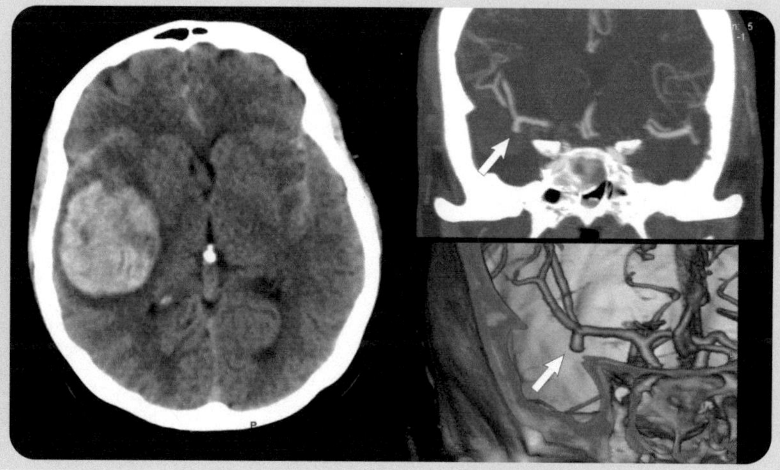

Figure 13.19

MCA aneurysm with parenchymal hemorrhage. 70-year-old patient. Sudden onset of right shoulder pain, radiating to the neck, followed by sudden left hemiplegia and dysarthria. The brain CT scan (top left) shows an intraparenchymal hematoma in the right temporo-parietal region and blood in the subarachnoid spaces. The angiographic CT scan (top right, with 3D reconstructions below) shows the presence of an aneurysmal dilatation at the bifurcation of the right ACM (arrow).

CT angiography or MR angiography can detect aneurysms with a diameter larger than 3 mm (Figure 13.19).

Larger AVMs can also be detected using CT angiography or MR angiography, but catheter angiography is the best technique for visualizing and studying their structure (Figure 13.20). However, hematoma can alter the hemodynamics of an AVM to the point that it becomes invisible on angiography.

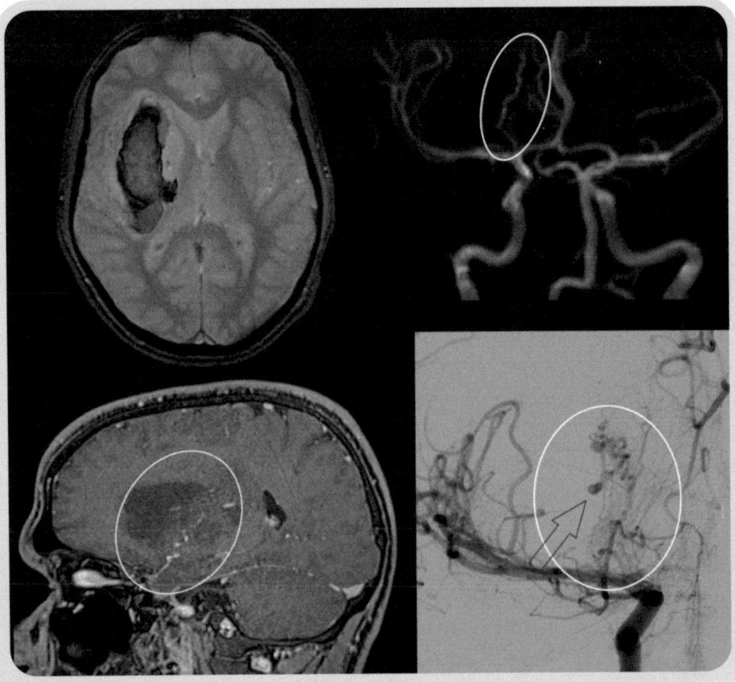

Figure 13.20

Arteriovenous malformation with aneurysm. 20-year-old patient. Sudden onset of dizziness, vomiting, and weakness in the left limbs. The MRI shows, in the GRE sequences (top left), a large hematoma in basal ganglia. In the TOF angiography reconstructions (top right) and sagittal acquisitions with gadolinium (bottom left), a tortuous vessel protruding into the hemorrhagic area is observed. Catheter angiography (bottom right) shows the presence of a small AVM nourished by a lenticulostriate artery, with a tiny nidus aneurysm (arrow).

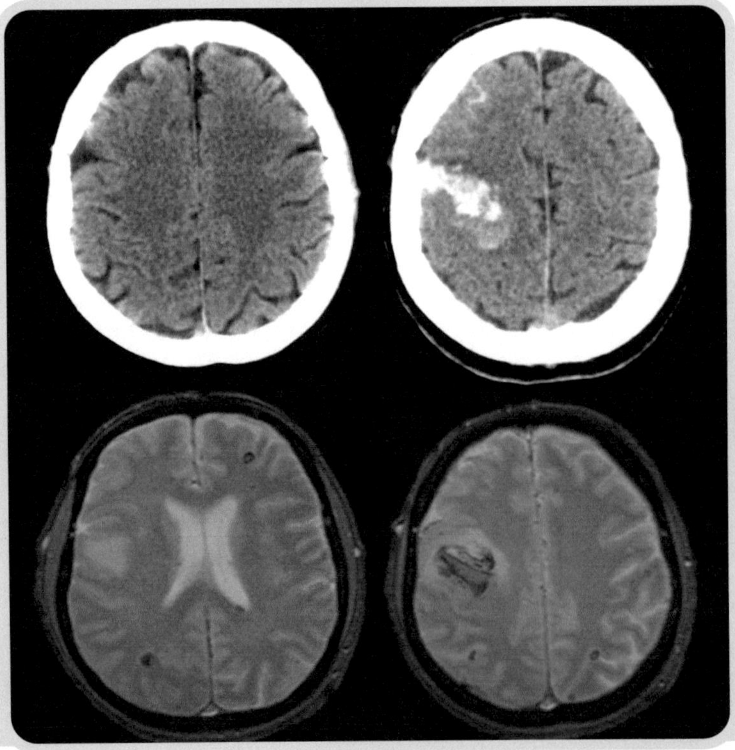

Figure 13.21

Cavernoma. 61-year-old patient, hypertensive. Sudden onset of weakness and hypoesthesia in the left hemisoma. Brain CT within normal limits (top left). Underwent thrombolytic treatment. At the end of the infusion, experienced headache and nausea with worsening of the weakness. Urgent brain CT: cortical hemorrhagic suffusion in the right frontal region (top right). Brain MRI: in the GRE sequences (bottom), there is a collection of blood in the pre-rolandic region of the right frontal lobe. Additionally, hypointense areas with a hyperintense central nucleus, attributable to cavernous angiomas, are evident.

Therefore, if the initial angiography is negative but there is a reasonable diagnostic suspicion, angiography should be repeated after a certain period of time (3-6 months).

Cavernous angiomas are recognized on MRI by the characteristic hypointense ring of hemosiderin surrounding an intense and irregular signal on T2-weighted images (Figure 13.21). They are typically isolated and supratentorial, but can be multiple, especially in familial cases. There are no angiographic abnormalities.

Dural fistulas can rarely be detected on brain CT, particularly when a dilated vein is present. MRI may reveal afferent vessels and dilated veins, but it is neither specific nor sensitive. The diagnosis is made with catheter angiography, which also involves the external carotid artery system.

13.7.6 Treatment

The general principles of stabilization treatment in stroke units, as already described for patients with ischemic stroke, also apply to patients with cerebral hemorrhage but with some noteworthy peculiarities. Regarding blood pressure management, in hemorrhagic stroke current guidelines recommend treatment when the systolic blood pressure is above 180 mmHg and/or the diastolic blood pressure is above 105 mmHg, setting a lower threshold for intervention compared to ischemic stroke. This is based on the assumption that high blood pressure levels can promote bleeding. Furthermore, as previously mentioned, more aggressive treatment of blood pressure, aiming to lower systolic pressure below 140 mmHg, has been shown to be effective in reducing the risk of hematoma expansion in the first 24 hours and, to a lesser extent, improving clinical outcomes.

Hemorrhage secondary to oral anticoagulant therapy with vitamin K antagonists and elevated INR upon admission continues to increase in volume until INR is normalized. Therefore, prompt administration of prothrombin complexes or, alternatively, fresh plasma is necessary, including co-administration of vitamin K. In the case of hemorrhage secondary to therapy with direct-acting anticoagulants, the use of prothrombin complex concentrates is suggested by the guidelines, which however recommend the use of specific available antidotes (reversal agents) as first choice treatment. In particular, the antidote for dabigatran (a direct thrombin inhibitor) is idarucizumab, which is a monoclonal antibody with very high affinity for the anticoagulant, and, when administered as an intravenous bolus, immediately blocks its activity. The antidote for rivaroxaban, apixaban, and edoxaban (direct factor Xa inhibitors) is andexanet, a molecule structurally similar to factor X but lacking of catalytic activity and with high affinity for the drugs. These latter are therefore displaced from factor X with an immediate anticoagulation reversal effect.

Resumption of anticoagulant therapy can be considered after approximately two to three weeks, during which the risk of cardioembolic stroke appears reasonably low, even in patients with valvular prostheses. However, in the presence of CAA, the resumption of anticoagulant therapy is not recommended. For patients with atrial fibrillation and a high risk of embolic events, percutaneous closure of the atrial appendage may be considered.

In patients with primary hemorrhage who are at risk of deep venous thrombosis (such as bedridden patients, obese patients, or those with a history of previous thrombophlebitis) and pulmonary embolism, prophylaxis is a concern. Given the ineffectiveness of elastic compressive stockings, various guidelines suggest the use of low molecular weight heparins at prophylactic doses starting 48 to 96 hours after symptom onset. Intermittent pneumatic compression of the lower limbs is also recommended.

The pharmacological treatment of cerebral edema in patients with cerebral hemorrhage does not differ from that indicated for patients with ischemic stroke, as there is no indication for the use of steroids. Finally, prophylactic antiepileptic treatment is not justified in cerebral hemorrhage, despite the potentially higher risk of seizures, especially in the case of extensive cortical hemorrhage. Therefore, the recommendation remains to treat individual epileptic seizures during the acute phase, reserving long-term antiepileptic therapy for those patients that develop epilepsyin the subacute/chronic phase.

13.7.7 Specific therapies

Early surgical evacuation of the hematoma (within 48 hours of symptom onset) does not appear to provide an advantage in terms of mortality and residual disability compared to conservative therapy, except in cases of more superficial hemorrhage. Currently, guidelines recommend surgical intervention in the following cases: a) cerebellar hemorrhages larger than 3 cm in diameter with neurological deterioration or signs of brainstem compression and hydrocephalus secondary to ventricular obstruction; b) lobar hemorrhages of medium(≥ 30 cm^3 e < 50 cm^3) or large (≥ 50 cm^3) size rapidly deteriorating due to compression of vital intracranial structures or herniation; c) intracerebral hemorrhages associated with surgically accessible aneurysms or AVMs.

Surgical removal of cavernous angiomas should be considered in cases of recurrent hemorrhage and sometimes in patients with drug-resistant epilepsy. Alternatively, radiosurgery can be considered. The observation that cavernous angiomas tend to bleed in clusters has led to perform stereotactic radiosurgery as the treatment of choice.

The choice between aggressive or conservative treatment for AVMs should be based on the angiographic study of the number and distribution of aferent arteries, venous drainage patterns, and flow through the lesion nidus. Other factors to consider include the patient's age, presence of comorbidities, possible evolution, and the presence of treatment-related risks. After the rupture of an AVM, the risk of early rebleeding is lower than that following an aneurysmal rupture, which allows to wait for patient clinical recovery in order to intervene under optimal conditions. Treatment options include surgical excision, embolization, or stereotactic radiosurgery, either individually or in combination. Surgical excision is the most definitive treatment and the preferred approach for smaller AVMs with a single feeder artery and a single venous drainage. Postoperative angiography should be performed to confirm complete excision.

Endovascular embolization using glue allows for complete eradication of approximately 20% of the AVM. However, there is a procedural risk, with a mortality rate of 14% and minor or major morbidity in 2-17% of cases. This includes a risk of cerebral ischemia in 20% of patients due to occlusion of a normal vessel or rupture of the AVM caused by glue deposition in a draining vein, which leadsto increased pressure within the nidus. Repeated embolization can also reduce the volume of the AVM, making it accessible to surgery or radiosurgery. Embolization may also be indicated in cases of medically refractory headaches or progressive neurological deficits. In the long term, embolized arteries may recanalize. Stereotactic radiosurgery, such as gamma knife, can be used in selected patients to deliver a high single dose of radiation stereotactically centered on the AVM nidus. Radiation causes endothelial damage, proliferation of smooth muscle cells, progressive sclerosis, and subsequent thrombosis of the AVM vessels. The success of treatment depends on the size of the AVM and the radiation dose delivered. Some AVMs may take 24-36 months to undergo a complete thrombization process, and during this period, the patient remains at risk of bleeding. Potential complications, such as radiation necrosis of healthy brain tissue or cranial nerve paralysis, depend on the radiation dose, treated volume, patient age, and AVM flow characteristics. Radiation-induced tumors are very rare.

13.8 Subarachnoid Hemorrhage (SAH)

13.8.1 Epidemiology and risk factors

SAH accounts forapproximately 3% of all acute cerebrovascular events, with an average incidence in Western countries of 6-16 new cases per 100,000 individuals per year, and in Italy of 8-10 new cases per 100,000 individuals per year. The incidence increases with age, being rare in individuals under 20 years old and peaking at the age of 55-60. The incidence in women is nearly double that in men. There are also geographical variations, with lower rates in the Middle East and higher rates in Scandinavian countries, particularly in Finland, where the incidence is three times higher than the rest of the world. Additionally, there are ethnic differences, as Afro-Caribbean individuals have a higher incidence compared to individuals of Caucasian ethnicity at the same age.

Cohort studies suggest that active or passive cigarette smoking, hypertension, and alcohol abuse are risk factors for SAH. Cigarette smoking, in particular, increases the risk of SAH by 3-10 times, with a clear dose-response effect, while smoking cessation reduces the risk within 2-4 years. The role of hypertension is less pronounced and less defined due to its high epidemiological co-occurrence. However, smoking and hypertension seem to act synergistically, with the risk of SAH in hypertensive smokers being 15 times higher than in non-smoking non-hypertensive individuals. Other risk factors include above-normal body mass index and the use of ilicit drugs and psychostimulants. Approximately 7-20% of SAH cases are related to familial aneurysms, with about one-third of asymptomatic family members showing aneurysms on neuroimaging. The relative risk of SAH in relatives of patients affected by SAH is six times higher than in individuals without a family history. Familial aneurysms tend to rupture at smaller sizes compared to non-familial cases, and there is an anticipation effect, with SAH occurring at increasingly younger ages in subsequent generations. Lastly, the presence of aneurysms in the same or mirror locations is more frequent in familial cases, and the frequency increases with closer degrees of kinship.

In a minority of cases, specific genetic factors may be involved. Approximately 5% of intracranial aneurysm cases are associated with an underlying hereditary connective tissue disorder, such as Marfan syndrome, Ehlers-Danlos syndrome, *pseudoxanthoma elasticum*, α1-antitrypsin deficiency, or autosomal dominant polycystic kidney disease.

The most important complications during SAH include:

- rebleeding, with around 50% of patients experiencing a recurrent hemorrhage within a month;
- vasospasm, which typically peaks at 7-10 days after SAH onset and can worsen the clinical picture by leading to widespread ischemic damage;
- hydrocephalus, resulting from obstruction of cerebrospinal fluid flow due to clots, which can occur even years after the initial SAH.

The prognosis of SAH remains quite severe, with an overall mortality rate (including pre-hospital mortality) of approximately 50-60% within the first month and severe residual disability in about 30% of surviving patients. Over 50% of survivors may experience memory impairments or mood disorders. The most important prognostic factors for an unfavorable outcome are age, level of consciousness at admission, and the extent of bleeding.

13.8.2 Pathogenesis

Spontaneous (non-traumatic) SAH is due to aneurysmal rupture in 85% of cases; idiopathic non-aneurysmal SAH accounts for 10% and usually has a perimesencephalic location and a benign prognosis; the remaining 5% are secondary to rare causes such as AVMs, vasculitis, neoplasms, dural arteriovenous fistulas, carotid or vertebral artery dissections (including those occurring in the context of connective tissue disorders such as Marfan syndrome, Ehlers-Danlos syndrome, Loeys-Dietz syndrome), coagulopathies, or the use of sympathomimetic substances like cocaine and methamphetamine.

An international multicenter registry on unruptured aneurysms revealed a higher prevalence among women (with a female-to-male ratio of 3:1) and at a younger age (mean age 51.4 years). The registry also showed a high percentage of current or former smokers (79%) and a positive family in 20% of cases, with a higher incidence in families with multiple aneurysms and a higher propensity for rupture. Familial cases suggest a genetic background in approximately 40% of cases, although no clear candidate genes have been identified so far, and the picture is further complicated by possible interactions with environmental factors.

The most common location for unruptured aneurysms is the middle cerebral artery, while the less frequent is the anterior communicating artery. The risk of rupture is related to the size and location of the aneurysm, with an annual rupture rate of 0.05% for aneurysms smaller than

7 mm of diameter in the anterior circulation. A higher risk of rupture is associated with aneurysms located in the midline (anterior communicating artery and basilar artery apex). Furthermore, the likelihood of an aneurysm rupture in patients with a history of previous SAH from another aneurysm is 11 times higher than in patients without a previous SAH. Lastly, the risk of complications from surgical treatment of unruptured aneurysms is elevated, especially in individuals over 60-70 years old, for aneurysms located in the posterior fossa and larger aneurysms, and in the presence of compressive symptoms.

13.8.3 Clinical aspects

The most indicative presenting symptom for an SAH diagnosis is a sudden, explosive headache described as a "thunderclap headache," occurring within seconds, intense, and unlike any previous headaches. It is present in 85-100% of SAH cases and may be the sole symptom in approximately one-third of patients. However, it should be noted that only 10% of patients presenting to the Emergency Department with this type and intensity of headache have an SAH, and there are no specific clinical features that allow distinguishing a benign "thunderclap headache" from a symptomatic SAH-related headache. Within minutes to hours, the pain tends to localize to the occipital and nuchal areas or the spine as the blood spreads along the lower subarachnoid spaces. The duration can be up to 12 weeks, but in cases of milder bleeding, it may last only a few hours. Around 25% of patients with SAH may have experienced a previous bleeding episode manifested as a headache diagnosed as migraines or "cervical arthrosis." These are known as "sentinel headaches" caused by aneurysm fissures, which can be followed, in the subsequent weeks, by a major rebleeding episode, often with dramatic outcomes. Therefore, all patients presenting to an Emergency Department with a headache of acute onset and unusual in terms of type and/or intensity should be carefully examined by a neurologist and, if necessary, undergo diagnostic imaging. Vomiting is generally present from the onset of the headache. Neck stiffness, on the other hand, is not an early sign and usually appears 3-12 hours after the onset of SAH, irrespective of its severity, so its absence does not rule out the diagnosis. Changes in the level of consciousness at onset or shortly after the onset of SAH are very common, with lethargy and confusion present in approximately one-third of cases, transient loss of consciousness in another third, and coma in approximately 17% of patients. Loss of consciousness can be due to the amount of blood in the subarachnoid space or complications of SAH, such as brain herniation due to hematoma or acute hydrocephalus. Seizures can occur as early as the first day in around 10% of patients with SAH, while up to 30% of cases may have seizures starting from 6 months after SAH onset. The presence of significant bleeding in the basal cisterns and the possibility of rebleeding are predictive variables for the occurrence of post-SAH seizures.

Focal neurological signs and symptoms are found in approximately 20% of cases and result from intraparenchymal extension of bleeding or vasospasm leading to cerebral ischemia in the 4-12 days following the hemorrhage. Sometimes, the symptoms allow to determine the localization of the aneurysm. For example, anterior communicating artery aneurysms may cause frontal symptoms such as bilateral lower limb weakness, bilateral extensor plantar reflexes, spincteric incontinence, and abulia. Aneurysms of the anterior choroidal artery and middle cerebral artery may present with hemiparesis, aphasia, or visuospatial neglect, while aneurysms of the pericallosal artery and distal anterior cerebral artery may result in monoparesis of the lower limb. Aneurysms of the posterior communicating artery and, less frequently, the carotid bifurcation, basilar artery apex, posterior cerebral artery, and superior cerebellar artery can cause compressive third cranial nerve palsy with unilateral mydriasis and loss of direct and consensual light reflexes, despite normal extraocular motility. Sixth cranial nerve palsy in the context of increased intracranial pressure is common and often bilateral in the acute phase due to nerve compression against the petrous ridge caused by a downward transtentorial herniation of the diencephalon. Occasionally, sixth cranial nerve palsy can result from direct compression by posterior circulation aneurysms. The Parinaud syndrome (fixed miosis, paralysis

Table 13.8 HUNT-HESS* SCALE

Grade		Survival %
Grade 0	silent aneurysm	
Grade I	asymptomatic or mild headache and mild neck stiffness	70%
Grade Ia	focal neurological deficits without meningeal signs	
Grade II	cranial nerve deficits, moderate to severe headache, neck stiffness	60%
Grade III	confusion/stupor, mild focal neurological deficits	50%
Grade IV	stupor, moderate to severe hemiparesis, stiffness	40%
Grade V	coma, decerebrate posturing	10%

Grade I-III: generally associated with a favorable clinical outcome; these patients are candidates for early surgical intervention. Grade IV and V: indicative of an unfavorable prognosis; these patients require stabilization and progression to Grade III before undergoing surgical or endovascular intervention.

* Adapted from: Hunt WE, Hess RM. "Surgical risk as related to time of intervention in the repair of intracranial aneurysms." Journal of Neurosurgery 1968 Jan;28(1):14-20

of downward gaze and convergence) usually indicates hydrocephalus, which, by dilating the Sylvian aqueduct, causes dysfunction of the pretectal area.

Based on the level of consciousness and the presence or absence of focal signs, the clinical severity can be quantified in terms of scores. by using the Hunt and Hess scale (Table 13.8), or the World Federation of Neurological Surgeons (WFNS) scale (Table 13.9), with higher scores indicating a more severe condition and predicting mortality and the risk of neurological complications. Retinal and preretinal hemorrhages (subhyaloid) occur in approximately 20% of SAH cases. The hemorrhage is believed to be caused by increased intracranial pressure on the optic nerve and the central retinal vein passing through it, impeding venous outflow from the retina. The resulting venous congestion can rupture the retinal veins. Blood streaks or flame-shaped hemorrhages appear in the preretinal layer (subhyaloid), usually near the optic nerve. In about 4% of SAH cases, the preretinal hemorrhage extends into the vitreous body (Terson syndrome). Subhyaloid and vitreous hemorrhages are negative prognostic factors, being often associated with extensive SAH. Surviving patients with Terson syndrome should undergo follow-up due to the risk of developing increased intraocular pressure and retinal detachment.

Table 13.9 WORLD FEDERATION OF NEUROLOGICAL SURGEONS (WFNS) SCALE

Grades	
Grade I	GCS 15, no motor deficits
Grade II	GCS 13-14, no motor deficits
Grade III	GCS 13-14, presence of motor deficits
Grade IV	GCS 7-12, motor deficits present or absent
Grade V	GCS 3-6, motor deficits present or absent

GCS = Glasgow Coma Score

13.8.4 Diagnosis

In cases of clinical suspicion, the first examination to be performed is a brain CT scan, which, if done within 24-48 hours, can detect blood in approximately 95% of cases, typically distributed symmetrically in the basal cisterns, Sylvian fissures, and cortical sulci (Figure 13.22). However, since the blood rapidly flows out the subaracnoid spaces, the diagnostic sensitivity of CT decreases over the days following symptom onset, reaching a minimum of 30% when performed after 2 weeks.

Asymmetric distribution of blood may suggest the location of the aneurysm, which is important, particularly in patients with multiple aneurysms, to identify the one requiring intervention. Anterior communicating artery aneurysms can often cause intraventricular hemorrhage, while concurrent intracerebral hemorrhage is common in cases of middle cerebral artery aneurysms (Figure 13.19) and posterior communicating artery aneurysms. CT can also reveal the presence of cerebral ischemia, hydrocephalus, mass effect with midline shift, or rebleeding.

Conventional MRI is not sensitive to blood in the acute phase, because there is little methemoglobin to differentiate hemorrhage from cerebrospinal fluid. However, in the following days, the breakdown products of blood become more evident on MRI, making it the preferred modality for demonstrating subacute or previous bleeding that CT may not detect. Diffusion-weighted MRI sequences can also be useful in identifying any associated cerebral ischemia in more detail. During the acute phase in cases of inconclusive CT and strong clinical suspicion of SAH, the next appropriate diagnostic investigation is not MRI but a lumbar puncture. The cerebrospinal fluid may be frankly bloody, but a traumatic tap can yield the same result, and a decrease in red blood cell count in subsequent tubes is not a reliable method to differentiate the two conditions. Only spectrophotometric examination of the supernatant of the centrifuged cerebrospinal fluid allows for a diagnosis of SAH by revealing characteristic xanthochromia, a yellowish color due to the presence of bilirubin, which becomes positive approximately 12 hours after bleeding and remains so for up to 2 weeks, even when the cerebrospinal fluid appears colorless at the time of extraction.

The diagnostic process then proceeds with angiographic studies, both in cases of confirmed SAH and in cases where previous investigations were inconclusive but there is a strong clinical suspicion. CT angiography with 3D reconstructions and MR angiography are accurate and non-invasive imaging techniques that are very useful for diagnostic purposes. However, catheter angiography is still necessary if these examinations are negative or as a preparatory step for intervention. Catheter angiography allows for the study of the aneurysm's location, size, orientation, the presence of any intraluminal thrombi or calcifications, its relationship with nearby vessels, and the presence of any additional aneurysms. In cases where an intraparenchymal hematoma is present, it can suggest which aneurysm has ruptured. In the absence of a concomitant hematoma or a diagnosis of SAH made through cerebrospinal fluid analysis, the general rule is that the most likely ruptured aneurysm is the largest, most irregular, with mass effect or associated vasospasm of surrounding arteries.

Catheter angiography may be negative in 10-15% of confirmed SAH cases. In approximately two-thirds of these cases, the bleeding is likely venous in origin, involving the prepontine or perimesencephalic regions and affecting younger individuals. These cases tend to have a better prognosis due to a lower tendency for rebleeding and secondary ischemia. However, a similar distribution of blood can also occur in 10% of vertebrobasilar aneurysms, which have a less favorable prognosis. The remaining cases of SAH with negative angiography may be due to immediate aneurysm thrombosis, small aneurysms (less than 2 mm in diameter) that rupture during bleeding, or generalized or local vasospasm. In these cases, repeat angiography performed after 2-4 weeks reveals aneurysms in 2-5% of cases.

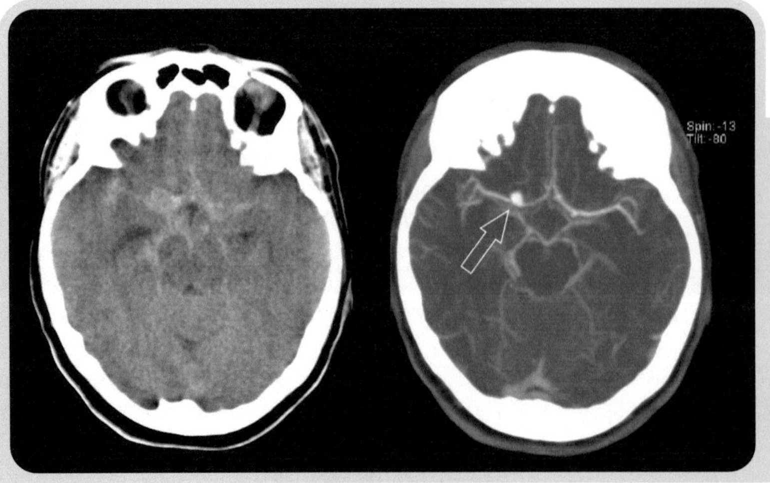

Figure 13.22

Subarachnoid Hemorrhage. 48-year-old patient with sudden onset of severe headache and vomiting, no neurological deficits. The CT scan (on the left) shows a subarachnoid hemorrhage in a bilateral location, predominantly involving the optic chiasm and the basal cisterns. The CT angiogram (on the right) reveals the presence of an aneurysm at the bifurcation of the right middle cerebral artery.

Finally, for the diagnosis and monitoring of vasospasm, the most appropriate diagnostic technique is transcranial Doppler, which has the advantage of being non-invasive and can be performed at the patient's bedside, although approximately 10% of patients may have a poor acoustic window.

13.8.5 Treatment

The general treatment of patients with SAH is similar to that described for patients with ischemic stroke or intracerebral hemorrhage, aimed at stabilizing neurological and cardiorespiratory function. The acute phase of SAH may be complicated by fever, arterial hypertension, and hyperglycemia. The most common medical complications are pulmonary edema (23%), both cardiogenic and neurogenic, cardiac arrhythmias (35%), including sudden death in up to 15% of cases, and electrolyte disturbances (28%), particularly hyponatremia. The latter can result from either cerebral salt-wasting syndrome with hypovolemia or syndrome of inappropriate antidiuretic hormone secretion with normo or hypervolemia. If not properly treated, both conditions are associated with high mortality, and intervention is warranted for sodium levels <125 mEq/L. The former condition requires administration of abundant sodium and fluids, while the latter necessitates fluid restriction. Fluid restriction in the setting of cerebral salt-wasting syndrome exacerbates hypovolemia, predisposing the patient to vasospasm.

Vasospasm is the most common neurological complication, occurring in approximately half of SAH cases and being symptomatic in 20-30% of patients. It is believed to result from the release of metabolites with vasoconstrictive effects during thrombus lysis in the basal cisterns and from impaired vasodilation of cerebral arteries due to endothelial dysfunction. Other pathogenetic hypotheses, such as spreading depression (see subsection 13.3.2 for further details), have been proposed. The peak of vasospasm occurs between 3 and 14 days after bleeding. The severity and distribution of vasospasm are greater in cases of blood in the basal cisterns than in diffuse bleeding in the ventricles or on the cortex. Older age, higher systolic blood pressure, reduced level of consciousness, and the presence of motor deficits or hydrocephalus are all variables associated with the risk of developing vasospasm. Patients with vertebral artery aneurysms, predominantly intraventricular blood, or negative CT findings have a lower risk of vasospasm. The diagnosis is challenging and is made after excluding other causes of neurological deterioration, such as hydrocephalus, electrolyte disorders, seizures, or rebleeding. Transcranial Doppler can confirm the diagnosis.

Elevation of blood pressure, expansion of blood volume, and hemodilution are not effective interventions for reducing vasospasm. Moreover, they expose the patient to the risk of cardiac decompensation, electrolyte disorders, and bleeding from untreated aneurysms. A clinical trial has shown the effectiveness of nimodipine (a calcium channel blocker) in reducing the risk of cerebral infarction by 34% and consequently improving clinical outcomes by 40% in patients with SAH. However, the mechanism by which the drug achieved these results is not clear. In fact, in patients undergoing angiographic follow-up several days after symptom onset, there was no difference in the incidence of vasospasm between those treated with nimodipine and those treated with a placebo. It is therefore possible that nimodipine acted more as a neuroprotective agent in patients who developed ischemia due to vasospasm rather than as a direct vasospasm antagonist. Regardless of the explanation, it is routine practice to administer 60 mg of nimodipine every 4 hours orally if the patient can swallow, or intravenously if not, from the start of hospitalization.

In case of pharmacologically intractable vasospasm, a possible option is endovascular angioplasty, which can achieve improvement in 60-80% of patients, with a 5% risk of complications such as bleeding due to vessel rupture or unclosed aneurysms. Concurrent endovascular administration of papaverine is effective in increasing vessel caliber and flow, but it may lead to increased intracranial pressure (which should be carefully monitored in these patients) and respiratory depression if administered in the inferior posterior cerebellar artery. The treatment is not indicated in patients who have not already undergone treatment for the ruptured aneurysm due to the risk of bleeding, and in patients with evident ischemic lesions on CT due to the risk of hemorrhagic transformation of the lesions. Symptomatic hydrocephalus occurs in 10-35% of patients as a result of mechanical obstruction by blood of the cerebrospinal fluid pathways in the cisterns or ventricles. External ventricular drainage for some days is indicated in cases of reduced level of consciousness; the intervention improves the clinical picture in 50-80% of patients but increases the risk of rebleeding and entails infectious complications in 5-10% of cases. A preliminary study has suggested the potential effectiveness of intraventricular application of t-PA to reduce bleeding and prevent hydrocephalus, but confirmation on a larger sample of patients is required before recommending its routine use. Only 10-15% of patients develop chronic hydrocephalus due to arachnoid adhesions with progressive dilation, which manifests clinically with spatial-temporal disorientation, urinary incontinence, ataxia, and spastic paraparesis. A permanent ventriculoperitoneal shunt can improve the clinical status of these patients.

Seizures can occur at onset or within the first 24 hours in 3-18% of cases, while 6-15% of surviving patients develop epilepsy. The risk of developing epilepsy is higher in the presence of intracerebral hematoma, vasospasm, systemic hypertension, greater clinical severity, perioperative complications, rebleeding, early seizures, and hydrocephalus requiring a permanent shunt.

If the ruptured aneurysm is not treated, the most serious risk is rebleeding, with a risk ranging from 20% within 14 days to 40% within 180 days. Subsequently, the probability of recurrent rupture is 3% per year. The incidence of recurrent rupture is significantly higher in the first 2 days and particularly within the first 24 hours. Rebleeding accounts for approximately 30% of unfavorable prognoses in terms of mortality and morbidity. The treatment of the aneurysm can include surgical clipping, which was the only possible treatment for many years, or endovascular coil embolization, in which coils are inserted into the aneurysm and detached from the guiding catheter. Coils of different length and thickness are often used to exclude the aneurysm from the circulation. The greater safety and efficacy of endovascular treatment for ruptured aneurysms compared to surgical clipping have been demonstrated. The clinical advantage of endovascular treatment varies according to the location of the aneurysms but is superior to traditional surgery in all locations. However, the occlusion rate achieved with surgery is higher.. Another advantage of endovascular treatment is the lower risk of developing epilepsy. However, in individual cases, , several factors need to be taken into consideration to decide which is the most appropriate treatment, such as the patient's age, the location and size of the aneurysm, its morphology and relationships with adjacent vessels, as well as the patient general clinical conditions.

13.9 Spinal cord vascular pathology

13.9.1 Vascular anatomy

The main arteries that vascularize the spinal cord are the anterior spinal artery and the two posterior spinal arteries.

The anterior spinal artery originates from the anastomosis of two branches coming from the vertebral arteries and runs for almost the entire length of the spinal cord, up to the apex of the conus medullaris within the anterior median fissure. The two posterior spinal arteries, much smaller in caliber than the anterior artery, originate as direct branches from the vertebral arteries and run parallel and longitudinally from the first segments of the cord to the apex of the conus medullaris. Along their course, these arteries give rise to anterior and posterior segmental arteries that, heading inferolaterally, penetrate the intervertebral foramina and anastomose in the cervical tract of the cord with the vertebral artery or the ascending or deep cervical artery, in the thoracic tract with the posterior intercostal arteries, in the lumbar tract with the lumbar arteries, and at the level of the cauda equina with the lateral sacral arteries.

The major segmental artery is called the artery of Adamkiewicz and usually branches off from the anterior spinal artery at the T7 level on the left side and anastomoses with the corresponding posterior intercostal artery between T9 and T10 after giving rise to a branch for the anterior spinal artery and another one for the posterior spinal artery. The anterior spinal artery supplies the anterior two-thirds of the cord, while the posterior spinal arteries supply the remaining posterior one-third.

Venous drainage of the spinal cord follows a course similar to the arterial supply, and the veins assume corresponding names. It should be noted that in the adipose tissue of the epidural space, there is the epidural venous plexus (anterior and posterior), which surrounds the meningeal dura mater and freely anastomoses, receiving part of the blood from the segmental veins. The blood from this plexus is drained by the intervertebral veins, which exit through the intervertebral foramina and converge into the azygos venous system.

13.9.2 Spinal cord infarction

Spinal cord infarction is a relatively rare event that can be caused by factors similar to those indicated for cerebral infarction (Table 13.10). However, among these, the most frequent causes are atherosclerotic pathology, pathology of the collateral extrathecal arteries, aortic dissections and rarely aneurysms of the vertebral arteries, surgerical interventions on the aorta, especially in the suprarenal tract with possible involvement of the artery of Adamkiewicz, or complications of aortic angiography. In at least 50% of cases, no cause can be identified. The spinal cord segment most commonly involved is the middle or lower thoracic region, and the most frequent clinical presentation is anterior spinal artery syndrome. Infarction in the territory of this artery is characterized by thermodolorific anesthesia below the level of the lesion, with preserved proprioceptive sensation, paraparesis or paraplegia, and loss of sphincter control. Sometimes, the onset is characterized by radicular chest pain, which can be very intense.

The cervical cord is highly vascularized, so it is rarely affected by infarction in other areas. However, vertebral artery dissection can, although rarely, lead to infarction of the cervical cord with cervical pain and brachial diplegia. The diagnosis is clinical, confirmed by the presence of hyperintense signal areas on T2-weighted MRI, predominantly located in the central cord (Figure 13.23).

Sometimes, vascular malformations or dural arteriovenous fistulas cause ischemia that presents as progressive or fluctuating myelopathy. The myelopathy can occur several segments away from the vascular nidus. The clinical picture may present with progressive and symmetrical weakness of the lower limbs and sensory disturbances of variable severity and distribution.

There are no specific therapies for spinal cord infarction. It is important to prevent deep venous thrombosis in patients with paraplegia by administering a prophylactic treatment with low-molecular-weight heparin.

Table 13.10 MAIN CAUSES OF SPINAL CORD INFARCTION

Atherosclerotic	Diabetes, hypertension, hyperlipidemia
Inflammatory	Sarcoidosis, arachnoiditis
Infectious	Syphilis, tuberculosis, herpes zoster, HIV, bacterial meningitis
Vasculitis	Systemic lupus erythematosus, giant cell arteritis, panarteritis
Aortic pathologies	Dissecting aneurysm, aortic occlusion, trauma, Takayasu's disease
Arteriopathies	Connective tissue diseases, Marfan syndrome, fibromuscular dysplasia
Embolic pathologies	Cardiogenic embolism, decompression sickness
Hypoperfusion states	Cardiac arrest, hypovolemia, cardiopulmonary bypass
Vertebral artery pathologies	Spontaneous or traumatic dissection
Prothrombotic states	Coagulation factor disorders, antiphospholipid antibodies
Drug abuse	Cocaine, heroin, MDMA
Various medical conditions	Anemia, sickle cell disease, Moya-Moya disease, CADASIL, Paget's disease
Iatrogenic	Vascular surgery, cardiac surgery, spinal surgery, diagnostic/interventional catheter angiography, spinal/epidural anesthesia, intrathecal medications

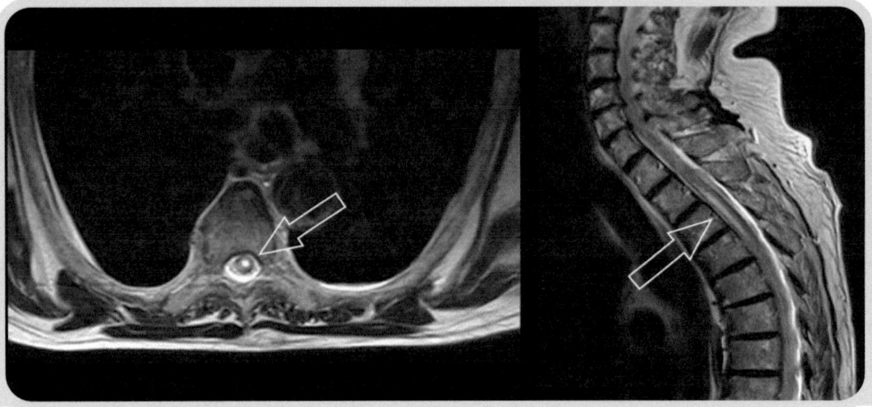

Figure 13.23

Spinal cord infarction. 71-year-old patient, sudden onset of right brachio-crural hemiparesis, with subsequent evolution into right upper limb paresis and paraplegia. MRI images show the presence of central spinal cord hyperintensity in the T2 sequences (arrows).

13.9.3 Spinal cord hemorrhage

Similar to the brain, hemorrhage in the spinal cord can occur, , as intramedullary, subarachnoid, epidural, or subdural hemorrhage. It presents clinically with severe pain, hypoesthesia, motor deficits below the level of the lesion, and loss of sphincter control.

Subarachnoid hemorrhage is characterized by particularly intense dorsal pain followed by neck stiffness. Myelopathy may be present, with sensory-motor deficits (less severe compared to intramedullary hemorrhage).

One possible cause of intramedullary hemorrhage is spinal cord cavernomas. However, they often present with a more gradual course of neurological symptoms.

13.9.4 Vascular malformations

Vascular malformations account for approximately 4% of space-occupying lesions in the spinal cord. They can be classified into four different types (Table 13.11); among these, dural arteriovenous fistulas are the most frequent. Clinically, they manifest as progressive myelopathy over months or years, due to venous congestion or spinal cord hypoperfusion caused by steal phenomena. Less frequently, they can present acutely with parenchymal hemorrhage, subarachnoid hemorrhage, or spinal cord infarction. In patients with suspected cerebral subarachnoid hemorrhage and normal angiography, the possibility of a spinal arteriovenous

Table 13.11 CLASSIFICATION OF SPINAL ARTERIOVENOUS MALFORMATIONS (AVMS)

Type	Structure	Localization
Type I: Dural arteriovenous fistulas	Without a nidus of abnormal vessels Direct connection between artery and vein, with single or multiple feeders Spinal draining veins intra- or extra-dural	Intervertebral foramen, more commonly at the thoracic level
Type II: Glomus AVMs	Compact nidus of malformed arteries and veins Supplied by normal arteries such as the anterior and posterior spinal arteries	Within the spinal cord
Type III: Juvenile or metameric AVMs	Voluminous, supplied by multiple vessels Often involve bone or adjacent soft tissues	Intra- or extra-dural
Type IV: Dural arteriovenous fistulas	Without a nidus of abnormal vessels Direct connection between artery and vein	Surface of the spinal cord Extra-medullary but intradural

malformation (AVM) should be considered, especially if there is neck stiffness and pain or headache.

The differential diagnosis includes other causes of progressive myelopathy, particularly spondylotic and demyelinating myelopathies. MRI may reveal the vascular structures of the malformation as serpentine "flow voids", but diagnosis requires expertise. Catheter angiography is generally necessary for definitive diagnosis and to perform intra-arterial occlusion through embolization or using clues.

Bibliography

AA.VV., SPREAD - Linee Guida Italiane per la prevenzione e il trattamento dell'ictus cerebrale (www.spread.it).

Astrup J., Siesjö B.K., Symon L.,Thresholds in cerebral ischemia the ischemic penombra. Stroke; 12:723-725, 1981.

Flossmann E., Schulz U.G.R., Rothwell P.M., Systematic review of methods and results of studies of the genetic epidemiology of ischemic stroke. Stroke; 35:212-227, 2004.

Hacke W., Kaste M., Bluhmki E., Brozman M., Dávalos A., Guidetti D., Larrue V., Lees K.R., Medeghri Z., Machnig T., Schneider D., von Kummer R., Wahlgren N. and Toni D. for the European Cooperative Acute Stroke Study (ECASS) investigators. Alteplase Compared with Placebo within 3 to 4.5 Hours for Acute Ischemic Stroke. N Engl J Med; 359:1317-29, 2008.

Wahlgren N., Ahmed N., Dávalos A., Ford G.A., Grond M., Hacke W., Hennerici M.G., Kaste M., Kuelkens S., Larrue V., Lees K.R., Roine R.O., SoinneL.,ToniD.,Vanhooren G. for the SITS-MOST investigators. Thrombolysis with alteplase for acute ischaemic stroke in the Safe Implementation of Thrombolysis in Stroke-Monitoring Study (SITS-MOST): an observational study. Lancet; 369:275-82, 2007.

We would like to thank our neuroradiology colleagues for providing the CT and MRI images, *Prof. Giulio Guidetti* for the catheter angiography images, and *Dr. Alessio Pieroni* for the selection and processing of the visual material.

14 NEUROSURGICAL APPROACH TO INTRACEREBRAL HEMORRHAGES

Antonio Santoro, Luigi Valentino Berra

Subarachnoid Hemorrhage (SAH) is characterized by bleeding within the subarachnoid space, which is located between the pia mater and the arachnoid membrane. Such bleeding can occur in various situations, such as cranial trauma. Spontaneous SAH is a very serious event resulting from the bleeding of a cerebral aneurysm or, less frequently, other cerebrovascular malformations (arteriovenous malformations or dural fistulas). In about 20% of cases, SAH from aneurysm rupture is associated with intraventricular hemorrhage.

The risk factors for SAH include cigarette smoking, hypertension, alcohol abuse, and the use of sympathomimetic drugs (cocaine, amphetamines). There are also genetic diseases associated with the presence and rupture of aneurysms, such as polycystic kidney disease and Ehlers-Danlos syndrome.

The incidence of SAH in Italy is 6-7 cases per 100,000 population annually, with slight interregional variability. Females are more frequently affected, with a ratio of 3:2 compared to males. The most affected age group is between 40 and 65 years, which accounts for 70% of cases. 15% of SAH cases occur in individuals between 20 and 40 years old. Only 5% of SAH cases affect individuals under 20 years old, and it is rare in children under 10 years old, representing only 0.5% of all cases.

14.1 Clinical presentation

The clinical presentation of SAH varies widely depending on the extent and location of the bleeding. It is estimated that about 15% of patients with SAH from aneurysm rupture do not seek medical attention and experience sudden death. Patients who survive the bleeding arrive at the hospital with clinical pictures ranging from mild headache to deep coma.

The Hunt-Hess classification divides the clinical presentations of SAH into 5 grades according to progressive severity.

- Grade I - Asymptomatic or mild headache and mild neck stiffness;
- Grade II - Cranial nerve palsy, moderate to severe headache, neck stiffness;
- Grade III - Moderate focal deficit, lethargy, or confusion;
- Grade IV - Stupor, moderate to severe hemiparesis, initial decerebrate rigidity;
- Grade V - Deep coma, decerebrate rigidity, moribund appearance.

In the Hunt and Hess classification, a lower grade corresponds to a better prognosis. In patients who arrive awake (Hunt-Hess 1-2), the most frequent symptom is a headache, which has peculiar characteristics. It is a violent headache with a sudden onset, localized in the frontal or occipital region, often described as the most severe ever experienced, and frequently associated with photophobia, nausea, and vomiting. Clinical signs include neck stiffness and signs of meningeal irritation, such as Kernig's sign and Brudzinski's sign. In some cases, focal neurological deficits may be present, related to the location of the aneurysm (e.g., diplopia due to compression of the 3rd cranial nerve in posterior communicating artery aneurysms) or associated intracerebral hematoma (e.g., hemiparesis in middle cerebral artery aneurysms).

In a variable number of cases (30-50%), aneurysm rupture is preceded by minimal bleeding called "warning leaks or sentinel headaches", which manifest as a sudden, violent, focal, or generalized headache. In some cases, they may present with neck pain, nausea, vomiting, photophobia, or general malaise and are rarely recognized due to the nonspecificity of the symptoms. Warning leaks occur several hours or days before the actual rupture of the aneurysm. In approximately 30-40% of patients, SAH occurs when the patient is at rest, while in 60-70% of cases, the patient is in a condition of physical exertion or under situations of high emotional stress.

Neurological examination may be normal in patients with moderate bleeding. In about half of the patients, there is a mild or moderate increase in blood pressure. Hyperpyrexia is common after the fourth day following the bleeding. Tachycardia may be present for several days after the occurrence of hemorrhage. Examination of the fundus oculi may reveal papilledema, and in 20-30% of cases, subhyaloid or subretinal hemorrhage is observed. Vitreous hemorrhage (Terson syndrome) occurs less frequently and is associated with copious subarachnoid bleeding. There may be a global depression of neurological function, with altered level of consciousness and the presence of a confused state up to deep coma. Focal or generalized epileptic seizures can occur. Focal motor neurological deficits are frequently associated with aneurysms of the middle cerebral artery, which can also manifest as aphasia, and are attributed to ischemia or hypoperfusion in the terminal vascular territory or the presence of an intraparenchymal hematoma. Cranial nerve paralysis is present in 25% of patients, and the most frequent is oculomotor nerve palsy with or without ipsilateral mydriasis, which is generally associated with the presence of a posterior communicating artery aneurysm. Abducens nerve palsy is generally due to increased intracranial pressure and does not constitute a true localizing sign. Monocular amaurosis can be caused by an aneurysm of the ophthalmic or anterior cerebral artery compressing the ipsilateral optic nerve.

14.2 Diagnosis

The diagnosis is based on the patient's clinical features and radiological confirmation using non enhanced computed tomography (CT), which should be urgently performed (Figures 14.1, 14.2). In cases of high clinical suspicion and negative CT findings, a lumbar puncture should be performed, even though with current high-resolution systems, the sensitivity of brain CT in detecting SAH is over 99%. After confirming the diagnosis of SAH, further imaging diagnostic tests are necessary to identify the source of the bleeding. The first choice is usually CT cerebral angiography with contrast medium, followed possibly by cerebral angiography or brain magnetic resonance angiography (MRA). Cerebral angio-CT can also use 3D vessel reconstructions and, in many cases, is sufficient for planning the subsequent treatment of the malformation (Figure 14.3).

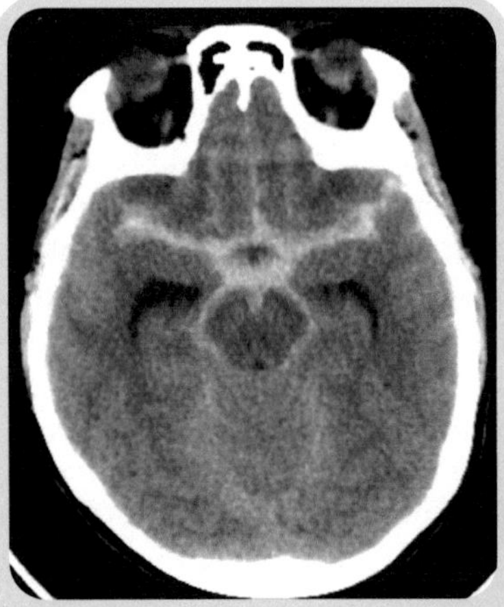

Figure 14.1

Brain CT of a patient with abundant subarachnoid hemorrhage, at high risk of developing vasospasm.

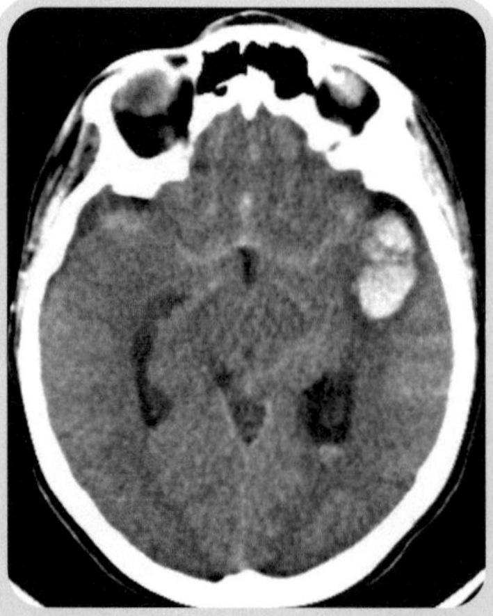

Figure 14.2

CT scan of the brain of a patient with subarachnoid hemorrhage due to rupture of the middle cerebral artery aneurysm. In this case, the cisternal bleeding is more limited, while there is an intraparenchymal hematoma present.

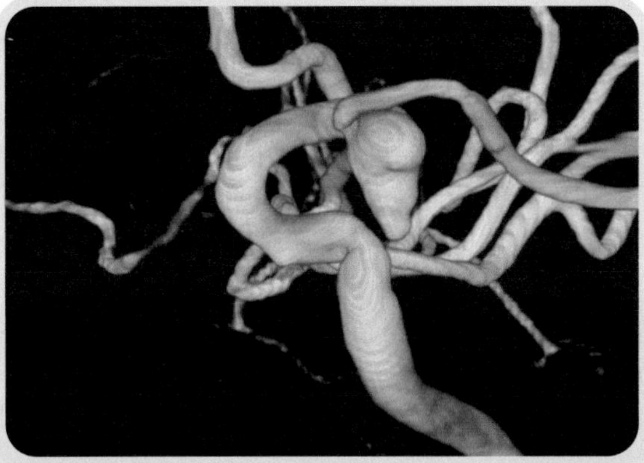

Figure 14.3

Angiography with 3D reconstructions of supraclinoid carotid siphon aneurysm.

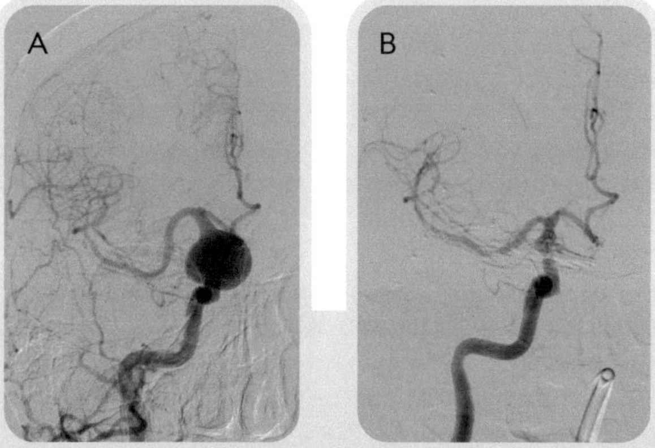

Figure 14.4

A) Anteroposterior carotid angiography showing the presence of a giant aneurysm of the carotid siphon. B) Post-operative follow-up showing the exclusion of the sac with numerous clips and patency of the distal branches.

In other cases, an digital subtraction angiography is necessary to accurately assess cerebrovascular anatomy, aneurysm size and shape, dome and neck orientation, the relationship of the aneurysm with the parent artery and perforating branches, and the presence of multiple aneurysms (Figure 14.4). During the angiographic examination, temporary balloon occlusion may be performed to evaluate collateral circulation, providing useful information for guiding surgical or endovascular planning.

The clinical manifestations of SAH encompass a wide spectrum of often nonspecific signs and symptoms, which can pose diagnostic challenges. The differential diagnosis of SAH includes various forms of headache such as migraine, cluster headache, ischemic events (TIA, stroke), meningitis and encephalitis, and other intracranial hemorrhages.

14.3 Complications and treatment

Subarachnoid bleeding can cause acute brain damage of variable severity, even leading to sudden death. In patients who survive the initial bleeding, various complications may arise, which should be prevented to the extent possible and, in any case, recognized and treated. The main complications of SAH include rebleeding, vasospasm, and hydrocephalus. Additionally, there are complications not strictly neurological but typically associated with SAH, such as hyponatremia and cardiac functional abnormalities.

The rupture of a cerebral aneurysm causes a brief episode of bleeding, followed by tamponade due to increased intracranial pressure and intra-aneurysmal coagulative mechanisms. However, in the hours and days following the initial bleeding, there is a high risk of rebleeding due to a new rupture of the aneurysm. *Rebleeding* generally has a poor prognosis, so once the diagnosis is made, it is necessary to secure the aneurysm with surgical or endovascular treatment as soon as possible, depending on the patient's clinical condition. The incidence of rebleeding is highest within the first 2 weeks, with a peak within 24-48 hours of the initial SAH (approximately 6%), and a daily rate of 1.5% for the subsequent 12-14 days. Clinical factors that increase the likelihood of rebleeding include hypertension, agitation, and seizures. In some cases, the use of antifibrinolytic drugs such as tranexamic acid (1 g IV every 6 hours) is recommended to prevent rebleeding while awaiting surgical treatment. The treatment should be continued until the aneurysm is treated but should not exceed 72 hours to avoid thrombotic complications.

Vasospasm is another feared complication of subarachnoid hemorrhage (SAH). It occurs as a result of bleeding in the subarachnoid space where cortical arterial branches run, and it is clinically relevant in approximately 30% of patients, constituting a major cause of disability in SAH patients. It is characterized by the narrowing of arterial vessels in the cerebral circulation and manifests as late ischemic events (Figure 14.5). Vasospasm typically occurs after the third day of bleeding, peaks between the sixth and eighth day, decreases dramatically after about 14 days, and resolves in the majority of cases by the third week of SAH. Overall, nearly 50% of patients develop vasospasm during the peak period. There is a clear correlation between the amount of blood in the basal cisterns as seen on the initial CT scan and the incidence of vasospasm. When the CT scan does not show bleeding or only shows a thin layer of blood in the cisterns, vasospasm is an unlikely event. However, if the CT scan reveals a thick layer of blood in the cisterns, severe angiographic spasms and clinical deficits occur in almost all cases.

The symptoms of vasospasm can vary, but patients typically present with a global decrease in the level of consciousness, moderate fever, and new-onset focal neurological deficits depending on the involved arterial territory. Conventional angiography is the gold standard imaging study for vasospasm. However, the diagnosis of vasospasm can also be reliably made noninvasively at the patient's bedside using transcranial Doppler. Other tests, such as single-photon emission computed tomography (SPECT), positron emission tomography (PET), xenon CT scanning, and radioactive xenon clearance, can be useful for evaluating regional cerebral blood flow in patients with vasospasm. However, these tests are often difficult to perform on critically ill patients. The treatment of vasospasm is primarily preventive and involves the use of calcium channel blockers (the first choice being nimodipine) and improving cerebral perfusion through blood pressure support, hemodilution (to improve blood rheology), and hypervolemia, known as triple-H therapy. The use of triple-H therapy has been questioned in recent years and is currently controversial. The only established efficacy in preventing vasospasm damage is the use of controlled hypertension. Once symptomatic vasospasm is identified, selective treatment may be performed through intrarterial administration of vasodilators or endovascular balloon dilatation in selected cases. Some data support the use of continuous spinal drainage, after aneurysm treatment, to accelerate cerebrospinal fluid clearance and removal of hemoglobin degradation products.

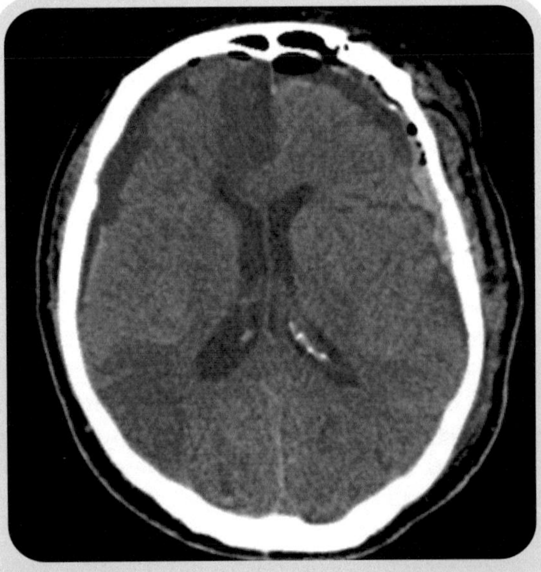

Figure 14.5

Patient underwent clipping of the left carotid siphon aneurysm. On the 6th day, contralateral hypodense ischemic lesions in the frontal and parietal regions due to vasospasm are observed.

Hydrocephalus can be an acute or delayed complication of SAH. Acute obstructive hydrocephalus complicates 20% of SAH cases. Clinical risk factors for the development of hydrocephalus include increasing patient age, use of antifibrinolytic drugs, left ventricular systolic dysfunction, and seizures. Acute hydrocephalus usually occurs within the first 24 hours after hemorrhage but can also occur after 7 days. It presents as a relatively abrupt change in the level of consciousness, progressing to stupor and coma. Acute hydrocephalus can lead to a potentially life-threatening increase in intracranial pressure and has a worse prognosis. Therefore, any change in the level of consciousness requires an urgent CT scan to assess ventricular size. If obvious ventricular dilation is present, emergency ventriculostomy should be performed.

Late or chronic hydrocephalus, caused by obstruction of the arachnoid granulations and alterations in the absorption of cerebrospinal fluid, occurs in 10-15% of patients with subarachnoid hemorrhage (SAH). Typically, chronic hydrocephalus is of the communicating type and develops from 10 days to a month or more after the bleeding. Patients may present with incontinence, gait instability, and progressive cognitive decline, sometimes with a subtle course. Once diagnosed, it is treated with a ventriculoperitoneal shunt.

Seizures occur in 13-24% of patients with SAH, often within the first 24 hours after the hemorrhage. They are more common after the rupture of middle cerebral artery aneurysms. Seizures can be focal or generalized. Generalized seizures can lead to increased cerebral blood flow, hypertension, and elevated intracranial pressure, thereby increasing the risk of rebleeding and secondary neurological deterioration.

A significant number of patients with SAH experience *cardiac dysfunction.* Neurogenic sympathetic hyperactivity and increased systemic catecholamine levels have been implicated in SAH-associated cardiac dysfunction. Arrhythmias occur in approximately 90% of patients and most commonly include premature ventricular complexes, bradyarrhythmias, and supraventricular tachycardia. Arrhythmias are more frequent in the first 48 hours following SAH, and only a small percentage (usually those associated with hypokalemia) are life-threatening.

Hyponatremia is frequently associated with SAH (10-34% of cases) and is associated with the release of high levels of atrial natriuretic factor.

Acute pulmonary edema and *hypoxia* are almost invariably present in patients with severe subarachnoid hemorrhage. Neurogenic pulmonary edema in SAH is believed to be of neurogenic origin and unrelated to triple-H therapy; however, the latter is associated with an increased risk of fluid overload. Similarly, neurogenic-induced hypoxemia in SAH is thought to be partially neurogenic in origin because it is disproportionate to what would be expected from heart failure or fluid overload.

The choice of *treatment* depends on the characteristics of the aneurysm and the patient's clinical condition. The therapeutic options for aneurysm closure are surgical and endovascular. Surgical treatment involves craniotomy, exposure of the inflowing vessel, dissection of the aneurysm, and exclusion by placing various shapes and sizes of metal clips to exclude the sac while maintaining the patency of the distal and perforating vessels. Endovascular treatment is performed through selective catheterization of the supplying artery and obliteration of the sac by filling it with metal coils or other devices to create *intrasaccular thrombosis*. Surgical treatment in some cases is superior because it results in the safe definitive exclusion of the aneurysm while in other cases endovascular treatment is less risky.

The decision on which method to use takes into account the location (aneurysms located in certain sites have a better prognosis with endovascular treatment, e.g., basilar artery aneurysms; others have a better prognosis when treated surgically, e.g., middle cerebral artery aneurysms), the size and morphology of the aneurysm (in some cases, endovascular treatment is not safely feasible, e.g., in the presence of a wide neck). Clinical grade, the presence of intraparenchymal hematoma or intracranial hypertension (that may benefit from a craniotomy or craniectomy), age, and the presence of comorbidities guide the choice of treatment.

14.4 Prognosis

The prognosis of subarachnoid hemorrhage (SAH) has improved in recent decades, thanks to more refined diagnosis, advancements in surgical and endovascular techniques, and more aggressive treatment of vasospasm, hydrocephalus, and other general complications. However, SAH remains an extremely serious event with high mortality and morbidity rates. Hunt-Hess grades 1-3 are generally associated with a favorable outcome, while grades IV and V have a generally poor prognosis. Survival is correlated with the degree of subarachnoid hemorrhage at the time of hospitalization. The reported data show a survival rate of 70% for Hunt-Hess grade I, 60% for grade II, 50% for grade III, 40% for grade IV, and 10% for grade V. The overall mortality rate is 45%, and a moderate to severe disability persists in one-third of the survivors in the long term.

Screening for the presence of aneurysms is not recommended in the general population. Even in high-risk populations, such as patients with polycystic kidney disease, no benefit has been demonstrated for screening. In patients who have had two or more first-degree relatives with radiologically confirmed intracranial aneurysms, screening with CT angiography or MR angiography may be individually advised.

Bibliography

Rosen D.S., Macdonald R.L. Subarachnoid hemorrhage grading scales: a systematic review. Neurocrit Care. 2005;2(2):110-8.

Long B., Koyfman A., Runyon M.S. Subarachnoid Hemorrhage: Updates in Diagnosis and Management. Emerg Med Clin North Am. 2017 Nov;35(4):803-824.

Cantore G., Santoro A., Guidetti G., et al. Surgical treatment of giant intracranial aneurysms: current viewpoint. Neurosurgery. 2008 Oct;63(4 Suppl 2):279-89; discussion 289-90.

Etminan N., Macdonald R.L. Management of aneurysmal subarachnoid hemorrhage. Handb Clin Neurol. 2017;140:195-228.

Bederson J.B., E. ConnollyJr S., Batjer H.H., et al. Guidelines for the Management of Aneurysmal Subarachnoid Hemorrhage. Stroke. 2009 Mar;40(3):994-1025.

15 MOVEMENT DISORDERS

Giovanni Fabbrini, Daniele Belvisi, Giorgio Leodori,
Alfredo Berardelli,

Movement disorders are neurological conditions characterized by alterations in voluntary movement and/or the presence of involuntary movements. Movement disorders are generally caused by anatomical or functional changes in the basal ganglia, cerebellum, connected cortical structures, and spinal cord. In this chapter, movement disorders are classified into hypokinesias (Parkinson's disease and atypical parkinsonism) and hyperkinesias (tremors, dystonia, athetosis, chorea, ballism, tic, myoclonus). Additionally, other disorders such as Wilson's disease, stiff-person syndrome, myoclonus and facial spasms, restless legs syndrome, and functional movement disorders will be addressed. Cerebellar ataxias will also be described in this chapter.

15.1 Hypokinetic syndromes

15.1.1 Parkinson's disease

Parkinson's disease (PD) is a chronic degenerative disorder of the central nervous system characterized by motor slowing (akinesia, bradykinesia, hypokinesia), muscle rigidity and tremor. The disease was first described in 1817 by James Parkinson in his treatise "*An Essay on the Shaking Palsy*".

Epidemiology

The prevalence of PD is approximately 0.3% of the entire population. It is relatively rare before the age of 50, with prevalence increasing to 1% in individuals over 60 years of age and 4% in those over 80 years of age. The incidence is also low before the age of 50 and reaches its highest values in the age groups between 70 and 79 years, with estimated rates of 8-18 cases per 100,000 people per year in the general population and 120 cases per 100,000 people per year at 70 years of age. It is estimated that there are currently around 250,000-300,000 people with PD in Italy. In approximately 90% of cases, the disease is considered sporadic, but in the remaining 10%, especially in early-onset forms, it is genetically determined. Men are affected by the disease with a slightly higher frequency than women (ratio of 3:2). This difference likely reflects variations in risk factors (less exposure to environmental chemical factors, reduced frequency of brain injuries) as well as differences in sex hormones. With the introduction of L-Dopa as a therapeutic treatment in the late 1960s, the survival of PD patients has increased, although the mortality rate remains approximately 1.6-2.9 times higher than the general population. The most common cause of death in Parkinson's patients is bronchopneumonia, resulting from the reduced mobility and dysphagia that characterize the advanced stages of the disease.

Pathological anatomy

The most characteristic neuropathological lesion of PD is the loss of pigmented cells in the substantia nigra *pars compacta* (SN), located in the midbrain, whose terminations in the striatum release dopamine, as well as other pigmented nuclei in the brainstem (*locus coeruleus*, raphe nucleus). Macroscopic examination reveals the typical pallor of the SN and *locus coeruleus*, while microscopic examination shows marked depletion of neurons in the pigmented nuclei. In some residual neurons, eosinophilic cytoplasmic inclusions are observed, characterized by a dense central nucleus surrounded by a pale halo, known as Lewy bodies, which represent the main histopathological feature of the disease. Lewy bodies are composed of α-synuclein filaments. The degeneration affects brainstem nuclei, basal ganglia, cerebral cortex, and structures of the autonomic nervous system. The reduction in dopamine concentration in the putamen and substantia nigra is correlated with the clinical severity of motor symptoms, and degeneration of the locus coeruleus appears to be associated with cognitive impairments. A reduction of at least 60-80% in putaminal dopamine concentration (or a loss of at least 60% of nigral dopaminergic neurons) is required for the disease to manifest clinically. Dopaminergic depletion triggers numerous mechanisms that can compensate, at least initially, for the loss of dopamine. In addition to the dopaminergic system, there is degeneration of the ascending noradrenergic monoaminergic systems originating from the pigmented neurons of the locus coeruleus, as well as the serotonergic systems originating from the raphe nucleus. The cholinergic transmission system, due to neuronal loss in the basal nucleus of Meynert, is particularly involved in the early stages of the neurodegenerative process of PD. Alterations in these anatomofunctional systems likely underlie the high frequency of autonomic disturbances, mood tone, and cognitive impairments observed during the course of the disease.

Etiopathogenesis and pathophysiology

In recent years, numerous studies have demonstrated how the accumulation of α-synuclein and its altered folding process lead to the formation of toxic protofibrils in dopaminergic cells. Some mutations responsible for genetic forms of Parkinson's disease (PD), such as mutations in the parkin gene (ubiquitin ligase protein), result in improper folding of alpha-synuclein or impairment of the protein degradation and clearance system, leading to the accumulation of alpha-synuclein within the cells. Recent studies have suggested that anatomopathological alterations and the accumulation of alpha-synuclein initially occur in the motor nuclei of the vagus and glossopharyngeal nerves and in the anterior olfactory bulb. According to this hypothesis, the degenerative process propagates in an ascending manner starting from the olfactory bulb or the gastrointestinal system, reaching the brainstem, particularly the substantia nigra (SN), and then progressing to cortical structures (especially the mesial temporal cortex, frontal associative areas, and primary sensorimotor areas). The propagation mechanism is believed to be similar to that of prion diseases. Other hypothesized mechanisms include processes related to inflammation, oxidative stress, mitochondrial dysfunction, and apoptosis.

Approximately 10-15% of PD patients have one or more affected family members. Genetic etiology is particularly important in early-onset forms with dominant or recessive inheritance (■ Table 15.1). Among the dominant inheritance forms, the first to be discovered was the mutation in the SNCA gene (α-synuclein gene), located on chromosome 4, identified in an Italian family. The "classic" mutation causes the substitution of the amino acid alanine with threonine at position 53, although other types of mutations have been found in other families. Amino acid substitutions in the chains of alpha-synuclein induce the formation of oligomers and fibrillar aggregates of the protein, which are likely toxic to the cell. The clinical phenotype is similar to that of PD but with a more rapid progression of symptoms. Among the dominantly inherited forms, there is the LRKK2 mutation located on chromosome 12, which is present in a significant percentage (up to 4%) of apparently sporadic PD cases. The prevalence of this mutation can be very high in genetically "isolated" populations, particularly in Ashkenazi Jews and Arab populations in North Africa. A number of studies conducted in different geographical areas have shown an increased risk of PD associated with mutations in the GBA gene (glucocerebrosidase), the enzyme that encodes the lysosomal enzyme glucocerebrosidase implicated in Gaucher's disease. The penetrance is incomplete and increases with age, reaching approximately

30% by 80 years old, and with the severity of the mutation. The motor phenotype is similar to that of idiopathic PD, while several studies have highlighted a higher frequency and severity of cognitive deficits, autonomic nervous system disturbances, and REM sleep disorder in individuals with GBA mutations. Among the recessively inherited forms there are the forms caused by mutations in the "parkin" gene, mutations in the PINK1 gene, and mutations in the DJ-1 gene. The common clinical characteristics of recessive forms are early-onset (even before the age of 30), a good therapeutic response to L-Dopa, early onset of dyskinesias, dystonias, and motor fluctuations, and a generally milder course compared to sporadic forms. From a pathogenetic point of view, it is believed that the genetic alterations

Table 15.1 GENETIC CAUSES OF PARKINSON'S DISEASE

Gene	Function	Onset	Phenotype	Additional signs	Pathology#
LRRK2	Lysosomal	Late/variable	Typical	-	±LB; ±tau
VPS35	Vesicle transport	Late	Typical	-	-
SNCA	Unknown	Late/early*	* Atypical/Typical*	D; PSI; PIR; MIO	LB
HTRA2	Mitochondrial	Late	Typical	-	Unknown
GIGYF2	Possible IGF-1 signaling	Late	Typical	-	Unknown
UCHL1	Ubiquitin-proteasome	Late	Typical	-	Unknown
EIF4G1	Protein synthesis	Late	Typical	-	Nn
CHCHD2	Mitochondrial	Variable	Typical	-	LB, tau
DNAJC13	Vesicle formation	Late	Typical	-	LB, tau
TMEM230	Vesicle transport	Late	Typical	-	LB, tau
RIC3	Formation/expression of AchR	Variable	Typical	-	Unknown
GBA	Lysosomal	Late/variable	Atypical/typical	D	LB
PRKN	Mitochondrial	Early/young	Typical	-	-
PINK1	Mitochondrial	Early	Typical	-	± LB
DJ-1	Mitochondrial	Early	Typical/typical	-	± LB
VPS13C	Mitochondrial/vesicle transport	Early	Atypical	D; PIR	LB
PTRHD1	Ubiquitin-proteasome	Early	Atypical	DI; PIR; PSI	LB
PODXL	Neurite growth	Young	Typical	-	LB
DNAJC6	Synaptic endocytosis	Young	Atypical	D; PSI; EP; PIR	LB
SYNJ1	Synaptic endocytosis	Young	Atypical	D; EP; DIST; MO	Unknown
ATP13A2	Lysosomal	Young	Atypical	D; PIR; MO; MIO	Lipofuscin
PLA2G6	Membrane homeostasis/ mitochondrial	Young	Atypical	D; PIR; AT; PSI; MO	LB
FBXO7	Ubiquitin-proteasome/ Mitochondrial	Young	Atypical	PIR; PSI	nn
RAB39B	Vesicle transport	Early in males	Atypical in males	DI; MC	LB

Genes responsible for monogenic forms of PD and their corresponding phenotypic characteristics. D = dementia; PSI = psychiatric disorders; PIR = pyramidal signs; MIO = myoclonus; DI = intellectual disability; EP = epilepsy; MO = ocular movement abnormalities; AT = ataxia; nn = unknown; LB = Lewy Bodies; * = in specific genetic alterations; # = in addition to the loss of dopaminergic neurons. Table created in collaboration with Dr. Simona Petrucci.

characterizing recessive PD interfere with the proper functioning of cellular proteasomal mechanisms and the autophagy system. Parkinsonism similar to PD can also be present in various neurodegenerative diseases in which the phenotype is dominated by involvement of other systems. These include diseases with DNA expansions (SCA2, SCA3, SCA7, Huntington's chorea), frontotemporal degenerations (MAPT, GRN, c9orf72), Wilson's disease, manganese transport disease (SLC30A10), neurodegeneration with iron accumulation (FTL, c9orf12, WDR45), hereditary spastic paraplegia (SPG11), some mitochondrial disorders (POLG), chorea-acanthocytosis, X-linked dystonia-parkinsonism, Niemann-Pick disease, and others.

PD is currently considered a condition with multifactorial etiology, meaning it is linked to the interaction between genetic predisposition and endogenous and exogenous risk factors. Since the monogenic forms of PD are rare, several studies have pursued the hypothesis of 'common disease-common variant,' in which the genetic component of the disease is considered the cumulative result of many common low-risk alleles. Genome-wide association studies (GWAS) have identified 90 independently associated genetic risk factors consistently linked to the pathology. Regarding exogenous risk factors, numerous studies have investigated the possible association between PD development and exposure to toxic substances or drugs, head trauma, surgical interventions, and lifestyle factors.

For instance, in the 1980s, it was demonstrated that a neurotoxin called 1-methyl-4-phenyl-1,2,3,6-tetrahydropyridine (MPTP), inadvertently synthesized during 'home' production of heroin and self-injected by drug addicts, induced irreversible parkinsonism and selective destruction of the cells in the substantia nigra pars compacta (SNpc). In line with this observation, recent studies have shown that exposure to certain pesticides like rotenone (which also shares structural similarities with the toxin MPTP) or specific hydrocarbons increases the risk of developing PD.

Regarding protective factors for PD, studies agree on the possible protective effect of smoking habits (likely due to a protective action exerted by nicotine), caffeine consumption (a competitive antagonist for adenosinergic receptors of subtype A1 and A2A, facilitating action on the striatal-pallidal GABAergic system), and physical activity (through plastic effects on the dopaminergic system). Similar to genetic factors, it has recently been suggested that environmental factors have a combined effect that reflects the coexistence of multiple risk factors in the same individual.

Parkinson's disease is primarily attributed to the progressive degeneration of nigrostriatal dopaminergic pathways and, consequently, functional alterations affecting the "motor system". The motor system (■ Figure 15.1) is composed of parallel circuits originating from primary and non-primary motor cortical areas and projecting to the basal ganglia, specific thalamic nuclei, and back to the same cortical areas of origin. Within the striatum, two types of dopaminergic receptors, D1 and D2, represent the origin of the two transmission pathways from the striatum to the thalamus: the direct pathway (striatum-internal globus pallidus (GPi)-substantia nigra pars reticulata (SNr)-thalamus) and the indirect pathway (striatum-external globus pallidus (GPe)-subthalamic nucleus (STN)-GPi/SNr-thalamus). Under physiological conditions, inhibitory GABAergic and excitatory glutamatergic connections between the various nuclei result in a reduction of inhibitory output from GPi and SNr, leading to increased thalamo-cortical drive in the direct pathway, and conversely, an increase in inhibitory output from GPi and SNr, resulting in reduced thalamo-cortical drive in the indirect pathway. The action of the direct and indirect pathways is modulated by the SNpc. Dopaminergic depletion, characteristic of Parkinson's disease, leads to a reduction in the inhibition of the indirect pathway and, simultaneously, reduced activation of the direct pathway. The consequence of these alterations is increased neuronal activity in GPi and STN, a reduction in thalamic activation, and therefore, reduced motor cortex activity.

However, recent studies have suggested that the pathophysiology of PD involves not only the dopaminergic circuits but also the cholinergic, GABAergic, serotoninergic, noradrenergic, and glutamatergic circuits.

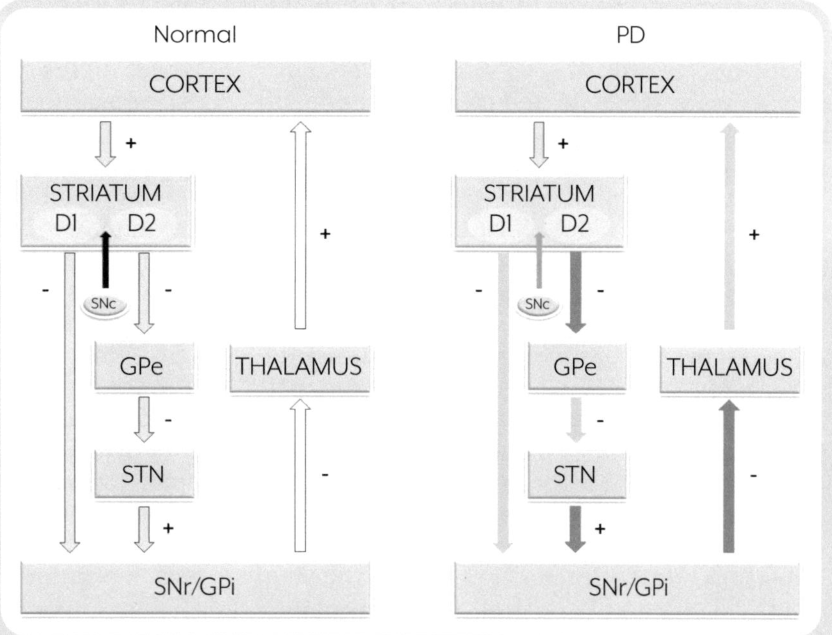

Figure 15.1

Schematic representation of the motor circuitry under physiological conditions and in Parkinson's disease. In Parkinson's disease, due to dopaminergic depletion, there is reduced activity in the direct pathway and reduced inhibition of the indirect pathway, resulting in reduced activation of the thalamus and motor cortex.

Studies of pathophysiology have demonstrated how bradykinesia is evident during the execution of simple movements, but even more so during the execution of complex movements, such as sequential and simultaneous movements. The predominant characteristic of bradykinesia in Parkinson's disease (PD) is its progressive worsening during the execution of repeated movements over time (sequence effect). The bradykinesia that correlates most with dopaminergic denervation appears to be caused by insufficient activation of cortical areas by the basal ganglia, resulting in excessive thalamic inhibition of the primary motor cortex. Numerous experimental studies have also shown altered integration of sensory stimuli and altered plasticity of neuronal structures at both subcortical and cortical levels. Changes in resting-state functional connectivity (which indicate intrinsic fluctuations of electrical signals in functional MRI) have been demonstrated. The most modern view is to consider bradykinesia as secondary to a network dysfunction (basal ganglia, integration of sensory information at subcortical and cortical levels, and based on recent evidence, the cerebellum as well).

Resting tremor appears to be related to pathological interaction between the basal ganglia and the cerebello-thalamo-cortical circuit. Re-emergent tremor (see section on clinical characteristics) is determined by the same mechanisms as resting tremor, while serotonin is thought to play an important role in postural tremor. For the pathophysiology of tremor, an alteration of the network composed of the thalamo-cerebello-cortical circuit and the internal globus pallidus is hypothesized. Rigidity also appears to be affected by basal ganglia alterations, as well as modifications of spinal circuits and altered integration of afferent sensory stimuli at the spinal level and trans-cortical circuits.

Clinical features

The clinical picture of PD is characterized by a slowly progressive course. Initial symptoms may be of modest magnitude and sometimes not immediately recognized as they are "nonspecific" or attributed to normal age-related changes (Table 15.2).

Bradykinesia, rigidity, and tremor are the main motor symptoms of the disease. At onset, motor symptoms and signs predominantly manifest on one side of the body, later spreading to the contralateral side over the years. However, a certain degree of asymmetry between the two sides persists throughout the disease. Patients with Parkinson's disease (PD) have various types of movement impairment. Bradykinesia refers to slowness in executing voluntary movements. Hypokinesia refers to reduced amplitude of movements, while akinesia refers to difficulty initiating the desired movement. The term bradykinesia is often used to encompass all three components described. Bradykinesia is evident in the execution of normal activities of daily living, such as slowed gait, reduced pendular movements of the upper limbs, reduced overall limb movements, difficulty performing complex movements of the upper limb, and progressively smaller handwriting (micrographia). The characteristic feature of bradykinesia in PD is the progressive reduction in amplitude (sequence effect) of voluntary movements (e.g., repeated movements of the index finger on the thumb or opening and closing of the hand when performed for 15 seconds). In the cranial region, bradykinesia manifests as reduced facial expression (hypomimia) and blink frequency, limitation of conjugate upward eye movements and convergence movements, alteration of voice tone (becoming hypophonic and monotonous), and excessive salivation (drooling) due to reduced frequency of spontaneous swallowing acts. Typical manifestations of akinesia include prolonged time required to initiate a voluntary movement (the patient hesitates for a few seconds before starting to walk) and the commonly known motor block called freezing. This phenomenon is characterized by a sudden and transient

Table 15.2 FREQUENCY OF INITIAL SYMPTOMS OF PARKINSON'S DISEASE

Symptom	Frequency
Tremor	60-65%
Slowness of movement	20%
Loss of dexterity/impaired handwriting	13%
Gait disturbance	11%
Pain, muscle cramps	8 %
Depression, anxiety	4 %
Speech difficulty	4 %
Fatigue, weakness	3 %
Excessive salivation (drooling)	2 %
Reduced facial expression (hypomimia)	1,5 %
Others	3 %

(usually lasting a few seconds) inability to move, mainly involving the lower limbs, which feel "stuck" to the ground at the initiation of a step, changing direction, or passing through narrow spaces (e.g., doorways). Rigidity or plastic hypertonia refers to increased muscle tone of the limbs and head during passive mobilization (resembling a "lead pipe" rigidity). Rigidity differs from "spastic" hypertonia, typical of pathologies involving the upper motor neuron, due to uniform involvement of both antigravity and gravity-dependent muscles, and the absence of changes in muscle tone with varying speed of passive movements. The *phenomenon of cogwheel rigidity* (rhythmic interruptions of rigidity perceived as joint "catches") may be present, but the presence of tremor can make it difficult to identify. Rigidity can be associated with postural deformities, predominantly affecting the neck and trunk, such as camptocormia, characterized by abnormal flexion of the thoracolumbar spine (beyond 45°), which disappears when the subject lies on a bed or *Pisa syndrome*, characterized by marked lateral deviation of the trunk. Tremor is the third fundamental motor sign. Parkinsonian tremor typically occurs at rest and has a frequency ranging from 4 to 6 Hz. If present, it is often one of the first symptoms perceived by the patient, especially when it affects the hand, and it is accentuated by emotions; it attenuates or disappears with voluntary movement and during sleep. Resting tremor in Parkinson's disease is characterized by repeated movements of supination-pronation of the hand (like rolling a pill or counting coins). Tremor can also involve the lips, chin, and lower limbs but not the voice or head. In patients with resting tremor, while keeping the upper limbs extended, a tremor of the limbs may appear after a few seconds (reemergent tremor), or the tremor may be present immediately after assuming a posture (postural tremor). Reemergent tremor is considered a form of resting tremor, while postural tremor has a higher frequency and a different pattern of muscle activation. Advanced stages of the disease are characterized by postural instability, which can be clinically assessed by giving a sudden backward push to the patient's shoulders to evaluate the normal postural response (recovery of balance in two steps or fewer) or the impairment of it (recovery of balance in two or more steps or complete absence of response). Postural instability is the main cause of falls in patients with advanced PD. The clinical picture is classified into progressive stages of disability (from I to V) according to the Hoehn and Yahr scale (■ Table 15.3). Other scales are used to assess symptom severity (such as the Movement Disorder Society Unified Parkinson's Disease Rating Scale: MDS-UPDRS) and quality of life (e.g., PDQ-39) or non-motor symptoms (Non-Motor Symptoms Rating Scale).

The disease is also characterized by the presence of non-motor symptoms that profoundly affect the patient's quality of life and often precede the onset of motor symptoms (premotor phase of the disease). In particular, sleep disturbances, mood disorders, constipation, and hyposmia can appear many years before the motor symptomatology. In the course of PD, depression frequently occurs, affecting up to 40% of patients, and is characterized by apathy, disinterest, reduced activities and social relationships, and anhedonia, or loss of pleasure and interest in performing common activities. Cognitive impairments, which are mild in almost all patients (alterations in executive and frontal functions), can progress to dementia in at least 30-40% of cases (dementia can be observed in 70% of patients over 80 years old). Frequent urinary disorders (increased urinary frequency, urgency, nocturia, sometimes incontinence), orthostatic hypotension, and erectile dysfunction in men are also common. Finally, sleep disorders (excessive daytime sleepiness, insomnia, parasomnias, particularly REM sleep disorders), anxiety disorders, gastrointestinal disorders (dysphagia, constipation), and pain can be observed. Olfactory disorders (hyposmia) are also very common and can manifest in a high percentage of patients even before the onset of motor symptoms.

The clinical presentation and progression of PD are characterized by high inter-individual variability. Several clinical subtypes have been identified, initially based on the presence of motor symptoms (tremor-dominant subtype vs. bradykinetic-rigid subtype). Clinical, neuropathological, and neuroimaging evidence has suggested that the tremor-dominant subtype is milder compared to the bradykinetic-rigid subtype, but this classification has been criticized because it applies a one-dimensional model based solely on motor characteristics and does not include the numerous non-motor symptoms that characterize the disease. More recently, statistical cluster analysis techniques have been used to identify three subtypes: mild motor-dominant subtype, intermediate subtype, and malignant subtype. The malignant subtype is characterized by the early onset of cognitive deficits, orthostatic hypotension, REM sleep disorder, and urinary dysfunctions.

Table 15.3 HOEHN & YAHR SCALE FOR DISEASE SEVERITY

Stage	Disease
1	Unilateral disease
2	Bilateral disease without balance impairment
3	Bilateral disease, postural instability, independent
4	Severe disease, still able to walk independently, postural deficits
5	Bedridden or wheelchair-bound patient

Diagnosis

The diagnosis is based exclusively on clinical evaluation; diagnostic criteria were updated in 2015 by a group of experts from the Movement Disorder Society (■ Table 15.4a and b).

The diagnostic criteria involve two distinct phases: in the first phase, the presence of parkinsonism must be identified by assessing the presence of the main motor symptoms; in the second phase, the application of the criteria suggests a useful pathway to identify whether the parkinsonism is due to PD or other causes. Morphological neuroimaging (particularly MRI) does not show specific aspects of the disease; however, it is useful for ruling out structural alterations due to vascular injuries, normotensive hydrocephalus, brain tumors, etc. It should be emphasized that high-field MRI (7 Tesla, currently only used for research purposes) can reveal specific morphological alterations of the *substantia nigra*. In some ambiguous clinical situations, such as in the case of atypical tremor, a brain scintigraphy (SPECT) with the use of dopaminergic reuptake markers (DAT-Scan) may be useful to assess the integrity or alteration of the nigrostriatal

Table 15.4a DIAGNOSTIC CRITERIA FOR PARKINSON'S DISEASE

1. Diagnosis of parkinsonian syndrome
- Bradykinesia (slowness of movement + decreased amplitude or velocity of movement) + 1 of the following - Muscular rigidity (like a "lead pipe") - Resting tremor 4-6 Hz (postural and kinetic tremors are possible but only if resting tremor is also present)
2. Absolute exclusion criteria
- Cerebellar signs - Downward gaze palsy - Diagnosis of frontotemporal dementia, behavioral variant, or primary progressive aphasia - Parkinsonism limited to the lower limbs - Possible drug-induced parkinsonism - Lack of response to high doses of L-Dopa - Presence of cortical sensory deficit, apraxia, or aphasia - Normal functional neuroimaging (DAT Scan) - Other known conditions causing parkinsonism
3. Supporting criteria for Parkinson's disease diagnosis
- Clear response to dopaminergic therapy - Presence of L-Dopa-induced dyskinesias - Resting tremor in one limb - Positive result in at least one ancillary test (reduced sense of smell, positive myocardial scintigraphy with Metaiodobenzylguanidine)
4. Red flags for Parkinson's disease diagnosis
- Rapidly worsening gait disturbance (e.g., wheelchair use within 5 years from onset) - Absence of progression - Early bulbar dysfunction (severe dysphonia, dysarthria, dysphagia) - Respiratory dysfunction - Severe autonomic deficits within the first 5 years of the disease (orthostatic hypotension, urinary retention/ incontinence) - Recurrent falls within 3 years from onset - Antecollis, severe hand/foot contractions - Absence of common non-motor symptoms within the first 5 years of the disease (sleep disorders, autonomic dysfunction, hyposmia, psychiatric disorders) - Unknown etiology of corticospinal signs - Bilateral parkinsonism

Table 15.4b DIAGNOSTIC CRITERIA FOR PARKINSON'S DISEASE

Definite parkinson's disease (clinically)
1. Diagnosis of parkinsonian syndrome 2. Absence of absolute exclusion criteria 3. Presence of at least two supporting criteria 4. No red flags
Probable parkinson's disease (clinically)
1. Diagnosis of parkinsonian syndrome 2. Absence of absolute exclusion criteria 3. Presence of red flags counterbalanced by the presence of supporting criteria (e.g., if a red flag is present, at least one supporting criterion must be present)

compartment (Figure 15.2). In patients with early-onset autonomic system disorders (e.g., symptomatic orthostatic hypotension) that pose differential diagnostic challenges with Multiple System Atrophy (MSA - see section on atypical parkinsonisms), myocardial scintigraphy with metaiodobenzylguanidine may be helpful as it often appears altered in PD and normal in MSA. The use of L-Dopa or other dopaminergic drugs (such as apomorphine) as an acute test to confirm the diagnosis is not considered useful and should be avoided. Studies have also demonstrated that the echogenicity of the *substantia nigra* measured by transcranial Doppler can be useful in differentiating normal subjects from patients with PD or other forms of parkinsonism. A comprehensive clinical assessment may require diagnostic investigations to evaluate cognitive, cardiovascular, urological, and psychiatric functions. In the differential diagnosis, essential tremor, other forms of degenerative parkinsonism, and secondary parkinsonisms should be considered (see further details). Recent studies have also shown that the presence of α-synuclein and structural modifications of this protein can be demonstrated in cerebrospinal fluid, saliva, and skin.

Treatment

Treatment is still primarily symptomatic since there is currently no possibility to interfere with the mechanisms of neuronal damage. The fundamental treatment aims to increase dopamine concentration in the basal ganglia (Table 15.5) using certain pharmacological agents described below (for rehabilitative therapy, see Chapter 30, Neurorehabilitation). However, regular exercise and proper nutrition undoubtedly play an important role in maintaining patient functionality.

Levodopa | Since dopamine is unable to cross the blood-brain barrier, except in minimal amounts, therapy is based on the use of its natural precursor, levodopa (or L-Dopa), an amino acid capable of crossing the blood-brain barrier. L-Dopa, administered orally, is transformed into dopamine by dopa decarboxylase at the peripheral level. For this reason, it is administered in combination

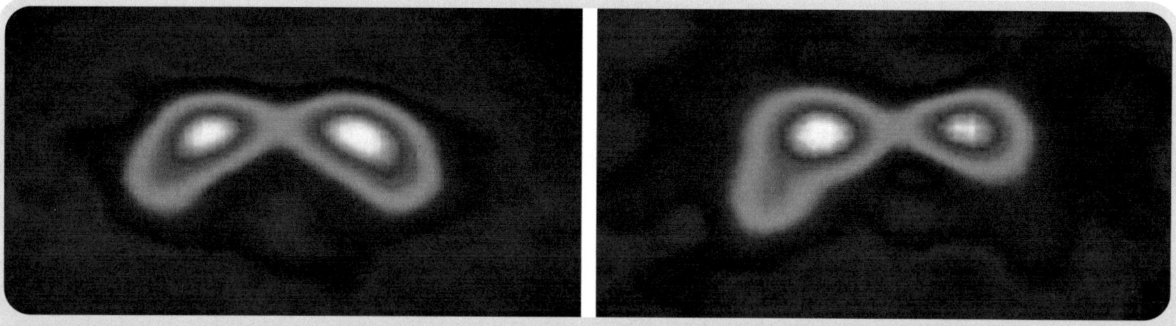

Figure 15.2

123I FP-CIT striatal uptake in a healthy subject (left) and in a patient with Parkinson's disease (right). Uptake is significantly reduced in the patient compared to the healthy subject. The reduction in uptake in the subject with Parkinson's disease is also asymmetric.

with carbidopa or benserazide, peripheral inhibitors of dopa decarboxylase (incapable of crossing the blood-brain barrier). L-Dopa, when administered orally in combination with one of the two inhibitors, is absorbed in the duodenal portion of the intestine, enters the bloodstream, crosses the blood-brain barrier, is taken up by the remaining efficient dopaminergic terminals (in advanced stages, also by serotoninergic terminals), and then transformed into dopamine. Intestinal absorption of L-Dopa can be limited by the presence of high concentrations of other amino acids in the intestine, as occurs, for example, after a high-protein meal. The most frequent side effects of L-Dopa treatment are gastrointestinal (nausea, vomiting), autonomic (postural hypotension), and sometimes neuropsychiatric (hallucinations and psychotic phenomena). Chronic treatment with L-Dopa can facilitate the onset of peripheral neuropathy.

Table 15.5 MAIN DRUGS FOR PARKINSON'S DISEASE THERAPY

Pharmacological class	Active ingredient	Indications	Daily dose	Side effects
Dopamine precursor	Levodopa (oral) Levodopa (intrajejunal gel infusion)	Motor symptoms	300-1200 mg	Dyskinesia, hypotension, nausea Technical issues with PEG; polyneuropathy
Dopamine Agonists	Pramipexole Ropinirole Rotigotine (transdermal)	Motor symptoms Motor symptoms Motor symptoms	1,05-3,15 mg 8-24 mg 8-16 mg	Nausea, vomiting, hypotension, hallucinations, impulse control disorder (pathological gambling, hypersexuality, bulimia, compulsive shopping), edema
	Apomorphine penjet (subcutaneous)	Delayed on	3-6 mg	Nausea, vomiting, hypotension
	Continuous subcutaneous apomorphine infusion	Fluctuations, dyskinesias	Individual	Subcutaneous nodules, hallucinations, hypotension
COMT Inhibitors	Entacapone Tolcapone Opicapone	Motor fluctuations Motor fluctuations Motor fluctuations	200 mg with levodopa 300 mg 50 mg	Dyskinesia, hypotension, nausea, urine discoloration, diarrhea, hallucinations, hepatotoxicity (tolcapone only)
MAO-B Inhibitors	Selegiline Rasagiline	Motor symptoms (initial, advanced)	10 mg 1 mg	Increased dyskinesia, hallucinations
MAO-B Inhibitors plus	Safinamide	Motor fluctuations	50-100 mg	Increased dyskinesia
NMDA Antagonist	Amantadine	Dyskinesia	200-400 mg	Edema, hallucinations, livedo reticularis

COMT: catechol-O-methyltransferase. MAO-B: monoamine oxidase-B.

L-Dopa, available in various types of rapidly absorbed and sustained-release formulations, is very effective in reducing bradykinesia and rigidity, but probably less effective in reducing tremor and unable to modify postural instability. A therapeutic response of at least a 20% improvement in the motor section of the MDS-UPDRS scale is considered as a good response to L-Dopa. L-Dopa has several primarily pharmacokinetic limitations, including its short plasma half-life (approximately 90 minutes) and not always complete absorption. In cases of advanced disease with severe motor fluctuations, L-Dopa can be administered continuously via intraduodenal route through percutaneous endoscopic gastrostomy.

Dopamine agonists (DA agonists) | Drugs that directly act on pre- and post-synaptic dopaminergic receptors. The most commonly used non-ergot derived DA agonists are pramipexole and ropinirole, administered orally, and rotigotine, administered transdermally. Apomorphine is a parenterally administered DA agonist (usually subcutaneous) and is only used in the advanced stages of the disease. While less effective than L-Dopa, DA agonists are useful both as monotherapy during the early stages of the disease and in combination with L-Dopa in later stages. The most frequent side effects of DA agonists include nausea, vomiting, orthostatic hypotension, excessive daytime sleepiness, sudden sleep attacks, hallucinations, psychosis, and impulse control disorders (pathological gambling, hypersexuality, hyperphagia, compulsive shopping), which are more common in younger male patients.

MAO-B inhibitors | These drugs inhibit the intracerebral metabolism of dopamine, thereby increasing its duration in the synapse. MAO-B inhibitors are used both in the initial phase as monotherapy and in later stages in combination with L-Dopa. Various MAO-B inhibitors are available, including rasagiline, selegiline, and more recently, safinamide. The latter molecule combines MAO-B inhibitory dopaminergic action with inhibitory action on glutamate release. These drugs are generally well-tolerated.

COMT inhibitors | These drugs inhibit the metabolism of L-Dopa by blocking its transformation into 3-O-methyldopa. Entacapone and opicapone act only peripherally (they are unable to cross the blood-brain barrier), while tolcapone acts both peripherally and centrally. COMT inhibitors increase the bioavailability of L-Dopa by approximately 50% by prolonging its plasma half-life. The use of tolcapone is limited by its potential hepatotoxicity. These drugs must be administered in combination with L-Dopa and may cause a significant increase in dyskinesias. In such cases, the dose of L-Dopa should be appropriately reduced.

Anticholinergics | (Biperiden and trihexyphenidil), the first drugs introduced in PD therapy, are currently less commonly used due to side effects such as increased intraocular pressure, acute urinary retention in patients with prostatic hypertrophy, confusion, and hallucinations, especially in elderly patients. Furthermore, there is no scientific evidence from randomized studies demonstrating their efficacy.

Amantadine | It is a drug with pro-dopaminergic action (inhibition of intrasynaptic dopamine reuptake) and anti-glutamatergic action. The latter has been found to be useful in the treatment of dyskinesias (see below).

Therapeutic Strategies | The choice of drug(s) to use in PD is based on the evaluation of several factors, including the patient's age, level of disability, presence of comorbidities, and the risk of long-term adverse events. In patients under 60 years of age, the initial therapy involves the use of DA-agonists or MAO-B inhibitors, with or without low doses of L-Dopa. In most cases, within 3 years of starting treatment, adding L-Dopa will be necessary to achieve better control of motor symptoms. In elderly patients (>70 years), those with significant comorbidities, or cases where functional disability is high from the beginning, L-Dopa is considered the first-choice medication, potentially combined with MAO-B inhibitors or low doses of DA-agonists. After several years (typically 5-10) of clinical well-being and stable clinical response, most patients develop motor complications. These are primarily represented by fluctuations in motor response and dyskinesias. The most frequent motor fluctuation is "wearing-off," characterized by alternating phases of good mobility (the "on" phase) and phases of motor block (the "off" phase). These phases are correlated with the timing of drug intake and thus the variations in plasma concentrations of L-Dopa (predictable motor fluctuations). Morning akinesia, as well as nocturnal akinesia, fall into this group of complications and are associated with a marked nocturnal reduction in plasma levels of L-Dopa. Sometimes, the patient can show a rapid transition between the on and off phases without predictability based on drug administration schedules (unpredictable motor fluctuations). Dyskinesias are involuntary choreoathetoid or dystonic movements affecting the limbs, trunk, and face, representing the most frequent side effect of chronic L-Dopa treatment. Dyskinesias are more common in patients with an early onset of the disease and are correlated with the duration and severity of the illness, as well as the duration and dose of dopaminergic treatment. They can be categorized as follows: *"off" dystonia*, characterized by involuntary and prolonged muscle contractions leading to abnormal postures (flexion attitudes of the foot or more frequently extension of the big toe); *peak-dose dyskinesias* (occurring at the peak plasma levels of L-Dopa), characterized by involuntary choreoathetoid movements mainly affecting the head, trunk, and upper limbs; *biphasic dyskinesias* or *on-off fluctuations* (occurring during the ascending or descending phases of plasma levels of L-Dopa), presenting as painful dystonias localized to the lower limbs. The pathogenesis of motor fluctuations and dyskinesias is linked, on one hand, to the progressive loss of dopaminergic terminals, which is accompanied by a reduced capacity to store and release dopamine constantly, and probably also to the use of short-acting drugs such as L-Dopa. The pulsatile and discontinuous stimulation of striatal dopaminergic receptors leads to molecular and neurophysiological changes within the corticostriatal circuits. The therapy for motor complications, particularly "wearing-off," is based on various strategies: a) increasing or fractionating doses of L-Dopa and/or adding controlled-release L-Dopa; b) adding a DA-agonist; c) adding a MAO-B inhibitor; d) adding a COMT inhibitor; e) surgical therapy.

The advanced stage of the disease is characterized by severe motor fluctuations and prolonged involuntary movements (generally >5 hours of OFF time per day and at least 2 hours of disabling dyskinesia), which are no longer controllable with modifications to oral therapy. In such situations, more invasive therapies are available. Strategies for continuous administration of dopaminergic drugs can be used, including continuous subcutaneous infusion of apomorphine or intraduodenal administration of a gel of L-Dopa/carbidopa via percutaneous endoscopic gastrostomy. Subcutaneous continuous L.-Dopa administration will also be available in the near future. The surgical therapy for Parkinson's disease is based on electrical stimulation of the subthalamic nucleus (STN) or the internal globus pallidus (GPi) using stereotactic techniques (deep brain stimulation or DBS). Stimulation leads to inhibition of STN and GPi activity. The improvement of symptoms after DBS primarily affects bradykinesia, rigidity, and tremor, while satisfactory results are not achieved for balance, postural deficits, and dysarthria. Significant adverse events, in addition to surgical complications (usually small intracerebral hemorrhages in about 1% of cases), include infection or displacement of the electrodes and sudden malfunctioning of the stimulator. Preliminary data are available for the possible benefit deriving from the use of Focussed Ultrasounds in the treatment of drug resistant tremor.

Treatment of non-motor complications

Hallucinations, especially visual ones, are frequently observed in patients with cognitive impairments and can be controlled with the use of atypical antipsychotics (such as clozapine and quetiapine; olanzapine and risperidone should be avoided because they can produce severe deterioration of motor symptoms). In the treatment of cognitive disorders, some studies have shown moderate efficacy of acetylcholinesterase inhibitors (such as rivastigmine and donepezil), typically used in the treatment of Alzheimer's dementia. Rivastigmine is also considered effective in the treatment of apathy, while selective serotonin reuptake inhibitors are recommended for depression. Orthostatic hypotension can be controlled by wearing compression stockings, increasing hydration and salt intake, and administering medications such as midodrine and fludrocortisone. Sleep disorders can be treated with slow-release L-Dopa in cases where the problem is related to nocturnal immobility, or with benzodiazepines such as clonazepam in cases of fragmented or interrupted sleep due to nightmares. Melatonin can also be useful. Urinary disturbances are usually treated with anticholinergic drugs, which reduce bladder hyperactivity. Chronic treatment with macrogol can be beneficial for constipation. For sexual disorders, phosphodiesterase type 5 inhibitors can be used with caution.

Future perspectives | In the symptomatic field, a soluble formulation of L-dopa administered subcutaneously and probably a sublingual formulation of apomorphine will be available. Numerous studies are underway to address the etiological treatment of the disease. The most promising prospects (based on animal studies) arise from interventions aimed at preventing the aggregation of α-synuclein and the formation of toxic α-synuclein oligomers. Such therapies are based on active and passive immunotherapy (including monoclonal antibodies) and the use of drugs capable of modulating the aggregation of α-ynuclein, along with gene silencing interventions to reduce α-synuclein mRNA levels. Precision medicine (i.e., therapeutic interventions targeted to the specific genotype/phenotype of PD patients) represents the future of PD therapy. A prime example of this approach is therapeutic protocols dedicated to PD patients carrying a GBA mutation through the administration of "chaperone" molecules that promote lysosomal translocation of glucocerebrosidase, facilitating the degradation of α-synuclein.

15.1.2 Atypical and secondary parkinsonisms

Atypical parkinsonisms are a group of sporadic neurodegenerative disorders characterized by the combination of parkinsonian motor signs and other neurological features. Secondary parkinsonisms, on the other hand, are those caused by a known (and sometimes reversible) cause (■ Table 15.6). Atypical parkinsonisms are much less common than PD and represent approximately 10-15% of hypokinetic syndromes. Atypical parkinsonisms are characterized by a faster clinical progression compared to PD and have a more disabling prognosis. The three main forms of atypical parkinsonism are multiple system atrophy (MSA), progressive supranuclear palsy (PSP), and corticobasal syndrome (CBS). Since there are no biological markers for a definite diagnosis of atypical parkinsonism, diagnosis primarily relies on the clinical picture, progression of clinical signs, and sometimes suggestive findings on neuroimaging. Confirmatory diagnosis can only be made through post-mortem neuropathological examination.

Table 15.6 PARKINSONISM CLASSIFICATION

Primary forms
Parkinson's disease
Other degenerative forms
• Classic sporadic forms Multiple system atrophy (MSA-P variant) Progressive supranuclear palsy Corticobasal degeneration • Dominant genetic forms Huntington's chorea Spinocerebellar ataxia type 2 (SCA2) and 3 (SCA3) Frontotemporal dementia (FTDP-17) • Recessive genetic forms Wilson's disease Neurodegeneration with brain iron accumulation • Uncertain genetic forms • Parkinsonism-dementia-ALS complex • Atypical PSP-like parkinsonism in guadeloupe • Parkinsonisms associated with dystonia
Secondary forms (symptomatic)
• Drug-induced (phenothiazines, butyrophenones, metoclopramide, tetrabenazine, α-methyldopa, calcium channel blockers, lithium) • Toxic (MPTP, carbon monoxide, carbon disulfide, hydrogen cyanide, manganese, mercury, methanol, ethanol, hexane) • Post-infectious (encephalitis lethargica, other viral encephalitis, AIDS, subacute sclerosing panencephalitis) • Whipple's Disease • Creutzfeldt-Jakob Disease • Metabolic (hepatocerebral degeneration, hypoxia, hypoparathyroidism) • Structural damage-related (brain tumor, trauma, punch-drunk encephalopathy, normal-pressure hydrocephalus, syringomyelia) • Vascular (multi-infarct encephalopathy, Binswanger's disease) • Functional

Multiple System Atrophy (MSA)

MSA is a disease characterized by neuronal loss and abnormal accumulation of α-synuclein (synucleinopathy) in the cytoplasm of oligodendrocytes (glial cytoplasmic inclusions) in specific areas of the central nervous system. Neuronal loss is prominent in the basal ganglia, brainstem, cerebellum, intermediolateral columns, and Onuf nucleus of the spinal cord. MSA is a neurodegenerative disease that typically begins after the age of 40, with a median age of around 57 years, and a median survival of 10 years. It is clinically characterized by a combination of parkinsonian signs, early autonomic dysfunction (orthostatic hypotension, syncope, urinary incontinence or retention, constipation, sweating disturbances, erectile dysfunction in men, anorgasmia in women), cerebellar dysfunction (ataxic gait, dysarthria, limb ataxia, nystagmus), and signs of impaired corticospinal function. MSA is classified as MSA-P when parkinsonian symptoms predominate, and MSA-C when cerebellar dysfunction is more evident. Patients with MSA-P have a faster disease progression compared to PD and show poor response to L-Dopa therapy, but the differential diagnosis with PD, especially in the early stages of the disease, can be very challenging even for experienced neurologists. Moreover, in forms with greater autonomic involvement, patients may initially consult other specialists (urologists, andrologists, cardiologists) long before a neurological evaluation. Cardiovascular tests (e.g., tilt-test), when they show severe involvement of the autonomic system, can provide additional support for an MSA diagnosis, although they are not absolute discriminatory factors, as both orthostatic hypotension and bladder disturbances can be present, especially in the advanced stages of PD. Patients with MSA may also exhibit other clinical features useful for diagnosis, such as early dysarthria and/or dysphagia, pronounced cold sensitivity, laryngeal stridor, myoclonus, emotional lability, limb contractures, severe truncal dystonia, and early postural instability, as well as sleep disturbances. Symptomatic therapy for MSA is based on the use of antiparkinsonian drugs (but only a minority of cases respond to this treatment), measures and medications for orthostatic hypotension (α-adrenergics, mineralocorticoids), and drugs for bladder disturbances (anticholinergics, α-blockers, botulinum toxin). Rehabilitation, speech therapy, and occupational therapy can be helpful.

Progressive Supranuclear Palsy (PSP)

PSP is a neurodegenerative disease characterized by the accumulation of Tau protein (tauopathy). This protein plays numerous roles, including regulating cellular transport systems and transmitting neuronal signals. During development, it also regulates myelination and axonal growth. In PSP, Tau protein undergoes phosphorylation and forms toxic oligomers for the cell membrane. Histologically, there is neuronal loss in several areas of the brainstem, cerebellum, basal ganglia, and frontal cortex, associated with the accumulation of hyperphosphorylated Tau protein. The average age of onset is just over 60 years, never before 40 years, and the average survival is around 7-8 years. PSP in its classical form (Richardson's syndrome or PSP-R) is a progressive sporadic disease characterized by parkinsonism with bradykinesia, early postural instability with a tendency to fall in the first year of symptom onset, cognitive deficits, and supranuclear gaze palsy, both vertically and horizontally, more often downward. There are also clinical forms with a slower progression. Some patients initially present with a clinical picture similar to classical Parkinson's disease but have a poor response to L-Dopa and a more rapid clinical course than Parkinson's disease (PSP-P). Others present with an isolated form of akinesia and freezing of gait ("pure akinesia"). More rarely, the clinical onset can be characterized by symptoms indicative of frontotemporal dementia or isolated language disorder (primary progressive aphasia). Symptomatic therapy for PSP is very limited and is based on antiparkinsonian drugs (L-Dopa and amantadine), selective serotonin reuptake inhibitors (for apathy and emotional incontinence), and atypical antipsychotics (for the treatment of behavioral and sleep disorders).

Corticobasal degeneration (CBD) and corticobasal syndrome (CBS)

CBD is a pathological condition characterized by the accumulation of hyperphosphorylated

Tau protein (tauopathy), swollen cortical neurons in the parietal and frontal areas, astrocytic plaques in the cortical region, neurofibrillary tangles, and often asymmetric frontal and parietal atrophy. Onset typically occurs around the age of 60, and the average survival is 8 years. Corticobasal syndrome (CBS), the most frequent clinical manifestation of CBD, is characterized by asymmetric rigidity and akinesia, postural instability, irregular postural and action tremor, myoclonus, dystonia, apraxia, alien limb phenomenon, cortical sensory deficits, and sometimes cognitive-behavioral disturbances. However, the clinical manifestations of CBD can be highly heterogeneous. Some patients may present with typical features of PSP or those of dementia or prion diseases. Differential diagnosis, often challenging, includes distinguishing corticobasal syndrome from PSP and various forms of dementia. There are no effective therapies for treating patients with CBD.

15.1.3 Secondary parkinsonisms

The correct differential diagnosis between PD and various secondary forms of parkinsonism (Table 15.6) is crucial for the clinical assessment of the patient, as it sometimes allows the initiation of potentially curative specific treatments. Therefore, in addition to a thorough medical history, all necessary diagnostic tests should be performed.

From medications | All medications blocking dopaminergic receptors or causing depletion of presynaptic dopamine can lead to symptoms typical of PD. Among these, typical neuroleptics (phenothiazines, butyrophenones, thioxanthenes, benzamides) are still the most common cause of iatrogenic parkinsonism. The onset of parkinsonian symptoms is related to the ability of these drugs to competitively inhibit dopaminergic D2 receptors with high binding potency. Atypical neuroleptics (particularly clozapine and quetiapine) can induce a parkinsonian syndrome, usually when used at high dosages (a condition that leads to increased binding with the D2 receptor). In cases of drug-induced parkinsonism, the distribution of symptoms is often bilateral, and the onset is subacute.

The therapy involves discontinuing or reducing the dosage of the responsible medication. Other drugs responsible for parkinsonism include lithium salts and some medications used in common clinical practice such as antiemetics (metoclopramide, clebopride), vasodilators (cinnarizine, flunarizine), and antihypertensives (e.g., methyldopa, now rarely used). Some antiepileptic drugs (e.g., valproate) can rarely cause parkinsonism.

From vascular causes | The classical clinical presentation of these forms is characterized by predominant, if not exclusive, involvement of the lower limbs, with gait disturbances, rigidity, and absence of tremor. Pseudobulbar signs, corticospinal dysfunction, and cognitive decline often coexist, indicating widespread vascular damage. The response to treatment with L-Dopa is usually minimal. This type of parkinsonism is observed in elderly patients with vascular risk factors, and MRI examination reveals multiple ischemic lesions in the subcortical structures and basal ganglia or deep vascular alterations of the white matter (see also the chapter on dementias).

From infectious causes | Various infectious diseases can be responsible for the onset of secondary parkinsonism, either as an acute complication or as a long-term condition. Among the latter, Von Economo's encephalitis lethargica (1916-1927) is a viral disease whose viral etiology is currently under intense debate. In addition to signs of parkinsonism, patients exhibited oculogyric crises, ophthalmoplegia, behavioral changes, severe autonomic symptoms, and various types of involuntary movements (tics, dyskinesias, dystonia). Other diseases that can be complicated by parkinsonism include American equine encephalitis, Japanese B encephalitis, and encephalitis caused by influenza viruses. Currently, the most common infectious cause of parkinsonism is AIDS, either due to the direct action of the virus or opportunistic CNS infections associated with this disease. Prion encephalopathy can lead to the acute or subacute onset of parkinsonian symptoms in combination with other characteristic signs of this condition (dementia, myoclonus, ataxia).

In hydrocephalus | Early alterations in gait and posture may be present in normotensive hydrocephalus, accompanied by sphincter disorders and cognitive decline. However, the gait is not typically parkinsonian but often characterized by a wide base and gait apraxia. The onset can be subacute or progressive. The clinical picture can be resolved with a cerebrospinal fluid shunting procedure.

From space-occupying lesions | Various types of space-occupying lesions (hemorrhages, benign and malignant tumors, abscesses) can cause a parkinsonian syndrome. Most frequently, these are midline tumors or supratentorial meningiomas, predominantly frontal.

From cranial traumas | Parkinsonism can be secondary to repeated and prolonged cranial traumas (e.g., in professional boxers). In this case, the most frequent neurological consequence is dementia, but signs of involvement of the pyramidal and extrapyramidal systems can also occur, either separately or in combination.

From toxic substances | Exposure to environmental toxins and drug abuse can be associated with the onset of parkinsonism. The most frequent form is the one that can affect certain professional categories such as miners and workers exposed to manganese. In this form, in addition to bradykinesia and rigidity, fatigue and cognitive and behavioral disturbances (aggressiveness and irritability) are also present. Furthermore, there is a characteristic gait disorder secondary to the appearance of action dystonia with forced plantar flexion of the foot (cock-walk gait). The compound MPTP (accidentally synthesized in domestic production of heroin) specifically affects the neurons of the substantia nigra and is capable of reproducing a syndrome very similar to idiopathic Parkinson's disease (PD). Therefore, MPTP intoxication represents the main experimental model of PD used in laboratory animals. Other toxic causes include intoxication with methanol and carbon monoxide.

15.2 Hyperkinetic syndromes

The most frequent hyperkinesias are tremors, dystonias, athetosis, chorea, and ballism, as well as tics. Proper identification of the type of movement is essential for formulating a diagnostic hypothesis, identifying possible etiology, and initiating the most appropriate therapeutic treatment. Figure 15.3 provides a useful framework for the clinical classification of hyperkinesias.

15.2.1 Tremor

Tremor is defined as an involuntary rhythmic oscillation of one or more body segments around one or more joints. The movement that characterizes tremor is defined based on various variables, particularly body location, frequency, amplitude, and mode of onset. The frequency of tremor remains stable in individual patients, while the amplitude is variable and increases during muscle fatigue or in a state of excessive emotionality. There is a tremor considered physiological that mainly affects the upper limbs and occurs during the maintenance of a posture. Typically, it is a low-amplitude tremor with a high frequency that is accentuated by fatigue, emotional states, and coffee consumption. Pathological tremor is generally constant, clearly visible, and is described based on clinical presentation characteristics (at rest, during a posture, or during an action) (Table 15.7). Among pathological tremors, resting tremor occurs when the patient is completely at rest (theoretically when the effect of gravity is eliminated) and does not perform active movements. Resting tremor usually has a frequency ranging from 4 to 6 Hz. The re-emergent tremor seen in Parkinson's disease is considered a form of resting tremor (as mentioned in the section dedicated to PD). Action tremor, on the other hand, appears during the execution of a voluntary movement and usually has a frequency ranging from 4 to 12 Hz. It can be classified as:

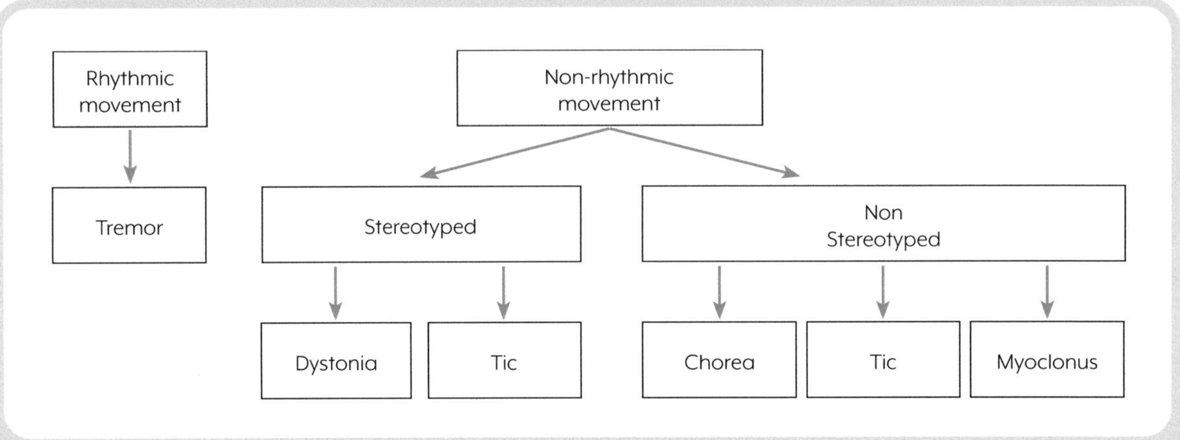

Figure 15.3

Classification of Hyperkinesias.

- *Postural tremor*, typically observed during the maintenance of a posture (e.g., extended position of the upper limbs).
- *Kinetic tremor*, present during the execution of a voluntary movement. Simple kinetic tremor usually remains constant during the movement, while intentional tremor intensifies as the affected segment approaches the intended target (e.g., in the finger-to-nose test).
- *Task-specific tremor*, which occurs only during the performance of specific motor acts (e.g., writing or voice tremor).
- *Isometric tremor*, which occurs when the limb contracts voluntarily against resistance.

Clinical phenotypes of tremor are usually associated with specific pathological conditions (Table 15.7). However, in various clinical conditions, the simultaneous presence of multiple types of tremor can be observed. The causes of tremor are numerous, and a selected list is shown in Table 15.8.

The new classification of tremor recently proposed by the Movement Disorder Society is based on two main axes. Axis I considers

Table 15.7 CLINICAL CLASSIFICATION OF TREMOR BASED ON ACTIVATION CONDITIONS

Onset time	Clinical aspects	Example of disease
At rest	Body segment at rest	Parkinson's disease
Action - Postural Dependent or independent of a position	When the body segment assumes an antigravity posture	Physiological tremor, accentuated physiological tremor, essential tremor, neuropathic tremor
- Kinetic Simple Intentional	During voluntary movement execution Increases during movement	Cerebellar diseases, multiple sclerosis, traumas, strokes, Wilson's disease, medications, toxic substances
Specific task	Only during the execution of specific activities	Writing tremor, voice tremor
- Isometric	In voluntary contraction against resistance	Writing tremor, voice tremor Physiological or associated with other types of tremor (essential)

Note: The translation provided is a general representation and may not capture the full context or nuances of the original text.

Table 15.8 CAUSES OF TREMOR

Neurodegenerative diseases
- Parkinson's disease - Multiple system atrophy - Progressive supranuclear palsy - Corticobasal degeneration - Genetic forms of parkinsonism and dystonia - Neuroferritinopathies - Spinocerebellar ataxias - Basal ganglia calcifications - Genetic forms of polyneuropathy causing tremor - Wilson's disease - Dystonia-parkinsonism in the Filipino population (DYT3, Lubag) - Fragile X premutation
Mitochondrial genetic diseases
Inflammatory and infectious diseases
- Multiple sclerosis and other demyelinating diseases - Subacute sclerosing panencephalitis - HIV - Tuberculosis, neuroborreliosis - Bacterial and viral encephalitis
Endocrine and metabolic diseases
- Liver and kidney failure - Hyperthyroidism
Neuropathies and spinal muscular atrophy
- Kennedy's disease - Guillain-Barre syndrome - Neuropathies
Toxins
- Mercury - Lead - Manganese - Arsenic - Toluene - Alcohol and alcohol withdrawal
Medications
- Antiepileptic drugs - Antidepressants - Beta stimulants - Lithium salts - Neuroleptics - Amiodarone - Thyroid replacement therapy - Antineoplastic drugs
Other
- Brain tumors - Brain damage from trauma, ischemia, hemorrhage - Anxiety and stress - Fatigue - Peripheral tissue injury - Functional tremor

Table 15.9 CLASSIFICATION OF DIFFERENT TYPES OF TREMOR

Axis I: Clinical features
Anamnestic factors - Age of onset (birth to 2 years, 3-12 years, 13-20 years, 21-45 years, 46-60 years, > 60 years) - Type of onset and progression - Remote pathological history - Familial history - Sensitivity to alcohol and medications
Characteristics of tremor - Body location (focal, segmental, hemi-tremor, generalized) - Triggering conditions (see Table 15.7) - Frequency
Associated signs - Signs of systemic illness - Other neurological signs
Ancillary tests - Neurophysiological tests - Structural imaging - Receptor imaging - Biomarkers
Axis II: Etiology
Acquired *Genetically defined idiopathic* - Familial - Sporadic

clinical characteristics, while Axis II assesses etiology (Table 15.9).

Essential tremor

It is the most common movement disorder in the general population. In fact, it is estimated that 5% of individuals over the age of 40 are affected by it. Essential tremor (ET) is defined as a bilateral postural and action tremor of the upper limbs, lasting for at least 3 years, associated or not with tremor in other body regions (e.g., head, voice, lower limbs), and in the absence of other neurological signs such as ataxia, dystonia, or parkinsonism. Therefore, isolated tremor of the head and voice, once considered focal forms of essential tremor, are now classified within the realm of dystonic tremor. ET presents considerable clinical heterogeneity and currently does not appear to be a single clinical entity. The frequency of ET ranges from 4 to 12 Hz, and its amplitude varies, tending to increase in stressful situations and states of anxiety. ET has a significant genetic component (autosomal dominant). Some studies conducted on twin populations have demonstrated a 93% concordance for tremor in monozygotic twins and a 29% concordance in dizygotic twins. Inheritance is characterized by significant genetic heterogeneity, and to this day, the responsible genes have not been definitively identified. The neuropathology of essential tremor is controversial. Some studies have shown pathological changes in the cerebellum, demonstrating a reduction in the number of Purkinje cells and other cerebellar structures. However, these alterations have not been confirmed by other studies. Regarding the pathophysiology, it is believed that ET derives by oscillations in a "network" comprising the cerebellum, basal ganglia, thalamus, and motor cortex. Many patients may have difficulty performing activities such as writing, eating, drinking, pouring liquids into a glass, and other occupational activities. One particular observable characteristic in some patients with ET is the improvement of tremor after consuming moderate amounts of alcohol. In the differential diagnosis, the following should be considered: exaggerated physiological tremor, usually characterized by smaller oscillations and lacking an important kinetic component; Parkinson's disease, when postural tremor is also present; tremor associated with hyperthyroidism; cerebellar tremor; dystonic tremor; functional (psychogenic) tremor; and tremor of Wilson's disease. In the recent classification proposed by the Movement Disorder Society, a new clinical entity has also been identified: essential tremor plus, characterized by the coexistence of essential tremor and subtle neurological signs. It is currently under study whether this condition presents different pathophysiological and clinical characteristics compared to classic ET. There are no specific therapies for ET, but medications such as beta-blockers (particularly propranolol), primidone, topiramate, clonazepam, or rarely, the administration of botulinum toxin in the muscles affected by tremor can be helpful. In selected cases resistant to pharmacological therapies and in which the tremor causes severe functional disturbances, deep brain stimulation with electrodes (DBS) placed in the thalamus or focused ultrasound therapy at the level of the thalamus (FUS) can be used.

Dystonic tremor | It is an undefined tremor that typically occurs in patients with dystonia (e.g., head tremor in patients with cervical dystonia). This tremor can also be present in segments unaffected by dystonia (e.g., hand tremor in patients with cervical dystonia). Isolated head and voice tremors, once considered focal forms of essential tremor, may also be forms of dystonic tremors. In general, these are tremors with variable frequency and amplitude.

Cerebellar tremor | It is a tremor caused by a lesion in the brainstem or cerebellar peduncle. It is an action tremor that worsens during the execution of voluntary movements. Multiple sclerosis is one of the most common causes.

Holmes tremor | It is a resting, postural, and action tremor caused by an alteration of the cerebellar-red nucleus-thalamus and nigrostriatal pathways.

Palatal tremor | It is caused by a lesion in the dentate nucleus-red nucleus-olivary nuclei.

Orthostatic tremor | It is a high-frequency tremor (13-16 Hz) of the lower limbs that occurs when the subject maintains an upright position. It sometimes improves with clonazepam therapy.

Finally, among the rare tremors, we can mention tremors occurring in neuropathies (particularly in demyelinating forms) and tremors present in patients with Fragile X Syndrome.

15.2.2 Dystonia

Dystonia is characterized by prolonged or intermittent muscle contractions that result in repetitive movements and/or abnormal postures, involuntary movements with a twisting appearance, and, in some cases, tremors. The involuntary dystonic movements are present at rest but can be triggered or worsened by the execution of voluntary movements. The prevalence of primary dystonias varies depending on the studies and the type of dystonia and appears to be approximately 150 cases per 1,000,000, a figure that is likely lower than the actual reality. From a pathophysiological perspective, it is believed that dystonias are caused by anatomical or functional alterations of the basal ganglia and functional modifications of the basal ganglia-thalamo-cerebral cortex sensorimotor circuit. It is also believed that the cerebellum may play an important role. The main altered physiological mechanisms are represented by a deficit in inhibitory mechanisms at various levels of the motor system, alterations in sensorimotor integration, and changes in cortical and subcortical plasticity mechanisms. In particular, for focal dystonias, it is believed that they are linked to common pathophysiological alterations of a circuit ("network") that includes the basal ganglia, sensorimotor cortex, cerebellum, and brainstem. For the various types of focal dystonia, it is believed that there is a different involvement of these structures. For example, brainstem structures would play a fundamental role in blepharospasm, while the cerebellum would be more involved in the appearance of tremor in patients with cervical dystonia.

Dystonias can be classified based on two axes: the first considers the set of phenomenological and clinical characteristics, while the second takes into account the etiology (Table 15.10). The first axis considers the age of onset, the body site of the dystonia, the coexistence of other movement disorders, and possibly other neurological or systemic manifestations. Onset of dystonia in the first year of life has a high probability of being associated with a congenital metabolic disorder, onset between 2 and 6 years is frequently related to infantile cerebral palsy, especially if accompanied by motor developmental delay, or due to genetic mutations. Late onset, between 30 and 60 years of age, is generally associated with sporadic forms and focal clinical manifestations. Based on body distribution, dystonias are classified as follows: *focal* when they affect a single body part, *segmental*, when they affect adjacent muscle groups, *multifocal* when two or more non-contiguous body segments are involved, *hemidystonia* when only one side of the body is affected (these forms are usually due to structural lesions, often vascular, located in the contralateral hemisphere), and *generalized* when the entire body is affected.

Focal dystonias are the most common dystonias in adults and are classified as follows: blepharospasm, characterized by prolonged involuntary bilateral contraction (lasting for several seconds) of the orbicularis oculi muscle, which can cause severe functional visual impairment; oromandibular dystonia, characterized by muscle contractions in the

Table 15.10 CLINICAL CLASSIFICATION OF DYSTONIAS

Axis I: Clinical features

Age at onset
- From birth to 2 years
- From 3 to 12 years
- From 13 to 20 years
- From 21 to 40 years
- After 40 years

Distribution
- Focal
- Segmental
- Multifocal
- Generalized
- Hemidystonia

Temporal pattern
- Course:
  - Static
  - Progressive
- Variability:
  - Persistent
  - Action-specific
  - Diurnal
  - Paroxysmal

Associations
- Isolated dystonia or associated with other movement disorders
- Dystonia associated with other neurological or systemic conditions

Axis II: Etiology

Neurological pathology
- Evidence of neurodegeneration
- Evidence of structural lesions
- Absence of neurodegeneration

Hereditary or acquired
- Hereditary
  - Autosomal dominant
  - Autosomal recessive
  - X-linked
  - Mitochondrial
- Acquired
  - Perinatal brain trauma
  - Infections
  - Medications
  - Toxic substances
  - Vascular
  - Neoplastic
  - Psychogenic

Idiopathic
- Sporadic
- Familial

lower half of the face; cervical dystonia, which variably affects different muscles of the cervical region (sternocleidomastoid, splenius capitis, trapezius, anterior scalene, supraspinatus, and others) and results in abnormal postures of the neck and head (torticollis, retrocollis, laterocollis, anterocollis); upper limb dystonia, including "writer's cramp," characterized by excessive contraction of the forearm and upper limb muscles during writing, sometimes making writing impossible, and other occupational cramps (pianists, violinists, guitarists, and typists may be affected); spasmodic dysphonia, which affects the adductor and abductor muscles of the larynx, causing severe difficulties in phonation.

A peculiar feature of focal dystonias is the presence of an antagonistic gesture, characterized by a reduction in dystonia following voluntarily performed movements by the patient (e.g., touching the chin in patients with cervical dystonia). Another clinical characteristic of focal dystonias is the presence of non-motor symptoms such as pain, sleep disturbances, cognitive impairments, and psychiatric disorders.

Dystonia can be isolated or associated with other movement disorders and may be observed in conditions such as Parkinson's disease, atypical parkinsonism, Wilson's disease, and many other conditions, without necessarily being the predominant movement disorder. Although rare, it is worth mentioning among these forms the *dystonia responsive to L-Dopa* (or *Dopa-responsive dystonia*, DYT-GCH1), an autosomal dominant disease with reduced penetrance (30%), characterized by childhood onset with lower limb dystonia causing walking difficulties, diurnal fluctuation of symptoms (worsening in the evening and improvement after overnight rest). The peculiarity of this condition is the excellent therapeutic response to low doses of L-Dopa. Most forms of Dopa-responsive dystonia are caused by a mutation in the GCH1 gene, which encodes GTP cyclohydrolase 1, an enzyme that catalyzes the first step in the formation of tetrahydrobiopterin, an essential factor in the synthesis of tyrosine hydroxylase and therefore dopamine.

Myoclonic dystonia (DYT-SGCE), an autosomal dominant condition due to a mutation in the epsilon-sarcoglycan gene, is characterized by a combination of dystonia and myoclonic movements of the neck, trunk, and sometimes the upper limbs, with onset in childhood or in the second and third decades of life. Symptoms may improve after alcohol intake.

The etiological classification (axis II, ▫ Table 15.10), divides dystonias on the base of the presence or absence of identifiable anatomical lesions or neurodegeneration and on a possible specific inheritance pattern. From a genetic point of view, there is a constant reclassification of various forms of primary dystonia. ▫ Table 15.11 lists the most frequent genetic forms of isolated dystonia or dystonia combined with other neurological disorders. Primary dystonias that begin in childhood in the lower limbs and subsequently tend to involve other parts of the body are frequently genetic in nature and largely secondary to alterations in the DYT-TOR1A gene on chromosome 9. On the other hand, primary dystonias that begin in adulthood, such as focal or segmental dystonias, lack a specific inheritance pattern (sporadic idiopathic forms). The continuous discovery of new genes involved in the pathophysiological process will likely lead to an increasing number of dystonias currently considered sporadic to be reclassified as genetically determined.

Genetic forms of dystonia also include *paroxysmal dystonias*, which are characterized by brief duration attacks of involuntary movements and a normal neurological examination between paroxysmal episodes. They represent a clinically heterogeneous group and are typically triggered by the execution of voluntary movement, prolonged physical exercise, and caffeine intake.

Secondary dystonias result from a wide range of causes: vascular (ischemic lesions, hemorrhages, arteriovenous malformations); perinatal (infantile cerebral palsy); infectious (viral encephalitis, lethargic encephalitis, subacute sclerosing panencephalitis, HIV infections, tuberculosis, syphilis, etc.); toxic (manganese, cobalt, carbon disulfide, cyanide, methanol intoxication, etc.); traumatic (mechanical and electrical trauma); neoplastic (brain tumors and paraneoplastic encephalitis); pharmacological (caused by the intake of L-Dopa and dopamine agonists, neuroleptics, anticonvulsants, and calcium channel blockers). Forms of likely psychogenic dystonia (functional dystonias) can also be observed with some frequency.

The administration of botulinum toxin in hyperactive muscles represents the most effective treatment for various forms of focal dystonia. Botulinum toxin reversibly blocks the release of acetylcholine at the presynaptic terminal of the neuromuscular junction, resulting in a reversible functional paralysis by blocking neuromuscular transmission. The effect typically lasts for 3 months, and subsequent administrations need to be repeated over time. High-dose anticholinergic medications can be useful in childhood dystonias, and modest benefits can be obtained with the use of benzodiazepines. Tetrabenazine can be used in multifocal or generalized forms. In cases of severe generalized or focal dystonia, deep brain stimulation (DBS) of subcortical brain structures, particularly the GPi, can be employed. The treatment of secondary dystonias is based on addressing the underlying cause of the dystonia.

Table 15.11 GENETIC FORMS OF DYSTONIA

Locus	Phenotype	Inheritance	Gene	Chromosome
DYT 1	Early-onset dystonia with initial involvement of the lower limbs and subsequent spread to other areas resulting in generalized dystonia	AD	TorsinA	9q34
DYT 2	Early-onset torsion dystonia	AR	HPCL	1p35
DYT 3	Dystonia with parkinsonism. Endemic in the Philippines, demonstrating the presence of neurodegenerative phenomena	X-linked	TAF1	Xq13.1
DYT 4	Severe generalized dystonia, lingual dystonia	AD	TUBB4	–
DYT 5a/b	Dystonia with onset in childhood, characterized by diurnal fluctuations, parkinsonism, and response to low doses of levodopa	AD	GCH1, TH, SPR	14q22.1
DYT 6	Dystonia with onset in adolescence and variable phenotype. Dysphonia, upper limb dystonia, followed by cranio-cervical involvement	AD	THAP1	8q21-q22
DYT 7	Familial cervical dystonia	AD	–	18p
DYT 8	Paroxysmal non-kinesigenic dystonia/choreoathetosis	AD	MR1	2q33-q35
DYT 9	Paroxysmal dyskinesias with spasticity	AD	GLUT1 (SLC2A1)	1p21
DYT 10	Paroxysmal kinesigenic dyskinesia	AD	PRRT2	16p11.2
DYT 11	Myoclonus-dystonia syndrome characterized by action-induced myoclonic jerks, responsive to alcohol, usually involving the neck and upper limb	AD	e-SG	7q21.3
DYT 12	Acute-onset dystonia associated with parkinsonism. Severity of dystonia with a rostro-caudal gradient	AD	ATP1A3	19q13
DYT 13	Craniocervical dystonia and upper limb dystonia	AD	–	1p36
DYT 15	Myoclonic dystonia	AD	–	18p11
DYT 16	Early-onset laryngeal, retrocollis, or generalized dystonia associated with parkinsonism	AR	PRKRA	2q31.2
DYT 17	Juvenile-onset torticollis and dysarthria	AR	–	20p11
DYT 18	Exercise-induced paroxysmal dystonia	AD	GLUT1 (SLC2A1)	1p31
DYT 19	Paroxysmal kinesigenic dystonia	AD	–	16q13
DYT 20	Paroxysmal non-kinesigenic dystonia	AD	–	2q31
DYT 21	Pure dystonia with mixed distribution	AD	–	2q14
DYT 23	Cervical dystonia and myoclonus	AD	CACNA1B	9q34
DYT 25	Variable-onset craniocervical dystonia	AD	ANO3	11p14
DYT 26	Segmental dystonia (cranial and cervical) with adult-onset	AD	GNAL	18p11
DYT 27	Cervical/dystonia generalized Cervical dystonia	AR AD	COL6A3 CIZ1	2q37 9q34
DYT 28	Early-onset generalized dystonia	AD	KMT2B	19p13

15.2.3 Chorea

Choreiform movements are involuntary, irregular, arrhythmic movements that are usually rapid, non-stereotyped, discontinuous, and can affect any body region, particularly the muscles of the limbs, trunk, and face. The most typical semiotic characteristic of choreiform movements is their random and non-stereotyped involvement of various body parts (chorea = dance). They are present at rest and accentuated during the execution of voluntary motor acts. Choreiform movements characterize numerous pathological conditions (Table 15.12). Among these, Huntington's disease (HD) is particularly important, as it is a characteristic and severe hereditary-degenerative disorder.

Huntington's disease

In George Huntington's 1872 description, all the main features of Huntington's disease (HD) can be recognized: its hereditary nature, onset in adulthood, choreic movements, cognitive deficit, presence of psychiatric and behavioral disorders with an increased risk of suicide, and a progressive course with a fatal outcome. It is an autosomal dominant inherited disease, with a worldwide prevalence of 5-10 cases per 100,000 population. The mutation responsible for the genetic defect, represented by the expansion of the CAG triplet on chromosome 4, results in the transformation of a ubiquitously expressed protein, with an unknown function and normally abundant in cortical and striatal regions (huntingtin), into an abnormal protein characterized by an excess of glutamine residues. The presence of the mutation can be easily determined in DNA samples. It is believed that 36 repetitions of the CAG triplet are the minimum threshold of CAG repetitions associated with the clinical manifestations of the disease. Penetrance is complete in patients with at least 42 repetitions. There is an inverse correlation between the age of onset of HD and the length (repetitions) of the CAG triplet expansion. Consequently, in juvenile-onset forms, the number of repetitions appears significantly higher. In the advanced stages of the disease, there is marked cortical atrophy with ventricular dilatation, atrophy of the caudate nucleus, internal segment of the globus pallidus, and substantia nigra. The biochemical alteration is characterized by an excess of dopaminergic activity, likely responsible for the appearance of involuntary movements; other biochemical/functional alterations underlie the cognitive and behavioral changes typical of the disease. Intranuclear inclusions of huntingtin and ubiquitin are present in striatal neurons and cerebral cortex. The mechanism of neuronal damage may be related to the presence

Table 15.12 ETIOLOGICAL CLASSIFICATION OF CHOREIC SYNDROMES

Chorea in infancy and the Elderly	
- Physiological infantile chorea - Cerebral palsy - Senile chorea	
Hereditary choreas	
- Huntington's disease - Benign hereditary chorea - Neuroacanthocytosis - Dentatorubral-pallidoluysian atrophy (DRPLA) - Paroxysmal forms - Other degenerative CNS disorders: SCA, ataxia-telangiectasia, tuberous sclerosis, PKAN, hereditary basal ganglia calcifications - Neurometabolic disorders: - Wilson's disease, Lesch-Nyhan syndrome - Lysosomal storage disorders, Leigh's disease, Porphyria	
Iatrogenic	**Toxic**
- Neuroleptics - Antiparkinsonian drugs - Amphetamines - Tricyclic antidepressants - Oral contraceptives - Anticonvulsants	- Alcohol - Carbon monoxide - Manganese - Mercury - Thallium - Toluene
Metabolic	
- Hyperthyroidism - Hypoparathyroidism - Pregnancy (Gravidarum chorea) - Hyper-hyponatremia, Hypocalcemia - Hypo-hyperglycemia - Acquired hepatocerebral degeneration - Nutritional (beriberi, pellagra, vitamin B12 deficiency in children)	
Autoimmune	
- Sydenham's chorea - Systemic lupus erythematosus (SLE) - Henoch-Schönlein purpura - Other rare causes: sarcoidosis, polyarteritis nodosa, Behçet's disease, myeloproliferative disorders	
Vascular	
- Cerebral infarction - Cerebral hemorrhage - Polycythemia vera - Arteriovenous malformations	
Tumors and Paraneoplastic Syndromes	
Post-traumatic	

of such aggregates. Following damage to striatal cells, functional changes occur in the circuits that connect the basal ganglia to the motor areas, resulting in a decrease in the discharge frequency of the globus pallidus and increased activation of cortical areas.

From a clinical point of view, Huntington's disease usually begins in adulthood and is characterized by the presence of neurological symptoms, cognitive deficits, and psychiatric symptoms, with a fatal outcome after 15-20 years of illness. Onset can be characterized by *choreic involuntary movements* that become increasingly prominent with disease progression. The visible effects of chorea depend on the affected body segments; involvement of the limbs and upper extremities leads to difficulty in performing daily activities, while involvement of the lower limbs causes difficulties in walking. Facial muscle involvement is common and can manifest as grimacing and excessive blinking (sometimes resembling motor tics); dysarthria and dysphagia are also common symptoms. In addition to choreic movements, dystonic movements and motor slowness during voluntary movements can also be present. Chorea increases with disease progression, but after years of illness, predominantly bradykinetic-rigid symptoms prevail. An akinetic-rigid syndrome may characterize juvenile-onset disease from the beginning (Westphal's rigid variant). Cognitive impairments are typical of so-called subcortical dementias, with bradyphrenia, compromised attentional capacities, deficits in executive functions (difficulty planning and executing complex tasks), and the absence of aphasia, apraxia, and agnosia, which are typical signs of cortical forms. Cognitive disturbances are secondary to damage to the fronto-striatal circuits. The most important psychiatric disorders are depression, present in 30-50% of patients during the course of the disease, apathy, and anhedonia, i.e., loss of pleasure and interest in performing common activities. The risk of suicide is about 5 times higher than that of the control population and is influenced not only by the severity of affective disorders but also by residual functional capacity, level of awareness of the illness, and the social support offered to the patient. Agitation and aggression are significant phenomena, with serious repercussions on the quality of life of family members, while frank psychotic manifestations are less frequent. In the advanced stages, the patient becomes completely dependent on others; death is usually due to complications related to immobility, weight loss, aspiration pneumonia, and opportunistic infections. Diagnosis is based on clinical history and genetic testing. CT and MRI of the brain can demonstrate progressive atrophy of the caudate nuclei. Symptomatic treatment aims to control motor, cognitive, and psychiatric symptoms. Reduction of choreic movements can be achieved with dopamine-depleting drugs such as tetrabenazine, while control of psychotic symptoms can be achieved with receptor-blocking agents for D2 dopaminergic receptors such as classical neuroleptics (phenothiazines, butyrophenones, thioxanthenes, diphenyl-piperidines) or atypical antipsychotics (clozapine, quetiapine, risperidone, and olanzapine). Possible new frontiers include basal ganglia cell transplantation or therapies capable of reducing the toxic effect caused by mutated huntingtin (antisense oligonucleotides).

The ease of performing genetic testing in an inherited disease with a dominant transmission pattern, characterized by a poor prognosis and without an effective therapy, makes it necessary to refer patients and strict relatives to specialized centers for genetic counseling. Genetic testing in the children of affected patients should always be agreed upon after careful assessment of the risks and benefits.

Other genetically determined choreas

Several studies have shown the existence of patients with clinical features (motor, cognitive, and psychiatric) typical of Huntington's disease (HD), but without the typical genetic alterations of Huntington's disease. These cases are considered phenocopies of HD and mimic the condition. Among these, *Dentatorubral-pallidoluysian atrophy* is an extremely rare autosomal dominant form characterized by ataxia, choreoathetosis, cognitive impairment, and predominantly myoclonic epileptic seizures. It is caused by a mutation in the CAG trinucleotide on chromosome 12. It is characterized by extensive cell loss and gliosis in the dentate nucleus, red nucleus, lateral portion of the globus pallidus, and subthalamic nucleus.

Benign Familial Chorea (BFC) | It is transmitted with incomplete penetrance through autosomal dominant inheritance and is caused by a mutation in the gene encoding a thyroid transcription factor (T1TF1). It has an onset in childhood, and the neurological picture is essentially non-progressive and usually not associated with cognitive impairment.

Neuroacanthocytosis | It is a condition in which chorea (and other movement disorders) is associated with the presence of acanthocytes in peripheral blood. The disease usually begins in early adulthood, mostly with autosomal recessive transmission, with a mutation in the CHAC gene (more rarely dominant or *X-linked*). Chorea is the most relevant clinical feature and can be associated with dystonia, motor and vocal tics, and parkinsonism. Hyperkinesias primarily involve the face and can sometimes cause self-injurious behaviors with damage to the lips and tongue. Involuntary movements are associated with a sensory-motor polyneuropathy, with amyotrophy and increased creatine phosphokinase (CPK) levels. Generalized epileptic seizures occur in about half of the cases, as well as mild cognitive impairment. Acanthocytic red blood cell alterations (spiny red blood cells) are a characteristic but not essential element for the diagnosis.

Secondary choreas

Drug-induced chorea | Chorea movements, especially affecting the orofacial region and less frequently the trunk and limbs, can be observed in patients undergoing chronic treatment with neuroleptics and are commonly referred to as "tardive dyskinesias." The syndrome predominantly involves the oro-linguo-mandibular segment and can cause chewing difficulties. Chorea movements are also common in patients with Parkinson's disease undergoing chronic treatment with L-Dopa or other dopaminergic drugs.

Vascular chorea | It represents 20-40% of non-genetic choreas, although it is a rare occurrence as it is found in no more than 1% of patients with cerebrovascular disease. Vascular-based chorea is usually hemichorea and is associated with ischemic or hemorrhagic lesions located in the basal ganglia or adjacent white matter. In some cases, spontaneous remission of involuntary movements can occur.

Infectious and immune-mediated choreas | *Sydenham's chorea* and PANDAS (Paediatric Autoimmune Disorder associated with Streptococcal infection) are the most common forms and occur in pediatric age. Patients present with choreic movements and neuropsychiatric manifestations. The use of antibiotic therapy has dramatically reduced the incidence of the disease in industrialized countries over the past 30 years. The pathophysiology of *Sydenham's chorea* remains unknown, although antibodies directed against striatal and subthalamic neurons have been identified. It is believed that there is a cross-reaction between antistreptococcal antibodies and basal ganglia neurons. Typically, chorea worsens over a period of 2-4 weeks, persists for a variable period of time, and resolves spontaneously within 3-6 months.

15.2.4 Ballism

Ballism is a condition similar to chorea, from which it differs because the involuntary movements predominantly involve the proximal segments of the limbs and are of considerable intensity, great amplitude, and almost always unilateral (hemiballismus). Hemiballismus is usually secondary to a vascular lesion of the contralateral subthalamic nucleus and is generally characterized by a good prognosis. Bilateral ballistic movements are rare and, if present, are usually due to metabolic disorders (e.g., severe hyperglycemia).

15.2.5 Tic

Tics are rapid, recurrent, involuntary movements. They are classified as motor or vocal, simple or complex. Typical examples of simple motor tics are "eye blinking, head turning, nose twitching, shoulder shrugging," while complex tics tend to simulate or imitate a complex voluntary movement, such as touching or smelling objects, imitating others' gestures (echopraxia), or jumping. Vocal tics involve the emission of sounds (simple vocal tics) or words or entire phrases (complex vocal tics). Sometimes complex motor tics can lead to self-injurious behaviors, and in cases of vocal tics, they can result in the production of involuntary vocalizations and echolalia, sometimes socially embarrassing (e.g., coprolalia). Tics can be voluntarily suppressed, at least for short periods of time. They can be preceded by a sensation described by patients as the need to perform the tic itself (*sensory urge*) and are sometimes accompanied by a feeling of tension reduction at the end of the tic. An important characteristic of tics is their variability in intensity and affected site over the years. Motor and vocal tics can be classified as follows: a) *transient*, when they last less than 1 year. These tics are frequently observed in children and adolescents; b) *chronic*, when tics last for more than 1 year. Finally, tics are the most characteristic manifestation of *Tourette's syndrome*. The diagnostic criteria for this condition are: onset of tics before the age of 18, coexistence of multiple motor tics and vocal tics for at least one year, and exclusion of other medical conditions that can cause the described symptoms. Tourette's syndrome is frequently associated with attention deficit hyperactivity disorder in children and obsessive-compulsive disorder in all age groups. The prevalence of Tourette's syndrome is relatively common, ranging from 0.5-1 cases per 1,000 individuals. The etiology is unknown, although a strong genetic component has been demonstrated. A possible role has been hypothesized for infectious factors (streptococci) with the formation of anti-basal ganglia antibodies. It is believed that tics and Tourette's syndrome, in particular, are caused by biochemical alterations (typically involving increased central dopaminergic activity and reduced GABAergic activity) and changes in the functional activity of the basal ganglia and cortical circuits, in which the primary motor cortex, premotor cortices, and parietal cortex are believed to play a relevant role. Therapy is based on the combined use of cognitive-behavioral psychotherapy techniques (*Habit Reversal Therapy* is widely used) and medications such as antipsychotics, both typical (pimozide, haloperidol) and atypical (aripiprazole, risperidone), adrenergic presynaptic blockers (clonidine), and benzodiazepines. In rare cases, botulinum toxin therapy can be useful, especially for facial tics. Surgical therapy using deep brain stimulation (DBS) can be used in severe and generalized forms, but there is no consensus on the most effective anatomical target.

15.2.6 Acathisia

Acathisia is defined as the need or urgency to move and is characterized by a subjective feeling of restlessness. It is usually a side effect of treatment with dopamine receptor-blocking drugs and can sometimes be observed in Parkinson's disease.

15.2.7 Athetosis

Athetoid movements are slower involuntary movements than choreic movements, sometimes with serpentine or dystonic characteristics. It should be noted that athetosis, chorea, and ballismus represent a continuum of a type of hyperkinetic movement, which is why they are often classified together (choreoathetosis, chorea-ballismus). Athetoid movements are typically present in patients with cerebral palsy.

15.2.8 Wilson's disease

Wilson's Disease, or hepatolenticular degeneration, is a rare genetic disease characterized by altered copper metabolism and pathological copper accumulation in various organs, which manifests in the first two decades of life. The autosomal recessive disease is caused by a mutation in the ATP7B gene, located on the long arm of chromosome 13, which encodes a membrane ATPase located in the Golgi apparatus of hepatocytes. This enzyme is crucial for the formation of ceruloplasmin, the protein that carries copper in the plasma. The faulty functioning of the enzyme leads to reduced copper excretion with bile and the consequent accumulation of the metal in hepatocytes. Once the copper storage capacity in the liver is exhausted, the proportion of "free" copper increases, distributing to other parts of the body, particularly in the central nervous system, kidney, ocular bulb, and bones. In Wilson's Disease, the pathological neurological alterations are represented by necrotic cavitation of the putamen and caudate, associated with neuronal loss, axonal degeneration, and astrocytosis. Cortical atrophy, cavitations in the subcortical white matter, and reactive protoplasmic astrocyte hyperplasia in response to liver failure and hyperammonemia can also be observed. The clinical presentation at onset can vary, affecting the liver in 40% of cases and the central nervous system (CNS) in 40% of cases. Liver abnormalities can manifest as acute hepatitis, active chronic hepatitis, cirrhosis, and fulminant liver failure. When the clinical presentation is neurological, it usually begins around the second or third decade of life with highly heterogeneous clinical manifestations: akinetic-rigid syndrome, dystonic syndrome, choreic syndrome, or simply postural or intentional tremor associated with ataxia and dysarthria (the latter present in 90% of cases) or with a combination of various movement disorders. The tremor is usually low frequency and of considerable amplitude, particularly visible in the proximal regions of the limbs (*wing-beating tremor*). Dystonia can be focal, segmental, multifocal, or generalized, but in many cases, it tends to involve the facial region, giving the typical fatuous expression to the face (*risus sardonicus*). Other characteristic features of the disease include slowed saccadic eye movements, ophthalmoplegia, dysphagia, and excessive drooling. Orthostatic hypotension, sweating abnormalities, as well as bladder, bowel, and sexual dysfunctions, can also be observed. The disease can also present with psychiatric disturbances such as personality and behavioral changes, irritability and depression, mania, catatonia, disinhibition, and rarely psychosis. Ocular involvement and the presence of the Kayser-Fleischer ring, observable with a slit lamp, characterized by a rust-brown semilunar discoloration of the corneal periphery caused by copper deposition in the Descemet membrane, are nearly constant. Finally, some patients may manifest renal impairment with proximal tubulopathy and osteoarthritis. In the differential diagnosis, essential tremor, early-onset Parkinson's disease, generalized dystonia, and other rarer genetic forms such as *Pantothenate kinase-associated neurodegeneration* (PKAN) should be considered. PKAN is a neurodegenerative disease characterized by intracerebral iron accumulation and linked to mutations in the PANK2 gene on chromosome 20, usually with onset around 3-4 years of age. It is characterized by a combination of gait disturbances, dystonia, spasticity, and cognitive deficits. Wilson's Disease should also be distinguished from *aceruloplasminemia*, an autosomal recessive disease associated with reduced ceruloplasmin, copper, and iron levels, increased serum ferritin, and iron deposition in the CNS.

The diagnosis of Wilson's disease is based on the demonstration of low levels of ceruloplasmin and copper in the serum, increased urinary copper excretion over 24 hours, the Kayser-Fleischer ring, quantitative evaluation of copper in liver biopsy specimens, and genetic analysis on chromosome 13. Brain MRI can show increased signal intensity in T2-weighted sequences of the lentiform nucleus and caudate nucleus, thalamus, pontine tegmentum, and substantia nigra. It is necessary to always exclude the diagnosis of Wilson's disease in young patients with various types of movement disorders, as Wilson's disease is treatable with specific pharmacological therapies.

The main therapeutic strategy is chelation therapy, based on the administration of D-penicillamine (associated with pyridoxine to prevent anemia) or alternatively triethylene tetramine (trientene). Medications that decrease copper absorption, such as zinc or ammonium tetrathiomolybdate, can also be used. It is helpful to reduce dietary copper intake by avoiding certain foods (liver, mushrooms, cocoa, chocolate, nuts, shellfish). Symptomatic medications such as L-Dopa, dopamine agonists, anticholinergics, and benzodiazepines may also be employed. In many patients with advanced liver disease, liver transplantation may be necessary, which often leads to an improvement in the neurological picture.

15.2.9 Stereotypies

Stereotypies are coordinated movements that repeat continuously and always in the same manner. Compared to tics, they last longer, are repetitive and continuous (not paroxysmal), serve no purpose, and may resemble ritualistic behaviors. Both simple (e.g., head rocking or banging) and complex stereotypies are typical of patients with autism, intellectual disability, Rett syndrome, psychosis, Tourette syndrome, and other conditions.

15.2.10 Myoclonus

It is an involuntary, rapid, and sudden movement caused by a brief muscle contraction (positive myoclonus) or inhibition of tonic muscle activity (negative or asterixis myoclonus). Myoclonus causes a displacement of the affected body segment. It can be classified based on spatial distribution (focal, segmental multifocal, generalized), temporal distribution (rhythmic/arrhythmic, synchronous/asynchronous), and mode of onset (spontaneous, action-related, reflex, stimulus-dependent). Based on etiology, it is classified as physiological (e.g., hypnic myoclonus), essential (idiopathic or hereditary), epileptic, and symptomatic (when secondary to a demonstrable pathology). There are numerous causes of myoclonus (Table 15.13). Myoclonus, both positive and negative, is characteristic of metabolic encephalopathies (particularly hepatic and uremic), while postanoxic myoclonus refers to myoclonus secondary to severe cerebral anoxia (usually resulting from respiratory failure) and manifests primarily as action-related myoclonus. Myoclonus can also be observed in patients with atypical parkinsonism (MSA, CBD).

Table 15.13 CLASSIFICATION OF MYOCLONUS

Physiological
- Hypnic (sleep-related)
- Exercise-induced
- Hiccups
Essential
- Sporadic
- Autosomal dominant
Epileptic
- Continuous partial epilepsy
- Stimulus-sensitive idiopathic myoclonus
- Photosensitive myoclonus
- Myoclonic absences
- Infantile spasms
- Lennox-Gastaut syndrome
- Cryptogenic myoclonic epilepsy
- Juvenile myoclonic epilepsy
- Benign familial myoclonic epilepsy
- Progressive myoclonic epilepsy (Unverricht-Lundborg)
Secondary
- Focal central nervous system lesions
- Storage diseases
- Spinocerebellar degenerations
- Dementias
- Multisystem degenerations
- Infectious or post-infectious
- Paraneoplastic
- Metabolic
- Toxic
- Drug-induced
- Physical agents-induced
- Malabsorption-related
- Hashimoto's encephalopathy

15.2.11 Stiff person syndrome

Stiff person syndrome is a rare adult-onset condition characterized by severe muscle rigidity (initially intermittent and then continuous), primarily affecting the paravertebral muscles and abdominal wall, but can also involve the proximal muscles of the limbs. In its most characteristic form, excessive activation of the paraspinal muscles can cause severe lordosis. Other clinical features include painful muscle spasms, the disappearance of muscle rigidity during sleep or under spinal or general anesthesia (suggesting a central origin of the pathology), and the frequent association with insulin-dependent diabetes mellitus. Less commonly, the syndrome may manifest with localized symptoms and signs in a single limb. Electromyographic recordings show continuous muscle activity in the paraspinal muscles, even when the subject is at rest. From a pathophysiological standpoint, it is believed that this syndrome is caused by altered control of GABAergic and glycinergic circuits, which normally exert inhibition on spinal motor neurons. In approximately two-thirds of cases, the syndrome is associated with the presence of anti-glutamic acid decarboxylase (GAD) antibodies, the enzyme responsible for GABA synthesis, and antiglycine receptor antibodies in the serum and cerebrospinal fluid. A paraneoplastic variety (usually associated with breast tumors) is present in about 5% of cases of Stiff Person Syndrome and is associated with the presence of anti-amphiphysin-I antibodies. It is an inflammatory encephalomyelitis with rigidity and a poor prognosis. Differential diagnosis should be made with benign fasciculation syndrome, which typically manifests in the lower limbs, and peripheral hyperexcitability syndromes (neuromyotonia). Treatment is recommended with plasmapheresis or intravenous immunoglobulin administration, as well as high doses of benzodiazepines and antispasmodics (particularly baclofen).

15.2.12 Myokimia

Myokimia is characterized by spontaneous, continuous muscle contractions often associated with a subcutaneous sensation of "movement." It is particularly common in the orbicularis oculi muscle and is mostly benign or associated with muscle fatigue. However, it should always be considered that it may represent the expression of localized lesions, especially at the pontine level (e.g., in multiple sclerosis), or peripheral nerve distress. Myokymia is generated by the hyperexcitability of peripheral axons. Electromyographic recording demonstrates the presence of brief discharges of single motor units at 5-150 Hz.

15.2.13 Facial spasm

Facial spasm is characterized by rapid and irregular paroxysmal clonic contractions of one or more muscle groups innervated by the facial nerve. It is a movement disorder of peripheral origin. It is a relatively common disorder and affects females more frequently. The average age of onset is between the fifth and sixth decade of life, but it can also occur in younger individuals. The contractions almost always involve the facial muscles on one side (bilateral facial spasm is extremely rare, less than 1%). The contractions typically start in the orbicularis oculi muscle and then spread to other facial muscles (particularly those in the perioral region). The contractions can persist for several minutes and are facilitated by stress, fatigue, or voluntary movements of the facial muscles. They can also persist during sleep. Facial spasm is divided into *primary* (or idiopathic, Figure 15.4) and *secondary*. In many cases of primary spasm, a "neurovascular conflict" can be demonstrated, represented by the compression or contact of the facial nerve along its course with an artery. The neurovascular conflict is highlighted by brain magnetic resonance imaging and brain angio-MRI (an examination that should

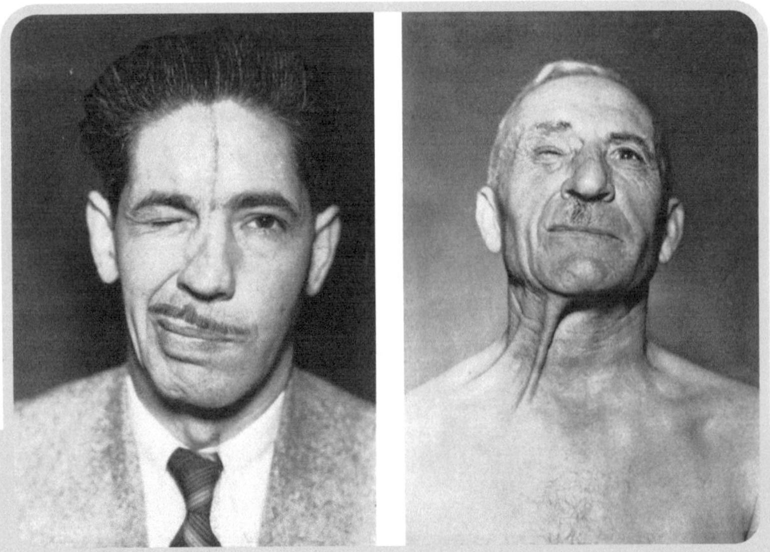

Figure 15.4

Patients affected by right primary hemifacial spasm. (Wartenberg, 1952).

always be performed in these patients). Secondary hemifacial spasm may occur after peripheral facial nerve paralysis (Bell's palsy) or due to compression by pathological intra- and extracranial processes, including tumors (usually of the ponto-cerebellar angle), vascular malformations, and infectious processes. From a pathophysiological perspective, the compression of the nerve root and the resulting segmental demyelination lead to the formation of artificial synapses and, therefore, ephaptic transmission. Electrophysiologically, facial spasm is characterized by a distinctive electromyographic pattern consisting of high-frequency (150-400 Hz), rhythmic, and synchronized discharges. The first-line treatment, which is generally very effective, consists of the injection of botulinum toxin into the affected facial muscles, resulting in clinical improvement for approximately 3-5 months. The treatment needs to be repeated thereafter. In patients resistant to treatment, surgical therapy may also be considered, performed through microvascular decompression of the facial nerve using a suboccipital lateral approach. Long-term recurrence of spasms has, however, been observed in some patients.

15.2.14 Restless legs syndrome

Restless Legs Syndrome manifests as restlessness and discomfort in the lower limbs, described by patients using various terms (tingling, pain, cramps, or other sensations). The symptoms improve with movement and walking, while they worsen when lying down. The symptoms typically occur in the evening during the early stages of nighttime rest or throughout the night, leading to insomnia. According to some epidemiological studies, this syndrome affects between 3% and 10% of the general population and generally affects adult individuals. The syndrome usually presents as a sporadic disorder, but in a significant percentage of cases, it can be genetically determined. Secondary cases, which are rarer, are usually associated with Parkinson's disease, iron deficiency, pregnancy, peripheral neuropathies, renal insufficiency, and the use of medications (particularly neuroleptics and tricyclic antidepressants). The pathophysiology is not known, but it is believed that there is an increased excitability of the spinal cord. The differential diagnosis should be made with the syndrome of periodic limb movements in sleep, characterized by repetitive movements of the lower limbs (usually 4 movements within 90 seconds), bilaterally, occurring during sleep and detectable through polysomnography. Dopamine agonist medications, administered at low doses before bedtime, are the most effective treatment. In some cases, levodopa, gabapentin, or clonazepam are used.

15.2.15 Functional Movement Disorders

Functional movement disorders are those disorders in which there is no evidence of demonstrable organic causes of the central and peripheral nervous system. They predominantly manifest as hyperkinetic disorders (tremor, dystonia, myoclonus), less frequently with hypokinetic manifestations (parkinsonism). They may or may not be associated with frank psychopathological alterations. A functional origin may be suspected when the onset of symptoms is acute/subacute, clinical characteristics are inconsistent and change over time, and when there is spontaneous remission of symptoms. Functionally based movements can appear "bizarre" and transiently improve with the administration of a placebo. Treatment is very complex and requires a combined pharmacological, psychotherapeutic, and rehabilitative approach carried out in specialized centers.

15.2.16 Cerebellar ataxias

The term ataxia refers to the impairment in the coordination of voluntary movements. Essentially, all body regions can be affected by ataxia, but in particular, the limbs, trunk, bulbar musculature, and ocular movements are affected. Gait ataxia is characterized by unsteady walking with a broadened base of support and balance deficits. Postural and truncal ataxia involves the inability to maintain a seated position. Limb ataxia may present with a variable combination of dysmetria, hypometria or hypermetria, asynergy or dyssynergy, dysdiadochokinesia, and postural and kinetic tremor. Speech ataxia presents with characteristic cerebellar dysarthria, and ocular movement ataxia presents with nystagmus and ocular dysmetria.

Cerebellar ataxias can be classified based on the mode of onset and clinical course or based on etiology. From an etiological perspective, cerebellar ataxias can be classified into three main groups: 1) acquired, due to endogenous and exogenous causes; 2) hereditary (dominant, recessive, X-linked); 3) degenerative (■ Table 15.14).

Acquired cerebellar ataxia

Ischemic and hemorrhagic lesions of the cerebellum | Manifest as acute ataxia (usually unilateral), often accompanied by headaches and other signs of increased intracranial pressure. Signs of brainstem involvement are also frequently present. Clinical diagnosis is confirmed through brain CT or MRI.

Table 15.14 CEREBELLAR ATAXIA CLASSIFICATION

Acquired Ataxias
- Cerebrovascular causes - Neoplasms - Toxic-metabolic causes - Paraneoplastic causes - Autoimmune causes - Infectious/post-infectious causes - Demyelinating diseases - Non-cerebellar ataxias
Genetically determined ataxias
- *Autosomal dominant* Spinocerebellar Ataxias (SCA) Episodic Ataxias - *Autosomal recessive* Friedreich's Ataxia Ataxia-Telangiectasia Ataxia with Isolated Vitamin E Deficiency Abetalipoproteinemia Early-Onset Ataxia with Oculomotor Apraxia and Hypoalbuminemia Recessive Spastic Ataxia of Charlevoix-Saguenay - *x-linked* Ataxia/Tremor Syndrome associated with X-Fragile premutation
Degenerative ataxias
- Multiple System Atrophy (MSA-C variant or olivopontocerebellar atrophy) - Late-Onset Idiopathic Ataxia - Myoclonic Epilepsy

Toxic and metabolic causes | Antiepileptic drugs (phenytoin, carbamazepine, phenobarbital) and other medications such as lithium and 5-fluorouracil can cause ataxia. Among toxic agents (mercury, toluene, solvents, pesticides), alcohol abuse is particularly significant. Alcohol can induce ataxia both in the context of acute ethyl intoxication and chronic abuse. Acute alcohol consumption interferes with the normal functional activity of the cerebellum, leading to ataxia, while chronic alcohol consumption results in irreversible cerebellar damage (particularly to the vermis) with progressive symptoms. The pathogenesis of alcohol-related cerebellar ataxia is attributed to both direct toxic action and thiamine deficiency. Thiamine deficiency causes metabolic acidosis, mitochondrial dysfunction, and neuronal loss due to the inability of brain cells to utilize pyruvic acid. In all cases of toxic-metabolic ataxia, a thorough medical history evaluation and laboratory tests such as measurement of liver enzymes, drugs, or vitamins (especially the B group) are essential for diagnosis. Treatment involves discontinuing alcohol or other potential toxins and administering vitamin B1, B6, B12.

Inflammatory or immunomediated diseases | Multiple sclerosis usually causes ataxia due to localized lesions in the cerebellar peduncles. Other immune-mediated causes of ataxia include lupus erythematosus (LES) and Sjögren's syndrome, ataxia with anti-GAD antibodies often associated with insulin-dependent diabetes mellitus, adult-onset celiac ataxia, and Hashimoto's encephalopathy. Guillain-Barré syndrome (or acute inflammatory demyelinating polyradiculoneuropathy) and its Miller-Fisher variant can also be associated with ataxia.

Acute-onset cerebellar ataxia can result from infectious diseases of the central nervous system (CNS). In children, it is most commonly caused by viral infections (*Echovirus, Coxsackie, Herpes Simplex, Epstein Barr*) while in adults, it can be caused by *Haemophilus influenzae*, *Mycoplasma pneumoniae*, or *Listeria monocytogenes infections*. Ataxia can also be observed in patients with Whipple's disease, a systemic disease caused by *T. Whipplei* primarily affecting the gastrointestinal system (with diarrhea, malabsorption, and weight loss), the osteoarticular system, and the nervous system, leading to diverse clinical manifestations. Lastly, in adults, progressive ataxia can be a symptom of prion diseases, particularly Gerstmann-Sträussler disease and Creutzfeldt-Jakob disease.

Cerebellar ataxia can result from *primary* or *metastatic neoplasms* or *paraneoplastic cerebellar degeneration*. The most common cerebellar tumors include medulloblastoma, astrocytoma, and hemangioblastoma. Paraneoplastic cerebellar degeneration is an autoimmune condition with subacute onset and rapidly progressive course, sometimes appearing before clinical manifestations of the primary tumor. The neoplasms most frequently associated with paraneoplastic cerebellar syndrome are small cell lung cancer, breast cancer, ovarian cancer, testicular cancer, and Hodgkin's lymphoma. The detection of antibodies in the serum, including anti-Yo, anti-Tr, anti-Hu, anti-Ri, and anti-mGluR1, is very useful for diagnostic confirmation. In such cases, the therapeutic approach involves treating the underlying neoplasm. Parenteral high-dose glucocorticoids, intravenous administration of immunoglobulins or plasmapheresis are essential therapeutic measures for controlling the symptoms.

Ereditary ataxias

Dominant autosomal ataxias | Dominant autosomal cerebellar ataxias (or spinocerebellar ataxias - SCAs) represent a group of rare diseases that are clinically and genetically highly heterogeneous (Table 15.15). The main clinical features common to most SCAs are onset between the third and fourth decades of life, although onset during adolescence or later adulthood is also possible, a progressive course, and the presence of signs of involvement of other neurological systems (pyramidal, basal ganglia, ocular, and cognitive) in addition to cerebellar involvement. Over 30 dominant ataxia loci have been identified, but not all responsible genes have been identified. SCAs can be classified based on the type of genetic mutation as follows:

a) SCAs caused by polyglutamine expansion
b) SCAs caused by conventional mutations
c) SCAs caused by non-coding expansion.

SCAs caused by polyglutamine expansion (SCA1, 2, 3, 6, 7, 17, and DRPLA: Dentatorubral-pallidoluysian atrophy) are caused by the expansion of the CAG triplet. Clinical manifestations appear when the number of triplets exceeds 37-40 repetitions.

Table 15.15 SPINOCEREBELLAR AUTOSOMAL DOMINANT ATAXIAS: GENES, MUTATIONS, AND CLINICAL PHENOMENOLOGY

Name	Locus/gene	Mutation/protein	Symptoms/signs in addition to ataxia
SCA 1	6p23/ATXN 1	Ataxin 1, CAG repeats 41-81	Pyramidal signs, amyotrophy, extrapyramidal signs, ophthalmoparesis
SCA 2	12q24/ATXN 2	Ataxin 2, CAG repeats 35-39	Slow saccades, extrapyramidal signs, rarely dementia, ophthalmoplegia, peripheral neuropathy, pyramidal signs
SCA 3 (Majado-Joseph disease)	14q24.3-q31 ATXN 3	Ataxin 3, CAG repeats 62-82	Pyramidal signs, amyotrophy, exophthalmos, extra-pyramidal signs, ophthalmoparesis
SCA 4	16q22.1	Unknown	Sensory axonal neuropathy, pyramidal signs
SCA 5	11q13/SPTBN2	III Spectrin	Pure cerebellar ataxia (late onset), pyramidal signs (early onset)
SCA 6	19p13.2/CACNAIA	Cav 2.1, CAG repeats 21-30	Pure cerebellar ataxia, onset >50 years
SCA 7	3p21.1-p12	Ataxin 7, CAG ripetizioni 38-130	Macular degeneration, ophthalmoplegia, pyramidal signs
SCA 8	13q21.33/ATXN8OS ATXN8	RNA Toxic; CAG repeats	Pyramidal signs, reduced vibratory sense, dysarthria
SCA 9	Unknown	Unknown	Central demyelination (1 patient), extrapyramidal signs, ophthalmoplegia, posterior column degeneration, pyramidal signs
SCA 10	22q13.31/ATXN10	Intronic repeats ATTCT	Epilepsy, cognitive deficits, psychiatric disorders, poly-neuropathy, pyramidal signs
SCA 11	15q15.2/TTBK2	Kinasi-2 TAU tubulin	Pure cerebellar ataxia

Name	Locus/gene	Mutation/protein	Symptoms/signs in addition to ataxia
SCA 12	5q32/PPP2R2B	Protein phosphatase PP2a, CAG repeats in 5'UTR 51-78	*Upper limb tremor*, hyperreflexia
SCA 13	19q13.3-13.4/KCNC3	Kv3.3	Intellectual deficit (French pedigree), pure ataxia (Filipino pedigree)
SCA 14	19q13.4/PRKCG	Protein kinase C gamma	*Pure cerebellar ataxia*, rarely chorea
SCA 15 SCA 16	3p26.1/ITPRI	Inositol 1,4,5-trisphosphate receptor	*Pure cerebellar ataxia*
SCA 17 (Huntington disease-like 4)	6q27/TBP	TATA box-binding protein, CAG repeats 46-63	*Chorea*, dementia, extrapyramidal signs, hyperreflexia, psychiatric symptoms
SCA 18 (neuropathy, sensorimotor, with ataxia)	7q22-q32	Unknown	*Posterior column deficit*, amyotrophy, early onset (< 20 years), hyporeflexia
SCA 19/SCA 22	1p13.3/KCND3	Kv4.3	*Pure cerebellar ataxia*, cognitive deficit, myoclonus, postural tremor
SCA 20	11p11.2-q13.3 Gene duplication	Unknown	*Spasmodic dysphonia* or *spasmodic cough*, palatal tremor
SCA 21	7p21.3-p15.1	Unknown	*Akinesia*, cognitive deficits, dysgraphia, early onset, hyporeflexia, postural or resting tremor
SCA 23	20p13/PDYN	Prodynorphin	*Late onset* (>50 years), reduced vibratory sensation
SCA 25	2p21-p15	Unknown	*Areflexia, sensory neuropathy*
SCA 26	19p13.3	Unknown	*Pure cerebellar ataxia*
SCA 27	13q34/FGF14	Fibroblast growth factor 14	*Orofacial dyskinesias*, cognitive deficits, tremor
SCA 28	18p11.22-q11.2/ AFG3L2	ATPase family gene 3	*Early onset* (<20 years), hyperreflexia, ophthalmoparesis, ptosis
SCA 29	3p26	Unknown	Congenital, non-progressive
SCA 30	4q34.3-q35.1	Unknown	*Pure cerebellar ataxia*, late onset (>50 years)
SCA 31	16q22/BEANI e TK2	NEDD4, thymidine kinase 2	*Pure cerebellar ataxia*, late onset (>50 years), deafness
SCA 35	20p13/NOP56	Transglutaminase 6	*Pyramidal signs, pseudobulbar paralysis*
SCA 36	20p13/NOP56	Nucleolar 56-kDa protein Intronic GGCCTG repeats	*Second motor neuron signs, tongue atrophy*
SCA 37	1p32.2-p32.1/ DABI	Unknown	*Progressive cerebellar ataxia and dysarthria*
SCA 38	6p12.1/ ELOVL5	Unknown	*Cerebellar ataxia, polyneuropathy*
SCA 40	14q32.11-q32.12 / CCDC88C	Missense c.1391G>A (pR464H)	*Cerebellar ataxia, hyperreflexia*
SCA 41	4q27/TRPC3	Missense c.2285G>A (pR762H)	*Cerebellar ataxia*
SCA 42	17q21.33 / CACNA1G	Missense c.5144G>A (pR1715H)	*Cerebellar ataxia*
SCA 43	3q25.2 /MME	Missense c.428G>A (p.C143Y)	*Cerebellar ataxia, polyneuropathy*
SCA 44	6q24.3/GRM1	Missense c.2375A>G (p.Y792C) c.785A>G (p.Y262C)	*Cerebellar ataxia, pyramidal signs*
SCA 45	5q33.1/FAT2	Missense c.10946G>A (p.R3649Q) c.10758G>C (p.K3586N)	*Cerebellar ataxia*
SCA 46	19q13.2/PLD3	Missense c.923T>C (L308P)	*Cerebellar ataxia, polyneuropathy*
SCA 47	1p35.2 /PUM1	Missense g.31414862 T>A (p.T1035S)	*Cerebellar ataxia*
DPRLA (dentatorubral-pallidoluysian atrophy)	12p13.31/ATN1	Atrophin-1, CAG repeats 49-75	*Myoclonic epilepsy, choreoathetosis, dementia*

Italicized symptoms/signs represent the most distinctive features of each form

A greater number of triplets corresponds to an earlier age of onset and greater severity of symptoms. The symptoms are characterized not only by ataxia but also by a variable combination of pyramidal signs, ocular disturbances, peripheral neuropathies, and other symptoms. A typical aspect of SCAs with polyglutamine expansion is the presence of cerebellar atrophy on MRI examination. SCAs associated with conventional mutations (SCA11, 13, 14, 15/16, 20, 27, 28) more often present during adolescence, have a purely cerebellar phenotype, and have a milder course than forms with polyglutamine expansion. SCAs caused by non-coding expansion are associated with a *gain-of-function* mechanism caused by the accumulation of genes containing CUG and CCUG expansions. The most common ones are SCA 8, 10, 12, and 31, and the clinical picture can range from pure cerebellar phenotype to more complex forms with epilepsy, peripheral neuropathy, and spasticity. SCA 1, 2, 3, 6, and 7 represent more than 50% of genetically determined ataxia cases.

Lastly, among the dominant ataxias, *episodic ataxias* should be briefly mentioned. They are rare forms characterized by the sudden onset of ataxic attacks, often associated with other neurological symptoms (particularly migraine, diplopia, and choreoathetosis). The attacks have variable durations (seconds, minutes, hours) and spontaneous remission. In many cases of episodic ataxia, mutations in genes encoding potassium and calcium ion channels have been demonstrated.

Recessive autosomal ataxias | This is a heterogeneous group of familial degenerative diseases. They primarily manifest during childhood and in young adults, typically before the ages of 20-30. In addition to cerebellar ataxia, peripheral neuropathies, movement disorders (chorea, dystonia), alterations in eye movements, pyramidal signs, mental retardation or cognitive disorders, epilepsy, and disorders of other organs and systems can be observed. The classification of these numerous forms of ataxia is continuously evolving. Among the most important recessive autosomal ataxias are Friedreich's ataxia and ataxia-telangiectasia.

Friedreich's ataxia | It is the most common cause of hereditary ataxia. The typical age of onset is between 10 and 20 years. Parental consanguinity is the major risk factor for the development of the disease. Friedreich's ataxia is clinically characterized by the presence of ataxia in the upright stance and gait, dysarthria, signs of corticospinal tract involvement (extensor plantar reflex), peripheral axonal neuropathy (with areflexia), optic atrophy, scoliosis, and sometimes cardiomyopathy and diabetes. In a significant variant of Friedreich's ataxia, tendon reflexes can be normal or even accentuated, and limb spasticity can be observed. The pathogenetic mechanism is a 'loss of function' due to interference from the expansion of the GAA triplet repeat in the transcription of the FXN gene. This gene encodes for a mitochondrial protein called frataxin, which is likely involved in iron transport within the mitochondria. The anatomopathological alterations begin at the level of the dorsal root ganglion with the loss of sensory neurons and subsequently spread to the spinocerebellar tracts and the posterior columns of the spinal cord. There are currently no effective therapies for this disease; however, it is believed that Idebenone (a short-chain analog of coenzyme Q10) may slow the progression of left ventricular hypertrophy, an important risk factor for arrhythmias and sudden death, without producing significant improvements in neurological symptoms. The differential diagnosis should be made primarily with vitamin E deficiency ataxia.

Ataxia telangiectasia | It is the second most common form of recessive inherited cerebellar ataxia. It begins before the age of 5 and has a progressive course (loss of walking ability around the age of 10 and death around the age of 20). It usually presents with trunk ataxia and dysarthria, often associated with conjunctival and auricular telangiectasias, chorea, dystonia, and sensorimotor axonal neuropathy. Patients with this condition also have immunodeficiency with reduced production of immunoglobulins and T cells, and therefore, the risk of recurrent infections and neoplasms, particularly lymphomas and leukemias, is high. The disease is caused by a mutation in the ATM gene, which encodes a protein kinase that plays an important role in the regulation of the cell cycle, apoptosis, and DNA repair mechanisms. These forms are associated with an increase in α-fetoprotein.

Ataxia associated with oculomotor apraxia

It is a very rare form characterized by ataxia and oculomotor apraxia (impairment of saccadic eye movements). Several subtypes of this condition are recognized.

X-Linked

X-linked tremor/ataxia syndrome associated with the premutation of the X fragile syndrome (FXTAS) is the most common cause of X-linked ataxia. It is a rare condition that typically affects males and less frequently female carriers of the FMR1 premutation. Cerebellar ataxia is associated with other neurological signs such as tremor, cognitive decline, parkinsonism, neuropathy, and autonomic dysfunction. It should be considered in the differential diagnosis of certain forms of adult-onset tremor. MRI shows a characteristic hyperintensity signal in T2-weighted sequences at the level of the cerebellar peduncle.

Ataxias caused by vitamin E deficiency

Among these, the most frequent is the one associated with abetalipoproteinemia, clinically characterized by predominantly sensory ataxia, areflexia, and retinopathy. Vitamin E deficiency is also associated with reduced blood cholesterol levels and the presence of acanthocytes in the blood.

Sporadic ataxias

Among sporadic degenerative ataxias, particular mention is made of *Multiple System Atrophy* (MSA), in its cerebellar variant (MSA-C), already described in this chapter, and *Late-Onset Idiopathic Cerebellar Ataxia* (ILOCA). This form of ataxia, also known as sporadic cerebellar ataxia, of unknown etiology, with onset in adulthood, starts around the age of 50 and has a progressive course, but less severe than that observed in MSA. It usually presents with clinical signs exclusive to cerebellar dysfunction, but sometimes sensory deficits or pyramidal signs (extensor plantar reflex) may be present. The diagnosis of ILOCA can only be made after excluding possible acquired and genetic causes of ataxia and MSA-C, which differs from ILOCA by the concomitant presence of autonomic dysfunction and a more rapid and aggressive course.

Bibliography

Albanese A., Bhatia K., Bressman S.B., et al. Phenomenology and classification of dystonia: a consensus update.Mov Disord. 2013 Jun 15;28(7):863-73.

Bhatia K., Peter Bain P., Nin Bajaj N. et al, and the Tremor Task Force of the International Parkinson and Movement Disorder Society Consensus Statement on the Classification of Tremors. Mov Disord 2018;33: 75-87.

Berardelli A., Rothwell J.C., Thompson P.D., Hallett M., Pathophysiology of bradykinesia in Parkinson's disease. Brain; 124:2131-2146, 2001.

Colosimo C., Bologna M., Lamberti S., Marinelli L., Fabbrini G., Abbruzzese G., Defazio G., Berardelli A. A comparative study of primary and secondary hemifacial spasm. Archives of Neurology; 63:441-444, 2006.

Defazio G., Berardelli A., Hallett M. Do primary adult-onset focal dystonias share aetiological factors? Brain; 130:1183-93, 2007.

Fabbrini G., Defazio G., Colosimo C., Thompson P.D., Berardelli A. Cranial movement disorders: clinical features, pathophysiology, differential diagnosis and treatment. Nature Clinical Practice Neurology; 5:93-105, 2009.

Fabbrini G., Brotchie J.M., Grandas F., Nomato M., Goetz C.G. Levodopa-induced dyskinesias. Movement Disorders; 22:1379-1389, 2007.

Postuma RD, Berg D, Stern M et al. MDS Clinical Diagnostic Criteria for Parkinson's Disease. Mov Disord 2015:30:1591-1599.

Van de Warrenburg BPC, van Gaalen J, Boesch S, et al EFNS/ENS Consensus on the diagnosis and management of chronic ataxias in adulthood. European Journal of Neurology 2014, 21: 552-562.

16 NEUROCOGNITIVE DISORDERS AND DEMENTIAS

Fabrizia D'Antonio, Marco Canevelli,
Alessandro Trebbastoni, Giuseppe Bruno, Carlo De Lena

16.1 Definition and theoretical background

The term "dementia" (or major neurocognitive disorder) defines an acquired syndrome that is not better explained by other psychiatric or systemic conditions. It is characterized by a noticeable and significant cognitive decline, with or without neuropsychiatric manifestations, of such severity that it interferes with the individual's usual daily functioning and independence (DSM-5).

The past twenty years of research in the field of neuroscience have led to the development of new biological, clinical, and instrumental knowledge, justifying a profound theoretical and clinical revision of dementias and a nosological redefinition of cognitive disorders. Recent studies have shown that dementias result from a slow and progressive accumulation of neuropathological damage, which begins in adulthood and becomes fully manifest with aging. Simultaneously, the clinical manifestations of these pathologies gradually evolve over time, initially presenting as subtle cognitive symptoms and eventually developing into confirmed dementia. As evidence of the widespread acceptance of this pathophysiological model of dementias, recent diagnostic criteria for Alzheimer's disease (AD), the most common clinical form of dementia, have included the definition of preclinical or prodromal stages (identifiable solely based on neurobiological abnormalities in asymptomatic individuals) and stages of pre-dementia (characterized by the onset of mild cognitive deficits).

The pre-dementia phase could be seen as the ideal stage for implementing treatments aimed at preventing or delaying the progression to confirmed dementia. Within this phase, two entities are of great interest in the scientific community: Subjective Cognitive Decline (SCD) and Mild Cognitive Impairment (MCI). SCD is defined as the subjective experience of a decline in cognitive efficiency that occurs in the absence of objectively observable deficits on neuropsychological assessment. More specifically, the terms that define this construct are as follows:

- *Subjective*: Refers to the individual's perception of their cognitive performance, independent of performance on cognitive tests (which are often not sensitive enough to detect subtle neuropsychological alterations).
- *Cognitive*: Pertaining to every domain of cognitive functioning (memory, language, attention, executive functions, visuospatial functions).
- *Decline*: Refers to the subjective experience of worsening cognitive abilities, emphasizing the progressive nature of the disorder.

SCD is a common condition in the general population, with estimated prevalence ranging from 25% to over 50%, depending on the age of the studied sample. Despite some conflicting results, SCD is now considered a potential risk factor for subsequent development of objective cognitive decline. Individuals with SCD have an increased risk (two to four times, according to available evidence) of developing MCI or dementia. Furthermore, some studies have shown that individuals with SCD may exhibit neuropathological alterations similar to those characteristic of AD in their brains.

Therefore, it has been hypothesized that SCD may represent the first true manifestation of an alteration from normal cognitive health. Consistent with this model, SCD is now considered a major criterion for the definition of MCI and a possible prodromal phase of AD. In light of these considerations, dementia prevention trials have recently been increasing the inclusion of participants reporting subjective disturbances. However, it should be noted that SCD may also be the expression of numerous potentially reversible clinical conditions (e.g., fatigue, pain, psychiatric comorbidities, physical frailty, concomitant therapies) and, therefore, may present complete clinical remission. Its exact nosological nature is still a subject of critical reflection.

Box 16.1 DEMENTIA PREVENTION

Dementia has been recognized as a public health priority. The progressive aging of the population and the lack of curative treatments are indeed contributing to a significant increase in the prevalence and socio-assistential impact of these conditions. In this scenario, there is a growing interest in the identification and implementation of effective preventive strategies. In this regard, epidemiological studies have identified a wide range of potentially modifiable risk factors for dementia. The most convincing evidence concerns cardiovascular risk factors, certain psychosocial determinants (e.g., depression), and unhealthy lifestyles/habits (e.g., reduced physical activity, smoking). On the contrary, engagement in mentally and physically stimulating activities, social relationships, high levels of education and professional complexity, adherence to specific dietary patterns (e.g., Mediterranean diet) have been found to be protective against dementia.

It has recently been estimated that a considerable proportion of dementia cases worldwide (about 40%) can be attributed to twelve potentially modifiable risk factors. Some of these factors, such as low education level, act in childhood/adolescence. Others, such as hearing loss, head injuries, hypertension, high alcohol consumption, and obesity, occur in early adulthood. Finally, factors like smoking, depression, social isolation, sedentary lifestyle, diabetes, and pollution occur in late adulthood and old age. The incidence of the disease could be significantly reduced by implementing public health strategies aimed at reducing the prevalence of these factors. This approach could be accompanied by a significant reduction in the prevalence of neurodegenerative, vascular, and mixed dementias (degenerative-vascular), considering that most of the risk and protective factors are shared by these conditions.

Box 16.2 FRAILTY AND COGNITIVE DISORDERS

The care and assistance models currently adopted in healthcare have been developed to meet the needs of a younger population compared to the current one, mainly focused on individual diseases with an acute or subacute onset. These approaches do not reflect the complexity of the aging process and age-related pathological conditions, characterized by the presence of multiple and interacting pathophysiological processes and morbid states. Therefore, it is necessary to develop new paradigms that capture the profound sociodemographic changes occurring and the resulting clinical and healthcare repercussions. In this scenario, the concept of *frailty* is attracting increasing interest in the scientific community. Frailty is defined as a condition characterized by a reduction in the organism's homeostatic reserves, resulting in a state of greater vulnerability to the action of both endogenous and exogenous stressors. It exposes the individual to an increased risk of adverse events (e.g., mortality, hospitalization, falls, functional decline). This concept can provide valuable assistance in addressing age-related conditions by supplementing the (outdated) criterion of chronological age with the more informative criterion of biological age. It is not surprising, therefore, that frailty has now transcended the boundaries of geriatric/gerontological disciplines and is increasingly being used in other medical fields, from cardiology to anesthesia, from infectious diseases to oncology.

The adoption of frailty measures in the context of dementia and cognitive disorders can have important clinical and research implications. It could promote a multidimensional approach to these pathological conditions, supporting a better understanding of the complex underlying pathophysiological processes, as well as the diverse clinical and biological factors that contribute to their onset and influence their clinical trajectories. Supporting this notion, available evidence shows that more frail individuals are at higher risk of developing dementia and exhibit more impaired cognitive performance compared to robust individuals. In patients already presenting cognitive disorders, the adoption of frailty measures (such as the Frailty Index) allows the prediction of unfavorable outcomes, such as mortality, institutionalization, and a more rapid progression of cognitive and functional impairment. The routine use of these measures could, therefore, improve clinical assessment and risk stratification profiles in individuals with cognitive disorders.

Mild Cognitive Impairment (MCI) is a clinical syndrome characterized by a decline in cognitive functions, as evidenced by neuropsychological tests, to an extent that does not result in any limitation of individual functional autonomy. It is a mild cognitive deficit that can affect different cognitive domains (not just memory) without impacting daily life functions, and therefore does not meet the diagnostic criteria for established dementia. Different forms of MCI can be distinguished based on the cognitive domains affected:

- *Amnestic MCI*: characterized by an exclusive memory deficit.
- *Non-amnestic MCI single domain*: characterized by an isolated non-memory cognitive deficit.
- *Multidomain MCI*: characterized by mild deficits involving multiple cognitive functions (including or excluding memory), which can further be divided into *amnestic* and *non-amnestic subtypes*.

The prevalence of MCI is estimated to be around 10-20% in the population over 65 years old. Numerous studies have shown that MCI is an important risk factor for the subsequent onset of dementia. Reviews conducted on the subject have demonstrated conversion rates to dementia ranging from 5% to 15% per year. There is currently significant attention focused on identifying factors that can predict the progression from MCI to established dementia. However, it should be noted that a considerable percentage of affected individuals do not exhibit significant clinical progression over time and may even return to normal. Furthermore, certain clinical studies have shown that specific interventions (e.g., physical activity and cognitive stimulation) can reduce the risk of progression from MCI to dementia and lead to significant improvements in cognitive performance.

16.2 Neurodegenerative dementias

16.2.1 Alzheimer's disease

Alzheimer's Disease (AD) is the leading cause of dementia, accounting for approximately 60% of all cases. In Italy, around 600,000 patients are affected by AD, and over 3 million people are directly or indirectly involved in their care.

Neuropathology

Macroscopically, the brain of a patient with AD shows varying degrees of atrophy depending on the clinical stage. Atrophy primarily affects the cerebral cortex and is more pronounced in the anterior and medial regions of the temporal lobes (particularly the hippocampus) and parietal lobes. Cerebral sulci and ventricles appear enlarged due to substance loss (ex vacuo dilation). The weight and size of the organ are severely reduced.

Microscopically, the brain exhibits characteristic extracellular deposits and intracellular inclusions known as senile plaques and neurofibrillary tangles, respectively. The main constituent of senile plaques is a 4kD protein with a β-sheet secondary structure called β-amyloid (Aβ).

Three types of plaques are described:

a) diffuse;
b) neuritic;
c) compact.

Neuritic plaques are most numerous in the brain affected by AD. They present a central core of radial arrangement of Aβ surrounded by abnormal, dystrophic neurites, around which microglia cells and reactive astrocytes accumulate, responsible for the production of inflammatory cytokines. Complement activation products are also present in neuritic plaques, confirming the presence of a localized inflammatory reaction. The presence, distribution, and number of neuritic plaques constitute the main neuropathological (autopsy) diagnostic criteria for AD. Diffuse plaques consist of Aβ deposits that appear amorphous and are not yet structured into fibers. There is no evidence of activated cells or dystrophic neurites (neuritic plaques) around diffuse plaques. Diffuse plaques represent the initial stage of neuritic plaque formation. Compact plaques are characterized by highly compacted fibrillar Aβ, significant cellular rarefaction, and the absence of reactive cellular species. These plaques represent the final evolution of neuritic plaques. Ab precipitates and accumulates inside the media of cerebral blood vessels. Most deposits are observed in the walls of small and medium arteries, leptomeningeal arterioles, and cortical capillaries, particularly in the posterior regions of the brain. This phenomenon, known as amyloid angiopathy, is found in over 80% of AD-affected brains. The presence of these deposits alters the structure of the vessel, increasing the risk of rupture. Microhemorrhages (asymptomatic) resulting from this condition are a frequent histological finding in the disease.

Neurofibrillary tangles are composed of intracellular accumulations of tau protein. Under normal conditions, tau protein is closely bound to microtubules, providing support and stabilization to the neuronal cytoskeleton. In AD, tau protein undergoes excessive phosphorylation, which alters its structure. This results in a loss of affinity for microtubules, causing detachment and precipitation into insoluble fibrillar aggregates inside the neuron. Neurofibrillary tangles occupy a significant portion of the pyreneophore and surround the nucleus, displacing it and giving the neuron its characteristic "flame-like" appearance. Accumulations in axons and dendrites are referred to as "neurofibrillary threads". The spatial distribution of neurofibrillary tangles within the brain follows a specific temporal order. This has allowed for the neuropathological staging of AD. The first neurofibrillary tangles can be observed in neurons of the second layer of the entorhinal cortex (stages I and II, trans-entorhinal); subsequently, they appear in the Ammon's horn (CA1), subicular regions of the hippocampus, and amygdala, eventually involving limbic areas (stages III and IV, limbic). Only in the later stages of the disease, neurofibrillary tangles localize in the neocortex (stages V and VI, isocortical).

Other histological alterations present in the brains of AD patients include granulovacuolar degeneration and Hirano bodies. Granulovacuolar degeneration is characterized by the presence of small vacuoles containing an argyrophilic granule. Although frequently found in the brain of healthy elderly individuals, this type of alteration is much more severe in AD, with pronounced vacuolization, particularly in the hippocampus. Hirano bodies are elongated, glassy, eosinophilic formations consisting of paracrystalline arrangements of granular filaments, primarily composed of actin. They are predominantly located in the pyramidal cells of the hippocampus (CA1 region).

Pathogenetic mechanisms | Among the most studied pathogenetic hypotheses in recent years, the so-called "amyloidogenic" hypothesis has found the most support. According to this theory, the primum movens of the neuropathological process lies in the abnormal degradation of amyloid precursor protein (APP), which leads to the production and accumulation of a neurotoxic polypeptide. In the healthy brain, almost all APP is degraded through the action of the α-secretase enzyme, resulting in the production of soluble catabolites with neurotrophic function. A second pathway for APP metabolism involves the involvement of a different enzyme, β-secretase. β-secretase enzyme cleaves APP, producing two fragments: a short soluble amino-terminal fragment and a longer carboxy-terminal fragment that remains anchored to the membrane. This second fragment is the target of γ-secretase. This enzyme is composed of a heteromeric complex that includes presenilin 1 and 2 (PS1 and PS2), which constitute its catalytic subunits. γ-secretase cleaves the carboxy-terminal fragment of APP in the transmembrane region of the glycoprotein, resulting in the release of two fragments. The first, intracellular fragment is degraded in lysosomes, while the second, a peptide consisting of 40-42 amino acids (Aβ), is released outside the cell. The 42-amino acid isoform of Aβ (Aβ-42), when newly produced, assumes a 'beta-sheet' conformation that makes it poorly soluble and resistant to proteases. Aβ-42 monomers begin to polymerize into more complex aggregates known as oligomers. These oligomers precipitate into insoluble clusters and assume the conformation of fibrils. Fibrillogenesis is a crucial step in the deposition process of Aβ-42 and leads to the formation of amyloid cores that constitute plaques. An imbalance favoring the activity of β-secretase and γ-secretase is believed to be responsible for the excessive production of Aβ-42. All forms of aggregation of this peptide (monomers, oligomers, and fibrils) exhibit high toxicity, both direct and indirect, underlying the neurodegenerative processes. The series of events starting with the production of Aβ-42 by γ-secretase, continuing with the production and accumulation of neurotoxic species, and ending with synaptic depletion and cell death is referred to as the "amyloid cascade". Confirmation of the central pathogenic role of Aβ-42 in AD development has been obtained by studying genetically determined forms of the disease. Causative mutations affecting the genes encoding APP, PS1, and PS2 lead to an over tenfold increase in the production of Aβ-42. In Down syndrome as well, the condition of trisomy of chromosome 21 and the resulting presence of three copies of the APP gene are associated with increased production of glycoprotein degradation products, including Aβ-42. Affected patients develop early and widespread amyloid deposits starting from childhood, which, after the age of 35, assume characteristics similar to those seen in AD patients.

A second pathogenetic hypothesis of AD focuses on the prominent role of the tau protein. According to the "tau-centric", theory, the initial alterations occur in this protein, which undergoes abnormal phosphorylation by cytoplasmic protein kinases. Tau hyperphosphorylation has dual consequences. On one hand, it leads to the structural collapse of the cytoskeleton due to the detachment of the protein from microtubules, and on the other hand, it promotes the precipitation of insoluble aggregates (neurofibrillary tangles) capable of directly damaging neurons mechanically. The central role of tau protein alterations in AD is further supported by evidence of the correlation between tau lesion load and clinical findings. The progression of the disease and worsening of symptoms occur in parallel with the spatial spread of neurofibrillary degeneration in the brain. Despite the numerous accumulated pieces of evidence, the causes leading to tau protein hyperphosphorylation remain largely unknown. The presence of Aβ-42 seems to stimulate tau phosphorylation through the modulation of cytoplasmic protein kinases and phosphatases.

Genetics

Approximately 90% of all AD cases are sporadic. In 10% of cases, the disease occurs in a familial form with the presence of at least two affected individuals among first-degree relatives. In 10% of familial cases, a causative mutation can be identified. In these cases, three genes have been associated with the determination of AD:

1) the gene encoding APP (chromosome 21, locus 21q21.2)
2) the gene encoding PS1 (chromosome 14, locus 14q24.3)
3) the gene encoding PS2 (chromosome 1, locus 1q31-q42).

Mutations in these genes are rare and affect approximately 5% of the affected population. They are transmitted in an autosomal dominant manner and are associated with almost complete penetrance. The clinical picture associated with these mutations is characterized by early onset and rapid progression. In these cases, the disease is linked to the massive increase in levels of Aβ-42 produced in the brain. Mutations in the APP gene, in fact, result in the production of a glycoprotein with an abnormal structure that is more easily targeted by beta- and gamma-secretases. This leads to an imbalance in the metabolism of APP in favor of the amyloidogenic pathway. The same result is achieved with mutations in the PS1 and PS2 genes. In this case, however, the excessive production of Aβ-42 depends on the increased efficiency of γ-secretase, of which PS1 and PS2 are cleavage sites, in cleaving APP. The newly discovered mutations are collected on a specific website for continuous updates (http://www.molgen.ua.ac.be/ADMutations).

In sporadic forms of AD, numerous polymorphisms and mutations with protective or favoring significance have been identified. The most studied example is the polymorphism of the gene encoding apolipoprotein E (APOE) on chromosome 19. The human APOE gene has three allelic variants called ε2, ε3 and ε4. The presence of the ε4 allelic variant in heterozygosity (ε2/ε4 and ε3/ε4), increases the risk of developing the disease by 2-3 times, while homozygosity for (ε4/ε4) increases the risk from 5 to 50 times.

Clinical picture

The clinical history of AD spans a long period of time. The progressive accumulation of damage and the consequent exhaustion of the brain's compensatory abilities occur very slowly. Therefore, there is a long period, estimated to be between 15 and 30 years by some studies, during which the pathology is present without any evidence of cognitive deficits. This means that the onset of symptoms in AD is a relatively late event in the course of the disease, preceded by a long asymptomatic phase. From this perspective, AD fits into a *cognitive continuum*, with dementia being the final stage (Figure 16.1).

The search for biological, genetic, biochemical, and neuroradiological markers related to the onset and development of AD has led to the identification of some biomarkers useful for in vivo diagnosis of the disease. The introduction of these biomarkers in the most recent diagnostic criteria proposed by the National Institute on Aging - Alzheimer's Association (NIA-AA) in 2011 has increased diagnostic accuracy in AD and identified three diagnostic categories corresponding to three different degrees of clinical expression of the disease:

1) *Preclinical AD*: corresponds to the asymptomatic phase of the disease in which all the pathogenic mechanisms are active, but the extent of damage is not sufficient to cause symptoms. This phase completely escapes diagnosis in clinical practice. However, it can be recognized in asymptomatic individuals carrying causative AD mutations (autosomal dominant).
2) *Prodromal AD*: corresponds to the early symptomatic phase of the disease. The pathology reaches a level of damage that mildly affects some cognitive functions without interfering with the overall functioning of the individual. This phase includes the previously mentioned mild cognitive impairment (MCI) associated with Alzheimer's pathology.
3) *AD Dementia:* corresponds to the established phase of the disease. The level of neuropathological alteration is severe enough to impair many cognitive functions. The individual experiences compromised levels of independence. Within this diagnostic category, three levels of clinical severity can be identified based on scores obtained by patients on tests such as the

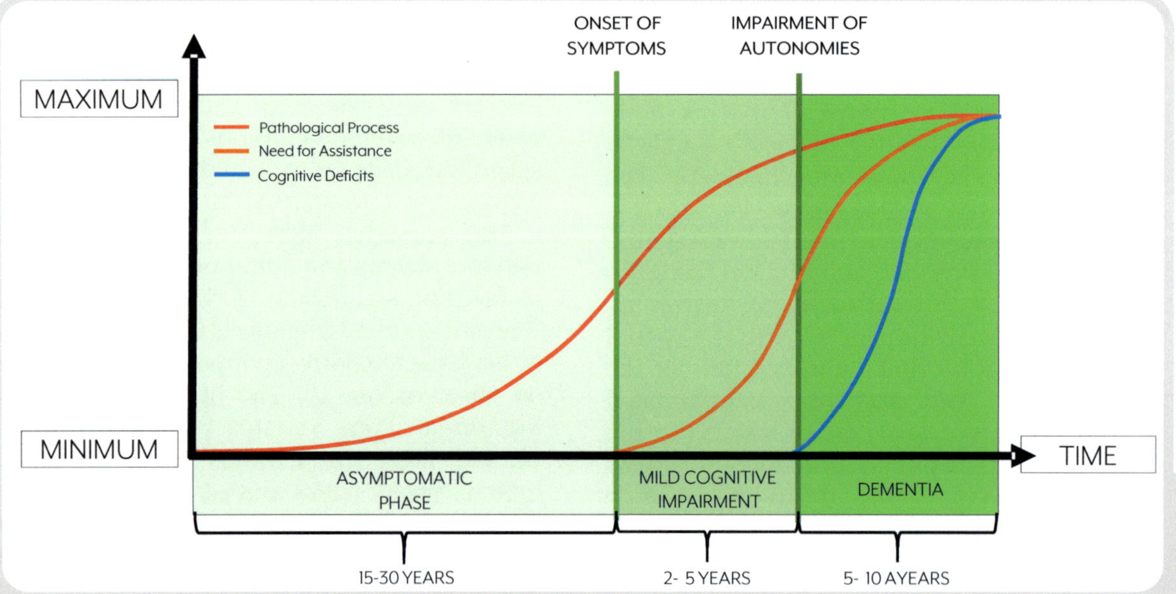

Figure 16.1

The Cognitive Continuum in Alzheimer's Disease. The pathological process is already active many years before the onset of symptoms (ASYMPTOMATIC phase). With the development of initial deficits, a mild cognitive impairment emerges that does not alter the functional abilities of the individual. Progressively, the severity of the clinical picture becomes such that it impairs autonomy and dementia appears. Below are approximate estimates of the duration in years of the various stages.

Box 16.3 BIOMARKERS

Over the last 30 years, numerous techniques have been developed to detect the pathological process in Alzheimer's disease (AD) in living subjects. The development of these techniques has led to the discovery of disease-specific biological markers (biomarkers) recently included in the NIA-AA diagnostic criteria for research. Biomarkers for AD can be classified based on the explored pathogenic mechanism, allowing them to be divided into two groups:

Amyloid deposition biomarkers:

a. Reduced levels of Aβ-42 in cerebrospinal fluid (CSF)
b. Positivity on PET images obtained with amyloid tracers

Neurodegeneration biomarkers:

a. Increased concentrations of tau protein and p-tau in CSF
b. Positivity on PET images obtained with tau tracers
c. Reduced uptake of 18-fluorodeoxyglucose in PET
d. Evidence of typical brain atrophy on MRI

The use of biomarkers in the study of preclinical and prodromal stages of AD has allowed the description of a disease-evolution model based on their progressive changes over time.

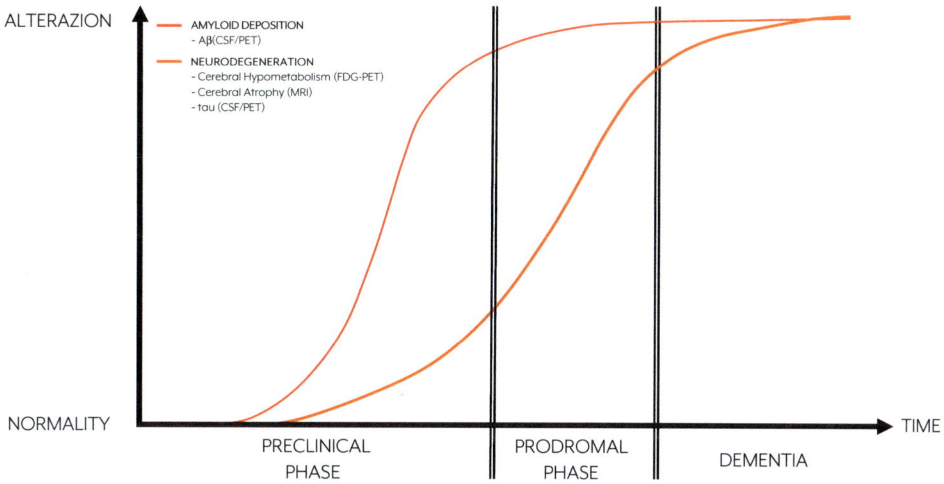

Biomarkers in Alzheimer's disease: the graph shows the temporal trend through which the main biomarkers can be identified and their dynamics as they evolve over time.

According to this model, alterations in biomarkers related to amyloid deposition are the first to appear. Neurodegeneration biomarkers, on the other hand, tend to become positive in the more advanced stages of the disease. At the same time, amyloid deposition biomarkers quickly reach a saturation level, so once they appear, their concentrations do not substantially change over time. In contrast, neurodegeneration biomarkers undergo slower changes that can be measured throughout the course of the disease. The characteristics of these two types of biomarkers (early but static for amyloid deposition and late but dynamic for neurodegeneration) differentiate their utility. The former (measurement of A in CSF/PET with amyloid tracer) are crucial for early diagnosis (e.g., in the preclinical phase) but are of limited use in monitoring the disease's progression. The latter (evaluation of brain atrophy and hypometabolism, quantification of cerebral tau deposits, and tau protein measurement in CSF) allow describing the disease's evolution, showing a significant correlation with symptom progression.

In pharmacological trials employing disease-modifying therapies, biomarkers for Alzheimer's disease are widely utilized. In these studies, their role is crucial. On one hand, the positivity of a biomarker (e.g., amyloid deposition) is the primary inclusion criterion for the experimentation, ensuring the enrollment of patients with high diagnostic accuracy. On the other hand, the repeated assessment of biomarkers over time allows for the evaluation of therapy effectiveness. For instance, a monoclonal antibody targeting Aβ can influence biomarkers related to amyloid deposition, and its efficacy can be measured by observing how these biomarkers change over time (reduction in Aβ-42 concentration in cerebrospinal fluid and/or reduced amyloid tracer uptake in brain PET scans).

MMSE: mild (22 ≤ MMSE ≤ 27), moderate (15 ≤ MMSE ≤ 21), and severe (MMSE ≤ 14). The three diagnostic categories identified by the NIA-AA criteria reflect the cognitive continuum of AD. However, since the procedures used to study biomarkers are often invasive, associated with high costs, and not widely available, their use is recommended exclusively within the scope of research.

The diagnosis of MCI is based on the identification of mild cognitive impairment that is greater than expected for the individual's age and education level but does not interfere with daily activities. MCI is considered a transitional phase between normal brain aging and pathological senescence. As previously described, MCI is a heterogeneous syndrome in which cognitive impairment can affect only memory (amnestic MCI) or other cognitive functions (non-amnestic MCI) and can involve a single domain (single-domain MCI) or multiple domains (multi-domain MCI).

Amnestic phenotypes (single- or multi-domain) are more frequently associated with the progression to Alzheimer's dementia. This phenomenon is referred to as "conversion." The annual conversion rates for MCI range from 6% to 20%, with estimates of 3-year conversion rates reaching up to 70%. Therefore, MCI is a clinically uncertain condition associated with an increased risk of developing dementia.

The clinical diagnosis of Alzheimer's dementia is based on the identification of cognitive impairment affecting memory and at least one other function. The cognitive deficit must have four characteristics:

a) Insidious onset
b) Gradual progression
c) Impairment of the individual's autonomy
d) Confirmation through neuropsychological evaluation with standardized tests.

Satisfying these criteria allows for a diagnosis of probable Alzheimer's disease (AD). If not all criteria are met, it is referred to as possible AD. This is the case, for example, when cognitive deficits exhibit atypical patterns or occur in the context of mixed etiology involving significant evidence of cerebrovascular disease (history of stroke, widespread vascular lesions in the white matter, etc.) or in conjunction with signs and symptoms suggestive of other neurological syndromes (parkinsonism, signs of motor neuron disease, etc.) other than AD.

The symptoms that manifest during AD can be grouped into two clusters: Cognitive Symptoms and Behavioral and Psychological Symptoms.

Cognitive symptoms of AD | The most frequently affected function in AD is memory. Deficits in recent memory are the prominent clinical feature and initial manifestation of the disease. Typical symptoms of early memory impairment include misplacing objects or repeatedly asking the same questions. Autobiographical memory and long-term historical memory remain intact. Disorientation (spatial and temporal) is a constant feature throughout the course of the disease. Initially, the problem may be limited to difficulty indicating the date, but as the disease progresses, the patient loses the ability to orient themselves in time and space. This can lead to getting lost outside the home and, in severe cases, even within their own residence. Such events increase the risk of wandering and elopement.

Deficits in concentration and attention are consistently reported by patients and caregivers as among the earliest symptoms. Their presence contributes to the development of learning difficulties, as the individual is unable to acquire and retain new information. Language impairment is common in AD. Although language function may initially be preserved, a reduction in vocabulary can be observed during early clinical interviews. Patients often experience difficulty retrieving words and the emergence of anomia, interrupting the flow of speech. They may complain of not being able to "find" the right word and resort to using alternative words (e.g., thing, stuff, etc.). In addition to anomia, phonemic and semantic paraphasias may occur, while a more complex aphasic syndrome with deficits in naming, repetition, and comprehension typically presents in the later stages.

More challenging to assess, especially outside highly specialized centers, are the disturbances in gnosis, praxis, and visuospatial abilities. Among the agnosias, anosognosia is very common in AD, and the lack of awareness of the illness greatly complicates its management for both the physician and family members. Visuospatial deficits are often confused with visual impairments, resulting in a delay in their identification. Impairment of visuospatial functions can lead to significant difficulties in interacting with space, including the ability to localize stimuli, appreciate distances, orientations, or relative and absolute dimensions. Difficulty recognizing bodily and extrabodily spatial coordinates can affect any action, including ambulation, with a higher risk of falls. Apraxias are functionally linked to visuospatial deficits. Constructive apraxia, in particular, can be evaluated using tests that assess the capacity for construction, composition, and drawing. Drawings by patients with AD generally exhibit simplifications, distortions, and a lack of perspective. In the early stage of the disease, copying simple figures may be relatively preserved, while copying complex figures, which is highly sensitive to disease progression, may already be impaired.

Executive dysfunctions and alterations in abstract thinking, which may be present at the onset of symptoms in some cases, progressively impair planning, critical thinking, and judgment with disease advancement. This raises important medico-legal issues in clinical practice as it affects the patient's decision-making capacities.

Behavioral and psychological symptoms of Alzheimer's disease | A relevant clinical aspect of Alzheimer's disease (AD) is the presence, varying but commonly observed throughout the course of the disease, of behavioral disturbances and psychiatric symptoms that manifest with a wide range of phenomenology. These "non-cognitive" symptoms often profoundly impact the progression of the disease, severely affecting the quality of life of patients and caregivers. The development of depression, anxiety, apathy, delusions, hallucinations, agitation, verbal and/or physical aggression, irritability, inappropriate social behaviors, aberrant motor activity, disinhibition, euphoria, sleep disturbances, eating disorders, and sexual disorders affects over 70% of patients, tending to manifest with different patterns and frequencies in various stages of the disease. The onset of these symptoms is the most common reason for medical intervention and pharmacological prescription. Furthermore, as these symptoms often lead to a considerable increase in caregiver burden, particularly those related to the psychotic sphere, they are the primary cause of institutionalization of the patient. The use of dedicated scales such as the Neuropsychiatric Inventory (NPI) can be useful in assessing the severity and frequency of these symptoms and the potential response to the therapy administered.

Although symptom fluctuations do not properly characterize the clinical picture of AD, the affected individual often experiences a "circadian" worsening that occurs in the late afternoon and evening hours. This phenomenon is known as "sundowning syndrome." This condition is characterized by the exacerbation of cognitive and behavioral disturbances (confusion, anxiety, restlessness, psychomotor agitation) that occur at dusk. Sundowning syndrome is found in up to 65% of AD patients. Two factors contribute to the determinism of this condition: on one hand, the increased fatigue and vulnerability that the patient may experience at the end of the day; on the other hand, the increase in misperceptive phenomena caused by the reduction of ambient light, which worsens the patient's visual abilities and promotes incorrect interpretations of environmental stimuli.

In the advanced stages of the disease, cognitive deterioration is so severe that the patient is no longer able to independently perform even basic activities of daily living such as dressing, washing, and attending to physiological needs. The appearance of incontinence due to the loss of voluntary control of the sphincters further compromises the picture. Over time, long-term memory is also impaired, as is language, leading the patient to exhibit severe aphasia with significant impairments in comprehension and expression. In the terminal phase, motor deficits and muscular tone disorders may also occur. Dysphagia can also manifest, being one of the main causes of complications such as malnutrition, dehydration, and aspiration pneumonia. Difficulties with ambulation can be complicated by falls and resulting fractures. Bedridden status can lead to the development of pressure ulcers, increase the risk of infections (urinary and respiratory tract), and worsen constipation, potentially leading to fecal impaction and intestinal blockage. The overlap of all these conditions significantly reduces the patient's life expectancy and quality of life. Generally, the patient's demise occurs due to concurrent internal pathologies, predominantly of infectious nature.

Diagnostic tools

The gold standard for diagnosing AD is based on post-mortem detection of typical neuropathological changes in the brain of affected individuals. The presence and distribution of amyloid plaques and neurofibrillary tangles allow for a definitive diagnosis of the disease and determination of its stage of progression. In living individuals, the diagnosis is based on a thorough collection of medical history, neurological and general physical examination, neuroimaging (CT and/or MRI of the brain), and assessment of cognitive function. Routine laboratory tests, thyroid hormone levels, and certain blood factors such as vitamin B12 and folate levels complete the diagnostic process. Gathering the medical history should involve both the patient and the caregiver, and should thoroughly investigate the onset characteristics of the symptoms, progression patterns, and the impact on the patient's level of autonomy. Neurological examination in AD may reveal reduced ideation speed and the presence of ideomotor and orofacial apraxia. Frontal release reflexes (snout reflex, palmomental reflex, and the grasp reflex) may be present even in the early stages of the disease. Evaluation of cognitive function is a central aspect of the diagnostic phase. Administering tests by qualified neuropsychologists in highly specialized facilities such as Centers for Cognitive Disorders and Dementia (CDCD) allows for an accurate neuropsychological profile of the patient and a qualitative and quantitative description of the deficits present. This approach ensures a diagnostic accuracy of 70-90% compared to histopathological diagnosis. The test battery used should assess all cognitive functions. Along with the use of fast screening tests such as the MMSE, Montreal Cognitive Assessment (MoCA), and the Clinical Dementia Rating Scale (CDR), it provides the necessary tools for diagnostic assessment and follow-up of deficits. The use of standard neuroimaging of the brain (CT and/or MRI) primarily helps exclude other causes of cognitive decline (space-occupying lesions, vascular lesions, etc.). More complex imaging techniques, such as high-resolution volumetric MRI, allow for the evaluation of regional atrophy patterns in the patient. In AD, cerebral atrophy affects the medial and basal regions of the temporal lobe, the hippocampus, entorhinal cortex, and parietal lobes. An increase in the size of the lateral ventricles (particularly the temporal horns) is another indirect sign of brain parenchymal degeneration (■ Figure 16.2).

Functional neuroradiological methods are generally employed as secondary examinations in the differential diagnosis of the disease or at the onset of symptoms. Positron emission tomography using 18F-fluorodeoxyglucose (FDG-PET) as a tracer and single-photon emission computed tomography using technetium-99 (SPECT) highlight metabolism and cerebral perfusion alterations primarily affecting parietal and temporal regions, particularly the posterior cingulate and precuneus. A significant advance in the diagnosis of AD has been achieved with the development of PET scans that use radiotracers capable of binding Aβ or tau in the brain in vivo. Amyloid PET is by far the most commonly used technique, employing radioactive tracers (florbetapir, flutemetamol, florbetapen) that bind to different Aβ, isoforms, particularly the species deposited in plaques. In AD, the typical distribution of uptake involves widespread cortical areas in the parietal, temporal, and frontal lobes (■ Figure 16.3).

Cerebrospinal fluid examination through lumbar puncture is also used in the in vivo diagnosis of AD. In addition to cytophysical and cytochemical analysis, it allows for the measurement of the concentration of different amyloid and tau species in the cerebrospinal fluid. The profile observed in AD includes reduced concentrations of Aβ (due to peptide deposition in plaques) and increased levels of total tau protein (t-tau) and phosphorylated tau (p-tau). The increase in t-tau and p-tau depends on the high release of both peptides by

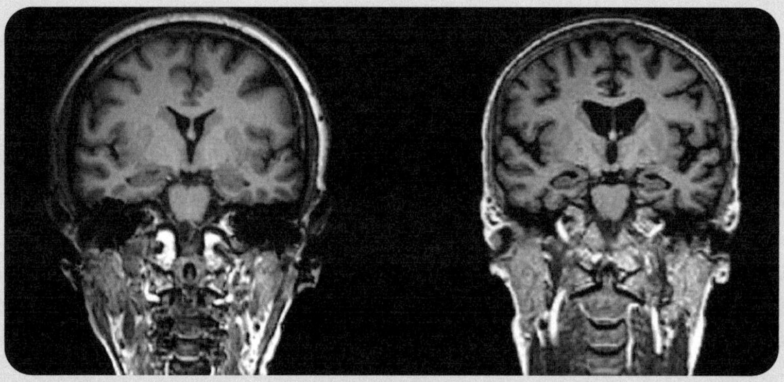

Figure 16.2

Coronal plane T1 images of a normal brain (left) compared to that of an age-matched patient with Alzheimer's disease (right). An increase in the width of the cortical sulci, Sylvian fissures, the third ventricle, and lateral ventricles can be observed. Additionally, there is a noticeable reduction in volume of the hippocampus and entorhinal cortex in both temporal-mesial regions.

damaged neurons. PET scans using radioactive tracers for amyloid or tau, volumetric MRI, cerebrospinal fluid analysis, and FDG-PET represent the currently employed techniques for studying AD biomarkers in vivo.

Clinical variants of Alzheimer's disease

Posterior cortical atrophy (PCA): Described as the posterior variant or visual variant of AD, it is characterized by the accumulation of neuritic plaques and neurofibrillary tangles in the posterior brain regions (including the primary visual cortex). Clinically, PCA manifests with symptoms related to damage in the dorsal occipitoparietal and ventral occipitotemporal tracts, initially resulting in visual agnosia and apraxia. Neurological examination may reveal typical signs of Balint's syndrome (optic ataxia and oculomotor apraxia), simultanagnosia, prosopagnosia, and sometimes hemineglect. Other observed symptoms include constructive apraxia, ideomotor and ideational apraxia, dressing apraxia, and elements of Gerstmann syndrome, such as agraphia, acalculia, left-right disorientation, and digital agnosia. Memory deficit is a common symptom. Neuroimaging shows atrophy, hypoperfusion,

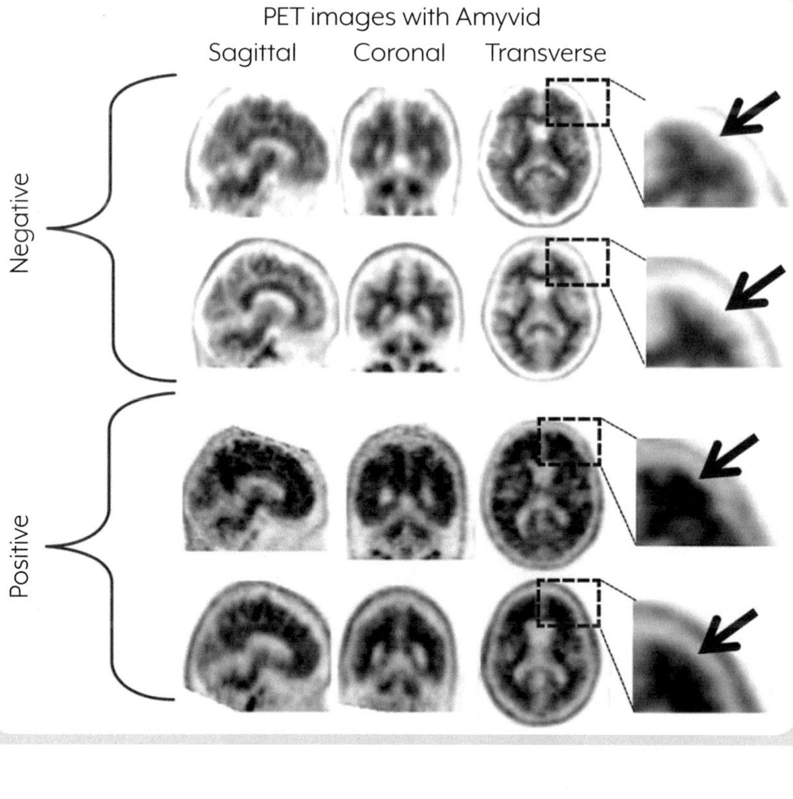

Figure 16.3

PET images with florbetapir (Amyvid) showing examples of negative scans (top two rows) and positive scans (bottom two rows). The two arrows at the top indicate the normal gray-white contrast preserved with cortical activity lower than that of the adjacent white matter. The two arrows at the bottom indicate areas with reduced gray-white contrast and increased cortical activity comparable to that of the adjacent white matter. Courtesy of Eli Lilly.

or hypometabolism in the posterior cortical areas, particularly in the occipitoparietal regions.

Anterior variant of AD | Patients with this variant, also known as the "frontal" variant, develop behavioral disturbances and an executive syndrome. Executive impairments appear to be more prominent at the onset, while behavioral symptoms become more significant as the disease progresses. Apathy is the most frequent symptom, while perseverative behaviors and obsessive-compulsive aspects are rarer. The clinical picture often overlaps with the behavioral variant of frontotemporal dementia. Neuropsychologically, the anterior variant of AD presents less severe memory deficits compared to the typical form, but the impairment of executive functions is much more severe. Neuroimaging reveals temporo-parietal atrophy, while postmortem examination shows the accumulation of neurofibrillary tangles in the frontal lobes.

Logopenic aphasia | This represents the rarest of the three clinical variants of primary progressive aphasia. The main cognitive deficit concerns language: patients have difficulty in word retrieval and repetition of phrases, with evident phonological errors in spontaneous speech in the absence of agrammatism. Neuroimaging shows predominant atrophy in the perisylvian and parietal areas of the dominant hemisphere.

Therapy

The treatment of AD is currently focused on the use of "symptomatic" drugs. These drugs aim to alleviate some symptoms of cognitive decline without directly targeting the underlying pathogenic mechanisms. Acetylcholinesterase inhibitors (AChEIs) act by increasing acetylcholine levels in the brain through competitive and reversible blockade of the main enzyme responsible for its catabolism. Acetylcholine is an important neurotransmitter for proper cognitive functioning. Early impairment of important cholinergic pathways has been demonstrated in AD. The action of AChEIs aims to compensate for the functional deficit associated with this impairment. Three molecules have been approved for use in our country: donepezil, rivastigmine, and galantamine. All of them are indicated for mild to moderate stages of the disease. Rivastigmine also inhibits a second enzyme that catabolizes acetylcholine in subcortical regions: butyrylcholinesterase. Galantamine, in addition to its inhibitory effect on acetylcholinesterase, can modulate nicotinic receptors present on cholinergic neurons, promoting the release of the neurotransmitter. The efficacy of these drugs in terms of improving cognitive functions is limited. Pharmacological trials have shown only temporary slowing of disease progression in a small percentage of patients. Memantine is used for the treatment of moderate to severe stages of the disease and acts as a competitive inhibitor of NMDA glutamate receptors. The inhibitory effect of memantine modulates the activity of glutamate on receptors that physiologically regulate calcium entry into the cell, facilitating *short-* and *long-term synaptic potentiation* underlying learning and memory processes. The partial blocking activity of NMDA receptors also counteracts calcium-dependent excitotoxic phenomena caused by their abnormal activation due to excessive glutamate release. Similar to AChEIs, clinical trials for memantine have demonstrated limited effectiveness in slowing symptom progression. Memantine is generally prescribed in combination with AChEIs.

In the last two decades, research has focused on studying drugs capable of interfering with the pathogenic mechanisms of the disease. Such drugs are not symptomatic but aim to change the course of the disease (*disease modifying therapies*). On June 7, 2021, the United States Food and Drug Administration (FDA) approved the drug aducanumab, a monoclonal antibody targeting β-amyloid, for the treatment of Alzheimer's disease (AD) through an accelerated procedure. This decision was primarily motivated by evidence that aducanumab reduces cerebral amyloid plaques in affected patients. However, post-approval studies will be necessary to clarify the real clinical benefit (as well as the biological effect) resulting from this therapy. In addition to the aducanumab protocols, numerous pharmacological trials are still ongoing to evaluate the effectiveness of passive immunization against β-amyloid and tau protein.Monoclonal antibodies directed against β-amyloid can bind to various forms of the peptide, promoting the breakdown of deposits, countering the formation of oligomers and fibrils, and stimulating phagocytosis by microglial cells. All these effects lead to a reduction in the amount of β-amyloid deposited in plaques and, consequently, its potential toxicity. Similar mechanisms are shared by monoclonal antibodies directed against the tau protein, which is of more recent synthesis. In this case, immunization counters the extracellular spread of the pathology. A second innovative approach involves the use of molecules capable of reducing the production of β-amyloid through enzymatic blockade. β-secretase inhibitors can reduce the amount of β-amyloid produced by countering the enzyme's activity on the neuronal membrane. Most of the experiments conducted so far have not demonstrated the efficacy of these new therapies. One of the main reasons for the failure of these trials lies in the choice of the included sample, consisting of patients with already evident cognitive decline. To be truly effective, monoclonal antibody therapy or β-secretase inhibitors should be administered in the early stages of the disease, before the pathogenic mechanisms have already caused irreversible damage. From this perspective, the importance of targeting an earlier diagnosis, even in the preclinical phase of the disease, is becoming increasingly clear.

Non-pharmacological therapies | The limited effectiveness of conventional pharmacological therapy and evidence that a lack of consistent cognitive stimulation throughout life reduces cognitive reserve and promotes deterioration have driven research to investigate the effects of non-pharmacological interventions in Alzheimer's disease (AD) as well. The principles underlying the various interventions are extremely diverse, as are the targets they aim to achieve: increasing cognitive performance, managing behavioral and psychological symptoms of dementia, and improving patients' quality of life. The effectiveness of these approaches is generally transient and of modest magnitude, but if prolonged over time, they can provide benefits similar to pharmacological therapy. Among the interventions primarily focused on cognition, cognitive stimulation is among the most commonly used. It consists of a wide range of structured activities aimed at overall improvement of social functioning and the maintenance of various functions. This approach places particular emphasis on social interactions and is generally implemented in group settings. Cognitive rehabilitation focuses on identifying goals to be achieved regarding the cognitive deficits presented by the individual. These deficits are treated by proposing a compensatory approach, where a preserved function becomes vicarious for the impaired one. This approach has shown significant efficacy in patients with dementia, resulting in improved overall cognitive performance and functional autonomy. This more frequently individual approach also involves family members and aims not so much at improving a "single" function but at enhancing the individual's overall functioning. For this reason, cognitive rehabilitation takes place in the real world, directly in the spaces where the patient lives. A completely different principle underlies *cognitive training*. It involves performing standard tasks designed for various cognitive functions. The exercises proposed can involve the use of pen and paper or be replicated on the computer. The difficulty of the exercise is determined based on the degree of impairment of the specific cognitive function and is modulated according to improvements. The underlying principle of cognitive training is that repeated exercise and practice can improve or maintain a compromised function.

16.2.2 Lewy body disease

Lewy body disease is characterized by cognitive deterioration, movement disorders, and neuropsychiatric disturbances. It is referred to as Lewy body disease rather than dementia because, like Alzheimer's disease (AD), it is preceded by a phase called mild cognitive impairment (MCI), in which cognitive decline is not severe enough to compromise the individual's independence. During this phase, impairment primarily affects visuospatial, executive, and attentional functions while sparing memory. Neuropsychiatric disturbances, which are part of the core and supportive criteria for dementia with Lewy bodies (DLB), can also coexist during this phase.

In recent years, the belief that Lewy body disease can be considered a spectrum of disorders (Parkinson's disease [PD], Parkinson's dementia [PDD], and DLB) sharing the same neuropathological process has been gaining ground. The clinical presentation differs depending on the region of the brain primarily affected by the accumulation of Lewy bodies.

Neuropathology

The neuropathological hallmark of the disease is represented by aggregates of α-synuclein and ubiquitin, which form eosinophilic cytoplasmic inclusions known as Lewy bodies. In DLB, Lewy neurites, which are abnormal neurites containing granular material and abnormal α-synuclein filaments, can also be observed. Lewy bodies deposit in the brainstem and have preferred sites of accumulation, including the substantia nigra, as seen in PD, as well as the olfactory nerve, vagus nerve, and locus coeruleus. Dysfunction of these structures leads to reduced or loss of sense of smell (hyposmia/anosmia), autonomic dysfunctions, alterations in wakefulness, and disruptions in rapid eye movement (REM) sleep and rapid eye movements, which are features observed in both PD and DLB. In DLB and PDD, α-synuclein accumulation is also observed in neocortical regions such as the temporal, parietal, and frontal cortices. From a neuropathological perspective, three variants of Lewy body disease are distinguished:

- The variant with predominantly Lewy body accumulation in the brainstem without involvement of neocortical regions. Deposits are found in the substantia nigra, nucleus of the vagus and glossopharyngeal nerves, reticular nuclei, and locus coeruleus. This form is associated with PD.
- The limbic variant, with predominant accumulation in the entorhinal cortex, cingulate gyrus, and amygdala.
- The neocortical variant, which is diffuse and characterized by widespread accumulation of Lewy bodies in neocortical regions.

The latter two variants are associated with cognitive manifestations and are characteristic of DLB and PDD. Lewy body disease has also been found to coexist with amyloid plaques and neurofibrillary tangles typical of AD. Unlike AD, the presence of Lewy bodies and neurites is not associated with neuronal loss and therefore cerebral atrophy.

Epidemiology

DLB is the second most common neurodegenerative dementia, in terms of incidence, after AD, accounting for an estimated 15-30% of all dementia cases. Onset typically occurs between the ages of 70 and 85, and it is more frequent in males.

Clinical picture

DLB is characterized by progressive cognitive deterioration associated with one or more main symptoms, such as recurrent visual hallucinations, fluctuations in attention and consciousness, movement disorders, and REM sleep behavior disorder.

The cognitive impairment presents with compromised attention, executive functions, visual perception, and visuospatial abilities. In the early stages, memory and language appear to be preserved. Attention deficits can be detected through tests that assess speed of reasoning, sustained and divided attention, and reaction times. Visuoperceptual disturbances characterize the neuropsychological profile of these patients, particularly with difficulties in discriminating the shape or size of objects and identifying ill-defined or incomplete figures. These disturbances are more pronounced in patients who also experience visual hallucinations. The predisposition to produce visual hallucinations can be revealed by the occurrence of pareidolia (tendency to perceive familiar shapes in random objects or patterns). Visuospatial alterations involve difficulties in perceiving depth and object relationships and can be detected in tests such as complex figure copying, the pentagon test, discriminating line orientations, or assembly tasks.

A characteristic feature of these patients is the spontaneous fluctuation in vigilance, attention, or cognitive states, which can occur over a period of hours or days. Episodes may manifest as incongruous behaviors, illogical speech, confabulations, attentional impairments, or alterations in consciousness (recognized by episodes of fixed gaze or moments of "absence" or drowsiness).

Movement disorders more commonly present as a parkinsonian syndrome with akinesia and rigidity rather than resting tremor, and they have a more symmetric presentation compared to Parkinson's disease (PD). These symptoms are often associated with severe postural instability, leading to frequent falls. Dopaminergic medication therapy is less effective in treating these symptoms compared to PD.

Visual hallucinations represent another major symptom of DLB. They are usually recurrent, well-formed, occur in the central visual field, and predominantly involve seeing insects, other animals, or people. In the early stages, patients may retain partial insight into their hallucinations, while in later stages, this capacity diminishes, and hallucinations are often accompanied by delusions. The exact mechanism responsible for the occurrence of visual hallucinations is still unclear. It is possible that there is a reduction in cholinergic subcortical projections from the brainstem to the visual system. Alternatively, there may be a specific dysfunction of the ventral visual system due to neuropathological changes. A 2011 study hypothesized an alteration in the integration between the dorsal attention network, ventral attention network, and the default mode network, in which the dorsal attention network fails to activate correctly in the presence of ambiguous visual stimuli, allowing intrusion of default mode network contents and the emergence of hallucinations.

REM Sleep Behavior Disorder (RBD) is characterized by vivid dreams and the absence of the typical muscle atonia during this sleep phase. In fact, patients "act out" their dreams by shouting and moving energetically, posing a risk of self-injury or injury to their bed partners. RBD can appear many years before cognitive impairment and seems to be associated with the accumulation of Lewy bodies in the brainstem, which damage the pontine cholinergic and noradrenergic cortical projections.

Other supportive features of DLB include: hypersensitivity to antipsychotic drugs, autonomic dysfunction, hypersomnia, hyposmia, hallucinations with sensory modalities other than visual, delusions, apathy, anxiety, and depression. Hypersensitivity to neuroleptic drugs manifests as severe paradoxical reactions, worsening of motor symptoms, and increased risk of mortality. The most frequent autonomic dysfunctions include orthostatic hypotension, syncope, postural instability with a history of frequent falls, urinary incontinence, constipation, and impotence.

In 2020, diagnostic criteria were defined for the prodromal phase of DLB, currently limited to research settings pending validation for clinical practice. Classically, the prodromal phase of DLB has been defined as mild cognitive impairment (MCI) associated with one or more main DLB symptoms. The mild cognitive alterations of MCI-DLB typically involve attentional, executive, and visuospatial abilities, with relative preservation of memory.

Diagnostic tools

Magnetic resonance imaging (MRI) shows a relative sparing of temporo-mesial regions compared to Alzheimer's disease (AD). However, a specific pattern of atrophy for this form of dementia has not yet been identified.

Functional neuroimaging techniques such as single-photon emission computed tomography (SPECT) or positron emission tomography (PET) with fluorodeoxyglucose show hypoperfusion/hypometabolism in posterior regions, particularly the occipital lobes.

Dopamine transporter (DAT) scan reveals reduced striatal uptake and has high sensitivity and specificity, proving useful in the differential diagnosis with AD.

Myocardial scintigraphy demonstrates reduced uptake of 123I-metaiodobenzyl-guanidine (MIBG), a norepinephrine analog, and is adequately sensitive in discriminating from other forms of dementia, although the same finding can be present in elderly patients due to cardiac comorbidities.

Polysomnography can be useful in documenting REM sleep disorder and lack of atonia.

Electroencephalogram (EEG) shows specific abnormalities in posterior derivations, including a slowing of background rhythm, pre-alpha activity with periodic theta and delta activity. This pattern of alterations is highly specific and has a high predictive value. It is related to symptom severity and cognitive fluctuations and can also be observed in the early stages of mild cognitive impairment (MCI).

The diagnostic criteria for DLB were recently redefined (2017) based on cardinal symptoms, suggestive features, and indicative/suggestive biomarkers. The probable diagnosis requires the presence of at least two cardinal symptoms with or without suggestive criteria, or one cardinal symptom associated with one or more suggestive criteria. Supportive criteria include hypersensitivity to antipsychotic drugs, postural instability, history of frequent falls, syncope, autonomic dysfunction, hypersomnia, hyposmia, hallucinations with sensory modalities other than visual, delusions, apathy, anxiety, and depression. Indicative biomarkers include reduced dopamine uptake in the basal ganglia demonstrated by SPECT or PET, reduced tracer uptake in myocardial scintigraphy, and polysomnography revealing REM sleep disorder. Other biomarkers include relative preservation of medial temporal lobe structures on MRI, reduced cerebral metabolism in posterior brain regions (occipital, cingulate cortex), and specific EEG alterations.

16.2.3 Parkinson's dementia

Parkinson's Dementia (PDD) is characterized by a progressive cognitive disorder that arises within the context of Parkinson's disease (PD): cognitive symptoms must, in fact, appear at least one year after the onset of motor symptoms. This "one-year rule" represents an arbitrary temporal criterion but is widely used to differentiate PDD from Dementia with Lewy Bodies (DLB), in which cognitive symptoms must appear concurrently or earlier than motor symptoms. However, the one-year criterion is currently under revision.

PDD has a high prevalence in PD, reaching up to 80%, and increases proportionally with the duration of the disease. Other risk factors include being over 70 years of age, having the akinetic-rigid phenotype, and experiencing severe motor symptoms.

Clinical picture

The cognitive impairment in this form is similar to that found in DLB and is characterized by impaired attention, executive functions, memory, visuospatial abilities, and the presence of neuropsychiatric disturbances. Two main neuropsychological profiles can be distinguished within PDD. The first profile shows pronounced difficulties in executive functions, planning abilities, and working memory. This profile, more common in the early stages of cognitive decline (Mild Cognitive Impairment - MCI), is associated mainly with the tremor-dominant phenotype of PD and reflects dopaminergic depletion not only in the nigrostriatal system, responsible for motor symptoms, but also in the frontostriatal circuit, resulting in cognitive dysfunction, emotional changes, and motivation. The second profile, characterized by deficits in visuospatial functions and semantic fluency, is associated with impairment in posterior cortical and temporal regions and is related to a more rapid cognitive decline.

Similar to DLB, visual hallucinations, REM sleep behavior disorder, and behavioral disturbances such as apathy, depression, anxiety, and autonomic dysfunction can be observed in PDD.

Treatment

For cognitive symptoms, acetylcholinesterase inhibitors (AChEIs) are used, which have shown efficacy in overall cognitive decline. Memantine can be used as monotherapy or in combination with AChEIs, with a good level of tolerability and moderate benefits.

For the treatment of neuropsychiatric disturbances, AChEIs are used, as they have demonstrated effectiveness in treating apathy, visual hallucinations, and delusions. Since anxiety and agitation often result from psychosis, the use of AChEIs can also secondary improve these symptoms.

Considering the hypersensitivity to neuroleptics, typical of this disease, such medications should be used with caution, at effective minimum doses and for short durations, with a preference for quetiapine and clozapine. The use of dopamine for the treatment of extrapyramidal symptoms is less effective compared to what is observed in PD and should be employed cautiously due to the risk of exacerbating psychotic symptoms.

16.2.4 Frontotemporal dementias

Frontotemporal dementias (FTDs) constitute a heterogeneous group of neurodegenerative diseases characterized by the following:

1) Frequent familial aggregation and early onset;
2) Predominant involvement, at a neuropathological level, of the frontal and temporal regions of both cerebral hemispheres;
3) Prevalence of affective-behavioral disturbances, language impairments, and executive function deficits;
4) Preservation of memory and visuospatial functions in the early stages of the disease;
5) Frequent association with motor neuron diseases (MND) and parkinsonism.

FTDs collectively represent the third leading cause of neurodegenerative dementia (after Alzheimer's disease and dementia with Lewy bodies) and account for a high percentage (up to 25%) of cases of presenile dementia. Onset typically occurs between the ages of 45 and 65.

Genetics and neuropathology

A family history of dementia is reported by 40% of patients with FTD, although a pattern of autosomal dominant inheritance is recognizable in only a small percentage of cases. Approximately 60% of all hereditary forms are supported by mutations in the C9orf72, MAPT (encoding the tau microtubule-associated protein), and GRN (encoding progranulin) genes.

From a neuropathological perspective, FTDs are macroscopically characterized by neuronal rarefaction and gliosis affecting the frontal and anterior temporal lobes, the anterior and insular cingulate cortex, often with asymmetric distribution (right vs. left forms). In some cases, a bilateral atrophy affecting the anterior cerebral regions, known as "knife-edge atrophy," can be identified instead. The combination of these neurodegenerative changes is often referred to as Frontotemporal Lobar Degeneration (FTLD) and can be found in other pathologically related conditions, clinically and neurobiologically associated with FTD, such as Progressive Supranuclear Palsy, Corticobasal Degeneration, and forms of FTD associated with motor neuron disease. FTLD can be further classified based on the immunohistochemical characteristics of the proteins composing the intracellular deposits found in neurons. The most common subtypes of FTLD are (■ Figure 16.4):

- FTLD-Tau: also known as taupathies. They are characterized by inclusions consisting of hyperphosphorylated forms of the tau

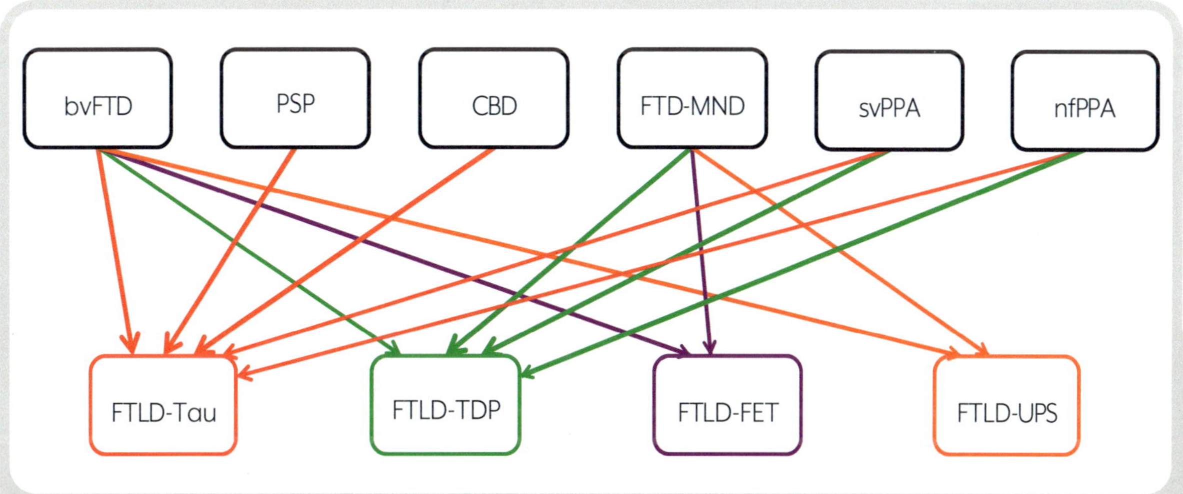

Figure 16.4

protein (known as "Pick bodies"), which differ in deposition pattern and organization from the neurofibrillary tangles typically observed in Alzheimer's disease. These findings are seen in the majority of cases of behavioral variant FTD, Progressive Supranuclear Palsy (PSP), and Corticobasal Degeneration (CBD), while they are less consistent in the language variants.

- FTLD-TDP: characterized by intracellular accumulation of TDP-43, a ribonucleoprotein involved in mRNA processing, stabilization, and transport. TDP-related pathology can be associated with phenotypic presentations of bvFTD, nfvPPA, svPPA, and CBD, and is commonly observed in forms associated with motor neuron disease.
- FTLD-FET: characterized by the presence of cytoplasmic inclusions of FUS protein, a DNA/RNA binding protein. It is predominantly associated with bvFTD and FTD with motor neuron disease.

Clinical presentation

FTDs are classified into three main variants based on clinical features (Figure 16.5):

Behavioural variant frontotemporal dementia (bvFTD) | This is the most common form characterized by changes in personality and behavior, which are present from the early stages. These changes primarily include emotional blunting, apathy/inertia, indifference, disinhibition, and irritability. Behavioral disinhibition can lead to inappropriate actions (such as approaching strangers without regard for physical and social boundaries), personal and interpersonal conduct disorders, impulsive behaviors, and occasionally, dangerous actions. Patients often exhibit a loss of understanding and empathy towards family and friends, as well as a lack of awareness of their own behaviors. Executive function deficits are also common, including easy distractibility, difficulties in planning

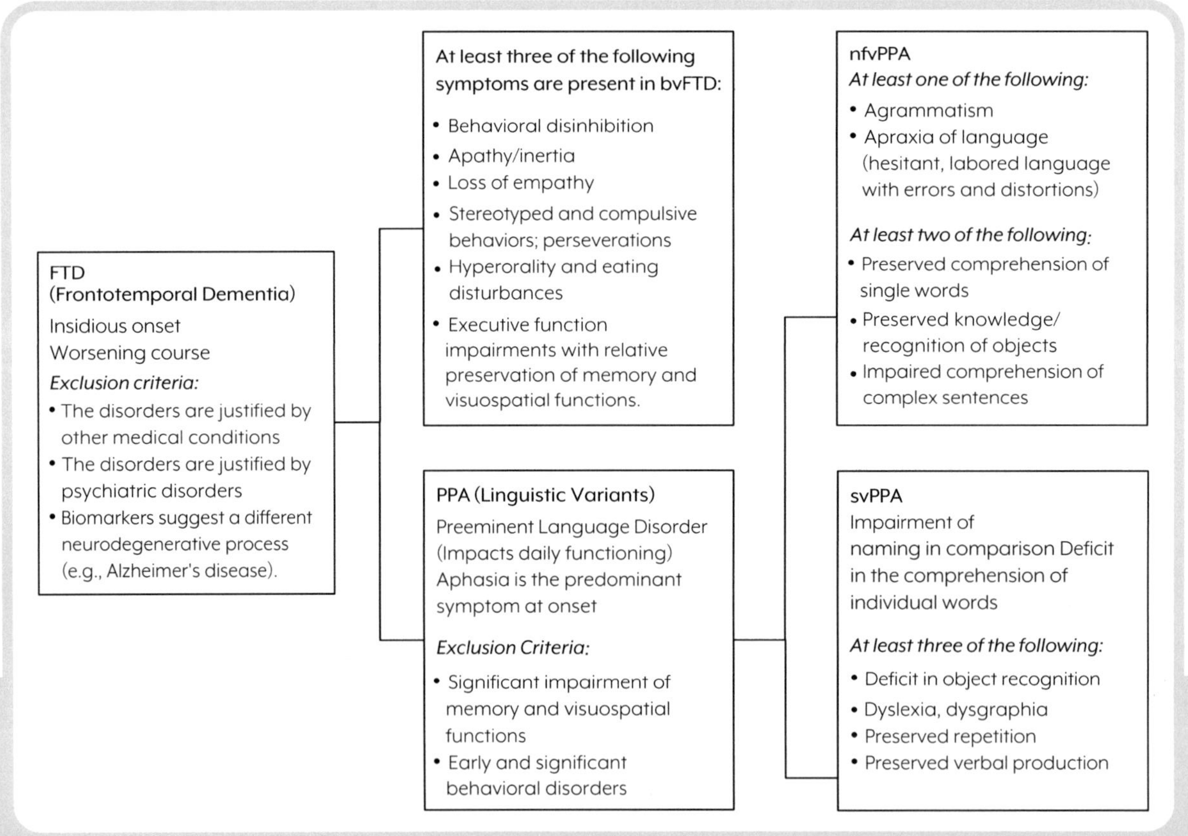

Figure 16.5

and organizing. Sensory disturbances, mainly alterations in pain perception, are frequently observed.

Non-fluent variant primary progressive aphasia (nfvPPA) | The most relevant clinical feature is a progressive language impairment characterized by reduced verbal fluency (leading to mutism), omission or reduction of grammatical structures (agrammatism), and phonemic paraphasias. Speech is slow, laborious, hesitant, with insertions, deletions, substitutions, transpositions, and distortions (language apraxia). Writing, reading, repetition, and naming may also be impaired, although comprehension, except for complex sentences, is generally preserved. Behavioral disturbances tend to occur later and are milder compared to bvFTD.

Semantic variant primary progressive aphasia | In this variant, language impairment predominates, but it is fluent (often verbose), poorly communicative, and characterized by paragrammatism, semantic paraphasias, neologisms, and a marked deficit in comprehension. Echolalia and palilalia may also be present. Behavioral and executive function impairments are more frequent than in the non-fluent variant and are associated with involvement of the non-dominant hemisphere.

The occurrence of motor neuron disease (MND), manifested by signs of involvement of the upper (hyperreflexia, Babinski sign, spasticity) and/or lower motor neurons (atrophy, fasciculations) and/or bulbar region (dysarthria, dysphagia), is documented in 10-15% of patients with bvFTD, while it is less commonly found in the language variants. Parkinsonism is described in 20% of cases.

The three variants of FTD can only be distinguished in the early stages of the disease. As the neurodegenerative process and cognitive decline progress (which also extends to mnemonic and visuospatial functions), the differentiation of the different clinical phenotypes becomes extremely complicated. The main problems of differential diagnosis at onset arise with psychiatric disorders (regarding bvFTD) and with the logopenic variant of AD (regarding nfvPPA and svPPA).

Instrumental exams

In bvFTD, a pattern of atrophy (via CT or MRI) and hypometabolism (PET) is observed, affecting the frontal and anterior lobes to varying degrees and distribution. The language variants, on the other hand, are characterized by the presence of atrophy/hypometabolism in the frontal and temporal regions of the dominant hemisphere (nfvPPA) and the temporal poles (svPPA).

Therapy

At the moment, there are no specific treatments for FTD. The management of affective and behavioral disturbances can rely, albeit with varying efficacy, on different classes of psychoactive drugs such as SSRIs, neuroleptics, and antiepileptics used as mood stabilizers.

16.2.5 Atypical parkinsonisms

This term defines a heterogeneous group of neurodegenerative disorders characterized by the association of parkinsonism, cognitive decline, and other signs and symptoms. Progressive supranuclear palsy and corticobasal degeneration, which neuropathologically belong to the group of tauopathies, and multiple system atrophy, which is a synucleinopathy, are considered (see also the chapter on movement disorders).

Progressive supranuclear palsy is characterized by oculomotor dysfunction, particularly vertical gaze palsy, postural instability, axial rigidity, and a pseudobulbar syndrome (dysarthria, dysphonia, dysphagia). This syndrome may exhibit cognitive decline characterized by ideational slowing, difficulties in processing information, deficits in attention, abstraction, and reasoning abilities, phonemic verbal fluency (letter-based), and executive functions. It may also be associated with neuropsychiatric disorders such as apathy, depression, dysphoria, anxiety, and irritability. These deficits can be attributed to alterations in frontostriatal networks.

Corticobasal degeneration involves the basal ganglia and cortical areas in the neuropathological process, often with a strong asymmetric presentation. A characteristic sign of this condition is the involvement of an upper limb, which appears apraxic in the absence of motor or sensory deficits. Ideomotor apraxia (inability to perform a task on command or imitation) and ideational apraxia (inability to use objects) predominantly affect the right limb. Other cognitive manifestations include acalculia, gaze apraxia, orofacial apraxia, non-fluent aphasia, and deficits in executive functions. Visuospatial function impairments can also be observed due to involvement of the dorsal visual pathway, sometimes presenting as Balint's syndrome (simultaneous agnosia, optic ataxia, optic apraxia). These disturbances reflect atrophy of the parietal and frontal regions, while the occipital and temporal regions may be spared.

Involvement of cognitive functions leading to a picture of frank dementia is unusual in MSA, where selective impairment of executive functions or the onset of behavioral disturbances may be observed. However, sleep disturbance with REM sleep behavior disorder is common in this syndrome, as well as in other synucleinopathies.

16.2.6 Huntington's disease

Huntington's disease is characterized by motor symptoms (chorea), cognitive symptoms (dementia), and neuropsychiatric symptoms. Cognitive impairments involve deficits in executive functions, planning and reasoning abilities, as well as attention deficits, especially in set-shifting tasks. Memory difficulties, particularly in recall capacity, prospective memory, and procedural memory, are also present. These deficits are caused by frontal dysfunctions and are attributed to alterations in the frontostriatal network. Language deficits manifest as a progressive loss of verbal fluency, with increasingly unintelligible speech, partly due to motor impairments. Deficits in visuospatial functions and perceptual integration may also occur. Emotional dysfunctions, particularly in interpreting facial expressions, have been reported. In terms of neuropsychiatric disturbances, apathy, irritability, depression, and loss of inhibitory control over impulses are typical. Aggression and personality changes may also be present.

16.3 Secondary dementias

16.3.1 Vascular cognitive disorders

Vascular cognitive disorders occur in patients with cerebrovascular diseases and can present as either mild cognitive impairment (MCI) or vascular dementia (VaD). VaD is the second leading cause of dementia in Western countries, accounting for approximately 15-20% of all cases as "pure" forms. Vascular damage, whether ischemic, hemorrhagic, or vasculitic, is the most important underlying pathogenic mechanism. Frequently, degenerative alterations resembling those found in Alzheimer's disease (AD) coexist with vascular damage. The coexistence of neurodegenerative and vascular pathogenic mechanisms forms the basis of mixed dementia, a condition that, based on autopsy studies, is estimated to have a prevalence of 10-30%.

VaD shares the same risk factors as cardiovascular diseases, including advanced age, hypertension, diabetes mellitus, dyslipidemia, obesity, smoking, cardiac rhythm abnormalities, prior ischemic or hemorrhagic cerebrovascular events, and hyperhomocysteinemia. According to the NINDS-AIREN international criteria, VaD is characterized by the presence of:

1) Cognitive deterioration not attributable to other causes;
2) Cerebrovascular disease defined by focal neurological signs and brain lesions visible on CT or MRI;
3) Temporal relationship between the cerebrovascular event and the onset of cognitive deterioration and/or sudden onset of deterioration and/or stepwise progression of deterioration.

Early development of gait disturbances, frequent falls, signs and symptoms of pseudobulbar syndrome, and executive function impairment are supportive clinical features for the diagnosis. Definitive diagnosis is achieved through autopsy, which reveals typical vascular damage, including infarcts, subcortical white matter changes (demyelination, axonal loss, fibrosis), and cortical-subcortical atrophy. In pure forms, histological alterations typical of other degenerative pathologies should be absent. In mixed forms, coexistence of Alzheimer's-type alterations (senile plaques and neurofibrillary tangles) may be observed.

VaD can be classified based on the type of causative vascular damage:

1) ***involvement of large arterial vessels***
   a) Multifocal infarction: The damage is caused by the involvement of medium and large-sized arterial vessels. VaD can occur as a result of single or multiple infarctions in territories directly supplied by a main arterial trunk or in the border zones between them. According to the NINCDS AIREN criteria, a diagnosis of VaD can be made for larger ischemic lesions if they are bilateral or located in the dominant hemisphere.
   b) Strategic infarcts: Vascular damage does not involve extensive areas of the brain but rather important areas that are crucial for proper cognitive functioning. Typically, it depends on the involvement of medium-sized arterial trunks. Infarcts in the thalamus can manifest with attentional disturbances, ideomotor slowing, aphasia, amnesia, and behavioral disorders, particularly affecting the emotional sphere. Involvement of the angular gyrus can result in a fluent aphasia syndrome, apraxia, memory deficits, and disorientation. Bilateral lesions of the hippocampus can lead to the sudden onset of an amnesic syndrome.
2) ***Subcortical ischemic VaD:*** The damage affects cerebral arterioles that branch off from major trunks near the basal ganglia and thalamus or arise from the pia mater to supply the cortex and underlying white matter. Neuroimaging reveals generally diffuse ischemic damage predominantly localized at the subcortical level. The lesions accumulate in the deep white matter and around the lateral ventricles (leukoaraiosis), usually starting from the poles. On MRI, the lesions appear hyperintense on FLAIR sequences, with a punctate appearance in mild forms. In moderate and severe forms, white matter changes progress and diffuse confluent lesions may occur. Lacunar infarcts may also be present. Subcortical ischemic VaD also encompasses nosological entities previously included under the term "Binswanger's disease".

Clinical picture

VaD can manifest with extremely heterogeneous clinical presentations depending on the cerebral areas involved in the vascular lesion. The onset of cognitive decline is often sudden and may be related to a previous cerebrovascular event. The course is typically "stepped," with alternating phases of stability, sometimes prolonged, and phases of worsening. This type of progression correlates with the progression of the disease and the accumulation of brain lesions. The clinical examination may reveal focal neurological signs due to involvement of the pyramidal or sensory system. If the basal ganglia and deeper subcortical regions are affected, movement disorders and pseudobulbar signs may occur. Often there are also alterations in gait and sphincter disturbances. Cognitively, the severity of deficits is typically related to the topography and extent of the vascular lesions: deficits in language and visuospatial skills, apraxia, and agnosia characterize forms with predominant cortical involvement, while in subcortical ischemic VaD, executive deficits (prefrontal) predominate. Less frequently, the patient may exhibit an amnesic syndrome similar to that found in AD. The presence of affective and behavioral disturbances is very common. These include depression, apathy, abulia, emotional lability, dysphoria, and aggression. The use of dedicated scales such as the Hachinski Scale (see Box 16.4) is very useful in the differential diagnosis with degenerative dementias.

Instrumental examinations

Neuroimaging plays a crucial role in the diagnosis. CT and MRI allow for the

Box 16.4 HACHINSKI SCALE AND FAZEKAS SCORE

The quantification of the "vascular component" in the determinism of cognitive deficits is essential in the diagnostic phase of dementia. Often, patients with a clinical diagnosis of Alzheimer's disease (AD) present chronic ischemic vascular lesions in the white matter of the brain on neuroimaging, which may require a differential diagnosis compared to Vascular Dementia (VaD) or mixed forms. In these cases, Hachinski's Ischemic Scale and Fazekas Score can be extremely useful tools.

Hachinski's Scale is calculated based on the collection of specific clinical information and the neurological examination of the patient. It consists of 13 items to which a score of 1 or 2 is assigned depending on the presence or absence of anamnestic data and signs and symptoms suggestive of cerebrovascular disease.

This scale is useful for making a differential diagnosis between degenerative and vascular genesis of cognitive decline. The higher the score, the greater the estimated weight of the vascular component. A diagnosis of AD is compatible with a score ≤ 4 on the Hachinski Scale, while higher scores suggest a vascular etiology of the disorders.

The Fazekas Score is assigned by visualizing MRI images acquired in transverse planes with FLAIR sequence. This score is used to quantify the extent of vascular alterations in the cerebral white matter. The absence of appreciable vascular lesions corresponds to a score of "0" on the scale. The presence of mild focal lesions is rated as "1," multiple lesions tending to coalesce are rated as "2" (moderate grade), and widespread involvement of the white matter corresponds to a score of "3" (severe grade). The absence of detectable vascular lesions or mild involvement (Fazekas score < 2) is compatible with the diagnosis of AD.

Hachinski Scale

- Acute onset (2 points) ☐
- Stepwise deterioration (1 point) ☐
- Fluctuation of symptoms (2 points) ☐
- Nocturnal confusion (1 point) ☐
- Relative preservation of personality (1 point) ☐
- Depression (1 point) ☐
- Somatic disturbances (non-focal neurological signs and symptoms) (1 point) ☐
- Emotional lability (spastic laughing and crying) (1 point) ☐
- History of hypertension (1 point) ☐
- Previous cerebral stroke (2 points) ☐
- Lateralized focal symptoms (2 points) ☐
- Lateralized focal signs (2 points) ☐
- Signs of atherosclerosis in other districts (e.g., heart, major arteries) (2 points) ☐

Total:

localization of lesions, distinction of their characteristics (ischemia, hemorrhage, vasculitis), and assessment of their size. FLAIR images, in particular, are used to estimate the cerebrovascular lesion burden in dementia patients and are extremely helpful in the differential diagnosis (Fazekas score). Functional investigations such as FDG-PET and SPECT are rarely employed in VaD. In the subcortical form, they may demonstrate heterogeneous cortico-subcortical hypometabolism/hypoperfusion ("leopard spot" pattern). In certain multi-infarct or strategic infarct forms, hypofunction may be more evident in the frontal region due to deafferentation caused by damage to subcortical gray structures (e.g., the thalamus).

Therapy

There is no specific therapy for VaD. Drugs used in AD such as AChE inhibitors and memantine have been tested in this type of dementia but with limited or no benefits. For this reason, none of these substances are indicated in this type of pathology. Control of cardiovascular risk factors remains the main therapeutic approach in VaD, aiming to achieve control and stabilization of the clinical picture.

16.3.2 Normotensive hydrocephalus

Normotensive Hydrocephalus (NPH) is a clinical syndrome characterized by a specific triad of symptoms:

1) Disturbance in gait;
2) Cognitive deterioration;
3) Urinary incontinence.

This triad is associated with the presence of marked dilation of the cerebral ventricular system and normal cerebrospinal fluid pressure. Epidemiologically, NPH has a low prevalence, accounting for approximately 1% of all dementias.

Pathogenesis

The pathogenetic mechanisms underlying NPH are related to an alteration in the cerebrospinal fluid circulation system, resulting in an imbalance between the production and reabsorption of cerebrospinal fluid, leading to an excessive accumulation of fluid within the ventricular system. NPH belongs to the group of communicating hydrocephalus.

Clinical presentation

The complete triad of symptoms is observed in 50-75% of cases. The most common symptom is cognitive deterioration, present in up to 95% of cases, while urinary incontinence occurs in up to 75%. Gait disturbance is the most frequent symptom at onset, followed by cognitive deficits. Finally, urinary incontinence appears, sometimes preceded by urgency. The gait disturbance is characterized by small, hesitant steps, difficulty in changing direction, resulting in instability and an increased risk of falls. This presentation shares similarities with Parkinson's disease. Additionally, apraxia of gait (likely due to frontal lobe dysfunction) and, in some cases, broad-based ataxia can often be observed in NPH. Cognitive deficits in NPH can range from mild ideational slowing to overt subcortical dementia. Memory, attention, and executive functions are predominantly affected, while the presence of apraxia, agnosia, and aphasia is rarer. These alterations are associated with difficulties in concentration, emotional instability, irritability, and apathy. Genuine urinary incontinence typically presents later, but signs of urgency may appear early. The cause of urinary incontinence is attributed to the mechanical effect exerted by cerebrospinal fluid on the periventricular nerve fibers, resulting in the loss of supraspinal (voluntary) control over bladder contraction.

Instrumental examinations

Neuroimaging is the most important tool in the diagnosis of NPH. CT, but particularly MRI, allows for confirming the presence of hydrocephalus, characterized by a marked enlargement of the cerebral ventricles that is disproportionate to the degree of atrophy (increase in subarachnoid spaces) that may be present. The calculation of the Evans index (the ratio between the size of the frontal horn of the lateral ventricle and the size of the intracranial cavity at the same level) enables the diagnosis of hydrocephalus for values above 0.30. Often, FLAIR scans reveal diffuse periventricular hyperintensity, partly due to transependymal resorption of cerebrospinal fluid. Lumbar puncture and cerebrospinal fluid withdrawal are useful to confirm normal pressure levels of the cerebrospinal fluid (between 18 and 20 cm of water) and to determine any improvement in the clinical picture associated with acute fluid subtraction (up to 100 ml). The evaluation of the effectiveness of the drainage procedure should be estimated by planning a clinical and neuropsychological assessment before the procedure and in the following hours. Significant improvement in gait or a significant increase in scores obtained from post-lumbar puncture tests would confirm the diagnosis of NPH.

Treatment

The treatment for NPH is surgical and involves two types of interventions:

1) ventriculoperitoneal shunting;
2) endoscopic ventriculostomy.

Shunting involves creating a communication between the lateral ventricles and the peritoneal cavity using a catheter with a valve. Ventriculostomy consists of surgically creating an opening in the floor of the third ventricle towards the prepontine cisterns. All these interventions aim to promote the drainage of cerebrospinal fluid outside the ventricular system in order to rebalance the production and absorption of the fluid.

16.3.3 Malattie da prioni

They are a heterogeneous group of rare pathologies characterized by the accumulation of abnormal proteins (Prion Protein, PrP) that are transmissible and clinically exhibit a rapidly progressive and fatal course. The estimated prevalence is 1 case per million inhabitants. Prion diseases can be classified into sporadic forms (Creutzfeldt-Jakob Disease, CJD), familial forms (Fatal Familial Insomnia, Gerstmann-Sträussler-Scheinker Syndrome, familial forms of CJD), and acquired forms (Kuru, Variant CJD or "Mad Cow Disease," also see Chapter on encephalitis).

Neuropathology

Prion diseases are characterized, from an anatomopathological perspective, by gliosis, neuronal loss, and a spongy appearance of the gray matter due to extensive microvacuolization. The distinctive feature of CJD is the presence of amyloid PrP plaques, which are more numerous in the frontotemporal cortex.

Clinical picture

CJD manifests between the fifth and seventh decade of life, with nonspecific psychiatric disorders (depression, apathy, anxiety disorders, emotional lability). Over the course of weeks, additional symptoms appear, including widespread cognitive decline that rapidly worsens, spontaneous or evoked myoclonus, cerebellar ataxia, pyramidal signs, movement disorders, and cortical visual disturbances (difficulties in recognizing three-dimensional objects, depth, and spatial relationships). The duration of the disease is approximately 6-12 months.

Gerstmann-Straussler-Scheinker syndrome is characterized by an earlier clinical onset and a predominance of dementia and ataxia. Unlike CJD, the clinical course is slowly progressive (the duration of the disease is about 7 years). The variant form of CJD, considered the human variant of bovine spongiform encephalopathy, affects individuals who are younger than those with CJD, presents with psychiatric manifestations that can be accompanied by significant sensory disturbances, and generally has a less rapid progression.

Fatal Familial Insomnia is characterized by the development of a progressive "malignant" form of insomnia, with a reduction, up to complete loss, of total sleep time. Severe dysautonomic disturbances are associated, including increased sympathetic activity, high levels of cortisol, and loss of circadian fluctuations in blood pressure and heart rate. Motor and balance disturbances occur, and in the terminal stages, dementia. This rare familial prion disease selectively affects the anteroventral and mediodorsal thalamic nuclei.

Diagnostic tests

In the case of CJD, MRI can reveal hyperintensity areas in the putamen and head of the caudate nucleus on T2-weighted sequences, which are associated with increased signal intensity, even in diffusion-weighted sequences, likely due to reduced water diffusivity caused by endoneuronal microvacuolization. CJD is characterized by EEG abnormalities that vary during the course of the disease, with the most characteristic findings being periodic sharp-wave complexes (1-2 cycles per second). Analysis of cerebrospinal fluid may show slight hyperproteinorrachia and, with specific methods, demonstrate the presence of the 14-3-3 protein (a neuronal cytoplasmic protein), whose detection in patients with clinical suspicion of CJD is associated with a high predictive value (97%) for the disease. However, it should be noted that this protein can also be found in other pathological conditions such as viral encephalitis, acute-phase ischemic strokes, certain metabolic encephalopathies, brain tumors, and paraneoplastic encephalopathies. The presence of the prion protein can also be detected from cells of the olfactory mucosa obtained through a brush test.

Therapy

Currently, there are no available treatments capable of modifying the natural history of these conditions or providing significant symptomatic benefit.

16.3.4 Alcohol-related dementia

It represents one of the most frequent causes of early-onset dementia and is classified among "reversible" dementias due to the possibility of partial remission, usually with abstinence. It often manifests as a dysexecutive syndrome or diffuse cognitive impairment and can be associated with other manifestations of alcohol abuse such as liver disease, peripheral neuropathy, and macrocytic anemia. In addition to alcoholic dementia, there are several clinical syndromes related to alcohol abuse: Wernicke's syndrome (caused by thiamine deficiency, with oculomotor disturbances), Marchiafava-Bignami disease (characterized by corpus callosum and cerebellar damage), and Korsakoff's psychosis (often associated with abstinence: characterized by recent memory disturbances, confabulations, and hypomania).

16.3.5 HIV/AIDS-related dementia

It is a complication that affects approximately one-third of HIV infection cases. It manifests as rapidly progressive cognitive decline (weeks or months) characterized by attention, abstraction, language, and memory deficits. Most cases also present with pyramidal signs, myoclonus, and behavioral disturbances (agitation, apathy, depression, anxiety, mania). MRI scans may show cortico-subcortical atrophy, subcortical white matter alterations, and features indicative of other HIV-related conditions (such as focal lesions from various opportunistic infections, progressive multifocal leukoencephalopathy, etc.).

16.3.6 "Reversible" dementias

This term is used to describe various forms of cognitive decline primarily caused by metabolic, nutritional, or organ insufficiency disorders. These conditions are characterized by the potential for clinical remission, although often incomplete, after the resolution of the underlying disease process (Table 16.1). Despite their low incidence, they should always be considered in the diagnostic evaluation of cognitive decline due to the potential response to timely treatments.

16.4 Behavioral disorders

Behavioral and psychological symptoms of dementia (BPSD) refer to a heterogeneous group of psychiatric symptoms and atypical behaviors that occur in patients with dementia. BPSD encompasses disturbances in perception, thought content, mood, and behavior. These disturbances are now considered an integral part of the natural course of the disease.

It has been estimated that over 80% of dementia patients develop BPSD during the course of their illness. BPSD are included in the central diagnostic criteria for degenerative dementias such as Dementia with Lewy bodies (DLB) and Frontotemporal dementia (FTD), and they are suggestive criteria for Alzheimer's disease (AD) and Vascular dementia (VaD). Although these disturbances often occur in advanced stages of dementia, longitudinal studies have shown that the presence of behavioral symptoms is not necessarily associated with the degree of cognitive decline. A new nosological entity called *Mild Behavioural Impairment* (MBI) has recently been proposed, characterized by changes in personality or behavior, which may manifest as reduced motivation, affective dysregulation, loss of impulse control, social relationship inadequacy, and alterations in thinking or perception. In MBI, the disturbance must be present for at least 6 months and can be associated with Mild Cognitive Impairment (MCI) but not with established dementia. Behavioral disorders are typically grouped into five clusters: psychosis, affective sphere disorders, apathy, agitation, and behavioral alterations (Table 16.2).

Psychosis includes disorders of thought (i.e. delusions) and disorders of perception (i.e. hallucinations). Delusions consist of a false belief. The content of delusions in dementias is varied but simple: they involve small distortions or reworkings of real experiences. They are differentiated into paranoid and misidentification delusions. Among the former, we distinguish delusions of theft, persecution, infidelity, abandonment, or those with specific contents, such as the belief that deceased people are still alive. Misidentification delusions are often associated with alterations in the recognition or identification processes of familiar places and subjects, and with phenomena of altered interpretation of reality, such as the belief that one's own home is not one's own, that a family member is not who they claim to be and has been replaced by an imposter (Capgras syndrome), that the

Table 16.1

Etiology	Clinical presentation
Depressive pseudodementia	The primary affective disorder causes attention and working memory impairments and ideational slowing. Although there are differential diagnostic features compared to degenerative dementias, such as the acute/subacute onset, subjective accentuation of symptoms, presence of psychiatric history, generally preserved functional status, and cognitive impairment variably related to emotional state, recent research indicates that over 70% of patients with depressive disorder associated with cognitive impairment develop degenerative dementia in subsequent years. This data highlights the possibility that psychiatric symptoms may constitute the clinical onset of dementia. In other cases, pharmacological treatment allows for the resolution of the affective/cognitive disorder.
Postoperative cognitive dysfunction	Cognitive deterioration that occurs weeks or months after surgery in elderly patients with reduced cognitive reserve, characterized by involvement of various cognitive domains, mainly short-term memory and executive functions. Generally resolves spontaneously over varying periods and does not require specific treatment according to recent studies.
Hypothyroidism	Prominent attention and vigilance disturbances (hypersomnia), psychomotor slowing, irritability, and apathy. Possible progression to myxedema coma (characterized by marked hypothermia) if not treated with appropriate replacement therapy. In the context of Hashimoto's encephalopathy, seizures may also be present.
Hyperthyroidism	Psychiatric manifestations such as depression of mood, hypomanic episodes, and hallucinations may be present. There is also involvement of executive functions.
Hypocalcemia	Cognitive deficits predominantly involving subcortical organization, extrapyramidal symptoms, and seizure episodes. Neuroimaging may reveal widespread calcifications affecting the basal ganglia (Fahr's Syndrome).
Renal insufficiency	Gradual onset of asthenia, apathy, irritability, confusion, hallucinations, delirium, and may progress to uremic coma. "Dialysis dementia" is characterized by behavioral and personality disturbances, speech disturbances (mild dysphasia, stuttering, irregularities in vocal rhythm), and movement disorders.
Irespiratory insufficiency	Cognitive decline is associated only in the advanced stages when significant hypoxemia and hypercapnia are present. Deficits generally affect memory and executive functions.
Hepatic insufficiency	Progressive onset of neuropsychiatric symptoms (apathy, restlessness, mood depression or euphoria, alterations in sleep-wake cycle), cognitive deficits (memory and orientation disturbances), and motor symptoms (flapping tremor). In the advanced stages, vigilance disturbances may lead to coma.
Vitamin B12 and folic acid deficiency	Neuro-hematological syndromic picture characterized by cognitive deficits (predominantly in attention and executive functions), sometimes severe enough to qualify as a full-blown dementia, and affective-behavioral disturbances (irritability, suspiciousness, apathy, emotional lability, major depression), which are entirely reversible with proper supplementation.
Medications	Benzodiazepines (especially those with long half-lives), antipsychotics with marked anticholinergic action, tricyclic antidepressants, dopaminergic agonists, and antihistamines. Reversibility depends on the duration of exposure and various individual biological factors (concomitant pathologies, other medications taken, etc.).

reflection in the mirror is not one's own, that there are ghosts present, or that the people on television are actually present in the house. It is believed that there is involvement of the frontal (orbitofrontal), temporal, and salience network regions, which is the functional network that selects salient stimuli, typically involved in attentional, motivational, and executive tasks.

Table 16.2 BEHAVIORAL DISORDERS IN DEMENTIA

Clusters	Symptoms
Psychosis	Delusions Hallucinations
Apathy	Loss of interests Emotional flatness
Disorders of affective sphere	Depression Anxiety
Agitation	Aggressiveness Irritability
Behavioral disinhibition	Aberrant motor activity Exaltation/euphoria Sleep disorders Appetite disorders Hypersexuality

Hallucinations in dementias are predominantly visual and sometimes auditory. Visual hallucinations have phenomenological characteristics that differ depending on the clinical context of presentation: in AD, for example, they are represented by familiar or unfamiliar human figures, animals (predominantly insects), or objects of various kinds, and are interpreted as secondary alterations due to perceptual disturbance or an inability to attribute the correct meaning to the perceived stimulus. In DLB, visual hallucinations and perceptual phenomena in

Box 16.5 COGNITIVE DISORDERS AND COVID-19

COVID-19 (Coronavirus Disease 2019) is a systemic illness caused by the SARS-CoV-2 virus, characterized by bilateral interstitial pneumonia in its most severe forms, which can lead to complications affecting multiple organs, including the nervous system. Neurological manifestations can occur during the acute phase, sometimes persisting, or manifesting at the end of the infection or even several weeks later. These manifestations can last for weeks or months or continue as long-term sequelae. Among the acute manifestations, alterations in consciousness or mental status and sudden personality changes have been described. "The dysexecutive syndrome" is one of the specific cognitive alterations observed during COVID-19 infection. This condition is characterized by attention deficits, disorientation, and difficulty in controlling voluntary movements. Complications during the acute phases may also include neuropsychiatric symptoms such as insomnia, anxiety, post-traumatic stress disorder, psychosis, and mood disorders. The condition where symptoms persist beyond recovery is called "long COVID". The most frequent manifestation here is the so-called "brain fog," which can present with multiple symptoms such as difficulty concentrating, disorientation, cognitive impairments, and associated psychiatric disorders. The main cognitive impairments consist of alterations in executive functions, processing speed, verbal fluency, and memory difficulties. The underlying pathogenic mechanisms are not yet fully understood. Among the hypothesized mechanisms are direct infection of the central nervous system (CNS) by the virus, which can reach nervous tissue through retrograde diffusion starting from the olfactory nerve, or through hematogenous spread. Other possible mechanisms include ischemic damage due to endothelial dysfunction or coagulation abnormalities, inflammation, acute respiratory distress syndrome (ARDS), and the use of invasive ventilation.

COVID-19 and DEMENTIA

Although the virus affects individuals of all ages, the elderly population has been most severely affected by the pandemic, especially if they already suffer from other chronic conditions, including dementia. Dementia, in fact, represents a risk factor for COVID-19. Patients with dementia are at higher risk of contracting the disease due to difficulties in adhering to measures to avoid contagion, such as social distancing, and the need for constant care that does not allow for physical distancing. COVID-19 can present with atypical symptoms in these patients, such as confusion, agitation, disorientation, and loss of appetite, leading to delays in timely diagnosis and consequently worse outcomes. Precautions taken to avoid contagion in people with dementia have also led to periods of social isolation, which have worsened both cognitive and neuropsychiatric symptoms. COVID-19 itself can contribute to pathological damage in dementia and worsen cognitive decline. This may happen as a consequence of ischemic vascular damage from small vessel involvement, due to the hypercoagulable condition induced by the virus, or as a consequence of the inflammatory state. It has also been hypothesized that vascular/inflammatory damage may, in turn, contribute to the accumulation of pathological proteins such as amyloid and tau, as well as the accumulation of alpha-synuclein, typical of DLB (Dementia with Lewy Bodies).

general vary in their phenomenology depending on the stages of the disease. In the early stages, illusions, pareidolia (the tendency to perceive familiar shapes, objects, or profiles in random stimuli), and minor hallucinations are common, including "passage"hallucinations characterized by indistinct objects rapidly crossing the periphery of the visual field, and "presence" hallucinations characterized by the perception of someone being present nearby. In this phase, hallucinations may be correlated with involvement of the brainstem in the neuropathological process, particularly with the impairment of subcortical and cortical control systems of eye movements, as well as involvement of the secondary visual areas in the parietal lobe. In the later stages, visual hallucinations become more complex and organized, with content usually represented by visions of living or deceased individuals or animals.

The psychotic cluster is more frequently found in DLB, where the presence of visual hallucinations is one of the main symptoms for diagnosis. However, visual hallucinations are also very common in AD.

The disturbances of the affective sphere include depressive symptoms and anxiety. Depression is a condition frequently associated with dementia and, when already present in the MCI phase, represents a risk factor for conversion to dementia. It can be one of the first onset symptoms and may initially mask the cognitive decline process.

Apathy is the most frequently encountered behavioral disturbance in all forms of dementia and constitutes a separate cluster from affective disorders. It is characterized by a lack of motivation, absence of spontaneous behaviors, and emotional blunting. Apathy and depressive symptoms often coexist. The most sensitive symptoms to differentiate apathy from depression are indifference, emotional blunting, and lack of social relationships. Apathy is very common in the preclinical stages of dementia and has a greater predictive value than depressive symptoms for the development of established dementia. It is frequently observed in AD and PDD. From a neurobiological perspective, it is associated with impairment of regions such as the anterior cingulate and subcortical frontal circuits. The anterior cingulate plays a role in integrating external and internal stimuli that, once processed, determine actions and behaviors aimed at achieving a goal and is involved in the brain network responsible for reward mechanisms, attentional functions, and goal-directed actions.

Agitation is a frequently encountered disturbance, particularly in Alzheimer's disease (AD), frontotemporal dementia (FTD), and dementia with Lewy bodies (DLB). Aggressive behavior, irritability, and loss of inhibitory control can also be present. Agitation is often associated with or a consequence of other behavioral disorders such as psychosis or depression. Dysfunction of the frontal regions appears to play an important role in its onset.

Among other behavioral disorders, sleep disturbances should be noted, especially rapid eye movement sleep behavior disorder (RBD), which involves active and physical participation of the individual in dreams (resulting in "acting out" of dreams). It is important to be aware of this disorder as it can precede the onset of DLB and Parkinson's disease (PD) by several years. Its presence has recently been included as a major diagnostic criterion for DLB and is correlated with the accumulation of Lewy bodies in the brainstem.

Bibliography

Spalletta G., Musicco M., Padovani A., Rozzini L., Perri R., Fadda L., Canonico V., Trequattrini A., Pettenati C., Caltagirone C., Palmer K. Neuropsychiatric Symptoms and Syndromes in a Large Cohort of Newly Diagnosed, Untreated Patients With Alzheimer Disease. Am J Geriatr Psychiatry. 2010;18:1026-35.

Trebbastoni A., Imbriano L., Podda L., Rendace L., Sacchetti M.L., Campanelli A., D'Antonio F., de Lena C. Cognitive Training in Patients with Alzheimer's Disease: Findings of a 12-month Randomized Controlled Trial. Curr Alzheimer Res. 2018 Mar 14;15(5):452-461.

Waters F., Collerton D., Ffytche D.H., Jardri R., Pins D., Dudley R., Blom J.D., Mosimann U.P., Eperjesi F., Ford S., Larøi F. visual hallucinations in the psychosis spectrum and comparative information from neurodegenerative disorders and eye disease. Schizophr Bull. 2014;40 Suppl 4:S233-45.

McKeith I.G., Ferman T.J., Thomas A.J., Blanc F., Boeve B.F., Fujishiro H., Kantarci K., Muscio C., O'Brien J.T., Postuma R.B., Aarsland D., Ballard C., Bonanni L., Donaghy P., Emre M., Galvin J.E., Galasko D., Goldman J.G., Gomperts S.N., Honig L.S., Ikeda M., Leverenz J.B., Lewis S.J.G., Marder K.S., Masellis M., Salmon D.P., Taylor J.P., Tsuang D.W., Walker Z., Tiraboschi P.; Prodromal DLB Diagnostic Study Group. Research criteria for the diagnosis of prodromal dementia with Lewy bodies. Neurology. 2020 Apr 28;94(17):743-755.

McKeith I.G., Ferman T.J., Thomas A.J., Blanc F., Boeve B.F., Fujishiro H., Kantarci K., Muscio C., O'Brien J.T., Postuma R.B., Aarsland D., Ballard C., Bonanni L., Donaghy P., Emre M., Galvin J.E., Galasko D., Goldman J.G., Gomperts S.N., Honig L.S., Ikeda M., Leverenz J.B., Lewis S.J.G., Marder K.S., Masellis M., Salmon D.P., Taylor J.P., Tsuang D.W., Walker Z., Tiraboschi P.; Prodromal DLB Diagnostic Study Group. Research criteria for the diagnosis of prodromal dementia with Lewy bodies. Neurology. 2020 Apr 28;94(17):743-755.

Hampshire A., Trender W., Chamberlain S., Jolly A., Grant J., Patrick F., Mazibuko N., Williams S., Barnby J., Hellyer P., Mehta M. Cognitive deficits in people who have recovered from COVID-19. EClinical Medicine. 2021;39:101044.

17 MULTIPLE SCLEROSIS

Marco Salvetti, Giulia Coarelli, Silvia Romano, Antonella Conte

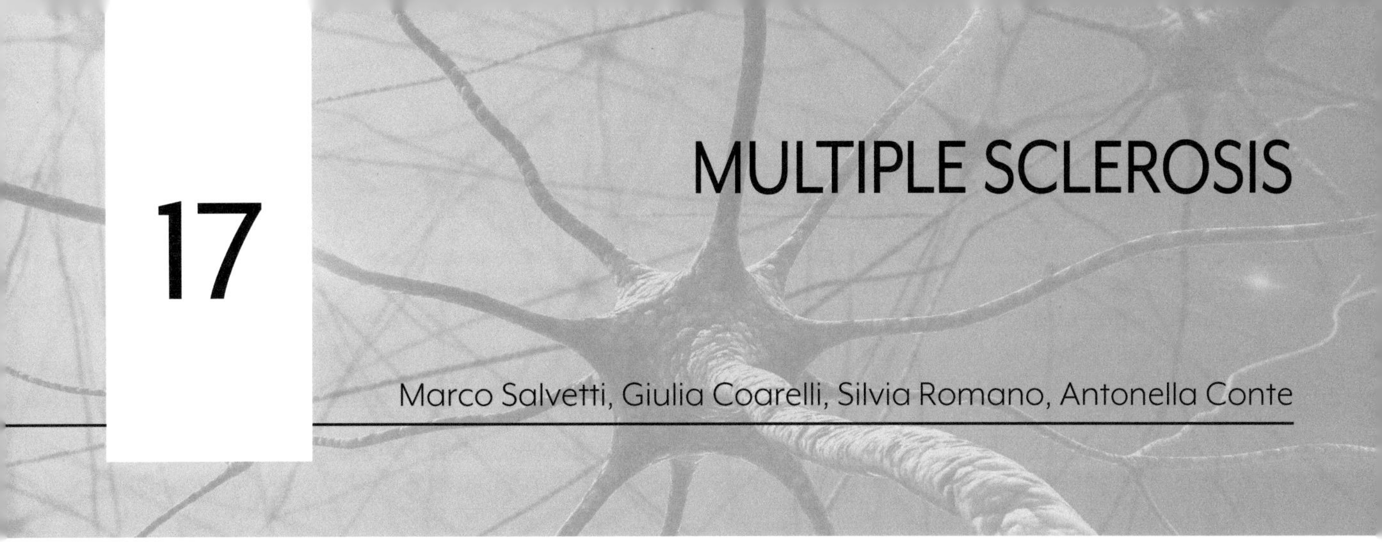

17.1 Etiology

Multiple Sclerosis (MS) is the leading cause of progressive neurological disability. It is a chronic inflammatory demyelinating disease that affects the central nervous system. The etiology likely involves environmental factors, genetic susceptibility, and stochastic events, making Multiple Sclerosis a multifactorial disease.

Environmental factors | The prevalence of the disease tends to increase with the distance from the equator in both the southern and northern hemispheres. It is more common in northern European populations, although the prevalence, in predisposed individuals, is influenced by the geographic area where they lived in childhood. The prevalence of the disease is not always homogeneous among populations living at the same latitude (for example, the prevalence is higher in Sardinia compared to Lazio). Several studies also show an increasing incidence of the disease over the past decades, especially in the female population, partially explained by diagnostic improvements. These studies suggest that improved hygiene conditions and the introduction of antibiotics may have favoured the development of predisposing immunological alterations, particularly in Western populations.

Epidemiological studies have suggested various environmental factors as possible risk factors. Among these, microbial agents, vitamin D, smoking, and obesity are the factors that currently receive the highest consensus among the scientific community. Among viral infections, the most recognized risk factor is Epstein-Barr virus (EBV) infection. The risk of developing Multiple Sclerosis is 15 times higher in individuals who contract this infection during childhood and 30 times higher during adolescence compared to non-infected individuals, especially when delayed exposure leads to infectious mononucleosis. Reduced vitamin D intake and/or reduced sunlight exposure are also potential risk factors, as cigarette smoking.

Genetic factors | The studies evaluating the disease concordance in monozygotic twins compared to dizygotic twins have been crucial to demonstrate the contribution of genetic factors in the development of MS. Relevant data, in this regard, have also come from comparisons between siblings and half-siblings, or between adopted individuals, or between children with parents affected by MS. In all cases, the risk of the disease increases with the degree of shared genetic background with an affected individual, not with the shared family "microenvironment".

Attempts to identify the genes responsible for the disease have been ongoing for about 40 years. Associations between MS and alleles of the major histocompatibility complex (MHC) were already identified in 1970 with the identification of DR15 and DQ6 and their corresponding genotypes DRB1*1501, DRB5*0101, DQA1*0102, and DQB2*0602 (DRB1*1501 being the allele with the strongest association with multiple sclerosis). These associations are mainly found in the northern European population but are present in most populations. Strong associations with DR4 (DRB1*0405, DQA1*0301, and DQB1*0302) are observed in Sardinia and other Mediterranean areas. Recently, with the advances in research such as the Genome Project and the development of new technologies for single nucleotide polymorphism analysis and DNA sequencing, the list of loci involved in individual genetic predisposition is growing. Currently, 110 genetic variants associated with the risk of MS have been identified, some are shared with other autoimmune diseases such as ulcerative colitis, Crohn's disease, primary biliary cirrhosis, celiac disease, rheumatoid arthritis, psoriasis, and autoimmune thyroiditis. Many of these genes are related to immune response control, involved in cytokine pathways (CXCR5, IL2RA, IL7R, IL7, IL12RB1, IL22RA2, IL12A, IL12B, IRF8, TNFRSF1A, TNFRSF14, TNFSF14), co-stimulatory signals (CD37, CD40, CD58, CD80, CD86, CLECL1), and signal transduction (CBLB, GPR65, MALT1, RGS1, STAT3, STAT4, TAGAP, TYK2), as well as genes related to risk factors such as vitamin D (CYP27B1, CYP24A1) and genes related to therapy responses such as Natalizumab (VCAM1) and Daclizumab (IL2RA). However, according to the most recent data, about 90% of the variants associated with MS, as well as other autoimmune diseases, are in "non-coding" regions regulating gene expression.

Possible stochastic events | Generally, these associations can only explain a small part of the overall risk. It is likely that a significant portion of the yet unidentified risk resides in the interactions between risk genes (epistatic interactions) or between genetic and environmental risk factors. Many of these interactions could be random and therefore difficult to identify. Much work remains to be done to identify additional loci, define potential epigenetic factors that can modify the expression of genes relevant to pathogenesis, and clarify whether the etiological mechanisms are the same for all forms of the disease.

17.2 Pathological anatomy

Macroscopically, the topography of the lesions is quite characteristic (see also Chapter 5 Neuroradiology), although it exhibits a certain degree of variability from patient to patient. Typical sites of the disease include regions adjacent to the lateral ventricles, the corpus callosum, the subcortical white matter, the optic nerves, the brainstem, and the spinal cord. Microscopically, different lesion patterns can be identified based on the predominant effector mechanisms within the demyelinating area: T lymphocytes and macrophages, or B lymphocytes and complement. In other cases, the damage appears to be less dependent on inflammation and more related to hypoxic/ischemic injuries or primary pathology of the oligodendrocyte. Regardless of the mechanism that seems to prevail in generating the damage, the sclerotic lesion is the end product of these processes. In some cases, remyelination attempts can also be observed; however, they are never complete, due to either the presence of astroglial scars or to the defective regenerative capacity of oligodendrocytes. In the primary progressive form, the lesion burden is on average lower, and the inflammation appears to be less pronounced (although this does not necessarily translate into a milder form of the disease).

It is believed that the pathogenesis of the lesions begins with the migration of pro-inflammatory lymphocytes across the blood-brain barrier. However, it is not fully clear whether the intrathecal recruitment of these cells occurs due to autoimmune activation against myelin antigens (or, in any case, of the nervous system) or towards microbial antigens or other as-yet undefined processes. The mechanisms that underlie the transition between different phases of the disease are equally unknown: relapse and remission of the acute phase and the shift from the acute phase to the progressive phase. In acute lesions, lymphocytic infiltrates and perivascular microglial activation can be associated with axonal transections. In progressive phases, demyelinating areas coexist with widespread axonal and neuronal degeneration, accompanied by the accumulation of hyperphosphorylated and insoluble Tau protein aggregates. Some alterations also appear to be present in normal appearing white matter, within an inflammatory context identifiable through widespread activation of parenchymal microglia.

17.3 Clinical aspects of multiple sclerosis

The signs and symptoms of MS vary depending on the location of the lesions, therefore a wide spectrum of clinical presentations can be observed. However, certain disorders recur more frequently than others, as demyelination areas tend to distribute in preferential sites. At onset, the disease can manifest with a single symptom (monosymptomatic onset) or a combination of symptoms (polysymptomatic onset) that occur acutely or subacutely. This event is known as *clinically isolated syndrome* (CIS). In approximately 10% of cases, the disease takes on a subtle and progressive course from the beginning, with or without relapses superimposed on the progression. Onset is more common between 20 and 40 years old, but there are forms with childhood or adolescent onset, as well as cases with a first clinical episode occurring after 50 years old. The disease affects women more frequently, with a ratio of about 2:1. The most common symptoms of MS are:

- *Motor symptoms* | They are present at the onset in 40% of cases and are due to involvement of the pyramidal tracts. They often manifest insidiously (for example, noticeable functional impairment only after fatigue). During the course of the disease, weakness and localized spasticity in one or more limbs, predominantly the lower limbs, are frequent and significant causes of disability. Neurological examination reveals hyperreflexia and pathological reflexes such as the Hoffman and Babinski signs. Spasticity, although affecting ambulation, can be useful in maintaining an upright posture in some cases where voluntary control of movement and paravertebral musculature are deficient.

- *Sensory symptoms* | They are present at the onset in approximately 20% of cases and result from lesions in the posterior columns, spinothalamic tracts, or the entry zones of the posterior roots. The site of the disorders varies: initially, involvement of the more distal parts (hands, feet) is common, while the involvement of the proximal parts of the limbs, perineum, trunk, or face is less pronounced. On general examination, marked alterations are generally not evident, but the patient may experience dysesthesias and paresthesias. Impairment of deep sensations due to involvement of the posterior columns of the spinal cord is frequently observed; neurological examination reveals hypopallesthesia, particularly in the lower limbs, position sense deficits, and a positive Romberg's sign. Pain or paroxysmal symptoms, characterized by sudden onset and high frequency of occurrence, often triggered by specific movements and sensory stimuli, are less common. *Lhermitte's sign*, belongs to this group of symptoms, it is the sudden sensation of an electric shock that extends down the spine and limbs upon flexion of the head.

- *Visual symptoms* | *Retrobulbar optic neuritis* (RBON), inflammation of the optic nerve, occurs at the onset in 20% of cases. The patient complains of a partial or total vision loss in one eye, and less commonly, there may be a bilateral involvement. Generally, the impaiment is described as "blurring," and the patient reports "seeing through a foggy glass." The onset of the disturbance occurs over a few hours or days and may be accompanied by retro-orbital pain worsening with palpation of the eyeball or eye movements. Ocular fundus examination may reveal oedema of the optic nerve head (papillitis), although the end of the optic nerve may appear normal since the inflammation affects the retrobulbar portion of the nerve. Visual field testing usually demonstrates the presence of a scotoma involving the macular area and blind spot, but a wide variety of visual field defects can be observed, and rarely, a hemianopsia. In over half of the cases, visual deficits resolve completely, but sequelae such as decreased color sensitivity may persist. Not every RBON represents the onset of MS. In adults, the risk of developing a definite form of the disease after RBON is estimated to be around 50% over 10-year period, but it is considerably higher (88%) when noticeable demyelinating lesions are present on magnetic resonance imaging (MRI). The case is different for RBON with childhood onset, where the risk of developing the disease in the future is more limited, suggesting a different aetiology (e.g., viral). Subclinical involvement of the optic pathways is also frequent: a pale and atrophic optic disc is commonly observed in advanced cases of the disease or in cases of previous RBON. A common phenomenon in patients with MS is the *Uhthoff's phenomenon*, characterized by a transient reduction in visual acuity following physical exercise or fever; this manifestation reflects worsened nerve conduction in demyelinated fibers, possibly due to increased body temperature.

- *Cerebellar symptoms* | Generally infrequent at onset, they often become severe in the later stages. They have a low tendency to regress, and if present in the early phase, they have a negative prognostic value. In the early phase of the disease cerebellar symptoms include limb dysmetria, intention tremor, and dysdiadochokinesia. Cerebellar dysarthria and ataxic-spastic gait are commonly found in later stages.

- *Truncal symptoms* | The most frequent symptoms include diplopia, usually with a favourable prognosis, and nystagmus, which often coexists with cerebellar symptoms and tends to persist over time. *Internuclear ophthalmoplegia*, resulting from a lesion in the medial longitudinal fasciculus (MLF) (see chapter on cranial nerves), is characteristic, although not pathognomonic, of MS. *Trigeminal neuralgia* is not uncommon, and when it occurs in an individual under the age of 50, it may suggest a demyelinating disease. It is caused by a pontine lesion in the area where the trigeminal nerve enters and is often associated with hypoesthesia and paresthesias in the trigeminal nerve distribution territory. Peripheral facial paralysis due to a brainstem lesion and vertigo may also be observed. In the advanced stages of the disease, dysarthria and dysphagia are often present, both for liquids and solid foods.

- *Sphincter and sexual symptoms* | Sphincter disturbances are widespread, particularly urgency in urination (urge incontinence), with or without incontinence. In other cases, there may be a retention with difficulty initiating micturition, leading to post-micturition residue and an increased frequency of urinary tract infections. In advanced cases, sphincter disturbances are mixed with detrusor sphincter dyssynergia. Sexual dysfunctions are also common due to lesions in the spinal centers, resulting in erectile dysfunction in men and anorgasmia in women, although psychological and depressive aspects are important contributing factors.

- *Affective and cognitive symptoms* | Depressive symptoms are often present, frequently reactive, especially in the early phases following the diagnosis. Cognitive deficits are also described in the early stages of the disease (mostly subclinical problems detectable in neuropsychological tests or of mild severity). The most affected domains are the frontal executive functions such as attention, working memory, and information processing speed. Deficits in long-term memory, calculation ability, and verbal fluency are also observed. However, overall intelligence (as measured by IQ) does not seem to be affected.

- *Other symptoms and complications* Approximately 80% of individuals with MS experience fatigue, defined as a sensation of continuous tiredness that interferes with normal activities of daily living. This disabling disorder must be distinguished from the more common symptoms associated with depression. Most MS patients also report excessive fatigue that occurs even after limited and usual activities (easy fatigability). Furthermore, it's important to know the association of three symptoms (nystagmus, scanning speech, and intention tremor) easily observed in the advanced stage of the disease, known as Charcot's triad, since, in the past, it was considered pathognomonic of MS. The prevalence of epilepsy in MS is around 2% and is caused by subpial, intracortical, or juxtacortical lesions, detectable through new imaging techniques. According to some studies, the presence of epileptic seizures may be an unfavorable prognostic factor.

Disability and EDSS | A common need for those involved in MS is the definition of a standardized assessment scale that, based on the neurological examination, allows to obtain a score indicative of the clinical disability degree. This enables comparison among different examiners and, above all, the evaluation of clinical progression over time. The most commonly used rating scale in outpatient evaluations is the Kurtzke (*Expanded Disability Status Scale* (EDSS). The scale is based on the assessment of "Functional Systems" (FS) (pyramidal, cerebellar, visual, sensory, bowel and bladder, and ambulation function), to which a score from 0 to 5 is assigned based on the degree of impairment. Considering the FS scores, a final score ranging from 0 (corresponding to a normal neurological examination) to 10 (indicating death due to MS) is assigned. For example, a score of 4 indicates a patient with moderate disability who, while retaining the ability to walk, has reduced autonomy (approximately 500 meters); a score of 6 indicates a patient who requires unilateral support to walk; and a score of 7 corresponds to a patient essentially confined to a wheelchair but with the ability to perform postural transitions independently. The main limitation of this scale is the predominant role of walking impairment compared to other FS, particularly beyond the value of 4.

17.4 Course and prognosis

Few diseases are as variable and unpredictable as MS. The age of onset, type of first symptoms, frequency of relapses, and disease course. in terms of progression and disability differ for each patient. Based on the course of the disease, several forms of MS can be distinguished:

- *Relapsing-remitting MS (RRMS)* | This form represents 80-90% of newly diagnosed cases. It is characterized by the onset of new neurological symptoms or worsening of preexisting symptoms (clinical relapses or poussée), with varying and unpredictable recovery, but with a repetitive pattern. During periods of clinical remission, there is no disease progression, although neurological deficits may fluctuate, especially during periods of psychological or physical stress or sudden temperature changes. Relapses can manifest and reach their peak within a few hours or days, and occasionally they can occur so acutely and prominently that the patient urgently seeks medical consultation. The regression of symptoms generally occurs within one or two months. The intervals between relapses are not constant; patients typically experience an average of one or more relapses per year during the early stages, but the frequency tends to decrease over time. Approximately one-third of relapses are preceded by a febrile episode (often a flu-like syndrome or respiratory tract infection).

- *Secondary progressive MS (SPMS)* | This form is characterized by the progression of clinical disability after an initial phase of RRMS. Relapses can still occur, but in these cases, recovery is often partial, and the worsening of symptoms is continuous even between relapses. Natural history data, referring to patients who have not received pharmacological treatment, indicate that 50% of patients with RRMS will develop SPMS within 10-15 years from the clinical onset.

- *Primary Progressive MS (PPMS)* | In 10-15% of cases, clinical disability progresses from the beginning. This form generally starts insidiously, with a slow and progressive disturbance of gait and balance. It is more common in men, especially those with an onset in late adulthood. Clinical relapses are absent, but progressive worsening can lead to severe disability.

- *Progressive-Relapsing MS (PRMS)* | This form is characterized by a combination of progression and relapses, with or without recovery. In recent years, this definition has been the subject of discussion because it may actually represent a transitional phase from RRMS with evident impairments to a truly progressive form.

- *Benign MS* | Although there is no complete consensus regarding this definition, it is generally considered a disease that, at least 15 years after onset, has not resulted in neurological disability, allowing the patient to be fully independent (Expanded Disability Status Scale score of 3 or lower).

Overall survival in an MS patient is only slightly compromised: in Western countries, it is only 5-7 years lower than that of the general population. The advent of disease-modifying therapies, such as beta interferon, copolymer, immunosuppressants, and more recently, the use of monoclonal antibodies, has altered the natural history of the disease by reducing the incidence of relapses and short- to medium-term disability. However, long-term disability remains the main challenge for clinicians. Although the prognosis for early exacerbations is generally good, as recovery appears to be more or less complete in most cases, deficits tend to accumulate in over 80% of patients over the years. While initially the disease symptoms generally manifest in an isolated manner, in advanced cases, spasticity, ataxia, sensory disturbances, visual deficits, and sphincter disorders coexist. Although it is essentially impossible to make a certain prognosis about the course of the disease at onset, some factors can be taken into consideration. Negative prognostic factors for all forms of MS include progressive course and greater disability reached at 2 and 5 years from onset. In RRMS, other negative prognostic factors include high frequency of relapses, short interval between onset and subsequent relapse, and multisystem involvement from the beginning.

17.5 Diagnosis

The key features of the diagnosis of MS have always been: 1) demonstrating dissemination in space (DIS) and time (DIT) of symptoms and clinical signs, and 2) excluding other conditions that could account for the observed clinical picture(Table 17.1).

Therefore, the diagnosis involves the evaluation of clinical and instrumental parameters to establish a correct diagnostic framework. Through medical history and neurological examination, the specialist can assess which functional systems have been involved and monitor the appearance of new clinical relapses over time.

Brain and spinal cord magnetic resonance imaging (MRI) and evoked potentials are additional tools that complement the clinician's ability to demonstrate dissemination in time and space of neurological involvement. Brain and spinal cord MRI is the preferred technique for highlighting areas of altered signal suggestive of demyelinating lesions in the white matter and, to a lesser extent, in the gray matter (Figure 17.1 and 17.2). In MRI, inflammatory lesions appear as hyperintense areas on T2-weighted, Proton Density (PD), and Fluid *Attenuated Inversion Recovery* (FLAIR) sequences.

The most frequently affected brain regions include the periventricular white matter, corpus callosum, corticospinal junction, internal capsule, and brainstem. The lesions are generally small, ovoid, and well demarcated, although in some cases, especially in the advanced stage of the disease, they may appear confluent and extend largely into the white matter. In the spinal cord, "plaques" are predominantly located in the posterolateral region and the cervical tract, and their extent usually does not exceed the length of a vertebral body. The visible lesions on T2-weighted sequences can indicate long-standing myelin damage or recent-onset inflammation. In the latter case, there is disruption of the blood-brain barrier (BBB). By performing a scan after gadolinium administration, a paramagnetic contrast agent, the lesions expressing ongoing inflammation become visible as hyperintense lesions on post-contrast T1-weighted sequences ("active lesions"). Sometimes, hypointense images can be observed on T1-weighted sequences, indicating recent edematous lesions or axonal loss, often irreversible (referred to as "black holes").

Over the years, clinical and instrumental criteria have been developed and subsequently modified, to achieve an early and accurate diagnosis of the disease from the first clinical event.

The internationally criteria currently used are those proposed by McDonald in 2001, revised by Polman in 2005, and Thompson in 2017. This diagnostic algorithm takes into account the occurrence of clinical episodes, the characteristics of MRI with the aforementioned DIS and DIT criteria for lesions, cerebrospinal fluid (CSF) analysis, and neurophysiological evaluation through evoked potentials (EP).

Table 17.1 ALGORITHM FOR THE DIAGNOSIS OF MULTIPLE SCLEROSIS

Clinical presentation	Additional data required for the diagnosis of MS
≥2 clinical attacks; clinical evidence of ≥2 lesions, or clinical evidence of 1 lesion + 1 attack reported in the medical history involving a different location.	None
≥ 2 clinical attacks; clinical evidence of 1 lesion.	DIS (Dissemination in Space)
1 clinical attack; clinical evidence of ≥ 2 lesions.	DIT (Dissemination in Time)
1 clinical attack; clinical evidence of 1 lesion (CIS - Clinically Isolated Syndrome).	DIS and DIT or DIS and the presence of OB (Bands in Cerebrospinal Fluid).
Insidious disease progression suggestive of MS (SM PP - Primary Progressive).	1 year of disease progression (retrospectively or prospectively determined) + 2 of the following 3 criteria: Evidence of DIS at the brain level based on ≥2 lesions in T2 in periventricular, juxtacortical, or infratentorial areas. Evidence of DIS in the spinal cord based on ≥2 lesions in T2 in the spinal cord. Positive cerebrospinal fluid (presence of Bands).

Legend - DIS: ≥1 lesion in T2 in at least 2 of the 4 typical regions of the central nervous system involved in MS (periventricular, juxtacortical or cortical, infratentorial, spinal cord) or an additional clinical episode in a different location of the central nervous system from the first. DIT: simultaneous presence of contrast-enhancing lesions and non-enhancing lesions at any time; or new lesions in T2 or contrast-enhancing lesions at a subsequent MRI regardless of the timing of its execution; or new clinical episode. BO: Oligoclonal Bands in the cerebrospinal fluid.

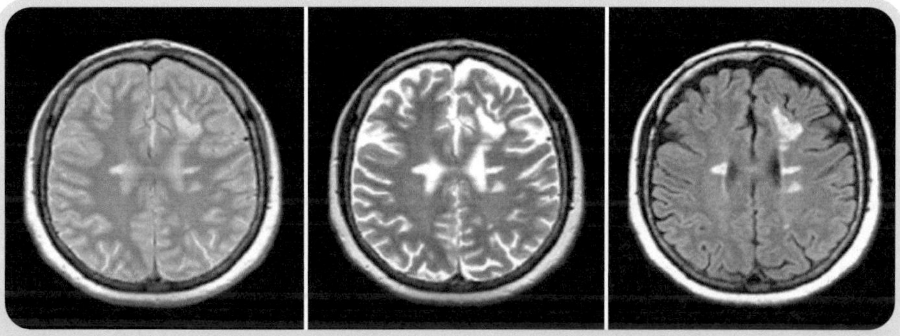

Figure 17.1

'Typical hyperintense MS lesions on DP-weighted, T2, and FLAIR images

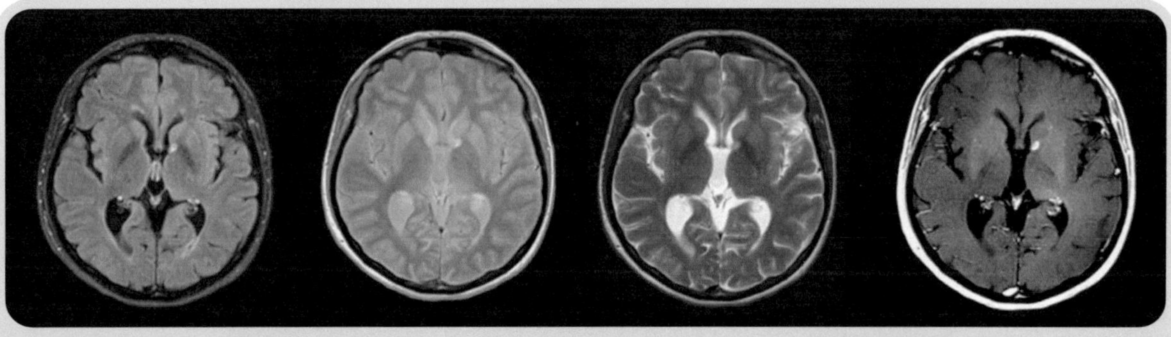

Figure 17.2

Left periventricular hyperintense lesion on FLAIR and DP-weighted and T2-weighted images, and hyperintense on post-contrast T1-weighted sequence after gadolinium administration (active lesion).

CSF analysis is performed to demonstrate the presence of IgG intrathecal synthesis, as indicated by an increase in the IgG index or the presence of oligoclonal bands (OB). This result is present in approximately 90% of patients with MS. EPs (visual, somatosensory, motor, and auditory) aim to evaluate any delayed wave latency along the explored pathways, indicating slowed nerve conduction due to demyelination of the fibers.

To enable the earliest possible diagnosis, increasing the sensitivity of diagnostic criteria without compromising specificity, a new algorithm was perfected in 2017. While maintaining the clinical criteria unchanged, it further simplified the definitions of DIS and DIT lesions, allowing for diagnosis with fewer MRI examinations compared to the past. It emphasized the importance of cortical lesions, while downsizing the role of CSF abnormalities and EPs (Table 17.1). *Oligoclonal bands in cerebrospinal fluid:* positive findings of oligoclonal bands in spinal fluid can substitute the dissemination of lesions in time in some cases.

Types of lesions | Both asymptomatic and symptomatic MRI lesions can be considered when determining dissemination in space or time. Optic nerve MRI lesions are not included in a person presenting with optic neuritis.

Location of the lesions | Cortical lesions have been added to juxtacortical lesions in the determination of MRI criteria for the dissemination of lesions in space. Despite conventional MRI being widely used in the study of MS, the correlation between the number of detected lesions and clinical disability is still limited. This appears to be due to the inability of MRI to determine damage in the so-called "normally appearing" areas of the CNS. These areas of white and gray matter, despite not showing evident lesions in common MRI scans, have been found to be extensively involved in the pathological process through anatomopathological studies and the use of different neuroimaging techniques. Therefore, within the field of MS research, there is a growing interest in the application of new MRI sequences and techniques, including *Double Inversion Recovery* (DIR), Magnetization Transfer MRI (MT-MRI), Diffusion MRI (DTI), Proton Magnetic Resonance Spectroscopy (H-MRS), and Functional MRI (fMRI). Research is also underway to find new biological markers in order to obtain increasingly accurate diagnostic and prognostic indicators.

17.6 Differential diagnosis

There are many diseases that can mimic the clinical and/or radiological course of MS. These can be systemic diseases complicated by involvement of the central nervous system with a relapsing course (e.g., systemic vasculitis) or a progressive course (haematological diseases, often lymphomas), degenerative neurological diseases many of which are hereditary such as cerebellar ataxias and leukoencephalopathies, monophasic diseases such as acute disseminated encephalomyelitis (ADEM), or non-organic pathologies such as somatizations (Table 17.2). It is often not possible to arrive at a definite differential diagnosis in the early stages of the disease. Therefore, it is essential

Table 17.2 DIFFERENTIAL DIAGNOSIS OF MULTIPLE SCLEROSIS

RRMS - Relapsing-Remitting Multiple Sclerosis
Inflammatory Conditions Systemic Lupus Erythematosus (SLE) Sjogren's Syndrome Behcet's Disease Susac Syndrome Cerebral Vasculitis Sarcoidosis Devic's Syndrome (Neuromyelitis Optica) Transverse Myelitis Leber's Hereditary Optic Neuropathy (LHON)
Infectious and Parainfectious Pathologies Lyme Disease Syphilis HTLV-1 (Human T-cell Lymphotropic Virus Type 1) JC Virus Encephalitis Acute Disseminated Encephalomyelitis (ADEM)
Progressive MS
Adrenoleukodystrophy Metachromatic Leukodystrophy Autosomal Dominant Cerebral Arteriopathy with Subcortical Infarcts and Leukoencephalopathy (CADASIL) Mitochondrial Disorders Hereditary Degenerative Diseases (including rare "periodic" forms) Brain and Spinal Cord Tumors

Note: The abbreviations used in the table are for convenience and easier reference.

to maintain an open-minded approach to consider alternative diagnostic possibilities, especially during the initial follow-up period. Equally important is explaining to the patient the reasons for maintaining a verifying attitude. Often, due to understandable anxiety in the early stages of the disease, the patient seeks certainties, and it is important for him to understand the difference between necessary investigations and doubt or excessive certainty.

In the differential diagnosis of MS, para-infectious inflammatory encephalopathies should be considered, including acute disseminated encephalopathy (ADEM) and acute hemorrhagic leukoencephalopathy (AHL). These are acute para-infectious encephalopathies characterized by multifocal inflammatory lesions primarily affecting the white matter of the central nervous system. ADEM mainly affects children and young adults and occurs in up to 80% of cases following a febrile episode (measles, rubella, chickenpox, and others) or vaccination (rabies, whooping cough, measles, etc., particularly HBV) with an interval of 1 to 4 weeks. Clinically, ADEM presents with an acute and rapid course and is often initially characterized by fever, headache, and drowsiness, leading to severe encephalopathy. Neurological deficits are typically multifocal (motor deficits, visual loss, sensory disturbances, cranial nerve palsy, movement disorders, and sphincter disorders). There may also be a coexisting acute polyradiculoneuropathy with a negative prognostic significance, occurring in 5% to 43% of cases, depending on the studies (rarely in cases with childhood onset). The mortality rate is 5% to 20%. On MRI, the lesions are generally large, supra- and infratentorial, and typically contemporaneous. Cerebrospinal fluid shows pleocytosis and increased protein, while the presence of oligoclonal bands, if present, can be transient. ADEM is considered an immunomediated condition rather than a direct expression of infection. From an anatomopathological perspective, it is characterized by multiple perivenous demyelinating areas located in the white matter. Recovery generally occurs in weeks or months in 50% to 70% of cases. The course is monophasic, but recurrent forms (same symptoms recurring 3 months or more later after onset) or relapsing forms (polysymptomatic features, but with symptoms different from the first episode and appearing at least three months after onset) exist. Treatment consists of cortisone administration or, alternatively, immunoglobulins and plasma exchange.

Acute hemorrhagic leukoencephalopathy (AHL) is a fulminant acute encephalopathy. The disease progresses rapidly and often leads to death. From an anatomopathological perspective, it is characterized by vasculitis of small vessels associated with hemorrhages and demyelination.

Finally, in the differential diagnosis, it is necessary to consider the neuromyelitis optica spectrum disorders (NMOSD). This group of diseases includes typical neuromyelitis optica (NMO or Devic's disease), optic neuritis, and acute transverse myelitis, a syndrome characterized by neuromyelitis optica with brain involvement.

NMOSD is considered an autoimmune disorder in which, with a certain frequency (seropositive forms), an antibody (anti-AQP4-Ab) can be identified, targeting the "aquaporin-4" antigen (with important functions for water homeostasis). Recently, even in seronegative forms, the presence of an antibody against oligodendrocyte glycoprotein (anti-MOG-Ab) has been identified. These two forms have different pathophysiological mechanisms, although the clinical manifestations can overlap. The presence of anti-AQP4 antibodies results in astrocyte damage, while anti-MOG antibodies appear to be responsible for a predominantly demyelinating pathology.

NMO represents the classic form of seropositive NMOSD. It is a demyelinating disease of the central nervous system, currently considered a distinct disease from MS, affecting young individuals, predominantly females (with a female-to-male ratio of up to 9:1), and clinically characterized by myelitis and optic neuritis (unilateral or bilateral). It has a relapsing course in 80-90% of cases, and a monophasic course in the remaining 10-20%.

Diagnostic criteria are evolving as the disease has only recently been identified as a nosological entity distinct from MS. NMO can be classified as "definite" in the presence of the two major criteria (optic neuritis and myelitis) and at least two of the three "supporting" criteria: spinal cord lesion demonstrated by MRI, extending over at least 3 vertebral segments, brain lesions not-characteristic for MS, and positivity for NMO-IgG antibodies. Other useful elements for differential diagnosis with MS include the absence of primary progressive forms (secondary progressive course is very rare), cerebrospinal fluid examinations sometimes showing pleocytosis, presence of neutrophils, and oligoclonal bands (only in 15-30% of cases).

17.7 Treatment

The treatment of MS involves relapse therapy, preventive therapy, and symptomatic therapy.

Relapse therapy is carried out using cycles of intravenous methylprednisolone (typically 1 gram per day for three or five days). In milder relapses, or following methylprednisolone, ACTH can be used. In case of persistent symptoms, plasma exchange (initiated no later than one month after symptom onset) can be attempted. The goal of these therapies is to reduce the clinical duration of relapse and any resulting outcomes.

Preventive therapy currently involves the use of first or second-line drugs. The predominantly used first-line drugs include interferon-beta (at different dosages), glatiramer acetate, teriflunomide, or dimethyl fumarate. Interferon-beta has been tested since the 1970s for its potential benefits related to antiviral effects. It is believed that the reduction in disease activity is linked to the immunomodulatory action of the cytokine. In recent years, a long-acting formulation, pegylated interferon-beta or peg-interferon, has also become available, allowing less frequent administration. Glatiramer acetate also acts through immunological mechanisms, possibly inducing anergy towards myelin antigens. As for teriflunomide and dimethyl fumarate, both orally administered drugs, the mechanism of action is only partially understood. Teriflunomide is a selective immunosuppressant that selectively and reversibly inhibits pyrimidine synthesis, thereby reducing the number of lymphocytes. Dimethyl fumarate activates the nuclear factor Nrf2 (nuclear factor erythroid 2-related factor 2) transcription pathway, resulting in immunomodulatory and anti-inflammatory actions.

In cases where these drugs are not effective (either from the beginning or over the years), or in rare situations of particularly aggressive disease, "biological" drugs such as natalizumab have been available for several years. Natalizumab is a monoclonal antibody against alpha-4 integrin that blocks the adhesion of inflammatory cells to the brain endothelium. It is a highly effective therapy (in registrational studies, it reduced the relapse rate by 68% after one year and the risk of disability acquisition at two years by 42%), but it is burdened by the risk of progressive multifocal leukoencephalopathy due to opportunistic JC virus infection. However, there is a blood test available to identify exposed patients and carriers of the virus. Through this test, it is possible to classify patients based on their risk and make the most appropriate therapeutic choice, considering the risk-to-benefit ratio (0.1/1000 in case of a negative test; from 0.5 to 3.9/1000, depending on the duration of less than or more than 24 months in patients with a positive test; from 1.5 to 10.6 in case of a positive test and a history of previous immunosuppressive therapy before starting natalizumab, again based on the duration of less than or more than 24 months). In addition to natalizumab, as a second-line therapy, there is also fingolimod, an orally administered drug. It has the ability to reduce inflammation of the central nervous system by suppressing the immune response through a new mechanism: the sequestration of lymphocytes within lymph nodes, achieved by the drug binding to sphingosine-1-phosphate receptors. Recently, ozanimod has also been approved by AIFA. Unlike fingolimod, it selectively modulates only subtype 1 and 5 of the sphingosine-1-phosphate receptors, reducing the potential cardiologic side effects. The siponimod also falls into this class of drugs and is the only one to have obtained indication for secondary progressive forms with disease activity.

Another option is alemtuzumab, a humanized monoclonal antibody that selectively binds to the CD52 protein on the surface of T and B cells, resulting in reversible depletion.

In 2018, two new treatments were approved: cladribine and ocrelizumab. Cladribine is an orally administered immunosuppressive drug that interferes with lymphocyte proliferation and leads to a reduction in circulating T and B cells. Ocrelizumab, on the other hand, is a monoclonal antibody, the first drug to be registered for the treatment not only of relapsing-remitting MS but also of primary progressive MS. It acts by selectively binding to the CD20 protein present on the surface of certain B cells.

Finally, there are symptomatic therapies that involve the use of pregabalin, gabapentin, and carbamazepine for neuropathic pain; alpha-lipoic acid, amantadine, and aminopyridine (fampridine) for fatigue; anticholinergics, intermittent catheterization, suprapubic catheterization, and intravesical botulinum toxin for bladder disorders; laxatives for constipation; sildenafil for impotence; and botulinum toxin, tizanidine, dantrolene, and baclofen (including intrathecal administration) for spasticity.

Bibliography

Ascherio A., Munger K.L., Simon K.C., Vitamin D and multiple sclerosis. Lancet Neurol; 9(6):599-612, 2010.

Ascherio A. Environmental factors in multiple sclerosis. Expert Rev. Neurother; 13(12 Suppl):3-9, 2013.

Compston A., Coles A., Multiple sclerosis. Lancet; 372(9648):1502-17, 2008.

Degenhardt A., Ramagopalan S.V., Scalfari A., Ebers G.C., Clinical prognostic factors in multiple sclerosis: a natural history review. Nat Rev Neurol; 5:672-82, 2009.

Hsu CL, Iwanowski P, Hsu CH, Kozubski W. Genetic diseases mimicking multiple sclerosis. Postgrad Med. 2021 Sep;133(7):728-749.

International Multiple Sclerosis Genetics Consortium (IMSGC), Wellcome Trust Case Control Consortium 2 (WTCCC2). Genetic risk and a primary role for cell-mediated immune mechanisms in multiple sclerosis. Nature; 476 (7359): 214-219, 2011.

International Multiple Sclerosis Genetics Consortium (IMSGC). Analysis of immune-related loci identifies 48 new susceptibility variants for multiple sclerosis. Nat. Genet.; 45(11): 1353-60, 2013.

Lublin F.D., Reingold S.C., Defining the clinical course of Multiple Sclerosis: results of an international survey. National Multiple Sclerosis Society (USA) Advisory Committee on Clinical Trials of New agents s in Multiple Sclerosis. Neurology; 46:907-911, 1996.

Polman C.H., Reingold S.C., Banwell B. et al., Diagnostic criteria for multiple sclerosis: 2010 revisions to the McDonald criteria. Ann Neurol; 69(2):292-302, 2011.

Salvetti M., Giovannoni G., Aloisi F., Epstein-Barr virus and multiple sclerosis. Curr Opin Neurol; 22(3):201-6, 2009.

Thompson A.J., Banwell B.L., Barkhof F., et al. Diagnosis of multiple sclerosis: 2017 revisions of the McDonald criteria. Lancet Neurol; 17:162-173, 2018.

Wingerchuk D.M., Banwell B., Bennett J.L., et al. International consensus diagnostic criteria for neuromyelitis optica spectrum disorders. Neurology 2015; 85(2):177-89.

18 SLEEP AND ITS DISORDERS

Carlo Di Bonaventura, Jinane Fattouch, Anna Teresa Giallonardo

The physiology of sleep and its disorders have always generated great scientific interest. The acquired knowledge has allowed for a better understanding of its phenomenology. In recent years, sleep medicine has accurately classified sleep disorders and discovered new nosological entities.

18.1 Definitions

Wakefulness is a physiological phenomenon that ensures full contact with the surrounding environment and a response to external stimuli with appropriate actions and reactions. It is strongly influenced by cognitive processes, including attention.

Sleep is a physiological phenomenon of a phasic nature characterized by:

1) Profound modification of cerebral electrical activity;
2) Reversible suspension of consciousness and of the critical and discriminative abilities characteristic of wakefulness. This can be modified by external stimuli, distinguishing it from states of consciousness.

18.2 Anatomic, physiological, and neurobiological bases of sleep

The regulation of wakefulness and sleep depends on complex neuronal and biochemical interactions involving the cortex, diencephalon (thalamus and hypothalamus), and brainstem.

Wakefulness is dependent on brainstem activation, particularly the tonic activation of numerous ascending parallel pathways organized into a complex cellular system located at the ponto-mesencephalic junction, called the *Ascending Reticular Activating System* (*ARAS*). Multiple neurotransmitters (glutamate, acetylcholine, and monoamines such as serotonin and norepinephrine) are involved in wakefulness control systems.

The main afferent pathways projecting from the brainstem to the thalamus and cortex are represented by:

1) Cholinergic pathways located in the lateral dorsal tegmentum and pontine tegmentum;
2) Glutamatergic and monoaminergic pathways from the *locus coeruleus* (norepinephrine) and dorsal raphe (serotonin);
3) The monoaminergic system (histamine) located in the tuberomammillary nucleus of the caudolateral hypothalamus;
4) The cholinergic system originating from the basal nucleus of Meynert.

Another element that plays an activating role is the orexin system (also known as hypocretin), located in the lateral hypothalamus, which sends diffuse projections throughout the nervous system. Orexin contributes to maintaining wakefulness through direct excitatory action on other components of the ascending system and contributes to the control of the transition from wakefulness to sleep. The cholinergic system, especially in its ascending component from the lateral dorsal tegmentum and pontine tegmentum, is active during wakefulness and REM sleep and reduces its activity during NREM sleep (Figure 18.1).

Sleep is stimulated by the activation of a specific cellular group called the hypothalamic preoptic area (Ventrolateral Preoptic

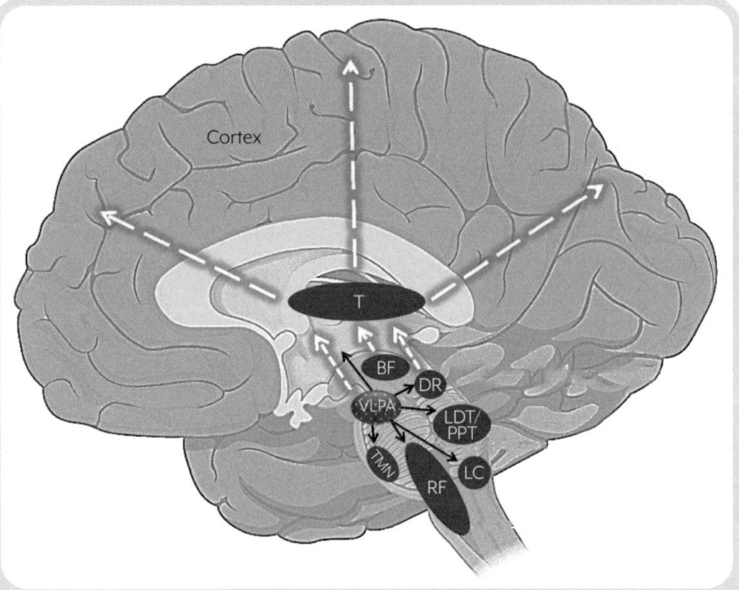

Figure 18.1

Schematic representation of the systems involved in wakefulness and NREM sleep. The activating systems of the brainstem and their projections (BF = basal forebrain; DR = dorsal raphe; LC = locus coeruleus; T = thalamus; LDT/PPT = laterodorsal and pedunculopontine tegmentum; RF = reticular formation; TMN = tuberomammillary nucleus) determine thalamic and cortical activation characteristic of wakefulness (white arrows). During NREM sleep, the activation of these systems is reduced by inhibitory influence from the ventrolateral preoptic area (VLPA) (black arrows).

Area, VLPO), which contains inhibitory neurotransmitters (GABA, galanin). The VLPO is inhibited by neurotransmitters from the ARAS and, at the same time, sends inhibitory projections to all elements of the ARAS. This functioning ensures stability to the wake-sleep system and the transition between different sleep stages.

Based on neurophysiological parameters, sleep can be divided into NREM sleep and REM sleep. NREM sleep depends on reduced activation of facilitating ascending systems and increased inhibitory action of the VLPO. REM sleep is mainly regulated by brainstem systems, particularly dependent on the inhibition of the activating monoaminergic system and simultaneous activation of the cholinergic system (LDT/PPT and BP) (Figure 18.1). The characteristic features of REM sleep include an EEG characterized by desynchronization of brain rhythms associated with rapid eye movements (REM) and muscle atonia.

NREM sleep is controlled by different neuronal groups located in the pontine reticular formation (RF), known as "effector neurons." EEG desynchronization (similar to wakefulness) is determined by neurons located at the pontomesencephalic level, including cholinergic neurons in the tegmentum. Eye movements are controlled by neurons in the medial pontine RF. Muscle tone is controlled by neurons in the lateral pontine RF (ventrolateral and dorsolateral), which send inhibitory projections to spinal motoneurons.

18.3 Sleep-wake cycle

Fluctuations and alternations between different states characterize the sleep-wake cycle. Sleepiness is determined by two factors: the *homeostatic factor* and the *circadian factor*. The homeostatic factor determines the amount of sleep in relation to the time spent in the wakeful phase; its action is mediated by adenosine, a substance that inhibits components of the ARAS. The circadian factor varies with a 24-hour periodicity, regardless of the time spent in the preceding wakefulness or sleep state, and is regulated by the suprachiasmatic nucleus, whose action inhibits components of the ARAS. Both the homeostatic and circadian factors modulate the need for sleep and influence the balance between wakefulness and sleepiness.

18.4 Functional significance of sleep

Sleep serves important functions, including control of certain metabolic processes (elimination of endogenous metabolites formed during wakefulness), endogenous stimulation (cortical maturation and synaptogenesis during development), homeostatic function (restorative processes), endocrine regulation (secretion of certain hormones closely dependent on the sleep-wake cycle, e.g., cortisol, sex hormones, etc.), and regulation of the immune system. Recently, it has been discovered that sleep also plays a crucial role in processes related to memory and other cognitive functions: resetting the system for recording irrelevant information to prepare the brain for new information, transferring recollections from short-term to long-term memory, consolidating or erasing mnemonic traces, and learning.

18.5 Sleep structure and instrumental investigations

There are three parameters used to define sleep and its structure: cerebral electrical activity (detected by EEG), muscle activity (detected by EMG), and eye movements (detected by EOG). Evaluating these parameters allows for the definition of the macrostructure of sleep and the distinction between NREM sleep (with its three stages) and REM sleep.

During sleep, the EEG is characterized by progressive slowing of brain rhythms and the appearance of specific graphical elements. Based on neurophysiological studies, the macrostructure of sleep and its potential alterations can be defined (Figure 18.2). NREM sleep consists of three stages that make up the macrostructure of sleep (N1, N2, N3 according to the American Academy of Sleep Medicine). Stage N1 represents about 2-5% of total sleep and is characterized by initial slowing or desynchronization of alpha rhythms and the appearance of vertex sharp waves and sleep spindles. Muscle tone is still present, and slow eye movements can be

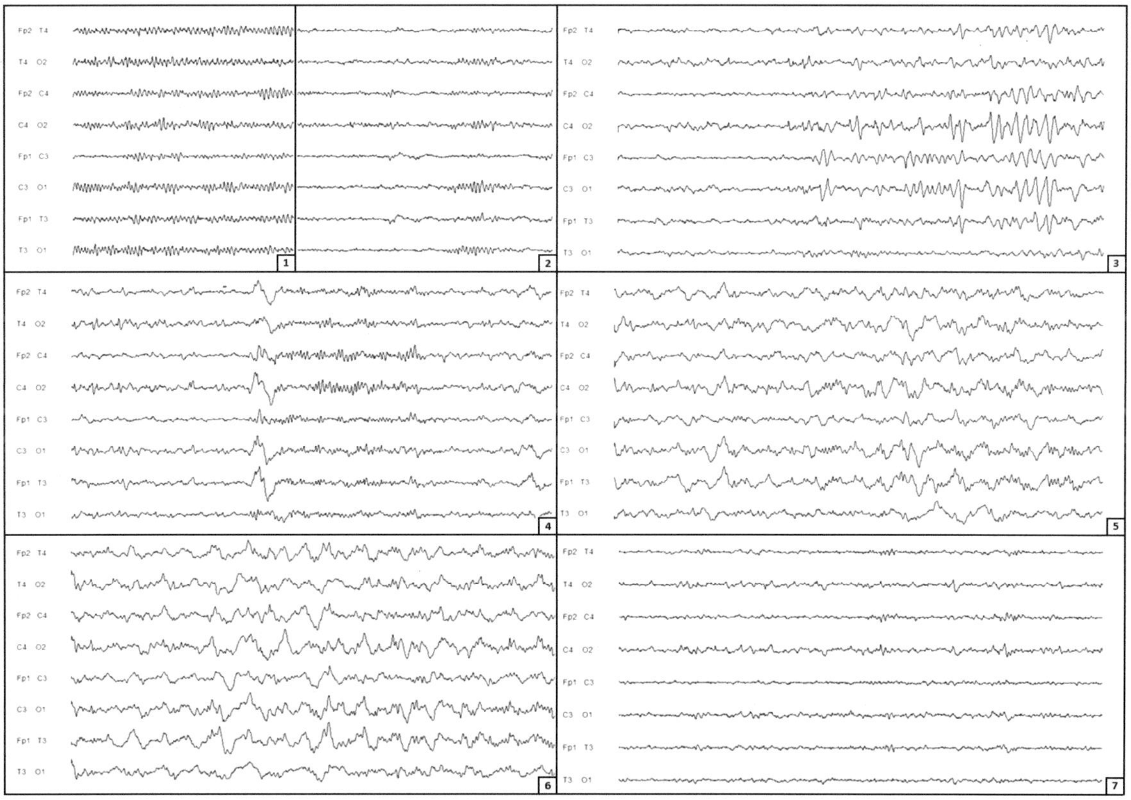

Figure 18.2

EEG recording of typical brain rhythms during different sleep stages. 1) Wakeful rest; 2) Drowsiness; 3,4,5,6) Respectively, stage I, II, III, IV of NREM sleep (NI, N2, and N3 according to the American Academy of Sleep Medicine); 7) REM sleep.

observed. Stage N2 represents 45-55% of total sleep and is characterized by the presence of sleep spindles and K-complexes. Muscle tone is reduced, and eye movements are absent. Stage N3 (which has replaced Stages III-IV as defined in the previous classification) represents about 25% of total sleep and is characterized by the presence of K-complexes and further slowing of electroencephalographic activity with the appearance of delta waves (≥ 20% of an epoch). Muscle tone remains reduced, and eye movements are absent. REM sleep, which constitutes 10-15% of total sleep, is characterized by an EEG pattern similar to wakefulness, reduced muscle tone, and rapid eye movements (Table 18.1).

Electroencephalographic recording of the different sleep stages allows for the assessment of quantitative aspects. The profile of sleep macrostructure changes over the course of life's different periods (Figure 18.3). In early childhood, the total time dedicated to sleep is equivalent to that of wakefulness but gradually decreases with age. The depth of sleep also progressively diminishes with age.

From a neurophysiological perspective, in addition to defining the macrostructure of sleep, it is possible to identify a microstructure that allows for a better assessment of qualitative aspects. Within the various stages of deep sleep, a particular type of EEG pattern called the Cyclic Alternating Pattern (CAP) can be recognized, characterized by alternating sequences of CAP cycles. Each CAP cycle consists of an A phase (arousal phase, with the reappearance of alpha rhythms, K-complexes, and large amplitude slow waves) and a B phase (return to deep sleep phase with typical elements of those stages). The duration of a CAP cycle (A+B phase) is approximately 1 minute, with the A phase lasting about one-third of the entire cycle. Evaluation of the microstructure of sleep (and the so-called CAP index) is usually used to define the quality or "goodness" of sleep.

18.6 Sleep disorders

Definitions and classification

The classification of sleep disorders, in its most recent formulation (International Classification of Sleep Disorders third edition

Table 18.1 NEUROPHYSIOLOGICAL PARAMETERS CHARACTERIZING THE DIFFERENT STAGES OF SLEEP

Stage	% of total sleep	EEG	EMG	EOG
I	2-5%	slowing of α, rhythm, vertex sharp waves	medium to high muscle tone occasional	slow eye movements
II	45-55%	sleep spindles and K-complexes	↓ muscle tone	absence of eye movements
III	3-8%	K-complexes δ waves	↓ muscle tone	absence of eye movements
IV	10-15%	δ waves	↓ muscle tone	absence of eye movements
REM	10-15%	similar to wakefulness	↓ muscle tone	rapid eye movements

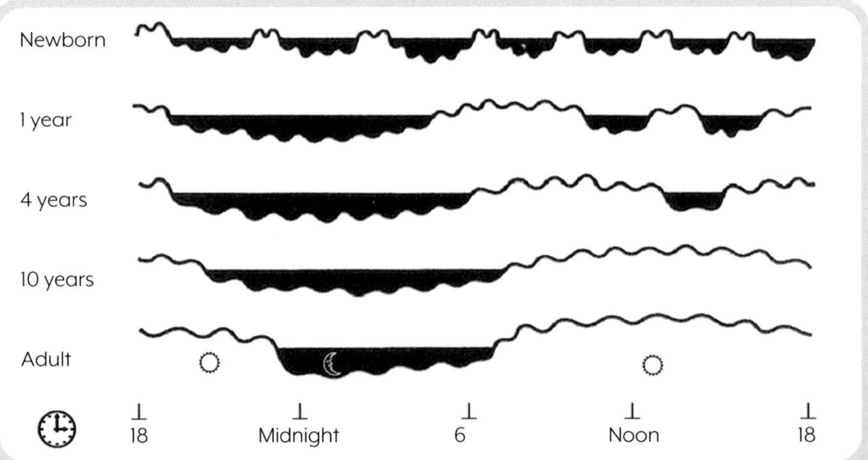

Figure 18.3

Course and duration of sleep. Schematic representation of the gradual transition of polyphasic wake-sleep alternations.

- ICSD-3, 2014) consists of 7 main groups: insomnia, sleep-related breathing disorders, central disorders of hypersomnolence, circadian rhythm sleep-wake disorders, parasomnias, sleep-related movement disorders, and other sleep disorders (Table 18.2, Classification).

18.6.1 Insomnia

Insomnia is a condition characterized by inadequate duration and quality of sleep, resulting in insufficient restorative sleep. The direct consequences are excessive sleepiness and excessive daytime fatigue. It is commonly reported by patients as "not getting enough sleep," and it requires specific treatment in 8-14% of cases. Insomnia can be idiopathic (intrinsic disorder) or secondary (extrinsic disorder). In the latter case, it can be caused by multiple conditions or situations, including psychiatric disorders (anxiety, depression, etc.), substance or medication use, inadequate sleep hygiene, cardiac or respiratory diseases. Certain neurological disorders can cause insomnia due to alterations in the sleep architecture resulting from nocturnal pain (multiple sclerosis, Parkinson's disease, etc.) or nocturnal paroxysmal events (epileptic seizures, parasomnias, etc.). In a rare clinical condition, such as fatal familial insomnia,

Table 18.2 SLEEP DISORDERS CLASSIFICATION

1. Insomnia	**4. Circadian rhythm sleep-wake disorders**
Chronic Insomnia Short-Term Insomnia Other Types of Insomnia	Delayed sleep-wake phase disorder Advanced sleep-wake phase disorder Irregular sleep-wake rhythm disorder Non-24-hour sleep-wake rhythm disorder Shift work sleep disorder Jet lag disorder Circadian rhythm sleep-wake disorder, unspecified
2. Sleep-related breathing disorders	**5. Parasomnias**

Obstructive sleep apnea (OSA)
  Adult OSA
  Pediatric OSA
Central sleep apnea syndromes (CSA)
  CSA with Cheyne-Stokes breathing
  CSA attributed to a medical condition without Cheyne-Stokes breathing
  CSA with high-altitude periodic breathing
  CSA related to medication or substance
  Primary CSA
  Primary CSA of infancy
  Primary CSA of prematurity
  CSA due to treatment
Sleep-related hypoventilation disorders
  Obesity hypoventilation syndrome
  Central alveolar hypoventilation, congenital
  Late-onset central alveolar hypoventilation with hypothalamic dysfunction
  Idiopathic central alveolar hypoventilation
  Sleep-related hypoventilation due to medication or substance
  Sleep-related hypoventilation due to a medical condition
Sleep-related hypoxemia disorder
	A. Non-REM sleep parasomnias
	  Confusional arousals
	  Sleepwalking
	  Night terrors
	  Sleep-related eating disorder
	B. REM sleep parasomnias
	  REM sleep behavior disorder
	  Isolated sleep paralysis
	  Nightmare disorder
	C. Other parasomnias
	  Exploding head syndrome
	  Sleep-related hallucinations
	  Nocturnal enuresis (bedwetting)
	  Parasomnia due to medical condition
	  Parasomnia due to medication or substance
	  Unspecified parasomnia

3. Central hypersomnia	**6. Sleep-related movement disorders**
Narcolepsy type 1 Narcolepsy type 2 Idiopathic hypersomnia Kleine-Levin syndrome Hypersomnia due to medical condition Hypersomnia due to medication or substance Hypersomnia associated with a psychiatric disorder Insufficient sleep syndrome	Restless legs syndrome Periodic limb movement disorder Sleep-related leg cramps Sleep-related bruxism Sleep-related rhythmic movement disorder Benign infantile hypnic myoclonus Propriospinal myoclonus of sleep onset Sleep-related movement disorder due to medical condition Sleep-related movement disorder due to medication or substance
	7. Other sleep disorders

American Academy of Sleep Medicine. International Classifi cation of Sleep Disorders . 3rd ed. Darien, IL : American Academy of Sleep Medicine; 2014.

the sleep disorder associated with cognitive decline represents the characteristic clinical core. The treatment of insomnia involves appropriate sleep hygiene (regular sleep schedules, elimination of napping or limitation of daytime sleep, avoidance of physical activity close to bedtime, etc.), abstaining from the use of stimulating substances or medications, and, finally, therapy with sleep-inducing medications. Among these, gamma-aminobutyric acid (GABA)ergic drugs (benzodiazepines) or the so-called *Z-drugs* (zolpidem, zaleplon, zopiclone), which are more selective for GABA-A receptor subtypes, can be used. In the case of chronic insomnia, antidepressant medications may be considered.

According to the latest classification of sleep disorders, insomnia is further divided into chronic insomnia disorder, short-term insomnia disorder, and other insomnia disorders (Table 18.2). The criteria for defining chronic insomnia include: 1) reported difficulties in sleep onset or maintenance; 2) adequate opportunities or circumstances for sleep; 3) daytime consequences; 4) insomnia duration of at least 3 months and frequency of at least 3 times per week.

18.6.2 Sleep-related breathing disorders

Sleep-related breathing disorders are divided into four sections: obstructive sleep apnea syndrome, central sleep apnea syndrome, sleep-related hypoventilation disorders, and sleep-related hypoxemia disorders.

Obstructive sleep apnea/hypopnea syndrome

This is a pathological condition characterized by repeated episodes of complete and/or partial and/or prolonged obstruction of the upper airways during sleep, typically associated with a reduction in blood oxygen saturation. Risk factors include secondary airway obstruction due to various causes, including hypertrophic tonsils and adenoids (in pediatric age), macroglossia, muscle hypotonia of the oropharyngeal area resulting in collapse of the soft tissues during sleep (in adults), and structural abnormalities of the mandible or airways. The main symptoms include excessive daytime sleepiness, frequent episodes of breathing cessation during sleep (apnea), snoring (intermittent due to interruptions by apnea), headache upon waking, concentration and memory disturbances, and libido disorders. This condition can lead to cardiovascular complications, including hypertension. Moreover, there is a correlation with cardiac and cerebrovascular disorders. In addition to clinical data, the diagnosis is based on polysomnography and ambulatory cardiorespiratory monitoring. Polysomnography shows the presence of numerous breathing pauses with a decrease in oxygen (O_2) and an increase in carbon dioxide (CO_2) in the blood. Apnea is considered complete cessation of airflow for at least 10 seconds, while hypopnea is a 50% reduction in airflow for 10 seconds or a 30% reduction with a decrease in oxygen saturation that tends to awaken the patient. The severity of apnea is determined by an index that correlates the number of events per hour, known as the "*apnea-hypopnea index*" (AHI), allowing an objective assessment of the disorder: AHI < 5 = normal, AHI between 5 and 15 = very mild, AHI 15-30 = moderate, AHI > 30 = severe.

Treatment is based on different approaches, including lifestyle changes (avoiding alcohol, smoking, sedative and muscle relaxant medications), weight loss, and surgical therapy for removable obstructions. Positive airway pressure devices are commonly used, with *continuous positive airway pressure* (CPAP) being the most common. Oral appliances can also be used. Medical therapy includes certain medications such as theophylline (to reduce central apneas) and stimulant drugs (amphetamines, modafinil, etc.).

Central sleep apnea syndrome

Central sleep apnea syndrome is a sleep-related disorder in which the ability to breathe is diminished or absent, typically for 10-30 seconds, in a cyclical or intermittent pattern. The respiratory pause is associated with a reduction in blood oxygen saturation. This condition is usually due to instability in the physiological feedback mechanisms that control breathing. In central sleep apnea, the brainstem respiratory control centers exhibit instability, failing to send the necessary signals to activate respiratory movements in response to hypoxemia or hypercapnia resulting from the pause. The disruption of feedback and the reduction or cessation of respiratory drive are clinically identifiable by the absence of activation of the respiratory muscles. Otherwise, the clinical symptoms are similar to those described for obstructive apneas. The diagnosis is based on clinical aspects as well as polysomnography or cardiorespiratory monitoring data. Central sleep apnea syndrome can be idiopathic or secondary to central nervous system (CNS) disorders and medications (e.g., opioids). If the diagnosis is confirmed, the therapy is based on the use of respiratory assistance with BiPAP (bilevel positive airway pressure).

18.6.3 Central disorders of hypersomnolence

These disorders are often caused by intrinsic alterations in the control of the sleep-wake cycle. According to the new and recent classification, this group includes narcolepsy (type 1 and type 2), idiopathic hypersomnia, Kleine-Levin syndrome, hypersomnia due to medical conditions, hypersomnia due to medications or substances, hypersomnia due to psychiatric disorders, and insufficient sleep syndrome.

Narcolepsy and cataplexy

Narcolepsy is a disease characterized by uncontrollable and sudden daytime sleepiness. It is a relatively uncommon condition (3-16 per 10,000 individuals in the USA) that affects both men and women equally. It typically manifests during puberty, with an onset age between 15 and 30 years. The cardinal symptoms include excessive daytime sleepiness, cataplexy, hypnagogic hallucinations, and sleep paralysis. During the onset of the disorder, the symptoms can be mild, often leading to a significant delay in diagnosis. Excessive daytime sleepiness is characterized by numerous episodes of daytime sleep that the patient cannot resist, lasting for about 10-20 minutes. Sleep attacks can occur regardless of the number of hours slept during the night. Cataplexy, which specifically characterizes narcolepsy and is the second most common symptom (present in approximately 80% of children with narcolepsy), is characterized by a sudden and transient loss of muscle tone, often triggered by strong emotions (laughter, sudden anger, physical exertion, or sexual activity). During a cataplectic episode, the individual does not lose consciousness and retains memory of the event. Episodes can last from a few seconds to several minutes, with complete resolution after the episode. The presence or absence of cataplexy distinguishes the subtypes of narcolepsy: type 1 (with cataplexy) and type 2 (without cataplexy). Hypnagogic hallucinations (auditory and visual hallucinations), often described as dreams, occur during the transition from sleep to wakefulness. Sleep paralysis prevents the patient from moving or speaking (during sleep onset and REM sleep) and can last from a few seconds to several minutes before spontaneously resolving.

From a pathophysiological perspective, narcolepsy appears to be caused by an alteration in the centers responsible for regulating the sleep-wake cycle, and the symptoms are related to an abnormality in REM sleep. Currently, narcolepsy is believed to be associated with an alteration in the hypocretin/orexin system due to the loss of neurons involved in its production in the hypothalamus. In some cases, with normal or increased hypocretin levels, the inefficiency of this system may result from "hypocretin resistance" secondary to altered receptor transmission, leading to an excess of hypocretin. Narcolepsy (or clinically similar conditions) can also be observed in neurological disorders (head trauma, encephalitis, tumors, etc.) or rare genetic disorders (Niemann-Pick disease type C, Prader-Willi syndrome, etc.).

Diagnosis is based on clinical and instrumental criteria. Neurophysiological investigations are necessary for diagnosis. Specifically, the *Multiple Sleep Latency Test* (MSLT) and polysomnography are essential diagnostic tests for narcolepsy. The MSLT consists of a series of five 20-minute EEG recordings performed at 2-hour intervals, evaluating the average sleep latency in resting wakefulness conditions. Polysomnography allows for an objective evaluation (quantitative and qualitative) of an individual's level of sleepiness. The presence of cataplexy and excessive daytime sleepiness, combined with abnormal MSLT findings, allows for a definitive diagnosis. Diagnosis can also be confirmed through genetic testing to determine HLA subtypes (a significant correlation has been demonstrated between narcolepsy and HLA DQB1*06:02 subtype).

New diagnostic criteria have been established by both the DSM-5 and ICSD-3. The criteria in both classification systems include excessive daytime sleepiness and the following elements: 1) cataplexy; 2) cerebrospinal fluid hypocretin deficiency; 3) ≤15-minute REM sleep latency on nocturnal polysomnography; 4) average sleep latency ≤8 minutes on MSLT with ≥2 REM sleep periods at sleep onset.

Treatment for this disorder includes proper sleep hygiene (including planned daytime naps) and the use of medications. Excessive daytime sleepiness can be treated with amphetamine-like medications (usually dextroamphetamine) or methylphenidate and modafinil. Modafinil has fewer side effects compared to amphetamine-like drugs. Tricyclic antidepressants (especially clomipramine) and selective serotonin reuptake inhibitors (SSRIs, especially fluoxetine) are indicated for cataplexy. Venlafaxine and sodium oxybate can be effective in some cases.

Hypersomnia

Hypersomnia is a condition characterized by excessive daytime sleepiness. Similar to insomnia, it can be either idiopathic or secondary. Idiopathic hypersomnia is a rare condition of unknown etiology, with an onset in adolescence and often a familial incidence. Diagnosis is based on polysomnographic findings, which include reduced sleep latency, increased total sleep time, and the absence of REM sleep periods at sleep onset. Recurrent hypersomnia can also be observed in a rare condition called Kleine-Levin syndrome, characterized by sleep disturbance and periodic behavioral changes with hyperphagia, aggression or depression, and hypersexuality. Causes of secondary hypersomnia include various neurological disorders such as head trauma, infectious or autoimmune conditions (e.g., encephalitis, immune-mediated encephalitis), and neurodegenerative diseases (Alzheimer's disease, Parkinson's disease, etc.).

18.6.4 Circadian rhythm sleep-wake disorders

This category encompasses different conditions including delayed sleep-wake phase disorder, advanced sleep-wake phase disorder, irregular sleep-wake rhythm disorder, non-24-hour sleep-wake disorder, shift work disorder, jet lag disorder, and unspecified sleep-wake rhythm disorders.

The main criteria for defining this specific category of disorders are: 1) a chronic or recurrent pattern of sleep-wake rhythm disturbance primarily caused by an alteration in the endogenous circadian factor or a misalignment between the circadian factor and the desired or required amount of sleep; 2) sleep-wake cycle disturbances (e.g., insomnia or excessive sleepiness); 3) associated distress or impairment; 4) duration of at least 3 months (this criterion does not apply to jet lag disorder).

18.6.5 Parasomnias

Parasomnias encompass various types of phenomena (motor, verbal, and experiential) that occur during sleep and can be considered as disorders of the transition between different sleep stages and arousal. They can be classified as primary (disorders of sleep stages) or secondary (symptomatic, i.e., specific to neurological disorders such as sleep-related headaches and internal medical conditions). Parasomnias can be divided into three main clusters: NREM-related parasomnias, REM-related parasomnias, and other parasomnias (Table 18.2).

NREM-related parasomnias

This group includes arousal disorders and phenomena characteristic of the transition from wakefulness to sleep (typically occurring during NREM sleep).

Arousal disorders, characteristic of NREM sleep, include *sleepwalking*, *sleep terrors* and *confusional arousals*. They are often observed in children (sometimes with a familial pattern) and are equivalent to incomplete awakening from deep sleep.

Sleepwalking is usually observed in the first part of the night and typically begins during deep sleep. The behavior can be calm or agitated, automatic, and sometimes stereotyped. Actions can be appropriate and purposeful or disorganized. The duration is usually 1-2 minutes, and when induced, awakening can be slow and confused (amnesia of the event is usually present).

Sleep terrors are characterized by sudden awakenings in which the individual (mostly children) appears fearful and panicked, often inconsolable. Motor activity, occasionally violent, can be associated with terror. Tachycardia, tachypnea, mydriasis, and increased muscle tone may be present. These episodes, lasting from 30 seconds to 3 minutes, usually occur in the first part of sleep (during deep sleep but occasionally during all NREM stages).

Confusional arousals typically manifest in childhood and are characterized by physiological movements typical of the waking phase (crying may be present) associated with confusion and altered ideation. Behavior is typically inappropriate and sometimes aggressive. Confusional episodes, which usually last a few minutes, can be associated with conditions that impair sleep, such as toxic-metabolic encephalopathies.

Transition disorders between sleep and wakefulness include some *manifestations considered non-pathological, including physiological hypnic myoclonus, sleep talking, nocturnal leg cramps,* and *hypnagogic hallucinations*.

REM-related parasomnias

This group includes nightmares, sleep paralysis, and REM sleep behavior disorder.

Nightmares are dreams with distressing content. They usually last a few minutes and can be accompanied by vocalizations, moaning, and motor activity. They typically occur in the latter part of the night and are favored by conditions that reduce REM sleep (stress, medications, medical conditions). Nightmares at sleep onset are characteristic of terrifying hypnagogic hallucinations, which can occur independently or be associated with narcolepsy.

Sleep paralysis refers to experiences that can occur both during the transition to sleep and upon awakening. It is characterized by the subjective sensation of being unable to activate muscles and move the body. It represents a conscious perception, in a state of incomplete wakefulness, of the muscle atonia typical of certain sleep stages.

REM sleep behavior disorder REM sleep behavior disorder (RBD) is a disorder typically observed in older individuals (predominantly men), characterized by the occurrence of altered, often violent, behavior during sleep, accompanied by motor activity. Behaviors can be simple (laughter, talking, shouting, etc.) or complex (gesturing, punching, kicking, sitting up, getting out of bed, running, etc.). *Vivid* and well-structured dream content is often present, which can lead to uncontrolled motor behaviors and occasionally cause accidents and injuries to the patient and/or partner. The duration can range from 2 to 10 minutes, and the frequency is usually several episodes per week. As to neurophysiological correlates, there is a lack of muscle atonia, which typically accompanies REM sleep, and an emergence of excessive motor activity. In some cases, this disorder may be the only symptom, but it often coexists with various neurological conditions (Parkinson's disease, multiple system atrophy, Lewy body dementia, Machado-Joseph disease, amyotrophic lateral sclerosis, etc.), sometimes preceding their onset by years. It can also be observed in other conditions, including epilepsy, multiple sclerosis, Guillain-Barré syndrome, cerebrovascular disorders, and the use or withdrawal of medications and substances (alcohol, sedatives, anticholinergics, drugs, etc.). The treatment involves the use of clonazepam and, alternatively, imipramine, carbamazepine, levodopa, and gabapentin.

18.6.6 Sleep-related movement disorders

These disorders are characterized by simple and stereotyped movements that occur during sleep. This category includes restless leg syndrome (RLS), periodic limb movement disorder (PLMD), sleep-related leg cramps, bruxism, sleep-related rhythmic movement disorder, benign sleep myoclonus of infancy, propriospinal myoclonus at sleep onset, sleep-related movement disorders secondary to internal medical conditions, sleep-related movement disorders secondary to medications or substances, and unspecified sleep-related movement disorders (▮ Table 18.2).

Restless leg syndrome

RLS is a condition characterized by the need to move the lower limbs, leading to restlessness that affects sleep quality. It is more prevalent in women aged 35 to 50, and in 60% of cases, there is a family history (with possible autosomal dominant transmission and variable penetrance). It usually affects the lower limbs but can also involve the arms and trunk. Movement of the limbs provides temporary relief. Patients report tingling or a sensation of needing to move their legs. The diagnostic criteria include:

1) An urge to move the legs, with or without paresthesias;
2) Relief with movement;
3) Worsening with rest;
4) Worsening in the evening or at night.

RLS can be either primary or secondary in terms of etiology. The primary form, considered idiopathic, typically has a subtle onset, possible progression, and a tendency to worsen over time. The secondary form often has a sudden onset, usually after the age of 40, and may be associated with specific clinical conditions or the use of certain medications. The most common condition associated with RLS is iron deficiency and related anemia (present in over 20% of RLS cases), but venous varicosities, folate or magnesium deficiency, metabolic disorders, autoimmune diseases, and neurodegenerative disorders (such as Parkinson's disease) can also be associated with RLS.

From a pathophysiological perspective, the dopaminergic system plays a central role, and there is a deficiency of iron in the substantia nigra (iron being an essential cofactor for the formation of L-dopa, a precursor of dopamine). Treatment includes behavioral measures such as avoiding alcohol consumption in the evening, stretching exercises, and applying alternating hot and cold showers to the limbs. Pharmacological therapy with low-dose dopaminergic agonists, benzodiazepines, sedatives, and opioid analgesics is highly effective.

Periodic limb movement disorder

PLMD is a very common disorder observed in 30% of individuals over the age of 65. It is characterized by the recurrence of rhythmic movements, described as "jerks" or "kicks," typically occurring in the lower limbs during sleep. These movements can vary in frequency and location. Although often asymptomatic, this disorder can cause difficulty in falling asleep, frequent awakenings, and excessive daytime sleepiness. It can occur in isolation or be associated with other sleep disorders such as restless leg syndrome, narcolepsy, sleep apnea syndrome, and REM sleep behavior disorder. The movements typically occur in stages N1 and N2 but are rarely documented during slow-wave sleep and REM sleep. If the disorder interferes with sleep quality, treatment with benzodiazepines can be helpful.

18.6.7 Other sleep disorders in neurological conditions and differential diagnosis

The sleep-wake cycle can be disturbed or compromised by numerous neurological alterations characterized, for example, by persistent involuntary movements during sleep. In some conditions (such as Parkinson's disease, Tourette syndrome, Huntington's disease, and dystonias), the typical motor alterations of these conditions and sphincteric disturbances (nocturia) can contribute to substantial sleep fragmentation and excessive daytime sleepiness. Another neurological condition with complex relationships with sleep is epilepsy. Sleep often facilitates the occurrence of ictal episodes (both in some focal and generalized forms) or triggers specific EEG abnormalities (in benign childhood epilepsy as well as encephalopathic conditions). Furthermore, certain types of seizures are difficult to differentiate from other sleep phenomena. Representative examples include hypermotor seizures typical of the frontal lobe (including autosomal dominant nocturnal frontal lobe epilepsy), which can resemble REM sleep behavior disorder, and dystonic seizures, which are difficult to differentiate from paroxysmal dystonia (another form of parasomnia characterized by sudden, stereotyped dystonic, choreoathetoid, or ballistic movements). Other sleep phenomena with similar semiology and challenging differentiation from seizures include confusional arousals, sleepwalking, and episodic sleep-related ambulation.

Bibliography

Sateia M.J. International Classification of Sleep Disorders-Third Edition. Highlights and Modifications CHEST 2014; 146 (5): 1387-1394.

The international classification of sleep disorders. In: Sateia M., editor. Diagnostic and coding manual. 2nd edition. Westchester (IL): American Academy of Sleep Medicine, p. 1-297, 2005.

Kryger M., Roth T., Dement W. Principles and practice of sleep medicine. 5th ed. New York: Elsevier Saunders, 2010.

Lesage S., Hening W.A., The restless legs syndrome and periodic limb movement disorder: a review of management. Semin Neurol; 24:249-260, 2004.

Mahowald M.W., Bornemann M.C., Schenk C.H., Parasomnias. Semin Neurol; 24:283-292, 2004.

Olson E.J., Boeve B.F., Silber M.H., Rapid eye movement sleep behaviour disorder: demographic, clinical and laboratory fi ndings in 93 cases. Brain; 123:331-339, 2000.

Panossian L.A., Avidan A.Y., Review of sleep disorders. Med Clin N Am; 93:407-425, 2009.

19 MOTOR NEURON DISEASES (MND)

Marco Ceccanti, Chiara Cambieri, Laura Libonati, Maurizio Inghilleri

Motor Neuron Diseases (MND) represent an heterogeneous group of disorders characterized by primary and progressive degeneration of upper and/or lower motor neuron. Four forms of MND can be identified: *amyotrophic lateral sclerosis* (ALS), *primary lateral sclerosis*, *progressive muscular atrophy* and *progressive bulbar palsy* (Table 19.1). Is distinguished by the simultaneous involvement of the upper and lower motor neurons. In primary lateral sclerosis degeneration is limited to the upper motor neuron, while progressive muscular atrophy is characterized by the exclusive involvement of lower motor neuron. In progressive bulbar palsy, degeneration is selective for the motor neurons in the lower portion of the brainstem (Figure 19.1).

Table 19.1 Classification of motor neuron diseases

Sporadic motor neuron diseases
1) Sporadic amyotrophic lateral sclerosis 2) Primary lateral sclerosis 3) Progressive muscular atrophy 4) Progressive bulbar palsy
Hereditary motor neuron diseases
1) Familial amyotrophic lateral sclerosis 2) Hereditary spinal muscular atrophy a) type I (Werdnig-Hoffmann disease) b) type II (intermediate form) c) type III (Kugelberg-Welander disease) d) type IV (adult form) 3) X-linked spinal bulbar muscular atrophy (Kennedy's disease) 4) Progressive bulbar palsy a) Infantile form (or Fazio-Londe disease) b) adult form associated with deafness (vialetto-van laere disease)

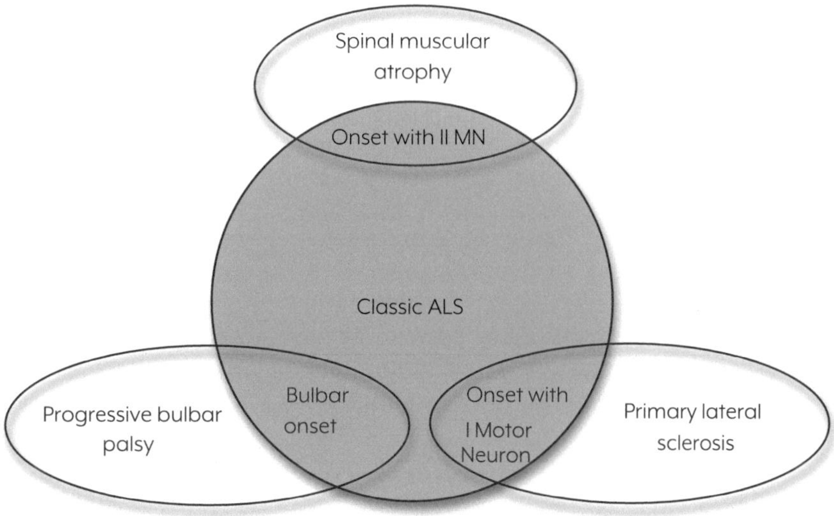

Figure 19.1

The types of onset in ALS.

The most common form of motor neuron disease is ALS. Progressive muscular atrophy represents about 10% of motor neuron diseases, primary lateral sclerosis accounts for 1-3%, and progressive bulbar palsy accounts for 1-2%. ALS has a prevalence of 2.7-7.4 per 100,000 and an incidence of 2.5 cases per 100,000 people per year, making it a rare disease with a prevalence of less than 5 per 10,000 individuals. In Western countries, this condition is evenly distributed in the population, while endemic groups have been found in the Kii Peninsula in Japan and Guam, associated with dementia and parkinsonism, likely linked to genetic and environmental factors, particularly dietary factors. Epidemiological studies have also shown that professional football players have a six-fold increased risk of developing ALS compared to the general population.

19.1 Etiology and pathophysiology

ALS is traditionally considered a "monosystemic" disease, specifically involving the motor system through specific degeneration of the upper and lower motor neurons. Although this view is clinically still valid, recent studies suggest a "multisystemic" degeneration that involves, among others, the sensory system and higher brain functions. The pathophysiological mechanisms underlying the development of ALS appear to be multifactorial, with increasing evidence of a complex interaction between genetic and environmental factors. One of the hypothesized pathogenic mechanisms is glutamate-mediated excitotoxicity in the motor cortex. Glutamate is the main excitatory neurotransmitter in the central nervous system, binding to the NMDA receptor and the post-synaptic AMPA receptor. Excessive activation of these receptors seems to trigger the process of neurodegeneration through calcium-dependent enzymatic pathways or the generation of free radicals with increased expression of inflammatory mediators. The reason why excitocicity causes motor neuron degeneration is not fully understood yet. Two models have been proposed: the dying-forward and the dying-back model. The dying-forward model suggests that the upper motor neuron determines the anterograde degeneration of the lower motor neuron through glutamate excitotoxicity. The dying-back hypothesis, on the other hand, proposes that the pathological process begins at the muscle cell or neuromuscular junction and then retrogradely affects motor neurons. Transgenic mice that overexpress the mutated SOD1 protein, one of the most common mutations responsible for ALS, only in skeletal muscle, develop atrophy, marked weakness, contractile apparatus alterations, and mitochondrial dysfunction, with some features similar to that of mice expressing the same mutation ubiquitously. This suggests a possible role of muscle in the neurodegenerative process. It has also been observed that mice with high levels of creatine kinase (CK), an enzyme involved in muscle energy production mechanisms, have a better prognosis, with greater metabolic reserve that prevents SOD1-mediated neurodegeneration. Furthermore, the functionality of nicotinic acetylcholine receptors (AChRs) in the muscle has been studied in ALS patients using a technique of muscle membrane microtransplantation onto African frog oocytes. This technique showed different electrophysiological properties of AChRs in ALS compared to AChRs from traumatic denervated muscles, with reduced affinity for acetylcholine in ALS AChRs, thus confirming a possible key role of the skeletal muscle in the pathogenesis of the disease.

There are two forms of ALS: sporadic and familial. Some mutations cause ALS with specific characteristics: mutations in the C9ORF72, TBK1, TARDBP, and FUS genes can be associated with cognitive decline. Other mutations may also show a phenotype indistinguishable from sporadic ALS. Sporadic ALS accounts for the vast majority of cases (90%), while familial forms in about 10% of cases, with high-penetrance Mendelian genetic transmission. More than thirty gene mutations associated with familial ALS have been identified (Table 19.2). Some of the involved genes have incomplete penetrance, and with some exceptions, the genotype does not necessarily predict the phenotype. Among the various genes responsible for familial ALS, the most relevant ones are Superoxide Dismutase 1 (SOD1), Alsin, FUS/TLS, TARDBP, and *C9orf72*. Approximately 15-20% of familial ALS cases are due to point mutations in the SOD1 gene located on chromosome 21q, which encodes the Cu/Zn SOD1 enzyme. These mutations were first identified in 1993, and more than 100 mutations in this gene have been identified so far. The mutation leads to an increased production of radicals and reactive oxygen species (ROS) that are harmful to cells. The SOD1 mutation also appears to be involved in 5% of sporadic ALS. It has recently been highlighted that the *C9orf72* gene is the main cause of ALS, with a double frequency compared to SOD1 gene (about 40% of familial and 20% of sporadic cases). The patogenetic mechanism of *C9orf72* is not clear yet. The mutation consists of a hexanucleotide repeat expansion (GGGGCC) in the first intronic sequence of the gene, which disrupts DNA transcription by sequestering normal proteins and RNA involved in transcriptional regulation, leading to the accumulation of RNA aggregates in the nucleus. The Alsin mutation shows recessive inheritance associated with the 2q33 chromosomal region (alsin) and is found in very early-onset ALS cases (< 25 years).

The hypothesis of alteration in glutamatergic homeostasis, with consequent excitotoxicity, is still the most widely supported in the pathogenesis of ALS. However, new evidence, including the abnormal accumulation of neurofilaments in the pyrenophore and axons of motor neurons, also suggests an alteration

Table 19.2

Gene	Localization	Protein function
ALS2	2q33	Vesicular trafficking
ANG	14q11	Angiogenesis
ATXN2	12q24	Endocytosis; RNA translation
C9ORF72	9p21	DENN protein (Differentially Expressed in Normal and Neoplasia)
CHMP2B	3p11	Vesicular trafficking
DCTN1	2p13	Axonal transport
ELP3	8p21	RNA metabolism
FIG4	6q21	Vesicular trafficking
FUS	16p11	RNA metabolism
HNRNPA1	12q13	Disregulation of protein polymerization
HNRNPA2B1	7p15	Disregulation of protein polymerization
NEFH	22q12	Axonal transport
NEK 1	4q33	Tyrosine kinase activity-related functions
OPTN	10p13	Vesicular trafficking
PFN1	17p13	Cytoskeletal proteins
SETX	9q34	RNA metabolism
SOD1	21q22	Superoxide metabolism
SPG11	15q14	DNA damage repair
SQSTM1	5q35	Ubiquitination; autophagy
TARDBP	1p36	RNA metabolism
UBQLN2	Xp11	Proteasome
VAPB	20q13	Vesicular trafficking
VCP	9p13	Proteasome; vesicular trafficking

Adapted from Renton AE, Chio A, Traynor BJ. State of play in amyotrophic lateral sclerosis genetics. Nat Neurosci. 2014; 17(1): 17-23. doi:10.1038/nn.3584 in axonal transport in affected motor neurons. This aspect could be related to the mutation in the TARDBP gene, which encodes the TDP-43 protein, a nuclear protein that regulates RNA transcription and splicing. The TARDBP and *C9orf72* genes have also been found in other neurodegenerative diseases, such as frontotemporal dementia (FTD), suggesting a common neurobiological basis between ALS and FTD. We highlight that the extreme phenotypic variability of ALS indicates the pleiotropy of all the genes so far associated with it. Finally, there would be an association with smoking and a diet rich in fats and low in proteins.

The increased incidence of ALS in professional soccer players was not confirmed in other categories of athletes. Hypothesized pathogenic mechanisms leading to a higher prevalence of ALS in soccer players include excessive physical activity, the use of anti-inflammatory drugs or branched-chain amino acids or performance-enhancing substances, trauma and microtrauma, and exposure to fertilizers or herbicides used in soccer fields.

19.2 Clinical aspects and classification

Amyotrophic lateral sclerosis | ALS reveals the degeneration of motor neurons at the cerebral cortex, brainstem, and spinal cord. The acronym "ALS" accurately describes the typical anatomopathological signs of the disease, which is characterized by sclerosis of the lateral cord of the spinal cord, where the pyramidal tracts run, associated to amyotrophy, i.e., the loss of muscle trophism, secondary to the degeneration of the lower motor neuron. The classic signs and symptoms of ALS are always attributable to the degeneration of the upper motor neuron (spasticity, increased deep tendon reflexes, reduced motor dexterity, overall weakness) and lower motor neuron (muscle atrophy, fasciculations, cramps, segmental weakness, reduced deep tendon reflexes, muscle hypotonia). A key feature of the clinical diagnosis is the weakness without a concurrent sensory deficit. The average age of disease onset is 55-65 years, and only in 5% of cases occurs before the age of 30. Men are predominantly affected, with a male-to-female ratio of 1.5:1. The average survival is 36 months. Paralysis is progressive and leads to death from respiratory failure within 2-3 years in the bulbar onset and 3-5 years for spinal onset ALS. Other possible causes of death are choking and aspiration pneumonia, both resulting from dysphagia.

ALS can show different phenotypic expressions, depending on the initial site of involvement, predominant involvement of the upper or lower motor neuron, and topographic or temporal distribution (■ Figure 19.2). According to the distribution of the first symptoms, a spinal- and bulbar-onset forms of the disease may be identified. The spinal form occurs in 2/3 of patients, while the bulbar form is more common in women. Spinal-onset forms usually show asymmetric involvement of the limbs with muscle weakness and atrophy in the upper and/or lower limbs, without sensory disturbances. Cases of ALS with bulbar onset present bulbar signs or symptoms (dysphagia, dysarthria, lingual atrophy and fasciculations, swallowing, breathing, and speech disorders) in the first three months after diagnosis, followed by spinal signs. The dysarthria and dysphagia in the bulbar form should not be confused with the pseudobulbar syndrome, where the loss of cranial motility is due to a bilateral degeneration of the cortical motor efferences (cortico-bulbar pathways) to the bulbar nuclei of the cranial nerves, while in the bulbar ALS a direct degeneration of bulbar nuclei is observed. Pseudobulbar syndrome involves a spastic dysarthria, dysphagia, sudden and involuntary episodes of laughter and crying, and the appearance of the jaw jerk reflex.

Despite the specific involvement of the motor system, not all motor nuclei responsible for voluntary movements are affected in ALS: voluntary control of the anal and urethral sphincters, controlled by the Onuf's nucleus, and control of eye movements, controlled by the brainstem oculomotor nuclei, are typically spared in ALS until extremely advanced stages of the disease. Recent studies have demonstrated subclinical involvement of the sensory nervous system in some ALS patients. In particular, some patients with dysphagia, which is more frequent in the bulbar-onset ALS, show a sensitivity deficit in the larynx. Histological examinations of the larynx have confirmed morphological changes in

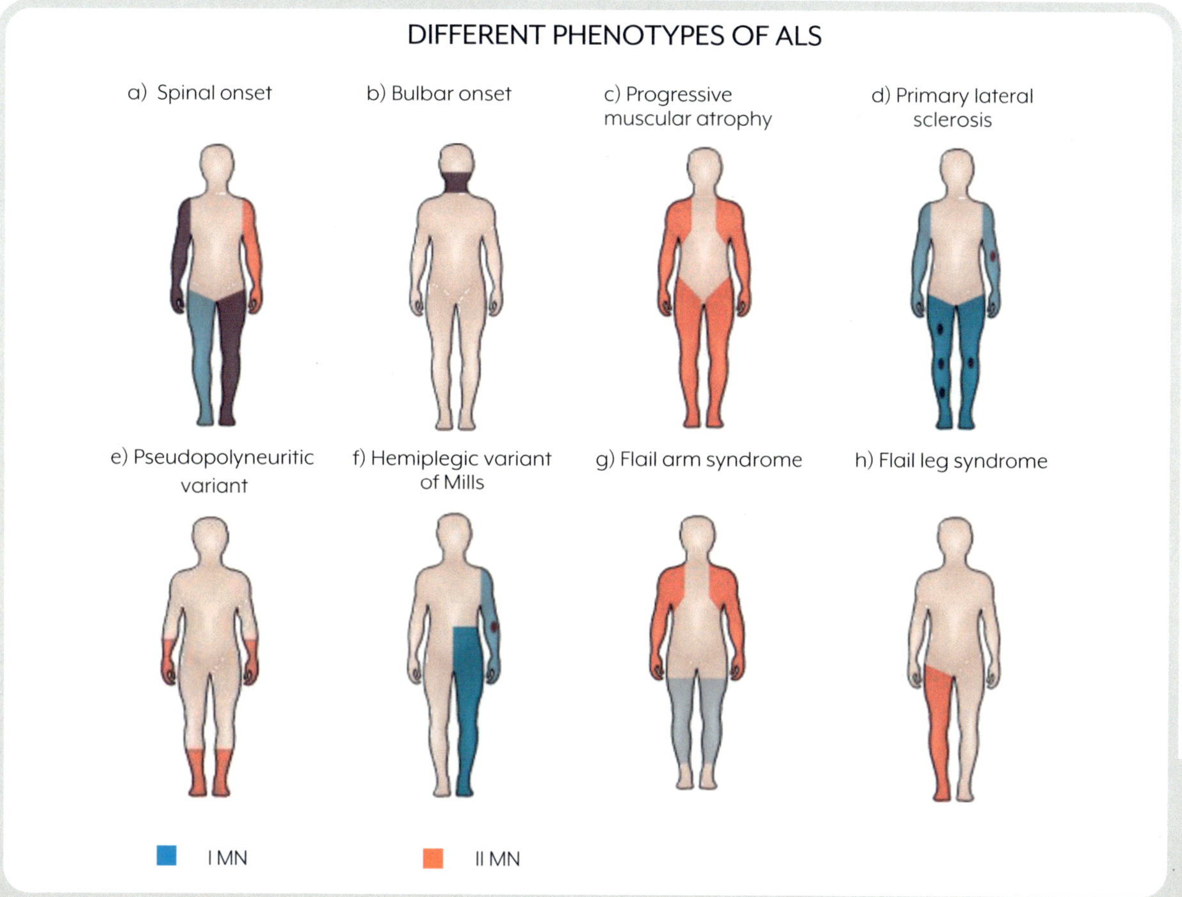

Figure 19.2

Motor disturbance distribution in different phenotypes of ALS. a) I and II MN observed in all limbs; b) I and II MN in bulbar muscles; c) II MN in the upper and lower limbs, generally in proximal location; d) I MN affecting the upper and lower limbs; e) II MN confined to the extremities of the limbs; f) unilateral involvement of I MN with sparing of the face; g) II MN affecting the upper limbs and less prominent involvement of I MN in the lower limbs; h) II MN confined to the lower limbs, often asymmetric. Adapted from Bart Swinnen and Win Robberecht. *The phenotypic variability of amyotrophic lateral sclerosis*, Nat Rev Neurol 2014.

intraepithelial nerve fibers, with evidence of increased branching and swelling of axonal components. In patients with spinal onset, concomitant distal sensory neuropathy of small sensory fibers responsible for thermo-pain sensitivity has been found. In the past, ALS was believed to be a selective pathology of the motor system, with the cognitive system spared and the diagnostic criteria for ALS in 1994 identified the cognitive deficits as an exclusion criterion. Currently, alongside the classification that takes into consideration the motor axis, a cognitive-behavioral axis is identified, which includes four different clinical profiles: ALS-dementia (meeting the criteria for a diagnosis of dementia but not FTD dementia), where dementia appears before motor symptoms; ALS with cognitive involvement without dementia (ALS-CI), where verbal fluency is predominantly affected; ALS with behavioral involvement without dementia (ALS-BI); ALS with frontotemporal dementia (ALS-FTD). In this way, frontotemporal dementia and ALS appear to be the extremes of a common pathogenetic mechanism, also sharing some pathogenic genes, as previously described. Cognitive impairment in ALS patients is associated with a worse prognosis.

The signs and symptoms of degeneration of the first motor neuron are characterized by increased osteotendinous reflexes, spasticity, weakness, the appearance of pathological reflexes (Babinski sign), and pseudobulbar syndrome. The symptoms and signs of the second motor neuron are muscle atrophy, fasciculations, reduced deep tendon reflexes, hyposthenia, and hypotonia. Therefore, deep tendon reflexes can be either brisk or diminished depending on the predominant degenerative phenomenon affecting the upper or lower motor neuron.

There are some clinical variants, depending on the predominant initial involvement of the first or second motor neuron in different areas. The hemiplegic form of Mills begins with unilateral involvement of the first motor neuron in the lower limbs, with a slow progressive involvement of the same-side upper limb while sparing the face. *Flail Arm Syndrome* (Vulpian-Bernard Syndrome or scapulohumeral form of ALS) involves the second motor neuron, limited to the upper limbs for at least 12 months, while the lower limbs remain unaffected, although they may present hyperreflexia and hypertonia. It has a male predominance with a ratio of 4:1, and after about 20 months, almost all patients develop a spread of weakness to the lower limbs. The pseudo-polyneuritic variant (Marie-Patrikios or peroneal form of ALS) is a form of *flail leg syndrome* predominantly affecting the distal and bilateral regions, to the extent that it can be initially mistaken for a motor polyneuropathy.

Primary lateral sclerosis | This form begins around the age of 50-60, involves the first motor neuron, and is characterized by spasticity in the lower limbs, initially unilateral, later involving the upper limbs and evolving into spastic paraparesis. Cranial nerve involvement is late. There are no signs or symptoms related to sensory system alterations, and muscle strength is generally preserved compared to patients with ALS. Approximately 30% of patients develop urinary disturbances (overactive bladder) during the course of the disease. According to recent diagnostic criteria, a definite diagnosis of Primary Lateral Sclerosis (PLS) requires clinical progression over time (two years) and the absence of signs and symptoms of the second motor neuron for an observation period of at least 4 years. Pharmacological therapy involves reducing spasticity with medications such as baclofen, tizanidine, and eperisone hydrochloride.

Progressive bulbar palsy | It is characterized by progressive weakness of the muscles innervated by the motor nuclei of the cranial nerves located in the lower portion of the brainstem. The degenerative process causes weakness in the bulbar muscles, with clinical manifestations including dysarthria, dysphagia, facial weakness, strength deficits, and tongue fasciculations; only the cranial region is clinically affected. The course is inevitably progressive, with subsequent involvement of the muscles involved in swallowing and breathing, leading the patient to rapidly become dependent on artificial nutrition and assisted ventilation. The clinical course is often complicated by the occurrence of pneumonia, and patients typically succumb to the disease within 3-4 years of symptom onset.

There are sporadic and familial forms of progressive bulbar palsy. The sporadic form rarely remains an independent syndrome: many cases initially presenting with isolated involvement of the motor neurons in the lower portion of the brainstem later evolve to affect both the upper and lower motor neurons, characteristic of ALS. Familial forms can have an onset in childhood (Fazio-Londe disease) or adulthood (Brown-Vialetto-Van Laere); the latter is associated with bilateral neurosensory deafness and recent identification of a mutation in a gene encoding a riboflavin transporter. Currently, some researchers tend not to consider progressive bulbar palsy, in its sporadic form, as a distinct nosological entity of motor neuron disease but rather as part of the bulbar-onset ALS.

Progressive muscular atrophy | This form involves the lower motor neuron and more commonly affects men than women, with a ratio of 4:1. The disease has a relatively early onset (before the age of 50) and a slow progression (10-15 years). Patients experience atrophy of the muscles in the limbs with a symmetric distribution, primarily affecting the distal muscles, progressing to the proximal segments. Additionally, fasciculations, weakness or absence of deep tendon reflexes, and absence of pyramidal signs are present. Superficial sensitivity is normal, while deep sensitivity is sometimes reduced or absent. This condition should not be confused with hereditary forms of adult-onset spinal muscular atrophy, and the differential diagnosis is primarily made with immune-mediated motor neuropathy with or without conduction blocks.

Spinal muscular atrophy | Spinal muscular atrophies (SMA) are a group of autosomal recessive hereditary diseases characterized by weakness and progressive atrophy primarily affecting the proximal muscles of the limbs and trunk. They are caused by degeneration of motor neurons located in the anterior horns of the spinal cord (lower motor neurons). Laboratory tests may show normal or slightly elevated levels of creatine kinase (CK) in the serum. Spinal muscular atrophies differ in terms of age of onset [infantile (I-II), juvenile (III), late-onset (IV)], clinical course, duration, and genetic alteration.

SMA Type I (Werdnig-Hoffmann disease) begins in the first six months of life and has a poor prognosis due to early involvement of bulbar functions. New genetic therapies have recently dramatically changed life expectancy and quality of life in these patients, thus changing the phenotype.

SMA Type II (intermediate form) has an onset between 7 and 18 months of age. Patients affected by the disease in early childhood are able to maintain a seated position without support but are unable to maintain an upright position, with a prognosis between Type I and Type III.

SMA Type III (Kugelberg-Welander disease) has a later onset, between 5 and 15 years of age. Generally, patients can acquire an upright position and walk without assistance. Bulbar muscles are rarely involved.

SMA Type IV has adult-onset, occurring afte the age of 25, and a milder course.

SMA Types I to IV are caused by mutations in the SMN1 gene, located on chromosome 5q13. Currently, therapies are available that ensure the production of the protein product of the SMN2 gene, a gene with a function similar to that of SMN1. These therapies have improved the disease course for patients with SMA.

Spino-Bulbar Muscular Atrophy (or Kennedy's disease) is an X-linked disease, exclusively affecting males with an adult-onset. It involves both skeletal and bulbar muscles. The disease has a slowly progressive course, characterized by reduced strength in bulbar and spinal muscles, muscle wasting, and fasciculations. The patient's tongue is almost always atrophic, accompanied by dysarthria with nasal speech. Diabetes mellitus, gynecomastia (50% of cases), and testicular atrophy are common, associated to reduced sensitivity of androgen receptors. The mutation affects the short arm of the X chromosome and is characterized by an expansion of the CAG triplet in exon 1 of the androgen receptor gene (Xq13). It is accompanied by a sensory axonal neuropathy, identifiable through electroneurography, and the diagnosis is confirmed by detecting the mutation through genetic testing.

19.3 Other forms of lower motor neuron (LMN) disease

Monomelic variant: benign focal amyotrophy (Hirayama's disease) | It is more common in young males. It is characterized by weakness and distal muscular atrophy in the upper limbs, usually unilateral, with onset in adolescence and subsequent clinical stabilization. The lower cervical territories (intrinsic hand muscles) are particularly affected. The diagnosis is made by electromyographic examination, which shows neurogenic involvement in the distal regions of the upper limbs, and by cervical MRI in a standard position and with maximum neck flexion, which shows compression of the anterior horn (snake-eye sign) cervical and dural detachment. Differential diagnosis includes multifocal motor neuropathy, syringomyelia, plexopathy, and poliomyelitis.

Poliomyelitis | It is an infectious disease that selectively affects the motor neurons of the anterior horns of the spinal cord. Currently, viruses other than the poliovirus can infect lower motor neurons.

19.4 Diagnosis

The diagnosis is based on the clinical history, neurological examination, and electromyographic (EMG) examination. Clinical suspicion arises whenever there is progressive motor disturbance without accompanying sensory deficit. The classification of ALS is based on the El Escorial international criteria, proposed in 1994 and revised in 2000. It is defined as "clinically definite," "clinically probable," "clinically probable with laboratory support," and "clinically possible." To make a definite diagnosis of ALS, signs of both upper and lower motor neurons degeneration must be present in at least three body regions, including the following areas: bulbar (muscle group: jaw, face, tongue, soft palate, larynx), cervical (neck, arms, hands, diaphragm), thoracic (back, abdomen), lumbosacral (lower back, legs, feet), with clear evidence of disease progression over time and absence of any other cause explaining the symptoms (Table 19.3). ALS can be suspected when there are signs of upper or lower motor neuron involvement in one or more areas, but this "suspected ALS" does not meet the revised El Escorial criteria. These criteria have a specificity of 100% and a sensitivity of 57%, being too restrictive to allow for an early diagnosis of ALS and enrolment in clinical trials. In order to facilitate the most accurate early diagnosis possible, new electromyographic diagnostic support criteria (Awaji criteria) were introduced in 2008. According to these criteria, fasciculations alone (without other signs of lower motor neuron degeneration) in a muscle with signs of chronic neurogenic damage is sufficient to establish lower motor neuron involvement, equating recorded fasciculations with electromyographic findings of fibrillations and positive sharp waves. The electromyographic examination may reveal signs of denervation (diffuse fibrillation potentials), fasciculations, changes in motor units (increased amplitude and duration, polyphasic morphology), and reduction in the number of motor units recruited during maximum effort. Nerve conduction study (NCS) is important for excluding peripheral nerve, neuromuscular junction, or muscle pathologies.

Currently, there is a proposal for new diagnostic criteria under review, aiming for greater simplification to enable an earlier diagnosis, also in view of possible new therapies (Table 19.3).

The study of Motor Evoked Potentials (MEPs) from transcranial magnetic stimulation

Table 19.3 PROPOSAL OF NEW CRITERIA FOR THE DIAGNOSIS OF ALS. THEY MUST OCCUR SIMULTANEOUSLY

1. Progressive motor impairment documented by medical history or repeated clinical assessments, preceded by normal motor function.
2. Presence of both upper motor neuron[1] and lower motor neuron[2] dysfunction in at least one region of the body (with upper and lower motor neuron dysfunction detected in the same body region in case of focal involvement) or lower motor neuron dysfunction in at least 2 regions of the body.
3. Appropriate diagnostic tests[4] to exclude other possible diseases.

Notes:

[1] Upper motor neuron dysfunction includes at least one of the following:
a. Increased deep tendon reflexes, including the presence of a reflex in a clinically weak and atrophic muscle, or with spread to adjacent muscles.
b. Presence of pathological reflexes, including the Hoffman sign, Babinski sign, crossed adductor reflex, or snout reflex.
c. Increased velocity-dependent muscle tone (spasticity).
d. Voluntary movement that is slow and poorly coordinated, not attributable to weakness from lower motor neuron involvement or with parkinsonian features.

[2] Lower motor neuron dysfunction in a given muscle requires:
a. Evidence from clinical examination of muscle weakness and muscle atrophy.
b. EMG abnormalities that must include:

Both signs of chronic neurogenic damage, defined by longer and/or larger motor unit potentials, with polyphasic and unstable motor units, considered supportive but not mandatory for the diagnosis, and signs of ongoing denervation, including fibrillation potentials, positive sharp waves, or fasciculation potentials.

[3] Body regions are defined as bulbar, cervical, thoracic, and lumbosacral. To be classified as a region involved in lower motor neuron involvement, abnormalities must be present in two muscles of the limbs innervated by different roots and nerves, or one bulbar muscle, or one thoracic muscle, both on clinical examination and EMG.

[4] Appropriate investigations depend on the clinical presentation and may include nerve conduction studies and needle EMG, MRI or other imaging, blood or cerebrospinal fluid analysis, or other clinically necessary modalities.

demonstrates a reduction in amplitude of potentials and an increase in central conduction time (alteration of the upper motor neuron). Muscle biopsy can be useful to exclude potential muscle pathologies with similar clinical presentation (e.g., inclusion body myositis). Magnetic Resonance Imaging (MRI) plays a fundamental role in the differential diagnosis with conditions that may "mimic" the clinical features of ALS (e.g., cervical myelopathy). MRI can show degeneration of the corticospinal tracts as hyperintensity on T2 and FLAIR imaging, located in the posterior limb of the internal capsule, descending motor tracts of the brainstem, and spinal cord.

Instrumental examinations commonly used in the study of dysphagia include fiberoptic laryngoscopy (which allows a dynamic visualization of swallowing, laryngeal penetration of the bolus, or the endotracheal aspiration), videofluoroscopy (to identify the presence, nature, and severity of dysphagia), and electromyography.

Differential diagnosis is considered with muscular diseases (inclusion body myositis, distal myopathies), nerve or root diseases (radiculopathies, diabetic polyradiculoneuropathy, plexopathies, predominantly axonal motor neuropathies, multifocal motor neuropathy), anterior horn diseases (adult-onset spinal muscular atrophy, paraneoplastic motor neuropathies, post-polio syndrome, Kennedy's disease), and spinal cord diseases (spondylotic myelopathy, syringomyelia, hereditary spastic paraparesis).

19.5 Therapy

The management of ALS is best achieved through a multidisciplinary approach, involving neurologists, psychologists, nutritionists, pulmonologists, physiotherapists, occupational therapist, speech therapists, and specialized nurses. Multidisciplinary care prolongs survival, reduces the number of hospitalizations, shortens hospital stays, and improves the quality of life (QOL) for ALS patients. This outcome is likely related to the optimization of pharmacological and non-pharmacological interventions and improved adherence to treatment guidelines. Despite more than 50 drugs with different mechanisms of action being studied, only two drugs have been approved for market use in sporadic ALS. Riluzole is the only drug that extend the survival of ALS patients, from 11.8 to 14.8 months in the absence of tracheostomy. Riluzole is a benzothiazole that blocks voltage-dependent sodium channels, reducing glutamate excitotoxicity by inhibiting presynaptic release. The drug-induced side effects may include nausea, abdominal pain, and hepatotoxicity. Hepatotoxicity is completely reversible upon discontinuation of the drug. In 2017, edaravone was included by the AIFA (Italian Medicines Agency) in the list of available drugs for ALS treatment (AIFA determination 1224 of 28/6/17; Official Gazette no. 153 of 3/7/2017). The drug induces a moderate slowdown in motor degeneration associated with the disease, resulting in a slight delay in the worsening of functional status in patients with specific characteristics such as disease onset not exceeding two years, moderate disability, and good respiratory function. However, further studies are needed to conclude the efficacy of this drug. In the US a new composite drug with sodium phenylbutyrate (PB) and taurursodiol (TURSO) was approved to slow-down ALS progression. Patients with SOD1 gene mutation can access therapies that reduce the translation of SOD1-mRNA, thus reducing the protein synthesis. This strategy, utilizing antisense oligonucleotide technology, has proven effective in maintaining muscle strength and respiratory function.

The excessive salivation is a common occurrence in ALS and is not caused by increased saliva production by the salivary glands but by reduced swallowing capacity (pseudosialorrhoea). To improve this symptom, the anticholinergic effect of certain medications can be used, such as tricyclic antidepressants (amitriptyline) or atropine, which cause xerostomia. If these measures are unsuccessful, injections of botulinum toxin can be performed into the salivary glands.

Nutrition is compromised when significant swallowing difficulties and weakness of the bulbar muscles occur. Dietary adjustments can be made, recommending a pureed diet with thickened liquids to prevent dysphagic episodes. As dysphagia worsens, artificial nutrition with a percutaneous endoscopic gastrostomy (PEG) or jejunostomy tube becomes necessary. This device improves quality of life and survival for several months but should be applied before respiratory function impairment increases the risks of the surgical procedure. However, PEG does not eliminate the risk of aspiration and pneumonia, which can occur through a gastroesophageal reflux. When dysarthria appears, the patient should undergo a speech evaluation.

Regular monitoring of respiratory function is necessary to assess respiratory function over time and delay the onset of acute respiratory failure, which can be fatal. This monitoring includes arterial blood gas analysis, nocturnal pulse oximetry, and spirometry. Parameters of interest are the partial pressure of carbon dioxide ($PaCO_2$), and oxygen (PO_2), forced vital capacity (FVC), forced expiratory volume in 1 second (FEV1), peak expiratory flow (PEF), and peak cough flow (PCF). In the case of orthopnea, $PaCO_2$ > 45 mmHg, FVC < 50%, or abnormalities in nocturnal pulse oximetry, non-invasive ventilation (NIV) therapy may be employed. Another important aid is the use of assisted cough devices. If non-invasive respiratory support is insufficient, tracheostomy becomes necessary.

The role of stem cells and neuroprotective therapies in ALS is still under study.

Bibliography

Brooks B.R., Miller R.G. et al., El Escorial revisited: revised criteria for the diagnosis of amyotrophic lateral sclerosis. Amyotroph Lateral Scler Other Motor Neuron Disord; 1:293-9, 2000. Inghilleri M., Iacovelli E., Clinical neurophysiology in ALS. Arch Ital Biol.; 149(1):57-63, 2011.

Ceccanti M, Pozzilli V, Cambieri C, et al. Creatine Kinase and Progression Rate in Amyotrophic Lateral Sclerosis. Cells 2020;9(5) doi: 10.3390/cells9051174.

Ceccanti M, Sbardella E, Letteri F, De Michele M, Falcou A, Romanzi F, Onesti E, Inghilleri M. Acute Flaccid Paralysis by Enterovirus D68 Infection: First Italian Description in Adult Patient and Role of Electrophysiology. Front Neurol. 2017 Nov 27; 8:638.

Dobrowolny G, Aucello M, Rizzuto E, Beccafico S, Mammucari C, Boncompagni S, Belia S, Wannenes F, Nicoletti C, Del Prete Z, Rosenthal N, Molinaro M, Protasi F, Fanò G, Sandri M, Musarò A. Skeletal muscle is a primary target of SOD1G93A-mediated toxicity. Cell Metab. 2008 Nov;8(5):425-36.

Heteronymous H reflex in temporal muscle as sign of hyperexcitability in ALS patients. Libonati L, Barone TF, Ceccanti M, Cambieri C, Tartaglia G, Onesti E, Petrucci A, Frasca V, Inghilleri M. Clin Neurophysiol. 2019 Aug;130(8):1455-1459.

Gilio F, Iacovelli E, Frasca V, Gabriele M, Giacomelli E, Picchiori F, Soldo P, Cipriani AM, Ruoppolo G, Inghilleri M. Botulinum toxin type A for the treatment of sialorrhoea in amyotrophic lateral sclerosis: a clinical and neurophysiological study. Amyotroph Lateral Scler. 2010 Aug;11(4):359-63.

Lorson C.L., Rindt H. and Shababi M., Spinal muscular atrophy: mechanisms and therapeutic strategies. Human Molecular Genetics; 19, 2010.

Miller R.G., Jackson C.E. et al., Practice parameter update: the care of the patients with amyotrophic lateral sclerosis: multidisciplinary care, symptom management, and cognitive/behavioral impairment (an evidence-based review). Neurology; 73:1227-33, 2009.

Onesti E., Schettino I., et al. Dysphagia in Amyotrophic Lateral Sclerosis: Impact on Patient Behavior, Diet Adaptation, and Riluzole Management. Front. Neurol.: 21; 8:94, 2017.

Palma E., Inghilleri M. et al., Physiological characterization of human muscle acetylcholine receptors from ALS patients. Proc Natl Acad Sci U S A; 13:20184-8, 2011.

Palma E., Reyes-Ruiz J.M. et al., Acetylcholine receptors from human muscle as pharmacological targets for ALS therapy. Proc Natl Acad Sci U S A; 15:3060-5, 2016.

Renton A.E., Chiò A., Traynor B.J. State of play in amyotrophic lateral sclerosis genetics. Nat Neurosci. 2014 Jan;17(1):17-23, 2014.

Rothstein J.D., Edaravone: A new drug approved for ALS. Cell; 2:725, 2017.

Ruoppolo G., Onesti E. et al., Laryngeal Sensitivity in Patients with Amyotrophic Lateral Sclerosis. Front Neurol; 28:212, 2016.

Mariani L, Ruoppolo G, Cilfone A, Cocchi C, Preziosi Standoli J, Longo L, Ceccanti M, Greco A, Inghilleri M. Progression of Oropharyngeal Dysphagia in Amyotrophic Lateral Sclerosis: A Retrospective Cohort Study. Dysphagia. 2021 Jul 23.

Ruoppolo G, Schettino I, Biasiotta A, Roma R, Greco A, Soldo P, Marcotullio D, Patella A, Onesti E, Ceccanti M, Albino F, Giordano C, Truini A, De Vincentiis M, Inghilleri M. Afferent nerve ending density in the human laryngeal mucosa: potential implications on endoscopic evaluation of laryngeal sensitivity. Dysphagia. 2015 Apr;30(2):139-44.

Swinnen B., Robberecht W. The phenotypic variability of amyotrophic lateral sclerosis. Nat. Rev. Neurol.; 10: 661-670, 2014.

Tiryaki E., Horak H.A. ALS and Other Motor Neuron Diseases. Continuum (Minneap Minn); 20(5):1185-1207, 2014.

Shefner JM, Al-Chalabi A, Baker MR, Cui LY, de Carvalho M, Eisen A, Grosskreutz J, Hardiman O, Henderson R, Matamala JM, Mitsumoto H, Paulus W, Simon N, Swash M, Talbot K, Turner MR, Ugawa Y, van den Berg LH, Verdugo R, Vucic S, Kaji R, Burke D, Kiernan MC. A proposal for new diagnostic criteria for ALS. Clin Neurophysiol. 2020 Aug;131(8):1975-1978. doi: 10.1016/j.clinph.2020.04.005. Epub 2020 Apr 19. PMID: 32387049.

Truini A., Biasiotta A. et al., Small-fibre neuropathy related to bulbar and spinal-onset in patients with ALS. J Neurol, 262:1014-8, 2015.

Wijesekera L.C., Leigh P.N. Amyotrophic lateral sclerosis. Orphanet J. Rare Dis.; 4:3,2009.

Writing Group; Edaravone (MCI-186) ALS 19 Study Group. Safety and efficacy of edaravone in well defined patients with amyotrophic lateral sclerosis: a randomised, double-blind, placebo-controlled trial. Lancet Neurol, 16:505-512, 2017.

20 PERIPHERAL NERVOUS SYSTEM DISEASES

Andrea Truini, Giulia Di Stefano, Giorgio Cruccu

20.1 Clinical overview

20.1.1 Overview of peripheral nerve anatomy

The peripheral nervous system begins a few millimeters after the spinal roots exit the spinal cord, with the myelin sheath formed by Schwann cells instead of oligodendrocytes. The anterior and posterior roots merge to form the spinal nerves. These nerves are surrounded by a dense and resistant connective tissue called epineurium, which sends connective tissue septa deep into the nerve and divides it into fascicles. Each fascicle is enveloped by the perineurium, a dense sheath that isolates the fascicles. In turn, the fascicles are traversed by a delicate connective tissue network called the endoneurium, which isolates the individual axons.

The arterial vessels (*vasa nervorum*) derive from regional arteries and terminate in an endoneurial capillary plexus. The capillary wall has limited permeability, forming a barrier between the blood and nerve fibers. Nerves also possess *nervi nervorum*, which originate from the nerve fibers themselves and provide nociceptive innervation. Nerve fibers can be myelinated or unmyelinated. Each myelinated fiber is wrapped in a sheath composed of Schwann cells that spiral around it, forming multiple layers of myelin. The myelin sheath is interrupted between adjacent Schwann cells at the node of Ranvier. At the node of Ranvier, the flow of current along the axon concentrates, and the nerve impulse propagates in a saltatory manner from node to node.

Unmyelinated fibers, on the other hand, are surrounded by a single Schwann cell that does not fold to form the myelin sheath. The impulse propagates at a slow speed along these individual axons.

The survival and proper functioning of the axon depend on the integrity of the cell body, which contains the ribosomes necessary for protein synthesis and where the synthesis of enzymes and structural proteins of the axon occurs. Molecules are transported along the axon through anterograde axonal flow. Metabolic waste products are transported back to the cell body through retrograde axonal flow for degradation in the lysosomes.

20.1.2 Symptoms and general signs of peripheral nervous system diseases

Symptoms of peripheral nervous system diseases can be sensory, motor, or autonomic. Traditionally, within the first two categories, *positive or negative disturbances are distinguished.*

Negative sensory disturbances | Involve hypoesthesia (reduced sensitivity) and anesthesia (loss of sensation). Damage to large-caliber myelinated fibers manifests as deficits in tactile, vibratory, positional, and movement sensation, leading to the development of ataxia. Osteotendinous reflexes are reduced or abolished. Damage to small-caliber myelinated fibers and unmyelinated fibers results in deficits in thermal and pain sensation. Typically, neuropathies cause homogeneous damage to small and large-caliber myelinated fibers and unmyelinated fibers. However, in some conditions, there may be predominant (sometimes exclusive) damage to specific afferent fibers.

Positive sensory disturbances | Include paresthesias, dysesthesias and neuropathic pain. Paresthesias are abnormal, spontaneous, non-painful sensations. The most common is a tingling sensation. Dysesthesias are unpleasant, spontaneous, or evoked sensations. A common form of dysesthesia is the spontaneous or evoked sensation of pins and needles. Neuropathic pain presents as burning sensations, electric shocks, and dynamic mechanical allodynia (pain evoked by light touch).

Negative motor disturbances | Consist of weakness (paresis) or absence of muscle contraction (paralysis). In traumatic mono-neuropathies, motor deficits usually manifest as paralysis affecting all muscles innervated by the nerve distally to the site of injury. In demyelinating inflammatory neuropathies, which sometimes have a predominant motor disturbance compared to sensory disturbances, severe symmetrical paresis occurs. In traumatic neuropathies, motor disturbances result from direct disruption of motor axons, leading to muscle atrophy. In demyelinating neuropathies, the axon remains intact, and the motor disturbance is caused by demyelination, which leads to conduction block. In this case, muscle atrophy does not develop. In common forms of neuropathy such as diabetic neuropathy or toxic neuropathies, motor disturbances are typically clinically mild and occur later than sensory damage.

Positive motor disorders | Positive motor manifestations include myokymia, fasciculations, and cramps. Myoclonus refers to repetitive contractions of the same motor unit, caused by focal damage to the motor axon. Fasciculations are contractions of individual motor units due to damage to the motor neuron or motor axon. They are particularly observed in patients with motor neuron diseases. Both myokimia and fasciculations can also occur in healthy individuals. Cramps are localized and painful contractions of a muscle or group of muscles, caused by focal damage to the motor axons. They frequently occur, especially at night, even in healthy subjects.

Autonomic disorders | These are due to damage to the unmyelinated fibers. In certain forms of neuropathy (such as amyloid neuropathy), autonomic symptoms predominate and manifest as gastrointestinal disturbances (e.g. nocturnal diarrhea), genitourinary disturbances (e.g. erectile dysfunction, sphincter dysfunction), cardiovascular disturbances (e.g. orthostatic hypotension, syncope), and anhidrosis.

20.1.3 Neuropathological classification of neuropathies

Neuronopathies | These involve damage to the cell body with secondary axonal degeneration. Sensory neurons in the ganglia are selectively affected because they are located outside the blood-brain barrier and are therefore susceptible to systemic pathogenic insults (autoantibodies, toxic substances). Examples of neuronopathies include paraneoplastic neuronopathy and neuronopathy due to Sjogren's syndrome.

Wallerian degeneration | This is a degenerative phenomenon that affects the axon and myelin and develops following nerve injury distal to the lesion. In the hours following nerve injury, degenerative processes occur in the myelin and axon (which becomes thinner and eventually fragments). These processes result in immediate loss of sensory and motor function in the territories downstream of the lesion, progressive disappearance of sensory and motor potentials of the nerve, and ultimately, non-excitability of the nerve trunk. The possibility of nerve regeneration depends on various factors, such as the integrity of the connective tissue structures of the nerve and Schwann cells. Wallerian degeneration typically occurs in focal traumatic neuropathies.

Axonal degeneration or distal axonopathy | This is characterized by degeneration of the distal part of the axon with a distal-to-proximal pattern. For this reason, this phenomenon is often referred to as "*dying back*". Both the axon and myelin are involved in the pathological process. Axonal degeneration is caused by toxic or metabolic damage that, although affects the entire peripheral nerve (including the cell body), results in more severe damage to the distal segments of the nerve, where axoplasmic transport has a lower "biological reserve." Clinically, it is characterized by sensory and motor disturbances with a distal, symmetrical distribution, progressive course, and distal-to-proximal gradient. Therefore, the sensory disturbance is usually referred to as a "stocking and glove" pattern.

Segmental demyelination | This involves primary damage to the Schwann cell and myelin, but not the axon (at least initially). Myelin regeneration is due to the proliferation of new Schwann cells. In genetically determined demyelinating neuropathies, the proliferation of Schwann cells is characterized by "onion bulb" formations, reflecting the processes of demyelination and remyelination. These formations consist of extensions of the Schwann cell cytoplasm around a demyelinated axon. Acute and chronic inflammatory neuropathies of autoimmune etiology are the most common forms of demyelinating neuropathy. Focal demyelinating damage also occurs in compressive neuropathies such as carpal tunnel syndrome. Clinically, they manifest as a deficit in sensory and motor function, along with mild muscle atrophy.

20.1.4 Topographic classification

Neuropathies can be focal (*mononeuropathies*), multifocal (*multineuropathies*) or systemic (*polyneuropathies*).

Mononeuropathies | Involve damage to a single nerve. One of the most common causes of mononeuropathy is compressive and traumatic injuries. Traumatic nerve injuries can result in the following conditions in increasing order of severity: neuropraxia, axonotmesis, and neurotmesis. Neuropraxia is generally caused by compressive damage that produces focal demyelination without interruption of nerve fibers. Therefore, the prognosis is benign and characterized by more severe motor impairment than sensory impairment, without atrophy. Recovery occurs relatively quickly and simultaneously in all muscle groups.

Axonotmesis refers to damage and/or interruption of nerve fibers while preserving the connective tissue structures of the nerve. The integrity of the connective tissue provides anatomical guidance for spontaneous axonal regeneration, which occurs at a rate of approximately 1 mm per day. Functional recovery varies and depends, in particular, on the distance that regenerating axons must travel to reach the distribution territory.

Neurotmesis involves complete nerve interruption, including the connective framework. It results in severe sensory and motor deficits. Prognosis for functional recovery is poor due to hindrances in axonal regeneration caused by the loss of the nerve's normal supportive connective structure and the formation of scar tissue.

Multineuropathies | Are characterized by damage that involves multiple nerve trunks asymmetrically, irregularly, and at different times. One of the most common causes of multineuropathy is vasculitis. In mono- and multineuropathies, sensory and motor disorders affect the territories of the affected nerves' distribution.

In *polyneuropathies*, the damage involves the nervous system bilaterally and symmetrically. They are caused by a systemic disease. They are generally classified into axonal and demyelinating forms. The most common form of axonal polyneuropathy is diabetic neuropathy, while the most common forms of demyelinating polyneuropathy are inflammatory neuropathies.

In axonal polyneuropathies, predominantly sensory disorders are bilateral and symmetrical from the beginning and are distributed along the length of the axon. In demyelinating polyneuropathies, sensory and motor disorders are bilateral, symmetrical, and generally involve proximal regions (including cranial nerves).

Following peripheral nerve damage, trophic alterations can also develop in the skin, bones, and connective tissues in general. The skin becomes thin, hyperkeratotic, inelastic, and ulcerated. Nails appear fragile with longitudinal ridges. The bones also undergo regressive processes, leading to osteoporosis and an increased risk of fracture. Unfortunately, precise epidemiological data on the prevalence of neuropathies do not exist to date. For example, the prevalence of traumatic-compressive neuropathies, which are probably the most common neuropathies, is unknown. The prevalence of polyneuropathies is 2.4% in the general population. However, this prevalence reaches 8% in individuals above the age of 55, likely due to the increased incidence of systemic diseases that cause polyneuropathies (such as diabetes, renal insufficiency, hypothyroidism, and neurotoxic substance therapies).

20.1.5 Diagnostic test examinations

Collecting medical history and conducting a clinical examination are fundamental elements in diagnosing peripheral nervous system diseases. *Diagnostic test* examinations help confirm a clinical diagnosis, determine the distribution and nature (axon or demyelinating) of the peripheral nerve damage, and are sometimes crucial in the etiological diagnosis of neuropathy.

Nerve conduction study (NCS) | Plays a crucial role in neuropathy diagnosis as it verifies the anatomical and functional integrity of large myelinated fibers. It evaluates two main types of parameters: the amplitude of sensory and motor nerve potentials and the sensory and motor conduction velocity. Axonal damage primarily leads to a reduction in the amplitude of sensory and motor potentials, with normal or slightly altered conduction velocity. Demyelinating damage, on the other hand, results in a significant reduction in conduction velocity and increased distal latency of potentials, with relatively preserved amplitude. In acquired demyelinating polyneuropathies, another sign of demyelination is temporal dispersion of nerve potentials, with an increase in their duration. This phenomenon is due to the non-uniformity of demyelination among various nerve fibers, leading to loss of synchrony in action potential conduction velocity. Such phenomena are quite rare in genetically determined demyelinating neuropathies because the demyelinating damage in these cases is homogeneous.

Electromyography (EMG) | Allows the study of muscle denervation phenomena, variations in motor units, and recruitment deficits resulting from motor axonal damage. In polyneuropathies, electromyographic exploration is of little use, both because they often primarily produce sensory damage and because the electrophysiological study of motor potentials provides clearer and more reproducible information about motor axonal damage. An exception may be acute inflammatory axonal neuropathies, where acute and abundant denervation phenomena occur. Electromyography, however, is highly useful in the diagnosis of mononeuropathies as it provides information about potential neurogenic damage to the muscles innervated by the affected nerve, allowing for a relatively precise determination of the site of damage.

Laser-evoked potentials (LEPs) | Electric nerve conduction studies do not provide information on the function of nociceptive fibers. Currently, the most reliable neurophysiological method for studying the nociceptive system is laser-evoked potentials. Laser stimulation selectively activates cutaneous nociceptors and elicits brain signals mediated by the activation of the pain pathway. Several studies have demonstrated that peripheral nervous system disorders result in a reduction in the amplitude of laser-evoked potentials due to damage to the nociceptive pathway.

Skin biopsy | is a morphometric method that uses a pan-neuronal marker (PGP 9.5) to study the density of cutaneous innervation, which consists predominantly of C fibers. It is currently indicated as the reference method for diagnosing small fiber neuropathies. These neuropathies are characterized by exclusive involvement of the unmyelinated C fibers and, consequently, no alterations are detected in the electroneurographic examination.

Nerve biopsy | This procedure is useful in the etiological definition of neuropathy. Generally, a sural nerve biopsy is performed. The outcome of the procedure is hypoesthesia in the territory of nerve distribution, which usually occurs subclinically. The diagnostic utility is significant in neuropathies secondary to vasculitis. In this case, the neuropathological results consist of necrotizing vasculitis of the *vasa nervorum*, with inflammatory infiltrate and axonal degeneration, and the uneven involvement of various fascicles within the nerve due to irregular vascular damage. Nerve biopsy is also useful in the diagnosis of amyloid neuropathy and neuropathies associated with storage diseases.

Nerve ultrasound | This diagnostic technique has recently gained prominence in the study of peripheral nervous system diseases. Ultrasound allows for the assessment of the anatomical integrity of the nerve along its accessible course and is particularly useful, especially in mononeuropathies, for accurately identifying the site of damage.

Magnetic resonance imaging | In selected cases, magnetic resonance imaging can contribute to the precise identification of the location and characteristics of lesions in larger nerve trunks (e.g., brachial plexus).

Cerebrospinal fluid | It is extremely useful in cases of inflammatory polyradiculoneuropathy, such as Guillain-Barré syndrome and chronic inflammatory demyelinating polyneuropathy (CIDP). These neuropathies result in a significant increase in cerebrospinal fluid proteins with a normal cell count. In particular, an increase in cerebrospinal fluid cellularity should raise suspicion of neuropathy associated with HIV, CIDP and Guillain-Barré syndrome may exhibit the presence of oligoclonal bands.

20.2 Mononeuropathies

20.2.1 Plexus pathology

Brachial plexus

The brachial plexus is formed by the primary ventral rami of the C5-T1 roots. It consists of a upper primary trunk (C5-C6), a middle primary trunk (C7), and an lower primary trunk (C8-T1). Between the clavicle and first rib, the primary trunks divide into anterior and posterior divisions. The first two anterior divisions give rise to the lateral cord, the anterior division of the inferior primary trunk gives rise to the medial cord, and the posterior divisions give rise to the posterior cord. The musculocutaneous, median, and ulnar nerves, which innervate the flexor muscles of the upper limb, originate from the lateral and medial cords, while the axillary and radial nerves originate from the posterior cord (Figure 20.1).

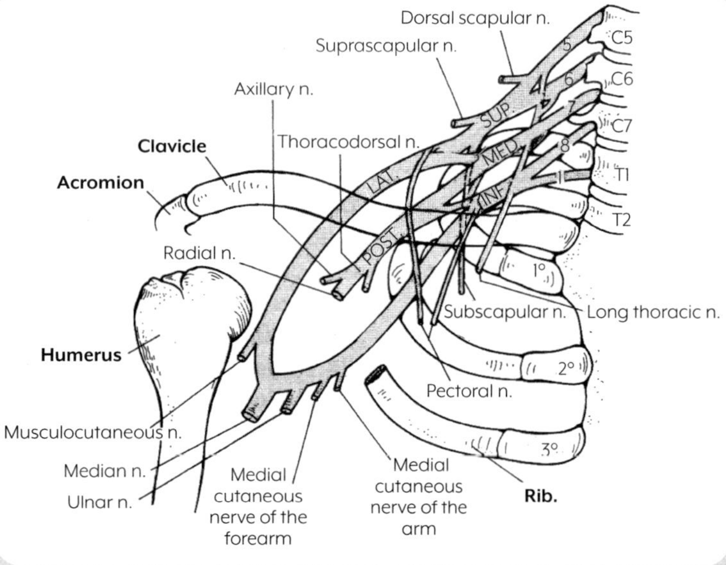

Figure 20.1

Brachial plexus. SUP, MED, INF: superior, middle, and inferior trunks. LAT, POST, MED: lateral, posterior, and medial cords (courtesy of Prof. Mario Manfredi).

Lesions of the brachial plexus | Can be global or selectively involve the upper, middle, or lower trunks or the secondary trunks. The most common is the upper lesion, which involves the C5-C6 fibers and presents with deficits in abduction, external rotation, arm extension, and forearm flexion. Other signs include the absence of biceps and brachioradialis reflexes and atrophy of the deltoid, supraspinatus, and biceps muscles. Sensory deficits may affect the shoulder, outer surface of the arm, and radial border of the hand. The middle lesion involves the C7 fibers, and it affects the extension of the forearm, hand, and fingers, abolishes the triceps reflex, and causes hypoesthesia on the back of the hand and the third finger. Differential diagnosis with a radial nerve lesion is based on the sparing of the brachioradialis muscle, which is innervated by C5-C6. The lower lesion involves the C8-T1 fibers and manifests as deficits in finger abduction, adduction, thumb opposition, and little finger opposition. The hands assume a characteristic claw-like appearance, with hyperextension at the metacarpophalangeal joint and flexion at the interphalangeal joints.

Selective lesions of the secondary trunks manifest as a combined lesion of some nerves of the upper limb. The differential diagnosis between plexus and radicular damage can be made through electrophysiological studies. In radicular damage, electromyographic studies show impairment of the paravertebral muscles, which are innervated by the posterior branch of the spinal nerve, while electroneurographic studies show normal sensory potentials. This is because the roots are usually damaged in the pre-ganglionic tract, with sparing of the axon downstream of the ganglion.

Causes of brachial plexus damage are diverse and include trauma, radiation therapy, neoplastic infiltration, compressive conditions (such as thoracic outlet syndrome), and inflammatory conditions (such as neuralgic amyotrophy). Traumatic damage to the brachial plexus can occur with penetrating wounds, direct stretching, anterior dislocation of the humeral head, clavicular fractures, and obstetric trauma.

In *traumatic brachial plexopathy*, the injury can be global, but in most cases, the upper part of the plexus is affected due to a violent displacement of the head and neck from the shoulder. Recovery depends on the extent of the damage, which is irreversible in the presence of root avulsion.

Radiation-induced brachial plexopathy | Typically begins in the lower portion of the plexus with a variable latency period after treatment, which can also be very long (radiation-induced brachial plexopathy is discussed in more detail in the section dedicated to neuropathies in oncological diseases).

The most common neoplastic conditions responsible for *neoplastic infiltration-induced brachial plexopathy* include primary tumors (neurinomas), infiltrating neoplasms originating in adjacent anatomical regions (apical lung carcinoma, lymphomas), or metastases from breast carcinoma. In cases of neoplastic invasion, the lower part of the plexus is more affected, and Horner's syndrome may be associated.

Thoracic outlet syndrome | Is due to compressive damage to the lower primary trunk of the brachial plexus, associated with compression of the artery and, less commonly, the subclavian vein. The most frequent causes are the presence of supernumerary cervical ribs, hypertrophic cervical transverse processes, and hypertrophy of the anterior scalene muscle. In addition to vascular symptoms (Raynaud's phenomenon, edema, cyanosis), the syndrome manifests with impairment of the lower portion of the plexus. Neurophysiological examinations show a reduction in sensory potential amplitude and increased F-wave latency after ulnar nerve stimulation, signs of denervation in the hand muscles, and absence of signal at the Erb's point during somatosensory evoked potential recording from ulnar nerve stimulation. To recognize thoracic outlet syndrome, it may be useful to look for the disappearance of the radial pulse during inspiration and rotation of the head toward the affected side with the neck extended and the arm adducted (Adson's maneuver). The therapy consists of surgical removal of the compression cause.

Neuralgic amyotrophy | also known as Parsonage-Turner syndrome or brachial plexitis, is a rare condition that develops acutely and primarily consists of pain, motor deficits, and atrophy affecting the muscles related to the brachial plexus. Although recovery occurs in variable times, most patients experience complete recovery. Only 5-10% of cases have persistent weakness. There are two main forms of neuralgic amyotrophy: an idiopathic form and a genetically determined form. The latter has an autosomal dominant inheritance with incomplete penetrance. In more than half of the families examined, the disease is associated with a point mutation or duplication of the SEPT9 gene, which maps to chromosome 17. The genetically determined form is earlier in onset, often results in bilateral and recurrent plexopathies, and has a less severe prognosis. In the idiopathic form, autoimmune processes likely play a determining role. Mechanical factors may also contribute to the development of the disease as the brachial plexus has a particular anatomical vulnerability. The detailed pathogenesis of the hereditary form is still unknown. The SEPT9 gene encodes 6 isoforms of septin 9, a cytoskeletal protein, through alternative splicing. The mechanism by which mutations in this protein can lead to brachial plexopathy is still unknown.

Lumbosacral plexus

The lumbosacral plexus, located in the retroperitoneal space, is formed by the roots L1-S4 and gives rise, through its anterior branches, to the lateral femoral cutaneous nerve, obturator nerve, and the tibial branch of the sciatic nerve. Through its posterior branches, it gives rise to the femoral nerve and the peroneal branch of the sciatic nerve (Figure 20.2).

Injuries to the lumbosacral plexus are much rarer than those of the brachial plexus, given its protected position in the pelvis and the lack of narrow anatomical passages that could lead to compression damage. However, the plexus can be damaged as a result of trauma, pelvic fractures, surgical procedures such as hysterectomy, tumors (carcinomatous or sarcomatous neuritis), exposure to radiation therapy, retroperitoneal fibrosis, hematomas in the context of the iliopsoas muscle or

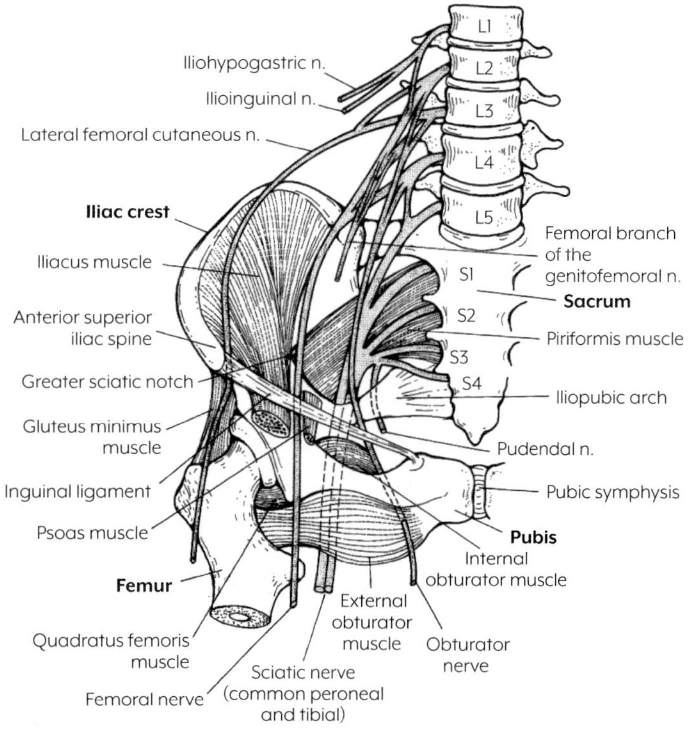

Figure 20.2

Lumbosacral plexus. L1, L2, L3, L4, L5: lumbar vertebrae and roots. S1, S2, S3, S4: sacral vertebrae and roots (by kind permission of Prof. Mario Manfredi).

during childbirth. In radiation therapy-induced plexopathy, the onset with weakness is typical, followed by pain, paresthesia, or hypoesthesia after months. There is also a rare possibility of idiopathic damage, similar to neuralgic amyotrophy, which manifests as pain, functional impotence, and muscle atrophy. A lesion involving only the lumbar plexus (L1-L4) presents with a deficit in flexion, external rotation, adduction of the thigh, and extension of the leg. A sacral plexus (L4-S3) lesion manifests as sensory disturbance on the posterior surface of the thigh, leg, and foot, along with paralysis of the femoral extensors, knee flexors, and all muscles of the leg and foot.

Lesions of the plexus must be differentiated from possible intraspinal expansive processes, characterized by progressive course, bilateral deficits, urinary alterations, and cerebrospinal fluid modifications, as well as from lumbar or sacral radiculopathies, recognizable by monoradicular deficits and the coexistence of vertebral symptoms.

20.2.2 Syndromes due to individual nerve trunk lesions

Median nerve | It is a mixed nerve originating from the roots C5-T1 and the lateral and medial cords of the brachial plexus. It courses in the arm at the medial bicipital groove, passes through the elbow between the two heads of the pronator teres muscle, continues in the forearm along the midline to the wrist, crossing the carpal tunnel, and then divides into its terminal branches at the palm of the hand. With its sensory component, it innervates the skin of the palm of the hand up to the middle of the fourth digit; with its motor component, it innervates the pronator teres and quadratus muscles, radial flexor of the wrist, superficial and deep flexors of the fingers (except for the ulnar heads for the fourth and fifth fingers), and the first and second lumbrical muscles, long and short flexors, abductor brevis, and opponens pollicis muscles (Figure 20.3).

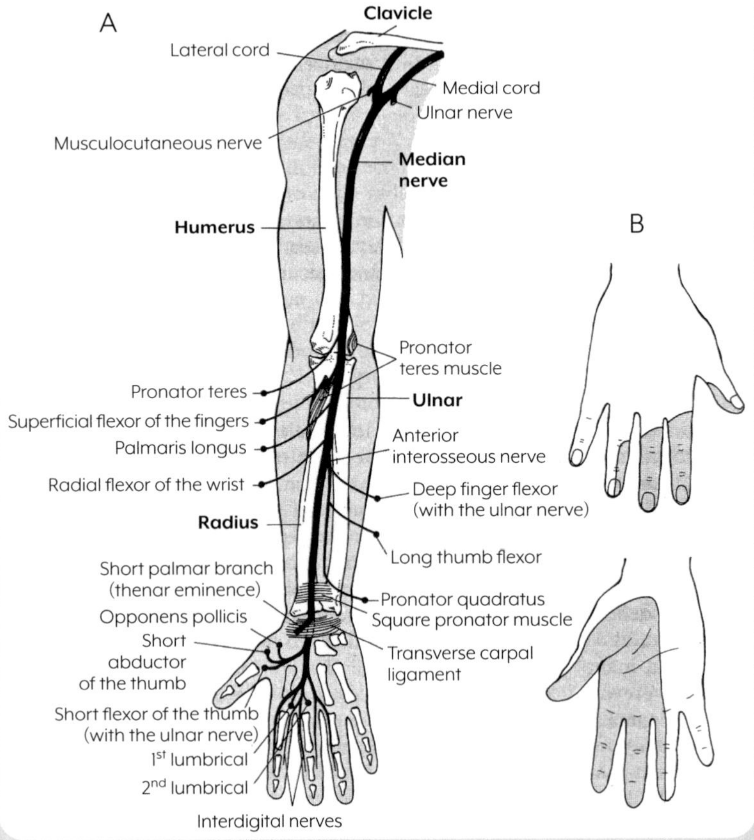

Figure 20.3

Median nerve.
A) Course, motor distribution, terminal cutaneous branches. B) Cutaneous distribution (with kind permission from Prof. Mario Manfredi).

The median nerve can be injured due to shoulder trauma, fractures or dislocations of the humerus, but by far the most common is its compression at the carpal tunnel.

The nerve injury compromises forearm pronation, wrist flexion, flexion of the second phalanx of the last four fingers, flexion of the distal phalanx of the second and third fingers, and abduction, opposition, and flexion of the distal phalanx of the thumb.

The most common form of mononeuropathy of the median nerve is carpal tunnel syndrome, which involves compressive damage to the median nerve within the carpal tunnel. Carpal tunnel syndrome is usually bilateral, more common in females, and in most cases, it is idiopathic. Secondary forms are associated with hypothyroidism, amyloidosis, renal insufficiency, and rheumatoid arthritis. It presents with paresthesia, predominantly at night, in the hand, in the territory of distribution of the median nerve, sometimes accompanied by pain that tends to radiate up the upper limb to the shoulder. In advanced cases, atrophy of the muscles of the thenar eminence and deficits in thumb opposition and abduction may be observed. The treatment of the idiopathic form involves surgical decompression. While waiting for the surgery, the use of a night splint may be helpful in alleviating symptoms (palmar splint).

Ulnar nerve | It is a mixed nerve that originates from the C8-T1 roots and the medial cord of the brachial plexus. It runs in the medial part of the anterior compartment of the arm, passes the elbow by traversing the groove between the medial epicondyle of the humerus and the olecranon of the ulna, and reaches the anterior part of the forearm on the medial side. It terminates at the palm of the hand after passing through the wrist at the Guyon's canal. With its sensory component, it innervates the skin of the ulnar half of the hand, and with its motor component, it innervates the flexor carpi ulnaris, deep flexors of the fourth and fifth fingers, interossei, third and fourth lumbricals, short flexor and adductor of the thumb, and the muscles of the hypothenar eminence (Figure 20.4).

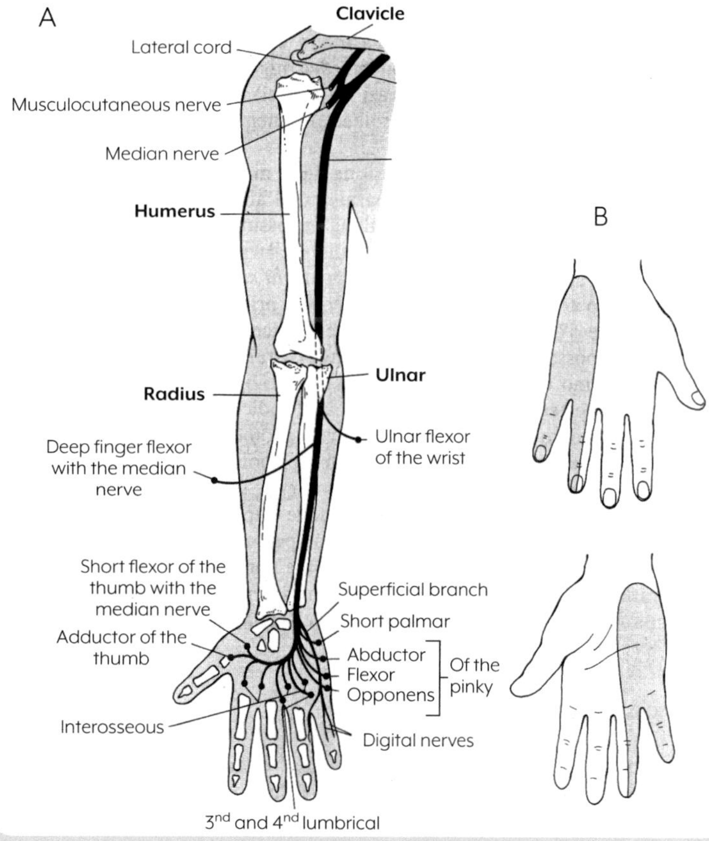

Figure 20.4

Ulnar Nerve.
A) Course, motor distribution, terminal cutaneous branches. B) Cutaneous distribution (courtesy of Prof. Mario Manfredi).

The ulnar nerve can be injured in fractures of the humerus, compression at the elbow, or entrapment at the Guyon's canal.

The injury affects the flexion of the wrist, flexion of the distal phalanx of the fourth and fifth fingers, flexion of the proximal phalanx, abduction and adduction of the fingers, and adduction of the thumb. Characteristic clinical findings include the "ulnar claw" hand deformity (hyperextended ring and little fingers at the metacarpophalangeal joints and flexed at the first interphalangeal joint) and Froment's sign (difficulty in grasping and holding a sheet of paper between the extended thumb and the base of the index finger). A lesion of the ulnar nerve, with atrophy of the hypothenar eminence and interosseous muscles, can be easily distinguished from a root injury by the sparing of the thenar eminence, which is innervated by the median nerve roots.

Radial nerve | It is a mixed nerve that originates from the C5-T1 roots and the posterior cord of the brachial plexus. It descends from the axillary cavity behind the axillary artery, then enters the spiral groove of the humerus and passes the elbow in front of the lateral epicondyle of the humerus. Above the radial head, it divides into its two terminal branches, the superficial sensory branch and the deep motor branch. With its sensory component, it innervates the skin on the dorsal side of the arm and forearm, and the cutaneous region on the back of the hand between the first and second metacarpals. With its motor branches, it innervates the triceps, supinator, brachioradialis, wrist extensors, extensor digitorum longus, extensor pollicis longus and brevis, and abductor pollicis longus muscles (Figure 20.5).

The most common causes of radial nerve injury include compression in the spiral groove of the humerus, humeral fractures, and elbow dislocations. The more proximal the site of the lesion, the more the extensor muscles are affected. Nerve section can compromise the extension, flexion, and supination of the forearm, as well as the extension of the hand

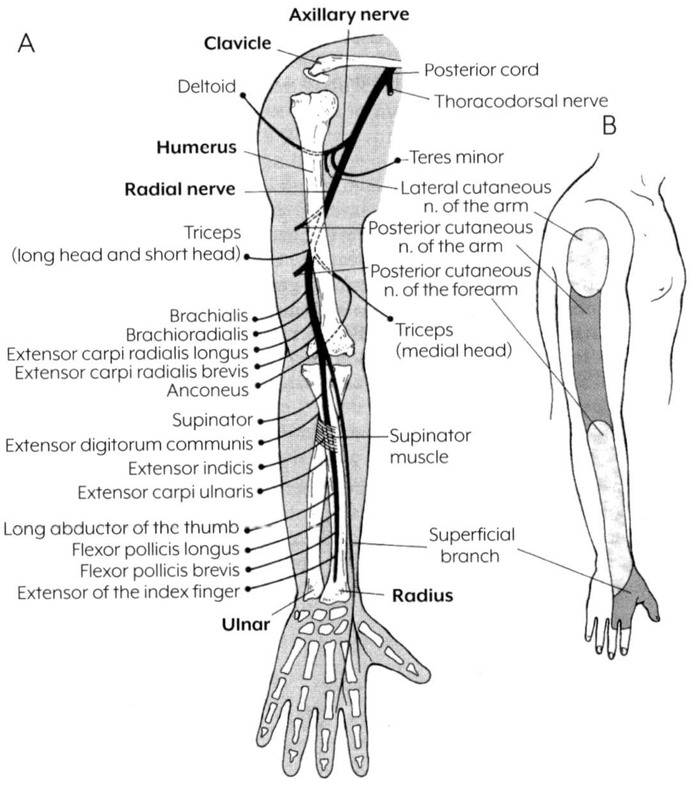

Figure 20.5

Axillary and radial nerves. A) Course, motor distribution, terminal cutaneous branches. B) Cutaneous distribution (courtesy of Prof. Mario Manfredi).

and fingers, resulting in the characteristic "wrist drop" sign.

Axillary nerve | It is a mixed nerve that originates from the C5-C6 roots and the posterior cord of the brachial plexus. It is responsible for the motor innervation of the deltoid and teres minor muscles, and the sensory innervation of the skin over the shoulder (Figure 20.5). It can be injured in cases of shoulder trauma, dislocation of the glenohumeral joint, surgical fractures of the surgical neck of the humerus or scapula. The injury manifests as a deficit in shoulder abduction, flexion, and extension, with atrophy of the deltoid muscle and decreased sensation in the outer proximal portion of the shoulder.

Dorsal scapular nerve | It is a motor nerve that originates from the C4-C5 roots and the upper trunk of the brachial plexus. It innervates the levator scapulae, rhomboid minor, and rhomboid major muscles, which elevate and adduct the medial border of the scapula. Isolated lesions are rather rare and may be associated with trauma in the posterior cervical region or costocervical malformations, as part of a thoracic outlet syndrome. Clinical manifestations are not very evident, except for difficulty crossing the arms behind the back and incorrect positioning of the scapula, which appears rotated outward at the lower angle.

Suprascapular nerve | It is a motor nerve that originates from the C5-C6 roots and the upper trunk of the brachial plexus. It innervates the supraspinatus and infraspinatus muscles. The injury can occur due to shoulder trauma and fractures of the humeral head, and it manifests as a deficit in abduction (for the first 15°) and external rotation of the arm, with a tendency for pronation and muscle atrophy, particularly evident in the infraspinatus muscle.

Subscapular nerve | It is a motor nerve that originates from the C5-C7 roots and the upper trunk and posterior cord of the brachial plexus, with two branches for the subscapularis and teres major muscles. The injury is quite rare, usually of traumatic origin, and impairs internal rotation of the arm.

Long thoracic nerve | It is a motor nerve that originates from the C5-C7 roots. It is responsible for innervating the serratus anterior muscle. Injuries are generally a result of shoulder trauma and manifest as a deficit in arm elevation beyond the horizontal plane, along with the characteristic winged scapula sign, which becomes more pronounced when the subject extends the upper limbs and forcefully leans against a wall.

Musculocutaneous nerve | It is a mixed nerve that originates from the C5-C7 roots and the lateral cord of the brachial plexus. It innervates the coracobrachialis, biceps brachii, and brachialis muscles, as well as a cutaneous area along the radial border of the forearm. The injury is relatively rare and can occur in cases of shoulder wounds or fractures of the humerus. It manifests as a deficit in forearm supination and flexion, partially compensated by the action of the brachioradialis and pronator teres muscles, along with atrophy in the anterior part of the forearm.

Lateral femoral cutaneous nerve | is a sensory nerve that originates from the L2-L3 roots. It emerges from the iliac fossa, crosses the inguinal ligament, and distributes to the lateral surface of the thigh (Figure 20.6). It can easily be compressed at the level of the ligament, leading to the development of a sensory neuropathy called "meralgia paresthetica." This condition manifests with paresthesia and pain, often described as burning or like pinpricks, in the distribution territory of the nerve. It is usually unilateral and commonly associated with weight gain. In most cases, it regresses spontaneously, but in the case of debilitating neuropathic pain, analgesic treatment may be necessary. Compression of this nerve can also result from abdominal tumors or hematomas in the iliopsoas muscle.

Femoral nerve | It is a mixed nerve that originates from the L2-L4 roots and exits the pelvis through the inguinal ligament. It provides sensory innervation to the skin on the anterior surface of the thigh, the medial aspect of the leg (saphenous nerve), and the root of the foot. Motor innervation is supplied to the iliopsoas, sartorius, and quadriceps femoris muscles (Figure 20.6). It can be injured

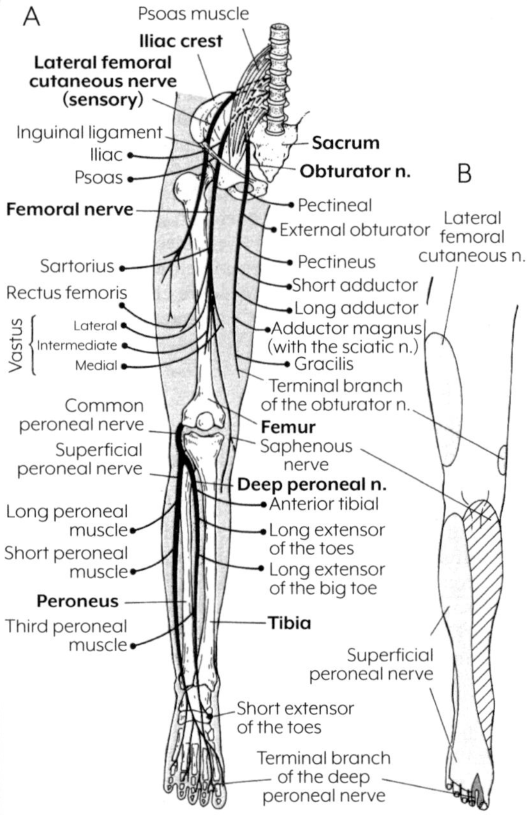

Figure 20.6

Femoral cutaneous nerve, femoral nerve, obturator nerve, and superficial and deep peroneal nerves. 11, 12: thoracic vertebrae. 1, 2, 3, 4, 5: lumbar vertebrae. A) Course, motor distribution, terminal cutaneous branches. B) Cutaneous distribution (courtesy of Prof. Mario Manfredi).

during surgical procedures involving the pelvis, tumors, fractures of the pelvis or femur, retroperitoneal hematomas, hematomas or abscesses of the psoas, aneurysms, or femoral artery catheterization. A femoral nerve injury presents with sensory deficit in the cutaneous distribution territory, weakness of thigh flexion at the hip (partially compensated by collateral innervation from direct branches of the L2 and L3 plexus), leg extension at the thigh, and quadriceps atrophy. The patellar reflex is either absent or diminished. As a consequence of saphenous vein surgery or secondary irritation from phlebitis, selective involvement of the saphenous nerve can occur, presenting with pain and a feeling of heaviness in the distal portion of the thigh and leg. Differentiating a L3-L4 root lesion from femoral nerve palsy can be easily done by sparing the adductor reflex.

Obturator nerve | is primarily a motor nerve that originates from the L2-L4 roots. It exits the pelvis through the obturator foramen and innervates the adductor muscles of the thigh and a small area of skin on the distal half of the medial surface of the thigh. It can be injured in cases of tumors, fractures of the pelvis, obturator canal hernias, or during childbirth. The injury manifests as a deficit in lower limb adduction, while sensory disturbances, typically inconsistent, include paresthesia in the cutaneous distribution territory of the nerve and knee pain (Howship-Romberg phenomenon) due to innervation by the posterior branch of the obturator nerve.

Sciatic nerve | Is a mixed nerve that originates from the L4-S3 roots. It exits the pelvis through the sciatic foramen, runs between the greater trochanter and the ischial tuberosity, separated from the hip joint by the gemelli muscles, and reaches the posterior thigh. It consists of two distinct branches, the tibial and the peroneal, which are surrounded by a common epineurium until the upper part of the popliteal fossa, where they separate (Figure 20.7). Therefore, even in cases of proximal sciatic nerve injuries, isolated paralysis of the tibial or peroneal nerve can occur. In the thigh, it innervates the semitendinosus, semimembranosus, long head of the biceps femoris, part of the adductor magnus (tibial nerve), and the short head of the biceps femoris (peroneal nerve). Injury to the sciatic nerve can occur due to pelvic tumors, dislocations of the femoral head, hip joint surgeries, femoral fractures, hematomas, or injuries resulting from injections in the gluteal region, as well as compression during prolonged bed rest or coma.

The injury presents with deficits in leg flexion at the knee, foot movements, and sensory disturbances in the anterolateral surface of the leg and foot (except for a small region below the medial malleolus, which is innervated by the saphenous nerve, a branch of the femoral nerve). While the patellar reflex is spared, the Achilles and plantar reflexes are lost.

Common peroneal nerve | (External Popliteal Sciatic Nerve). It is a mixed nerve that originates from the L4-S2 roots (predominantly L5). It branches off from the sciatic nerve trunk at the popliteal fossa level and, in the anterolateral compartment of the leg, divides into a superficial branch and a deep branch. The superficial branch innervates the peroneal muscles and the skin on the lateral surface of the leg and dorsum of the foot, while the deep branch innervates the anterior tibial muscle, extensor digitorum longus, extensor hallucis longus, short extensors of the toes, and a restricted cutaneous region between the hallux and the second toe (Figure 20.7).

The common peroneal nerve can be damaged in cases of fibular fractures, knee dislocations, compression due to prolonged bed rest, or the application of plaster casts. Significant weight loss or a state of vitamin deficiency can increase susceptibility to damage to this nerve, as it is particularly sensitive to ischemic injury due to the superficial course of the nutrient vessels, which are prone to compression. Common peroneal nerve injury presents with a deficit in foot extension and eversion, toe extension, a characteristic "steppage" gait, and sensory impairment in the cutaneous territory supplied by the nerve. Differential diagnosis from an L5 root lesion is based on the presence of signs of denervation in the posterior tibial muscle, which is innervated by the tibial nerve.

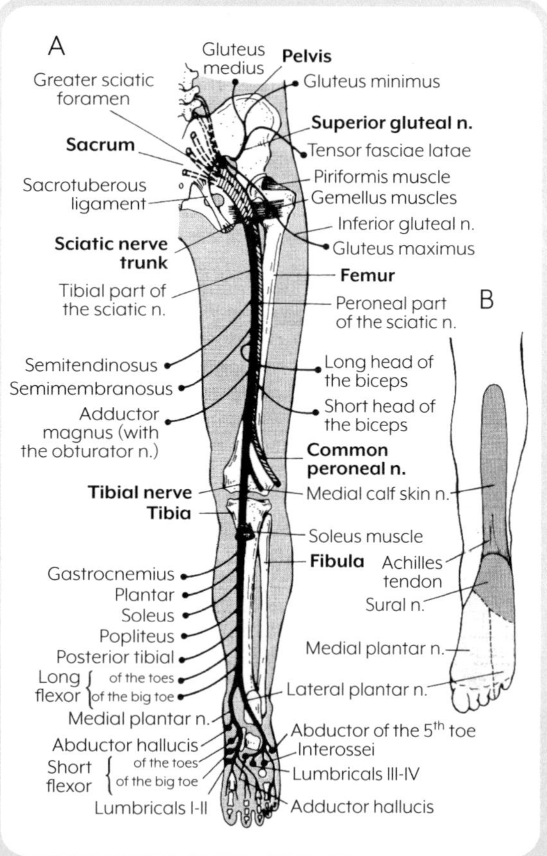

Figure 20.7

Gluteal, sciatic, common peroneal, and tibial nerves. A) Course, motor distribution, terminal cutaneous branches. B) Cutaneous distribution (by kind permission of Prof. Mario Manfredi).

Tibial Nerve | (Internal Popliteal Sciatic Nerve). It is a mixed nerve that originates from the L4-S3 roots and branches off from the sciatic nerve trunk at the popliteal fossa level. It runs deep in the posterior compartment of the leg, beneath the gastrocnemius muscle, reaches the ankle, passes through the tarsal tunnel, and terminates by dividing into its terminal branches, the medial and lateral plantar nerves. The motor component innervates the soleus, gastrocnemius, posterior tibial, long flexors of the toes and hallux, and the small muscles of the plantar surface of the foot. The sensory component innervates the skin on the posterior surface of the leg and the plantar surface of the foot. One of its branches, the medial sural cutaneous nerve, along with a branch of the peroneal nerve, gives rise to the sural nerve, which supplies the skin on the lateral border of the foot and the lateral aspect of the heel (Figure 20.7).

A tibial nerve injury is rather rare due to its deep course and can occur as a result of tibial fractures, fractures of the talus or medial malleolus, or compression beneath the flexor retinaculum (tarsal tunnel syndrome). A complete tibial nerve lesion presents with deficits in plantar flexion and inversion of the foot, deficits in toe flexion, abduction, and adduction, absent Achilles and medio-plantar reflexes, reduced patellar reflex, calf atrophy, and hypoesthesia on the posterior surface of the leg and the plantar surface of the foot. Tarsal tunnel syndrome manifests with ankle and plantar foot pain, predominantly at night, associated with deficits in toe flexion and abduction. Supporting the diagnosis are increased latency of the motor potential upon stimulation of the tibial nerve at the medial malleolus and signs of neurogenic damage in the abductor hallucis muscle.

Cauda equina | The cauda equina consists of the roots from L2 to S5 that, below the terminal cone, obliquely traverse the vertebral canal from top to bottom and from the inside to the outside. A bilateral lesion of these roots is responsible for complete cauda equina syndrome. This condition manifests with radicular distribution pain, hypoesthesia involving the lower limbs up to the root of the thighs (with a typical saddle distribution), flaccid paraplegia, absent medio-plantar and Achilles tendon reflexes, reduced patellar reflex, absence of bulbocavernous, anal, and cutaneous plantar reflexes. Impairment of urinary function, typically presenting as urinary retention, as well as genital and rectal functions, is also characteristic. Occasionally, the lesion may be incomplete, affecting only some roots, or it may be unilateral, resulting in the so-called hemi-cauda syndrome. Common causes include intradural tumors, L4-L5 or L5-S1 disc herniations with medial extrusion, and, less commonly, aneurysms within the sacral canal. Cauda equina syndrome can have an acute onset requiring urgent surgical intervention or a slowly progressive onset, as in the case of compression by ependymomas, metastases, or neurinomas. Bladder and anorectal disturbances may not be present at the onset in these latter cases. Differential diagnosis between conus medullaris lesions and cauda equina syndrome relies on the preservation of osteotendinous reflexes and the predominance of bladder disturbances over sensory and motor impairments in the lower limbs. The presence of pain or asymmetry of symptoms would be indicative of cauda equina syndrome.

20.3 Polyneuropathies

20.3.1 Hereditary neuropathies

These are a heterogeneous group of neuropathies characterized by insidious onset and a chronic course. They are generally distinguished from acute or subacute forms by marked muscular atrophy, the presence of trophic skin alterations, and osteoarticular deformities. Traditionally, they were classified based on the category of fibers involved, including *sensory-motor, sensory-autonomic,* and *purely motor forms*. However, this classification has been largely overcome thanks to recent advances in molecular biology and retains meaning only for the last two categories.

The sensory-motor forms are currently identified with the eponym Charcot-Marie-Tooth disease (CMT), which encompasses the largest group, accounting for approximately 90%, with a prevalence of 1 in 2500 and autosomal dominant, recessive, or X-linked inheritance. The classification is continuously evolving due to the discovery of new genes involved (Table 20.1). These neuropathies can be distinguished, based on neuropathological and electrophysiological characteristics, into demyelinating forms (CMT1, CMT4, Dejerine-Sottas syndrome, NIC, HNPP) and axonal forms (CMT2, AR-CMT2). This classification has always been based on the electrophysiological finding of motor conduction velocity values being either lower or higher than the cutoff value of 38 m/sec for the upper limb. However, recently, some subtypes of dominantly inherited CMT (IDCMT) have been identified with intermediate conduction velocity values between axonal and demyelinating forms. The high number of genes involved in hereditary neuropathies sometimes makes it challenging to direct the patient towards a specific genetic investigation. Therefore, molecular diagnosis cannot be separated from adequate clinical and electrophysiological evaluation.

Charcot-Marie-Tooth disease (CMT) and related neuropathies

CMT1 | Is an autosomal dominant or X-linked demyelinating neuropathy. Molecular biology studies have revealed mutations involving different gene loci. CMT1A is the most common form (40-50% of cases) and is associated with a duplication of a 1.5 Mb region on chromosome 17p11.2, where the gene for peripheral myelin protein 22 (PMP22) is located. A less frequent form, CMT1B (3-5%

of cases), is instead linked to point mutations of the myelin protein zero (MPZ). The second most common form of CMT1, CMT1X, has an X-linked inheritance and is associated with a mutation in the GJB1 gene (gap junction B1), which encodes for connexin 32. Despite genetic heterogeneity, the different subtypes of CMT1 do not differ significantly from a clinical standpoint. Characteristically, onset occurs between the second and third decades of life, with motor deficits starting from the distal extremities of the lower limbs, slowly worsening, accompanied by muscular atrophy, and followed by sensory disturbances. The most affected muscles include the anterior tibialis, toe extensors, and gastrocnemius. The sparing of the proximal two-thirds of the thigh gives the lower limbs a typical appearance. Sensory disturbances particularly affect deep sensations and can lead to an ataxic gait. Rarely, there may be involvement of small fibers resulting in thermal and pain hypoesthesia. Another typical feature is the presence of skeletal deformities such as pes cavus, hammer toes, claw hands, and scoliosis. Osteotendinous reflexes are weak or absent. 60% of affected adults complain of asthenia; tremors, mainly in the hands, can also be associated. Rare cases with associated non-progressive sensorineural hearing loss and vestibular abnormalities have been described. As it is a demyelinating condition, the electrophysiological examination shows markedly reduced sensory and motor conduction velocities. Nerve biopsy, which is generally rendered unnecessary by genetic tests, shows signs of hypertrophic neuropathy with onion bulb formations due to attempts at remyelination and areas devoid of myelin. The spectrum of clinical manifestations is heterogeneous, even within the same family, ranging from debilitating forms to asymptomatic forms characterized only by pes cavus and reduced osteotendinous reflexes. This phenotypic variability is dependent on genetic and environmental factors. In some debilitating forms, the simultaneous presence of two mutations in different genes associated with CMT has been identified. Recent evidence suggests the role of muscle magnetic resonance imaging, with measurement of the fraction of adipose tissue in the calf, as a sensitive biomarker capable of determining the progression of CMT1 during the disease.

CMT2 | It is a predominantly autosomal dominant axonal neuropathy. It represents about one-third of CMT cases; 20% are associated with mutations in the MFN2 (mitofusin 2) gene, 5% with mutations in MPZ, and, in rarer cases, involvement of other genes such as NEFL (neurofilament light chain) or GDAP1 (ganglioside-induced differentiation-associated protein-1). Onset occurs between the third and fourth decades of life, with distal motor deficits, usually limited to the lower limbs, and depressed osteotendinous reflexes. Sensory disturbances are generally mild or absent. Electrophysiological examination typically reveals reduced amplitude of motor and sensory action potentials and normal or slightly reduced conduction velocity in the median and ulnar motor nerves. Nerve biopsy lacks clear signs of demyelination and the so-called "onion bulbs" images. The course and prognosis do not differ from CMT1.

Dejerine-Sottas syndrome (DSD) | It is a demyelinating form with autosomal recessive or dominant inheritance involving several genes. It begins in childhood with severe motor developmental delay, atonia, and depression of osteotendinous reflexes. These are severe and disabling forms that impair walking. Electrophysiological examination shows the absence of sensory action potentials and significantly reduced motor conduction velocity. Cerebrospinal fluid examination shows increased protein levels, while nerve biopsy reveals nerve hypertrophy with reduced myelin fibers and the characteristic "*onion bulbs*" images.

Tomaculous neuropathy | Also known as HNPP (*Hereditary Neuropathy with Liability to Pressure Palsies*), it is a demyelinating neuropathy with autosomal dominant transmission, characterized by a defect in myelin repair mechanisms. It is associated with an 85-90% deletion of a 1.5 Mb region on chromosome 17p-11.2 (the same region duplicated in CMT1A), resulting in reduced expression of the PMP22 gene. In rare cases, it is associated with PMP22 gene mutations leading to non-coding stop codons. It has a prevalence of 7.3-16:100,000. Peripheral nerve fibers show a typical appearance, characterized by multiple nodular thickening of the myelin alternating with focal demyelination areas. It usually manifests during adolescence with recurrent focal demyelinating neuropathies triggered by minor trauma or physiological nerve compression, most commonly affecting the peroneal nerve and ulnar nerve (30-48% and 21-28% respectively), brachial plexus (12-27%), radial nerve (4-13%), and median nerve (4-11%). Symptoms usually regress within a few days or weeks, with complete recovery in about 50% of cases. However, the phenotypic spectrum of the disease is heterogeneous, including asymptomatic forms and severe forms that can mimic CMT. Nerve conduction studies show a characteristic pattern with increased distal motor latencies, particularly in the median and peroneal nerves. Focal motor slowing at entrapment sites (ulnar nerve at the elbow, peroneal nerve at the fibular head) is also common. In other segments, motor conduction velocity may be normal. Sensory conduction velocity is often reduced, as well as the amplitude of sensory potentials. A diagnosis of HNPP should always be considered in the presence of recurrent focal compressive neuropathies. A family history indicative of autosomal dominant inheritance is a characteristic feature, although de novo occurrence is possible (20%). In the differential diagnosis, compression mononeuropathies caused by neoplasms, hematomas, and abscesses must be considered. In suspected HNPP cases, clinical and neurophysiological data should be supported by genetic testing to detect the deletion of the PMP22 gene; if negative, genetic sequencing may be indicated.

Treatment | Currently, there are no effective treatments for CMT, except for traditional therapeutic approaches such as physiotherapy and surgical correction of skeletal deformities.

Hereditary sensory neuropathies (HSNs) and sensory-autonomic neuropathies (HSANs)

These are hereditary neuropathies characterized by sensory disturbances, sometimes associated with autonomic impairment. The classification is constantly evolving based on the identification of new loci and different genes involved. Type I is the most common form, characterized by autosomal dominant inheritance and associated with point mutations in the gene encoding the SPTLC1 protein (*serine palmitoyltransferase long-chain base one*). It manifests between the second and fourth decades of life with thermal-pain hypoesthesia, sparing of tactile, vibratory, and proprioceptive sensitivity, depression of osteotendinous reflexes, trophic disorders in the soles of the feet, ulcerations, and moderate autonomic disturbances such as hypohidrosis. These patients may develop neuropathic pain described as stabbing or burning. The selective impairment of small-caliber myelinated fibers (Adelta) and unmyelinated C fibers can be documented through laser-evoked potentials recording and skin biopsy.

Hereditary motor neuropathies (dHMN)

These are a rather heterogeneous group of neuropathies, difficult to distinguish from spinal muscular atrophies, characterized by the selective involvement of motor fibers. They differ, therefore, from CMT, in which sensory deficit is a key element for diagnosis. However, this distinction is not so clear-cut when considering some intermediate forms with minimal sensory involvement, overlapping with forms of CMT2. There are also subtypes characterized by the involvement of the first motor neuron, overlapping with juvenile forms of amyotrophic lateral sclerosis or hereditary spastic paraplegia. Eleven genes and four loci responsible for these neuropathies have been identified, showing autosomal dominant, recessive, or X-linked inheritance. Some genes, including BSCL2, are also involved in the onset of CMT2. Despite recent advances in molecular biology, the mutation remains unknown in 80% of cases. Onset generally occurs between the first and second decades of life with a slowly worsening distal motor deficit starting from the lower limbs, except for dHMN5, which primarily involves the upper limbs. Muscle atrophy and depression of osteotendinous reflexes are associated. Characteristic elements are vocal cord paralysis in dHMN7 and diaphragmatic paralysis in dHMN4. Electrophysiology confirms the clinical suspicion by showing a reduction in motor action potential amplitude and signs of neurogenic damage in the distal muscles. Electromyographic examination can also allow differential diagnosis with forms of distal myopathy.

Involvement of cranial nerves

Involvement of the cranial region can help direct toward a specific genotype. Optic atrophy has been described in patients with involvement of the MFN2 gene in CMT2A2. Involvement of the oculomotor nerve, instead, is associated with a mutation in the EGR2 gene. Hearing loss, although found in various subtypes of CMT, is characteristic of CMT4D. Vocal cord paralysis is more frequently associated with CMT2C (12q 23-24), AR-CMT2, or CMT4A (GDAP1) and dHMN7 (DCTN1).

Hereditary metabolic neuropathies

Fabry disease | Is a lysosomal storage disorder, X-linked, caused by a deficiency of the enzyme alpha-galactosidase A. The enzymatic defect leads to an accumulation of globotriaosylceramide (Gb3) in the lysosomes of endothelial cells, renal cells, myocardial cells, and spinal ganglia. The spectrum of symptoms varies from mild forms in heterozygous females to severe cases in hemizygous males who have no residual alpha-galactosidase A activity. The disease, which begins in childhood and adolescence, causes kidney damage, cardiomyopathy, cerebral stroke, and neuropathy. A characteristic clinical feature is diffuse angiocheratoma. Regarding the peripheral nervous system, the accumulation primarily affects the ganglion cells of small-diameter sensory and autonomic fibers. Clinical manifestations include neuropathic pain, which mainly affects the distal extremities of all four limbs, hypohidrosis, and gastrointestinal disturbances. Instrumental examinations show predominant damage to small-diameter fibers. Enzyme replacement therapy (recombinant alpha-galactosidase A) has been available for many years. Replacement therapy significantly improves clinical symptoms and potentially alters long-term prognosis.

Hereditary amyloid neuropathies | Are a heterogeneous group of diseases characterized by the accumulation of amyloid protein and inherited in an autosomal recessive manner. Four main clinical variants are described based on the ethnic origin of affected families: Portuguese type (the most common), Swiss type, Iowa type, and Finnish type.

In the Portuguese type, the abnormal amyloid protein that deposits in peripheral nerves is an abnormal transthyretin. Transthyretin is a soluble tetramer. In this disease, the protein dissociates into 4 monomers that aggregate into insoluble fibrils, infiltrating various organs. The manifestations of the disease are highly variable and depend on the specific mutation. The phenotypic expression ranges from almost exclusively neurological involvement (Val30Met mutation, valine-to-methionine substitution at position 30) to exclusively cardiac involvement (Thr60Ala, Leu111Met, Ile68Leu, and Val122Ile mutations). Other mutations are associated with a mixed phenotype with variable degrees of neurological and cardiac involvement.

Neurological symptoms typically begin around the ages of 25-35, although later onsets are not uncommon. The predominantly affected fibers are the small-diameter unmyelinated and myelinated fibers. Sensory thermosensitive disorders prevail, primarily in a deficit type, along with autonomic disturbances. The latter usually represent the most prominent clinical manifestation. Patients experience orthostatic hypotension, impotence, diarrhea, and pupillary motility alterations. The disease progresses slowly, with a survival rate of approximately 10 years. Death is usually secondary to renal or cardiac failure due to amyloid accumulation.

The diagnosis of amyloidosis is based on genetic testing, which has progressively replaced previous diagnostic tests (detection of amyloid protein in tissues through specific staining with Congo red). Therapeutically, various treatment approaches are now available: tafamidis, which stabilizes transthyretin polymers and reduces the formation of insoluble monomers, patisiran, and inotersen, which reduce transthyretin production.

Porphyric Polyneuropathy | Refers to a group of diseases caused by defects in heme metabolism, the prosthetic group of hemoglobin, myoglobin, cytochrome C, and catalase peroxidase. The most common form is acute intermittent porphyria, resulting from a deficiency of porphobilinogen deaminase, leading to the accumulation of porphobilinogen.

The disease generally manifests during adolescence with recurrent attacks of colicky abdominal pain (with a treatable abdomen) and involvement of the central and peripheral nervous systems. Crises can be triggered by drugs (including barbiturates, phenytoin, sulfonamides) or other conditions. The neuropathy is predominantly characterized by motor impairment, symmetrically starting distally. In some cases, due to the severity of hyposthenia and cranial nerve involvement, it may mimic Guillain-Barré syndrome. Involvement of respiratory muscles is not uncommon. Manifestations affecting the central nervous system include seizures, restlessness, confusion, and visual field defects. Generally, after an attack (which can last for weeks), symptoms resolve completely. In addition to typical clinical manifestations, the diagnosis is based on increased porphobilinogen and aminolevulinic acid in the urine. Urine left at rest assumes a reddish-brown color due to the conversion of porphobilinogen into porphobilin. Treatment for an attack is aimed at inhibiting heme synthesis through glucose infusion and hematin administration.

Genetically determined small fiber neuropathies

Genetically determined small fiber neuropathies refer to mutations involving genes encoding for voltage-gated sodium channels, which are associated with neuropathies affecting small fibers (i.e., diseases of the peripheral nervous system characterized by involvement of small-caliber myelinated A-delta fibers and unmyelinated C fibers). Particularly, the most commonly involved genes are those encoding for Nav1.7, Nav1.8, and Nav1.9 isoforms. These are generally point mutations that result in a gain of function in the voltage-gated channel. As a result, the predominant symptoms in patients with small fiber neuropathies are neuropathic pain and autonomic disturbances such as hyperhidrosis. The level of penetrance of the involved mutations is still unclear at present.

20.3.2 Neuropathies associated with systemic disease

Diabetic neuropathies

These are the most common forms (and the most extensively studied) of peripheral nervous system diseases. They can be classified into symmetric and asymmetric forms (focal and multifocal) (Table 20.1).

Table 20.1 DIABETIC NEUROPATHY CLASSIFICATION

Symmetrical diabetic neuropathies

- Acute sensory neuropathy
- Chronic sensorimotor neuropathy
  · Mixed form (involving both myelinated and unmyelinated fibers)
  · Small fiber neuropathy
- Autonomic neuropathy

Symmetrical and focal diabetic neuropathies
- Cranial neuropathies - Proximal motor neuropathy (diabetic amyotrophy) - Truncal radiculoneuropathy

Chronic sensorimotor neuropathy | Represents the most common form of polyneuropathy. It affects approximately 35% of patients with diabetes. It is more frequent in type II diabetes mellitus compared to type I diabetes mellitus. It is strongly associated with other complications of diabetes such as retinopathy and nephropathy. It presents as a length-dependent sensory-motor polyneuropathy. Sensory symptoms are generally predominant (often representing the only manifestation). Hypoesthesia has a stocking-glove distribution and typically involves all sensory modalities. It is accompanied by a reduction in osteotendinous reflexes, predominantly in the distal ones. Debilitating ataxia rarely occurs. Neuropathic pain is common (approximately 15% of patients with diabetes). Although in most cases, both painful and non-painful sensory fibers are involved relatively symmetrically, in some cases, there may be a preponderant or exclusive involvement of one of the two groups of afferent fibers. When the non-painful fibers are involved, the predominant sensory disturbances will be represented by tactile hypoesthesia, reduced sense of position, and movement. Painful sensory disturbances will be absent. On the other hand, when there is a preponderant or exclusive involvement of the painful fibers, the deficitary disturbances will only affect thermal-pain sensitivity. Osteotendinous reflexes will be spared or mildly reduced, and neuropathic pain will be constant. This clinical picture characterizes small fiber neuropathy, of which diabetes is the most common cause. In these patients, ENG (electroneurography) examination is normal, and to objectively demonstrate the selective damage of thermo-dolorific afference, diagnostic tests for assessing nociceptive pathways, such as laser-evoked potentials or skin biopsy, will be necessary.

Regarding diabetic polyneuropathy, there are two different and partly conflicting pathogenetic hypotheses: the vascular hypothesis and the metabolic hypothesis. The vascular hypothesis is based on histological evidence of microangiopathy damage to the vasa nervorum, which leads to nerve ischemia. However, this hypothesis does not explain the perfectly symmetrical course of diabetic polyneuropathy.

The metabolic hypothesis is based on clinical evidence that in diabetic neuropathy, many clinical parameters, including pain, significantly improve with glycemic control. According to the metabolic hypothesis, due to hyperglycemia, an accumulation of polyols, such as sorbitol and fructose, occurs within the nerve. Polyols can cause structural damage to the nerve fiber by functional interference with the Na-K pump, endoneurial edema, and production of free radicals. Persistent elevation of blood glucose also promotes increased non-enzymatic glycosylation of proteins, resulting in increased glycosylation end products. These alterations affect the anatomo-functional integrity of the extracellular matrix, the endothelial wall, and modulate tissue degranulation of macrophages. All these phenomena can damage the nerve directly or through microvascular damage resulting in ischemia.

Autonomic neuropathy | Autonomic neuropathy can occur in isolation or more commonly within the context of a sensory-motor polyneuropathy. It can present with cardiovascular, gastrointestinal, genitourinary, sweating, and pupillary motility disorders. Cardiovascular disorders affect a significant percentage of diabetic patients (up to 50% in some studies). They manifest as orthostatic hypotension and resting tachycardia. In many studies, autonomic neuropathy, as a cause of cardiovascular disorders (including subclinical ones), has been associated with silent myocardial infarction, coronary artery disease, and sudden cardiac death.

Gastrointestinal disorders manifest as atony of the gastrointestinal tract musculature, resulting in postprandial nausea, vomiting, and nocturnal diarrhea. Genitourinary disorders mainly present as erectile dysfunction and bladder atony. Bladder atony initially presents as reduced urinary frequency and later progresses to urinary retention and paradoxical incontinence. Sweating disorders involve hypo-anhidrosis and are due to damage to postganglionic unmyelinated fibers supplying the sweat glands. Pupillary motility disorders present as pupillary hyporeflexia in a generally miotic pupil.

Acute sensory neuropathy | It is a rare form of acute-onset, painful sensory neuropathy associated with cachexia. The predominant symptom of this condition is often debilitating pain that is poorly responsive to pharmacological therapy. It is associated with excessively rapid reduction of blood glucose following treatment with insulin or oral hypoglycemic agents. The most plausible pathogenic hypothesis is that the acute reduction of glucose may affect epineural vasculature, resulting in nerve ischemia. Treatment is based on maintaining stable blood glucose levels and managing pain. The condition resolves spontaneously.

Thoracoabdominal Radiculoneuropathies | These manifest with deficient sensory and painful disturbances affecting multiple thoracic dermatomes. Abdominal muscle weakness with secondary abdominal distension is common. The condition resolves spontaneously within varying timeframes (3 months to 2 years). The pathogenesis is unclear, with many researchers suggesting it is dependent on ischemic damage to the thoracic roots. Diagnosis is based on clinical evidence and electromyographic examination, which shows signs of neurogenic damage in the abdominal and paravertebral muscles of the affected dermatomes.

Proximal diabetic neuropathy | This condition, also known as diabetic amyotrophy, lumbosacral radiculoplexus neuropathy, or Garland's amyotrophy, affects individuals with type II diabetes, mostly males, in their fifth to sixth decade of life. It often overlaps with pre-existing diabetic polyneuropathy. It presents acutely or subacutely with sensory deficits, pain, weakness, and atrophy involving the thigh unilaterally. The symptoms may then extend beyond the thigh and also affect the contralateral lower limb. The condition is severely disabling, both due to the strength deficit and the pain. It is self-limiting and resolves spontaneously over variable periods (from 1 to 12 months) with only partial recovery. Neuropathological studies have shown that this condition is a microvasculitis, an ischemic nerve damage caused by occlusion of small vessels with particularly abundant inflammatory infiltrates. The diagnosis is based on clinical findings and electrophysiological tests (nerve conduction studies and electromyography). Therapy is based on the use of corticosteroids or intravenous immunoglobulins. Symptomatic pain management is usually necessary in addition to causal therapy.

Focal neuropathies | The most common form of focal neuropathy is third cranial nerve palsy, with sparing of the autonomic component. This occurs because the nerve damage is due to an ischemic lesion involving the central portion of the nerve (autonomic fibers are external). The sixth cranial nerve is less frequently affected. The prognosis is generally favorable. Although less common than third and sixth cranial nerve involvement, any nerve trunk can be affected by ischemic damage in the course of diabetes. Typically, the clinical picture resolves within a few months.

Neuropathy secondary to hypothyroidism

The most common forms of neuropathy secondary to hypothyroidism are carpal tunnel syndrome and polyneuropathy. The former is due to thickening of the transverse carpal ligament caused by the accumulation of myxedematous tissue. Polyneuropathy manifests as a mild sensory polyneuropathy. Electroneurographic examination shows a picture of axonal damage. Hormone replacement therapy significantly improves the clinical picture of this neuropathy.

Secondary neuropathy due to acromegaly

Acromegaly is frequently accompanied by carpal tunnel syndrome. Less commonly, it can cause a mild sensorimotor polyneuropathy secondary to endoneurial edema.

Peripheral nervous system diseases in the course of renal failure

Polyneuropathy | Uremic polyneuropathy has a prevalence of 60-90% in patients with renal failure. It presents as a length-dependent neuropathy, primarily sensory, with impaired tactile and vibratory sensitivity, loss of position and movement sense, and disappearance of osteotendinous reflexes. Clinically significant motor impairment only appears in the later stages. Uremic polyneuropathy is correlated with the duration and severity of uremia. Toxic substances play an important role, as they are only partially removed by dialysis due to their size (300-2,000 Daltons). Among these molecules, advanced glycation end products and myo-inositol likely contribute to neurotoxicity. Electrophysiological studies also suggest the accumulation of potassium as a relevant factor in axonal damage. Electroneurographic examination shows predominantly distally distributed sensory axonal damage. Long-term dialytic treatment can stabilize the clinical picture, while kidney transplantation, especially if performed early, can lead to significant improvement in clinical disturbances.

Autonomic neuropathy | In patients with renal failure, autonomic neuropathy can occur in association with somatic polyneuropathy or in an isolated manner. The most common clinical manifestation is impotence. Other manifestations involve cardiovascular autonomic function, which exposes the patient to sudden cardiac death, as well as gastrointestinal tract disorders. Kidney transplantation can considerably improve the clinical picture in this case as well.

Focal neuropathies | The most common form of focal neuropathy is carpal tunnel syndrome. It is believed that in patients undergoing dialytic treatment, carpal tunnel syndrome is due to the accumulation of beta-2 microglobulin at the level of the transverse carpal ligament, leading to secondary compression of the median nerve at the wrist.

20.3.3 Neuropathies in the course of infectious diseases

HIV | Neurological complications are very common during HIV infection and involve the nervous system at every level. The most frequent neurological complication of HIV is sensory axonal polyneuropathy. This neuropathy can be secondary to antiviral therapy, which can potentially be neurotoxic, or it can be caused by the virus itself. Since the discontinuation of the use of nucleoside reverse transcriptase inhibitors, such as stavudine, the neurotoxicity of therapy has significantly decreased. These drugs have significant neurotoxicity, probably due to damage to neuronal mitochondria. However, it should be noted that they are still widely used in developing countries, resulting in a higher prevalence of neuropathy compared to wealthier nations.

Regarding the neurotoxic effect of the virus, the pathogenic mechanisms are not yet fully understood. It is believed that the damage is likely due to immune-mediated processes, possibly triggered by viral proteins, primarily gp120. Indeed, gp120 is capable of activating macrophages, which in turn release potentially neurotoxic cytokines such as α-TNF. In laboratory animals, the administration of gp120 alone can induce neuropathy.

Despite potentially different mechanisms, neuropathy in the course of HIV tends to manifest in a fairly homogeneous manner. It consists of sensory axonal polyneuropathy, clinically presenting with predominantly sensory disturbances, in which "positive" symptoms such as paresthesia and neuropathic pain usually predominate. These sensory disturbances are predominantly localized distally, with a typical stocking distribution, and are accompanied by a reduction in osteotendinous reflexes.

Although sensory axonal polyneuropathy is the most common form of neuropathy in HIV, other conditions such as acute and chronic inflammatory demyelinating polyneuropathies and isolated and multiple mononeuropathies are frequently observed.

Demyelinating polyneuropathies in the course of HIV can occur acutely or, more commonly, chronically. They generally appear in the early stages of infection, in patients with a normal CD4 count. Clinically, they are indistinguishable from Guillain-Barré syndrome or chronic inflammatory demyelinating polyradiculoneuropathy (CIDP). Examination of the cerebrospinal fluid can be helpful because these patients do not exhibit the classic albumin-cytological dissociation, with an increase in cerebrospinal fluid cells (lymphocytic pleocytosis).

Cranial mononeuropathies are particularly common in HIV-infected patients. Facial nerve mononeuropathies, unilateral or bilateral, isolated or recurrent, are the most common forms and can occur at any stage of the disease. In some cases, they occur at seroconversion, related to a meningitis with clear cerebrospinal fluid. In other cases, they manifest as idiopathic forms similar to Bell's palsy. However, they are often due to opportunistic diseases, such as reactivation of varicella-zoster virus affecting the geniculate ganglion and mycobacterial infections, which cause skull base meningitis with involvement of cranial nerves.

In patients with severe immunosuppression, severe multiple mononeuropathies caused by cytomegalovirus (CMV) have been described. In these patients, neuroperipheral damage sequentially and progressively affects multiple nerve trunks. The diagnosis is based on the patient's medical history, physical examination, positive CMV PCR in the cerebrospinal fluid, and the presence of CMV in sural nerve biopsies. CMV infection can also involve the cauda equina, causing inflammation and necrosis of the lumbosacral roots. Clinical symptoms consist of a severe sensorimotor deficit affecting the territories supplied by the last lumbar and sacral roots (including sphincter disturbances).

Leprosy | Although the incidence of leprosy is progressively decreasing, it still remains a significant problem in many geographical areas such as India, Brazil, Nepal, and central Africa. Approximately 5-10% of leprosy patients have exclusive involvement of the nervous system without any cutaneous manifestations. Leprosy is caused by *Mycobacterium leprae*, which has a strong tropism for the peripheral nerves, colonizing Schwann cells.

Leprosy can manifest in three main forms. Often (indeterminate leprosy), it presents solely as a light-colored, anesthetic patch or papule. The disease may either not progress and remain at this stage, or the mycobacteria may show some local invasiveness, forming an epithelioid granuloma that affects subcutaneous nevi (sometimes enlarged and palpable), leading to an area of hypoesthesia (tuberculoid leprosy). In this form, the granuloma can affect larger nerve trunks, resulting in sensory-motor deficits consistent with nerve trunk involvement in addition to the anesthetic area. The granulomas undergo caseous necrosis, causing extensive tissue loss. The third form (lepromatous leprosy) is due to hematogenous dissemination of the mycobacteria, which localize in multiple areas, extensively involving the peripheral nervous system. Gradually, there will be widespread hypoesthesia, predominantly affecting temperature and pain sensations, with relatively preserved sensations mediated by larger fibers (often deep tendon reflexes are intact). Motor involvement is only present after a particularly prolonged course. In this form of the disease, the skin lesions are particularly extensive and diverse. Additionally, due to the anesthesia, the skin lesions go unnoticed, increasing the risk of infections, trophic changes, and tissue loss. The therapy is based on prolonged administration of dapsone, rifampicin, and clofazimine.

Lyme disease | Lyme disease is caused by the spirochete *Borrelia burgdorferi* and is transmitted to humans through the bite of a tick. The disease manifests in three stages, which include cutaneous, articular, cardiac, and neurological manifestations. Neurological manifestations occur in the second and third stages. In the second stage, several weeks after the bite, cranial neuropathies can occur (most commonly facial paralysis, sometimes bilateral) or painful asymmetric radiculopathies associated with clear cerebrospinal fluid meningitis. In these cases, the radicular pain in the lower back or neck can mimic compressive radiculopathy caused by a herniated disc.

In the third stage, demyelinating polyneuropathies with inflammatory cerebrospinal fluid mimicking Guillain-Barré syndrome and sensory polyneuropathies of an axonal nature have been described, as demonstrated by electrophysiological studies and nerve biopsies.

HCV | HCV infection is one of the most common viral infection worldwide. One of the most important extrahepatic manifestations is polyneuropathy. Although many studies have shown that polyneuropathy in the course of HCV is usually due to the concomitant presence of cryoglobulins, about 13% of HCV patients develop polyneuropathy in the absence of cryoglobulinemia. In patients with cryoglobulins, the mechanism causing nerve damage is likely attributed to vasculitis, which in turn causes ischemic damage to the nerve. Conversely, in patients without cryoglobulinemia, it is hypothesized that HCV itself is capable of autonomously causing nerve damage. The mechanisms that cause HCV-related neuropathy are not yet fully understood. Some data, such as the presence of viral RNA in nervous tissue, suggest a direct action of the virus, while others demonstrate that there is no correlation between HCV RNA and neuropathy, suggesting that this virus acts through an autoimmune mechanism. Although some patients with cryoglobulinemia may develop multiple neuropathies due to the vasculitic mechanism of damage, in most cases, a distally distributed polyneuropathy occurs. This is likely because cryoglobulins precipitate at low temperatures, and therefore, the nerves that distribute to distal areas such as the feet and hands are mainly damaged. In patients without cryoglobulinemia, HCV-related neuropathy always presents as a polyneuropathy. Regardless of the presence or absence of cryoglobulinemia, neuropathy in these patients manifests with sensory deficits involving all sensory modalities in a distal distribution. Neuropathic pain is common.

Diphtheria | The toxin produced by *Corynebacterium diphtheriae* has a particular affinity for the peripheral nerve, which it reaches through contiguity and the bloodstream, causing segmental demyelination. Diphtheric neuropathy manifests approximately 1-2 weeks after pharyngitis, with pharyngeal and palatal paralysis. Accommodation paralysis follows 1-2 weeks later. One month later, a sensory-motor neuropathy with an ascending course occurs. Since the introduction of mandatory vaccination, it has become exceptionally rare.

Zoster | *Herpes zoster* is an infection that arises from the reactivation of the varicella-zoster virus from its latent state in a dorsal root ganglion. The virus replicates within the ganglion cells, damaging them and producing the characteristic vesicles whose cutaneous localization follows the affected dermatomes. The most common locations are the thoracic and trigeminal (usually the first division). Clinical symptoms include hypo/anesthesia and neuropathic pain. In the majority of patients, these sensory disturbances resolve within 30 days. However, in a minority of patients, postherpetic neuralgia develops, characterized by neuropathic pain that responds poorly to pharmacological therapy.

Rarely, the varicella-zoster virus can spread through transynaptic transmission, leading to focal myelitis or selective damage to the anterior horns at the corresponding level of the affected segments.

SARS-CoV-2 | SARS-CoV-2 is frequently associated with neurological manifestations (NeuroCOVID). Many patients develop loss of smell and taste as initial symptoms of the infection. Hyposmia suggests the nasal route of infection as a potential mechanism for the virus to directly access the central nervous system. However, it is not possible to exclude that NeuroCOVID represents the consequence of immunomediated mechanisms triggered by a complex interaction between the virus and the host. It should also be noted that the ACE2 receptor, the virus's entry point into human cells, is also expressed by neurons in the sensory ganglia.

The direct impact of the virus on the peripheral nervous system is not yet known; however, there is clear association with inflammatory neuropathies, likely with an immune-mediated mechanism.

20.3.4 Neuropathies in oncological diseases

Neoplasms can cause peripheral nervous system disorders through various mechanisms. They can cause a sensory polyneuropathy through immune-mediated mechanisms (paraneoplastic neuropathy), or they can invade and compress nerve trunks. However, the most common forms of peripheral nervous system disorders in the course of oncological diseases are those related to chemotherapy treatment and, less commonly, radiation therapy.

Paraneoplastic neuropathy | The most common form of paraneoplastic neuropathy is an exclusively sensory neuronopathy that often precedes the diagnosis of a neoplasm. It is often associated with lung tumors (typically small-cell lung carcinoma), but it can potentially occur with any type of cancer. It is generally associated with serum and cerebrospinal fluid anti-Hu antibodies (anti-neuronal nuclear antigen of the central and peripheral nervous system), whose pathogenic role is possibly secondary to the direct attack by CD8+ T lymphocytes, which directly attack ganglion cells, leading to their destruction. Neuropathological data have shown that inflammation and degeneration extend from the ganglion to the roots and posterior columns.

Clinically, it manifests with a sensory disturbance involving all sensory modalities, with a subacute course, often following a distal gradient (often predominantly affecting large-caliber myelinated fibers). There is a consistent reduction in osteotendinous reflexes, and ataxia is frequent and disabling. The diagnosis is usually very insidious. Electroneurographic examination shows a sensory axonal neuropathy, in which the reduction in sensory potentials does not follow a proximal-to-distal gradient, as the damage primarily involves the ganglion cell and does not act according to a length-dependent mechanism. The paraneoplastic etiopathogenesis can be hypothesized based on data from the general physical examination, the presence of anti-Hu antibodies or tumor markers. It should be noted, however, that the absence of tumor markers and anti-Hu antibodies does not exclude the possibility of a paraneoplastic neuropathy. In cases of clinical suspicion of a paraneoplastic neuropathy, whether supported by laboratory tests or not, the most appropriate radiological examinations should be performed.

Less common forms of paraneoplastic neuropathies include autonomic neuropathy, which develops in 25% of anti-Hu positive patients. The most common form of autonomic neuronopathy manifests as severe gastrointestinal motility disorders due to a loss of enteric plexus neurons. This condition presents with nausea, loss of appetite, constipation, and abdominal distension. It is typically associated with small-cell lung carcinoma.

More rarely, a paraneoplastic neuropathy may present as a demyelinating neuropathy. Clinically, this condition is associated with anti-CV2 antibodies that are indistinguishable from Guillain-Barré syndrome or chronic inflammatory demyelinating polyneuropathy (CIDP).

Other neuropathies due to oncological diseases | Although less commonly, oncological diseases can cause peripheral nervous system damage by infiltrating and directly damaging nerve trunks. The most representative example is Pancoast syndrome. In this condition, a tumor at the apex of the lung compresses and damages the lower trunk of the brachial plexus. Therefore, in addition to potential general signs of neoplasia, sensory-motor disturbances (neuropathic pain is common) will be associated with C8-T1 distribution and a Horner's syndrome.

Another characteristic example is tumors of the skull base, such as infiltrating carcinomas of the nasopharynx that compress cranial nerves. In this case, the damaged nerve trunks, due to greater proximity, will be the second and third divisions of the trigeminal nerve. However, potentially, tumors of the skull base can damage any cranial nerve, leading to Garcin syndrome (unilateral paralysis of cranial nerves III to XII).

Neuropathies secondary to chemotherapy treatment | The peripheral nervous system can be damaged by chemotherapy through various mechanisms. Antineoplastic drugs easily reach the sensory and autonomic neurons, which lack the blood-brain barrier.

Most chemotherapeutic drugs cause peripheral nervous system damage that is dependent on the cumulative dose administered. However, the individual patient's characteristics also play a crucial role in the development of neuropathy. For example, advanced age or the presence of other risk factors (such as diabetes) are associated with a higher likelihood of developing neuropathy. Additionally, in recent years, several genetic studies have demonstrated that neurotoxicity is also influenced by polymorphisms in genes involved in the absorption, distribution, metabolism, and excretion of chemotherapeutic drugs.

Among chemotherapeutic drugs, platinum compounds (particularly cisplatin and oxaliplatin) are among the most commonly used. They act as DNA alkylating agents, thereby inducing apoptosis of the cell.

For cisplatin, manifestations of peripheral nerve damage are closely related to the cumulative dose. It affects dorsal root ganglia, predominantly those of larger-caliber myelinated fibers, producing a sensory polyneuropathy that frequently presents with distal sensory deficits and a "stocking and glove" distribution.

Oxaliplatin causes an acute and a chronic form of neuropathy. The chronic form is identical to that caused by cisplatin. The acute form is characterized by intense dysesthetic and allodynic manifestations upon exposure to cold, which appear extremely rapidly (even in the early treatment cycles). This phenomenon is likely dependent on chelation phenomena on the voltage-gated sodium channels induced by the drug, leading to hyperexcitability, predominantly in A-delta fibers. Regarding the prognosis of sensory disturbances induced by platinum compounds, although there is progressive improvement in sensory disorders upon discontinuation of therapy, since the dorsal root ganglion has been lost, functional recovery can only be partial.

Vinca alkaloids (vincristine and vinblastine) and taxanes (paclitaxel and docetaxel) act on microtubules. These drugs likely hinder axonal transport (mediated by microtubules) and damage all types of fibers, including motor fibers. Taxanes, widely used in breast cancer treatment, predominantly cause a distal sensory neuropathy. Vincristine, widely used in hematological malignancies, produces a distal sensorimotor neuropathy. More rarely, patients undergoing vincristine treatment develop autonomic neuropathy, which manifests as orthostatic hypotension, constipation, and impotence. Since the dorsal root ganglion remains intact, the prognosis for improvement of the symptoms is better compared to platinum compounds.

Bortezomib is a proteasome inhibitor currently used in the treatment of multiple myeloma. By modulating the activity of the proteasome, it is believed to alter the breakdown of many proteins and thus indirectly promote cellular apoptosis. Bortezomib induces a predominantly sensory, distally distributed axonal neuropathy in which clear signs and deficit symptoms are present, with neuropathic pain being the predominant feature.

Thalidomide, currently used in the treatment of various solid and hematological neoplasms, causes a predominantly sensory, distally distributed axonal neuropathy in which sensory deficits predominate over neuropathic pain. Lenalidomide, an analog of thalidomide, does not have clinically significant neurotoxicity.

Discontinuation of treatment generally has a beneficial effect on chemotherapy-induced neuropathy, sometimes resulting in complete, albeit slow, remission of symptoms. However, in some patients, neuropathy may manifest or worsen upon drug discontinuation. This phenomenon, known as coasting, is especially evident with platinum derivatives and vincristine.

There are various drugs and substances used for prophylaxis or treatment of chemotherapy-induced neuropathies. Some of these substances (alpha-lipoic acid, acetyl-L-carnitine, palmitoylethanolamide) have shown some efficacy in various clinical studies. However, as of now, due to the lack of controlled randomized trials, it is not possible to establish their potential effectiveness with certainty.

Other neuropathies secondary to oncological treatment | Include post-surgical mononeuropathies. Virtually any nerve trunk can be involved. The most common one is the mononeuropathy of the intercostobrachial nerve, which is frequently damaged during breast tumor surgeries, particularly when the procedure extends to the axillary cavity. Since the nerve is exclusively sensory, its damage results solely in sensory deficit and often neuropathic pain in the nerve's distribution territory.

Radiation-induced plexopathy most commonly affects the brachial plexus and is often a complication of radiation therapy for breast cancer. It can appear long after radiation therapy (over a year later). Neuropathological data demonstrate the presence of abundant fibrous tissue that envelops and destroys nerve fibers. It progresses slowly, initially affecting the lower components of the brachial plexus before relatively symmetrically involving the remaining parts. It causes severe sensory and motor deficits.

20.3.5 Monoclonal gammopathy-associated neuropathies

Monoclonal gammopathies encompass a highly heterogeneous group of conditions that include monoclonal gammopathy of undetermined significance, amyloidosis, multiple myeloma, Waldenstrom's macroglobulinemia, POEMS syndrome, and cryoglobulinemia. All these conditions are characterized by the production and deposition of a paraprotein consisting of a single heavy chain (M, G, or A) or light chain (kappa or lambda). Diagnosis is based on the detection of monoclonal protein through protein electrophoresis and immunofixation.

Monoclonal gammopathy of undetermined significance | Monoclonal gammopathies are a very common condition, affecting approximately 3% of individuals over the age of 70. The most common form of monoclonal gammopathy associated with neuropathy is the one in which the monoclonal component is IgM. In patients with IgM monoclonal gammopathy, neuropathy is usually caused by anti-MAG (myelin-associated glycoprotein) antibodies. This type of neuropathy primarily affects males starting in their sixth decade of life. It is characterized by predominantly distal sensory disturbances, ataxia, and tremor. The electrophysiological findings show a sensorimotor demyelinating neuropathy.

Neuropathies associated with IgG and IgA paraproteinemias have a less stereotyped clinical course. There are sensory, sensorimotor, axonal, and demyelinating polyneuropathies. Patients with demyelinating neuropathies associated with IgG and IgA paraproteinemias exhibit clinical and electrophysiological features indistinguishable from chronic inflammatory demyelinating polyradiculoneuropathy (CIDP).

Multiple myeloma | Neuropathy is associated with multiple myeloma in 13-14% of patients. The neuropathy is due to perineuronal or perivascular deposition of IgG kappa chains. Electroneurography reveals sensory axonal damage.

POEMS syndrome | POEMS syndrome (Polyneuropathy, Organomegaly, Endocrinopathy, Monoclonal gammopathy, and Skin changes) is a rare condition that predominantly affects males and manifests as a neuropathy causing sensory and motor disturbances with a predominantly distal distribution. The neuropathy is associated with monoclonal gammopathy, with or without osteosclerotic myeloma and multisystem involvement. This multisystem involvement includes organomegaly (most commonly involving lymph nodes, liver, or spleen), endocrine abnormalities (frequently resulting in hypothyroidism and adrenal insufficiency), and skin changes. Electroneurography shows a demyelinating damage with severe axonal loss superimposed.

Waldenstrom's Macroglobulinemia |

Approximately 5-10% of cases of Waldenstrom's Macroglobulinemia are accompanied by neuropathy. It is associated with IgM kappa with or without anti-MAG, which influences its manifestations. In patients with anti-MAG, it presents as a demyelinating neuropathy, while in patients without anti-MAG, its manifestations are more heterogeneous.

Amyloidosis | This condition is due to the production of IgG or IgA lambda with deposition of light chains in organs. Neuropathy can be caused by a direct toxic effect of deposited amyloid or vascular damage produced by the amyloid itself. The neuropathy manifests with a predominant involvement of unmyelinated fibers. Therefore, there are sensory disturbances related to temperature and pain, both deficits and painful, as well as autonomic disorders, including impotence, diarrhea, and orthostatic hypotension. Sensory disturbances affecting tactile and proprioceptive sensitivity, as well as motor disturbances, appear only at a later stage. The prognosis, especially due to amyloid deposition in the heart and kidneys, is poor and typically results in a relatively short period of time (average survival of 12-24 months).

20.3.6 Secondary neuropathies associated with autoimmune diseases

Vasculitis | Vasculitis is a heterogeneous group of diseases characterized by the involvement of organs and blood vessels of varying sizes. They are generally classified into systemic forms (primary and secondary) and non-systemic forms. Over 30% of patients with systemic vasculitis develop neuropathy. The primary systemic vasculitis most frequently associated with neuropathy are Churg-Strauss syndrome, polyarteritis nodosa, Wegener's granulomatosis, and microscopic polyangiitis (all vasculitides involving small- to medium-sized arterial vessels, 75-300 mm in diameter). The secondary systemic vasculitis most frequently associated with neuropathy are those occurring in connective tissue diseases and cryoglobulinemia. Non-systemic vasculitis (involving smaller vessels, < 40 mm in diameter, often referred to as microvasculitis) are characterized by a vasculitic process confined to a nerve or muscle.

Primary systemic vasculitides | Polyarteritis nodosa can be associated with active HBV infection. It manifests with skin lesions, arterial hypertension, and renal artery aneurysms. Approximately 70% of patients experience a multifocal distribution neuropathy.

Churg-Strauss syndrome presents with asthma, eosinophilia, and, in 60-70% of patients, a multifocal distribution neuropathy.

Wegener's granulomatosis, typically associated with high levels of ANCA antibodies, is a disease characterized by granulomatous infiltrates involving the respiratory system. Neuropathy manifests in approximately 15-25% of patients and generally occurs in those with more severe disease.

Microscopic polyangiitis is a systemic necrotizing inflammatory vasculitis that affects small vessels and is often associated with high levels of ANCA antibodies. It presents with renal, pulmonary, and cutaneous involvement. Neuropathy affects up to 50% of patients.

Secondary systemic vasculitis | Sjögren's syndrome is frequently the cause of peripheral nervous system diseases. Although the most common forms of neuropathy in Sjögren's syndrome are neuronopathies, in a small percentage of patients, this syndrome produces multifocal neuropathies dependent on vasculitis involving vessels with a diameter less than 40 μm.

Cryoglobulinemia is the presence of immunoglobulins, usually IgG or IgM, that precipitate at low temperatures. It can be an essential condition, but in most cases, it is secondary to oncological or infectious diseases. HCV infection is the most common cause of cryoglobulinemia. The peripheral nervous system is involved in the majority of patients. Neuropathy usually presents as a predominantly sensory disorder (neuropathic pain is common) with multifocal or distal distribution.

Non-systemic vasculitis | These conditions differ from the previous ones because the vasculitic process is isolated and produces a multifocal involvement of nerve trunks without systemic symptoms (or when present, they are less severe). They involve small-caliber arteries, arterioles, capillaries, and venules.

In vasculitis involving larger arterioles, the vessels of the epineurium and perineurium are primarily affected. In microvasculitis, the microvessels of the endoneurium (microarterioles, capillaries, and venules) are affected. In both cases, there are inflammatory infiltrates in the vessel wall and necrosis of the media and intima. Fibrinoid necrosis of the media and intima occurs. Furthermore, the nerve is affected multifocally (alongside affected fascicles, there will be unaffected ones).

Despite their extremely diverse etiopathogenesis, vasculitis tend to involve the peripheral nervous system quite homogeneously. They all cause secondary axonal damage due to ischemia. Therefore, vasculitis-related neuropathies manifest as mono- or multifocal neuropathies. They develop acutely or subacutely, resulting in sensory and motor deficits in the territories supplied by the affected nerves. Neuropathic pain is common. As involvement of multiple nerve trunks tends to occur over time, it is not uncommon (occurs in approximately 25% of patients) for a neuropathy in the course of systemic vasculitis to evolve into a polyneuropathy, with clinical evidence of symmetrical neuroperipheral damage. Additionally, in about 20% of patients, the clinical picture is that of a polyneuropathy from the onset.

The electrophysiological findings generally show asymmetric axonal damage affecting the nerves of all four limbs. The diagnosis of secondary neuropathy due to vasculitis is based on clinical and instrumental evidence of multifocal neuroperipheral damage. Nerve biopsy is often necessary to confirm the vasculitic process. Treatment involves the use of corticosteroids and immunosuppressants (such as cyclophosphamide, azathioprine, methotrexate).

Connective tissue diseases | Are a heterogeneous group of diseases characterized by autoimmune and inflammatory phenomena involving various organs. They include rheumatoid arthritis, systemic lupus erythematosus (LES), and Sjogren's syndrome. In rheumatoid arthritis, due to joint distortion and tendon thickening, the most frequent manifestations of neuroperipheral damage are entrapment mononeuropathies, such as carpal tunnel syndrome. A predominantly sensory, distally distributed, axonal polyneuropathy rarely occurs, likely due to occlusion of small-caliber vessels from the accumulation of immune complexes. In LES, the most common form of neuroperipheral damage (occurring in nearly 10% of patients) is a predominantly sensory axonal neuropathy with distal symptoms, which often develops subclinically. The most likely cause of secondary neuropathy in LES is occlusion of small-caliber vessels due to immune complex accumulation.

Neuropathy is frequent in Sjogren's syndrome and occurs in approximately 50% of patients. It often precedes the diagnosis of connective tissue disease and can have disabling symptomatic manifestations. In most patients, a sensory axonal neuropathy develops. Sometimes, predominantly unmyelinated fibers are involved, resulting in deficient thermosensitive sensations, neuropathic pain, and sensory deficits. In other patients, the sensory disturbances primarily affect large myelinated fiber-mediated sensations, resulting in tactile hypoesthesia and, above all, ataxia. Although in some patients, neuropathy is due to axonal damage secondary to vasculitis, neuropathological studies have shown the presence of inflammatory infiltrates affecting the spinal ganglia (ganglionopathy). Autonomic neuropathy in Sjogren's syndrome can manifest in association with sensory neuropathy or in isolation. Subacute demyelinating polyradiculoneuropathy indistinguishable from chronic inflammatory demyelinating polyneuropathy (CIDP) can occur in Sjogren's syndrome. Bilateral trigeminal neuropathy, exclusively sensory, due to ganglion cell damage, occurs in almost 20% of patients. Sensory deficits are frequently associated with pain.

Sarcoidosis | Is a systemic granulomatous disease that affects the lungs, skin, eyes, and lymph nodes. Involvement of the peripheral nervous system generally manifests as facial nerve mononeuropathy. Other cranial nerves may also be affected, or there may be a multineuropathy with thoracic and abdominal sensory disturbances. An association between sarcoidosis and small fiber neuropathy is characteristic. Peripheral nervous system damage is caused by granulomatous infiltration of meninges and nerve roots.

20.3.7 Toxic neuropathies

These neuropathies are caused by toxic substances such as heavy metals (arsenic, thallium, lead), industrial toxic substances (organic solvents and organophosphorus esters), certain medications, and alcohol (Table 20.2).

In general, all these neuropathies are secondary to the accumulation of the toxic substance, which results in a length-dependent axonal damage primarily involving large-caliber myelinated fibers. They manifest as sensorimotor polyneuropathies with distally distributed sensory and motor disturbances and a reduction in osteotendinous reflexes. Heavy metal neuropathies often develop concurrently with encephalopathy, and in cases of ingestion, they are preceded by gastrointestinal disorders.

Numerous medications are capable of causing neuropathy, including antineoplastic drugs, antiretrovirals, and isoniazid, which causes a deficiency neuropathy by interfering with the metabolism of vitamin B6. Supplementation with vitamin B6 prevents its development.

Table 20.2 MAJOR TOXIC SUBSTANCES AFFECTING THE NERVES

Industrial toxicants
Acrylamide
Hexacarbons
Organophosphorus esters
Heavy Metals
Arsenic
Lead
Mercury
Thallium
Medications
- *Chemotherapeutics*
Bortezomib
Carfilzomib
Platinum derivatives
Vinca Alkaloids (vincristine, vinblastine)
Taxoids
Thalidomide
Eptolonides
- *Antimicrobials*
Triazole antimycotics
Chloroquine
Dapsone
Isoniazid
Ethambutol
Nitrofurantoin
Metronidazole
Chloramphenicol
Dideoxynucleotide Inhibitors
Reverse Transcriptase Inhibitors
- *Other Drugs*
Amiodarone
Disulfiram
Nitrous oxide
Gold salts
Suramin

More than half of alcoholic patients present with neuropathy characterized by distally distributed sensory and motor disturbances. Sensory disturbances include hypoesthesia involving all sensory modalities, ataxia, and neuropathic pain. Electroneurographic examination reveals axonal damage. It is believed that neuropathy secondary to chronic alcohol abuse is dependent on the involvement of various factors, such as genetic susceptibility, thiamine deficiency, and malnutrition. Additionally, several studies indicate that ethanol can directly damage the nerves.

20.3.8 Deficiency neuropathies

Deficiency neuropathies are generally rare in Western countries. Beriberi is caused by a deficiency of vitamin B1. It manifests as a sensorimotor neuropathy with frequent cranial involvement, associated with congestive cardiomyopathy and generalized edema. Pellagra, caused by a deficiency of nicotinic acid, presents with the triad of dermatitis, diarrhea, and dementia, which is often associated with a sensorimotor polyneuropathy. Deficiency of vitamin B6 causes predominantly sensory polyneuropathy. The deficiency of this vitamin is usually due to pharmacological treatments with isoniazid or hydralazine. Vitamin B6 therapy during these treatments prevents the development of neuropathy. However, it should be noted that excessive intake of vitamin B6 itself can potentially cause neuropathy.

A deficiency of vitamin E can be a complication of cystic fibrosis and abetalipoproteinemia. It primarily affects large-caliber myelinated fibers, resulting in hypoesthesia, reduced osteotendinous reflexes, and especially severe ataxia. It can be associated with retinitis pigmentosa and spinocerebellar degeneration.

A deficiency of vitamin B12 can be due to gastric pathologies that cause an intrinsic factor deficiency, intestinal malabsorption, or gastric interventions for obesity. Vitamin B12 deficiency causes a predominantly sensory neuropathy with distal distribution, involving large-caliber myelinated fibers. There is a consistent association with combined degeneration of the dorsal and lateral columns of the spinal cord.

20.3.9 Critical illness neuropathy

It occurs in patients hospitalized in intensive care units. It manifests as a severe sensorimotor axonal polyneuropathy in patients with sepsis or multiorgan failure. It typically becomes evident during weaning from assisted ventilation when the patient fails to regain normal ventilatory activity despite the resolution of the condition that necessitated assisted ventilation.

This peripheral nervous system disease presents with severe sensorimotor deficits affecting all four limbs, accompanied by muscle wasting. Muscle tissue damage is commonly associated with the peripheral nerve damage. The etiopathogenesis of this condition has not been precisely identified to date. Gradual, albeit partial, improvement in sensitivity and strength is possible over a period of 6-12 months.

20.3.10 Inflammatory neuropathies

Guillain-Barré syndrome

Inflammatory demyelinating polyradiculoneuropathies are a group of acquired disorders of the peripheral nervous system with an immunomediated pathogenesis. Based on the clinical course, they can be classified into acute and chronic forms.

The acute form is typically referred to as Guillain-Barré syndrome, named after the first description by Guillain, Barré, and Strohl in 1916. In approximately two-thirds of patients, the development of this disease is preceded by respiratory or gastrointestinal tract infections. Specifically, various studies have found an association between Guillain-Barré syndrome and previous infections of the respiratory tract caused by Mycoplasma pneumoniae, Hemophilus influenzae, CMV, Epstein-Barr virus, and especially gastroenteritis caused by Campylobacter jejuni. It is also potentially associated with vaccinations. For example, the association with influenza vaccination has been extensively studied. Although there is an increased risk of developing Guillain-Barré syndrome following influenza vaccination, this risk is significantly lower compared to the risk following the actual influenza infection. More recently, a probable association with SARS-

CoV-2 has emerged. In this case as well, the peripheral nervous system damage does not appear to be directly caused by the virus (viral RNA is not present in the cerebrospinal fluid of patients with inflammatory neuropathy caused by SARS-CoV-2).

The relationship with previous infectious diseases and vaccinations reflects the likely underlying pathogenic mechanism of this acute demyelinating neuropathy. A contact with an infectious agent probably triggers a cell-mediated immune attack against Schwann cell antigens through cross-reactivity. From a neuropathological standpoint, Guillain-Barré syndrome is comparable to animal models of experimental allergic neuritis. T lymphocytes from patients are capable of attacking myelin in vitro. Subepineural injections of serum from Guillain-Barré syndrome patients into the sciatic nerve of rats can induce focal demyelination. Most experimental evidence shows that the damage is predominantly mediated by T lymphocytes and macrophages, which initially cause pure demyelination with axonal sparing. Neuropathological studies consistently demonstrate a perivascular lymphocytic inflammatory infiltrate. The infiltrates are widely distributed in the cranial nerves, spinal ganglia, ventral and dorsal roots, and throughout the course of the peripheral nerve.

Guillain-Barré syndrome manifests with sensory deficits and paresthesia, as well as motor deficits (which generally predominate over sensory disturbances) that have an acute onset and symmetric distribution. By definition, the time interval between symptom onset and their nadir is within 4 weeks.

Respiratory and pharyngeal muscles can also be affected. Involvement of the facial nerve is common, often asymmetrically. Less frequently, other cranial nerves are involved. Sensory deficits and positive sensory symptoms are a constant phenomenon but usually do not have significant clinical relevance. Osteotendinous reflexes are consistently absent. Autonomic dysfunctions, albeit mild, are very frequent. Urinary retention occurs in approximately 10% of patients. The symptomatic course completes within two to four weeks.

The diagnosis is based on clinical manifestations, as well as electrophysiological and cerebrospinal fluid findings. Electroneurography reveals a demyelinating neuropathy. There is a consistent reduction in motor conduction velocity and an increase or absence of F waves. Conduction blocks (absence of motor potential following proximal stimulation) are very common. Cerebrospinal fluid examination shows the characteristic albumin-cytological dissociation. Around one week after onset, there is a significant increase in protein levels, with a normal cell count 10/ mm^3). Increased cell count occurs in forms of acute demyelinating neuropathy secondary to HIV.

Although Guillain-Barré syndrome resolves spontaneously in approximately 80% of patients, with motor deficits tending to regress, the mortality rate can reach 10%. In most cases, death is directly or indirectly due to respiratory complications resulting from paralysis of respiratory muscles. Therapy is based on managing general conditions and immunomodulation. Despite being an immune-mediated disease, corticosteroids are ineffective. The elective treatment consists of plasmapheresis or immunoglobulins, and both treatments have shown comparable efficacy.

Some forms of Guillain-Barré syndrome are caused by axonal damage rather than demyelination. This is probably linked to the infectious agent responsible for triggering the immune response, *Campilobacter Jejuni*. This form usually presents with sensory and motor manifestations, although purely motor forms have also been described. These forms are frequently associated with anti-ganglioside antibodies (GM1 and GD1a).

Axonal damage is highlighted in electrophysiological examinations. Electroneurography shows an early disappearance of sensory and motor potentials. Electromyography reveals abundant denervation activity in the examined muscles. The clinical course overlaps with the demyelinating form of the syndrome, although a higher frequency of severe cases, a lesser response to plasmapheresis or immunoglobulin treatment, and a poor prognosis regarding motor recovery have been described.

Miller Fisher syndrome and clinical variants

Miller Fisher syndrome is an acute inflammatory neuropathy with a benign prognosis, first described by Fisher in 1956. It represents about 5% of acute neuropathies and, in its classic form, manifests as ophthalmoplegia, ataxia, and absence of reflexes. The presence of anti-ganglioside GQ1b antibodies is constant. The prognosis is invariably benign, with a course of approximately four weeks.

Bickerstaff's brainstem encephalitis is a variant of Miller Fisher syndrome involving the central nervous system. It shares similarities with Miller Fisher syndrome, including ataxia, absence of osteotendinous reflexes, and ocular motility disturbances. Patients with Bickerstaff's encephalitis also experience hypersomnolence, likely due to the expression of ganglioside GQ1b in the reticular formation, and potentially other signs of central nervous system involvement.

Another variant of this syndrome is acute ataxic neuropathy (previously defined as "Ataxic Variant of Guillain-Barré Syndrome"). This condition is also associated with anti-GQ1b ganglioside antibodies. It manifests with ataxia, absence of osteotendinous reflexes, but preservation of ocular motility.

Chronic demyelinating polyradiculoneuropathy

It is a chronic immune-mediated inflammatory demyelinating neuropathy. It can have a relapsing-remitting or chronic progressive course (with gradual or stepwise worsening). Less commonly, it has a monophasic course with complete remission.

Unlike Guillain-Barré syndrome (of which it does not represent the chronicization), there are no clear associations with previous infectious diseases. The myelin damage is likely mediated by humoral and cell-mediated mechanisms. These patients often show the presence of antibodies against various myelin antigens (P0, P2, GM1), but their importance in the pathogenesis of myelin damage is still unknown. Neuropathological studies show a perivascular inflammatory infiltrate composed of lymphocytes, macrophages, and plasma cells affecting the spinal roots and the entire course of the nerve. There are demyelination and remyelination processes, which indicate the chronic course of the disease. In patients with a more prolonged course, secondary axonal damage is the norm. The disease presents with a symmetric sensory and motor disturbance. One of the predominant symptoms is hyposthenia, involving both proximal and distal muscles. Absence of reflexes is the rule and ataxia is common. Cranial nerves are spared. Neuropathic pain is rare. Respiratory or autonomic impairments are usually not observed.

The diagnosis is based on clinical manifestations, electrophysiological findings, and cerebrospinal fluid analysis. Electroneurography examination shows demyelinating damage (reduction in motor conduction velocity, temporal dispersion phenomena). Axonal loss phenomena (reduction in amplitude of sensory and motor potentials) are also very common. Cerebrospinal fluid analysis shows a significant increase in proteins, with a normal cell count. Unlike Guillain-Barré syndrome, corticosteroid therapy (prednisone 1 mg/kg of body weight) is effective. Various studies have demonstrated the efficacy of plasmapheresis and intravenous immunoglobulins.

Clinical variants, rarer than the classic sensorimotor form of chronic demyelinating polyradiculoneuropathy, include the purely sensory form, the purely motor form, and the focal form. Patients with the purely sensory form exclusively present sensory deficits. However, electrodiagnostic examinations typically reveal damage to motor fibers in the majority of cases. The purely motor form is extremely rare and its identification remains uncertain. It manifests with exclusive motor disturbances and does not respond to corticosteroid therapy. For this reason, according to some researchers, this condition may actually represent a widespread variant of multifocal motor neuropathy.

The focal form is a rare variant characterized by involvement of one or both upper limbs. This condition is still a subject of discussion. Currently, it is included within the spectrum of chronic demyelinating polyradiculoneuropathy, primarily because the few cases described in the literature showed a good response to therapy with immunoglobulins or corticosteroids.

Multifocal motor neuropathy

This rare form of inflammatory neuropathy is characterized by a motor conduction block. In approximately 70% of cases, anti-GM1 ganglioside antibodies are present, likely playing a direct pathogenic role in disease development. It more frequently affects males. It manifests with motor deficits affecting the muscles supplied by the nerve involved in the conduction block (usually a nerve in the upper limbs). There are no sensory disturbances. The onset is gradual, slowly progressive, and accompanied by muscle atrophy over time. Due to the absence of sensory disturbances and the presence of atrophy, this condition can sometimes be misdiagnosed as a motor neuron disease. Diagnosis is based on clinical features and evidence of a motor nerve conduction block on electroneurographic examination (defined as a reduction of at least 50% in the proximal motor potential compared to the distal potential) with normal sensory nerve conduction. Cerebrospinal fluid examination shows a modest increase in cerebrospinal fluid proteins, with a normal cell count. Multifocal motor neuropathy responds excellently to intravenous immunoglobulin treatment.

Lewis Sumner disease

Unlike multifocal motor neuropathy, this condition presents with both sensory and motor multifocal conduction blocks. Neuropathic pain is often one of the initial symptoms. The weakness typically affects the dorsal extension of the wrist and fingers. Sensory disturbances, which may also include pain, involve the distribution territory of the affected nerve. Cerebrospinal fluid examination shows normal or modestly increased cerebrospinal fluid proteins. The response to corticosteroid or immunoglobulin therapy is similar to that of chronic demyelinating polyradiculoneuropathy. According to many researchers, this peripheral nervous system disease should be considered a variant of chronic demyelinating polyradiculoneuropathy.

Bibliography

Biasiotta A., Casato M., La Cesa S., Colantuono S., Di Stefano G., Leone C., Carlesimo M., Piroso S., Cruccu G., Truini A. Clinical, neurophysiological, and skin biopsy findings in peripheral neuropathy associated with hepatitis C virus-related cryoglobulinemia. J Neurol; 261(4):725, 2014.

Briemberg HR. Peripheral nerve complications of medical disease. Semin Neurol; 29(2):124, 2009.

Diezi M., Buclin T., Kuntzer T. Toxic and drug-induced peripheral neuropathies: updates on causes, mechanisms and management. Curr Opin Neurol; 26(5):481-8, 2013.

Feldman EL., Callaghan BC., Pop-Busui R., Zochodne DW., Wright DE., Bennett DL., Bril V., Russell JW., Viswanathan V. Diabetic neuropathy. Nat Rev Dis Primers; 13;5(1):41, 2019.

Graus F., Dalmau J. Paraneoplastic neuropathies Curr Opin Neurol; 26(5):489-9, 2013.

Guillain-Barré and Miller Fisher syndromes--new diagnostic classification. Nat Rev Neurol.; 10(9):537, 2014.

Gwathmey KG., Burns TM., Collins MP., Dyck PJ. Vasculitic neuropathies. Lancet Neurol; 13(1):67-82, 2014.

Li T., Mizrahi D., Goldstein D., Kiernan MC., Park SB. Chemotherapy and peripheral neuropathy. Neurol Sci.; 42(10):4109-4121, 2021.

Palaiodimou L., Stefanou MI., Katsanos AH., Fragkou PC., Papadopoulou M., Moschovos C., Michopoulos I., Kokotis P., Bakirtzis C., Naska A., Vassilakopoulos TI., Chroni E., Tsiodras S., Tsivgoulis G. Prevalence, clinical characteristics and outcomes of Guillain-Barre syndrome spectrum associated with COVID-19: A systematic review and meta-analysis. Eur J Neurol.; 28(10):3517-352, 2021.

Ramchandren S., Lewis RA. An update on monoclonal gammopathy and neuropathy. Curr Neurol Neurosci Rep; 12(1):102-10, 2012.

Wakerley BR., Uncini A., Yuki N.; GBS Classification Group; GBS Classification Group.

Shahrizaila N., Lehmann HC., Kuwabara S. Guillain-Barre syndrome. Lancet; 397 (10280):1214-1228, 2021.

21 MYOPATHIES AND DISEASES OF THE NEUROMUSCULAR JUNCTION

Matteo Garibaldi, Laura Fionda, Stefania Morino, Giovanni Antonini

21.1 Myopathies

The term "myopathy" refers to a pathological condition affecting the structural or functional aspects of skeletal muscle tissue.

The diagnosis of myopathy is based on a combination of medical history, clinical examination, and instrumental evaluations that define the phenotypic characteristics of the patient, providing insights into the etiopathogenic mechanisms of the disease.

Functional and metabolic organization of skeletal muscle

Skeletal muscle is a complex anatomical structure responsible for converting electrical impulses received from motor neurons at the neuromuscular junction into mechanical energy. Skeletal muscle fibers are syncytia formed by the fusion of multiple myocytes, mononuclear cells derived from myoblasts. During embryogenesis, myocytes come together to form myotubes, which, during the maturation process, undergo nuclear migration from the center to the periphery, acquire supportive connective tissue (basal lamina and endomysium), and become innervated by motor axon branches, transforming into myofibers or independent muscle fibers. Multiple muscle fibers grouped together form muscle fascicles, surrounded by connective tissue (perimysium), and held together by abundant loose connective tissue (epimysium) (Figure 21.1).

Muscle tissue is supplied with a vascular network distributed within the interstitial tissue, ensuring oxygenation and the delivery of metabolic substrates. Nerve fibers destined to innervate individual myofibers and neuromuscular spindles are also contained within the interstitial tissue. Each muscle fiber is innervated by a single motor neuron, while a motor fiber innervates multiple muscle fibers, forming a motor unit.

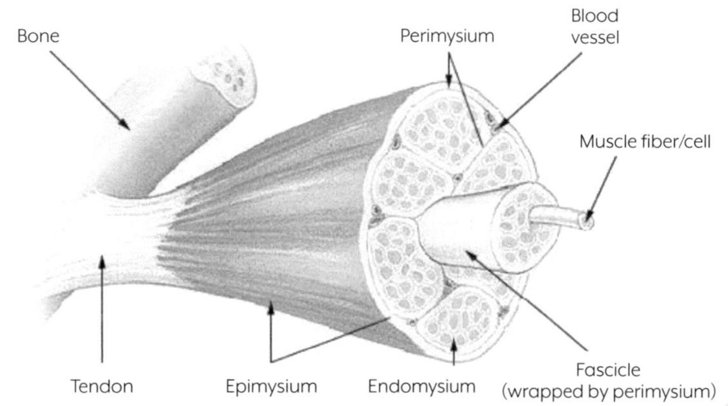

Figure 21.1

Muscle Structure in Cross-Section and Longitudinal Section from AR Gillies and RL Lieber. Structure and Function of the Skeletal Muscle Extracellular Matrix. Muscle Nerve. 2011 September 1; 44(3): 318–331. Note that the perimysium may be continuous with the tendon and delimits the muscle fascicles, while the endomysium separates the muscle fibers contained within the fascicles.

Muscle fibers are differentiated based on their preferred metabolic pathway, which influences their histochemical characteristics. It should be noted that muscle fibers belonging to the same motor unit and thus innervated by the same motor neuron are all of the same type. Type I fibers (red fibers) predominate in postural muscles that need to sustain prolonged efforts; they have predominantly oxidative metabolism and are "slow" fibers resistant to fatigue. Type IIA and IIB fibers (white fibers) predominate in muscles dedicated to rapid and precise movements (e.g., hand muscles or extraocular muscles); they have predominantly anaerobic metabolism and are "fast" fibers. Type IIC fibers have intermediate histochemical characteristics and constitute 15-20% of muscle fibers in neonates and 3-5% in adults. Additionally, skeletal muscle is equipped with undifferentiated cells (satellite cells) arranged along the basal lamina. These cells are believed to have a reparative function in muscle injuries due to their ability to fuse with adjacent muscle fibers.

The anatomofunctional structure of a muscle fiber can be schematically divided into three fundamental parts: the contractile system, membrane proteins, and ion channels (Figure 21.2). Alterations in each of these components correspond to different categories of myopathies.

a) The contractile apparatus | The muscle fiber contracts through the simultaneous sliding of numerous thick myosin filaments on thin actin filaments. This process occurs in each sarcomere, which represents the functional contractile unit of the muscle fiber itself. Sarcomeres are arranged in series, and their extension forms the myofibril.

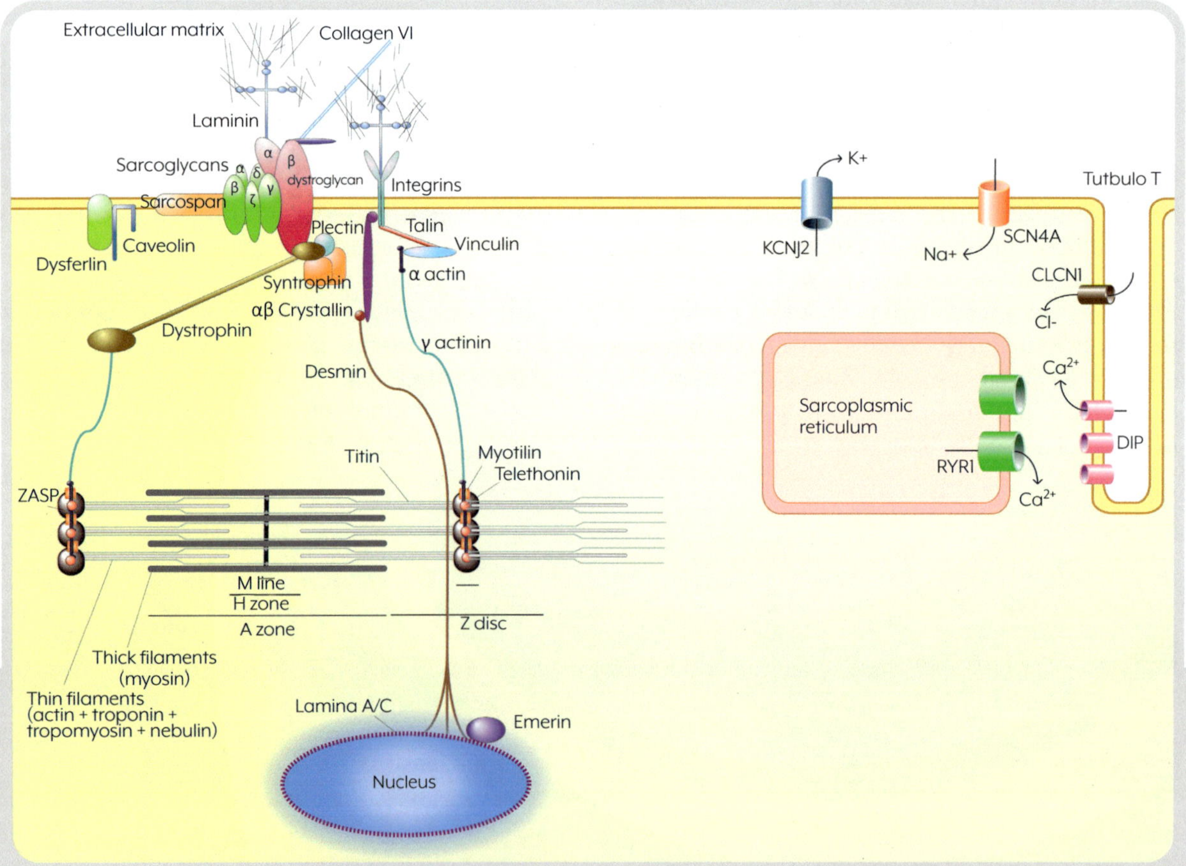

Figure 21.2

Contractile system, membrane proteins, and ion channels of the muscle fibrocell.

At the ultrastructural level, each sarcomere consists of two Z discs at its ends, a central A (anisotropic) band, and two peripheral I (isotropic) bands. The A band is composed of thick myosin filaments, which are anchored to the Z disc by elastic titin filaments. The I band is composed of thin actin filaments, which are surrounded by nebulin filaments and associated with troponin and tropomyosin. The Z discs are composed of a cluster of anchoring proteins necessary for maintaining the sarcomeric structure, including the myofibrillar structure. Alterations in the Z discs are the cause of numerous forms of myopathies (e.g., congenital myopathies, myofibrillar myopathies, limb-girdle myopathies, distal myopathies, etc.). Myofibrils are in close anatomical relation to T-tubules, invaginations of the sarcolemma that penetrate into the muscle fiber, allowing the diffusion of depolarization electrical events to the sarcomeres at the triad level. Triads are anatomical structures composed of a T-tubule and two cisternae of the sarcoplasmic reticulum, where the electro-mechanical signal transduction occurs.

b) Membrane proteins | The sarcomere is connected to the sarcolemma and the extracellular matrix by proteins essential for the stability of the muscle fiber's cytoskeleton. In particular, actin filaments are anchored to the basal lamina by a membrane protein complex consisting of dystrophin, Dystrophin-Associated-Proteins (DAPs), and laminins. The DAP complex, in turn, includes three groups of proteins: dystroglycans, sarcoglycans, and syntrophins. The actin-dystrophin-dystroglycan-laminin system constitutes the so-called "dystrophin-glycoprotein complex," which plays a crucial role in the mechanical stabilization of the sarcolemma, preventing its rupture during muscle fiber contraction and relaxation. Additionally, two transmembrane proteins (caveolin-3 and dysferlin) not directly associated with dystrophin also contribute to sarcolemma stability. Mutations in genes encoding this complex protein system are responsible for various types of muscular dystrophies.

c) Ion channels | Ion channels are transmembrane macromolecular proteins essential for maintaining the hydroelectrochemical homeostasis of all eukaryotic cells. In nerve and muscle cells, ion channels are also responsible for their excitability. They can be categorized into three major types based on the nature of the stimulus that activates them: 1) voltage-gated channels, 2) neurotransmitter-gated channels, and 3) mechanically gated channels (stretch/pressure activation).

There are four types of voltage-gated ion channels involved in regulating neuromuscular excitability, resting potential, and action potential: sodium, potassium, chloride, and calcium channels. Their alterations lead to myopathies characterized by abnormal neuromuscular excitability (periodic paralysis and myotonic syndromes). In addition to these, there are a series of channel proteins responsible for the release of intracellular calcium following sarcolemma depolarization at the triad level (*DHPR* and *RyR1*) and its reuptake into the sarcoplasmic reticulum (*SERCA1, ORA1* and *STIM1*), which are necessary for proper electro-mechanical coupling underlying the contraction and relaxation mechanism. Mutations in genes encoding these channels are responsible for certain Congenital Myopathies (Central Core Malignant Hyperthermia), Tubular Aggregate Myopathies (TAM), or conditions of impaired muscle relaxation (Brody syndrome).

Neurophysiology of muscle contraction

When the postsynaptic potential at the neuromuscular junction reaches the threshold value, it generates an action potential that propagates throughout the sarcolemma and reaches the depth of the muscle fiber through the T-tubules, which are contiguous with the sarcoplasmic reticulum, forming an anatomical system called the triad (Figure 21.3). Here, the action potential causes the opening of dihydropyridine calcium channels of the L-type (DHPR), resulting in a flow of small amounts of Ca2+ ions into the muscle fiber and, at the same time, a conformational change of the RyR1 channel located on the sarcoplasmic reticulum, leading to its opening and massive release of Ca2+ from the reticulum into the cytoplasm. The released calcium then binds to troponin, which modifies the conformation of actin filaments, exposing the binding sites for

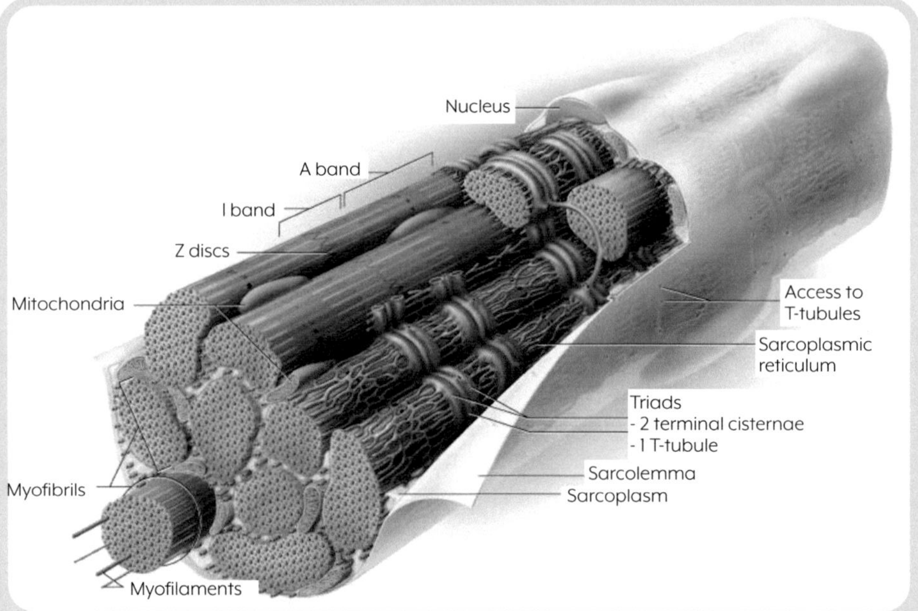

Figure 21.3

Arrangement of the sarcoplasmic reticulum and T-tubules around the myofibrils of skeletal muscle fibers in amphibians (in humans, the triads are located at the junction of the A band and I band).

myosin. The myosin molecules, when bound to actin molecules, undergo a rotation of their terminal portion, which, in the presence of ATP, causes the sliding of the filaments, resulting in the shortening of the sarcomere and contraction of the muscle fiber. When the intracellular calcium level decreases, the interaction between actin and myosin diminishes, allowing the elongation of the sarcomere and the relaxation of the fiber. At the same time, the depletion of sarcoplasmic calcium stores leads to the dimerization of STIM1, a protein located on the sarcoplasmic reticulum membrane that is sensitive to changes in calcium concentration. This dimerization, on the cytosolic side, leads to the binding and opening of the CRAC channel (Ca2+ release-activated Ca2+) located on the sarcolemma, which is composed of six monomers of ORAI1. The opening of this channel results in a flow of extracellular calcium into the cell, called SOCE (store-operated calcium entry), with subsequent restoration of intrasarcoplasmic calcium reserves through the reuptake of calcium into the reticulum via the SERCA1 channel. Inside the sarcoplasmic reticulum, calcium molecules are then bound by a molecule called calsequestrin (CASQ1), restoring the initial condition for a new excitation-contraction cycle. The proper functioning of this mechanism (SOCE) ensures cellular calcium homeostasis, which is necessary not only for muscle contraction but also for the maintenance of many other biological functions in different types of cells (mitochondrial function, gene expression modulation, cell growth and differentiation, nerve conduction, coagulation, hormonal release, etc.).

Muscle metabolism

Muscle activity involves a high energy consumption that is mainly produced using two main energy substrates (glycogen and fatty acids), which are metabolized under aerobic or anaerobic conditions, depending on the mode of muscle exertion (Table 21.1).

Glycogen constitutes the energy reserve of the muscle; it is synthesized during rest and transformed into glucose during muscle activity. Glucose metabolism occurs in the cytoplasm through glycolysis, which, under aerobic conditions, produces pyruvate, and under anaerobic conditions, produces lactate. Pyruvate diffuses along an electrical gradient into the mitochondria, where it is converted to Acetyl-CoA. Lactate is transported out of the muscle and, upon entering the bloodstream, reaches the liver, where it is metabolized in the Cori cycle.

Fatty acids are transported into the cell by specific transporters or can freely diffuse through the plasma membrane. From the cytoplasm, fatty acids are actively transported into the mitochondria, where they undergo

Table 21.1 METABOLIC PATHWAYS USED BY SKELETAL MUSCLE FOR ENERGY PRODUCTION

	Rest	Onset of movement	Intense isometric exercise (< 3 minutes)	Initial light to moderate exercise	Prolonged light to moderate exercise
Energy substrate	- Fatty acids	- CK/PFK - MADA - Glucose	- Glycogen - Glucose	- Glycogen - Glucose - (Fatty acids)	- Fatty acids - Glycogen - Glucose - (Amino acids)
Metabolism	Aerobic	Anaerobic	Anaerobic	Aerobic	Aerobic

CK: Creatine Kinase; PFK: Phosphofructokinase; MADA: Myoadenylate Deaminase

beta-oxidation, progressively reducing their length and producing Acetyl-CoA molecules.

The common product of glucose and fatty acid metabolism, Acetyl-CoA, is oxidized in the Krebs cycle. The products derived from beta-oxidation and the Krebs cycle are ultimately oxidized in the mitochondrial respiratory chain.

In a resting state, the energy used by muscle tissue is mainly derived from fatty acid beta-oxidation. At the onset of muscle exercise, the rapid decrease in ATP levels triggers the activation of anaerobic energy pathways (myoadenylate kinase/myoadenylate deaminase (MADA), phosphocreatine-creatine, and glycolysis). When the exercise is intense and of short duration or during intensity increments of moderate exercise, endogenous glycogenolysis is activated to produce glucose, which is metabolized through anaerobic glycolysis with lactate production. In mild to moderate exercise, muscle tissue tends to use a combination of circulating glucose (derived from the diet and hepatic glycogenolysis) and fatty acids, in varying proportions depending on the duration and intensity of the exercise, training status, and gender. Circulating glucose and hepatic glycogen reserves are sufficient to support exercise for a maximum of 1-2 hours. In prolonged exercises, by far the most important energy reserve is constituted by fatty acids. Amino acids, mainly branched-chain amino acids, are oxidized only to a limited extent and can only minimally supplement the muscle's energy needs.

Diagnosis of myopathies

The diagnosis of a myopathy is made based on a thorough patient history, clinical examination, laboratory tests, and, if necessary, targeted genetic tests.

Clinical evaluation | A careful collection of patient history is the first step in evaluating a patient with suspected myopathy. It is necessary to establish the precise onset of clinical history, the temporal relationship with any triggering causes (infections, exposure to toxic substances, medication use), the course of symptoms (acute, subacute, or chronic), and the presence of symptoms related to the involvement of other organs or systems. Family history plays a particularly relevant role in identifying other affected family members to determine potential hereditary factors.

Clinical symptoms and signs suggestive of a muscular disease |

Muscle Weakness. Weakness, although not always present, is the most common symptom in myopathic patients and can affect all muscle districts, leading to different symptoms. It can be assessed during the physical examination by evaluating the strength of individual muscles using the Medical Research Council (MRC) scale, which assigns a score from 5 to 0 to muscle strength, with 5 indicating normal strength against resistance, 4 indicating reduced strength against resistance, 3 indicating reduced strength against gravity, 2 indicating movement possible with gravity eliminated, 1 indicating contraction without movement, and 0 indicating complete absence of contraction.

The distribution of muscle weakness, both at the onset of the disease and during its course, is crucial for diagnostic orientation (Figure 21.4).

Most myopathies are characterized by a symmetric and proximal muscle weakness of the limbs. Weakness of the shoulder girdle muscles can cause difficulty in raising the arms and may result in winged scapula (scapular winging) (Figure 21.5). Involvement of the

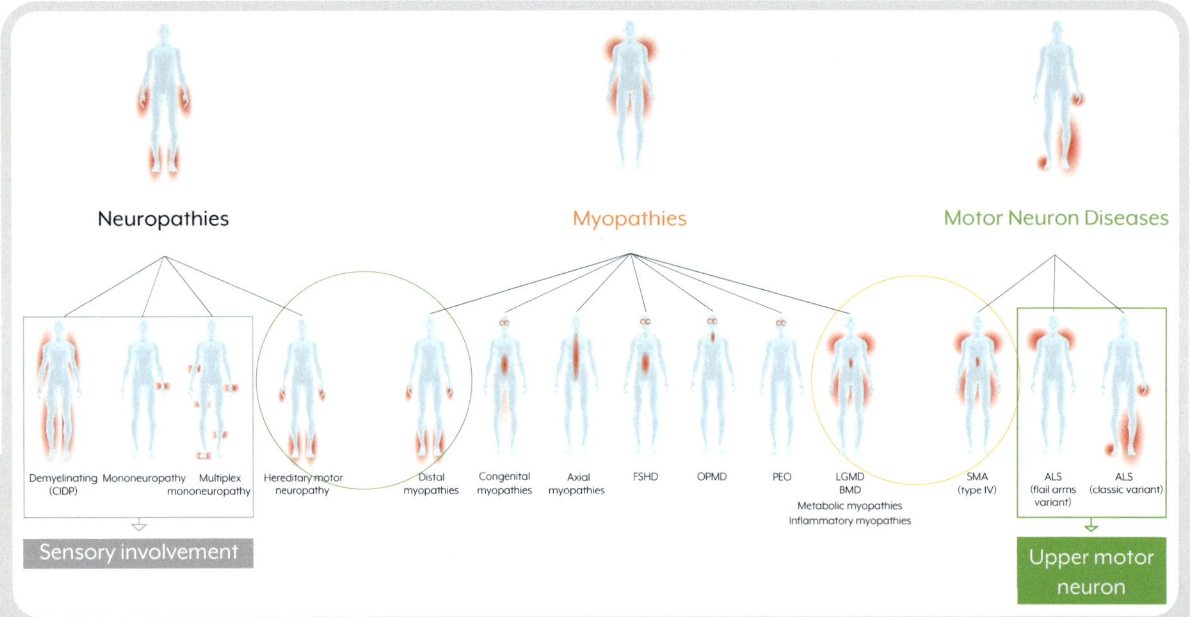

Figure 21.4

Muscle involvement distribution in different neuromuscular diseases, divided into major groups (neuropathies, myopathies, and motor neuron diseases). Note the potential phenotypic overlap (circles) even among diseases belonging to different major groups for the differential diagnosis of myopathies.

pelvic girdle can make it difficult to rise from the ground without the assistance of the arms (Gowers' maneuver) or climb stairs.

Weakness of the gluteus medius muscle alters the stability of the pelvis during walking, leading to hip swinging (Trendelenburg sign) and waddling gait. Weakness of the quadriceps can cause hyperextension of the knee during walking (genu recurvatum) (Figure 21.6).

Asymmetric weakness is characteristic of certain myopathies (facioscapulohumeral dystrophy, some metabolic myopathies, dysferlinopathies, anoctaminopathies, FHL1-related disorders, symptomatic carriers of myotubular myopathy, certain cases of inclusion body myositis, and focal myositis).

In some myopathies, weakness predominantly affects the distal muscles of the limbs. Weakness of the anterior muscles of the leg leads to foot drop and a "steppage" gait (Miyoshi myopathy, certain distal and myofibrillar myopathies), while weakness of the posterior leg muscles causes difficulty in standing on tiptoes (Miyoshi myopathy, certain distal myopathies). Distal weakness of the upper limbs results in difficulties with gripping, finger

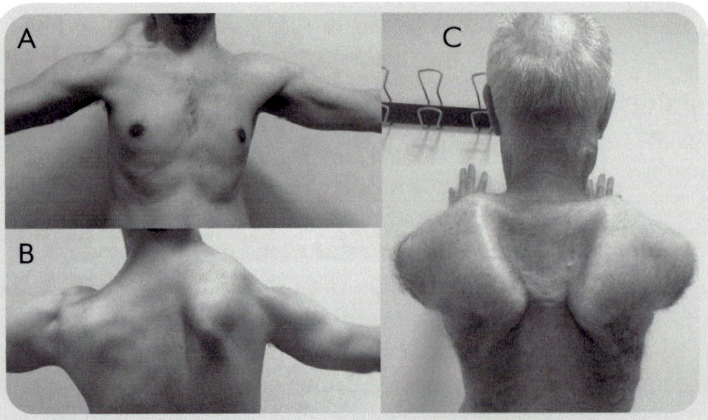

Figure 21.5

In (A, B), asymmetric winged scapula, or symmetric (C).

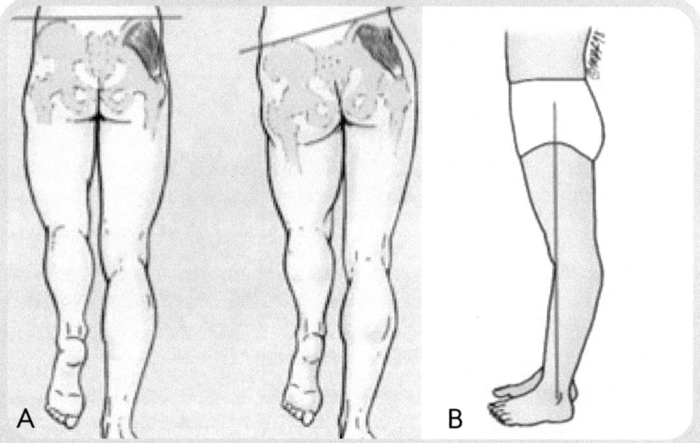

Figure 21.6

Trendelenburg sign (A) and genu recurvatum (B).

and hand extension (dropped hand), and finger movements (myotonic dystrophy, Welander distal myopathy, inclusion body myositis).

Weakness of the facial muscles can involve the muscles of the face (facioscapulohumeral dystrophy, myotonic dystrophy, nemaline myopathy), extraocular muscles (mitochondrial myopathies, certain congenital myopathies), masticatory muscles (myotonic dystrophy), pharyngeal and laryngeal muscles (oculopharyngeal dystrophy, myotonic dystrophy), and neck flexor muscles (myotonic dystrophy). Weakness of the neck extensor muscles leads to forward head drop (*dropped-head*) (Figure 21.7).

Weakness can involve the respiratory muscles, leading to restrictive ventilatory insufficiency, which is one of the most serious complications in a patient with myopathy. Respiratory insufficiency usually becomes symptomatic later in the disease but can be detected in the early stages through spirometry. In some myopathies, respiratory insufficiency may be an early symptom (glycogen storage disease type II).

The presence of generalized muscle weakness in infants results in the so-called *floppy baby syndrome*, characterized by generalized hypotonia and asthenia, reduced voluntary movements, frog-leg posture (hips in external rotation), and head lag (Figure 21.8).

Muscle fatigability. Muscles, especially when affected by a metabolic disorder that impairs energy availability, have reduced resistance to exertion. Fatigability is constantly present, along with weakness, in almost all forms of myopathy. Moreover, muscle fatigability is characteristic of neuromuscular junction disorders (*myasthenia gravis*).

Muscle pain and cramps. Muscle pain (myalgia) can occur at any stage of a myopathy and is more common in certain forms (inflammatory myopathies, facioscapulohumeral dystrophy,

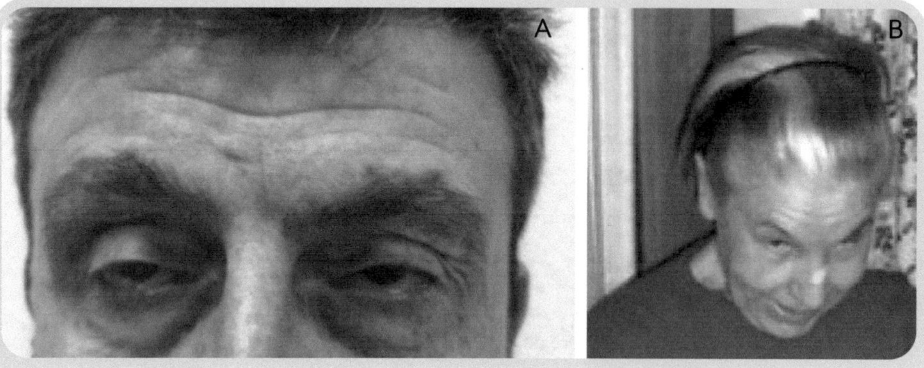

Figure 21.7

Bilateral eyelid ptosis in a patient with mitochondrial myopathy (A): note the compensation of ptosis with the corrugator. A case of dropped head (B).

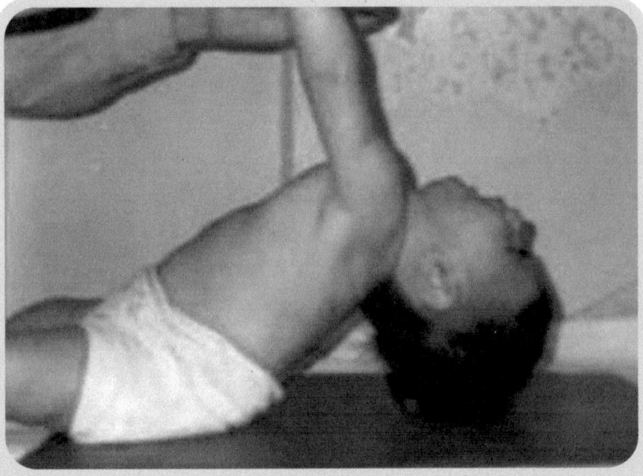

Figure 21.8

Floppy baby. Note the outward rotation of the hips and the weakness of the neck muscles.

myotonic dystrophy type II). Myalgia and cramps that occur after exertion suggest a possible metabolic disorder (glycogen storage diseases, mitochondrial myopathies). Cramps at rest are characteristic of neuromuscular diseases with a neuropathic pathogenesis.

Altered muscle trophism (atrophy, pseudo-hypertrophy, hypertrophy). Patients with muscle diseases may present with muscle atrophy, pseudohypertrophy, or muscle hypertrophy. Atrophy can be generalized or, more frequently, selectively affect certain muscles, defining characteristic phenotypes (muscles of the posterior compartment of the leg in Miyoshi myopathy, quadriceps in inclusion body myositis). Pseudo-hypertrophies are characterized by volumetric increase in muscles due to abundant fatty tissue replacement, which also leads to retraction (calf muscle in Duchenne muscular dystrophy). Muscle hypertrophy can be observed in the early stages of muscular dystrophies as a compensatory mechanism of synergistic muscles spared by the pathological process or, characteristically, in certain channelopathies (congenital myopathies) where there is a characteristic hypertrophy of all muscle masses, giving the patient a "Herculean" appearance (Figure 21.9).

Myotonia. It is a specific phenomenon, typical of muscle diseases caused by alterations in sarcolemmal ion channels, characterized by difficulty in relaxing muscles after forced contraction. The phenomenon improves with repeated contraction (warm-up), unlike paramyotonia, where difficulty in relaxation occurs during repeated contraction. The myotonic phenomenon can be stimulated by percussion of the muscles (mechanical myotonia) or recorded by electromyographic examination (electrical myotonia) (Figure 21.10).

Contractures, muscle contractures, and Joint deformities. The replacement of degenerated muscle tissue by connective tissue, which has less elasticity, promotes the development of retractions and muscle contractures,

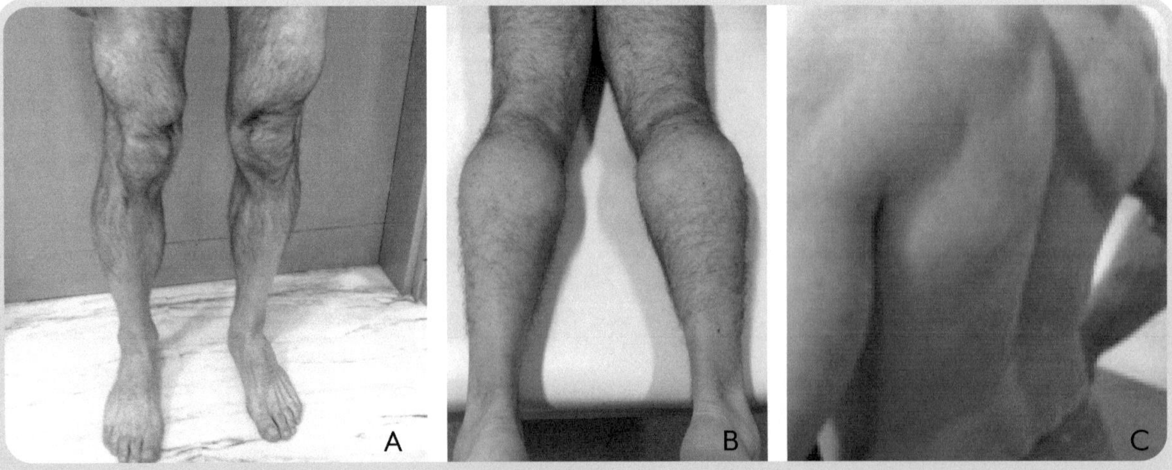

Figure 21.9

Muscular trophism alterations: atrophy (A); pseudohypertrophy (B); hypertrophy (C).

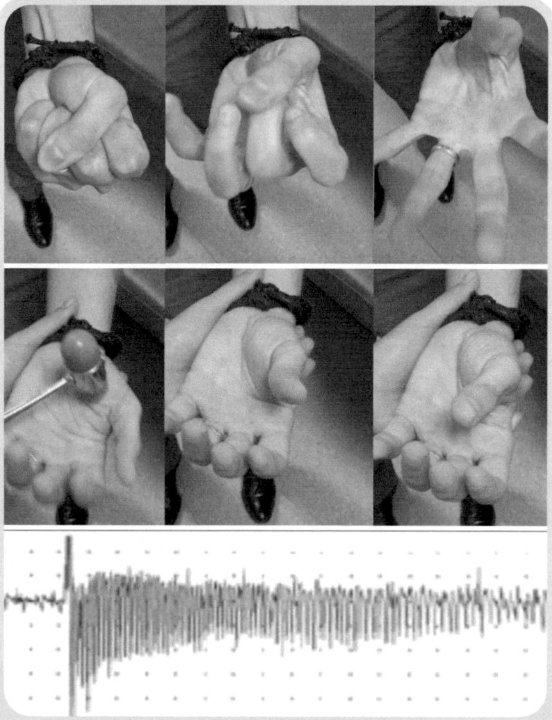

Figure 21.10

Myotonic phenomenon after maximal contraction (top images) and after percussion (bottom images). Graphic representation of the myotonic phenomenon recorded electrically during electromyography.

resulting in subankylosis and joint ankylosis, especially in dystrophic patients with limited autonomy. In some myopathies, contractures (or ligamentous laxities) may represent the predominant component of the clinical picture (Emery-Dreifuss dystrophy, laminopathies, collagenopathies). Additionally, weakness of the paravertebral muscles and abnormal postures contribute to the development of spinal deformities (kyphoscoliosis, hyperlordosis, etc.), which are very common in congenital myopathies.

Involvement of Other Extramuscular Areas. Some myopathies are characterized by multi-system involvement, where, in addition to muscle tissue, there is frequent involvement of the heart, brain, and other organs and systems (myotonic dystrophy, mitochondrial myopathies, dystrophinopathies, congenital muscular dystrophies).

Laboratory tests

Hematological tests | The measurement of creatine kinase (CK) is a simple but fundamental laboratory test in the diagnosis of myopathies. CK is an enzyme that plays a key role in the transport and storage of energy in skeletal, cardiac, and cerebral muscle cells. CK is a dimer composed of two monomers, muscle (M) and brain (B), which combine to generate three measurable isoenzymes (MM, MB, and BB), which are present in different proportions in different tissues. In skeletal muscle, MM isoenzyme represents 97-99% of CK, while MB isoenzyme represents 1-3%. The blood level of CK increases in most patients with muscle fiber degeneration or necrosis. However, there is also significant individual variability in CK levels in normal individuals, with higher values observed in Afro-Caribbean and Asian populations, individuals engaged in intense muscle activity, or those exposed to muscle trauma.

Metabolic myopathies can be assessed through the measurement of lactate and ammonia. Excessive increases in these metabolites during muscle exercise (>3-5 times the normal level) suggest disorders of the respiratory chain (mitochondrial myopathies) or glycogen metabolism.

The search for autoantibodies is useful in inflammatory myopathies, for which more detailed information can be found.

Urine analysis | Urine analysis can reveal pigmenturia in cases of massive muscle necrosis (rhabdomyolysis). The urine appears reddish-brown, resembling "coke" when urinary myoglobin levels, the muscle protein necessary for efficient oxygen diffusion in muscles, exceed 1g/L. The most common causes of rhabdomyolysis and myoglobinuria are metabolic myopathies (CPTII deficiency, myophosphorylase deficiency, phosphofructokinase deficiency, myoadenylate deaminase deficiency), as well as muscular dystrophies, channelopathies, toxic myopathies, inflammatory myopathies, and traumatic injuries (*crush syndrome*). Myoglobin, when precipitated in the renal tubules, can cause acute renal failure due to tubular necrosis. This can be prevented through hydration and diuretic support. The measurement of urinary organic acids is useful in the diagnosis of myopathies associated with mitochondrial beta-oxidation disorders.

Neurophysiological tests | Electromyography (EMG) is predominantly useful in the diagnosis of myopathies for determining the myopathic nature of muscle weakness (early recruitment, reduced duration and amplitude of motor unit potentials), differentiating it from neuropathic weakness, and identifying the presence of resting electrical activity, indicative of electrical instability in diseased muscle fibers (fibrillations and high-frequency discharges in inflammatory myopathies and certain muscular dystrophies; myotonic discharges in myotonic dystrophies). Repetitive stimulation and single-fiber electromyography are useful for defining the myasthenic nature of muscle weakness. Nerve conduction studies usually do not show significant abnormalities, except in distal myopathies where there may be a reduction in compound muscle action potential (CMAP), mimicking a motor neuropathy. Sensory and motor nerve conduction studies are also applicable in myopathies associated with neuropathic involvement (mitochondrial myopathies). For neurophysiological tests, see the chapter on EMG/ENG.

Muscle biopsy | Muscle biopsy is essential in the diagnosis of myopathies. The sample should be taken from the muscles affected by the myopathic process, under local anesthesia, through open surgery or with a biopsy needle. Various histological, histochemical, and immunohistochemical stains allow the characterization of the numerous alterations encountered, which will be discussed in detail for each specific disease. Ultrastructural examination using electron microscopy is employed to study alterations that cannot be characterized by light microscopy.

Neuroimaging | Muscle imaging is becoming increasingly important in clinical practice as different sequences can characterize and quantify muscle damage. MRI, in particular, evaluates T1 sequences for identifying fat replacement of muscle and STIR sequences for identifying muscle edema and indirectly inflammation. Muscle MRI has various implications in clinical practice. It allows for a more accurate selection of the muscle to be biopsied, highlighting muscles that are affected by the pathological process but not yet completely replaced by fat. It also enables better characterization of the clinical phenotype by evaluating muscles that are difficult to assess clinically. Neuroimaging studies have shown that the distribution of muscle damage tends to reproduce characteristic patterns in different myopathies. Therefore, identifying different patterns of fat replacement in muscles can be helpful in the diagnostic process, especially in myopathies where the same clinical phenotype can be caused by mutations in different genes (congenital myopathies, congenital muscular dystrophies, myofibrillar myopathies, limb-girdle muscular dystrophies, etc.). In recent years, quantitative muscle imaging has also become valuable for assessing disease progression and treatment response (▪ Figure 21.11).

Genetic testing | Genetic testing is a crucial step in the diagnostic process of a significant percentage of myopathy cases. For certain myopathies with highly characteristic phenotypes (such as myotonic dystrophy or facioscapulohumeral dystrophy), genetic testing is often the first diagnostic step after clinical examination. In other cases, genetic testing may be performed based on the results of muscle biopsy and other investigations. In recent years, advancements in technology have led to the development of massive sequencing techniques (Next Generation Sequencing, NGS) that allow for parallel sequencing of many genes or the entire exome or genome, making the diagnostic confirmation process much faster and more cost-effective than in the past.

Classification of myopathies

The list of known myopathies is continuously evolving, and several classifications have been proposed over the years in an attempt to organize the different forms into clinical, histological, or pathophysiological groups. However, the increasing complexity of this field has made it difficult to establish a definitive unified and comprehensive classification

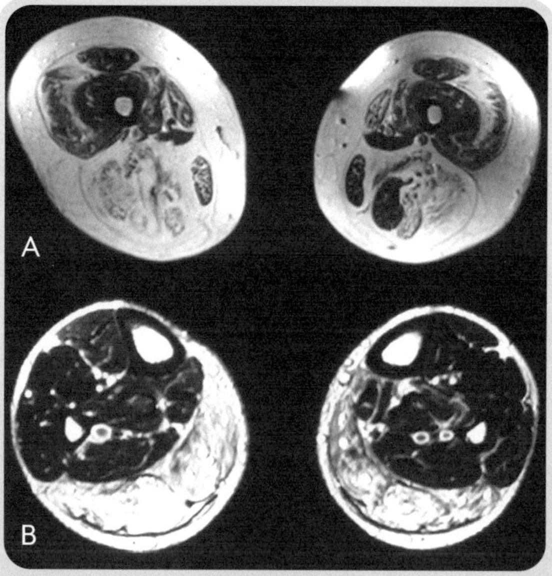

Figure 21.11

Muscle MRI in two patients with muscular dystrophy. Note the signal alteration of the posterior muscles (gracilis and biceps femoris) and the anterior muscles (vastus medialis and vastus lateralis) of the thighs (A) and the posterior muscles of the legs (gastrocnemius) (B).

according to any specific criterion. This complexity arises from the observation that the same phenotype (*clinical* or *histological*) can be caused by different genetic mutations (*genetic heterogeneity*), and conversely, mutations in the same gene can lead to different phenotypes (*phenotypic heterogeneity*).

The proposed organization (rather than classification) aims to respect this complexity, limiting the subdivision of myopathies into two main areas: genetic and acquired (Table 21.2).

Acquired myopathies are further divided into two major groups: inflammatory and non-inflammatory.

In clinical practice, genetic myopathies are classified into different groups based on the distribution of muscle involvement (facioscapulohumeral dystrophy, oculo-pharyngeal dystrophy, limb-girdle muscular dystrophies, distal myopathies, myotonic dystrophies), histopathological changes (myofibrillar myopathies, congenital myopathies), age of onset (congenital muscular dystrophies, congenital myopathies), or biochemical or protein defects (metabolic myopathies, muscular channelopathies). However, as mentioned earlier, a single disease (caused by mutations in a specific gene) can exhibit a wide phenotypic variability (e.g., desminopathies can present as myofibrillar myopathy, distal myopathy, limb-girdle muscular dystrophy, scapuloperoneal dystrophy). Conversely, a specific clinical or histological phenotype can have multiple genetic causes. This implies that the same gene can be found in different clinical forms and different genes can be associated with the same clinical form, resulting in a certain complexity of classification and categorization.

21.2 Genetic myopathies

Genetic myopathies of a dystrophic nature (muscular dystrophies) are progressive muscle diseases in which the muscle tissue, due to the processes of necrosis and fiber regeneration, shows characteristic variability in the caliber of the fiber cells, centralization of nuclei, increased endomysial and perimysial fibrous tissue, and replacement of muscle tissue with fatty tissue (Figure 21.12). Non-dystrophic genetic myopathies, on the other hand, are characterized by non-destructive alterations in muscle biopsy and a non-degenerative

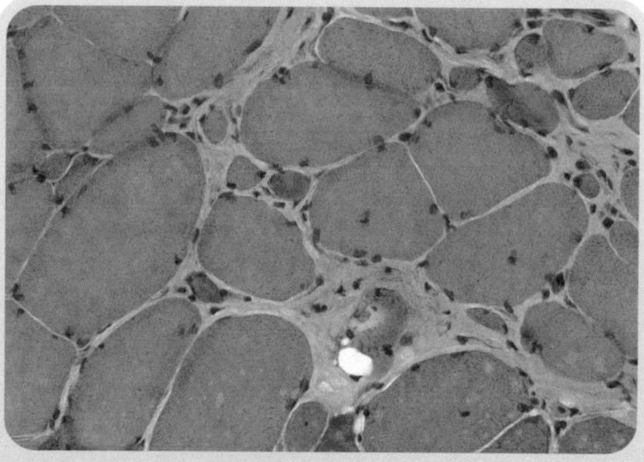

Figure 21.12

Histological preparation (Hematoxylin Eosin) of a muscle biopsy from a patient with muscular dystrophy (Becker Muscular Dystrophy). Notice the abundant connective tissue, atrophic fibers, hypertrophic fibers, and the presence of centrally positioned nuclei (centralized nuclei).

Table 21.2 CLASSIFICATION OF MYOPATHIES

Genetic

- Dystrophinopathies (DMD, BMD)
- Myotonic dystrophies (DM1, DM2)
- Facioscapulohumeral dystrophy (FSHD)
- Oculopharyngeal muscular dystrophy (OPMD)
- Limb-Girdle muscular dystrophies (LGMD)
- Congenital muscular dystrophies (CMD)
- Myofibrillar myopathies (MFM) and distal myopathies
- Congenital myopathies (CM)
- Tubular aggregate myopathies (TAM)
- Metabolic myopathies (glycogen storage diseases, mitochondrial myopathies, lipid myopathies)
- Channelopathies (non-dystrophic myotonic syndromes, periodic paralyses)

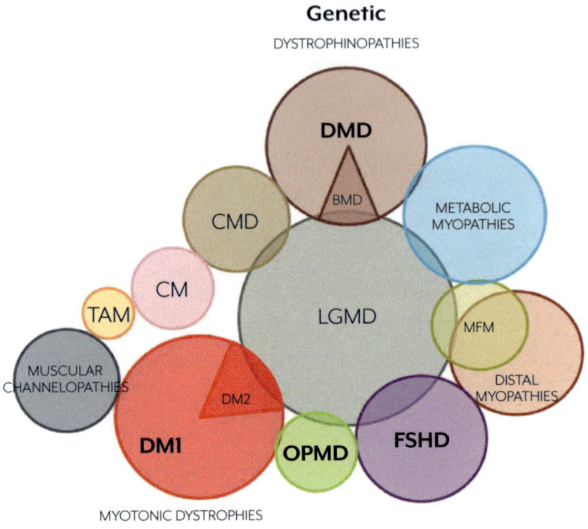

Acquired

Inflammatory Myopathies

Idiopathic Inflammatory Myopathies (IIM)
- Dermatomyositis (DM)
- Autoimmune Necrotizing Myopathies (NAM)
- Anti-synthetase Syndrome (ASS)
- Inclusion Body Myositis (IBM)

Other Inflammatory Myopathies
- Overlap Myositis (associated with other autoimmune diseases) and Myositis and Myasthenia
- Cervicobrachial Inflammatory Myopathy (BCIM)
- Inflammatory Myopathy with Mitochondrial Pathology (PM-mito)
- Immune Checkpoint Inhibitors (ICIs)- related Myositis
- Nonspecific Myositis
- Infectious Myopathies and COVID-19 Myositis
- Sarcoidosis
- Focal Myositis
- Miofasciitis

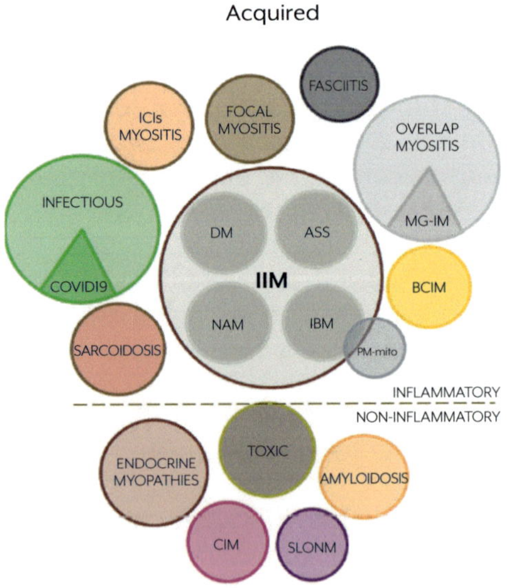

Non-inflammatory myopathies

Systemic diseases
Sporadic Late Onset Nemaline Myopathy (SLONM)
- Critical Illness Myopathy (CIM)
- Paraneoplastic myopathies
- Polymyalgia rheumatica

Endocrine myopathies
- Thyroid-related
- Parathyroid-related

Toxic myopathies
- Drug-induced
- Substance abuse-related

course of the muscle. However, as mentioned earlier, some muscular dystrophies may exhibit histological characteristics of the non-dystrophic type, and vice versa, blurring the boundary between dystrophic and non-dystrophic myopathies in some cases.

21.2.1 Dystrophinopathies

Dystrophinopathies are recessive dystrophic myopathies linked to the X chromosome, caused by a mutation in the gene located on the short arm of the X chromosome at the Xp21.2 site, which encodes dystrophin, one of the largest proteins in the body responsible for the structural integrity of muscle fibers. Generally, males are affected, and females are asymptomatic carriers. However, in some cases, female carriers may manifest muscular symptoms of varying severity.

Epidemiology | Two clinical forms of dystrophinopathy are distinguished, differing in severity: a) Duchenne Muscular Dystrophy (DMD), the more severe form (with an incidence of approximately 1 in 3,500 live male births and a prevalence of 3 in 100,000), which represents the most common form of childhood muscular dystrophy; b) Becker Muscular Dystrophy (BMD), a less severe form, with an incidence of 3 in 30,000 live male births.

Etiology and pathophysiology | All dystrophinopathies are allelic and result from different mutations of the same Xp21 gene. The Xp21 gene, composed of 79 exons, encodes several tissue-specific isoforms of dystrophin. In DMD, three isoforms are involved: the muscular isoform (expressed in striated and smooth muscle), the cerebral isoform (expressed in the cortex and hippocampus), and the Purkinje isoform (expressed in the Purkinje cells of the cerebellum).

The different phenotype of DMD compared to BMD is correlated with different mutations (more frequently deletions or duplications) that can occur in the Dystrophin gene. The production of dystrophin depends on the impact of the mutation (in-frame or out-of-frame) on the reading frame. In DMD, dystrophin is almost or completely absent (classically <5%), while in BMD, it is >5%. However, 10% of cases present an exception to this rule, due to phenomena of spontaneous exon skipping of the mutation, restoring the reading frame, or due to somatic mosaicism in which not all cells express the same mutation. Furthermore, the impact on the functionality of the produced protein depends on the site where the mutation occurs. In-frame deletions in different sites of the gene produce different phenotypes (DMD or BMD).

The amount of dystrophin expressed in the muscle can be evaluated using Western blot. Histological and experimental evidence has shown that quantitative or qualitative alterations of dystrophin are crucial for the mechanical stability of the sarcolemma, a mechanism that underlies progressive muscle degeneration.

Clinical aspects and classification | The predominant symptoms of dystrophinopathies are symmetric weakness, primarily affecting the limb girdles (with a marked increase in CK levels), accompanied by muscle atrophy, pseudohypertrophy, contractures, and skeletal deformities. There is significant clinical heterogeneity in severity.

Duchenne Muscular Dystrophy (DMD) | It is the most severe clinical form of dystrophinopathy. At birth, newborns with DMD do not exhibit motor deficits, but CK levels are already elevated (5.000-20.000 UI/L). Muscle weakness is usually noticed around 2-3 years of age. It initially affects the proximal lower limbs, making activities like climbing stairs, rising from the floor (Gowers maneuver), running, and jumping difficult for the child. Achilles tendon retraction with a tendency to walk on tiptoes may be present. Between 3 and 6 years of age, goose-like gait, lumbar hyperlordosis, and calf hypertrophy become evident. Later on, hypertrophy also affects the quadriceps, glutes, deltoids, and occasionally the masseter muscles, eventually leading to pseudo-hypertrophy due to connective tissue replacement of degenerated muscle tissue. Unlike in Becker Muscular Dystrophy (BMD), the flexor muscles of the neck are weak. Weakness also affects the extensors of the foot, while flexors remain intact and tend to develop contractures, causing toe-walking and foot deformity (equinovarus). Weakness of the shoulder girdle muscles, particularly the serratus anterior, causes the characteristic winging of the scapulae during upper limb movements. Children may complain of leg pain. Contractures progressively involve the hip, knee, wrist, and elbow, with shoulder contracture appearing later. Around the age of 10, the child loses the ability to walk without assistance from crutches, and around the age of 12, they become wheelchair-bound. With disease progression, CPK levels tend to decrease due to muscle depletion. Prolonged sitting position promotes the development of scoliosis, thoracic deformity, and subsequent respiratory problems. DMD also involves the heart, brain, and smooth muscle. 90% of DMD patients develop rhythm, conduction, and contractility abnormalities in the heart. DMD patients may also exhibit mild to moderate cognitive impairment. Smooth muscle involvement can lead to hypomobility or pseudo-intestinal obstruction. In the natural course of the disease, most patients die in the late second or early third decade, usually due to respiratory infections or progressive cardiomyopathy.

Becker muscular dystrophy (BMD) | BMD is characterized by extreme clinical variability, ranging from muscular dystrophy involving the limb girdles to asymptomatic or paucisymptomatic presentations. Symptoms typically onset between 7 and 15 years of age, but occasionally later (up to 40 years). Patients usually present with slowly progressive weakness of the pelvic girdle, thigh atrophy with calf pseudohypertrophy, and very high CK levels. Weakness of the shoulder girdle, symmetric scapular winging, and weakness of the tibialis and peroneal muscles appear later. Contractures may be present, mainly affecting the ankle. Unlike DMD, the neck muscles are generally spared. Loss of ambulation is proportional to clinical severity and can occur between 16 and 80 years of age. Cardiomyopathy can be a significant complication or even the presenting symptom, but it is rarer than in DMD. Rarely, BMD patients may present with exertional intolerance and rhabdomyolysis (pseudometabolic phenotype).

Symptomatic carriers | Female carriers of DMD mutations can exhibit symptoms. Clinical presentation varies considerably, ranging from asymptomatic CK elevation to cramps, calf hypertrophy, or isolated cardiomyopathy, to more severe clinical pictures. In most cases, weakness is mild, proximal, often asymmetric, with a predominant involvement of the pelvic girdle. Apart from extremely rare cases of DMD in patients with Turner syndrome (X0), different mechanisms, such as X-autosomal translocations with breakpoints in the Xp21 region and/or skewed inactivation of the normal X chromosome during early development, may underlie the expressivity of the disease in carriers.

Instrumental diagnosis

Electromyography | Myopathic pattern associated with fibrillations and positive potentials.

Muscle biopsy | Dystrophic histopathological pattern. Immunohistochemistry for dystrophin shows abnormal (BMD) or absent (DMD) representation of dystrophin at the sarcolemma. Quantification of dystrophin content in muscle tissue using Western blot.

Molecular diagnosis | Deletion/duplication screening, point mutation screening, haplotype analysis.

Therapy | The use of corticosteroids, ventilatory support, treatment of scoliosis and cardiomyopathy has improved the survival of DMD patients, extending it from less than 20 to over 30 years of age. ACE inhibitors are often associated with the disease course to prevent cardiac remodeling and delay heart failure. Significant progress has been made in the field of gene therapy for DMD in recent years. Currently, there are four drugs available based on exon skipping, a technique that allows skipping a specific exon during translation to restore the correct reading frame and production of a functional protein. Antisense oligonucleotides (ASOs) are used to improve disease symptoms. Molecules (e.g., Ataluren) that promote mRNA translation despite the presence of stop codons have also been identified, allowing protein synthesis. Another phase 3 gene therapy trial is underway, based on gene delivery techniques. Through a viral vector, a gene for the production of a mini-dystrophin capable of restoring dystrophin expression in muscle biopsies of these patients is introduced into muscle fibers. Approximately 30 trials using different therapeutic approaches, including exon skipping of other exons, gene editing, gene delivery, factors promoting muscle fiber growth and protection, calcium homeostasis regulation, and reduction of inflammation, are currently ongoing. For updates on available therapies, please consult the website https://www.parentprojectmd.org.

21.2.2 Myotonic dystrophies (DM1, DM2)

Myotonic dystrophy (DM1 and DM2) is an autosomal dominant disease characterized by the association of muscle weakness, myotonia, and multisystem involvement. Despite their name, both forms of myotonic dystrophy do not exhibit the muscle necrosis and regeneration processes typical of muscular dystrophies.

Epidemiology | There are two genetically defined forms of myotonic dystrophy: type 1 (DM1) and type 2 (DM2). First described in 1909 in Germany by Steinert, DM1 has an incidence of approximately 1 in 8,000 live births and a prevalence of 1-10 per 100,000, making it the most common myopathy in adulthood. DM2, first described in the 1990s, has a significantly lower prevalence and is more common in Europe.

Etiology and pathophysiology | DM1 is caused by an expansion of the CTG trinucleotide repeat (Cytosine-Thymine-Guanine) in the 3' untranslated region (transcribed but not translated) of the gene encoding myotonic dystrophy protein kinase (*DMPK*), or myotonia protein kinase, located on chromosome 19q13.3. The function of this protein is not entirely clear, but it appears to be involved in the regulation of early events in excitation-contraction coupling in skeletal muscle. The pathogenic mechanism of the disease is not related to protein insufficiency of this gene. Rather, it is primarily linked to the expansion of the CTG triplet repeat. In 90% of healthy individuals, the repeat is present below 35 repetitions. The threshold for defining the disease is above 50 repetitions. The disease is always present, even asymptomatic, in all carriers of an expansion greater than 50 repetitions (*complete penetrance*). The severity of the clinical phenotype tends to worsen from generation to generation (*anticipation phenomenon*) and in relation to the size of the expansion. The pathogenic mechanism by which the CTG expansion causes the disease appears to be related to the gain of function of the transcribed messenger RNA, which forms loops and impedes its nuclear export due to steric hindrance. This pathogenic transcript binds to various transcription factors, cascading into altered splicing of numerous other genes, which underlies the multisystem involvement of the disease.

DM2 is caused by the expansion of a CCTG repeat in intron 1 of the gene encoding Zinc Finger Protein 9 (ZNF9) on chromosome 3q21. In the healthy population, the average number of CCTG repeats is 15-30. The disease manifests with repeats exceeding 75 quadruplets, but large expansions of up to 10,000 (average of 5,000 repeats) are more frequently observed. The phenomenon of anticipation is less evident than in DM1, and there is no clear correlation between the size of the expansion and the clinical severity. However, the pathogenic mechanism appears to be very similar to that of DM1.

Clinical aspects | As multisystem diseases, DM1 and DM2 exhibit extreme heterogeneity in their manifestations, involving multiple organs and systems (Figure 21.13).

Myotonic dystrophy type 1 (DM1) | In the classic form, the disease begins between 20 and 50 years of age and is characterized by muscle symptoms and signs such as atrophy, weakness, and myotonia. Myotonia (which can precede weakness by many years) is most evident in the muscles of the hand, eyes, and tongue. Weakness and atrophy, in the most common form, consistently affect the distal muscles of the limbs (brachial extensors, small hand muscles [interossei], and anterior leg muscles, causing a "foot drop"), facial muscles (orbicularis oculi, levator palpebrae), masticatory muscles (masseters and temporals), and neck muscles (sternocleidomastoids with swan-like neck). Overall, the smoothing of wrinkles, mild ptosis, and enophthalmos give the face a typical "gloomy" expression. Pharyngolaryngeal muscle involvement results in a nasal, monotonous voice and dysphagia. Extramuscular manifestations include ocular disorders (early cataracts, retinal degeneration, reduced intraocular pressure), cutaneous features (frontal baldness), cardiac involvement (conduction disturbances, arrhythmias, and risk of sudden death), respiratory issues (restrictive patterns leading to respiratory failure or complications such as aspiration pneumonia, hypoventilation), gastrointestinal problems (megaesophagus, altered colonic motility, anal sphincter laxity), cerebral involvement (temporal and frontal changes with personality disorders, hypersomnia, non-progressive congenital mental retardation), endocrine abnormalities (hypogonadism, reduced libido, erectile dysfunction, testicular atrophy, spontaneous abortions), metabolic disturbances (insulin resistance, diabetes), bone alterations (cranial hyperostosis, reduction of the sella turcica), and immune abnormalities (reduced serum immunoglobulins). DM1 patients also have a higher risk of developing neoplasms compared to the general population. The congenital form is characterized by marked generalized hypotonia and facial diplegia. The absence of myotonia at birth becomes evident from the second or third year of life. Suckling and feeding difficulties are often present due to pharyngeal muscle weakness, along with respiratory deficits and joint deformities, especially of the foot (talipes). Surviving patients commonly exhibit mental retardation in 75% of cases, along with motor and language function impairments.

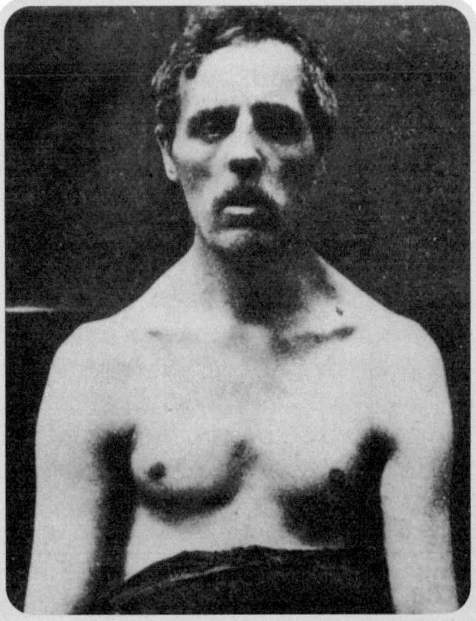

Figure 21.13

The first historic photograph of a subject affected by myotonic dystrophy. From *Myotonic Dystrophy*, 3rd edition By Peter S. Harper 2001.

Myotonic dystrophy type 2 (DM2) | Unlike DM1, DM2 presents a phenotype characterized by predominantly proximal limb muscle weakness associated with myotonia. For this reason, it was originally described as *Proximal Myotonic Myopathy* (PROMM). Involvement of facial muscles is less pronounced or absent, and myotonia is often clinically absent. Calf hypertrophy and muscle pain are frequently observed. Multisystem involvement is very similar to DM1, except for less frequent involvement of the central nervous system (CNS), although sensorineural hearing loss can occur. Congenital forms have not been described.

Diagnosis | CK levels can be normal in DM1 and DM2, particularly in mild clinical forms, but more often they are moderately elevated (<1000 IU/L). Electromyography (EMG) is useful for detecting myopathic damage and is particularly valuable for detecting myotonic discharges, which can be present even in paucisymptomatic or asymptomatic forms. Muscle biopsy shows nonspecific alterations, particularly an increase in centrally located nuclei with nuclear clumps. In clinically evident forms or in the presence of a family history, the diagnostic gold standard is molecular genetic testing, which evaluates the expansion of CTG or CCTG repeats and achieves a diagnostic sensitivity of 100%. Prenatal diagnosis of the congenital form is possible through prenatal molecular analysis conducted on chorionic villus samples collected in the eleventh week of gestation or, alternatively, in the sixteenth week on samples of amniotic fluid.

Treatment | Currently, therapy for DM1 and DM2 is solely symptomatic and aims to prevent and treat the various possible complications of the disease. The use of orthoses for foot drop can significantly aid in walking, as can collars to support the head in cases of severe weakness of the neck muscles. Blepharoplasty for ptosis is a useful intervention when ptosis obstructs vision. Pacemaker and defibrillator implantation should be considered for patients with cardiac rhythm disorders at risk of developing fatal arrhythmic events. Mexiletine, administered under cardiac supervision, can be useful in reducing myotonia in patients in whom this symptom is particularly disabling. In the last years, the development of gene therapy has shown promising results for DM1, and phase 2/3 clinical trials are underway, primarily with small molecules targeting the expanded transcript responsible for the disease. For updates, please consult the website https://www.myotonic.org.

21.2.3 Facioscapulohumeral muscular dystrophy (FSHD)

Described in 1884 by Landouzy and Dejerine, facioscapulohumeral muscular dystrophy, commonly referred to as FSHD, is an autosomal dominant inherited muscular dystrophy.

Epidemiology | After myotonic dystrophy and Duchenne muscular dystrophy, it is the third most common form of muscular dystrophy. Its prevalence is 4-10 per 100,000.

Etiology and pathophysiology | The molecular pathogenesis of FSHD is complex, and only recently have some of the mechanisms underlying the disease been partially elucidated. The most common form of FSHD (FSHD1) is associated with a pathological deletion of a D4Z4 repeat in the subtelomeric region of chromosome 4. When the repeat number falls below 10 (<43 kb) and is associated with a permissive haplotype, gene transcription occurs at this locus, leading to the expression of a toxic product (DUX4), which is normally repressed. However, a contracted D4Z4 allele has also been reported in the healthy population. Additionally, not all patients with a typical FSHD phenotype have a contracted D4Z4 allele. In these patients, referred to as FSHD2, DNA hypomethylation mechanisms caused by mutations in various genes (SMCHD1, DNMT3B, and more recently LRIF1) have been implicated. In the presence of a permissive haplotype, these mechanisms can also allow transcription of the gene locus and the expression of the toxic product DUX4, resulting in the disease, even in carriers of normal-sized D4Z4 alleles. These genes also act as modifiers of the clinical phenotype, influencing the severity of FSHD1.

Clinical aspects | The disease typically begins around 20 years of age (range: 10 to 50 years). Muscular involvement is typically asymmetric. Initially, there is weakness of the facial muscles (difficulty whistling, puckering lips, and closing eyelids) and weakness of the periscapular muscles (trapezius, rhomboids, serratus anterior), resulting in winged scapula and a characteristic triangular shape of the shoulders when the patient attempts to lift the upper limbs (Figure 21.14). Rarely, the onset can be distal (foot drop) or accompanied by muscle pain, which is characteristic of the disease. Marked weakness and atrophy of the brachial muscles (biceps and triceps) with sparing of the forearm muscles give the upper limbs an appearance resembling "Popeye's arms." Later, weakness of the abdominal muscles, especially the lower muscles, manifests with a protruding abdomen, hyperlordosis, and the Beevor's sign (cranial displacement of the umbilical scar when the patient attempts to flex the neck from the supine position) (Figure 21.15). Weakness of the anterior leg muscles, foot drop, and a steppage gait also occur. Loss of motor autonomy can occur in approximately 20% of cases. In some patients, weakness may extend to the proximal muscles of the lower limbs. Bulbar muscles, extraocular muscles, deltoids, and respiratory muscles are usually spared. Severe cases with childhood onset may present with sensorineural hearing loss and severe spinal deformities.

Diagnosis | Serum CK levels can be normal or moderately elevated. CK levels greater than 1500 IU/L should raise suspicion of a different diagnosis. EMG shows myopathic signs. Muscle biopsy is performed in patients in whom the clinical suspicion has not been confirmed by molecular genetic testing.

Treatment | The use of leg-foot orthoses is helpful in preventing falls and sprains in patients with foot drop. Moderate aerobic exercise contributes to improving muscle performance. The use of tear inserts helps reduce the incidence of keratitis due to partial eye closure. Surgical fixation of the scapula to the chest wall can improve upper limb mobility. In 2018, promising preliminary data on preclinical gene therapy were presented, based on gene silencing of the toxic product DUX4 in cultures of myoblasts from these patients.

In 2021, the results of the phase 2b ReDUX4 trial with Losmapimod, an MAPKs inhibitor that modulates DUX4 expression, were presented. Although the trial did not achieve the primary endpoint (reduction of DUX4 levels), it showed an effect on reducing the progression of muscular adipose replacement and partial clinical improvement. Other phase 1/2 therapeutic trials based on DUX4 inhibition are underway for FSHD. For updates on gene theraphies, please consult the website https://www.fshdsociety.org.

21.2.4 Oculopharyngeal muscular dystrophy (OPMD)

It is a rare form of adult-onset muscular dystrophy with autosomal dominant transmission, caused by the expansion of a small nucleotide repeat sequence GC(N) (where N indicates any type of nucleotide) within exon 1 of the poly(A)-binding protein 2 (PABP2) gene located on the long arm of chromosome 14 (14q11.1). The disease manifests with 12 to 17 GC(N) repeats. Typically, the disease onset occurs between the ages of 30 and 50 and is characterized by slowly progressive weakness of the pharyngeal and laryngeal muscles (resulting in dysphagia) and bilateral, symmetric ptosis

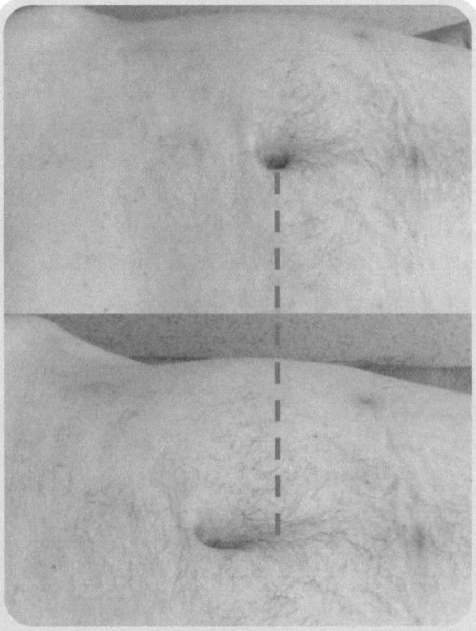

Figure 21.15

Beevor's sign: lifting of the umbilical scar during head elevation in supine position, due to a deficit of the rectus abdominis muscle with predominant involvement of the lower part compared to the upper part.

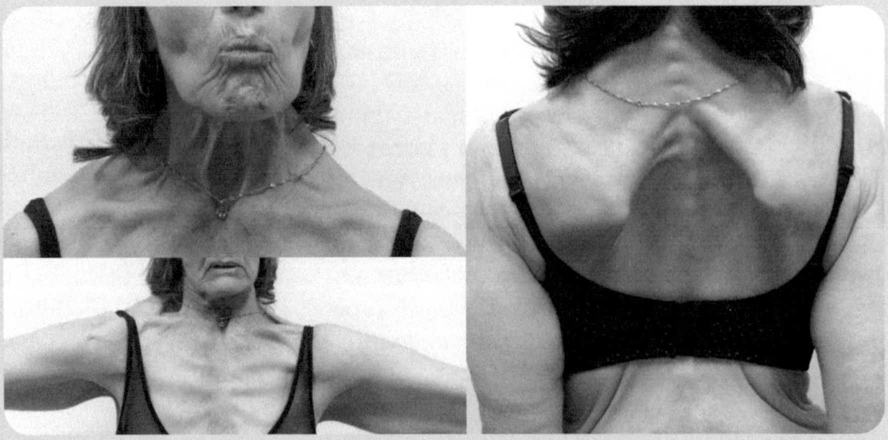

Figure 21.14

Patient with FSHD. Note the deficit of the orbicularis oris muscle, resulting in difficulty whistling, the characteristic triangular shape of the shoulders, the straight position of the clavicles, difficulty in abducting the arms with asymmetric elevation of the scapulae, and bilateral resting winged scapulae with atrophy of the trapezius and paraspinous muscles.

without variations related to fatigue, with sparing of ocular movement. Ptosis is compensated by contraction of the frontal muscles, leading to a characteristic prominence of forehead wrinkles. Swallowing difficulties expose these patients to the risk of recurrent respiratory complications (aspiration pneumonia). Later in the disease course, weakness of the pelvic and scapular girdles may occur. Rarely, head drop can be present. Muscle biopsy typically shows signs of myopathic involvement with rimmed vacuoles and tubulofilamentous nuclear inclusions visible under electron microscopy. The confirmatory diagnosis is based on the presence of at least one allele with CG(N) triplet repeat expansion.

21.2.5 Limb girdle muscular dystrophies (LGMD)

Under the term limb-girdle muscular dystrophy, commonly referred to as LGMD, there is a broad and heterogeneous group of muscular dystrophies characterized by slowly progressive and symmetrical weakness of the proximal muscles of the limbs (scapular and pelvic girdles). LGMD can have an onset in childhood or adulthood. Rarely, asymptomatic CK elevation can occur. They can be transmitted as autosomal dominant (LGMD1) or recessive (LGMD2) traits. Each group includes numerous distinct forms classified according to alphabetical letters. To date, 8 dominant forms (LGMD1A-H) and 24 recessive forms (LGMD2A-Z) have been described. However, as the number of clinical forms within each group is continuously expanding, particularly for the recessive forms, a revision of the nomenclature became necessary, resulting in the 2018 modification to LGMDD for dominant forms (LGMDD1-5) and LGMDR for recessive forms (LGMDR1-24).

Epidemiology | The frequency of different forms of LGMD is influenced by the existence of clusters in certain populations. There is limited epidemiological data on LGMD due to its heterogeneity. The estimated incidence is 1:14,500-123,000. However, the incidence of individual forms can vary significantly from the general data and vary widely in different regions of the world.

Etiology and pathophysiology | The majority of LGMDs are due to mutations in genes that encode different membrane proteins (sarcoglycans, caveolin), structural and contractile proteins (titin, myotilin, desmin, telethonin), nuclear lamina (lamin), proteins involved in protein glycosylation in the Golgi apparatus (α-dystroglycanopathies), and others (ANO5, plectin).

Clinical features | In addition to progressive weakness of the limb girdles, LGMD are clinically characterized by facial muscle integrity, elevated CK levels, and association with cardiomyopathies and varying degrees of respiratory impairment. Pseudohypertrophy is uncommon, and contractures usually appear late in the disease course.

Diagnosis | The classification of LGMD types is based on laboratory tests, including CK measurement and histological examination, particularly the identification of protein deficiency through immunohistochemical diagnosis on muscle biopsy, which should be confirmed by protein Western blot analysis and subsequently by molecular genetic analysis.

Treatment | Although specific therapies for LGMD are currently unavailable, certain general treatments can help prolong autonomy and improve patients' quality of life. These include prevention of obesity, physical therapy and stretching for maintaining mobility and preventing contractures, the use of orthotic supports to maintain motor autonomy, orthopedic monitoring and surgical treatment for skeletal complications (scoliosis, foot deformities), respiratory function monitoring with potential respiratory gymnastics or ventilation aids, cardiac monitoring (especially in forms with known cardiac involvement), and social and psychological support to encourage social participation and productivity. Gene therapy studies are currently underway for some forms of LGMD.

21.2.6 Congenital muscular dystrophy (CMD)

CMD comprises a broad and heterogeneous group of muscular dystrophies and is one of the most common causes of recessive neuromuscular diseases in children. They are all characterized by early onset (congenital or within the first year), diffuse weakness (*floppy baby*), contractures, skeletal deformities (kyphoscoliosis, rigid spine), and variable severity central nervous system disorders due to defects in myelination or neuronal migration. Despite severe muscle alterations (similar to Duchenne muscular dystrophy), the course of CMD is highly variable, ranging from forms with unfavorable outcomes in early childhood to stabilized forms that remain mildly symptomatic in adulthood and give rise to LGMD phenotypes.

Epidemiology | The incidence of all forms of CMD is 1:16.000-21.500, and their prevalence is 0.68-2.5:100.000.

Classification, clinical characteristics, and pathophysiology | CMD is caused by various types of mutations in different genes and is predominantly transmitted as an autosomal recessive trait. Within this group, several categories of diseases are distinguished:

- CMD with merosin deficiency (or laminin α2, LAMA2), which is the most common form of CMD in Europe and is characterized by severe muscle weakness associated with white matter abnormalities in the brain, very high CK levels, and reduced or absent merosin expression on muscle biopsy.
- CMD with muscle contractures and ligament laxity or rigid spine, which includes early-onset selenoprotein deficiency (SEPN2) with rigid spine and spinal deformities, *Emery-Dreifuss muscular dystrophies* (EDMD) characterized by widespread contractures and retractions and autosomal dominant (lamin A/C, LMNA) or X-linked (emerin deficiency) cardiac involvement, and collagenopathies due to collagen 6 deficiency (COL6A1,2, or 3) with proximal retractions and distal ligament laxity and the absence of cardiac involvement, known as *Ullrich* or *Bethlem Muscular Dystrophy* (the former with neonatal or early-onset, more severe symptoms often transmitted recessively, and the latter with later onset, milder symptoms often transmitted dominantly).
- α-dystroglycanopathies (α-DG) which represent a group of diseases related to glycosylation defects of alpha-dystroglycan due to mutations in genes (currently 16 known) encoding enzymes involved in protein glycosylation in the Golgi apparatus. These diseases affect muscle, the eyes, and the central nervous system. The phenotypic spectrum is highly variable, ranging from severe conditions such as Walker-Warburg syndrome (WWS), characterized by muscular dystrophy associated with severe eye and CNS malformations (including anencephaly), or Muscle-Eye-Brain disease (MEB), characterized by neonatal hypotonia, myopia, glaucoma, hydrocephalus, and cognitive delay, to milder forms of early-onset muscular dystrophy, to late-onset conditions with minimal or absent extramuscular involvement, such as LGMD due to FKRP or ISPD deficiency. Cardiac and respiratory involvement is common in these cases.

Diagnosis | Diagnosis is based on the clinical presentation, neuroimaging of the brain, muscle biopsy, muscle and skin immunohistochemistry, and genetic testing. Brain MRI can reveal diffuse white matter abnormalities, including severe brain involvement (Figure 21.16). Muscle histology shows features of a dystrophic myopathy with partial α-dystroglycan deficiency.

Treatment | Due to the complexity of the clinical picture, a multidisciplinary team is often necessary to manage respiratory disorders, swallowing difficulties, nutrition, speech, orthopedic abnormalities, and symptoms related to central nervous system involvement. Currently, there is no specific therapy for these diseases, although preliminary gene therapy trials are underway for some forms.

21.2.7 Myofibrillar myopathies (MFM) and distal myopathies

MFM encompasses a heterogeneous group of myopathies characterized by the presence of cytoplasmic deposits of granulofilamentous aggregates (myofibrillar) and *rimmed vacuoles* on muscle biopsy. They are caused by mutations in genes encoding various sarcomeric proteins (desmin, myotilin, αB-crystallin, ZASP, etc.) and have an autosomal dominant pattern of inheritance. Clinically, they are predominantly characterized by initially or predominantly distal and symmetric weakness with late onset (> 40 years), typically affecting the extensor or flexor muscles of the foot or, less commonly, the extensor muscles of the fingers. Cardiac involvement is often present in all forms (more frequent with desmin mutations), and additional features may include cataracts (αB-crystallin), and peripheral neuropathy (filamin C, BAG3). The muscle biopsy findings are similar among the different forms, and muscle MRI can provide useful distinctive *patterns* for differential diagnosis.

Distal myopathies are more of a clinical entity than a nosological one, encompassing numerous distinct clinical forms characterized by muscle weakness onset in distal regions. Most distal myopathies are either myofibrillar myopathies or atypical variants (with distal presentation) of other myopathies (such as FSHD or Myoshi myopathy due to dysferlin deficiency responsible for LGMDR2). An exception to this is GNE myopathy, caused by recessive mutations in the GNE gene encoding an enzyme responsible for sialic acid synthesis. The disease has multiple eponyms: Nonaka myopathy, hereditary inclusion body myopathy type 2 (HIBM or IBM2), quadriceps sparing myopathy (QSM), and distal myopathy with rimmed vacuoles (DMRV). It is classified as a distinct distal myopathy and is characterized by foot dorsiflexion deficit that begins in the second decade of life and rapidly progresses to widespread weakness in all limbs, with selective sparing of the femoral quadriceps, in advanced stages of the disease. Muscle biopsy typically shows a vacuolar myopathy pattern, and muscle MRI exhibits a characteristic pattern. Several therapeutic trials are currently underway for this disease.

21.2.8 Congenital myopathies

Congenital myopathies are a heterogeneous group of muscular diseases characterized by specific histopathological alterations observed in muscle biopsies. Typically, symptoms are present at birth or within the first year of life and include hypotonia (*floppy infant*), delayed motor milestones, and muscle weakness. However, the phenotypic spectrum is broad, ranging from severe neonatal lethal forms (sometimes with fetal akinesia) to mild adult-onset presentations. Muscle weakness is classically stable over time or slowly progressive. In neonatal or infantile cases, the strength deficit is often generalized, affecting the muscles of the limbs (proximal-distal), face (facial muscle weakness, ptosis), and axial muscles (spinal deformities). Difficulties in swallowing or sucking may necessitate parenteral nutrition or nasogastric tube placement. Respiratory muscle involvement is common and may require assisted ventilation, while cardiac involvement is rare. Cognitive development is always normal. Dismorphic

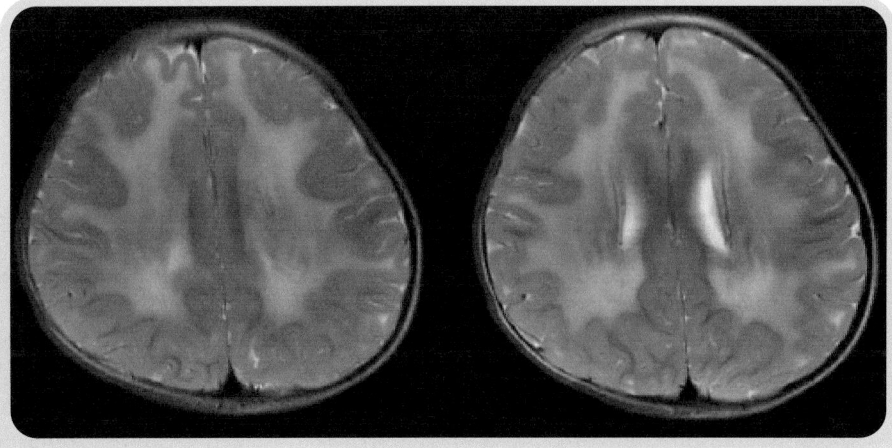

Figure 21.16

Brain MRI (T2 sequences) in a child with congenital muscular dystrophy due to merosin deficiency. Diffuse hyperintensity of the white matter in the cerebral hemispheres.

features (elongated face, high-arched palate, microretrognathia), skeletal abnormalities (congenital clubfoot, congenital hip dysplasia, arthrogryposis), and contractures are often present. In adult-onset cases, a detailed medical history is important to exclude mild signs of the disease that may have been unnoticed in infancy because they were non-disabling (see also Chapter 32 - Pediatric neurology).

Creatine kinase (CK) levels are often normal or slightly elevated. Electromyography (EMG) can be entirely normal or show mild myogenic changes. Muscle magnetic resonance imaging (MRI) can be helpful in differential diagnosis.

Inheritance patterns can be autosomal dominant, recessive, or X-linked.

The most important characteristic underlying the classification of different forms is the presence of specific alterations observed in muscle biopsies. The main types of congenital myopathies include:

1) Core myopathies (areas of myofibrillar disorganization depleted of mitochondria). They represent the most common form and are caused by dominant or recessive mutations in the *RYR1* gene, which encodes the ryanodine receptor expressed on the sarcoplasmic reticulum membrane and involved in muscle excitation-contraction mechanisms.
2) Centronuclear myopathies (fibers with centrally located nuclei).
3) Nemaline myopathy (areas of cytoplasmic rods likely derived from Z discs).

Among congenital myopathies, there is also the nosological entity of malignant hyperthermia susceptibility (MHS), a severe clinical condition (sometimes lethal) characterized by severe generalized muscle contraction crises, hyperthermia, and metabolic disturbances triggered by certain drugs used in anesthesia (such as ether, halothane, isoflurane, sevoflurane, desflurane, enflurane, and depolarizing muscle relaxants like succinylcholine). MHS is caused by a mutation in the RYR1 gene. It is characterized by persistent opening of the ryanodine receptor channel, leading to massive release of calcium from the sarcoplasmic reticulum, resulting in hypercontraction of muscles, secondary hyperthermia, and lactic acidosis. In most cases, symptoms manifest already in the operating room with tachycardia and tachypnea. The overt phase is characterized by widespread muscle contracture, high fever, acidosis, muscle cytolysis with hyperkalemia and arrhythmias, possible cardiac arrest, myoglobinuria, potential renal failure, and increased CK levels. Treatment involves discontinuing the triggering agent and administering intravenous dantrolene sodium. As a precaution, it is advisable to use "safe" anesthesia procedures and avoid these drugs in surgical interventions for all patients with myopathies or elevated CK levels without a precise diagnosis.

21.2.9 Tubular aggregate myopathies

Tubular aggregate myopathies (TAM) are a group of myopathies characterized by the presence of intensely eosinophilic material aggregates in muscle biopsies, as seen in Gomori trichrome staining, with intense NADH enzymatic activity and negative succinate dehydrogenase (SDH). Ultrastructurally, they exhibit a characteristic appearance of numerous concentric double-membrane structures organized in aligned hexagonal geometries. It is believed that they arise from proliferation of the sarcoplasmic reticulum. The disease, which has an autosomal dominant inheritance pattern, has been associated with mutations in three genes (*STIM1*, *ORAI1* e *CASQ1*) to date. Mutations in *STIM1* and *ORAI1* are gain-of-function mutations, resulting in a stable opening of the ORAI1 channel and subsequent increase in store-operated calcium entry (SOCE). The clinical presentation varies, ranging from pauci-symptomatic forms with mild elevation of creatine phosphokinase (CPK) to overt myopathic pictures with proximal limb weakness presenting later in life. Associated findings with the myopathy may include congenital miosis (sometimes with limitation of upward gaze), thrombocytopenia or thrombocytopathy with a bleeding diathesis (York-platelet Syndrome). Less commonly, it can be associated with hypocalcemia, hyposplenism, short stature, mild cognitive delay, hypocalcification of tooth enamel (Stormorken Syndrome). Tubular aggregates, however, have also been described in cases of muscle channelopathies (particularly periodic paralysis), Duchenne muscular dystrophy (DMD), congenital myasthenic syndromes due to gene mutations causing glycosylation defects, and rarely in certain metabolic disorders. Recessive mutations in *STIM1* and *ORAI1* are loss-of-function mutations, responsible for more severe and complex clinical syndromes characterized by neonatal hypotonia, congenital immunodeficiency, mydriasis, osteopetrosis, imperfect amelogenesis, dyshidrosis, splenomegaly, lymphocytic anomalies, and bleeding diathesis.

21.2.10 Metabolic myopathies

Metabolic myopathies represent a heterogeneous group of muscular diseases characterized by abnormalities in glucose and lipid metabolism (glycogen storage diseases and fatty acid oxidation defects) or oxidative phosphorylation (mitochondrial myopathies) (Table 21.2). Metabolic myopathies share an inability to perform the metabolic processes necessary for proper ATP production, which is essential for muscle activity. This results in two main types of muscle symptoms that can overlap to varying degrees in different clinical forms:

1) Muscular exertion intolerance associated with cramps, myalgias, and episodes of myoglobinuria.
2) Stable muscle weakness.

The first group of symptoms occurs in different situations depending on the type of metabolic deficit. Patients with glycogen storage diseases typically experience symptoms during intense exercise, with muscle symptoms affecting the muscles used in the exercise itself. In lipid metabolism disorders, exertion intolerance, myalgias, and myoglobinuria occur in relation to moderate and prolonged exercise, fasting, and are not accompanied by painful cramps. The relationship between exertion intolerance and the type of muscle exercise is less distinctive in mitochondrial myopathies, where the common final pathway for ATP production is impaired.

Mitochondrial myopathies

Mitochondria are cytoplasmic organelles responsible for energy production and cellular respiration. Mitochondria possess their own DNA (mtDNA), although during evolution, most of the genes necessary for mitochondrial functions have been transferred to nuclear DNA (nDNA). Mitochondrial myopathies are part of the mitochondrial disorders, which are systemic diseases caused by genetically determined disorders of the respiratory chain.

Mitochondrial disorders, in general, can be caused by mutations that occur directly on mtDNA (point mutations or single deletions) or by mutations in nuclear genes (nDNA) encoding mitochondrial proteins or transcription factors (multiple deletions) involved in maintaining mtDNA (depletions). The majority of mitochondrial disorders, due to the ubiquity of mitochondria, are characterized by multisystem involvement with damage to organs predominantly reliant on oxidative metabolism, such as the brain and muscles (hence the term encephalomyopathies).

Prevalence | In the United Kingdom, the estimated prevalence of all mtDNA mutation-related diseases is 6.5 per 100,000. Of these, approximately 20% are due to deletions and 80% to point mutations.

Etiology and pathophysiology | mtDNA consists of approximately 16,000 base pairs and is inherited entirely through the maternal lineage. Moreover, lacking introns or sophisticated genetic repair mechanisms, mtDNA more frequently accumulates mutations during cell replication compared to nuclear DNA (nDNA). For this reason, after repeated cell divisions, daughter cells will have a slightly different set of mtDNA among them. This characteristic, known as "heteroplasmy," explains the variable involvement of various tissues in mitochondrial diseases. Furthermore, for the disease to manifest, a certain number of mutated mtDNA copies are required to reach a specific threshold, which varies for each pathology. The majority of mitochondrial disorders are estimated to be due to mutations in nuclear DNA.

Mitochondrial diseases can, therefore, be classified into the following groups:

a) Defects in mtDNA (single deletions, point mutations).
b) Defects in nuclear DNA encoding mitochondrial proteins, proteins involved in

the assembly of respiratory chain complexes, or proteins involved in maintaining mtDNA (depletions or multiple deletions).

Clinical aspects and classification | Since muscles and the brain are the most commonly and frequently affected organs, the terms mitochondrial myopathies or encephalomyopathies are used. The common clinical features of encephalomyopathies include ptosis, external ophthalmoplegia, proximal muscle weakness, exercise intolerance, pathologically increased blood lactate levels after muscle activity, cardiomyopathies, sensorineural hearing loss, optic atrophy, retinitis pigmentosa, and diabetes mellitus. Symptoms affecting the nervous system mainly consist of fluctuating encephalopathy, epilepsy, dementia, migraines, stroke, ataxia, and spasticity.

Table 21.3 represents the phenotypic characteristics of some major mitochondrial encephalomyopathies caused by mtDNA mutations.

Diagnosis | Creatine kinase (CK) levels are often normal or slightly elevated. Serum and cerebrospinal fluid lactate levels may show elevated values or remain within the normal range at rest. During sustained muscle exercise, there is an abnormal increase in lactate and lactate/pyruvate ratio between 25 and 250:1 (in healthy individuals, it is <25:1). Electromyography (EMG), often normal, may reveal myopathic signs as well as signs of peripheral neuropathy.

Brain magnetic resonance imaging (MRI) may show altered signals in the putamen, caudate nucleus, and globus pallidus or ischemic lesions, often localized in the occipital region in MELAS (Figure 21.17), or diffuse signal alterations in the white matter in KSS. Brain spectroscopy may show lactate peaks.

Muscle biopsy is the most important examination to confirm the suspected diagnosis of mitochondrial myopathy and guide further genetic investigations. Appropriate staining allows the identification of *ragged red fibers* muscle fibers with subsarcolemmal accumulations of mitochondria) and fibers negative for cytochrome c oxidase (COX) and intensely positive for succinate dehydrogenase (SDH), demonstrating active mitochondrial proliferation despite deficient enzymatic activity (Figure 21.17). Enzymatic assays of various respiratory chain complexes should be conducted on muscle biopsies and other tissues (skin) and may show a reduction in individual complexes.

Molecular biology enables genetic typing of mitocondriopathies. In the case of suspected mitocondriopathy due to mtDNA defects, molecular genetic analysis should be performed on tissue affected by the disease due to heteroplasmy. In cases of suspected mitochondrial disorders with autosomal inheritance and multiple nDNA depletions or deletions, mutations in nDNA need to be investigated.

Therapy | The treatment of mitochondrial encephalomyopathies is largely symptomatic, including diabetes therapy, pacemaker implantation, surgical correction of ptosis, and cataract treatment. Patients with complex I and II deficiencies may benefit from oral administration of riboflavin. Coenzyme Q10 replacement therapy can be beneficial for deficiencies of this enzyme, with excellent response to treatment. Two synthetic analogs, idebenone and parabenzoquinone, appear to be promising therapies and have shown experimental efficacy in Leber's optic neuropathy and Leigh syndrome. Another therapeutic approach that has shown effectiveness, particularly in MNGIE (mitochondrial neurogastrointestinal encephalomyopathy), is allogeneic hematopoietic stem cell transplantation, which restores proper thymidine phosphorylase enzyme activity to normalize circulating toxic levels of thymidine and deoxyuridine. Gene therapies for specific forms of mitochondrial disorders due to nDNA defects are currently being studied.

Glycogen storage diseases (GSD)

These are diseases caused by defects in enzymes involved in glycogen metabolism, particularly in the glycolytic pathway. These disorders can affect the liver, leading to cirrhosis and hypoglycemia, as well as skeletal muscle, causing myopathies.

Etiology and pathophysiology | Glycogen plays a crucial role during intense muscle

Table 21.3 PHENOTYPIC CHARACTERISTICS OF mtDNA MUTATIONS

Mutation type	Disease	Clinical
mtDNA deletion	*Progressive External Opthalmoplegia (PEO) with ragged-red-fibers (RRF)*	Slowly progressive ptosis and paralysis of the extraocular muscles. Mild scapular girdle weakness. Myalgia, especially during physical exercise. Benign course.
	Kearns-Sayre Syndrome (KSS)	Onset before 20 years of age with PEO + retinitis pigmentosa + cardiac conduction disturbances or cerebellar ataxia or elevated cerebrospinal fluid protein. Additional features may include: juvenile dementia, hearing impairment, myopathy, and endocrinopathies.
Point mutations in tRNA encoding genes	*MERRF (Myoclonic Epilepsy; Ragged Red Fibers)*	Epilepsy, myoclonus, cerebellar syndrome, optic atrophy, dementia, polyneuropathy, myopathy, hearing loss.
	MELAS (Mitochondrial Encephalomyopathy; Lactic Acidosis; Stroke)	Onset in childhood: rare, less than 10% of cases. Onset in adolescence and adulthood: encephalopathy (juvenile strokes, headache, vomiting, loss of consciousness, seizures, dementia, mental retardation, sensorineural hearing loss, ataxia, extrapyramidal disorders); myopathy (proximal and symmetrical, ptosis, ophthalmoparesis); polyneuropathy (sensory axonal); oculopathy (optic atrophy, retinitis pigmentosa, macular dystrophy, hypertelorism); lactic acidosis, hypertrophic cardiomyopathy, diabetes, gastrointestinal disorders, endocrine disturbances, nephropathy.

activity, both aerobic and anaerobic. It is synthesized (glycogenesis) and stored in muscle fibers as a branched structure composed of long chains of glucose molecules. Its breakdown (glycogenolysis) is triggered by calcium released from the sarcoplasmic reticulum during muscle contraction, through the activation of glycogen phosphorylase and the debranching enzyme. These enzymes break the bonds between glucose molecules, allowing them to enter the glycolytic metabolic process. The removal of calcium at the end of contraction stimulates the synthesis of new glycogen molecules. To date, 17 forms of glycogen storage diseases have been described, mostly designated by Roman numerals and/or eponyms. All glycogen storage diseases have autosomal recessive inheritance, except for two X-linked forms (phosphorylase b kinase deficiency and phosphoglycerate kinase deficiency).

Clinical aspects | The most common glycogen storage diseases include GSD-V (McArdle's disease), due to myophosphorylase deficiency, an enzyme responsible for initiating glycogenolysis by detaching glucose-1-phosphate fragments from glycogen, and GSD-II (Pompe's disease) due to acid maltase (alpha-glucosidase acid) deficiency, a lysosomal enzyme that hydrolyzes α1-4 glycosidic bonds of glycogen during glycogenolysis. Glycogen

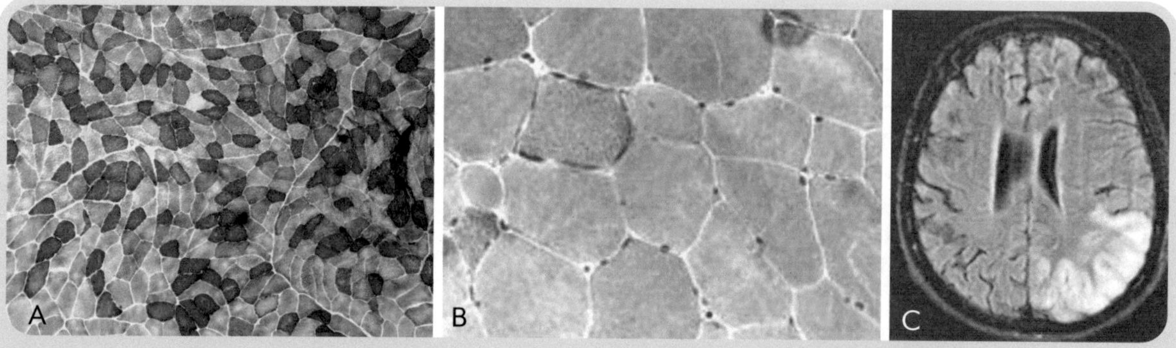

Figure 21.17

Fibre COX negative/SDH positive (A), ragged red fibres (B), and parieto-occipital ischemia in a case of MELAS (C).

storage diseases typically affect metabolically active muscles. The phenotype varies, ranging from exercise intolerance with cramps and rhabdomyolysis (with possible myoglobinuria) triggered by intense exercise, to forms with muscle weakness already present at rest, often progressive, mimicking dystrophic pathologies. In McArdle's disease, the phenomenon known as the "second wind" is characteristic, characterized by a recovery of strength, reduction in dyspnea, tachycardia, fatigue, cramps, and muscle pain after 6-8 minutes of physical activity. Pompe's disease often involves the respiratory muscles and tongue. Infantile-onset forms (GAA < 1%) may involve cardiac and hepatic manifestations. Late-onset forms (GAA 1-30%) typically present symptoms between the ages of 30 and 40, progressively manifesting as a predominantly pelvic girdle myopathy that is bilateral and symmetrical. Respiratory failure may sometimes be the initial symptom. Dolichoectasia and cerebral vessel aneurysms can also be associated.

Instrumental diagnosis | CK levels are elevated at rest in many glycogen storage diseases. In McArdle's disease, CK values increase significantly after exertion (rhabdomyolysis), as well as uric acid and ammonia levels. However, there is no physiological increase in lactate after exercise due to the lack of glycogenolysis activation.

Electromyography (EMG) may show signs of myopathic involvement but can also be entirely normal. McArdle's disease may exhibit fibrillations and positive potentials. Pompe's disease is characterized by myotonic discharges and complex repetitive discharges, most evident in proximal and paraspinal muscles.

Muscle biopsy in McArdle's disease reveals glycogen accumulations in muscle fibers, predominantly located subsarcolemmally, which can be visualized with periodic acid-Schiff (PAS) staining. Pompe's disease is associated with vacuoles positive for acid phosphatase and glycogen accumulations. However, in adult-onset cases, muscle biopsy may appear normal. Biochemical analysis, including enzyme activity assays in muscle tissue, allows for the diagnosis of different forms of glycogen storage diseases. In Pompe's disease, enzymatic activity measurement of acid maltase (GAA) can be performed on a small amount of blood collected on filter paper (dry-blood spot, DBS).

Therapy | Some lifestyle modifications are likely the best treatment for certain glycogen storage diseases. Short, intense physical exercises should be avoided, while progressive and aerobic exercise improves the functional abilities of individuals with GSD and prevents metabolic crises. Oral intake of glucose (35-40 g) just before exercise (5-10 minutes) represents a form of exogenous compensation that provides the necessary glucose in glycogenolysis defects. Vitamin B6 (pyridoxine) has been proposed as a supplement in McArdle's disease due to its conjugation with phosphorylase, but there are no clinical trials confirming its efficacy. A high-protein diet may enhance an alternative energy source. Low-dose creatine also appears to improve muscle performance, while medium and high doses may worsen it. Finally, in Pompe's disease, replacement therapy with recombinant human acid alpha-glucosidase (ERT) has shown significant therapeutic effects.

Fatty acid oxidation disorders (FAOD)

This group includes a series of metabolic myopathies caused by disorders in fatty acid metabolism. They can be divided schematically into two major groups:

- Myopathies with massive lipid accumulation.
- Myopathies with mild or absent lipid accumulation.

Etiology and pathophysiology | Fatty acids are the primary source of energy for resting muscles during fasting and non-intense exercise. Disorders in lipid metabolism can be due to: 1) impaired transport of long-chain fatty acids across mitochondrial membranes (as in CPT deficiency); 2) impaired carnitine transport into the cell (carnitine transporter deficiency); 3) defects in beta-oxidation, which represent the majority of FAODs but are very rare in adults. All genetic defects underlying FAODs have autosomal recessive inheritance.

Clinical features | Similar to glycogen storage diseases, FAODs can manifest clinically with cramps, myalgia, and myoglobinuria, or with phenotypes characterized by stable muscle weakness. In the former case, unlike glycogen storage diseases, symptoms occur after mild-to-moderate, prolonged muscle activity (e.g., long walks), especially if performed while fasting. These patients can often perform intense and short-duration exercises without issues, but as exercise continues, cramps and weakness develop, making it impossible to continue exercising. After exercise or in the hours following exercise, episodes of pigmenturia associated with muscle pain can occur and may persist for several days. In some cases, myalgia and rhabdomyolysis may be the only clinical manifestations of FAODs. CPTII deficiency is the most frequent cause of rhabdomyolysis in adults. FAODs can also affect other tissues besides skeletal muscle, particularly the heart and liver, as well as the central nervous system (epilepsy, mental retardation), skin (ichthyosis), eyes (retinitis pigmentosa), and nerves (neuropathy).

Instrumental diagnosis | Measurement of carnitine, CPTII, serum acylcarnitine profile, and urinary organic acid analysis can be helpful for diagnosis. Blood tests (CK, lactate, and glucose) may be normal in asymptomatic individuals. During metabolic crises, however, hypoketotic hypoglycemia often occurs with increased serum CK levels. Hyperkalemia can also be observed during rhabdomyolysis. If rhabdomyolysis leads to acute renal failure, an increase in creatinine and azotemia with metabolic acidosis can occur. EMG is often normal, but in some cases, it may show a myopathic pattern with small, brief-duration potentials. Fibrillation potentials, positive waves, and complex repetitive discharges may be present in the days following an episode of rhabdomyolysis. A mixed myopathic and neuropathic pattern may be present in certain forms of beta-oxidation defects. Muscle biopsy may show increased intracellular lipids with specific staining techniques (Oil Red O/Sudan Black). The confirmatory diagnosis is achieved through biochemical measurement of the involved factors (e.g., carnitine, CPT, etc.) and genetic testing to identify specific mutations.

Therapy | Avoiding prolonged exertion, particularly during fasting periods, and infections, is the first-line therapy for FAODs. A high-carbohydrate and low-fat diet (<30% of calories) is recommended. Multiple acyl-CoA dehydrogenase deficiency (MADD) responds to riboflavin (vitamin B2) supplementation. Oral carnitine supplementation is beneficial for patients with systemic carnitine deficiency.

21.2.11 Channelopathies

Skeletal muscle channelopathies are characterized by a disorder of sarcolemma excitability due to mutations in genes encoding muscle ion channels. These conditions predispose the muscle to conditions of hyperexcitability or inexcitability of the membrane, resulting in a clinical spectrum ranging from delayed muscle relaxation after contraction and stiffness (myotonia) to flaccid muscle paralysis. From a nosographic perspective, they can be divided into non-dystrophic myotonias (congenital myotonia, paramyotonia congenita, sodium channel myotonias) and periodic paralyses (hypokalemic, hyperkalemic, Andersen-Tawil syndrome) (Figure 21.18 and Table 21.2).

Epidemiology | The overall prevalence is approximately 1 in 100,000. Among non-dystrophic myotonias, the most common is congenital myotonia (with a prevalence of up to 1 in 10,000 in certain regions of northern Europe), and among periodic paralyses, it is hypokalemic periodic paralysis.

Etiology and pathophysiology | Congenital myotonia (CM) is caused by a mutation in the CLCN1 gene on chromosome 7q (encoding voltage-gated chloride channel proteins), resulting in altered sarcolemmal chloride ion conductance. The inheritance pattern can be autosomal dominant (Thomsen's disease) or autosomal recessive (Becker's disease).

Myotonias related to mutations in the *SCN4A* gene on locus 17q23 encode the alpha subunit of the sodium channel. The mutations cause a *gain-of-function* in the channel, leading to persistent sodium ion influx into the cell and thus persistent depolarization. The inheritance pattern is autosomal dominant. They represent a heterogeneous group of clinical forms, including paramyotonia congenita (PC), *sodium channel myotonia* (SCM), and hyperkalemic periodic paralysis (HyperPP), which differ in the presence or absence of episodic muscle weakness (absent in SCM, present in PMC and HyperPP).

Hypokalemic periodic paralysis (hypoPP) is an autosomal dominant disease linked to mutations in the CACNA1S gene on chromosome 1q32, which encodes the calcium channel. However, in 10% of cases, it can also be caused by mutations in the *SCN4A* gene.

Andersen-Tawil syndrome (ATS) is due to mutations in the KCNJ2 gene, which encodes the inward rectifier potassium channel (Kir2.1), responsible for maintaining the resting membrane potential.

Clinical features | *Non-dystrophic myotonic syndromes* are all characterized by the presence of myotonia (impaired muscle relaxation after contraction), stiffness, and muscle hypertrophy, often accompanied by a deficit of strength, mainly in a specific muscle group.

In CM, myotonia improves with repeated movement (*warm-up phenomenon*). Patients have difficulty initiating muscle activity (e.g., climbing stairs), which improves or disappears during exercise. Symptoms are often more pronounced in the lower limbs. The disease usually begins in the first decade of life but can sometimes manifest during adolescence. Aggravating factors include rest, emotional stress, cold (although to a lesser extent than in PC), and pregnancy.

In PC, myotonia is paradoxical because, unlike in CM, it occurs during repetitive movement. It most frequently affects the muscles of the face (orbicularis oculi), hands, and tongue. Weakness may persist for days. Cold is a typical exacerbating factor (causing a drastic worsening), along with fasting and pregnancy.

SCM is a heterogeneous entity that includes acetazolamide-responsive myotonia, myotonia fluctuans, and myotonia permanens. All forms are characterized by the absence of cold sensitivity, absence of weakness, and worsening of symptoms with potassium administration or consumption of potassium-rich foods. Myotonia in the fluctuans form is highly variable. Myotonia permanens is characterized by severe myotonia, which also affects respiratory muscles. Aggravating factors, in addition to potassium intake, include fasting or pregnancy.

Periodic paralyses are characterized by episodes of flaccid paralysis of variable severity (up to tetraplegia) without involvement of respiratory and cardiac muscles. The duration and frequency of attacks vary, with a tendency to decrease in older patients.

HypoPP typically begins in the first two decades of life, and attacks of paralysis are triggered by hypokalemia. The duration of attacks can vary from 2 hours to several days. Attacks are precipitated by carbohydrate-rich meals and rest after physical exercise. They typically occur during nighttime and upon awakening in the morning. Some patients may experience persistent focal muscle weakness.

HyperPP usually begins in the first decade, and attacks of paralysis are triggered by hyperkalemia. Generally, the attacks are shorter in duration than in hypoPP (< 2 hours) and occur throughout the day. Generalized muscle weakness is less frequent than in hypoPP.

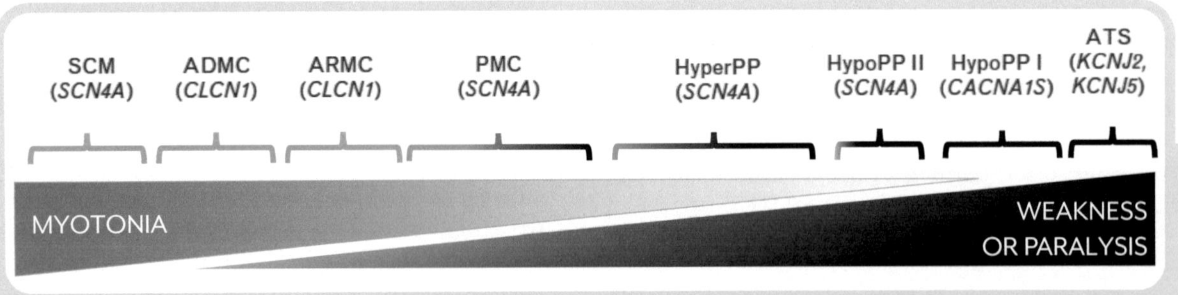

Figure 21.18

Overlap between myotonic phenotype and periodic paralysis in muscle channelopathies.

ATS is characterized by a triad of periodic paralysis, cardiac abnormalities (particularly long QT syndrome), and dysmorphism. Paralytic attacks typically start in adolescence and are more frequently associated with low serum potassium levels (but can also occur with hyperkalemia). Cardiac involvement is characterized by conduction abnormalities, especially long QT syndrome. Dysmorphic features include hypertelorism, low-set ears, microretrognathia, dental anomalies, and skeletal abnormalities (syndactyly, clinodactyly).

Instrumental diagnosis | Myotonic discharges are found in 100% of non-dystrophic myotonias and in 50% of hyperPP, but not in hypoPP, on electromyography (EMG). A useful test for differentiating the various forms of myotonia and periodic paralysis is the Fournier test. This electrophysiological examination evaluates the variation in amplitude of the compound motor potential over a specific time frame following short and prolonged muscle exertion, at room temperature and after cooling. The test results can provide valuable information in defining the clinical form of myotonia.

For periodic paralyses, measuring serum potassium levels during episodes of weakness is essential. A few hours after the attacks, potassium levels tend to return to the normal range.

Induction tests for periodic paralyses, such as the potassium loading test or the cold test, can be performed to trigger a crisis. These tests should be conducted in a hospital setting as they require simultaneous clinical and cardiac monitoring.

Therapy | The most effective drug for myotonia is mexiletine (300-900 mg/day), which should be prescribed after adequate cardiac screening. Alternatively, some efficacy has been demonstrated with procainamide (125-1000 mg/day), quinine (200-1200 mg/day), phenytoin (300-400 mg/day), and flecainide. Therapeutic effects have also been observed with carbamazepine, dantrolene, and acetazolamide. Myotonia can be aggravated by depolarizing muscle relaxants (e.g., succinylcholine), adrenaline, beta-adrenergic agonists, propranolol, and colchicine. The use of neuromuscular blockers should be avoided in myotonic syndromes.

In all cases of periodic paralysis, prolonged immobility after excessively intense efforts should be avoided. Triggering factors, such as carbohydrate-rich meals in hypoPP, fasting, or exposure to extreme cold in hyperPP, should also be avoided. Treatment for crises involves potassium administration for hypoPP and carbohydrate intake for hyperPP. Prevention of crises in both forms involves daily acetazolamide administration, as well as potassium supplementation and potassium-sparing diuretics for hypoPP.

21.3 Acquired myopathies

21.3.1 Inflammatory myopathies

Inflammatory myopathies are acquired muscle diseases characterized by primary muscular inflammation. This distinguishes them from muscular dystrophies, where dystrophic changes can be associated with inflammatory phenomena (e.g., DMD, FSHD, dysferlinopathies), or from diseases where inflammation affects anatomical structures associated with muscles rather than the muscles themselves (e.g., fasciitis)(Table 21.2).

Classification

Inflammatory myopathies are classified into idiopathic inflammatory myopathies (IIMs), which include well-defined nosological forms where the autoimmune mechanism is primarily directed against muscle tissue, and other forms of inflammatory myopathies where muscle tissue is affected by inflammatory processes in the context of other autoimmune diseases (overlap myositis, MG-PM), drug-induced (ICIs-related myositis), partial (focal myositis, fasciitis), or cases where the nosological entity is not universally recognized and excluded from idiopathic forms. Polymyositis is slowly disappearing as a distinct nosological entity, and currently, the term nonspecific myositis (NSM) is preferred when the inflammatory muscle picture cannot be classified into other specific forms of myositis (Table 21.4):

1) Idiopathic inflammatory myopathies (IIM)
   a) Dermatomyositis (DM)
   b) Anti-synthetase syndrome (ASS)

c) Necrotizing Autoimmune Myopathy (NAM)
d) Inclusion Body Myositis (IBM)

2) Other inflammatory myopathies
   a) *Overlap Myositis*: Inflammatory myopathies associated with autoimmune diseases (SLE, Scleroderma, Rheumatoid arthritis, Mixed connective tissue disease, Sjögren's syndrome, Systemic sclerosis, Myasthenia-myositis (MG-IM))
   b) Cervicobrachial inflammatory myopathy (BCIM)
   c) Inflammatory myopathy with mitochondrial pathology (PM-mito)
   d) Immune checkpoint inhibitors (ICIs) - related myositis (ICIs-related)
   e) Nonspecific myositis (NSM)
   f) Sarcoidosis
   g) Focal myositis and fasciitis
   h) Infectious and Post-infectious Myopathies
   i) Viral (HIV, EBV, CMV, HTLV-1, COVID-19), Bacterial (*Staphylococcus, Borrelia burgdorferi, Mycobacterium tuberculosis*), Parasitic (*nematodes, cestodes, protozoa*).

In this chapter, we will focus on idiopathic inflammatory myopathies, while discussions of other forms will be referred to specialized texts.

Idiopathic inflammatory myopathies (IIM)

Idiopathic inflammatory myopathies are the most common types among inflammatory myopathies and include dermatomyositis (DM), anti-synthetase syndrome (ASS), necrotizing autoimmune myopathies (NAM), and inclusion body myositis (IBM).

Epidemiology | The incidence of DM is around 0.5-1:100,000, with an approximate prevalence of 1:100,000. They are more common in non-Caucasian races and in females. DM is the most common form of inflammatory myopathy in children (juvenile DM). It has a bimodal distribution concerning age: between 5-14 years (juvenile DM) and between 45-64 years (DM).

ASS has a prevalence of 1-9/100,000 inhabitants. It is more common in women, with a male-to-female ratio of 2:3. The onset is typically in adulthood.

NAM, recognized as a specific nosological entity only in the last decade, is characterized by muscle necrosis and regeneration that predominate over the inflammatory picture on histological examination. Their incidence is increasing, and recent studies have shown that many cases previously classified as polymyositis can now be classified as NAM. NAM typically occurs between the ages of 40 and 70, but pediatric cases have also been described.

IBM represents the most common acquired myopathy in adults. Its frequency is probably underestimated. It is more prevalent in males and usually presents after the age of 50 (onset before the age of 30 is exceptional).

Etiology and pathophysiology | Idiopathic inflammatory myopathies have different etiopathogenic mechanisms. DM is caused by immune-mediated microangiopathy with a humoral mechanism, the etiopathogenesis of which is still unknown, but recent evidence suggests an interferon-mediated mechanism (interferonopathies). The inflammatory process is believed to be induced by complement activation. Complement deposition leads to thrombosis of capillaries, arterioles, and venules, primarily located at the periphery of muscle fascicles, causing ischemic damage, destruction of muscle fibers, and perifascicular atrophy (histopathological characteristics of DM). Due to the humoral nature of the underlying immunological process, the inflammatory infiltrates consist predominantly of B and CD4+ T lymphocytes. Recent research has also implicated the interferon pathway in the pathogenesis of DM, classifying it as a true interferonopathy.

ASS is due to the production of antibodies directed against specific tRNA synthetases for a particular amino acid substrate.

NAM shows histological similarities to toxic myopathies but with altered expression of major histocompatibility complex class I (MHC-I). In some forms, there is complement deposition (C5b-9) on the muscle fiber membrane in the absence of significant inflammatory infiltrates as observed in DM, ASS, and IBM.

The etiopathogenesis of IBM remains uncertain. Despite being classified as an idiopathic inflammatory myopathy, the presence of rimmed vacuoles, the accumulation of amyloid material in cytoplasmic inclusions, mitochondrial pathology characterizing the disease, as well as the poor response to immunosuppressive therapies, suggests a multifactorial and degenerative pathogenesis contributing to muscle damage.

Clinical aspects | Subacute and symmetrical muscle weakness associated with an increase in CK levels characterize DM, ASS, and NAM. IBM, on the other hand, is characterized by frequent asymmetric muscle weakness with a chronic course, often starting in the antibrachial volar regions (finger and wrist flexors) and quadriceps, and is associated with normal or slightly elevated CK levels.

Cutaneous symptoms are a characteristic feature of DM and anti-synthetase syndromes but are absent in IBM and NAM. They often precede myopathy and can sometimes be present without muscular symptoms (amyopathic DM). The classic cutaneous symptoms include:

a) Erythematous heliotrope rash, extending to the face (especially eyelids), anterior chest (V sign), knuckles, elbows, photosensitivity, often associated with edema and telangiectasias.
b) Gottron's papules: thickening on the dorsal surface of the interphalangeal joints.
c) Raynaud's phenomenon.
d) Mechanic's hands: coarseness and skin lesions on the fingertips.
e) Altered periungual capillaries (Figure 21.19).

In DM and anti-synthetase syndrome (rarely in NAM but not in IBM), involvement of other organ systems and associations with other diseases (Table 21.4) and tumors are frequently observed.

In children and late stages of DM, subcutaneous calcium deposits frequently form and can be detected through palpation or radiographic examination.

Instrumental and laboratory diagnosis | CK levels are usually elevated in DM, unless it involves cases with minimal muscle involvement. CK is also elevated in ASS. In NAM, CK levels are often markedly elevated. In IBM, CK levels are either normal or slightly altered.

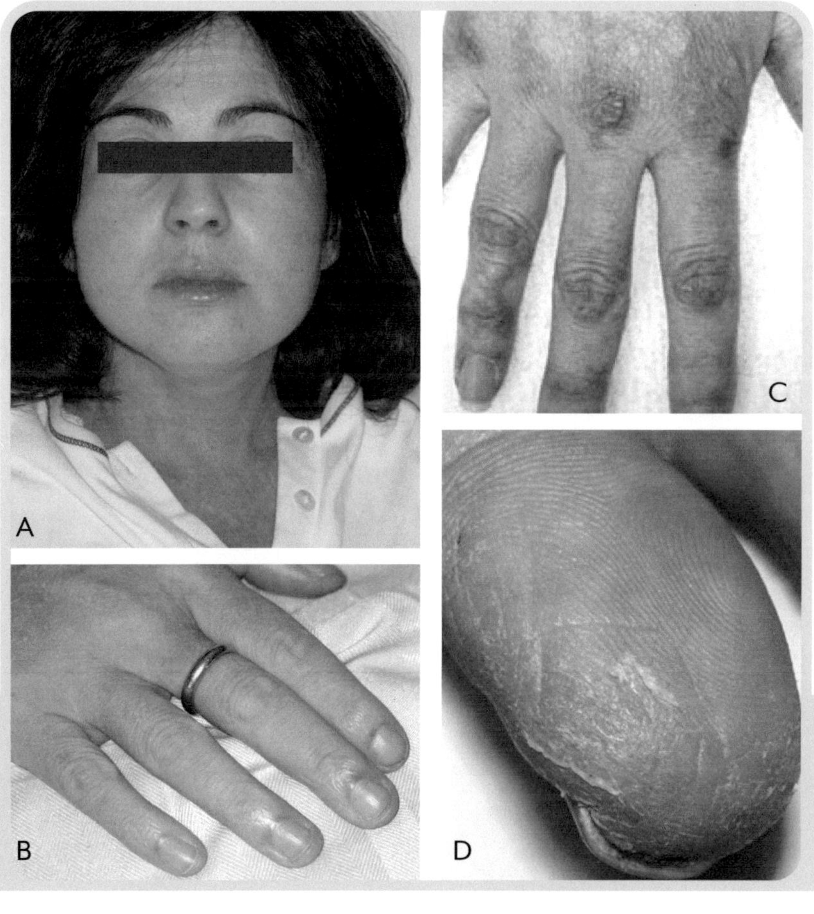

Figure 21.19

Heliotrope rash (A), erythema of the nail fold (B), Gottron's papules (C), and mechanic's hands (D) in patients with dermatomyositis.

Table 21.4 CHARACTERISTICS OF MAJOR INFLAMMATORY MYOPATHIES

	DERMATOMYOSITIS	ANTI-SYNTHETASE	NAM	INCLUSION BODY MYOSITIS
Onset age	Children-Adults	>40	>40	>50
Gender	F>M	M=F	F=M	M>F
Immunopathogenesis	Humoral	Cellular	Cellular	Unknown
Progression	Weeks/Months	Weeks/Months	Weeks	Years
Muscle weakness	Symmetrical (may be absent)	Symmetrical	Symmetrical (severe)	Often asymmetric
Muscles affected				
Proximal	Pelvic and scapular girdle	Pelvic and scapular girdle	Pelvic and scapular girdle	Quadriceps
Distal	Possible late	Possible	Possible	Frequent, finger flexors, wrist flexors, foot extensors
Respiratory	Late in severe forms	Frequent	Possible	Absent
Pharynx-esophagus	30%	Possible	30%	10-30%
Neck Flex/Ext	Common	Common	Common	Common
Facial	Occasional	Rare	Rare	Occasional
Extraocular	Absent	Absent	Absent	Absent
Cutaneous symptoms	Present	Frequent	Absent	Absent
Other associated diseases	Frequent	Frequent	Unusual	Unusual
Lung disease	Possible	Frequent	-	-
Heart disease	Possible	Rare	-	-
Tumors	Possible (up to 40%)	Rare (10-15%)	Rare	-
CK	Low / elevated	Elevated / very elevated	Very elevated	Normal / low elevated
Biopsy				
Degeneration	Possible perifascicular atrophy	Possible perifascicular necrosis	Necrotic and regenerating fibers	Necrotic and regenerating fibers
Inflammation	Perivascular and interfascicular CD4 > CD8. Without cellular invasion	Endomysial CD3, without cellular invasion	Absent or few CD68 > CD4/CD8	Few endomysial CD8 > CD4 With cellular invasion
HLA expression	Perifascicular/diffuse	Perifascicular/diffuse	Inconstant	Diffuse
Complement damage	Present. Complement deposits in capillaries	Perifascicular	Absent. Complement deposits on the membrane	Absent
Inclusions	Tubuloreticular inclusions in endothelial cells of vessels	Absent	Absent	Rimmed vacuoles. Intracellular amyloid deposits
Response to immunosuppression	Good	Good	Inconstant	Poor/absent

Inflammatory myopathies can present with IgG antibodies directed against cytoplasmic, nucleolar, and nuclear antigens, referred to as "myositis-specific antibodies" (MSAs). The percentage of patients positive for anti-MSA antibodies varies considerably among different cases. The most common are anti-Jo-1 antibodies, present in 20% of patients with anti-synthetase PM. In DM, anti-Mi-2 antibodies are present in 15-20% of patients with classic DM, anti-TIF-1g and NXP2 antibodies are often associated with neoplasms, and anti-MDA5 antibodies are associated with "amyopathic" forms characterized by ulcerative skin lesions and interstitial lung disease. Anti-SAE antibodies are typically not associated with neoplasms. In NAM, the most frequently detected antibodics arc anti-SRP and anti-HMGCR. The former is associated with more aggressive forms of necrotizing myositis, sometimes with associated myocarditis, and rarely with neoplasms. Cases of anti-SRP associated with non-necrotizing myositis have been described. The latter is associated, in approximately 50% of cases, with statin use, which acts as a trigger for the development of persistent autoimmune disease despite discontinuation of therapy. The presence of anti-HMGCR antibodies is more commonly associated with neoplasms. Lastly, a third group of NAM consists of seronegative forms (without anti-HMGCR or anti-SRP antibodies), which have been found to be more frequently associated with neoplasms. In IBM, anti-cN1A antibody positivity is present in 50% of cases.

Electromyographic examination in inflammatory myopathies reveals myopathic damage (low-amplitude, reduced-duration, and polyphasic potentials) and the presence of spontaneous activity indicating sarcolemmal irritability (fibrillations, positive sharp waves, and paroxysmal discharges) in the affected muscles.

Muscle MRI in the early phase shows muscle edema and inflammation on STIR sequences, and in untreated or therapy-resistant forms (more commonly NAM), it may show fibrofatty replacement on T1 sequences. MRI can also help in selecting the muscle for biopsy and therapeutic monitoring.

Muscle biopsy is the gold standard for the diagnosis of inflammatory myopathy and for distinguishing different clinical forms, although false negativity occurs in approximately 12% of patients, mostly due to the random distribution of lesions within the muscle tissue. The histological characteristics include perifascicular atrophy with perivascular and perimysial inflammation, primarily CD4 lymphocytes in DM, along with increased MxA expression (an interferon pathway activation marker); perivascular and perimysial inflammation with necrotic perifascicular areas and increased expression of major histocompatibility complex class II (MHC-II) in ASS; necrosis and regeneration with minimal inflammatory infiltrate, sarcolemmal complement (C5b-9) deposition, and reduced MHC-I expression in NAM; and the triad characterized by predominantly CD8 inflammatory infiltrates, rimmed vacuoles, and COX-negative fibers in IBM.

Therapy | Immunosuppressive therapies are considered the treatment of choice in DM, ASS, and NAM. Corticosteroids are the first-line therapy, and they can be combined with other immunosuppressive drugs such as azathioprine, methotrexate, or cyclosporine. In cases resistant to therapy, high-dose human immunoglobulins or Rituximab can be used. NAM often requires early triple therapy with corticosteroids, immunosuppressants, and immunoglobulins. It has been observed that the early use of IVIG (within 3 months of onset) improves long-term outcomes. Therapies should then be adjusted based on the clinical response, with a slow and gradual dose reduction after satisfactory improvement and stabilization of the clinical picture.

In IBM, immunosuppressive treatment has limited efficacy. However, considering the modest inflammation observed in the disease, patients with IBM are sometimes treated with a course of prednisone for 3-4 months. A recent trial showed some efficacy of Rapamicine for disease stabilization.

Because of interferon alfa pathway activation in DM, Janus-Kinase inhibitors (anti-JAK) have been used for refractory cases. In all cases, along with pharmacological treatments, patients should be advised to undergo physiotherapy and occupational therapy.

21.3.2 Toxic myopathies

Muscles can be damaged by drugs and toxic substances, which act on muscle fibers (necrotizing toxic myopathies) or by electrolyte imbalances, muscle ischemia, and excessive muscle activity. The damage can be local (e.g., at the injection site) or systemic. The toxic effect of the substance can manifest acutely or require chronic exposure. The main substances capable of causing muscle damage are: hypolipidemic drugs of the statin category (atorvastatin, cerivastatin, fluvastatin, lovastatin, pravastatin, simvastatin) and fibrates category (clofibrate, bezafibrate, fenofibrate, and gemfibrozil); corticosteroids (particularly fluorinated corticosteroids); amphiphilic drugs (chloroquine, amiodarone, quinacrine, chlorpromazine, imipramine, procainamide, doxorubicin, plasmocid); antimicrotubular agents (colchicine and vincristine); alcohol. The histological appearance is characterized by muscle necrosis and regeneration in which the presence of inflammatory infiltrates (mostly macrophages) is secondary to necrosis, and MHC-I is not overexpressed. CK levels are often elevated. The therapy is etiological and aims to eliminate the cause.

21.4 Neuromuscular junction disorders (NMJD)

This term refers to all diseases caused by a disorder of the mechanisms regulating neuromuscular transmission. Despite the various causes (congenital disorders of the protein structures involved in neuromuscular transmission, toxins, and humoral factors interfering with normal junction functioning), NMJDs share the same clinical symptom: loss of muscle strength (paresis or paralysis) resulting from the inability of the motor axon to correctly induce depolarization of the sarcolemma and muscle fiber contraction.

The neuromuscular junction

The neuromuscular junction or motor endplate is a morphofunctional unit composed of motor axons and muscle fibers, which are contiguous but separated by the synaptic cleft. There are three main anatomical regions of the neuromuscular junction:

1) The presynaptic membrane, consisting of the axolemma of the nerve terminal.
2) The synaptic cleft.
3) The postsynaptic membrane, consisting of the specialized region of the muscle fiber sarcolemma (Figure 21.20).

The most important anatomical and functional elements of the presynaptic nerve terminal are synaptic vesicles, a protein complex called "SNARE," and voltage-gated calcium and potassium channels. Synaptic vesicles are of different sizes and are located in different sites within the presynaptic terminal. The most abundant vesicles are small (50-60 nm) and are mainly concentrated at the synaptic terminal, where they are transported by rapid axoplasmic flow. At this level, they undergo further maturation: they are filled with the neurotransmitter synthesized in the cytoplasm of the nerve terminal and positioned at the "active zones" of the presynaptic membrane. The functions of the vesicles include:

1) *uptake* and *storage* of acetylcholine (ACh);
2) Movement and attachment to the "active zones";
3) Fusion with the presynaptic membrane and release of ACh into the synaptic cleft through exocytosis;
4) Recycling of the vesicles themselves. Each vesicle contains approximately 500,000 ACh molecules, called "quanta".

The SNARE complex is a multiprotein complex consisting of synaptobrevin (located in the membrane of synaptic vesicles), syntaxin (located in the "active zones" of the presynaptic membrane), and SNAP-25. These proteins, by interacting with each other under the action of calcium ions, allow synaptic vesicles to approach the presynaptic membrane, fuse with it, and undergo exocytosis.

Voltage-gated calcium channels are located adjacent to the "active zones." They consist of four subunits and are opened by the depolarization of the presynaptic membrane, allowing massive entry of calcium ions into the presynaptic terminal. By activating the SNARE complex, calcium ions enable the exocytosis of synaptic vesicles. Downregulation of

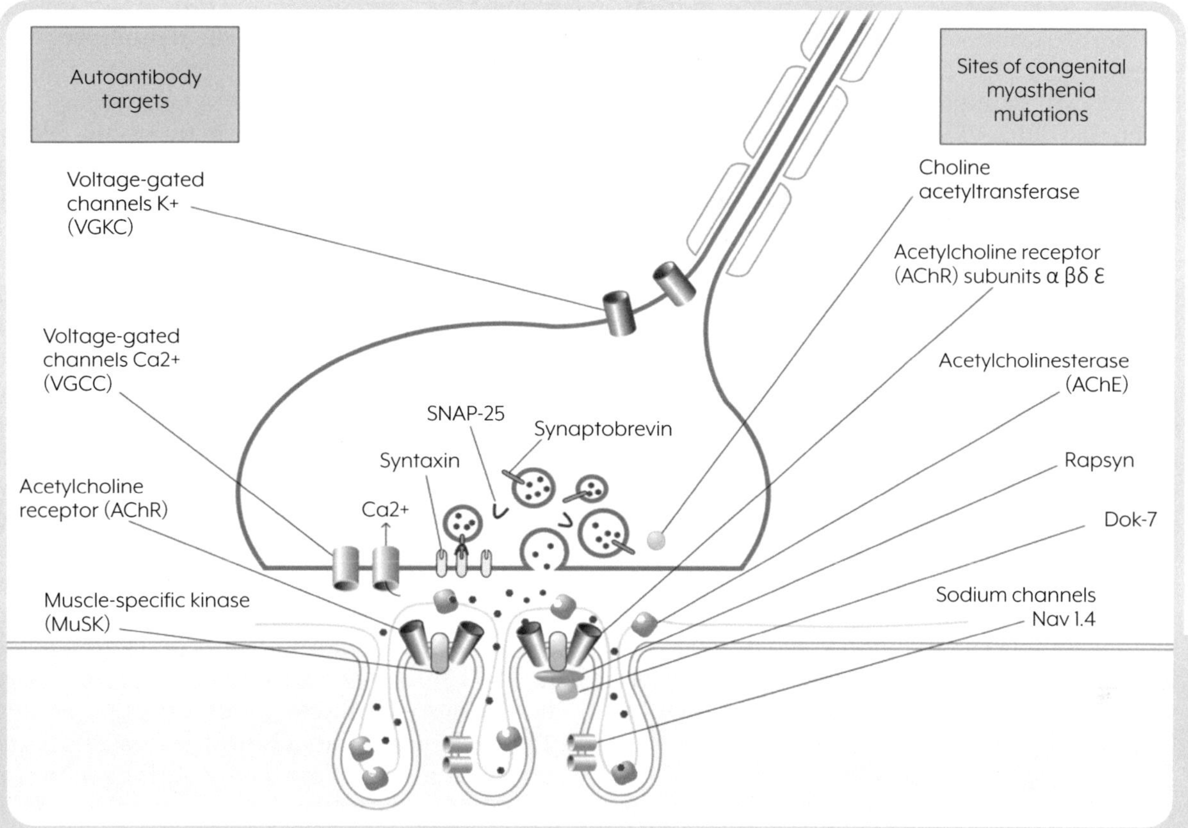

Figure 21.20

The neuromuscular junction and its "critical" sites.

calcium channels is observed in Lambert-Eaton myasthenic syndrome.

Voltage-gated sodium channels are not expressed at the presynaptic membrane, where only voltage-gated potassium channels, along with calcium channels, are present. The potassium channels are activated by the action potential and, by restoring the resting potential at the presynaptic level, lead to the inactivation of calcium channels. An alteration in potassium channels, as observed in neuromyotonia, or their pharmacological blockade with 3,4-diaminopyridine, prolongs the opening time of voltage-gated calcium channels, thereby increasing calcium entry into the nerve terminal and enhancing ACh release.

In the synaptic cleft, located between the presynaptic and postsynaptic membranes, the basement membrane is located. The Acetylcholinesterase (AChE) binds to the basement membrane through collagen filaments (ColQ). AChE is a protein consisting of multiple subunits and is responsible for hydrolyzing the molecules of ACh released into the synaptic cleft. ACh released into the synaptic cleft is hydrolyzed by AChE, and the produced choline is subsequently taken up by the synaptic terminal, acetylated, and stored in vesicles, which are made available for new exocytosis. The basement membrane, through its protein constituents (laminins, agrin, neuroregulins, collagen, proteoglycans), plays a fundamental role in the development and regeneration processes of the neuromuscular junction. The motor axonal terminal secretes agrin, a protein that activates a muscle-specific tyrosine kinase (MuSK) expressed on the postsynaptic membrane through a co-receptor called lipoprotein-related receptor 4 (LRP-4). MuSK, through an intracellular pathway, interacts with another postsynaptic protein called rapsyn, leading to the clustering of acetylcholine receptors (AChR). The postsynaptic membrane consists of multiple invaginations that form junctional folds. This particular conformation allows for a large postsynaptic surface area in a small space. AChRs are transmembrane protein complexes concentrated at the ends of junctional folds, with a density of 15,000/μm^2. AChR is composed of 5 subunits (2 alpha subunits, 1 delta, 1 beta, 1 epsilon in adults or gamma in fetuses) that form an ion pore. The extracellular part of the receptor has ACh binding sites located on the two alpha subunits and, in its outermost part, an amino acid sequence (from alpha-71 to alpha-76) called the Main Immunogenic Region (MIR), which serves as the target site for anti-AChR antibodies in myasthenia gravis and experimental autoimmune myasthenia. AChRs undergo continuous turnover dependent on their stability. Under normal conditions, the half-life of AChRs in an adult is 8-11 days, while the fetal form of AChR has a half-life of 24 hours.

Voltage-gated sodium channels are concentrated in the deepest part of the synaptic folds. Their density is inversely proportional to the excitability threshold of the postsynaptic membrane.

Function of the neuromuscular junction

The function of the neuromuscular junction is carried out through the interaction of ACh with its receptor. This process begins with the depolarization of the presynaptic membrane, which, by opening calcium channels, allows calcium ions to enter the axonal terminal. Calcium ions, by activating the SNARE complex, enable the mobilization and exocytosis of ACh vesicles located near the postsynaptic membrane. The simultaneous opening of potassium channels leads to the closure of calcium channels, returning the membrane to its resting state. The interaction of ACh with AChRs results in the opening of the channel, causing a flow of sodium ions and a local electrical event. This, in turn, triggers the opening of sodium channels located in the postsynaptic folds, generating an end-plate potential (EPP). When the EPP reaches the threshold potential of the membrane, it generates an action potential that propagates along the sarcolemma, initiating muscle contraction. Under normal conditions, the amount of ACh released and the number of AChRs and sodium channels exceed the minimum required to generate an action potential. As a result, the amplitude of the EPP is always greater than the threshold potential for generating the end-plate potential. This difference is referred to as the "safety factor of the end-plate" (SFP). Practically speaking, the SFP allows for prolonged muscle contraction, even during the physiological consumption of ACh that occurs during exertion, without signs of muscle weakness appearing. Any pathological condition that alters the processes and factors involved in the functioning of the neuromuscular junction (amount of released ACh, density, distribution, and kinetic properties of AChRs, density of sodium channels in the postsynaptic membrane) leads to a reduction in SFP. The consequence is the failure to depolarize a progressive percentage of muscle fibers during exertion. This phenomenon clinically manifests as progressive muscle weakness during prolonged contraction (abnormal fatigue), which is a characteristic feature of NMJD.

Classification of neuromuscular junction disorders

NMJD can be classified based on the site of alteration in the processes involved in neuromuscular transmission and their etiopathogenesis (Table 21.5).

21.4.1 Myasthenia gravis

Myasthenia Gravis (MG) is an acquired disease, where symptoms result from altered neuro-muscular transmission due to immune-mediated damage to the postsynaptic side of the neuromuscular junction. It is worth noting that the term "gravis", historically coined by Friedrich Jolly in 1895 when myasthenia was a highly fatal disease (with about half of the cases resulting in mortality), appears anachronistic today in light of the radical change in its clinical course thanks to available treatments.

Epidemiology | MG is the most common disease of the NMJ, with an incidence of 0.25-

Table 21.5 CLASSIFICATION OF NEUROMUSCULAR JUNCTION DISEASES

Neuromuscular junction diseases	Acquired	Congenital
From presynaptic defect	Myasthenic Syndrome (LEMS) Botulism	Choline Acetyltransferase (*ChAT*) deficiency (5%) Deficiency in synaptic vesicle quantity/quantal release (*SNAP25B*), choline transport (*SLC5A7*) (<0.5%) Impaired inactivation of the SNARE complex (*MUNC13-1, VAMP1, SYT2*) (<0.5%) Deficiency in proteins involved in NMJ development (*MYO9.4*) (<0.5%)
From synaptic defect		Basal lamina acetylcholinesterase (*COLQ*) deficiency (12%) Basement membrane beta-2-laminin deficiency (*LAMB2*)
From postsynaptic defect	Myasthenia Gravis (MG) - AChRab-MG - MuSKab-MG - LRP4ab-MG - Seronegative MG (SNMG)	Mutations in AChR subunits (50%): 1. AChR deficiency (33%) - Epsilon subunit deficiency (CHRNE) 2. AChR kinetic abnormalities (17%) - *Slow channel syndrome* - *Fast channel syndrome* Mutations in proteins involved in neuromuscular junction formation and maintenance (25%) - Rapsin (RAPSN) (14%) - Docking protein 7 (DOK7) (10%) - Lipoprotein-receptor related protein (LRP4) - Muscle-specific kinase (MUSK) - Agrin (AGRN) Sodium channel mutations Mutations in glycosylation proteins, involved in the regulation of solubility, stability, assembly, and intracellular transport of nascent peptides (4%)

2/100,000 and a prevalence of 5-40/100,000. MG can affect individuals of all ages (from childhood to old age), all races, and both sexes. Based on the age of onset, two groups can be distinguished: the first group, with early onset (< 50 years, peaking between 20-30 years), is characterized by a predominance of female patients, a higher frequency of thymic hyperplasia (80%), and an association with HLA B8 and DR3; the second group, with late onset (50-65 years) or very late onset (> 65 yrs), peaking between 60-70 years, predominantly affects male patients, shows a higher frequency of thymic atrophy, and is associated with HLA B7 and DR2. There is also a third group of patients (10-15%) in whom MG is associated with thymoma, with an incidence peak around 50 years of age and an equal frequency in both sexes.

Etiology and pathophysiology | MG is an autoimmune disease caused, in most cases, by IgG antibodies that interact with AChR (acetylcholine receptor), which can be detected in the blood of approximately 85% of patients. This form is referred to as AChRab-MG. AChR antibodies are directed against the Main Immunogenic Region (MIR) of the alpha subunit of AChR.

AChR antibodies, which are predominantly IgG1 and IgG3, exert their pathogenic effect through three main mechanisms:

1) Acceleration of AChR degradation by forming antigen-antibody complexes that are internalized and destroyed within the muscle fiber.
2) Activation of the complement cascade, resulting in lytic damage and structural simplification of the postsynaptic membrane, leading to reduced density of AChR and sodium channels.
3) Blockage of ACh binding sites on AChR.

Approximately 5-8% of myasthenic patients (40% of patients without AChR antibodies) have anti-MuSK (muscle-specific tyrosine kinase) antibodies, defining the anti-MuSK-MG form, which is characterized by a strong prevalence in females and an incidence peak around the fourth decade of life. MuSK is activated by neural agrin through its co-receptor LRP4 (lipoprotein-related receptor 4) and regulates AChR clustering through an intracellular pathway. Anti-MuSK antibodies are predominantly IgG4 and do not interact with the antigen through complement activation. Instead, they exert their pathogenic effect by blocking the MuSK-LRP4 binding.

A very low percentage of patients without AChR antibodies have anti-LRP4 antibodies. These antibodies are IgG1 and exert their pathogenic effect by activating the complement cascade and inhibiting AChR clustering through blocking the LRP4-agrin binding.

Other patients are negative for AChR, MuSK and LRP4 antibodies and they are referred to as having seronegative myasthenia gravis (SNMG). Using cell-based immunoassay (CBA) techniques, it has been shown that many patients with SNMG are actually carriers of AChR antibodies (which cannot be detected by radioimmunoassay techniques but have similar characteristics to AChRab-MG antibodies). However, a small percentage of patients with "seronegative" MG remains. Anti-Agrin antibodies have been detected in some of these patients, but their pathogenetic role is debated.

Autoimmune myasthenia has a significant correlation with certain thymic pathologies. Approximately 15% of MG patients have thymoma (more commonly cortical and well-differentiated), while around 50% of thymoma patients develop MG. In approximately 80% of MG patients without thymoma and with early onset, the thymus shows hyperplasia with inflammatory infiltrates, germinal centers, and B and T cells. The myoid cells (which are normally part of thymic tissue) are closely associated with or completely engulfed by inflammatory infiltrates. In contrast, thymus involvement is not observed in patients with anti-MuSK-MG.

The thymus plays a fundamental role in the development of immunocompetence in healthy individuals. It is believed that in MG without thymoma or anti-MuSK antibodies, the thymus plays a pathogenic role due to an inflammatory process that leads to the loss of tolerance towards AChR, which is expressed by myoid cells, similarly to skeletal muscle fibers. This results in an immune response that activates B cells against AChR, leading to the production of AChR antibodies. The cause of thymic inflammation is unknown, although a role of Epstein-Barr virus has recently been hypothesized. However, MG associated with thymoma, like other neuromuscular syndromes (neuromyotonia with antibodies against the potassium channel, rippling muscle syndrome, inflammatory myopathies, autonomic neuropathies) or central nervous system syndromes (cerebellar syndromes, Morvan's fibrillary chorea, encephalopathy) associated with this tumor, constitutes a distinct clinical form known as a paraneoplastic syndrome. Defective intratumoral thymocyte selection with export of autoreactive T lymphocytes is thought to be responsible for the development of MG in these patients. Except for rare exceptions, all patients have a high titer of AChR antibodies, often associated with positivity for titin antibodies (66%) and RyR antibodies (83%).

Symptomatology: | The cardinal symptom of MG, as well as other NMJDs, is progressive muscle weakness during exercise (Figure 21.21) that improves with rest. Equally characteristic is the fluctuation of muscle symptoms, which show significant temporal variations, sometimes on a daily basis. In some cases, especially in more severe patients, muscle weakness may be evident even at rest (and worsen with muscle exercise). Muscle trophism is usually unaffected, as are deep reflexes, although they can become hypoexcitable in cases of severe weakness. Clinical exacerbations are possible during the course of the disease, often triggered by events. All skeletal muscles can be involved in MG.

Weakness of the extraocular muscles manifests as eyelid ptosis and ophthalmoparesis, which cannot be attributed to deficits in individual cranial nerves. Patients may complain of blurred vision or frank diplopia. Although ocular symptoms are among the most common, they remain confined to the ocular muscles in only 15-20% of cases, tending to spread to other muscles within two years of onset.

Facial muscles are equally affected, causing weakness of the orbicularis oculi muscles, making it difficult for patients to forcefully close their eyelids, and weakness of the lower facial musculature, leading to difficulty inflating the cheeks and lifting the corners of the mouth to smile (vertical smile). Fatigability of the masticatory muscles results in progressive difficulty in chewing food and, in severe cases, jaw drooping.

Bulbar symptoms are due to the deficit of muscles innervated by the bulbar cranial nerves. Dysphagia is more pronounced

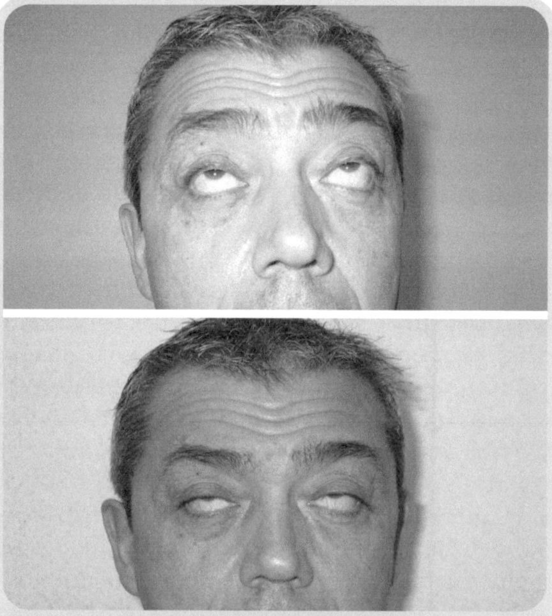

Figure 21.21

Appearance of evident eyelid ptosis during prolonged activation of the levator palpebrae.

for liquids (especially when hot) and may be accompanied by nasal regurgitation. In severe cases, it may require nasogastric tube placement. Dysarthria, which usually occurs during prolonged conversation, gives a nasal quality to the voice and can make speech unintelligible. It is caused by weakness of the lingual and pharyngeal-laryngeal muscles. Weakness of the neck flexor and extensor muscles can result in head drop or difficulty holding the head up from the bed surface. Patients with neck muscle fatigue often complain of retrocervical discomfort from the effort exerted by the posterior muscles to keep the head lifted.

In generalized forms, symptoms involve limb muscles, especially at the level of the girdles, causing difficulty in holding the arms up, supporting weights, and climbing stairs. Among distal muscles, the extensor muscles of the fingers are often asymmetrically affected. Involvement of the dorsiflexors of the foot, which can lead to diagnostic errors with polyneuropathies, is rarer.

Weakness of the pelvic muscles in women or the external urethral sphincter in men can cause episodes of urinary incontinence.

Respiratory muscle involvement occurs in 15-20% of patients within two years of onset and represents a sign of myasthenic crisis. It causes a restrictive type of ventilatory failure, which needs to be carefully monitored with gas exchange evaluation and promptly treated. Weak cough should be considered an early warning sign of respiratory muscle weakness. Respiratory failure is caused by diaphragmatic paralysis, weakness of other respiratory muscles, upper airway obstruction by secretions, and aspiration of saliva or other fluids. Myasthenic crises are mainly precipitated by respiratory infections, surgical procedures, over- or under-dosage of anticholinesterases, initiation of steroid treatment, sedation, and administration of medications that interfere with the NMJ.

Anti-MuSK-MG is characterized by predominant involvement of bulbar and axial muscles, with dysphagia, dysarthria, weakness of facial and neck muscles, frequent respiratory disturbances, and limited ocular involvement. Girdle and limb muscles are often spared.

The natural history of MG has undergone significant changes with the introduction of symptomatic therapy (anticholinesterases) and immunosuppressive and immunomodulatory treatments. Approximately 20% of patients experience improvements and spontaneous remissions of symptoms during the course of the disease. Mortality from MG is currently less than 5%, with the highest mortality rate occurring between 40 and 50 years of age.

Neonatal transient MG affects 10-30% of infants born to mothers with AChR antibodies and is caused by the transfer of antibodies through the placenta. It manifests at birth with dysphagia, weak crying, and hypotonia. Treatment is rarely required as the symptoms are transient and resolve within 1-4 weeks with the elimination of maternal antibodies. Transient neonatal MG is exceptional in infants born to patients with MuSK-Ab-associated MG, likely due to structural characteristics of these antibodies that prevent transplacental passage.

Different clinical forms can be recognized based on the groups of muscles affected by the symptoms. Historically classified by Osserman, they were reclassified in 2000 by

Table 21.6 MGFA CLASSIFICATION

I	Pure ocular (ptosis, ophthalmoplegia, weakness of the orbicularis oculi)
II	Mild weakness affecting muscles other than ocular muscles - IIa - Predominantly affecting limb, axial muscles, or both - IIb - Predominantly affecting oropharyngeal, respiratory muscles, or both
III	Moderate weakness affecting muscles other than ocular muscles - IIIa - Predominantly affecting limb, axial muscles, or both - IIIb - Predominantly affecting oropharyngeal, respiratory muscles, or both
IV	Severe weakness affecting muscles other than ocular muscles - IVa - Predominantly affecting limb, axial muscles, or both - IVb - Predominantly affecting oropharyngeal, respiratory muscles, or both
V	Need for mechanical ventilation

the MGFA (MG Foundation of America) into five groups of increasing severity (Table 21.6).

Diagnosis | The diagnosis of a neuromuscular transmission disorder is based on clinical evaluation, but clinical suspicion requires confirmation through diagnostic tests, including pharmacological tests, neurophysiological tests, and measurement of anti-AChR, anti-MuSK, and anti-LRP4 antibodies.

Pharmacological tests involve evaluating the variation of clinical symptoms after administration of anticholinesterase drugs (e.g., neostigmine, pyridostigmine, edrophonium chloride). These drugs prolong the half-life of ACh in the synaptic cleft and result in clinical improvement by allowing ACh to repeatedly bind to receptors. The most sensitive pharmacological test is the edrophonium chloride test (Tensilon test), administered intravenously as a slow bolus at a dose of 10 mg. This drug has a potent anticholinesterase effect and a duration of action of a few minutes, making it particularly suitable for diagnostic purposes. Approximately 90% of patients with Anti-AChR antibodies exhibit a positive response to anticholinesterases. In patients with anti-MuSK antibodies, anticholinesterases are usually ineffective and may worsen symptoms. A positive response can be observed in congenital myasthenias and Lambert-Eaton syndrome. A falsely positive response has been described in ALS and Guillain-Barré syndrome.

Neurophysiological tests involve repetitive stimulation and EMG study of single fibers. The first test assesses the compound muscle action potential (CMAP) amplitude during repetitive supramaximal stimulation at low frequency (2-3 Hz) at rest, immediately after a 10-second maximal effort, and during repetitive low-frequency stimulation at 1-3-5 minutes after maximal effort. The CMAP amplitude depends on the number of activated muscle fibers. In MG, a decrement in CMAP amplitude exceeding 10% between the first and fourth stimuli can be observed; the CMAP after maximal contraction does not exceed 25%; repetitive stimulation after 1-3 minutes from maximal contraction shows a more pronounced decrement in CMAP between the first and fourth stimuli (Figure 21.22). This test has good specificity but poor sensitivity, as it is altered in only 70% of patients with MG. Single-fiber EMG allows for the evaluation of temporal variability (jitter), which normally exists in the depolarization of two muscle fibers belonging to the same motor unit when it is activated continuously. Due to the increased excitability threshold of the postsynaptic membrane, the depolarization times of muscle fibers in MG lengthen or depolarization does not occur, resulting in increased jitter and blocking phenomena. This test has high sensitivity (90-95%) but modest specificity, as it is altered in any neuromuscular disorder with immature newly formed endplates (e.g., including motor axon damage or myopathies).

Measurement of antibodies plays a fundamental role not only in diagnosis but also in the classification of NMJ pathology. Anti-AChR and anti-MuSK antibodies are measured using radioimmunoprecipitation techniques (RIA). In cases of clinical suspicion of MG, anti-AChR antibodies should be tested for, and in case of negativity, anti-MuSK antibodies should be sought. The diagnostic accuracy of RIA is 97-99%. Antibodies directed against two intracellular muscle proteins, titin and ryanodine, can also be detected in MG. These antibodies are strongly associated with thymoma (95% for anti-titin and 70% for anti-ryanodine).

In patients with eyelid ptosis, the ice-pack test (application of an ice pack to the orbit for 2 minutes) can be a useful diagnostic aid, as it can improve ptosis in cases of myasthenia.

Mediastinal CT is essential for anatomical evaluation of the thymus, particularly for

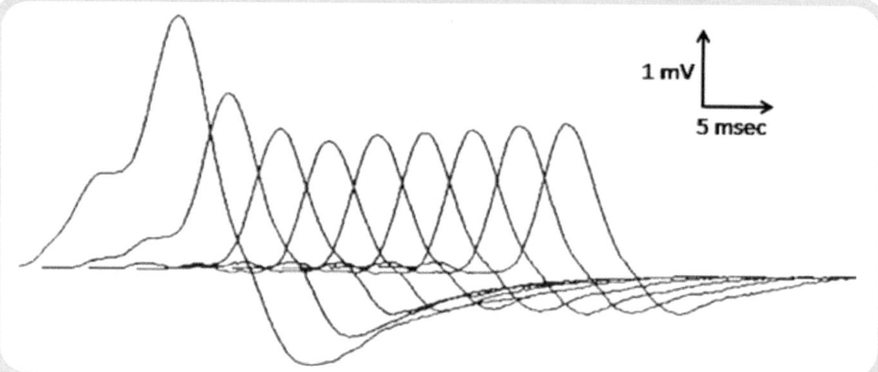

Figure 21.22

Repetitive stimulation in a myasthenic patient. The train of stimulations at 3Hz shows a decrease in cMAP of more than 10% between the first and fourth stimulation.

thymoma identification in patients with MG. CT should be performed with contrast medium. At present, chest MRI, although more expensive, is not more informative than CT.

Therapy | MG therapy involves symptomatic treatments, immunosuppressive treatments, and thymectomy. Symptomatic therapy aims to treat abnormal muscle fatigue using acetylcholinesterase inhibitors, which prolong the activity of ACh molecules in the synaptic cleft, improving neuromuscular transmission. The most commonly used drug is pyridostigmine bromide (Mestinon). The dosage should be adjusted based on the patient's clinical status and needs, considering that the average duration of action of 60 mg of Mestinon (1 tablet) is approximately 4 hours. In children, the dosage is established at 1 mg/kg. The latency between intake and therapeutic effect is approximately 1 hour. Overdosing with acetylcholinesterase inhibitors can cause a cholinergic crisis, characterized by muscarinic phenomena and weakness due to hyperpolarization of the postsynaptic membrane. These medications have limited efficacy in anti-MuSK-MG, and the risk of cholinergic crises is higher.

Immunosuppressive therapy involves oral prednisone (0.75-1 mg/kg/day). Prednisone is often combined with other immunosuppressants such as azathioprine (2.5 mg/kg/day), cyclosporine A (3 mg/kg/day), tacrolimus (3 mg/kg/day), mycophenolate (1 g twice daily) to reduce the steroid dose. Cyclophosphamide (500 mg/m^2/month) is used only in cases resistant to other therapies due to its toxicity and side effects. The utility of monoclonal antibodies, particularly particularly anti-CD20 (Rituximab), anti-C5 complement fraction (eculizumab, ravulizumab, zilucoplan) and anti-neonatal Fc receptor of IgG fraction antibody (efgartigimod, rozanolixizumab), has recently been demonstrated in generalized MG resistant to other immunosuppressive treatments. Rituximab has shown particular effectiveness in anti-MuSK-MG.

Plasmapheresis (3-6 exchanges of 1-1.5 plasma volumes on alternate days) aims to remove antibodies and inflammatory factors involved in the pathogenesis of the disease. It is indicated especially in patients with acute and generalized symptoms (myasthenic crises) but is also used as preparation for thymectomy in patients with significant symptoms. Intravenous human immunoglobulins (2 g/kg administered over 2-5 days) have the same indications as plasmapheresis.

Thymectomy is performed based on the correlations observed between thymic pathology and MG. The procedure traditionally performed via median sternotomy is now mainly done using VATS (video-assisted thoracoscopic surgery) and robotic procedures. In cases of MG associated with thymoma, thymectomy is mandatory. Surgical resection is combined with chemotherapy and radiotherapy based on the invasiveness of the thymoma (capsule, thymic fat, pleura, or pericardium). In MG not associated with thymoma, thymectomy is currently indicated for patients with AChR antibodies, symptoms not limited to the ocular area, and clinical onset of the disease before the age of 50. The absence of thymic tissue on CT does not exclude the indication for thymectomy due to the low sensitivity of CT in thymic hyperplasia. Thymectomy is not currently indicated in patients with onset of MG after the age of 60 or, regardless of the age of onset, in patients with symptoms limited to the ocular area, those without AChR antibodies, and those with MuSK antibodies. Children and adolescents are not subjected to thymectomy.

21.4.2 Lambert-Eaton Myasthenic Syndrome (LEMS)

LEMS is a presynaptic disorder of the neuromuscular junction, often associated with neoplasms, and characterized by weakness and muscle fatigue caused by impaired acetylcholine (ACh) release.

Epidemiology | LEMS is a rare disease, with an estimated prevalence of around 1/100,000. Both sexes can be affected. The disease can occur at any age, including in children, but is more common after the age of 40. In over half of LEMS patients, and with a clear predominance in men (70% vs. 30%), there is an association with malignancies. However, these malignancies may not become clinically apparent until up to 4 years after the onset of LEMS. The most frequently associated tumor is small cell lung carcinoma, observed in over 80% of cases, but LEMS has also been reported in association with lymphoproliferative diseases, malignant thymoma, and, more rarely, breast, stomach, colon, prostate, kidney, and bladder tumors. In 40% of LEMS patients, no neoplasms develop. In this form, there is no sex predominance, and one-third of these patients show an association with other autoimmune diseases such as myasthenia gravis (MG), thyroiditis, autoimmune diabetes, vitiligo, pernicious anemia, and celiac disease.

Etiology and pathophysiology | LEMS, in its various forms, is an autoimmune disorder caused by antibodies directed against voltage-gated calcium channels (VGCC-ab), which can be detected in 85-90% of patients. Calcium channels located in the presynaptic membrane allow the entry of calcium ions into the synaptic terminal, initiating the processes necessary for acetylcholine vesicle exocytosis. Their impairment reduces the safety factor of neuromuscular transmission by decreasing the availability of ACh. In LEMS associated with tumors, the production of antibodies is believed to result from molecular mimicry between tumor proteins and VGCC proteins. However, it is unclear what mechanism regulates antibody production in forms not associated with neoplasms.

Symptoms | Muscle fatigue and weakness are the predominant symptoms of LEMS. Weakness primarily affects the limbs, especially the lower limbs (80%). Involvement of the extraocular muscles and eyelid ptosis is less common (20%). Deep tendon reflexes are often weak or absent. Muscle strength and reflexes sometimes improve with physical exercise, which represents the clinical equivalent of the post-tetanic potentiation observable in neurophysiological examinations. Autonomic dysfunction symptoms are frequent in LEMS (85%), such as xerostomia, erectile dysfunction, and constipation. LEMS symptoms can be exacerbated by the use of calcium antagonists. In the form associated with neoplasms, there may be overlapping paraneoplastic syndromes (sensory neuropathy, subacute cerebellar ataxia, etc.) and positivity for other antibodies against onconeural antigens (anti-Hu, anti-Yo, etc.).

Instrumental diagnosis | Neurophysiological examination typically shows a low-amplitude compound muscle action potential (CMAP) with supramaximal nerve stimulation, further decrement with low-frequency stimulation (2-5 Hz), and a marked increase in CMAP (>100%) with tetanic stimulation (20-50 Hz) or after maximal contraction for 10 seconds (post-tetanic potentiation). This is due to the reduced release of ACh, which lowers the safety factor of neuromuscular transmission and reduces the number of muscle fibers capable of depolarizing in response to nerve stimulation. With continued maximal contraction, calcium channels remain open longer, allowing for the release of a larger quantity of ACh and an increase in the number of muscle fibers capable of depolarizing. VGCC antibodies can be detected in 85-90% of LEMS patients and are diagnostic of the disease. Once the diagnosis is established, patients should undergo oncological screening with total-body CT and FDG-PET. Patients with negative oncological screening should be carefully monitored, considering that the neoplasm can become apparent even after long periods of time.

Therapy | The treatment of the tumor, which is obviously a priority in LEMS patients, sometimes leads to an improvement in the symptoms of the disease. Symptomatic therapy is based on the use of 3,4-diaminopyridine, which blocks voltage-gated potassium channels in the presynaptic membrane, prolongs depolarization, and delays the closure of calcium channels, thereby increasing ACh release. Immunosuppressive therapy with prednisone, azathioprine, or cyclosporine is effective in LEMS. However, it should be used with caution in the form associated with neoplasms to avoid unmasking the tumor. The response to plasmapheresis and intravenous immunoglobulins is still controversial.

21.4.3 Botulism

Botulism is a severe intoxication of the neuromuscular junctions and autonomic nervous system caused by a potent neurotoxin produced by *Clostridium botulinum*, a gram-positive anaerobic bacterium that survives in the soil as spores.

Epidemiology | Botulism is primarily reported in geographical areas where home-made foods are consumed.

Etiology and pathophysiology | There are seven known types of botulinum toxin, each produced by a different bacterial strain. The toxin, usually ingested through contaminated food preserved in anaerobic conditions (favorable for the growth of toxin-producing bacteria), is absorbed in the gastrointestinal tract, spreads hematogenously, and irreversibly binds to neuromuscular junctions and autonomic nervous system, where it acts by cleaving proteins of the SNARE complex, blocking ACh release. Rarely, botulinum spores can also be ingested through inhalation or wound infection.

Clinical features | The disease usually begins 1-3 days after toxin ingestion with neuromuscular and cholinergic neurovegetative symptoms. Neuromuscular symptoms are characterized by paralysis of limb, trunk, bulbar, ocular, and respiratory muscles. Cholinergic neurovegetative symptoms initially manifest as constipation, pupillary dilation, bradycardia, hypotension, and hypohidrosis.

Instrumental diagnosis | Instrumental diagnosis of botulism is based on neurophysiological evidence of a presynaptic disorder of the neuromuscular junction, showing similarities to Lambert-Eaton syndrome, and the detection of botulinum toxin in feces.

Therapy | The prognosis of botulism is spontaneously favorable if the patient receives adequate supportive care (ventilatory support, treatment of autonomic disturbances, enteral nutrition). The duration of the illness can be significantly shortened by administering antitoxin.

21.4.4 Congenital myasthenic syndromes (CMS)

CMS encompasses numerous clinical forms caused by impaired neuromuscular transmission due to various types of mutations in genes encoding structures involved in the functioning and organization of the neuromuscular junction.

Epidemiology | Although the prevalence of CMS is estimated to be around 10% of that of MG, it represents the most common cause of NMJD in the first year of life and is likely underdiagnosed among patients with seronegative myasthenia onset before the age of 20.

Etiology and pathophysiology | CMS is caused by an abnormality in neuromuscular transmission due to a mutation in proteins involved in the development and function of the NMJ. All CMS forms are inherited as autosomal recessive traits, except for *slow-channel CMS*, which is transmitted in a dominant manner. Thirty genes have been described, and their mutation leads to a form of CMS. Based on the localization of the mutated protein, CMS can be classified as presynaptic, synaptic, or postsynaptic defects (Table 21.5).

The defect in choline acetyltransferase (CHAT), which represents the most common form of presynaptic CMS, accounts for 5% of all CMS cases. Deficiency of acetylcholinesterase function at the basal lamina caused by a mutation in the COLQ protein, which anchors acetylcholinesterase to the basal lamina filaments, is the most common form of synaptic CMS (12% of all CMS cases). However, the most common forms of CMS are postsynaptic and are caused by mutations that result in a quantitative deficit of AChR subunits (primarily the epsilon subunit) (50% of all CMS cases) or mutations that cause kinetic abnormalities of AChR (*slow-channel CMS* and *fast-channel CMS*) (17% of all CMS cases). Finally, 25% of all CMS cases are caused by mutations in proteins involved in the formation and maintenance of the neuromuscular junction. The most common of these are CMS due to mutations in Rapsin (14%) and Docking Protein 7 (DOK-7) (10%). In practice, the most common mutations are CHRNE, RAPSN, DOK7, and COLQ.

Clinical features | CMS can manifest in newborns or within the first months of life with hypotonia, altered development, delayed motor milestones, and unexplained episodes of apnea. In other cases (e.g., in *slow-channel syndrome*), the onset can be later (childhood, adolescence, or adulthood), requiring a differential diagnosis with acquired forms. In these cases, the clinical picture manifests as abnormal fatigability or fluctuating weakness of the ocular, facial, bulbar, truncal, and limb muscles. Sometimes, especially in CMS due to alterations in proteins involved in the normal aggregation of AChR, the clinical picture resembles a myopathy with muscular atrophy, similar to limb-girdle myopathy. Weakness tends to progress during adolescence, then stabilize, although episodic exacerbations can occur in conjunction with intercurrent events.

Instrumental diagnosis | The diagnosis of CMS is often complex and can be confirmed by genetic-molecular testing, which, however, only identifies the pathogenic mutation in less than half of cases. The diagnosis should always be suspected in patients with neuromuscular deficits who exhibit a decremental muscle response to low-frequency repetitive stimulation or an abnormality in single-fiber electromyography (SFEMG), negative AChRab and MuSKab, and lack of clinical response to immunological therapies. Neurophysiological examination in slow-channel syndrome is characterized by a compound muscle action potential (CMAP) followed by a second muscle potential.

Therapy | The response to therapy is often partial. The following treatments can be used: anti-acetylcholinesterase drugs (pyridostigmine bromide) to prolong the presence of ACh in the synaptic space (in AChR deficiency forms) or 3,4-diaminopyridine to increase ACh release (in *fast-channel syndrome*); drugs that block the ion pore opening, such as fluoxetine and quinidine, used in slow-channel syndrome; beta-adrenergic drugs (salbutamol, ephedrine) that are particularly effective in DOK7 and COLQ mutations. Anti-acetylcholinesterase drugs can be used prophylactically to prevent respiratory crises in specific conditions (e.g., fever, intercurrent infections) where it is important to monitor the respiratory function of patients.

Bibliography

Engel G. and Franzini-Armstrong C., Myology, Basic and Clinical, 3rd Edition. New York McGraw-Hill, 2004.

Di Mauro S., Tay S., Mancuso M., Mitochondrial encephalomyopathies: diagnostic approach. Ann N Y Acad Sci; 1011:217-231, 2004.

Dubowitz V., Muscle Biopsy: A Practical Approach, 3rd Edition, 626 pp. Saunders, 2007.

Karpati G., Hilton-Jones D., Griggs R. eds., Disorders of voluntary muscles, 7th edition. Cambridge: Cambridge University Press; 660-675, 2001.

Lunn M., Hanna M., Howard R., Parton M., Reilly N., Nerve and muscle diseases in: Neurology. A Queen Square textbook. Clarke C., Howard R., Rossor M., Shorvon S. WileyBlackwell; 383-410, 2009.

Mastaglia F.L., Drug induced myopathies. Pract Neurol; 6:4-13, 2006.

Ryan A., Matthews E., Hanna M.G., Skeletal muscle channellopathies. Curr Opin Neurol; 20:558-563, 2007.Weller R.O. e coll. Diseases of Muscle. Greenfield's Neuropathology. Graham D.I. e Lantos P.L.

Weller R.O. e coll. Diseases of Muscle. Greenfield's Neuropathology. Graham D.I. e Lantos P.L. Vol. II, Oxford University, Press; 489-581, 1997.

22 DISEASES OF THE AUTONOMIC NERVOUS SYSTEM

Antonella Conte, Alfredo Berardelli

The main function of the autonomic nervous system is to maintain internal homeostasis through the integrated and coordinated control of numerous bodily functions. The autonomic system regulates temperature variations, cardiovascular functions, bronchial activities, intestinal processes, metabolic and endocrine functions that accompany emotional states. It enables the organism to cope with situations such as exploration, social interaction, concentration, physical exertion, pain, cold/hot sensations, attack, defense, escape, rest, and reproduction. It consists of a sympathetic component and a parasympathetic component that have opposite effects on the innervated organs (Table 22.1). Specifically, the effects of the sympathetic system occur in emergency and stress conditions associated with *fight or flight* responses: it increases heart rate, blood pressure, blood flow, catabolic processes, and inhibits gastrointestinal functions. The effects of the parasympathetic system predominate in stable and resting conditions: it promotes digestive functions, reduces heart rate, blood pressure, and overall plays an anabolic role. The autonomic nervous system is connected to the organs and tissues on which it exerts its control functions and at the same time is in contact with the structures of the central nervous system that also control the autonomic system. The central components of the autonomic nervous system include certain areas of the cerebral cortex (frontal premotor, hippocampal cortex, insular cortex, anterior cingulate gyrus, anteromedial prefrontal cortex), the hypothalamus, the amygdala, the diencephalon, the brainstem (periaqueductal gray nuclei in the midbrain, pontine parabrachial nucleus, solitary tract nucleus in the medulla, reticular substance of the medulla). The hypothalamus integrates autonomic and endocrine functions and controls biological rhythms, thermoregulation, sexual function, and behavior. The central and peripheral structures of the autonomic nervous system are interconnected (sympathetic and

Table 22.1 FUNCTIONS REGULATED BY THE SYMPATHETIC AND PARASYMPATHETIC SYSTEMS ON TARGET ORGANS

Structure	Sympathetic system	Parasympathetic system
Eye	Dilation of the pupil	Constriction of the pupil
Salivary glands	Reduced salivation	Increased salivation
Heart	Increased heart rate and contractility	Reduced heart rate and contractility
Lungs	Bronchodilation	Bronchoconstriction
Stomach	Reduced gastric motility	Increased production of gastric juices and gastric motility
Small intestine	Reduced peristalsis	Increased digestive processes
Large intestine	Reduced motility	Increased motility
Liver	Increased glycogenolysis	
Adrenal medulla	Secretion of adrenaline and noradrenaline	
Kidneys	Reduced diuresis	Increased diuresis
Bladder	Relaxation of the detrusor muscle and contraction of the internal urethral sphincter	Contraction of the detrusor muscle and relaxation of the internal urethral sphincter

parasympathetic ganglia with their respective preganglionic and postganglionic fibers) through ascending and descending pathways.

22.1 Functional organization

The sympathetic and parasympathetic systems are organized into a cholinergic preganglionic neuron located in the central nervous system (spinal cord, brainstem) and a cholinergic or noradrenergic postganglionic neuron in the peripheral nervous system. Sympathetic fibers consist of short preganglionic fibers and long postganglionic fibers that originate from the paravertebral ganglia, while parasympathetic fibers are characterized by long preganglionic fibers and short postganglionic fibers that originate from ganglia located near the target organs (Figure 22.1). The activation of the sympathetic system results in diffuse responses in multiple body regions, while activation of the parasympathetic system elicits more localized responses. The sympathetic system is composed of a chain of ganglia located on each side of the vertebral column, as well as other more peripheral ganglia such as the celiac ganglia and the superior and inferior mesenteric ganglia. In contrast to the sympathetic system, the ganglia of the parasympathetic system are located near or in the walls of the innervated organs (Figure 22.2). Cholinergic preganglionic fibers of the sympathetic system originate in the thoracolumbar spinal cord and connect to cholinergic postganglionic fibers (which go to sweat glands and smooth muscle of the vascular network in skeletal muscles) or noradrenergic fibers in the paravertebral ganglia, celiac and mesenteric plexuses. The adrenal medulla is part of the sympathetic nervous system, and its function is to produce and release adrenaline and noradrenaline into circulation. Cholinergic preganglionic fibers of the parasympathetic system originate in the nuclei of cranial nerves in the brainstem (III, VII, IX, and X) or in the sacral segments of the spinal cord (S2-S4) and connect to cholinergic postganglionic fibers located in tissues and organs.

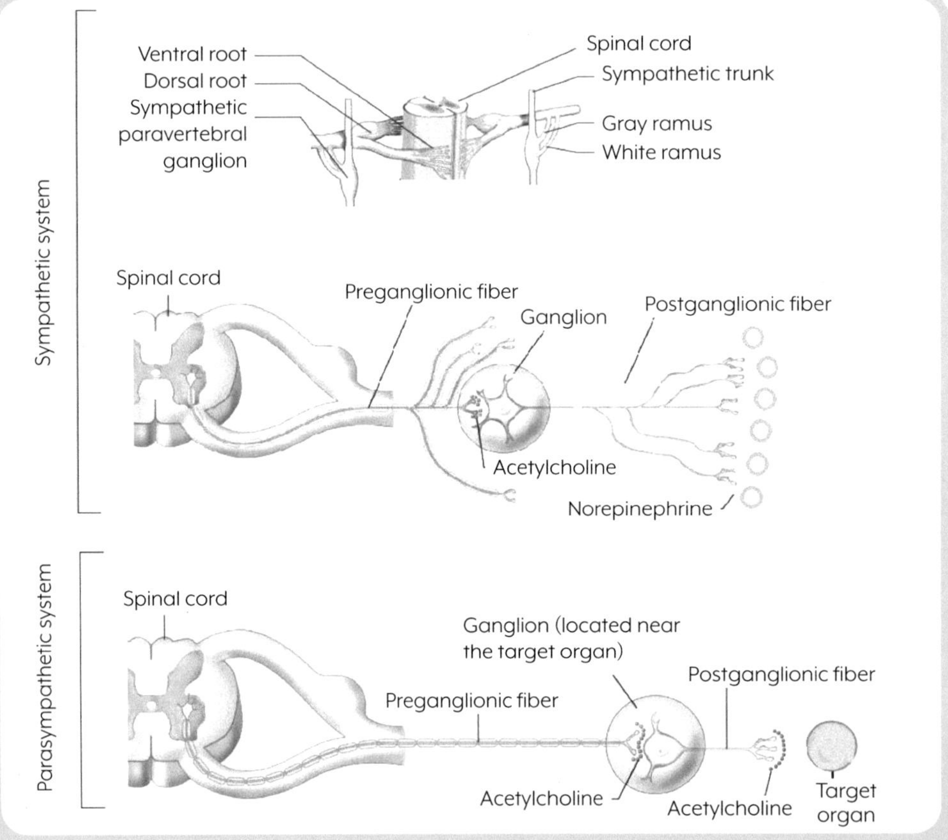

Figure 22.1
Autonomic nervous system.

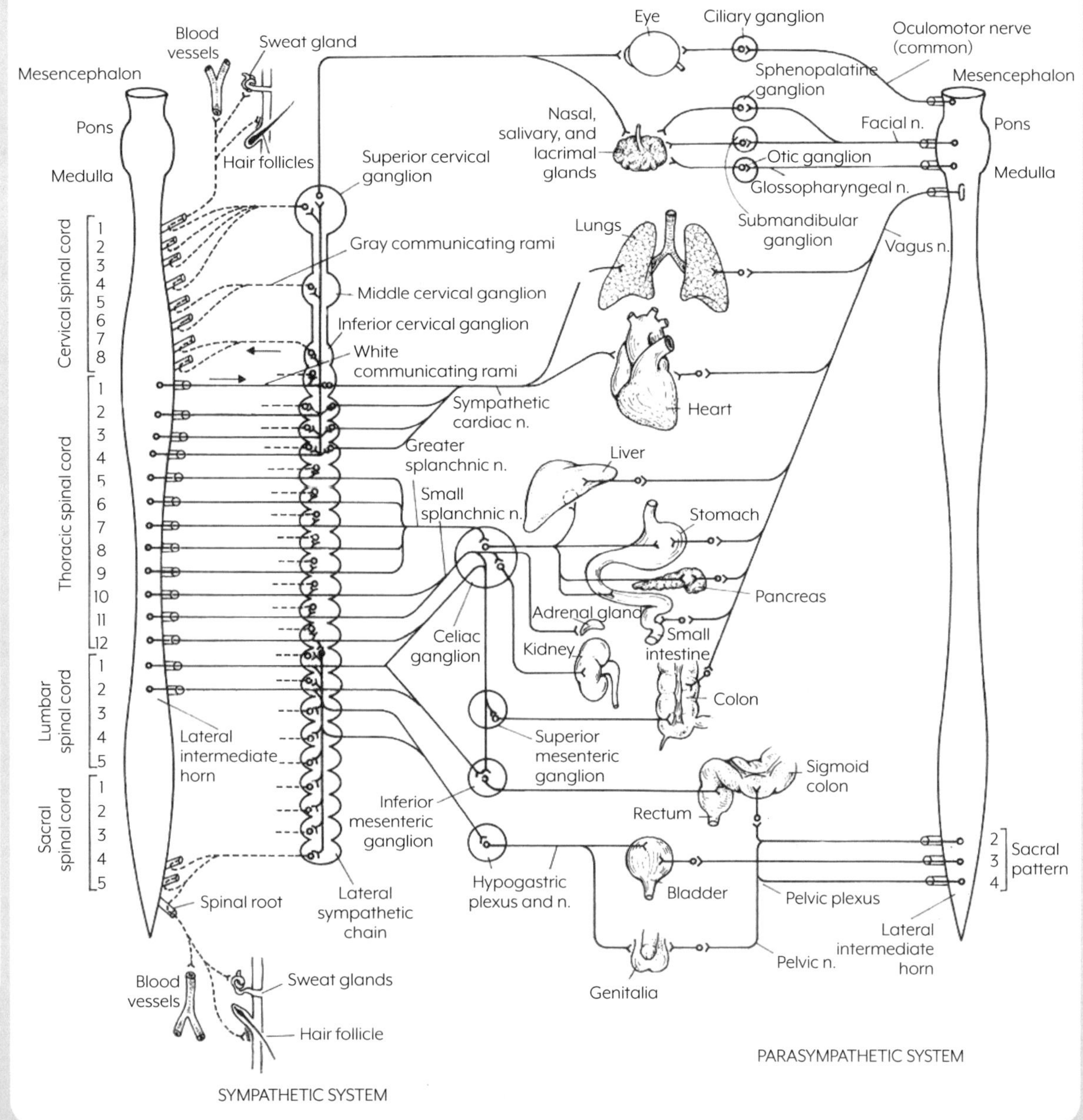

Figure 22.2

Fibers of the sympathetic and parasympathetic system (courtesy of Prof. M. Manfredi).

The enteric nervous system is considered the third part of the autonomic nervous system. Neurons of the enteric nervous system are interconnected and organized into reflex circuits capable of controlling various digestive activities (motility, secretion/absorption, circulation).

The autonomic nervous system produces its effects through the release of neurotransmitters. The preganglionic neuron of the sympathetic and parasympathetic systems releases acetylcholine, parasympathetic postganglionic fibers utilize acetylcholine, while sympathetic postganglionic fibers use norepinephrine, ATP (Adenosine 5-triphosphate), and numerous other neuropeptides.

22.2 Functions regulated by the autonomic nervous system

Thermoregulation | The regulation of body temperature involves a control system equipped with sensors and effectors. Body temperature sensors are located in the skin, deep tissues, and within the central nervous system. Warmth receptors are free unmyelinated C fibers activated by skin temperatures ranging from 30 to 50°C. Cold receptors are A-delta and C fibers activated by temperatures ranging from 10 to 40°C. The hypothalamus utilizes endocrine, behavioral, and autonomic systems to modify heat flow to and from the external environment.

Cardiovascular activity | The heart receives both parasympathetic and sympathetic innervation. The cell bodies of parasympathetic neurons that innervate the heart are located in the nucleus ambiguus and the dorsal motor nucleus of the vagus in the bulb region. Axons from the vagus nerve nucleus become part of the cardiac plexus at the thoracic level and form synapses with neurons in the intracardiac ganglia. Short parasympathetic postganglionic neurons then emerge from the intracardiac ganglia and innervate the myocardial muscle tissue. Sympathetic innervation of the heart originates from neurons in the intermediolateral columns of the spinal cord at the T1-T4 levels. Axons from sympathetic neurons form synapses with sympathetic postganglionic neurons at the stellate ganglion, which join with preganglionic parasympathetic neurons to form the cardiac plexus. Sympathetic neurons innervate the sinoatrial and atrioventricular nodes, the conduction system, and the cardiac muscle fibers at the ventricular level. Arteries, veins of the systemic circulation, as well as the adrenal glands and kidneys, are primarily under the control of the sympathetic system. Therefore, the sympathetic system exerts widespread control over vascular and cardiac activity.

Respiratory system | The autonomic system controls the caliber of the respiratory airways and regulates the tone of smooth muscles, blood flow in the airways, and bronchial mucus secretion. The innervation of the respiratory airways consists of cholinergic transmission in parasympathetic nerves, noradrenergic transmission in sympathetic nerves, and glutamatergic transmission in sensory fibers. Afferent nerve pathways of the respiratory tract pass through the vagus nerve. The cell bodies of these fibers are located in the nodose and jugular ganglia, which transmit information to the nucleus of the solitary tract in the brainstem. Sensory fibers exhibit baseline tonic activity that regulates respiratory function and plays a primary role in reflex defense mechanisms in response to inhaled noxious agents, foreign bodies, or inflammatory mediators.

Gastrointestinal tract | The dorsal nucleus of the vagus innervates the entire gastrointestinal tract, except for the proximal esophagus, distal colon, and rectum. The vagus nerve increases propulsive motility, sphincter relaxation, and secretion from the exocrine and endocrine glands of the stomach, intestine, pancreas, and liver. The sympathetic system consists of preganglionic nerves originating from the T1-L1 segments of the spinal cord, which, through the splanchnic nerves, reach the mesenteric and celiac ganglia and exert an inhibitory action on intestinal motility. The modulatory actions of the sympathetic and parasympathetic systems occur through the enteric nervous system, which is located in the intestinal wall.

Bladder, rectum, and sexual organs | Bladder function is controlled by three segmental circuits: the sacral parasympathetic system, the lumbar sympathetic system, and the somatic system. Sacral parasympathetic action (S2-S4) is carried out by pelvic nerves and mediated by cholinergic muscarinic receptors. Parasympathetic nerves promote bladder emptying by contracting the detrusor muscle and relaxing the internal urethral sphincter. Lumbar sympathetic fibers (T11-L2) relax the detrusor muscle and contract the internal urethral sphincter, thereby promoting bladder filling. The sacral somatic system (S2-S4, Onuf's nucleus) consists of pudendal nerves, which contract the external urethral sphincter and promote bladder filling. In healthy individuals, the segmental circuits mediating the micturition reflex are under the control of brainstem structures through a spinopontospinal circuit. The spinopontospinal circuit's function is to coordinate the simultaneous activation of the sacral parasympathetic system and inhibition of somatic neurons for the external urethral sphincter, allowing synergistic contraction of the detrusor muscle and relaxation of the external urethral sphincter during micturition. The control of micturition also relies on the integrity of a complex neural circuit, including the Pontine Micturition Center (located in the pontine reticular formation), the L-region, the periaqueductal gray matter, the hypothalamus, the insula, the cingulate gyrus cortex, the prefrontal cortex, the inferior frontal gyrus, and the preoptic nucleus. Bladder filling information is transmitted from bladder afferents to the periaqueductal gray matter, which informs the Pontine Micturition Center about the degree of bladder filling, serving as an important integration and control station for micturition. The periaqueductal gray matter is also connected to the thalamus, cingulate gyrus, insula, and prefrontal cortex, which are involved in conscious visceral sensation processing and responsible for the "social" behavior of micturition control (Figure 22.3). Afferents from the sigmoid colon and rectum pass through the pelvic nerves to the sacral center (S2-S4), while the anal mucosa

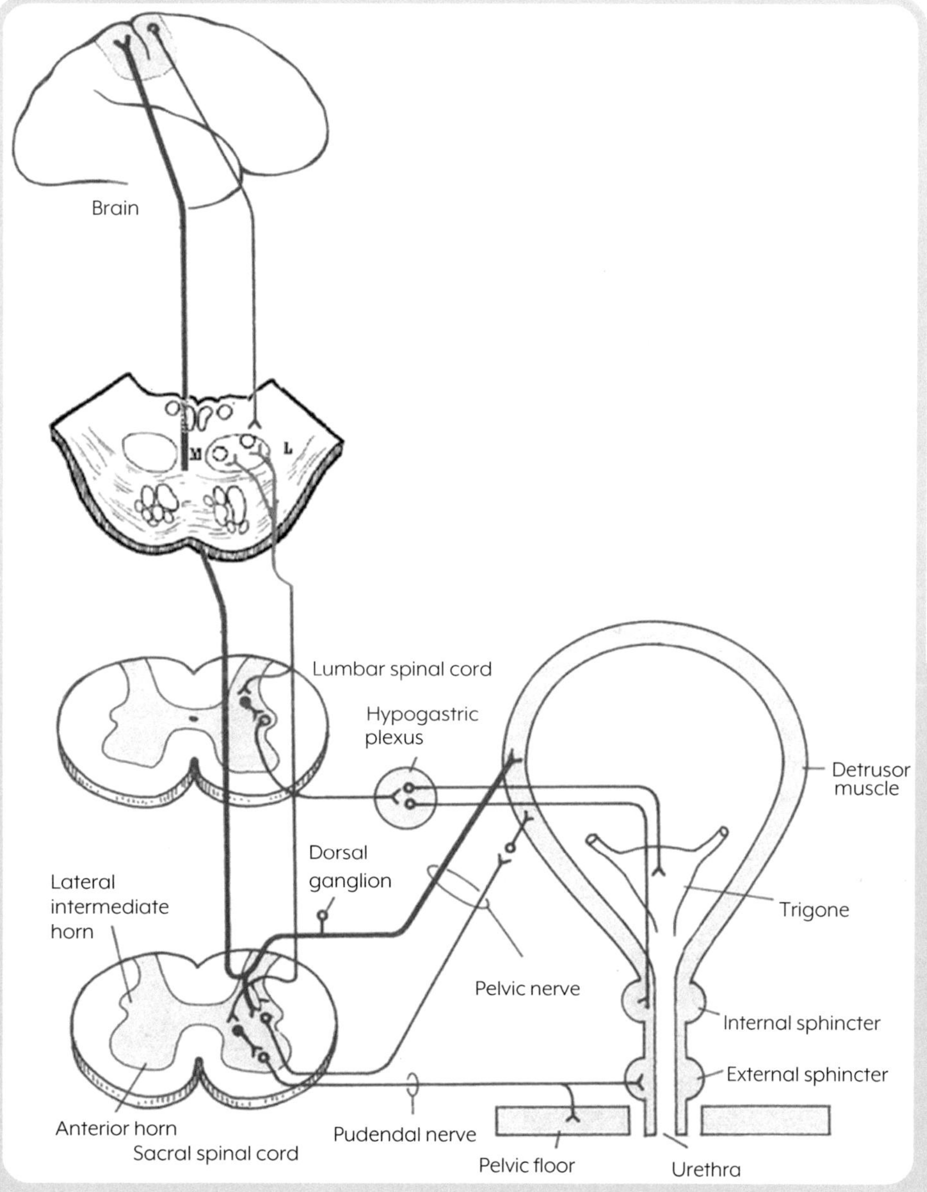

Figure 22.3

Nervous circuits for the control of micturition. Thick lines represent the nerve pathways that transmit information from the bladder afferents to higher centers (cerebral areas and brainstem nuclei). Thin lines represent the descending nerve pathways from cerebral areas to the detrusor muscle and external urethral sphincter muscle.

is innervated by the somatic system through the pudendal nerves. The motor innervation of the rectal walls and internal anal sphincter is dual and represented by the S2-S4 segments of the parasympathetic system, through the pelvic nerves with synapses in the parietal ganglia of the myenteric plexus, and the L1-L2 sympathetic system, through the hypogastric plexus with synapses in the inferior mesenteric ganglion. The parasympathetic system activates parietal peristalsis and inhibits the tone of the internal anal sphincter, while the sympathetic system produces opposite effects. The external anal sphincter is innervated by the somatic system through the pudendal nerves (S2-S4). Under normal conditions, sigmoid colon and rectal filling occur due to colonic peristalsis. Evacuation occurs under voluntary control through the activation of the abdominal wall muscles and the relaxation of the external anal sphincter.

In men, penile erection is a neurovascular phenomenon consisting of two mechanisms: psychogenic erection, initiated in supraspinal centers in response to visual, auditory, olfactory stimuli and generated by imagination, mediated by autonomic stimuli, and reflex erection, facilitated by tactile stimulation in the genital area and mediated by the reflex arc composed of somatic afferent and parasympathetic efferent fibers (S2-S4). The autonomic nervous system modulates the relaxation of intracavernous smooth muscle fibers and plays a fundamental role at the onset and during the maintenance of erection. The somatic nervous system is necessary for the perception of sensory stimuli and the completion of penile rigidity through the contraction of the ischiocavernosus and bulbocavernosus muscles. Seminal emission is mediated by the thoracolumbar sympathetic system, which activates the peristaltic contraction of the epididymis, vas deferens, and seminal vesicles, and by the somatic system (pudendal nerve), which, through the contraction of the pelvic floor muscles, expels the seminal fluid from the urethra. In women, afferent innervation from the clitoral mucosa, external genitalia, and anterior vaginal wall is mediated by the somatic system, as is the efferent innervation of the pelvic floor musculature. Efferent innervation related to tubal, uterine, and vaginal muscular structures is mediated by the thoracolumbar sympathetic system and the hypogastric plexus, while vaginal glands and blood vessels are innervated by the sacral parasympathetic system and pelvic nerves.

22.3 Clinically relevant autonomic symptoms

Alterations in the autonomic nervous system typically manifest with symptoms and signs related to both the sympathetic and parasympathetic systems. Generally, alterations in sweating, lipotimic manifestations, or syncope during postural changes predominantly indicate sympathetic dysfunction, while ocular and oral dryness, nausea, vomiting, constipation, and diarrhea predominantly indicate parasympathetic dysfunction. Sphincter and erectile alterations involve both the sympathetic and parasympathetic systems, as well as disruptions in control mechanisms within central nervous system structures.

In summary, symptoms and signs related to different systems and suggestive of a primary autonomic nervous system disorder include:

- Cardiovascular System: dizziness, blurred vision, and in severe cases, reduced or loss of consciousness; clinostatic hypertension partly due to baroreceptor hypersensitivity; and arrhythmias.
- Respiratory System: bronchospasm and sleep apnea.
- Genitourinary System: nocturia urgency, urinary incontinence, retention, impotence, and anorgasmia.
- Gastrointestinal System: constipation, diarrhea, and fecal incontinence.
- Skin: hyperhidrosis, hypohidrosis, anhidrosis, trophic disorders, and vasomotor disorders.
- Eyes: alterations in pupillary diameter and lacrimation disturbances.

22.4 Investigative methods

Regarding the *cardiovascular system*, the functionality of the sympathetic system is primarily assessed by monitoring blood pressure changes during postural modifications

(*Head-up tilt* and active orthostasis), exercise (*hand grip*) and temperature changes (*cold pressor test*). *Head-up tilt* involves passively tilting the patient to an inclination of 60-70° and maintaining this position for a variable duration of approximately 3 to 30 minutes. The active orthostatic test is performed with the patient in an upright position with the feet resting on the examination table. *Hand grip* is a test of sympathetic system function in which the patient is asked to forcefully grip a pressure cuff with their hands for about one minute, while blood pressure is monitored. Blood pressure is measured before and after the exercise. The *cold pressor test* is less commonly used in clinical practice and involves applying ice to the patient's hand for one minute while measuring blood pressure before and after the application.

Assessment of parasympathetic function is performed by monitoring heart rate during respiratory maneuvers (deep breathing, Valsalva maneuver, and hyperventilation). Deep breathing involves instructing the patient to inhale deeply for approximately 6 seconds and exhale for another 6 seconds, with a total duration of one minute. Under normal conditions, deep inhalation reduces the RR interval on the ECG, while exhalation increases it. Changes in heart rate induced by breathing reflect vagal tone. The Valsalva maneuver involves asking the patient to forcefully exhale against a closed glottis using a mouth-piece connected to a sphygmomanometer, maintaining a pressure of approximately 40 mmHg for about 10-15 seconds. Under normal conditions, the Valsalva maneuver results in reduced blood pressure, reflex tachycardia, and peripheral vasoconstriction followed by bradycardia. Heart rate is recorded at rest, during the strain, and for the 45 seconds following the maneuver, and the Valsalva ratio (maximum frequency during Valsalva/ minimum frequency recorded during the subsequent 45 seconds) is calculated. During hyperventilation, the patient is asked to hyperventilate for one minute, and the increase in heart rate is recorded.

There are other instrumental investigation methods available for the cardiovascular system. Nuclear imaging techniques use various radiotracers, including beta emitters for positron emission tomography (PET) and gamma emitters for scintigraphic studies (SPECT), such as 123I-MIBG. PET provides regional quantification of tracer uptake and has higher spatial and temporal resolution compared to SPECT. MIBG is readily available in all nuclear medicine centers for routine clinical use. These techniques are currently used in the differential diagnosis of parkinsonian syndromes.

A standardized test used in clinical practice to evaluate the *thermoregulatory function* of the autonomic nervous system is the sympathetic skin response (SSR). It measures the integrity of the sympathetic circuitry involved in sweating. The SSR is recorded using surface electrodes placed on the palm of the hand or sole of the foot (active electrode) and on the back of the hand or foot (reference electrode). It is typically evoked by sudden electrical stimuli, with an interval of more than 30 seconds between stimuli to account for habituation. The presence or absence of the response is evaluated. The thermoregulatory sweating test, performed using the colorimetric method of Minor, provides qualitative information about the distribution and extent of sweating. A solution of iodine and alcohol is applied to the patient's body, and rice starch powder is spread on the moist areas. The patient is placed in a warm environment to induce generalized sweating. The increase in sweating is evaluated, and pathological findings may include distal anhidrosis, segmental anhidrosis, loss of local sweating, global anhidrosis, and regional anhidrosis.

Respiratory system | Abnormalities can be investigated using laryngoscopy and sleep studies to detect any apnea or oxygen desaturation phenomena.

For the evaluation of the *genitourinary system's integrity* laboratory tests (such as daytime and nighttime fractional diuresis, sodium and potassium excretion), radiological tests (ultrasound of the kidneys and urinary tract, urography), and functional tests (urodynamic examination, electromyography of the anal sphincter, penile plethysmography) are used. Urodynamic examination is a diagnostic test that allows the analysis of filling volumes and pressures during the cystomanometric phase and emptying during the voiding phase. This examination helps differentiate bladder dysfunction due to central nervous system or peripheral nervous system pathologies.

Gastrointestinal disorders | They can be investigated using radiological studies with barium meal, videocinefluoroscopy, endoscopy, and gastric emptying studies.

In cases of *sexual dysfunction*, it is advisable to evaluate the profile of sex hormones (androgens, prolactin, LH, FSH) and perform more in-depth instrumental examinations, such as monitoring of nocturnal erections, transrectal prostate ultrasound, electromyography of the cavernous bodies, and penile arterial-venous Doppler. Erectile dysfunction can have organic causes (vascular diseases, diabetes, medications, endocrine imbalances, neurological conditions, trauma) and psychological causes.

Finally, the Schirmer test and pharmacological tests are useful for evaluating pupillary innervation.

22.5 Diseases of the autonomic nervous system

Disorders of the autonomic nervous system can be classified as primary when no specific cause is identified or secondary when there is an underlying pathology responsible for the autonomic dysfunction. An alternative classification distinguishes dysautonomic syndromes as acute, subacute, or chronic. Autonomic nervous system dysfunctions can also be either diffuse or limited to a specific region of autonomic innervation.

22.5.1 Primary autonomic nervous system diseases

Primary autonomic dysfunctions can be further categorized into acute-subacute and chronic forms. Acute and subacute forms include pure cholinergic dysautonomia, pure pandysautonomia, and pandysautonomia with neurological deficits. The etiology is not well understood, but there is evidence suggesting a post-viral autoimmune pathogenesis. Pure cholinergic dysautonomia is characterized by clinical signs resulting from dysfunction of the cholinergic transmission of the sympathetic and parasympathetic nervous systems, such as alacrimia, xerostomia, dysphagia, atonic colon, anhidrosis, urinary disturbances, and in males, erectile dysfunction. The two forms of pandysautonomia involve the global dysfunction of both sympathetic and parasympathetic pathways, with the form accompanied by neurological deficits showing signs of peripheral nerve involvement.

Chronic primary autonomic dysfunctions include pure autonomic failure (PAF), a chronic disease involving the sympathetic and parasympathetic nervous systems without other neurological symptoms; multiple system atrophy (MSA); and autonomic failure associated with Parkinson's disease, where autonomic dysfunction coexists with dysfunction of other neural circuits. The common pathophysiological element in these three forms is the degeneration of sympathetic nervous system cells in the intermediolateral column of the thoracic and lumbar spinal cord. PAF also shows degeneration of cells in the sympathetic paravertebral ganglia. Lewy bodies have been found in surviving ganglion cells, which is not observed in MSA cases. The clinical manifestations of PAF, primarily due to peripheral dysfunction, include orthostatic syncope, sweating disorders, urinary urgency, sphincter incontinence, male impotence, and female anorgasmia, which are generally stable. In MSA, the degenerative process primarily affects brain structures, along with the degeneration of the intermediolateral column of the thoracic-lumbar spinal cord and neurons of the sacral II and III anterior horn (Onuf's nucleus). In MSA, widespread cerebral alterations are observed, including involvement of the putamen, substantia nigra, and *locus coeruleus* in the parkinsonian form, as well as the pons and middle cerebellar peduncle in the olivopontocerebellar form. Additionally, the thalamus, vestibular nuclei, hypothalamus, and dorsal motor nucleus of the vagus are affected. MSA is characterized by the presence of glial cytoplasmic inclusions originating from alpha-synuclein-containing proteins. Clinical manifestations in MSA are progressive, with autonomic dysfunction typically appearing in the early stages of the disease. Autonomic dysfunction associated with Parkinson's disease can affect various systems, although it primarily affects the cardiovascular system.

22.5.2 Secondary autonomic nervous system diseases

Secondary autonomic nervous system diseases are due to associated or causal pathologies. Manifestations of secondary autonomic dysfunction can result from involvement of central nervous system structures (hypothalamus, brainstem, and spinal cord) and the peripheral nervous system. Diseases affecting the autonomic structures in the central nervous system include hypothalamic dysfunctions caused by primary hypothalamic disorders or focal lesions in the hypothalamic region (cranial trauma, pituitary surgery, tumors in the sellar region, hydrocephalus, basal meningitis, encephalitis, Hand-Schuller-Christian disease). Among the hypothalamic syndromes with effects on the autonomic nervous system, we have diabetes insipidus, characterized by altered antidiuretic hormone secretion leading to polyuria (daily diuresis up to 3-15 liters) and increased thirst; the syndrome of inappropriate antidiuretic hormone secretion, characterized by decreased diuresis, hypertonic urine, water retention, weight gain, and hyponatremia (< 130 mEq/L); and eating disorders resulting from hypothalamic organic pathologies, characterized by decreased or increased thirst (adipsia, polydipsia) or hunger (anorexia, bulimia). The posterior hypothalamus controls thermoregulation through heat production and dissipation. The upper limit of tolerable body temperature for a few hours (causing a confused state) is 42°C. Beyond this limit, irreversible damage to the central nervous system occurs. The lower limit is 26°C, below which death from ventricular fibrillation occurs. Hypothalamic lesions, particularly those following neurosurgical interventions, can cause fluctuations in body temperature. Lesions in the anterior hypothalamic region result in a lack of heat dissipation mechanisms (central neurogenic hyperthermia), while lesions in the posterior hypothalamic region can lead to hypothermia.

Pathologies of the brainstem can affect the nucleus tractus solitarius and its connections and can be secondary to brainstem tumors, Arnold-Chiari malformations, and syringobulbia. The typical clinical manifestation is postural hypotension or syncope following coughing or sneezing.

Acute spinal cord injuries involving the segments above D6 can result in alterations in blood pressure regulation, most commonly hypotension, and urinary disturbances. In chronic phases of spinal cord injury, hypertensive crises induced by painful stimuli may occur.

Secondary autonomic syndromes associated with peripheral nervous system diseases include neuropathies, both hereditary and acquired. Hereditary neuropathies are rare conditions characterized by alterations in sensory and autonomic fibers. Patients may experience ulcers, mutilations, fractures (due to lack of pain sensation), orthostatic hypotension, reduced sweating, and absence of tear production. Among the hereditary forms is familial amyloid neuropathy, which involves autonomic fiber dysfunction (diarrhea, impotence, etc.). Acquired neuropathies include diabetic neuropathy, alcoholic neuropathy, neuropathy in patients with amyloidosis, Sjogren's syndrome, systemic lupus erythematosus, rheumatoid arthritis, paraneoplastic syndromes (associated with anti-Hu antibodies), and those receiving chemotherapy. Involvement of autonomic fibers in secondary neuropathies due to infections can occur in conditions such as AIDS (HIV-1) and Chagas disease. More recently, autonomic symptoms have been observed during and up to six months after SARS-CoV-2 infection. The most frequently reported symptoms include dizziness, orthostatic headache, syncope, hyperhidrosis, and burning pains.

Autonomic fiber alterations can also be observed during immunomediated inflammatory processes such as acute inflammatory polyradiculoneuropathies (e.g., Guillain-Barré syndrome), which present clinical manifestations related to the cardiovascular (tachycardia, transient hypertension, cardiac arrhythmias), sudomotor, and gastrointestinal systems. Autonomic fiber involvement is generally observed in the later stages of acquired neuropathies.

22.5.3 Diseases of the autonomic nervous system: district disorders

Cardiovascular system dysfunction

Orthostatic hypotension | Orthostatic hypotension is defined as a sustained reduction in systolic blood pressure of at least 20 mmHg or diastolic blood pressure of at least 10 mmHg, within 3 minutes of assuming an upright position from lying down (or during prolonged orthostatic position or *during neurovegetative tests* in a head-up tilt of at least 60° on a tilting bed). The severity of orthostatic hypotension depends on the baseline blood pressure. Under physiological conditions, immediately after assuming the upright position, there is a redistribution of plasma volume due to gravity, resulting in an accumulation of approximately 300-800ml of blood in the lower limbs and splanchnic venous system. Venous return to the heart and cardiac filling pressure decrease, leading to a reduction in cardiac output. Consequently, sympathetic activity in the heart and blood vessels increases, while vagal cardiac activity decreases. These autonomic mechanisms increase vascular tone, heart rate, and cardiac contractility, stabilizing blood pressure. In cases of orthostatic hypotension, there is a dysfunction in the vasoconstrictor mechanisms or an excessive reduction in blood pressure. Orthostatic hypotension syndrome is observed in patients with multiple system atrophy (MSA), Parkinson's disease, and pure autonomic failure (PAF), and can be caused by certain medications (such as L-dopa and alpha-blockers). Orthostatic hypotension can also occur in patients with peripheral neuropathies secondary to conditions such as diabetes mellitus, liver cirrhosis, and alcoholism. Clinical symptoms of orthostatic hypotension are related to reduced cerebral blood flow and can range from mild dizziness, blurred vision, and sweating (lightheadedness) to loss of consciousness (syncope). These symptoms can occur suddenly and transiently, leading to falls. Orthostatic hypotension often occurs in the morning (due to increased nighttime diuresis and depletion of intravascular volume during sleep), after large carbohydrate-rich meals, after alcohol consumption, due to age-related changes in baroreceptor sensitivity, and as a side effect of certain medications (such as sympatholytic agents, tricyclic antidepressants, antiparkinsonian drugs, diuretics, and vasodilators). In some cases of orthostatic hypotension associated with dysautonomic syndromes, there may be the occurrence of hypertension in the supine position due to impaired baroreceptor control. In such cases, treatment for orthostatic hypotension may worsen blood pressure values in the supine position. The therapeutic approach to orthostatic hypotension involves the administration of fludrocortisone to increase salt and water retention, midodrine, pyridostigmine, sympathomimetic drugs, and, in cases of inadequate response to the first two, desmopressin. Octreotide, a somatostatin analogue, inhibits the release of certain intestinal peptides that mediate postprandial hypotension due to splanchnic blood pooling. In addition to pharmacological treatment, the use of compression stockings, abdominal binders, and moderation in meal size is recommended.

Postural orthostatic tachycardia syndrome (POTS) | Postural orthostatic tachycardia syndrome is characterized by a sustained increase in heart rate of ≥30 beats per minute (≥40 beats per minute for individuals under 20 years of age) or a heart rate of ≥120 beats per minute within the first 10 minutes of assuming an upright position or during a tilt test, without classic orthostatic hypotension. There may be a slight decrease in blood pressure. The etiology and pathophysiology of this disorder are unknown. It can occur following viral infections, such as SARS-CoV-2 infection, and chronic fatigue syndrome. Differential diagnosis should exclude tachycardia due to hyperthyroidism, cardiac rhythm disturbances, pheochromocytoma, adrenal insufficiency, anxiety disorder, dehydration, and medications (vasodilators, beta-adrenergic agents, diuretics). Symptoms include blurred vision, palpitations, tremors, weakness, exercise intolerance, shortness of breath, chest pain, nausea, tachypnea, cool extremities, and difficulty concentrating. These symptoms worsen with minimal physical exertion and resolve in the supine position. Treatment of postural orthostatic tachycardia syndrome includes the use of fludrocortisone, midodrine, and cardioselective beta-blockers (such as bisoprolol). Ephedrine is contraindicated due to its tachycardic effects.

Syncope | Syncope is defined as a transient loss of consciousness and postural tone, usually associated with falling to the ground, due to global and sudden cerebral hypoperfusion (reduction in cerebral blood flow below 30 ml/100 g/min) with spontaneous and complete recovery without neurological sequelae. Syncope is typically preceded by prodromal symptoms and signs that occur within 60 seconds of loss of consciousness and include pallor, sweating, nausea, yawning, and hyperventilation. These symptoms are followed by visual and auditory disturbances, difficulty concentrating, and ideomotor slowing.

Syncope can be classified based on the underlying pathophysiological mechanism as *neurally mediated syncope*, *cardiogenic syncope* due to arrhythmic or structural heart diseases, and *orthostatic syncope*. Neurally mediated syncope can occur during various conditions where the triggering factor can be central (emotions, pain, fear of blood) or peripheral (prolonged standing, increased carotid sinus stimulation, peripheral vasodilation due to heat exposure). Neurally mediated syncope can also occur in healthy individuals; therefore, it should be distinguished from syncope occurring in patients with orthostatic hypotension due to chronic autonomic failure. Specific forms of neurally mediated syncope include situational syncope that occurs during specific situations such as urination, defecation, or coughing, as well as during prolonged upright posture. Vasovagal syncope is more common in young individuals than in the elderly. Causes include pain, intense emotional situations, and certain gastrointestinal conditions (e.g., fecal impaction and diarrhea). Cardiogenic syncope is caused by cardiovascular disorders (cardiac arrhythmias, valvular heart diseases, myocardial infarction, obstructive cardiomyopathies). In cases of cardiogenic syncope, which is associated with cardiac rhythm disturbances, prodromal lightheadedness may not occur, and the patient may experience an immediate loss of consciousness. Differential diagnosis should consider other causes of loss of consciousness, such as epilepsy. Orthostatic syncope occurs when there is a failure of cardiovascular adjustment during the transition from lying down to standing up. The normal response to assuming the upright position is characterized by a slight reduction in systolic blood pressure (approximately 10mmHg), a slight increase in diastolic blood pressure, and an increase in heart rate (10-20 beats per minute). In patients with orthostatic hypotension due to neurodegenerative diseases, syncope episodes may not be preceded by the clinical manifestations associated with the normal sympathetic adrenergic discharge, and they are referred to as fixed-rate syncope. For neurally mediated syncope in healthy individuals with isolated and sporadic episodes, treatment is not indicated. Patients should be instructed to recognize the symptoms and perform maneuvers to prevent syncope or reduce its duration (e.g., assuming the Trendelenburg position). In cases of recurrent syncopal episodes, vasoconstrictor medications (midodrine, ephedrine), theophylline, selective serotonin reuptake inhibitors (fluoxetine, paroxetine, droxidopa, pyridostigmine) are useful in clinical practice. For cardiogenic syncope, treatment aims to correct the underlying cardiac disorder. In the treatment of orthostatic syncope, in addition to the medications used for orthostatic hypotension, the placement of an on-demand cardiac pacemaker may be indicated in cases where a cardioinhibitory component predominates.

Genitourinary dysfunction

Neurogenic Bladder | Neurogenic bladder refers to the alteration of bladder-sphincter regulation mechanisms caused by documented neurological pathology. The severity and characteristics of urinary dysfunction are determined by the location and extent of the neurological lesion. Neurogenic bladder can result from suprapontine, suprasacral-subpontine, or sacral/peripheral spinal cord lesions.

Suprapontine neurogenic bladder | It is the consequence of lesions in both cerebral hemispheres, particularly in the frontal lobes (multi-infarct encephalopathy, cerebral atrophy, tumors, brain trauma, hydrocephalus) or basal ganglia (Parkinson's disease and multiple system atrophy [MSA]). Cerebral involvement leads to a reduction in inhibitory control exerted under normal conditions on the pontine micturition center, resulting in uncontrolled detrusor activity known as "neurogenic detrusor overactivity." Patients experience uninhibited detrusor contractions that lead to increased frequency of micturition, reduced ability to delay micturition after the initial urge (urgency), and urgency urinary incontinence. The post-void residual volume, i.e., the amount of urine remaining in the bladder after urination, is absent or insignificant (less than 80 ml). Urinary disturbances in patients with Parkinson's disease generally occur in the later stages of the disease and are related to depletion of dopaminergic neurons in the substantia nigra and subsequent reduction in striatal dopamine. This results in detrusor overactivity secondary to reduced tonic D1-mediated inhibitory activity. An alternative hypothesis is the presence of a neurotransmitter imbalance in neurons that facilitate the pontine micturition center, such as the ventral tegmental area, leading to pollakiuria (urination at low bladder volumes), nocturia (repeated nighttime urination), and urinary urgency. In addition to detrusor overactivity, patients with Parkinson's disease also exhibit delayed relaxation of the perineal muscles at the beginning of micturition (bradykinesia of the striated external urethral sphincter) and impaired detrusor contractility, secondary to antiparkinsonian pharmacotherapy, which can cause partial urinary retention. In patients with MSA, urinary dysfunction is generally present from the onset of the disease. In MSA, structures such as the pontine micturition center, striatum, substantia nigra, cerebellar vermis, lateral intermediate sacral nucleus, Onuf nucleus, and postganglionic cholinergic fibers are believed to be damaged. Urinary disturbances in patients with MSA are characterized by detrusor hyperactivity in the early stages of the disease, reflecting central damage, and detrusor hypocontractility in the advanced stages of the disease, reflecting peripheral damage. Patients experience urinary urgency, urge urinary incontinence, and incomplete bladder emptying, progressing to complete urinary retention. In the early stages of the disease, the post-void residual is usually low, but it often exceeds 100 ml as the disease progresses, surpassing the threshold value for considering urinary catheterization.

Suprasacral-subpontine neurogenic bladder | Suprasacral-subpontine neurogenic bladder can result from spinal cord lesions above the sacral segments and is seen in demyelinating lesions associated with multiple sclerosis or transverse myelitis, traumatic or vascular injuries (due to arteriovenous malformations and spinal cord ischemia), neoplasms, and spondylogenic spinal cord lesions. Urinary dysfunction, regardless of the etiology of the spinal cord lesion, clinically manifests differently in the various phases of the disease. During the acute phase, known as spinal shock (up to 6-12 weeks after the injury), urinary retention occurs due to the lack of detrusor contractility. In this phase, the patient is unable to empty the bladder, and overflow incontinence may occur. Following the spinal shock phase, a chronic suprasacral-subpontine neurogenic bladder develops, characterized by detrusor hyperactivity, detrusor-sphincter dyssynergia, and a significant post-void residual. If the spinal cord lesion is above the D6 level, bladder emptying may be associated with neurovegetative symptoms of sympathetic hyperactivity, such as autonomic dysreflexia (sweating, piloerection, hypertensive crisis). The presence of detrusor-sphincter dyssynergia leads to high-pressure bladder filling and possible vesicoureteral reflux, hydronephrosis, and urosepsis.

Sacral and/or peripheral neurogenic bladder | Spinal cord lesions affecting the sacral segments result in complex clinical manifestations. Symptoms can resemble those of a suprasacral neurogenic bladder (neurogenic detrusor overactivity) or more commonly, they can reflect involvement of the S2-S4 reflex integration center at the spinal cord level, as well as the peripheral afferent and efferent fibers (detrusor underactivity). All lesions that damage the afferent and efferent pathways of the bladder lead to urinary retention due to the absence of sensory information regarding bladder filling, resulting in an inability to initiate voluntary and reflex voiding or insufficient detrusor contractility. Neurological conditions that affect the sacral reflex arc (afferent and efferent pathways and sacral segments) include trauma, myelodysplasia, diabetes, disc herniation, and neuropathies. The most common clinical manifestation is urinary retention, with possible overflow incontinence due to bladder distention and overcoming the resistance offered by the often hypotonic external urethral sphincter, which may be affected by concomitant involvement of the sacral somatic system. Bladder distention can also lead to renal dilatation, even in the absence of vesicoureteral reflux, due to bladder overdistention. Excessive bladder distention causes detrusor muscle fatigue and increased susceptibility to recurrent urinary tract infections due to urine stasis. In cases where sacral neurogenic bladder occurs as part of cauda equina syndrome and S2-S4 root involvement, urinary disturbances may be accompanied by painful symptoms, such as dolorific and tactile anesthesia in the perineal and urethral regions, as well as muscle weakness in the lower limbs innervated by the cauda equina roots.

The *first-line therapeutic* approach for detrusor overactivity involves the use of antimuscarinic drugs that block parasympathetic innervation at the M2 and M3 muscarinic receptors of the detrusor muscle. The central nervous system side effects of anticholinergic drugs are limited when tolterodine and trospium chloride are administered, as they have lower lipophilic activity compared to traditional antimuscarinics (thus, they are not expected to pass the blood-brain barrier). Recently, intradetrusor injection of botulinum toxin has been introduced for patients who have an inadequate clinical response to conventional antimuscarinic therapy. Botulinum toxin appears to improve detrusor overactivity by acting on bladder efferent and afferent pathways. In cases of underactive detrusor in patients with a post-void residual greater than 100 ml, intermittent catheterization is the treatment of choice.

Bowel dysfunction

Neurological causes of fecal incontinence can result from alterations in the central nervous system (multi-infarct and degenerative encephalopathy, demyelinating diseases, spinal cord lesions, neoplasms) and the peripheral nervous system (pudendal neuropathy, neuropathies in diabetes mellitus). Unlike urinary control, in cases of spinal cord lesions and cauda equina root involvement, the intrinsic activity of the peristaltic muscles is able to maintain

Table 22.2 CLINICAL AND URODYNAMIC PATTERNS ASSOCIATED WITH NEUROLOGICAL BLADDER

Circuit involved by the neurological pathology	Clinical picture	Urodynamic pattern	Treatment
Suprapontine cerebral circuit	Increased urinary frequency, pollakiuria, nocturia, urgency, urgency incontinence	Detrusor overactivity with detrusor-sphincter synergy, reduced bladder capacity	Behavioral therapy; antimuscarinics; desmopressin; Intradetrusor botulinum toxin type A; β3 adrenergic agonists (limited evidence); Neuromodulation through tibial nerve stimulation (limited evidence)
Spino-ponto-spinal circuit (subpontine-suprasacral level)	Increased urinary frequency, pollakiuria, urinary urgency, incontinence due to low bladder filling levels, abdominal straining incomplete bladder emptying	Detrusor overactivity with detrusor-sphincter dyssynergia	Intermittent catheterization, Alpha-blockers; botulinum toxin type A in the external urethral sphincter
Sacral segmental circuit	Urinary retention, overflow incontinence, abundant postvoid residual volume	Detrusor underactivity	Intermittent catheterization

adequate continence/evacuation function. In cases of suprasacral spinal cord lesions, automatic intestinal activity maintains continence, but loss of voluntary control over the external anal sphincter leads to spontaneous defecation. In cases of bilateral somatic system lesions (pudendal nerves), fecal incontinence occurs due to insufficient function of the external anal sphincter.

Sexual dysfunction

Erectile dysfunction is defined as the inability to achieve and/or maintain an erection sufficient for satisfactory sexual intercourse. Warning signs for the onset of likely sexual impotence include poor or absent morning or nocturnal erections, occasional sexual failures, the need for increasingly intense sexual stimuli, a long interval between sexual stimulation and erection, unstable erection during intercourse, poor rigidity, premature ejaculation, and penile pain during erection. Neurological causes of erectile dysfunction can be categorized as lesions of the central nervous system (intracranial: hypothalamic dysfunction, cortical atrophy, degenerative diseases of the basal ganglia; suprasacral spinal cord: multiple sclerosis, compressive lesions, trauma) and the peripheral nervous system (cauda equina syndrome from disc herniation, caudal dysraphism, vascular malformations, pelvic pathologies secondary to trauma or surgery; peripheral neuropathy from diabetes, alcohol abuse, autonomic neuropathies, etc.). Sexual dysfunction is also present in patients with basal ganglia disorders (Parkinson's disease and MSA). The most common sexual dysfunctions in these cases include decreased libido and frequency of sexual intercourse, reduced orgasm, erectile dysfunction, and ejaculation disorders. Treatment involves the use of phosphodiesterase type 5 inhibitors (such as sildenafil citrate, vardenafil, and tadalafil), which inhibit the enzyme responsible for cGMP degradation.

In women, sexual dysfunction is manifested by orgasmic disorders, which can be caused by psychogenic and neurological factors related to central nervous system diseases (e.g., multiple sclerosis, MSA, Parkinson's disease, myelopathies) and peripheral nervous system neuropathies. In patients with Parkinson's disease, therapy with dopamine agonists appears to improve sexual life, although symptoms of hypersexuality may occasionally occur.

Bibliography

Bolis C.L., Licinio J., Govoni S., Handbook of the Autonomic Nervous System in Health and Disease. Informa Healthcare, 2002.

Clarke C. (Editor), Howard R. (Editor), Rossor M. (Editor), Shorvon S.D. (Editor), Neurology: A Queen Square Textbook. Wiley Blackwell, 2009.

Manfredi M., Neurologia. Editore UTET Collana Medicina interna, 1994.

Conte A., Giannantoni A., Proietti S., Giovannozzi S., Fabbrini G., Rossi A., Porena M., Berardelli A., Botulinum toxin A modulates afferent fibers in neurogenic detrusor overactivity. Eur J Neurol.; 19(5):725-32, 2012.

Freeman R., Wieling W., Axelrod F.B., Benditt D.G., Benarroch E., Biaggioni I., Cheshire W.P., Chelimsky T., Cortelli P., Gibbons C.H., Goldstein D.S., Hainsworth R., Hilz M.J., Jacob G., Kaufmann H., Jordan J., Lipsitz L.A., Levine B.D., Low P.A., Mathias C., Raj S.R., Robertson D., Sandroni P., Schatz I., Schondorff R., Stewart J.M., Van Dijk J.G., Consensus statement on the definition of orthostatic hypotension, neurally mediated syncope and the postural tachycardia syndrome. Clin Auton Res; 21(2):69-72; 2011.

Guerra V.P., Evangelista L., Poloni M., L'imaging funzionale delle disautonomie. Neurovegetativo News, Volume 3, 2009.

Panicker JN, Fowler CJ, Kessler TM. Lower urinary tract dysfunction in the neurological patient: clinical assessment and management. Lancet Neurol.;14(7):720-32, 2015.

Shouman K., Vanichkachorn G., Cheshire W.P., Suarez M.D., Shelly S., Lamotte G.L., Sandroni S, Benarroch E., Berini S.E., Cutsforth-Gregory J.K., Coon E.A., Mauermann M.L., Low P.A., Singer W., Autonomic dysfunction following COVID-19 infection: an early experience Clin Auton Res. ;16: 1-10, 2021.

23 CEPHALALGIAS

Laura Di Clemente, Marta Altieri, Vittorio Di Piero

The term "cephalalgia" is used to designate any type of pain located in the head. It is a very common symptom, with a high incidence in the population, and in the majority of cases, it is harmless. Cephalalgia is secondary only in a small percentage of cases, meaning it can be attributed to an underlying organic pathology. More frequently, it presents as an occasional symptom or, if the episodes are repeated over time, as a clinical correlate of a primary headache syndrome. It is therefore essential to recognize warning signs and, if there is suspicion of secondary cephalalgia, conduct further diagnostic investigations.

In Italy, cephalalgia affects approximately 50% of the population, thus its impact is significant not only on individuals but also on society as a whole in terms of costs due to lost working days and diagnostic and therapeutic expenses.

23.1 Classification

Cephalalgia is a highly heterogeneous nosological entity, with different types characterized by different signs and symptoms. To make a correct diagnosis, it is crucial to obtain accurate medical history information with a detailed description of the episodes. Cephalalgias are classified according to the criteria of the International Headache Society, which divides cephalalgias into 14 main groups, further subdivided into different subgroups. The first four groups define primary cephalalgias, groups 5 to 12 involve secondary cephalalgias, while the last two groups refer to various cranial neuralgias and central or primary facial pains (Table 23.1).

Among primary cephalalgias, the following are distinguished: migraine with and without aura (Group 1), tension-type headache (Group 2), and autonomic trigeminal cephalalgias, including cluster headache (Group 3).

Secondary cephalalgias are symptoms of underlying conditions such as meningitis, sinusitis, dental or ophthalmological disorders, brain tumors, and psychiatric disorders. This group also includes medication-overuse headaches, which often evolve from chronic forms of primary cephalalgias and are extremely challenging to treat and increasingly prevalent in the population.

Finally, cranial neuralgias include trigeminal neuralgia, the most common one, as well as glossopharyngeal neuralgia, occipital neuralgia, and others. These can be either primary or secondary to compression, distortion, or irritation of nerve fibers caused by structural lesions, inflammations, or various types of neuropathies (neurovascular conflict, neuropathies).

23.2 Primary cephalalgias

23.2.1 Migraine

Pathogenesis

According to the recognized trigemino-vascular theory, the pain during a migraine attack is caused by sterile neurogenic inflammation of the meninges. Within the skull, pain sensitivity is limited to meningeal blood vessels and the dura mater, which are densely innervated by sensory nociceptive

Table 23.1 INTERNATIONAL CLASSIFICATION OF HEADACHE DISORDERS III EDITION

PART I - PRIMARY HEADACHES
1. Migraine
1.1. Migraine without aura 1.2. Migraine with aura 1.3. Chronic migraine 1.4. Migraine complications 1.5. Probable migraine 1.6. Episodic syndromes that may be associated with migraine
2. Tension-type headache
2.1. Sporadic episodic tension-type headache 2.2. Frequent episodic tension-type headache 2.3. Chronic tension-type headache 2.4. Probable tension-type headache
3. Cluster headache and other autonomic trigeminal cephalalgias
3.1. Cluster headache 3.2. Paroxysmal hemicrania 3.3. Short-lasting Unilateral Neuralgiform headache attacks (SUN) 3.4. Hemicrania continua 3.5. Probable autonomic trigeminal cephalalgia
4. Other primary headaches
4.1. Primary cough headache 4.2. Primary exertional headache 4.3. Primary headache associated with sexual activity 4.4. Primary thunderclap headache 4.5. Cold-stimulus headache 4.6. External-pressure headache 4.7. Primary stabbing headache 4.8. Nummular headache 4.9. Hypnic headache 4.10. New Daily-Persistent Headache (NDPH)
PART II – SECONDARY HEADACHES
5. Headache attributed to cranial and/or cervical trauma
6. Headache attributed to cranial or cervical vascular disorders
7. Headache attributed to non-vascular intracranial disorders
8. Headache attributed to substance use or withdrawal
9. Headache attributed to infection
10. Headache attributed to disorders of homeostasis
11. Headache or facial pain attributed to disorders of the cranium, neck, eyes, ears, nose, paranasal sinuses, teeth, mouth, or other facial or cranial structures
12. Headache attributed to psychiatric disorder
PART III – CENTRAL FACIAL PAIN, CRANIAL NEURALGIAS, AND OTHER HEADACHES
13. Central facial pain and other facial pains of central origin
14. Other headaches

afferent fibers of the ophthalmic division of the trigeminal nerve. The activation of these trigeminovascular afferents leads to the release of vasoactive substances (CGRP, calcitonin gene-related peptide, substance P, nitric oxide) that promote vasodilation, plasma extravasation, mast cell degranulation, and a process of neurogenic inflammation that gradually amplifies during the attack. The signals are conducted orthodromically and antidromically along the trigeminovascular fibers, thus spreading the inflammatory response to adjacent tissues. Nociceptive information projects to the *caudal part* of the trigeminal nucleus and upper segments of the cervical spinal cord (from the caudal bulb to C2), and from these functionally assembled structures, known as the "trigeminocervical *complex"*, second-order neurons convey the impulses rostrally to encephalic structures involved in pain perception and modulation, such as thalamic nuclei and the periaqueductal gray matter (PAG). Collateral branches also originate from the second-order neurons of the trigeminal nucleus, projecting to autonomic nuclei in the brainstem and the hypothalamus, causing the autonomic symptoms associated with cephalalgia. Nociceptive information directed to the parietal and insular cortex is involved in the representation of the discriminative component of pain (modality-specific), while projections to the anterior cingulate cortex play a role in the affective component of pain. The primary cause of migraine could be a transient dysfunction of brainstem nuclei involved in the central control of nociception. An alteration of these functionally related nuclei may be responsible for the onset of the migraine attack through direct activation of the trigeminovascular system (trigeminal generator hypothesis) or may have a permissive role, favoring a modification of trigeminal and cortical central excitability (Figure 23.1). On the other hand, migraine aura is related to a cortical electrical phenomenon called *cortical spreading depression*. A wave of neuronal depolarization progressively involves the cerebral cortex, starting from the occipital region (with the possibility of stopping or spreading anteriorly), giving rise to visual, sensory, or motor aura phenomena depending on the cortical areas affected by the phenomenon. The depolarization generates an initial excitatory potential, followed by a transient depression of neuronal activity. These electrical phenomena are associated with regional cerebral blood flow changes, characterized by an initial phase of focal hyperemia during depolarization and a second phase of cerebral hypoperfusion coinciding with reduced neuronal activity. Alternatively, these phenomena may be responsible for the activation of the trigeminovascular system, generating the migraine attack.

Clinical and diagnostic aspects

Migraine without aura | Is a widespread form of primary cephalalgia, with a prevalence of approximately 12% in the general population, three times more common in females. This prevalence gradually increases from the age of 12 to 40, beyond which there is a progressive decrease. Therefore, it is a pathology of young

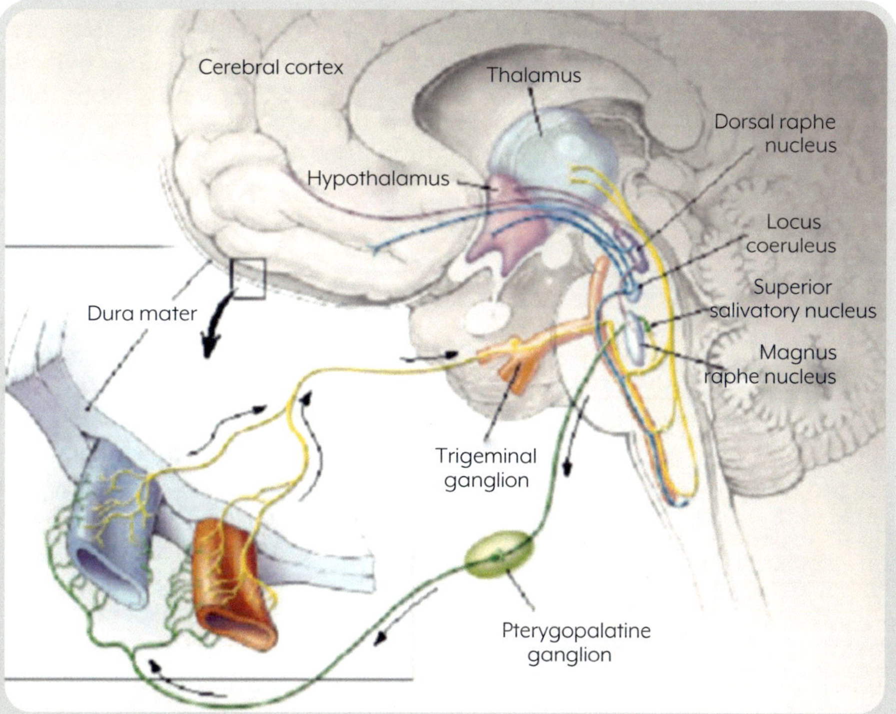

Figure 23.1

The pathophysiology of migraine (modified from Goadsby (2002), NEJM 364 (4), 257-270).

age that manifests in the majority of cases before the age of 30.

It is characterized by a symptom triad: pain, neurovegetative symptoms, and sensitivity to sensory stimuli. Migraine without aura typically presents with recurrent and disabling attacks of unilateral pulsating headache, of severe intensity and variable duration from 4 to 72 hours if left untreated, often accompanied by significant accompanying symptoms (photophobia, phonophobia, nausea, vomiting). In about half of the cases, the pain may be bilateral or variable in location, and it may not be pulsating in nature (Table 23.2).

The intensity of the pain, if the attack is inadequately treated, is often so severe that it prevents the patient from carrying out normal daily activities, exacerbated by physical activity or movement in general. Often, prodromal symptoms manifest as mood changes or behavioral alterations (irritability, euphoria, depression, hyperactivity, apathy), or neurological or systemic symptoms (difficulty concentrating, hypersensitivity to smells, fatigue, yawning, anorexia). The neurovegetative symptoms accompanying the migraine attack and associated with hypersensitivity to environmental stimuli occur with high frequency (in more than 80% of cases) and are as distressing for the patient as the pain itself. During the attack, the patient tends to remain still, lying down in the dark, avoiding any environmental stimuli, whether auditory, visual, or olfactory. In the resolution phase of the attack, feelings of fatigue, irritability, difficulty concentrating, or, conversely, euphoria and hyperactivity may occur.

Migraine is a clinically heterogeneous condition, in which a polygenic multifactorial hereditary component seems to interact significantly with triggering environmental factors. Alterations in the sleep-wake cycle, psychophysical stress, hormonal fluctuations, irregularities in meals, consumption of specific foods, or alcoholic beverages can play an important role in triggering migraine attacks. Given the high prevalence of migraine onset in the female population, hormonal factors often play a crucial role. In fact, migraine attacks often coincide with ovulation or the menstrual cycle. Oral contraceptives worsen the course of the condition, while pregnancy and menopause generally lead to an improvement in the frequency and intensity of the attacks.

Migraine should be considered a chronic condition, despite episodic painful manifestations, and it is comorbid with other neurological disorders such as cerebrovascular disorders, psychiatric conditions, autoimmune diseases, other pain syndromes, and epilepsy.

Migraine with aura | In approximately 20% of patients, migraine attacks are preceded by transient focal neurological symptoms (migraine aura). The frequency of attacks is often more irregular compared to migraine without aura, with long periods of remission. Frequently, both forms coexist in the same patient. The symptoms develop gradually over 5-20 minutes, with a maximum duration of 60 minutes for each symptom, and they are completely reversible. The typical aura consists, in the majority of cases, of visual symptoms such as an initial scintillating scotoma, which is a small monochromatic or multicolored luminous dot that expands like an oil spot, sometimes involving a large part of the visual field. The scotomas can be multiple and pulsating, and sometimes they take on peculiar shapes, jagged and colorful, or like zigzag lines resembling medieval fortification battlements, known as "fortification spectra." In other cases, visual perception may be distorted, for example, mosaic-like or as if filtered through frosted glass. All visual disturbances can be followed by sensory symptoms such as paresthesia, tingling or pins and needles, usually cheiro-oral or

Table 23.2 MIGRAINE WITHOUT AURA

Diagnostic criteria
A. At least 5 attacks fulfilling criteria B-D
B. Headache attacks lasting 4-72 hours (untreated or unsuccessfully treated)
C. Headache has at least two of the following characteristics: 1. Unilateral location 2. Pulsating quality 3. Moderate or severe pain intensity 4. Aggravation by or causing avoidance of routine physical activity (e.g., walking or climbing stairs)
D. During the headache, at least one of the following: 1. Nausea and/or vomiting 2. Photophobia and phonophobia
E. Not attributed to another disorder or diagnosis according to ICHD-3.

affecting the upper limb on the same side as the visual disturbance, with an extension starting from the fingertips. Sometimes, there may be a language disturbance, often of a dysphasic type (Table 23.3).

The progression of symptoms is called "migrainous march" (Table 23.4). Since the aura is a cortical phenomenon, its presence indicates the initial involvement of posterior cerebral areas with subsequent and gradual progression to more anterior areas. Less common symptoms include blurred vision, homonymous lateral hemianopsia or quadrantopsia, and hypoesthesia. Unilateral visual disturbances should be distinguished from monocular symptoms such as phosphenes, scotomas, or visual blurring (up to blindness), which characterize retinal migraine, a rarer form of aura that the patient is unlikely to recognize unless well informed. The characteristics of the aura are usually constant in the same patient. At the end of the aura, sometimes during or after an interval period that can last up to 60 minutes, headache occurs, which in most cases presents the previously described migraine characteristics. Sometimes, however, the aura is followed by headache with atypical features or even occurs without subsequent headache. There are also special types of aura, such as brainstem aura and hemiplegic aura. In the former case, the aura symptoms originate from the brainstem and include at least two of the following symptoms: dysarthria, dizziness, tinnitus, hearing loss, diplopia, ataxia, and decreased level of consciousness. Hemiplegic migraine, on the other hand, is characterized by, in addition to visual, sensory, or dysphasic symptoms, a completely reversible motor deficit within 72 hours, which is always absent in typical aura. Hemiplegic migraine can be sporadic or familial, meaning that a first- or second-degree family member also has the same disorder.

Table 23.3 MIGRAINE WITH AURA

Diagnostic criteria
A. At least 2 attacks that meet criteria B-D
B. Aura characterized by at least one of the following symptoms, in the absence of motor deficits: 1. Fully reversible visual symptoms, positive (such as flickering lights, spots, lines) and/or negative (e.g., loss of vision) 2. Fully reversible sensory symptoms, positive (e.g., "pins and needles") and/or negative (e.g., numbness) 3. Speech and/or language disturbances 4. Motor disturbances 5. Brainstem disturbances 6. Retinal disturbances
C. At least two of the following four characteristics: 1. At least one aura symptom develops gradually over ≥5 minutes and/or two or more symptoms occur in succession 2. Each individual aura symptom lasts 5-60 minutes 3. At least one aura symptom is unilateral 4. The aura is accompanied by, or occurs within 60 minutes of, headache
D. Not otherwise specified by another ICHD-3 diagnosis, and a transient ischemic attack (TIA) has been excluded

Chronic migraine | This is a highly disabling form of migraine characterized by at least 15 days of headache per month (of which at least 8 days are migraine) for at least 3 consecutive months. It often follows untreated episodic migraine, with a progressive and gradual increase in the frequency of attacks and a possible gradual loss of the typical accompanying symptoms of the episodic form. A sudden change in the frequency or presentation mode of the typical migraine attack in an individual patient is considered an alarming symptom.

Migraine complications | These are relatively rare and include status migrainosus, which is a completely disabling migraine attack lasting for more than 72 hours; persistent aura without

Table 23.4 KEY DIFFERENTIAL DIAGNOSIS ELEMENTS FOR PAROXYSMAL FOCAL NEUROLOGICAL SYMPTOMS

	TIA	Epileptic seizure	Migraine aura
Onset	rapid	fast	progressive
Progression	none	quick	slow
Symptom onset	simultaneous	successive	successive
Type of symptoms (if visual)	negative	positive/colorful	negative/positive black and white
Territory	vascular	cortical	cortical
Duration	short 10-15 minutes	short minutes	long 30-60 minutes

infarction, if focal symptoms persist for more than 7 days; migrainous infarction, which occurs when an ischemic stroke presents with the typical features of a migraine attack in a patient who already has migraine; and finally, migraine-induced epilepsy, if a seizure that meets the diagnostic criteria for epilepsy occurs during or within an hour after a migraine aura.

Treatment

The treatment of migraine involves the use of symptomatic medications to be taken during the actual migraine attack in order to reduce or eliminate the symptoms. It also includes preventive therapy, which the patient takes daily for a variable period of time, but not less than 3 months, with the aim of reducing the frequency, severity, duration, and overall impact of the attacks and improving the effectiveness of symptomatic therapy (Table 23.5).

Symptomatic therapy | This includes simple analgesics, nonsteroidal anti-inflammatory drugs (NSAIDs), and specific therapies for migraine, such as triptans. Adjuvant therapies for gastrointestinal disorders can also be used.

Simple analgesics and NSAIDs: These drugs work by inhibiting prostaglandin synthesis and reducing pain and inflammation in processes involving tissue damage. They are nonspecific for migraine but can be a useful resource for mild attacks, particularly in young patients or when triptans are intolerable or ineffective. The most commonly used ones are aspirin (500-1000 mg), naproxen (500 mg), ibuprofen (400-800 mg), indomethacin (25-100 mg), diclofenac (50-100 mg), and paracetamol (500-1000 mg). When using these medications, it is crucial to use the correct dosage and advise the patient to take them early. They can be administered in combination with antiemetics or caffeine, and there are various highly effective combined formulations available. The most common

Table 23.5 ALL ORAL MEDICATIONS FOR WHICH EFFICACY HAS BEEN DEMONSTRATED VERSUS PLACEBO OR OTHER PREVENTIVE THERAPY THROUGH AT LEAST ONE RANDOMIZED CONTROLLED TRIAL

The specified doses are those that have shown efficacy in clinical trials

Pharmaceutical class/mechanism	Drug	Average daily dose (mg)
Adrenergic receptor modulators		
- α2-agonists	Clonidine	0,1 - 0,3
	Tizanidine	2 - 24
- β-blockers	Atenolol	50 - 200
	Metoprolol	50 - 200
	Nadolol	40 - 240
	Propranolol	40 - 320
	Timolol	10 - 20
Angiotensin modulators		
- ACE inhibitors	Lisinopril	20
- AT blockers	Candesartan	16
Antidepressants	Amitriptyline	10 - 150
	Venlafaxine	75 - 150
Antiepileptics	Gabapentin	600 - 2400
	Topiramate	50 - 200
	Valproate	500 - 1500
Calcium channel blockers	Verapamil	240 - 320
	Flunarizine	5 - 10
5-HT2 antagonists	Methysergide	3 - 6
	Pizotifen	1,5 - 4,0
NSAIDs (Nonsteroidal Anti-Inflammatory Drugs)	Aspirin	1300 - 1500
	Flurbiprofen	200
	Ketoprofen	150
	Naproxen	500 - 1100
Others	Magnesium	360 - 600
	Riboflavin	400
	Botulinum Toxin	155 - 195 unit
	CoQ10	150

side effects are epigastric pain and diarrhea. NSAIDs are contraindicated in patients with gastritis or peptic ulcer and in patients taking anticoagulant therapy (for whom paracetamol or COX-2 inhibitors, which are safer but less effective, can be used).

Triptans: Triptans are specific medications for migraine that act as agonists of serotonin 5HT1B/1D receptors. They work both centrally and peripherally by causing vasoconstriction in the craniocephalic region, where 5HT1B receptors are more abundant, and by inhibiting sterile perivascular inflammation through selective action on presynaptic 5HT1D receptors, which are also present centrally. They are considered first-line drugs for the treatment of migraine attacks, with evidence of efficacy in treating multiple attacks and in the long term. Due to their unique mechanism of action, triptans not only relieve pain but also alleviate accompanying symptoms (photophobia, phonophobia, nausea, and vomiting) and overall functional disability. They often do not require combination with antiemetics, and their effect is rapid. Triptans are contraindicated in patients at risk of cardiovascular or cerebrovascular disease and in uncontrolled hypertensive patients. Possible side effects include asthenia, drowsiness, nausea, and a mild, transient sensation of chest tightness that can alarm patients if not properly informed.

Ditans: Ditans are a new class of drugs that act as agonists of the 5-HT1F receptor, present both centrally and peripherally. They work by reducing neuropeptide release and influencing pain pathways without causing vasoconstriction. Lasmiditan is the first approved ditan in this class, and it does not have contraindications for patients with vascular diseases. The most common side effects reported in studies are dizziness, fatigue, paresthesia, and sedation. For this reason, patients should be advised not to drive or operate machinery for at least 8 hours after taking the medication.

Gepants: Gepants are receptor antagonists of calcitonin gene-related peptide (CGRP) used for symptomatic treatment of migraine as an alternative to triptans, primarily due to their lack of vascular effects. The first molecules studied were abandoned due to hepatotoxicity. Recently, promising new molecules (ubrogepant and rimegepant) have shown good results and do not exhibit toxic effects on the liver. The most common side effects are nausea, dizziness, fatigue, xerostomia, and drowsiness.

Anti-emetics: Anti-emetics can be effectively used to reduce the neurovegetative symptoms associated with migraine attacks, which can be highly disabling. Additionally, when taken in combination with other analgesics, they improve absorption by promoting gastric motility. The most commonly used ones are domperidone, which has exclusively peripheral action, and metoclopramide, a phenothiazine neuroleptic analog with primarily central action. The main side effect is sedation and the occurrence of extrapyramidal effects, so these drugs should be used with caution.

Ergot derivatives: Ergotamine, an alkaloid derived from rye ergot, and its derivative dihydroergotamine are the oldest anti-migraine drugs. They act as agonists of alpha-adrenergic, serotoninergic, and dopaminergic receptors, causing marked vasoconstriction in all districts. Due to their nonselective, widespread, and long-lasting action, they can cause significant and severe side effects (nausea, vomiting, paresthesia, cerebrovascular or cardiovascular disorders). As a result, they have been almost completely replaced by triptans.

Preventive therapy | In cases of high frequency and intensity of monthly migraine attacks (at least 3 attacks causing disability lasting 3 or more days) or when the response to symptomatic therapy is no longer effective, it is important to propose daily pharmacological preventive therapy to the patient. Preventive therapy should be taken for at least 3 months and is considered effective if it reduces the monthly number of attacks by at least 50%. An improvement in intensity, duration, and effectiveness of symptomatic medications is also considered a positive outcome. Generally, preventive therapy is used in cycles, with a new treatment period required after a few months of discontinuation, during which the same previously effective medication is taken.

Table 23.5 lists all the medications used for migraine prophylaxis. First-line drugs include beta-blockers, antiepileptics, calcium channel blockers, and tricyclic antidepressants.

Antiepileptics: The efficacy of antiepileptic drugs has been extensively demonstrated in numerous studies, particularly valproate at a dosage of 500-1000 mg and topiramate at a dosage of 50-200 mg. Gabapentin and lamotrigine are valid alternatives to be used as second-line choices. The efficacy of antiepileptics in migraine therapy is likely related to the stabilization of cortical excitability through GABAergic action and inhibitory effects on glutamatergic transmission. However, these medications can have various side effects that are often poorly tolerated by patients (weight gain or loss, drowsiness, asthenia, gait disturbances, paresthesia, nausea, skin rashes, hepatotoxicity, and hematological disorders). Therefore, careful titration and continuous medical monitoring are important.

Beta-blockers: Beta-blockers are also a first-line class of drugs for migraine prevention. The most commonly used active ingredients are propranolol, atenolol, and metoprolol. These drugs can cross the blood-brain barrier and exert their anti-migraine effect centrally by inhibiting beta-adrenergic receptors, resulting in reduced norepinephrine release, as well as interacting with serotonin receptors. Possible side effects include drowsiness, asthenia, hypotension, bradycardia, impotence, and mood changes. They are contraindicated in patients with asthma, diabetes mellitus, or severe bradycardia.

Calcium channel blockers: Flunarizine is the leading drug in this class, at a dosage of 5-10 mg. Verapamil or cinnarizine can be used as alternatives, although they are not as effective. These medications have anticonvulsant activity, modulate vascular tone, and have inhibitory effects on dopaminergic and serotoninergic tone. Additionally, their direct blocking action on calcium channels has shown promise based on recent findings regarding their involvement in the pathophysiology of familial hemiplegic migraine. Calcium channel blockers are generally well tolerated without the need for titration, but they can occasionally cause weight gain, drowsiness, gastrointestinal disorders, ankle edema, and extrapyramidal effects (particularly in elderly individuals). Therefore, calcium channel blockers should be used under close clinical supervision and for short periods.

Antidepressants: Amitriptyline is the only first-line antidepressant for migraine prevention. It is a tricyclic antidepressant used in the treatment of various types of chronic pain. Its efficacy in migraine does not appear to be related to the antidepressant effect itself. Amitriptyline blocks the reuptake of norepinephrine and serotonin, increasing their availability, reduces the density of beta-adrenergic and histaminergic receptors, and increases the density of GABAergic receptors. However, it is still unclear which of these mechanisms is involved in migraine prevention. Amitriptyline also has antihistaminergic and antimuscarinic activity, which is responsible for most of its side effects such as sedation, orthostatic hypotension, constipation, and xerostomia. Therefore, it is advisable to administer it in the evening, gradually increasing the dosage from low levels. Other selective serotonin reuptake inhibitors (SSRIs) can be used as an alternative, but their efficacy in migraine prophylaxis remains anecdotal, despite being better tolerated than tricyclics. Examples of SSRIs include fluoxetine, paroxetine, and sertraline.

Monoclonal antibodies: Recently, monoclonal antibodies targeting calcitonin gene-related peptide (CGRP) or its receptor have been studied, and their action appears very promising in the treatment of both chronic and episodic migraine. Due to their large size, they do not cross the blood-brain barrier and therefore have minimal effects on the central nervous system. It is supposed that their main site of action is peripheral, specifically on the trigeminovascular system's sensory endings, which innervate meningeal arterioles. Monoclonal antibody administration is usually monthly, and it requires subcutaneous injection using a prefilled syringe. The strength of these medications lies in their efficacy, rapid onset of action, and high levels of safety and tolerability. Blood pressure monitoring is a precaution to take. These drugs are contraindicated in patients with major cardiovascular diseases (e.g., uncontrolled hypertension, unstable angina or myocardial infarction, TIA or cerebral ischemia, thromboembolic events, recent aortocoronary bypass or other revascularization procedures).

Botulinum toxin: In chronic migraine, a positive effect of botulinum toxin administration in the cranial muscles of patients with chronic migraine has been demonstrated. The proven efficacy, even in forms resistant to other traditional therapies, is believed to depend on a central action, through the inhibition of trigeminal nociceptors on the meningeal surface. Each treatment session, lasting 10-15 minutes, consists of 31 injections, according to a fixed injection site and dose scheme, each containing 5 units of onaBoNT-A for a total of 155U, distributed among seven muscle groups (bilateral) including the procerus, frontal, corrugator supercilii, temporal, occipital, cervical, and trapezius muscles, with the possibility of additional administrations of up to 40U (between the temporal, occipital, and trapezius muscle groups) at the discretion of the administering physician and based on the sites of greatest pain perceived by the patient. The treatment involves a session every 3 months for a total of 5 sessions in 15 months. In some patients, benefits may become evident after 10-14 days from the first session, while others may not experience improvement after the first session but may require the second or third application to achieve results.

Other therapies: In addition to traditional medications, the effectiveness of alternative therapies such as magnesium, riboflavin, coenzyme Q10, and feverfew has been demonstrated. These therapies are less effective but have practically negligible side effects.

23.2.2 Tension-type headache

Pathogenesis

Various peripheral and central factors are involved in the pathogenesis of tension-type headache, with the peripheral factors playing a fundamental role in episodic headache, while the central factors are believed to be the main contributors to the chronicization of the condition.

The increased sensitivity of pericranial myofascial structures commonly found in affected patients appears to be the main peripheral factor, which in turn is related to local anatomical conditions such as poor posture or temporomandibular disorders. Increased nociceptive input from muscle origins can be responsible for the headache and can be influenced by affective-emotional factors that temporarily reduce central pain control. A multifactorial genetic component may make the patient particularly susceptible to these peripheral and central alterations, possibly through predisposition to specific personality traits. Emotional factors can increase muscle tension through the limbic system while simultaneously reducing endogenous nociceptive activity.

Clinical and diagnostic aspects

Tension-type headache is the most common form of primary headache, with an incidence in the population ranging from approximately 30% to 78%. It appears to be more frequent in women, while both sexes experience a gradual reduction in frequency with increasing age. Despite being a widespread condition, the impact on quality of life varies greatly depending on the frequency of attacks. In the current classification, tension-type headache is therefore divided into chronic (more than 15 headache days per month) and episodic. The latter is further divided into two subtypes: infrequent (less than one headache day per month) and frequent (between 1 and 15 headache days per month). Frequent episodic tension-type headache can cause considerable disability, including the chronicization of the disorder, which occurs in 5% of patients.

Tension-type headache is a heterogeneous condition diagnosed mainly based on the absence of characteristic accompanying symptoms of other primary headaches. Additionally, this headache typically does not worsen with physical activity. The diagnostic criteria are detailed in Tables 23.6A and B. The attacks vary in duration, from 30 minutes to 7 days, and present with bilateral localization, often described as a constrictive or pressing pain, never throbbing, of mild to moderate intensity, with a "band-like" or "hat-like" distribution. Both the episodic and chronic forms can be distinguished as headaches with or without muscle contraction, depending on the presence or absence of increased pain in the pericranial muscles, assessed through manual palpation or functional tests. Tenderness increases in parallel with the intensity and frequency of the headache and is further

Table 23.6A	EPISODIC TENSION-TYPE HEADACHE
(to be distinguished as sporadic or frequent based on the number of monthly episodes)	
Diagnostic criteria	
A. At least 10 episodes occurring for at least 3 months and meeting criteria B-D	
B: Headache duration ranging from 30 minutes to 7 days	
C. The headache exhibits at least two of the following characteristics: 1. bilateral localization 2. quality described as pressing or tightening (non-pulsating) 3. mild or moderate intensity 4. not worsened by routine physical activity, such as walking or climbing stairs	
D. Both of the following conditions are present: 1. absence of nausea and vomiting 2. photophobia may be present, or phonophobia may be present, but not both	
E. Not otherwise specified by another ICHD-3 diagnosis	

Table 23.6B	CHRONIC TENSION-TYPE HEADACHE
Diagnostic criteria	
A. Headache is present for at least 15 days per month for at least 3 months (≥180 days per year) and meets criteria B-D	
B. Headache lasts for hours or days and may be continuous	
C. The headache exhibits at least two of the following characteristics: 1. Bilateral localization 2. Quality described as pressing or tightening (non-pulsating) 3. Mild or moderate intensity 4. Not worsened by routine physical activity, such as walking or climbing stairs	
D. Both of the following conditions are present: 1. No more than one of the following symptoms: photophobia, phonophobia, and mild nausea 2. Absence of moderate or severe nausea and vomiting	
E. Not otherwise specified by another ICHD-3 diagnosis	

heightened during the pain phase. Identified triggering factors include psychophysical stress and mental effort, anxiety or depression, lack of rest, poor posture, oromandibular dysfunctions or bruxism, and, in general, anything that can cause excessive contraction of the pericranial muscles.

Therapy

The first therapeutic measure consists of identifying and eliminating, as much as possible, any individual triggering factors. If behavioral modifications are not sufficient, symptomatic medications can be used, and when necessary, preventive therapies. While sporadic tension-type headache is a relatively easy disorder to treat, frequent and chronic tension-type headache can pose a challenging task for the physician, who often needs to employ different approaches sequentially or in combination.

Symptomatic therapy | The first-line medications for tension-type headache attacks are salicylates (aspirin 500-1000 mg) or NSAIDs (mainly ibuprofen, naproxen, ketoprofen, diclofenac). However, selective cyclooxygenase-2 (COX-2) inhibitors or acetaminophen can be used if there is intolerance or gastric disturbances. If these analgesics are not fully effective, combination medications (such as analgesic with a sedative, muscle relaxant, or caffeine) or other types of analgesics (such as opioids like codeine) can be used, with particular attention to the potential for patient abuse in these cases.

Preventive therapy | The therapeutic approach for high-frequency tension-type headache is often multidisciplinary. There are no specific drugs for prophylaxis, but as first-line medications, tricyclic antidepressants (amitriptyline is particularly effective, even at low doses) and SSRIs (fluoxetine, paroxetine, sertraline), can be used, either alone or in combination with alternative therapies. Among these, cognitive-behavioral therapies, biofeedback, and relaxation techniques have shown to be particularly effective.

In general, similar to migraine, preventive therapies for tension-type headache are administered for several months and then gradually reduced until discontinuation. Often, the clinical benefit persists for long periods of time after the therapy is discontinued, although in the majority of cases, new therapeutic cycles may be necessary.

23.2.3 Cluster headache and other autonomic-trigeminal headaches

In this subgroup of primary headaches, activation of the trigemino-vascular nociceptive pathways occurs, but there are distinctive features related to the pronounced reflex activation of the cranial autonomic nervous system. These syndromes include cluster headache, paroxysmal hemicrania, SUN (*Short-lasting Unilateral Neuralgiform headache attacks*), and hemicrania continua. These pathological conditions share some common characteristics: unilateral pain, severe headache episodes accompanied, on the same side as the pain, by typical symptoms mediated by the autonomic nervous system, and, in the first three cases, a short duration of individual attacks.

23.2.4 Cluster headache

Pathogenesis

The trigemino-vascular system is likely responsible for the pain manifestations of cluster headache. The clinical manifestation of the attack involves the nociceptive structures of the skull and the neurogenic inflammatory mechanisms already described for migraine. However, peripheral trigeminal activation is believed to be linked to the dysfunction of different central structures that contribute to the pathology through modulatory connections with the trigeminal caudal nucleus.

The periodic characteristics of cluster headache, with circadian rhythms of attacks and circannual rhythms of cluster periods, clearly suggest the involvement of a central biological clock. Functional neuroimaging studies have recently confirmed this hypothesis, indicating the posterior hypothalamus as the "*cluster generator*". Furthermore, alteration of the hypothalamic-pituitary-adrenal axis has been observed even during remission of the disease, providing further evidence of an underlying hypothalamic dysfunction. The hypothalamic-diencephalic area appears to play a central role, periodically permissive and inhibitory on the trigemino-vascular system and the trigemino-parasympathetic circuits responsible for the pain and autonomic disturbances of the pathology, respectively. Recent studies have also demonstrated the involvement of other pain control and modulation areas that allow for disinhibition of the hypothalamic-trigeminal circuit.

The typical autonomic phenomena of the condition appear to be caused by the activation of efferent parasympathetic fibers of the superior salivatory nucleus. Additionally, the incomplete Horner syndrome (miosis, ptosis) observed in many patients may be caused by compression and irritation of pericarotid sympathetic fibers due to vasodilation and perivascular edema in the cavernous sinus.

Although cluster headache was not considered a hereditary condition for a long time, recent studies have shown that approximately 10% of cases present in a familial form. Genetic factors, therefore, appear to play a significant role in individual susceptibility to this type of headache, although environmental factors remain fundamental.

Clinical and diagnostic aspects

Cluster headache is a relatively rare condition, with an estimated prevalence of around 0.1% in the population. It predominantly affects males, with a male-to-female ratio of approximately 3:1, which is the opposite of what is observed in migraine. This headache can occur at any age, although the peak onset is between 20 and 50 years old.

Among primary headaches, cluster headache is perhaps the one with the most stereotypical clinical features. It is characterized by extremely intense pain (often described as unbearable), always strictly unilateral in the orbital, supraorbital, and temporal regions, accompanied by marked ipsilateral autonomic symptoms such as conjunctival injection, tearing, nasal congestion, rhinorrhea, sweating, and redness of the forehead and face, miosis, ptosis, and eyelid edema. During a cluster headache attack, patients are typically restless and agitated, often pacing or repeatedly shaking their heads, contrary to what happens in a migraine attack. The attacks typically last between 15 and 180 minutes and occur with a frequency varying from once every two days to eight or more times a day, with circadian rhythmicity, dramatically impairing the patient's quality of life.

The diagnostic criteria are presented in Table 23.7, while the typical clinical characteristics useful for the differential diagnosis with other major primary headaches are summarized in Table 23.8.

Table 23.7 CLUSTER HEADACHE

Diagnostic Criteria
A. At least 5 attacks that meet criteria B-D
B. Severe or very severe unilateral pain in the orbital, supraorbital, and/or temporal region, lasting 15-180 minutes (untreated).
C. One or both of the following: 1. The headache is associated with at least one of the following symptoms or signs: a. Conjunctival injection and/or lacrimation b. Nasal congestion and/or rhinorrhea c. Eyelid edema d. Facial and forehead sweating e. Facial and forehead flushing f. Sensation of a blocked ear g. Miosis and/or ptosis 2. Restlessness or agitation
D. Attack frequency is between one every two days and up to 8 per day for more than half of the time the disorder is active
E. Not otherwise specified by another ICHD-3 diagnosis

In approximately 70-80% of cases, cluster headache presents in the episodic form. In these cases, painful attacks occur in specific periods called "cluster periods," which can vary from weeks to months and often repeat cyclically in the same month of the year, with periods of complete freedom from attacks in between. The onset of a cluster period often coincides with moments of particular stress, and certain factors can trigger attacks during the cluster phase (usually alcoholic beverages, but also strong odors). In severe and highly debilitating cases where cluster headache becomes chronic, the patient experiences attacks for more than a year without remission, or with remission periods lasting less than a month. These patients often had a previous episodic form, although in rare cases, chronic cluster headache presents as an initial manifestation.

Therapy

Symptomatic therapy | Due to the immediate exacerbation of pain, with the peak reached within a few minutes, medications for treating cluster headache attacks must act rapidly. Therefore, the first-line therapy for the acute phase includes triptans, particularly subcutaneous sumatriptan (6 mg), or high-flow inhaled oxygen (O_2 100% at a rate of 7 l/min for about 15 minutes). Nasal spray formulations of sumatriptan or zolmitriptan are valid alternatives but have a slower onset of action. Indomethacin, preferably given intramuscularly, and dihydroergotamine, administered intravenously, intramuscularly, or subcutaneously, are also effective in treating cluster headache attacks. The mechanisms of action and possible side effects are described in the section on migraine therapy.

Preventive therapy | During the cluster period, preventive therapies are used to reduce the frequency of attacks and, if possible, terminate the cluster period. The treatment should be gradually reduced after the cluster period ends, while continuous use of preventive therapies is recommended for chronic cases.

The first-choice drug for both episodic and chronic forms of cluster headache prevention is verapamil, a calcium channel blocker typically used at a daily dose of 240-360 mg. The most common side effects are fatigue, drowsiness, constipation, hypotension, and ankle edema, while rare effects include potential effects on cardiac conduction with prolongation of the PR interval. Verapamil is generally well-tolerated and does not have interactions

Table 23.8 TYPICAL CLINICAL CHARACTERISTICS OF THE MAJOR PRIMARY HEADACHES IN COMPARISON

	Migraine	Tension-Type Headache	Cluster Headache
Location	Unilateral	Bilateral	Unilateral
Type of pain	Throbbing	Pressing or tightening	Piercing-stabbing
Intensity	Moderate to severe	Mild to moderate	Extremely high
Duration of attacks	4-72 hours	30 minutes to 7 days	15-180 minutes
Temporal pain profile	Variable	Continuous	Paroxysmal
Main associated symptoms and signs	Photophobia, phonophobia, nausea, vomiting	None - possible photophobia or phonophobia	Tearing, conjunctival injection, nasal congestion, rhinorrhea, eyelid edema, miosis, ptosis
Patient behavior	Isolation and rest	None or mild alteration	Restlessness or agitation

with sumatriptan, corticosteroids, or other prophylactic medications.

Steroids have also shown efficacy in preventing cluster headache, but they are considered second-line treatments due to potential side effects and are not recommended for chronic cases. Prednisone, administered orally at a dosage of 50-60 mg/day, methylprednisolone given intravenously, or dexamethasone administered intramuscularly or intravenously can be used.

Lithium is effective at a dose of 600-900 mg per day, showing results within a few days of treatment. It is primarily used for chronic forms and has a narrow therapeutic window, requiring regular monitoring of lithium levels to prevent potential side effects such as tremors, diarrhea, confusion, insomnia, and nausea. As third-line options, antiepileptic drugs like topiramate, valproate, and gabapentin can be used, with reported side effects including drowsiness and cognitive disturbances.

23.2.5 Paroxysmal hemicrania

This syndrome is characterized by unilateral attacks of high-intensity pain in the orbital, supraorbital, and/or temporal regions, lasting from 2 to 30 minutes. The headache is always accompanied by at least one ipsilateral cranial autonomic symptom, including conjunctival injection or tearing, nasal congestion or rhinorrhea, eyelid edema, facial sweating or flushing, miosis, and/or ptosis. The frequency of attacks is usually more than five times a day, although there may be periods with a lower frequency. There are both episodic and chronic forms.

Indomethacin is considered the treatment of choice, starting at an initial dosage of 75-150 mg divided into three daily doses, which can be gradually reduced to the lowest effective maintenance dose.

23.2.6 SUNCT syndrome

This rare syndrome is characterized by unilateral attacks of stabbing pain in the orbital, supraorbital, or temporal regions, with a duration much shorter than observed in any other trigeminal-autonomic headache, ranging from 5 seconds to 10 minutes. The different accompanying symptoms allow for the distinction of two subtypes: SUNCT (intense ipsilateral tearing and conjunctival injection accompanying the pain) and SUNA (when the symptoms include previously described cranial autonomic features). The attack frequency is often very high. Only preventive therapy is used, as the attacks are too brief to be treated. Indomethacin and other treatments are often ineffective, while lamotrigine therapy has shown promising results.

23.2.7 "Hemicrania continua"

It is a persistent unilateral headache associated with at least one of the typical cranial autonomic symptoms found in other trigeminal-autonomic headaches. In this case as well, the patient is restless or agitated. Complete remission is achieved only with adequate doses of indomethacin.

23.2.8 Other primary headaches

This paragraph includes clinically heterogeneous headaches, characterized by a specific pathogenesis that is currently poorly understood, and treatment based on anecdotal reports rather than controlled clinical trials. This group includes primary cough headache, primary exercise headache, primary headache associated with sexual activity, primary thunderclap headache, cold stimulus headache, external pressure headache, primary stabbing headache, nummular headache, and "New Daily Persistent Headache (NDPH)".

The onset of some forms is particularly acute and often leads the patient to seek emergency care. In almost all of these headaches, however, it is advisable to subject the patient to careful clinical evaluation and appropriate instrumental investigations to exclude symptomatic forms. Table 23.9 provides the main warning signs that should prompt clinicians to conduct further diagnostic investigations, especially through neuroimaging tests.

Table 23.9 WARNING SIGNS IN THE CLINICAL PRESENTATION OF A HEADACHE THAT REQUIRE DIAGNOSTIC INVESTIGATION THROUGH NEUROIMAGING

- Presence of focal neurological signs
- Sudden change in the pattern of a recurrent headache (frequency or characteristics of pain)
- Sudden onset
- Late onset age
- Onset of a headache as chronic
- Association with physical exertion (coughing, sneezing, sexual activity, etc.)
- Headache or aura always on the same side
- Prolonged duration of aura
- Headache in patients with known neoplastic or infectious pathology

23.3 Secondary headaches

In cases where the patient presents with neurological signs accompanying the headache that differ even slightly from the classic features of primary headaches, a sudden change in the frequency, type, or location of recurrent headache pain, a late onset of symptoms, and, in general, when the characteristics of the headache do not fully fit the classification criteria for a primary form, diagnostic investigations are necessary to exclude a secondary headache. Differential diagnosis can be challenging in some patients and requires a detailed understanding of the clinical spectrum and characteristics of primary headaches.

23.3.1 Headache attributed to cranial and/or cervical trauma

All cranial and cervical traumas, even mild ones, can be followed by a newly onset headache or exacerbate pre-existing primary headaches. Often, this symptomatology persists for weeks or months, but in most cases, it is temporary. Generally, the headache has subcontinuous characteristics and is of moderate intensity, without particular focal accompanying symptoms. It may be associated with localized muscle pain in the neck and shoulders, especially in cases of whiplash. In the case of subdural hematoma, the headache can develop chronically in the weeks or months following the trauma. In cases of developing epidural hematoma, the headache often represents an acute symptom and is crucial for prompt intervention.

23.3.2 Headache attributed to cranial or cervical vascular disorders

Cerebrovascular disorders can often be accompanied or followed by headaches. In the case of ischemic stroke, headaches occur more frequently due to large artery thrombosis (large artery disease) rather than lacunar or embolic lesions, and their characteristics can vary significantly. Headaches can occur in cases of intraparenchymal or subarachnoid brain hemorrhage. In the former case, the intensity of the symptom often depends on the size of the affected area and the possible surrounding edema, which causes mechanical compression on surrounding structures. It is less frequently observed in cases of small-sized and typical hemorrhages. In subarachnoid hemorrhage, headache often constitutes the first and often the only symptom, assuming significant diagnostic relevance. It appears suddenly and is described as a "stabbing" or "worst-ever experienced" pain, often localized in the occipitonuchal region and sometimes associated with nausea and vomiting. Headache is also one of the possible symptoms of vasculitis. The most characteristic association is with temporal arteritis (giant cell arteritis), which is characterized by inflammation of the cranial arteries, primarily the branches of the external carotid artery and typically the temporal arteries. The headache is most frequently localized in the frontotemporal-orbital region and occurs in close temporal relation with other signs and symptoms of the condition (amaurosis fugax, polymyalgia rheumatica, claudication of the jaw, etc.). Increased inflammation markers such as ESR and CRP are essential for diagnosis. High-dose steroid therapy can halt the arteritic process and prevent irreversible damage. Definitive diagnosis is achieved through biopsy of the involved temporal artery. Additionally, although less frequently, a nonspecific headache can be associated with 25-30% of cases of any vasculitis involving the central nervous system (e.g., Wegener's granulomatosis, systemic lupus erythematosus, polyarteritis nodosa). Headaches originating from the epiaortic vessels occur in cases of arterial dissection or following surgical or endovascular procedures. In the case of dissection, the pain often precedes the onset of neurological deficits. The headache is of moderate to severe intensity, with variable characteristics and is more often localized in the frontoorbital region for carotid dissection, and in the occipitonuchal or cervical region for vertebral artery dissection. In cases of cerebral venous thrombosis, headache is present in 75% of cases and often represents the first of a series of subsequent, sometimes severe, symptoms related to increased intracranial pressure and possible venous infarction.

23.3.3 Headache attributed to nonvascular intracranial disorders

Alterations in cerebrospinal fluid pressure can cause headaches. Increased intracranial pressure manifests as diffuse headache, with intensity varying according to the patient's position. It is usually most intense upon awakening, after a long period of lying down, and after Valsalva-like maneuvers (coughing, abdominal straining). Headache is often associated with vomiting, and in severe cases, it can be projectile. Prolonged increased intracranial pressure can cause papilledema, progressive visual field deficits, cranial nerve VI palsy, altered consciousness, and postural instability. Benign intracranial hypertension, also known as "pseudotumor cerebri," is more commonly observed in young obese women. It is important to investigate possible metabolic, toxic, or endocrine causes that may increase intracranial pressure, as well as hydrocephalus. In all these cases, the headache improves after cerebrospinal fluid drainage and diuretic therapy such as the use of acetazolamide. On the other hand, low cerebrospinal fluid pressure manifests as orthostatic headache, often associated with neck stiffness, tinnitus, hearing loss, photophobia, and nausea. This condition can occur after lumbar puncture, immediately or up to a maximum of 5 days later, and typically resolves spontaneously within a short time. All intracranial neoplasms can cause headaches, often persistent and subcontinuous, with varying characteristics and frequently related to increased intracranial mass causing compression of surrounding structures and consequent increased intracranial pressure. It will be crucial, however, to distinguish these symptoms from the aforementioned causes of increased cerebrospinal fluid pressure. Less commonly, the tumor can cause headaches through carcinomatous meningitis or altered hypothalamic or pituitary secretion.

23.3.4 Headache attributed to substance use or withdrawal

Headache can be induced by the acute use or exposure to a specific substance. It is a common side effect observed with the use of vasoactive medications such as nitroderivatives (nitric oxide donors) and phosphodiesterase inhibitors, or after the consumption of alcohol and drugs such as cocaine or cannabis.

More complex and challenging to manage is the chronic headache associated with the excessive use of symptomatic medications. It represents one of the most difficult therapeutic challenges in the field of headache disorders. This condition is becoming increasingly prevalent and is found in 5-10% of individuals in specialized migraine centers. The diagnostic criteria are provided in Table 23.10.

The first step in treating this condition is discontinuing the abuse of medications, although this often leads to an initial rebound headache of even more unbearable intensity. Subsequently, a prophylactic therapy will be initiated, followed by frequent medical visits to prevent the patient from relapsing into medication overuse (which occurs in the majority of cases over time). Therefore, the patient's involvement in pain management and understanding the triggering mechanisms is crucial to achieve full compliance and the complete and long-lasting cessation of medication overuse. A multidisciplinary approach, involving professionals such as psychologists and physiotherapists, is often necessary.

23.3.5 Headache attributed to infection

All intracranial infectious processes (meningitis, encephalitis, brain abscesses, subdural empyema) can cause headaches due to the inflammatory process, with direct stimulation of meningeal sensory nerve endings or increased intracranial pressure.

23.3.6 Headache attributed to homeostatic disturbances

When a new headache begins or when a pre-existing headache worsens in close temporal relation to a homeostatic disturbance, it is attributed to that disturbance, even if it exhibits characteristics of migraine, tension-type headache, or cluster headache. A fundamental requirement for a definite diagnosis is the disappearance of the headache or the return to the original pattern after effectively treating the underlying disturbance.

Headache can be associated with hypoxia or hypercapnia, as seen in high-altitude environments, sleep apnea syndrome, and divers during diving. These homeostatic changes lead to relaxation of the smooth muscles of the cerebral vessels, resulting in vasodilation and increased intracranial pressure.

A syndrome characterized by headache, sometimes accompanied by nausea, muscle cramps, and potentially progressing to impaired consciousness and coma, can occur following hypotension and dialysis disequilibrium syndrome.

Table 23.10 MEDICATION-OVERUSE HEADACHE

Diagnostic criteria
A. Headache present for ≥15 days per month in a patient with pre-existing headache
B. Regular overuse for >3 months of one or more drugs that can be taken for acute and/or symptomatic headache treatment (ergotamine, triptans, opioids, or combination drugs for >10 days per month, analgesics for >15 days per month)
C. Not otherwise specified by another ICHD-3 diagnosis

Headache can also be caused by severe arterial hypertension, such as in idiopathic hypertensive crisis or hypertension triggered by an exogenous agent, pheochromocytoma, hypertensive encephalopathy, preeclampsia, or eclampsia. In chronic arterial hypertension, the pain is often diffuse throughout the head and pulsating in nature, but often lacks specific characteristics for etiological diagnosis. In the case of hypertensive crisis, however, regardless of the cause, a headache with migrainous characteristics usually occurs.

Finally, headache can be related to endocrine dysfunctions, such as hypothyroidism, prolonged fasting-induced hypoglycemia, and alterations in blood gas analysis, as in cardiovascular disorders.

23.3.7 Headache or facial pain attributed to cranial, neck, eye, ear, nasal, paranasal sinus, dental, oral, or other facial or cranial disorders

This category includes headaches whose origin is related to cranial or cervical bone abnormalities and soft tissue abnormalities in the neck.

Headaches can also be attributed to ocular pathologies such as acute glaucoma, refractive errors, heterophoria, and inflammatory disorders of the eye, or to ear disorders such as organic lesions of the auricle, external auditory canal, tympanic membrane, or middle ear. In all these cases, the headache develops simultaneously with the ocular or ear pathology and disappears once the underlying condition is treated.

Frontal headache, often accompanied by pain in one or more regions of the face, ears, or teeth, and accompanied by clinical, endoscopic, neuroradiological, and/or laboratory signs of acute or exacerbation of chronic sinusitis, suggests a diagnosis of headache attributed to rhinosinusitis. This condition is frequently overestimated by patients and clinicians. Many patients with chronic sinusitis are incorrectly attributed with migraine or tension-type headaches. Clinical signs of acute or exacerbation of chronic sinusitis include the presence of purulent nasal discharge, nasal obstruction, hyposmia or anosmia, and fever.

Rarely, headache can be caused by periodontitis or pericoronitis, as a complication of infection or traumatic irritation from dental practices. In this case, both the headache and dental pain resolve within a few months after effective treatment of the underlying dental condition.

Finally, headache can be caused by temporomandibular joint disorders, characterized by spontaneous pain localized in one or more regions of the head or face, or pain provoked by jaw movements and/or chewing. Radiography, magnetic resonance imaging, or bone scintigraphy can demonstrate any abnormalities of the temporomandibular joint.

23.3.8 Headache attributed to psychiatric disorders

Although headache frequently occurs comorbidly with various psychiatric disorders, possibly reflecting a common biological substrate, in the vast majority of cases, there is no causal relationship between headache and these disorders. Therefore, this category includes only headaches directly caused by somatization disorders or psychotic disorders. It should be noted, however, that in any case of headache diagnosis, the clinician should be vigilant for major depressive disorder, panic disorder, generalized anxiety disorder, and vice versa. Additionally, the presence of comorbid psychiatric disorders often worsens the course of migraine and/or tension-type headache, increasing their frequency and severity and making them less responsive to treatment. Identification and treatment of any coexisting psychiatric conditions are therefore essential for the appropriate management of headaches.

23.3.9 Cranial neuralgias

Cranial neuralgias refer to paroxysmal head pain with specific clinical characteristics, including unilateral symptoms, recurrent attacks, electric shock-like pain, and the presence of specific trigger factors. The most common condition within this category is trigeminal neuralgia, and it is discussed in Chapter 3 - Cranial nerves.

Bibliography

Cutrer F.M., Pathophysiology of migraine. Seminar Neurology; 30:120-130, 2010.

Edvinsson L. et al., CGRP as the target of new migrainetherapies - successful translation from bench to clinic. Nature Reviews Neurology volume 14, 338-350, 2018.

Eigenbrodt AK, et al., Diagnosis and management of migraine in ten steps. Nature Reviews Neurology volume 17, 501–514, 2021.

Fumal A., Schoenen J., Tension-type headache: current research and clinical management. The Lancet Neurology; 7:70-83, 2008.

Garza I., Schwedt T.J., Diagnosis and management of chronic daily headache. Seminar Neurology; 30:154-166, 2010.

Headache Classification Committee of The International Headache Society. The International Classification of Headache Disorders, 3rd edition. Cephalalgia; 38(1) 1-211, 2018.

Leone M., Bussone G., Pathophysiology of trigeminal autonomic cephalalgias. The Lancet Neurology; 8:755-164, 2009.

May A., Leone M., Afra J., Linded M., Sandor P.S., Evers S., Goadsby P.J., EFNS guidelines on the treatment of cluster headache and other trigeminal autonomic cephalalgias. European Journal of Neurology; 13:1066-1077, 2006.

Ramadan N.M., Current trends in migraine prophylaxis. Headache; 47(Suppl1): 52-57;2007.

24 MENINGITIS AND OTHER INFECTIONS OF THE NERVOUS SYSTEM

Giovanni Fabbrini, Maria Ciardi, Paolo Vassalini, Alfredo Berardelli

Meningitis is an inflammatory process of the leptomeninges (pia mater and arachnoid), secondary to infections, intoxications, traumas, physical agents (heat stroke), and other causes. Since the brain and spinal cord are in communication through the subarachnoid space, meningitis can simultaneously affect both the brain and the spinal cord (meningoencephalitis). Infectious agents reach the meninges through the systemic circulation, direct spread from contiguous infections (such as otitis, mastoiditis, sinusitis), from the external environment in the presence of cranial lesions (congenital, traumatic, or post-surgical), and through the ethmoid bone along the fibers of the olfactory nerve. Meningitis can be a complication of brain or spinal neurosurgical procedures or of a lumbar puncture performed with a non-sterile technique (iatrogenic meningitis). They are classified, based on the mode of presentation and clinical course, as acute meningitis and subacute/chronic meningitis. Acute meningitis is characterized by a sudden onset (hours to days) and a very rapid course, while subacute/chronic meningitis has a slower onset and evolution (weeks/months). They can also be further classified based on the etiological agent (bacterial, viral, fungal, and protozoal meningitis).

24.1 Acute meningitis

24.1.1 Bacterial meningitis

Epidemiology

Epidemiological data vary according to the socioeconomic level of the geographical area considered and the age of the patient. Bacterial meningitis has an incidence of approximately 0.5-4 cases per 100,000 in Western countries and about 50 cases per 100,000 in developing countries. 70% of bacterial meningitis cases occur in children under 5 years of age. There is a slight male predominance. In Italy, since 1994, a dedicated surveillance system for bacterial meningitis has been active. In 2015, 196 cases of meningococcal meningitis, 1,256 cases of invasive pneumococcal disease, and 131 cases of *Haemophilus influenzae* infection were reported.

Etiology and pathogenesis

Streptococcus pneumoniae (Pneumococcus) is responsible for 50% of meningitis cases, *Neisseria meningitidis* (Meningococcus) for 20%, group B streptococci for 10%, *Listeria monocytogenes* for 10%, while the incidence of *Haemophilus influenzae*, thanks to the availability of vaccines, has been reduced to less than 10%. Pneumococcal meningitis is more common in adults and often occurs in conjunction with other pneumococcal infections such as pneumonia, acute or chronic sinusitis, middle ear infections, and in debilitating conditions such as alcoholism, diabetes, hypogammaglobulinemia, complement deficiency, and basal skull fractures. Meningococcal meningitis is very common in children (it accounts for 60% of meningitis cases in children under 2 years old) and young adults (< 20 years old), while it is rare in adults over 50 years old. Pneumococcus and meningococcus often naturally inhabit the nasopharynx, and the risk of meningitis depends on both the virulence of the bacterium and the reduced immune defense capabilities of the host. Meningitis is often preceded by a simple infection of the upper respiratory tract. The infection begins when bacteria invade the intravascular space, crossing the apical junctions of the epithelial cells of the nasopharynx and entering the bloodstream. From there, the bacteria reach the choroid plexus and the cerebrospinal fluid, where they can further multiply as these structures are devoid of antibodies. *Listeria monocytogenes* is a significant cause of acute bacterial meningitis in newborns, pregnant women, individuals over 60 years of age, and immunocompromised individuals. The infection is usually caused by the ingestion of contaminated food. *Haemophilus influenzae* is more common in cases of middle ear infections, cranial trauma, or previous surgical interventions. Group B streptococci are an important cause of neonatal sepsis and meningitis (especially in premature and underweight infants) and in adults with conditions such as diabetes, cirrhosis, and malignant neoplasms. Gram-negative bacteria (particularly *Klebsiella pneumoniae, Escherichia coli, Pseudomonas aeruginosa*) can cause meningitis in individuals undergoing surgical procedures (craniotomies) and in patients with chronic debilitating diseases. *Staphylococcus aureus* and coagulase-negative staphylococci should also be considered in cases of meningitis following neurosurgical interventions (including shunt placement for hydrocephalus) and cranial thrombophlebitis.

In general, inflammation of the meninges is characterized by an accumulation of neutrophils and exudate on the surface of the leptomeninges and is due to the release of toxins and inflammatory cytokines in the cerebrospinal fluid. These substances increase the permeability of the blood-brain barrier and cause vasogenic edema with the passage of proteins into the subarachnoid space. The subarachnoid spaces become invaded by purulent exudate due to bacterial lysis, which hinders the normal reabsorption of cerebrospinal fluid through the ventricular system and dural sinuses, leading to hydrocephalus and interstitial edema. The resulting intracranial hypertension is the main element in the clinical course of meningitis. Meningitis is characterized by evident involvement of the cerebral arteries and veins. Cortical vasculitis, thrombosis of branches of the middle cerebral artery and major venous sinuses, and altered parenchymal perfusion with consequent ischemic changes can occur. Involvement of the cerebral microcirculation is responsible for alterations in the blood-brain barrier, with the opening of the "tight junctions" of the vascular endothelium. These processes contribute to the formation of cerebral edema, which further hinders the physiological drainage of cerebrospinal fluid.

Symptoms

Bacterial meningitis, particularly meningococcal meningitis, can be fulminant, with such a rapid clinical progression that it can lead to death within a few hours, or it can have a subacute course lasting a few days. Bacterial meningitis are characterized by common symptoms: fever, headache, and muscle stiffness (resistance to flexion of the neck), sometimes seizures, and alterations in consciousness. The headache can be very intense and worsens with exposure to sensory stimuli (light, noise). The muscle stiffness of the neck (*nuchal rigidity*) is caused by the reflex contraction of the paravertebral muscles induced by meningeal inflammation. Other signs of meningeal irritation include flexion of the hip and knee in response to neck flexion (Brudzinski's sign) and the inability to extend the legs with the hips flexed (Kernig's sign). In severe cases, the patient assumes a typical position called "opisthotonus," characterized by lateral decubitus, flexion of the legs on the thighs, and flexion of the thighs on the pelvis. The absence of signs of meningeal irritation does not exclude the diagnosis of meningitis. It should also be noted that signs of muscle stiffness are less frequent in patients with alterations in the level of consciousness, neonates, children, and the elderly. Patients with acute bacterial meningitis can experience confusion, delirium, and impaired consciousness. One-third of patients may experience projectile vomiting without preceding nausea, seizures (often partial type or even status epilepticus usually due to ischemic or hemorrhagic lesions of the brain parenchyma), and, in 10-20% of cases, focal neurological signs. Increased intracranial hypertension resulting from meningitis is a typical complication.

Based on the etiological agent, specific clinical and laboratory signs can be observed. Meningococcal meningitis should be suspected in the presence of an extremely rapid clinical course (alteration of consciousness within a few hours). Additionally, septic shock, disseminated intravascular coagulation (due to the release of endotoxin that forms the meningococcal cell wall), and the appearance of petechiae, particularly on the trunk and extensor surfaces of the lower limbs, as well as in the conjunctiva and pressure-prone areas of the skin (e.g., elastic bands or belts), may be observed. Pneumococcal meningitis is frequently preceded by lung infections or infections in other areas (such as middle ear infections), affects alcoholics, splenectomized or asplenic patients, and often involves cranial nerves.

Different age groups exhibit different clinical features. Acute meningitis in neonates often presents with lethargy, hypothermia, and seizures. In infants, tension of the bulging fontanelle and the presence of Lesage's sign (lifting the child's armpits, the child does not "kick" but the lower limbs remain flexed and inert) can be observed. Finally, in the elderly, the onset can be insidious, signs of meningeal irritation may be absent, and the fever may not be very high, while the presence of confusion is frequent.

Diagnosis

The essential test for the diagnosis of acute bacterial meningitis is the examination of cerebrospinal fluid obtained through lumbar puncture (also see Chapter 6, Cerebrospinal Fluid Diagnostics). Lumbar puncture should be performed after a CT or MRI scan of the brain to exclude the risk of brain herniation due to decompression, particularly in the presence of focal neurological signs or seizures. The classic cerebrospinal fluid abnormalities in bacterial meningitis are: neutrophilic pleocytosis (more than 100, but up to 5,000 leukocytes/mm^3), reduced glucose concentration (<40 mg/dL or two-thirds of blood glucose level), and increased protein level (>50 mg/dL). The initial cerebrospinal fluid pressure is very high (>180 mmH_2O). Cerebrospinal fluid culture is positive in approximately 80% of cases, and Gram staining shows the presence of microorganisms in 60% of cases. Culture is also important for in vitro antibiotic susceptibility testing. The presence of ongoing antibiotic therapy at the time of lumbar puncture reduces the chances of bacterial recognition through microscopic and culture examination in 40-60% of patients. In cases with negative microscopic and culture examination, the execution of specific immunological tests (latex agglutination test, immunoenzymatic test) to determine the presence of microbial antigens for *S. pneumoniae*, *N. meningitidis*, *H. Influenzae* type B, group B *Streptococcus*, and *E. coli*, in cerebrospinal fluid can help identify the pathogen. Molecular tests for bacterial DNA detection using Polymerase Chain Reaction (PCR) have high sensitivity and specificity values. In particular, a new molecular technology increasingly used for cerebrospinal fluid analysis in suspected meningitis is the FilmArray system: it is a multiplex PCR that allows simultaneous detection of the most common pathogens causing central nervous system infections (bacteria, viruses, or fungi) in the same cerebrospinal fluid sample. It has high diagnostic accuracy and enables species-specific diagnosis within a few hours. Finally, if bacteremia is suspected, serial blood cultures, which are positive in 60% of cases of H. influenzae meningitis, can be useful.

Neuroradiological investigations, especially MRI, can show widening of the cerebral sulci and signs of vascular congestion in the pia mater and arachnoid. After contrast administration, meningeal enhancement can be observed. However, the result is nonspecific and can be present in all conditions with altered blood-brain barrier permeability (see Chapter 5 Neuroradiology).

Bacterial meningitis can be recurrent, especially in patients with ventriculoperitoneal shunts for the treatment of hydrocephalus. In rare cases, it may be due to the presence of a fistula between the paranasal sinuses and the subarachnoid space, usually following traumatic injuries. These post-traumatic meningitis cases can be accompanied by rhinorrhea (cerebrospinal fluid leakage from the nasal cavity).

Differential diagnosis

The differential diagnosis of bacterial meningitis should consider other infectious diseases of the central nervous system, such as viral encephalitis (especially *herpes simplex virus encephalitis*), which, however, exhibit different cerebrospinal fluid abnormalities (lymphocytic pleocytosis with normal glucose levels), and MRI shows cerebral tissue involvement (predominantly in the temporal lobe). Other considerations include rickettsial infections, which are associated with rash (which can progress to gangrene), and non-infectious clinical conditions that can resemble acute bacterial meningitis, such as subarachnoid hemorrhage, chemical meningitis, and meningitis associated with systemic inflammatory diseases such as systemic lupus erythematosus, Behçet's disease, and uveomeningitis syndromes (e.g., Vogt-Koyanagi-Harada syndrome).

Prognosis

Acute bacterial meningitis, particularly in neonates, presents a high mortality rate. Meningococcal meningitis, in particular, is characterized by a mortality rate of 5-18% of cases.

Certain clinical characteristics (advanced age, presence of otitis and mastoiditis, low Glasgow Coma Scale score, seizures at onset, signs of intracranial hypertension, shock) and delayed administration of antibiotic therapy are associated with a worse prognosis. The most common and frequent clinical sequelae in childhood include impairment of higher mental functions, memory deficits, epilepsy, hydrocephalus, deafness, and gait and balance impairments.

Treatment

The first element of the treatment of bacterial meningitis is prevention. The National Vaccination Prevention Plan 2017-2019 in Italy, approved by the State-Regions Conference, includes a national immunization program that includes meningococcus B and C vaccines for newborns, tetravalent anti-meningococcus Acwy135 vaccine for adolescents, and anti-pneumococcal vaccination (conjugate PCV13 + polysaccharide PPV23) for individuals over 65 years of age.

Meningitis is considered a medical emergency, and in addition to the treatment of septic shock and control of vital parameters, therapy involves initiating pharmacological treatment with antibiotics as soon as possible. Even in the absence of a definite etiology, an empirical treatment model based on demographic factors and the presence of comorbidities should be implemented (see Table 24.1). Once the infectious agent is identified, the antibiotic therapy will be adjusted accordingly (see Table 24.2). Antibiotic therapy should be administered intravenously and continued for at least 10-14 days. In addition to antibiotic therapy, it is essential to use medications that reduce intracranial hypertension and its complications. Dexamethasone inhibits the production of inflammatory factors such as IL-1 and TNF and stabilizes the blood-brain barrier, making it useful in the treatment of acute bacterial meningitis.

Prophylaxis | Prophylaxis is particularly indicated for meningococcal meningitis in individuals who have had contact with the patient within the preceding 10 days. Rifampicin (600 mg orally twice daily) is usually used, or alternatively, ceftriaxone and ciprofloxacin can be administered as a single dose.

Table 24.1 EMPIRICAL THERAPY FOR ACUTE BACTERIAL MENINGITIS BASED ON AGE OF ONSET

Indication	Antibiotic choices
Up to 3 months of age	Ampicillin + cefotaxime
> 3 months < 18 years	Cefotaxime or ceftriaxone + vancomycin
> 55 years or younger age but with debilitating diseases	Ampicillin + cefotaxime + vancomycin
Compromised patients, meningitis from neurosurgical procedures, post-traumatic meningitis	Ampicillin + ceftazidime + vancomycin

Table 24.2 THERAPY FOR THE MOST COMMON ACUTE BACTERIAL MENINGITIS BASED ON THE IDENTIFIED PATHOGEN

Pathogens	Antibiotic choices
Neisseria Meningitidis	Penicillin G or ampicillin Ceftriaxone or cefotaxime
Streptococcus pneumoniae	Penicillin G Ceftriaxone or cefotaxime Ceftriaxone or cefotaxime + vancomycin
Gram-negative bacteria	Ceftriaxone or cefotaxime
Listeria monocytogenes	Ampicillin + gentamicin
Haemophilus influenzae	Ceftriaxone or cefotaxime

24.1.2 Viral meningitis

Epidemiology

Acute viral meningitis is a relatively common clinical event, but due to the non-mandatory reporting of the disease, it is difficult to obtain an accurate estimate of cases. Some epidemiological studies have documented an incidence of 10-25 cases per 100,000 people per year. Viral meningitis is more common in the summer months and early autumn, suggesting an etiology primarily related to enterovirus and arbovirus infections. Viral meningitis falls into the category of aseptic meningitis, defined by the absence of bacteria in the cerebrospinal fluid culture.

Etiology

The most common causative agents are enteroviruses (group A and B coxsackieviruses, echoviruses), arboviruses, herpes simplex virus type 2 (HSV-2), cytomegalovirus, mumps virus, and lymphocytic choriomeningitis virus (Table 24.3). Viruses usually reach the meninges through hematogenous spread, crossing the choroid plexus or endothelial cells of the capillaries, or they become pathogens through reactivation processes in the nervous system. It should be noted that in many cases of viral meningitis, the causative agent is not identified.

Table 24.3 CAUSES OF ASEPTIC MENINGITIS (CLEAR CEREBROSPINAL FLUID)

Viral infections	
Enteroviruses Echovirus Coxsackie A, B Measles Mumps Herpes Simplex Virus 2 Varicella-Zoster Virus	Cytomegalovirus Human Herpesvirus 6 Arboviruses Human Immunodeficiency Virus (HIV) Adenovirus West Nile Virus
Bacterial infections	
Partially treated bacterial meningitis Brucellosis Listeria Mycoplasma pneumoniae	Syphilis Leptospirosis Lyme disease Whipple's disease Endocarditis
Rickettsial infections	
Fungal infections	
Parasitic infections	
Vasculitis	
Sarcoidosis Behcet's disease Lupus Rheumatoid arthritis	Polyarteritis nodosa Mixed connective tissue disease Sjogren's syndrome Wegener's granulomatosis
Carcinomatous	
Leukemia Lymphomas	
Chemical-induced	
Contrast media	
Drug-induced	
NSAIDs (Non-Steroidal Anti-Inflammatory Drugs) Antineoplastics Immunosuppressants	Antibiotics Intravenous immunoglobulins Valacyclovir

Symptoms

Patients with acute viral meningitis usually present with a sudden onset of headache, often with frontal or retro-orbital localization, associated with photophobia, fever, and signs of meningeal irritation. The symptoms are typically less severe than those present in bacterial meningitis. Patients may also exhibit systemic symptoms such as malaise, pharyngodynia, muscle pain, nausea, vomiting, and drowsiness, while severe alterations of consciousness are rather rare. Seizures and focal neurological signs are relatively uncommon and, if present, should raise suspicion of a process involving the brain parenchyma (such as encephalitis).

Enterovirus meningitis (coxsackievirus A and B, echovirus 1-9, 11-25, 30-31) is the most frequent type (80% of cases of aseptic meningitis with documented etiology and 40-60% of viral meningitis cases) and can also occur in small epidemic outbreaks. Children, especially in the first year of life, are most commonly affected. Patients may exhibit characteristic systemic signs such as roseola-like rash, conjunctivitis, lymphadenopathy, herpangina, pericarditis, or pleurisy. Mumps virus meningitis occurs more frequently in males and typically appears about 5 days after the onset of parotitis; it is more common in the winter and spring months. Arbovirus meningitis is typical in the summer and autumn months and can occur in epidemic outbreaks in specific geographic areas. HSV-2 meningitis can occur concurrently with the initial (primary) episode of genital herpes; however, a significant percentage of cases do not exhibit signs of genital herpes at the time of meningitis. It can have a recurrent course.

HIV-related meningitis should be suspected in every patient with HIV (or with risk factors for HIV) who presents with signs of viral meningitis. Involvement of cranial nerves V, VII, or VIII is common.

Diagnosis

The essential diagnostic test for viral meningitis is cerebrospinal fluid analysis. The cerebrospinal fluid appears clear, flows under normal or slightly increased pressure. The cytological profile shows lymphocytic pleocytosis (25-500 cells/mL; neutrophils may predominate in the first 48 hours), with normal or slightly elevated protein levels (20-80 mg/dL) and normal or slightly reduced glucose levels. No microorganisms are detected. Amplification of specific viral DNA or RNA using PCR is currently the most useful method for diagnosing viral meningitis. PCR is available for all arbovirus infections. Given its limited diagnostic capacity, it has been suggested to implement molecular diagnostics using Multiplex PCR, which allows for simultaneous testing for multiple viruses. Viral cultures are not very useful for diagnostic purposes.

Differential diagnosis of aseptic meningitis

Lymphocytic pleocytosis and normal glucose levels in cerebrospinal fluid can characterize numerous conditions (Table 24.4). These include acute bacterial meningitis already under antibiotic treatment (which may alter the typical cerebrospinal fluid profile of these forms) and non-viral infections such as rickettsial infections (typhus, Q fever), spirochetal infections (syphilis, Lyme disease, leptospirosis), fungal infections, protozoal infections, and certain bacterial infections (tuberculosis, brucellosis, and some cases of listeriosis). Non-infectious etiologies such as neoplastic meningitis, sarcoidosis, systemic lupus erythematosus (SLE), rheumatoid arthritis, granulomatous arteritis, Behçet's disease, and oculocerebrofacial syndromes should also be considered. Additionally, some drugs can cause aseptic meningitis (drug-induced aseptic meningitis), including nonsteroidal anti-inflammatory drugs (NSAIDs), cotrimoxazole, immunoglobulins, antiepileptics (e.g., lamotrigine), and monoclonal antibodies (e.g., cetuximab, infliximab). In these cases, the symptoms overlap with those of classic meningitis, and cerebrospinal fluid examination typically (but not exclusively) shows lymphocytic pleocytosis, normal glucose levels, slightly increased protein levels, and negative microbiological tests.

Table 24.4 MOST COMMON INFECTIOUS CAUSES OF CHRONIC MENINGITIS

Immunocompetent patients	Immunocompromised patients
Bacteria *Mycobacterium tubercolosis* *Treponema Pallidum* Parameningeal infections From focal lesions (sinusitis, otitis, mastoiditis) Viruses Mollaret's meningitis (Herpes Simplex Virus II) Measles	Bacteria *Mycobacterium tubercolosis* Viruses Cytomegalovirus Fungi *Cryptococcus neoformans* Candida Protozoa *Toxoplasma gondii* *Acanthamoeba*

Treatment

The treatment of viral meningitis is primarily symptomatic, using analgesics, antipyretics, antiemetics, and maintaining the patient's fluid and electrolyte balance. Aciclovir is indicated in herpes simplex virus (HSV) meningitis (administered orally or intravenously, depending on the severity of the case), although clear evidence of efficacy in randomized trials is lacking.

Prognosis

The prognosis is generally good in adults. In neonates and children, there may be cognitive sequelae (learning difficulties) and hearing loss.

Coronavirus infection and neurological disorders

Coronavirus disease 2019 (COVID-19) is a global pandemic caused by SARS-CoV-2 infection and is associated with both acute and chronic neurological disorders.

Acute neurological disorders

Anosmia and ageusia were among the earliest reported symptoms in patients with

COVID-19. The hypothesized pathogenic mechanism is infection of the nasal mucosa and support cells of the epithelium with subsequent dissemination through the olfactory nerve.

At least one-third of COVID-19 patients admitted to intensive care units may experience altered mental status. Changes in mental status are associated with various pathogenic factors such as respiratory failure with hypoxia, renal failure, electrolyte disturbances, and pre-existing neurological and systemic comorbidities triggering a non-inflammatory encephalopathy in which COVID-19 infection is a co-factor but without a direct effect of the virus on the central nervous system. However, in a small percentage of COVID-19 patients, encephalopathy may develop in the absence of severe respiratory failure, suggesting a direct effect of the virus on vascular endothelial cells. Inflammatory encephalitis, either directly caused by the virus or secondary to para-infectious or autoimmune mechanisms, is rarer. This type of encephalitis can manifest in various ways, ranging from typical viral encephalitis to a presentation resembling acute disseminated encephalomyelitis (ADEM) or necrotizing hemorrhagic encephalitis.

Some studies have demonstrated an increased incidence and severity of stroke in COVID-19 patients compared to a control population with stroke in the absence of COVID-19 infection. Potential pathogenic mechanisms responsible for acute neurological vascular complications of COVID-19 include coagulopathies leading to hypoxic-ischemic brain damage and abnormalities in the blood-brain barrier with endotheliopathy. Hypercoagulability (induced by focal and systemic inflammation) may also underlie cases of cerebral deep venous thrombosis, which are more frequent in COVID-19 patients than in the control population and are characterized by high mortality. However, it should be noted that primary high-dose antithrombotic prophylaxis protocols have not shown greater efficacy than the use of standard doses in reducing mortality or thromboembolic events.

Cases of acute polyradiculoneuropathy (Guillain-Barré syndrome or Miller Fisher syndrome) have been described in COVID-19 patients. Neurological symptoms typically occur 5 to 10 days after infection and have a clinical course and response to treatment similar to classical forms. Many COVID-19 patients report myalgia and muscle weakness. Myositis and rhabdomyolysis with marked elevation of creatine phosphokinase (CPK) may be present in hospitalized COVID-19 patients and represent negative prognostic markers for mortality. Similar to other patients with prolonged hospitalization, COVID-19 patients may develop *critical illness polyneuropathy*.

Chronic neurological disorders

There is no complete consensus yet on the chronic neurological and psychiatric sequelae of COVID-19 infection, referred to as "Long COVID" syndrome. The signs and symptoms of this condition are diverse and include neurocognitive problems (particularly memory disturbances), headache, mood alterations usually in the depressive spectrum, apathy, fatigue, reduced quality of life, and autonomic dysfunctions (hypotension, hypertension, sexual dysfunctions). The diagnosis, pathophysiology, and treatment of these disorders remain an interesting area of study that requires further research.

24.2 Chronic meningitis

Chronic meningitis is defined as meningitis with a insidious onset, progressive course, symptoms lasting more than 4 weeks, and persistent inflammatory reaction in the cerebrospinal fluid. It is a rare condition in immunocompetent individuals, but the incidence significantly increases in the presence of conditions that impair the immune response. Chronic inflammation of the meninges is a severe condition that, if left untreated, can lead to death. The causes of chronic meningitis are diverse, with the most common ones including infections, malignant neoplasms, non-infectious inflammatory diseases, chemical meningitis, and parameningeal infections. The etiology may vary depending on the presence or absence of immune system alterations (Table 24.4). Infectious causes can be bacterial, with *Mycobacterium tuberculosis*, *Borrelia burgdorferi* (Lyme disease), and *Treponema pallidum* (*syphilis*) being the most common agents. Less frequently, *Actinomyces, Nocardia, Brucella,* and *Trophirema whipplei* (causative agent of Whipple's disease) can be involved. Chronic meningitis can also be caused by fungal infections (*Cryptococcus neoformans, Mononuclear Coccidioides immitis, Candida spp., Histoplasma capsulatum, Blastomyces dermatitidis, Aspergillus spp., Sporothrix schenckii*), protozoal infections (toxoplasmosis, trypanosomiasis), and parasitic infections such as cysticercosis. Additionally, viral infections such as mumps, HIV, and HSV can cause chronic meningitis. Non-infectious causes include sarcoidosis, recurrent arteritis, Wegener's granulomatosis, and Mollaret's meningitis.

Chronic meningitis may also be characterized by periods of exacerbation alternating with periods of spontaneous symptom remission. The most common causes of relapsing forms are HSV-2 infection, chemical meningitis (resulting from the passage of substances contained in epidermoid tumors, craniopharyngiomas, cholesteatomas, or drugs such as nonsteroidal anti-inflammatory drugs, sulfonamides, isoniazid, azathioprine, among others), and inflammatory conditions such as Vogt-Koyanagi-Harada syndrome, Behçet's syndrome, and systemic lupus erythematosus (SLE).

The symptoms of chronic meningitis depend on the anatomical location of the inflammatory process. Persistent headache, neck or trunk pain, cranial neuropathies, cognitive disturbances, behavioral changes, hydrocephalus, and radiculopathies are very common. Systemic signs of non-infectious etiology or associated with neoplasms may also be observed. The essential diagnostic test is cerebrospinal fluid analysis, which will show various abnormalities depending on the etiology. Contrast-enhanced brain MRI may reveal thickening of the meninges and meningeal nodules. Occasionally, a meningeal biopsy is necessary for etiological diagnosis.

Among the most important types of chronic meningitis, we will discuss tuberculous, syphilitic, and Lyme meningitis.

24.2.1 Tuberculous meningitis and other forms of central nervous system tuberculosis

Central nervous system tuberculosis (TB) is caused by the extrapulmonary localization of *Mycobacterium tuberculosis* (5-15% of cases). It is more common in children but can also occur in adults, especially in those with HIV infection and immunocompromised individuals. In these cases, the etiology may also involve atypical mycobacteria. The most frequent clinical manifestation of central nervous system TB is tuberculous meningitis. Tuberculous meningitis originates from the hematogenous spread of primary or post-primary pulmonary TB or from the rupture of a tuberculoma into the subarachnoid space. Meningitis predominantly affects the cranial base, with inflammatory exudates extending from the brainstem to the optic chiasm and enveloping the adjacent cranial nerves. In children, tuberculous meningitis presents with nonspecific symptoms such as anorexia, weight loss, low-grade fever, apathy, and headache. Paralysis of the ocular motor nerves, particularly the abducens nerve, is frequent (30-70% of patients) and occurs early. Tuberculous meningitis can be accompanied by vasculitis and subsequent cerebral infarctions. If left untreated, the disease progresses with typical signs of fulminant meningitis, such as severe headache, seizures, mental deterioration, hydrocephalus, intracranial hypertension, brainstem involvement, and coma, and is associated with high mortality rates. Cerebrospinal fluid analysis reveals pleocytosis (usually lymphocytic, with an average of 1000 cells/ mm^3 and occasionally a neutrophil predominance in the early stages), increased protein content (150-400 mg/dL), and reduced glucose levels (15-30 mg/dL). After being kept at 37°C for a few hours, the cerebrospinal fluid may show the formation of a thin fibrin network (Mya's reticulum). Culture tests may be negative in over 20% of cases, while the identification of mycobacterial DNA using PCR is rapid and reliable in terms of sensitivity (80%). Brain MRI can reveal hydrocephalus, contrast enhancement in the basal cisterns and ependyma, or small round lesions, single or multiple, showing contrast enhancement, which may indicate evolving tuberculosis.

Tuberculous meningitis is fatal if left untreated. Treatment involves a combination of isoniazid, rifampicin, pyrazinamide, and ethambutol (or streptomycin) for the first 2 months, followed by rifampicin and isoniazid for a total duration of 9-12 months. The use of steroids increases the likelihood of survival but does not reduce the frequency of reported sequelae in at least 25% of cases treated appropriately. Central nervous system TB can also manifest as brain parenchymal granulomas (tuberculomas), which predominantly localize in the brain, cerebellum, brainstem, and spinal cord. These granulomas can be single or multiple (in most cases) and occasionally coexist with meningeal involvement. Tuberculomas are rare in children with HIV infection but can occur in adults undergoing combined antitubercular and antiretroviral therapy, a condition known as immune reconstitution inflammatory syndrome. Clinical signs of tuberculomas include those of space-occupying lesions (headache, seizures, increased intracranial pressure). Finally, TB can also affect the vertebral bodies, leading to abscess formation. Vertebral collapse resulting from vertebral body involvement can be complicated by spinal cord compression, most commonly at the thoracic level.

24.2.2 Neurosyphilis

Caused by *Treponema pallidum*, neurosyphilis was long considered a late manifestation of syphilis; however, involvement of the nervous system can occur in all stages of the disease. The incidence of neurosyphilis is increasing, especially in individuals with HIV, with a prevalence rate of 1-2% among HIV-positive patients.

Neurosyphilis can be asymptomatic or give rise to various forms of nervous system impairment. *Asymptomatic neurosyphilis* is present in 25% of untreated syphilis patients and is characterized solely by abnormalities in cerebrospinal fluid parameters (pleocytosis, increased protein levels, reactive VDRL). Symptomatic forms of neurosyphilis include early manifestations and late complications. *Syphilitic meningitis*, the earliest form of neurological complication in syphilis, is characterized by headache, nausea, vomiting, neck stiffness, involvement of cranial nerves (especially optic, facial, and acoustic nerves), seizures, and mental status changes. It usually occurs within the first year after primary infection. Late neurosyphilis can be divided into meningovascular syphilis and parenchymal neurosyphilis. The characteristic feature of *meningovascular syphilis* is the presence of obliterative endarteritis in small vessels, leading to the development of multiple infarct areas and focal neurological signs (hemiplegia, aphasia, seizures). *Parenchymal neurosyphilis* is characterized by neuronal degeneration and presents with two rare clinical pictures: tabes dorsalis (demyelination of the dorsal roots and posterior columns of the spinal cord, mainly at the dorsal level) and general paresis (cortical degeneration with a dementia syndrome). Both complications occur more than 20 years after primary infection. It should be noted that the natural history of neurosyphilis can be significantly modified by the coexistence of HIV infection. The diagnosis of neurosyphilis is based on positive VDRL (possible false positives), intrathecal synthesis of anti-Treponema antibodies, IgM antibodies against *Treponema pallidum*, and PCR detection of mycobacterial DNA. The treatment of choice is intravenous benzylpenicillin for 10-14 days.

24.2.3 Neuroborreliosis (Lyme Disease)

Lyme disease is a zoonosis caused by the spirochete *Borrelia burgdorferi*, and is transmitted to humans through the bite of ticks or lice. The disease is particularly common in certain geographical areas (especially Austria, Germany, France, Switzerland, and Sweden in Europe, with an incidence of up to 100-300 cases per 100,000) and is more prevalent during the summer months. It can affect individuals of any age, particularly those who work outdoors. From a clinical perspective, the disease is divided into different stages. The incubation period can last from 3 to 32 days, followed by the appearance of a characteristic erythematous skin lesion (erythema migrans), which is usually painless or pruritic and tends to expand over several days. It may be accompanied or not by fever, malaise, and muscle pain. Subsequently, often weeks or months after the cutaneous manifestations, hematogenous dissemination occurs, which can be associated with cardiac and neurological complications (in approximately 15% of cases). The mechanism of neurological damage includes ischemic damage secondary to vasculitis, cytotoxic damage, immune reactions due to antigenic mimicry, and the release of neurotoxic mediators. Neurological manifestations vary widely. The most frequent neurological manifestation in children is facial nerve palsy (including bilateral palsy), while in adults, it is a combination of radicular pain (100% of cases), headache (44%), facial nerve palsy (33%), and meningeal signs (20%). Untreated patients can progress to the chronic phase or late neuroborreliosis (defined as active disease for at least 6 months), characterized by chronic arthritis, chronic axonal neuropathy, meningitis or chronic encephalomyelitis, and acrodermatitis. The diagnosis of neuroborreliosis can be challenging because the clinical manifestations of the disease are nonspecific. A thorough medical history and clinical examination may reveal possible exposure in endemic areas and the presence of erythema migrans. Laboratory diagnosis is based on culture, but it is positive in less than 40% of cases. Serological tests can yield false-positive results. The antigenic determinants of *B. burgdorferi* are complex and can vary depending on the stage of the disease. Therefore, the identification of specific antibodies against *B. burgdorferi* is usually performed using a two-step method, initially an enzyme immunoassay followed by confirmation with a Western blot test. Cerebrospinal fluid analysis usually shows lymphocytic pleocytosis (up to several hundred cells) and increased protein levels, with normal glucose levels. Therapy, which is usually highly effective, is based on intravenous ceftriaxone for 2-4 weeks or, alternatively, oral doxycycline.

24.3 Focal infections of the central nervous system

24.3.1 Cerebral abscess

Cerebral abscess is a focal suppurative process localized in the brain parenchyma, usually surrounded by a vascularized capsule. It is a rare condition (incidence < 1.5/100.000 for year). Cerebral abscess can originate from contiguous infections (otitis, mastoiditis, sinusitis, dental infections), hematogenous spread, localized infections in other body sites (particularly the lungs), and post-traumatic or post-surgical complications. In 25% of cases, the source of infection cannot be identified. Abscesses originating from ear and mastoid infections are predominantly located in the temporal lobe and cerebellum and are generally caused by *Bacteroides*, *Enterobacteriacee*, or *Pseudomonas aeruginosa*. Abscesses resulting from sinus infections are primarily located in the frontal lobe, with streptococci, *Haemophilus*, *Pseudomonas* and *Staphylococcus aureus* being the most implicated bacteria. Abscesses caused by hematogenous spread (often from a pulmonary infectious focus, bacterial endocarditis, or congenital heart diseases) are generally multiple, favor the territory of the middle cerebral artery, and tend to localize at the junction of gray and white matter. Post-traumatic abscesses are often due to *Staphylococcus aureus* and *Staphylococcus epidermidis infections*.

Cerebral abscess typically develops in the presence of pre-existing brain tissue damage (ischemic, necrotic, or hypoxic), which increases susceptibility to infections. Initially, a focal area of edema and inflammation (cerebritis) occurs, followed by the formation of a necrotic-purulent central area delimited by the development of a capsule characterized by newly vascularized tissue.

Symptoms primarily depend on the presence of a space-occupying lesion. The most common symptoms are headache (75% of cases), fever (50% of cases), and variable focal neurological dysfunction depending on the location. Critical episodes are also frequent. Brain MRI is the essential diagnostic tool,

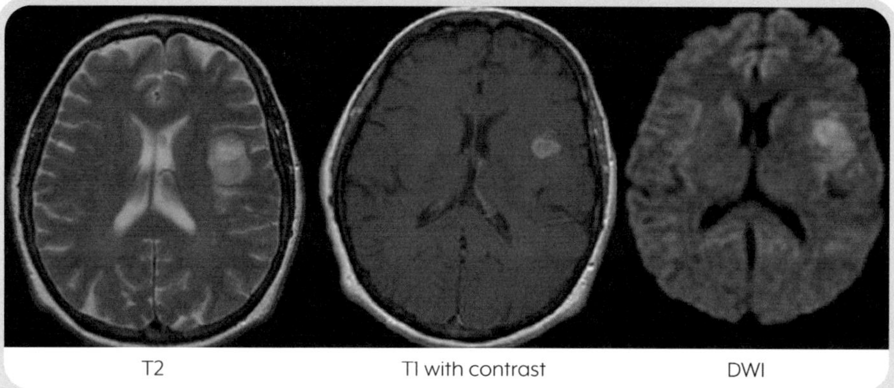

Figure 24.1

Brain MRI: the presence of an inflammatory signal alteration secondary to cerebritis is observed.

allowing visualization of the initial stages of abscess formation. The abscess appears as a central hypointense area with peripheral contrast enhancement, surrounded by cerebral edema (Figure 24.1). Lumbar puncture usually does not provide particularly useful information (positive cerebrospinal fluid culture in less than 10% of cases). Etiological diagnosis (microbiological and histological) is made from a brain tissue sample obtained through stereotactic biopsy, drainage, or excision of the abscess. Treatment involves the immediate evacuation of the purulent collection in larger abscesses and antibiotic therapy (third-generation cephalosporins, vancomycin, and metronidazole). Small abscesses (diameter less than 2.5 cm) are usually treated with antibiotic therapy alone. Prophylactic anticonvulsants are always recommended.

24.3.2 Non-bacterial focal infections

The most frequent causes of non-bacterial focal infections of the central nervous system are neurocysticercosis and toxoplasmosis. Neurocysticercosis mostly presents with new-onset epileptic seizures, usually partial seizures with or without secondary generalization. Toxoplasmosis is often asymptomatic but becomes symptomatic in the course of HIV infection, causing headache, fever, seizures, and focal neurological deficits. The diagnosis for both conditions is based on MRI. Neurocysticercosis lesions typically appear as cystic areas enhancing with contrast and surrounded by a significant amount of edema, along with the presence of calcifications. Toxoplasmosis usually manifests as multiple contrast-enhancing lesions distributed in the deep white matter and surrounded by edema.

24.3.3 Subdural empyema

Subdural empyema is a rare condition characterized by a collection of pus between the dura mater and arachnoid membrane. It predominantly affects young adult males. The most important risk factor is frontal sinusitis (including ethmoidal and maxillary sinuses), but it can also be associated with cranial trauma and neurosurgical interventions. Subdural empyema is caused by streptococci, staphylococci, and anaerobic bacteria. The infection likely occurs through retrograde spread from the cranial venous sinuses in the presence of osteomyelitic foci or thrombophlebitis of the venous sinuses. The most significant symptoms are fever and progressively worsening headache. As the infection progresses, focal signs (contralateral hemiparesis to the site of the empyema), seizures, and signs of increased intracranial pressure can occur. MRI is the diagnostic modality of choice, especially after contrast administration, which allows differentiation between the purulent collection and the underlying brain parenchyma. Lumbar puncture usually does not provide particularly useful information (positive cerebrospinal fluid culture in less than 10% of cases). The etiological diagnosis (microbiological and histological) is established by obtaining a sample of purulent material through drainage or excision. The treatment of subdural empyema involves immediate evacuation of the purulent collection and antibiotic therapy (third-generation cephalosporins, vancomycin, and metronidazole).

24.3.4 Epidural abscess

Epidural abscess is a rare condition characterized by the collection of pus in the space between the inner table of the cranial bones and the dura mater. It can occur following a neurosurgical procedure, cranial trauma, or be a complication of frontal sinusitis or infections of the middle ear, mastoid, or orbit. The etiology is very similar to that described in subdural empyema. The clinical presentation is characterized by fever, headache, neck stiffness, epileptic seizures, and focal signs. MRI is the diagnostic modality of choice (appears as a hyperintense fluid collection compared to cerebrospinal fluid on T2-weighted images). Therapeutically, epidural abscess requires the immediate evacuation of the purulent collection associated with antibiotic therapy (third-generation cephalosporins, vancomycin, and metronidazole).

Epidural abscess can also occur in the spinal region and in this case, it is usually secondary to osteomyelitis. It can be associated with skin wounds and septicemia and rarely be a complication of spinal surgery. Spinal epidural abscess is commonly due to *Staphilococcus aureus* infection. The most important symptoms are fever and localized pain in the spine or radiating along the nerve root. Rapid progression to spinal cord compression is possible. Surgical intervention with laminectomy and drainage of the abscess is usually necessary.

24.3.5 Intracranial thrombophlebitis

Intracranial thrombophlebitis refers to septic thrombosis of the cortical veins and venous sinuses. It often represents a complication of other CNS infections such as meningitis, subdural empyema, epidural abscess, or sinusitis, otitis, or mastoiditis. Cerebral veins and venous sinuses do not have valves, allowing blood to flow in both directions, facilitating the spread of thrombosis. The symptoms vary depending on the affected venous sinus. In the case of thrombophlebitis of the superior sagittal sinus, there is headache, fever, nausea, vomiting, epileptic seizures, and alterations in consciousness (up to coma). In the case of cavernous sinus thrombophlebitis, there are signs of involvement of cranial nerves III, IV, VI (with diplopia, ptosis, chemosis) and the ophthalmic and maxillary branches of the same side cranial nerve V (with hyperesthesia in the corresponding territories and reduced corneal reflex) along with headache, fever, frontal and retroorbital pain. Thrombophlebitis of the transverse sinus can present with headache, ear pain, paralysis of the cranial nerve VI, and retro-orbital or facial pain (Gradenigo's syndrome). The diagnosis of intracranial thrombophlebitis is essential with an angio-MRI study of the venous phase, which may show the absence of flow in the affected venous sinus. The treatment is based on the use of antibiotics (the choice of antimicrobial therapy is based on the identification of the responsible bacteria), hydration, and when possible (cavernous sinus or lateral sinus thrombophlebitis) surgical removal of the thrombus and infected tissue. Anticoagulant therapy with heparin is recommended if there are no major contraindications to the use of anticoagulants.

24.4 Other infections of the nervous system

24.4.1 Poliomyelitis

Poliomyelitis is an infectious disease caused by *poliovirus hominis* (serotypes 1, 2, 3) belonging to the family *Picornaviridae*, genus Enterovirus. The disease has practically disappeared in the Western hemisphere thanks to extensive vaccination. In areas where access to vaccination is more difficult and its effectiveness can be compromised by endemic intestinal infections, there are still outbreaks of infection (Asia, the Indian subcontinent, and some areas of Africa). The transmission of the disease occurs through the fecal-oral route. Once polioviruses enter the body, they multiply in the lymphoid tissues of the oropharynx and intestine and reach the CNS through transcapillary passage or direct migration from the pharynx via axonal transport. Poliovirus infection is subclinical in more than 90% of cases or may exhibit nonspecific characteristics of other viral infections (fever, headache, pharyngodynia, anorexia, vomiting, abdominal pain) with spontaneous resolution within a few days. Neurological manifestations are the result of selective involvement of the motor neurons in the anterior horns of the spinal cord, leading to peripheral-type paralysis (loss of strength, atrophy, fasciculations, reduced muscle tone). The lower limbs are most commonly affected (60% of cases), followed by the upper limbs (20-30% of cases), diaphragm, and intercostal muscles. The limbs are often asymmetrically involved. If bulbar regions are affected, cranial nerve paralysis predominates, particularly the IX and X pairs. The diagnosis is primarily based on clinical manifestations, and cerebrospinal fluid shows findings compatible with aseptic meningitis. The inflammatory process and neuronal destruction mainly occur in the motor neurons of the spinal cord's anterior horns, motor nuclei of the brainstem and pons, reticular substance, thalamus, and motor cortex. Electromyography will show signs of second motor neuron distress. There is no specific therapy, but prevention is achieved through the use of trivalent vaccine. Post-polio syndrome is a clinical entity that can occur in about 20% of patients, typically 20-40 years after the acute episode of poliomyelitis. It is characterized by pain and worsening of weakness and atrophy in the segments affected by the acute episode.

24.4.2 Tetanus

Tetanus is an acute, sporadic, but often lethal toxin-mediated infection caused by *Clostridium tetani's*, tetanospasmin exotoxin, a habitual resident of the intestinal tract of herbivores. Currently, it is rather rare in our country due to the availability of the vaccine, but it is very common in tropical areas, mainly affecting newborns and children. *C. tetani* is an obligate anaerobic, Gram-positive bacillus without a capsule, and its spores are highly resistant to chemical and physical agents, able to survive for years in soil, water, and atmospheric dust. Infection occurs through the penetration of spores or vegetative forms through cutaneous and mucosal breaks (wounds, burns, pressure ulcers, sores, animal bites, puncture wounds, injections). Spore germination occurs only under anaerobic conditions, with an oxygen tension lower than that normally present in tissues. The highly virulent and neurotropic tetanospasmin is released in the cutaneous or mucosal lesion, binds to peripheral motor neuron terminals, enters the axon, is retrogradely transported to the cell body located in the spinal cord and brainstem, and reaches the presynaptic terminals where it blocks the release of inhibitory neurotransmitters glycine and GABA. The reduction of inhibitory activity results in pathological increase of alpha-motoneuron firing, causing muscle hypertonia and spasms. Tetanospasmin also has a direct inhibitory action on preganglionic sympathetic neurons located in the gray matter of the spinal cord, leading to sympathetic hyperactivity. Lastly, tetanospasmin has a direct action on the neuromuscular junction, partially similar to that exerted by botulinum toxin.

Generalized tetanus, the most common form resulting from toxin release in the lymphatic system and blood, typically manifests with trismus, caused by masseter muscle contraction. The face assumes the characteristic expression of *risus sardonicus* due to persistent contraction of the facial muscles. Muscle rigidity extends cranio-caudally, affecting the skeletal muscles of the trunk and causing opisthotonus (hyperextension of the trunk), hyperextension of the lower limbs, and flexion of the upper limbs. Some patients experience violent and generalized spasms that can cause laryngospasm and interfere with breathing. Spasms can be spontaneous or triggered by voluntary movements and sensory stimuli. Dysphagia is common, and an increase in body temperature may occur. Autonomic changes due to sympathetic hyperactivity can cause hypertensive crises, hyperpyrexia, peripheral vasoconstriction, and profuse sweating. Cognitive functions are preserved. Localized tetanus, which is rarer, involves only specific muscle groups and is not associated with systemic symptoms or paroxysms. Neonatal tetanus is a generalized form that is usually fatal.

Tetanic spasms should be distinguished from spasms caused by rabies virus (which does not cause persistent contractions), nuchal rigidity accompanying meningitis (where cerebrospinal fluid examination will be abnormal, whereas it is usually normal in tetanus), strychnine poisoning (lack of fever and trismus), acute dystonias (or dystonic status), usually secondary to the use of drugs blocking dopaminergic receptors.

Evolution can be favorable in cases with a long incubation period (healing within 2-4 weeks). In severe tetanus (incubation period less than 48 hours), evolution is often rapid and fatal due to respiratory failure and cardiac arrhythmias. Therapy, carried out in intensive care units, involves general measures aimed at cardiopulmonary monitoring and reducing environmental stimuli; wound care is essential. The use of antibiotics, particularly penicillin G or metronidazole, aims to eliminate vegetative cells (the source of the toxin). Antitoxin (human immunoglobulins, 3000-6000 units) is used to neutralize circulating toxin that is not yet bound to nerve cells. Barbiturates, benzodiazepines (diazepam or lorazepam intravenously), meprobamate, or phenothiazines are used to treat contractions and spasms. Prophylaxis involves vaccination (active immunization) with tetanus toxoid and passive immunization with specific immunoglobulins in case of a dangerous wound. Vaccination provides complete immunity for a period of approximately 5 years, with subsequent doses recommended every 10 years.

24.4.3 Botulism

Botulism is a severe illness caused by the neurotoxin produced by *Clostridium botulinum* and characterized by rapidly progressive flaccid paralysis. *C. botulinum* is an anaerobic, Gram-positive bacillus whose spores are ubiquitous in soil, marine and lake waters and are highly resistant to heat. The spores can contaminate agricultural and fishery products. Spores can germinate under anaerobic conditions. Following germination and multiplication, exotoxin is produced. Botulinum toxin is the most potent toxin known, easily inactivated by heat (100°C for 20 min). The disease can result from the ingestion of contaminated food (foodborne botulism), often homemade preparations (particularly vegetables, fruits, condiments, less frequently meat or fish) or improperly preserved. It can rarely be a consequence of a wound. Intestinal botulism affects children under 12 months of age and is due to toxin production following ingestion of spores contained in food that undergo germination within the intestinal canal. Once absorbed, botulinum toxin reaches peripheral cholinergic nerve endings hematogenously, penetrates the neuron, is internalized into endocytic vesicles, and blocks the release of acetylcholine at neuromuscular junctions, postganglionic parasympathetic fibers, and peripheral ganglia. The synapse is irreversibly damaged, and recovery is related to the sprouting of new terminals. Symptoms can vary greatly. After a prodromal phase characterized by asthenia, nausea, vomiting, and diarrhea, a symmetrical descending paralysis occurs, involving the oculomotor nerves and resulting in ophthalmoplegia, diplopia, ptosis, accommodation paralysis, mydriasis, and anisocoria. Other symptoms may then appear, such as dysphagia, dysphonia, xerostomia, facial muscle weakness, and sometimes symmetric paralysis of the limbs, neck muscles, and trunk. Autonomic involvement can also cause constipation, urinary retention, reduced salivary and lacrimal secretions, and decreased sweating. In addition to the clinical and anamnestic data (with particular attention to possible ingestion of contaminated food), the diagnosis is based on neurophysiological tests, especially electromyography (EMG), which shows decreased muscle action potential following repetitive stimulation of the motor nerve at low stimulation frequencies and increased action potential for high frequencies. Botulism should be distinguished from Guillain-Barré syndrome, myasthenia gravis, Lambert-Eaton syndrome, stroke, and intoxication with substances that depress the nervous system (alcohol, organophosphates, CO, nerve gas). Definitive diagnosis is made by demonstrating the presence of the toxin in the patient's serum, feces, or gastric juice and, when possible, in the contaminated food. The course of botulism can vary depending on the type and amount of ingested toxin. It can rapidly lead to death due to respiratory failure or cardiac arrest caused by bulbar paralysis. In cases that evolve favorably, neurological disorders resolve within weeks or months, sometimes leaving residual accommodation and respiratory mechanical alterations. Treatment involves admission to the intensive care unit for respiratory control. Equine antitoxin serum must be administered intramuscularly and intravenously, preceded by a sensitivity test for equine serum. In infant botulism, a single dose of human immunoglobulins is indicated.

Bibliography

Deigendesch N., Stenzel W. Acute and chronic bacterial infections and sarcoidosis. Handbook of Clinical Neurology, 145 (3rd series). 217-225.

Deigendesch N., Stenzel W. Acute and chronic viral infections. Handbook of Clinical Neurology, 145 (3rd series). 227-242.

McGill F., Griffith M.J., Solomon T. Viral meningitis: current issues in diagnosis and treatment. Curr Opin Infect Dis, 30:248–256, 2017.

25 ENCEPHALITIS

Silvia Romano, Marco Salvetti

The term "encephalitis" is used to indicate a group of diseases characterized by an inflammatory process involving the brain parenchyma and can be triggered by a viral, bacterial, fungal, or parasitic infection. When the inflammatory process also involves the meninges, it constitutes the picture of meningoencephalitis; if, instead, the spinal cord is also involved, it is referred to as encephalomyelitis.

The definition of encephalitis does not necessarily imply the presence of the infectious agent within the brain tissue. In approximately one-third of encephalitis cases, an immune-mediated pathogenesis has been identified.

25.1 Epidemiology

Encephalitis manifests with a variable incidence ranging from 3.5 to 7.4 cases per 100,000 population. In Italy, according to ISTAT data from 2003 on infectious diseases, the incidence is approximately 1.26 cases per 100,000 population (695 cases of viral encephalitis were reported in 2009).

Encephalitis can occur at any age, although, like most infectious diseases, it is more common in children, elderly, and immunocompromised patients. Generally, there are no differences between genders, although there is a higher incidence in males with an M:F ratio of 1.3-1.4:1.

Over 100 different pathogens have been described as causing encephalitis. However, in many cases (32-85%), the etiological agent remains unidentified. In the last two decades, the introduction of vaccination against measles, mumps, and rubella has led to a drastic reduction in incidence. However, at the same time, there has been an increase in cases caused by new agents such as West Nile virus, enterovirus 71, Australian Lyssavirus, and Nipah virus. Significant epidemics caused by emerging viruses have occurred in the last two decades: West Nile virus (New York 1999), Nipah virus (Malaysia 1998-99), and Usutu virus (Emilia Romagna 2009).

Among viral agents, *Herpes Simplex Virus* (HSV) is considered the most common cause of sporadic encephalitis in Western countries, while in some countries in Central Europe or in Sweden, the most common encephalitis is arbovirus-related, transmitted by tick bites. Regarding the age of onset, in neonates and children under 2 years of age, enterovirus infections (Coxackie), associated with myocarditis and hepatitis, HSV type 2 infections, characterized by genital skin eruptions and transmitted to the neonate during childbirth, and Mycoplasma pneumoniae infections generally causing meningoencephalitis are more frequent. The mode of transmission is important, especially for certain viruses such as arboviruses, which are transmitted by arthropods (ticks and mosquitoes) and whose spread depends on the vector life cycle (seasonality) and colonization areas (specific geographic distribution). In Italy, the most common arbovirus encephalitis is caused by tick bites endemic in alpine areas.

Recently, following the coronavirus 2 (SARS-CoV-2) pandemic, cases of COVID-19-associated encephalitis have been described, characterized by a wide spectrum of clinical presentations, both concurrent with the infection and with a later onset (after 7-8 days).

Risk factors have not been identified specifically in the general population. However, certain groups, such as immunocompromised patients, are more predisposed to develop the disease, as are individuals engaged in agricultural activities associated with a higher risk of developing arbovirus encephalitis. Immunocompromised individuals have a high risk of developing encephalitis following opportunistic infections due to Toxoplasma, Cytomegalovirus (CMV), and JC Virus. With the introduction of new immunosuppressive drugs and selective monoclonal antibodies for the treatment of some autoimmune diseases (multiple sclerosis, Crohn's disease, etc.), there has been an increase in the incidence of progressive multifocal leukoencephalopathy due to JC virus, initially described only in patients with AIDS, hematological diseases, or organ transplantation.

25.2 Clinical aspects and classification

Regardless of the triggering etiological agent, acute encephalitis presents with an onset characterized by symptoms indicative of an acute inflammatory process associated with signs and symptoms indicating alteration of brain functions. Over 90% of patients experience fever, headache, general malaise, and diffuse muscle pain to varying degrees. Involvement of the brain parenchyma leads to focal and diffuse neurological symptoms. Typically, complex symptomatology can be characterized by cognitive dysfunction (memory disturbances up to cognitive impairment), behavioral changes (disorientation, restlessness, hallucinations, psychosis, personality changes), neurological deficits (motor and sensory disturbances, visual and cranial nerve deficits, etc.), and epileptic seizures. The presence of certain neurological symptoms can indicate an anatomical localization of the process: the presence of involuntary movements associated with behavioral and language disorders may indicate involvement of the basal ganglia, while cognitive dysfunction and behavioral changes may indicate involvement of the frontal and temporal lobes. Diffuse involvement inevitably leads to altered consciousness, ranging from stupor to coma. Epileptic seizures, both generalized and focal, are also common. Occasionally, autonomic disorders such as hypothermia may occur, indicating hypothalamic dysfunction. The presence of fever associated with headache and neck stiffness, indicative of meningeal involvement, suggests a diagnosis of meningoencephalitis. Clinical manifestations alone do not allow for an etiological diagnosis; however, in some cases, specific signs (e.g., skin rashes in exanthematous diseases) can provide significant support. The evolution and severity of symptoms are closely dependent on the patient's age and immune system status; in general, symptoms are more severe in children and in adults over 65 years of age.

25.3 Diagnosis

The diagnosis of encephalitis is based on several fundamental features for differential diagnosis. The clinical history and diagnostic tests should aim to identify the possible etiological agent, ruling out encephalopathy due to metabolic causes (renal failure, liver failure, hypoxia, diabetes, etc.) or immune-mediated causes (acute disseminated encephalomyelitis, paraneoplastic encephalitis). A detailed medical history is the first step in evaluating a patient with suspected encephalitis. The clinical history, often obtained with the help of family members (due to the patient's altered consciousness), should inquire about any travel to foreign countries (if the patient has been in Asia, Japanese encephalitis can be considered) or possible animal contacts (tick-borne encephalitis), gathering all relevant information, including the patient's immune status. The description of the onset is also important: a sudden onset of symptoms with rapid progression may indicate HSV infection, while a biphasic course suggests enterovirus encephalitis.

General examination of the patient is useful in detecting respiratory tract infections (influenza virus) or gastrointestinal infections (enterovirus). Blood tests (complete blood count and electrolytes) and evaluation of liver and renal function can be supportive in differentiating viral from bacterial forms and ruling out metabolic causes. Chest X-ray can detect pulmonary localizations of tuberculosis, Legionella, or Mycoplasma. Electroencephalography (EEG) is currently considered a non-specific investigational tool. In general, it is possible to establish that encephalitis involving the white matter shows EEG patterns characterized by diffuse slow activity, while forms involving the gray matter exhibit rhythmic slow activity. However, this distinction is not always easy to determine. Eighty percent of patients with Herpes Simplex encephalitis have abnormal EEG findings, including background slowing and the presence of Periodic Lateralized Epileptiform Discharges (PLEDS) in the temporal region. This periodic EEG pattern can be detected between the 2nd and 14th day from the onset of the disease, most commonly between the 5th and 10th day. Another characteristic pattern is described in subacute sclerosing panencephalitis, where EEG reveals periodic activity repeating at regular intervals every 4-15 seconds, synchronous with the patient's myoclonus. Magnetic Resonance Imaging (MRI) has higher sensitivity and specificity compared to CT and should be the first examination to be performed in the evaluation of a patient with suspected encephalitis. A basic MRI protocol requires T1-weighted, T2-weighted, and FLAIR (fluid-attenuated inversion recovery) sequences, with FLAIR being extremely sensitive in detecting even subtle abnormalities. CT scans may be normal in the early stages of herpes simplex encephalitis, while MRI can demonstrate areas of edema with altered signal intensity, primarily in the temporal lobes (especially in adults), orbital areas of the frontal lobes, insular cortex, and angular gyrus. Cases with marked cerebral edema may exhibit midline shift. Neuroimaging often reveals necrotic-hemorrhagic foci. All patients with clinical suspicion of CNS infection should undergo lumbar puncture with cerebrospinal fluid (CSF) examination, after ruling out intracranial hypertension or space-occupying lesions with marked cerebral edema. In viral encephalitis, lymphocytic pleocytosis (10-200 lymphocytes/mm3) associated with variable protein elevation (0.6-6 g/L) may be observed. In bacterial infections, generally associated with meningitis, an increase in neutrophils and a decrease in glucose are observed. Cultures should be performed in cases of suspected bacterial or fungal infections. The search for antibodies directed against certain viruses (HSV1, HSV2, VZV, CMV, HHV6, HHV7, CMV, EBV, RSV, HIV, adenovirus, influenza A and B, rotavirus, coxsackie) or against Mycoplasma pneumoniae can be useful, using enzyme assays capable of detecting even small amounts of antibodies. PCR (polymerase chain reaction) has significantly facilitated the diagnostic pathway for viral encephalitis, allowing for the direct detection of viral nucleic acids in the cerebrospinal fluid. Real-time PCR can identify and quantify the genomes of a panel of viruses (with their serotypes), amplifying multiple viral genomes simultaneously. This technique has reduced the turnaround time of the test, increased sensitivity (>99%), and achieved high specificity (>99%). Quantitative determination of the virus in the CSF is important as it provides an indirect parameter of the extent of infection that can be monitored over time to assess treatment response. PCR is currently considered the gold standard for detecting HSV1 and 2, HHV6, EBV, CMV, adenovirus, and influenza viruses in the cerebrospinal fluid. For enteroviruses and Parvovirus B19, PCR is the only available technique.

25.4 Classification

There are different classifications of encephalitis based on epidemiological aspects (sporadic and epidemic), anatomopathological features, course (acute, subacute, and chronic), pathogenetic mechanism (primary and secondary), and etiological agentl (▪ Tablel 25.1).

Sporadic encephalitis, such as HSV encephalitis, occurs in the absence of clusters, epidemic infections, or a previous systemic infection. Epidemic encephalitis, such as arbovirus encephalitis, is seasonal and occurs during specific periods of the year depending on the implicated etiological agent.

According to the anatomopathological classification, different types of encephalitis exist based on involvement of the gray matter and/or white matter:

- forms with exclusive involvement of the gray matter (polioencephalitis) caused

Table 25.1 PRIMARY CAUSES OF ENCEPHALITIS

Viral		Bacterial		Rickettsial
Herpesviruses - HSV 1 and 2 - VZV - EBV - CMV - Human herpesvirus 6 Enteroviruses - Poliovirus Coxsackievirus Echovirus Enterovirus 70 and 71 Paramyxoviruses - Measles (Morbillivirus) - Mumps (Rubulavirus) - Parainfluenza - Nipah Virus	Adenovirus Rubivirus - Rubella (German Measles) Orthomyxovirus - Influenza A and B Flavivirus - Dengue - Japanese encephalitis - ESt. Louis Encephalitis - West Nile Virus Tick-Borne Encephalitis Rabies HIV JC Virus	Neisseria meningitis Streptococcus pneumoniae Haemophilus influenzea Mycoplasm pneumoniae Streptococco group A	Listeria Mycobacterium Chlamydia Borrelia Brucella Leptospira Treponema pallidum Bartonella	Rickettsia rickettsi Coxsiella burnetii Ehrlichia **Parasitic** Toxoplasma gondii **Autoimmune** Paraneoplastic Non-paraneoplastic

by poliovirus, coxsackievirus, echovirus, enterovirus, rabies virus, arboviruses, paraneoplastic encephalitis, and Rasmussen encephalitis;
- forms with exclusive involvement of the white matter (leukoencephalitis) caused by JC virus, HIV, acute disseminated encephalomyelitis (ADEM);
- forms with involvement of both the white matter and gray matter (panencephalitis) caused by HSV1 and HSV2, varicella-zoster virus, CMV, HIV, measles, arboviruses, rickettsiae, Lyme disease, Rasmussen encephalitis, and paraneoplastic encephalitis.

According to the pathogenetic classification, encephalitis can be categorized as primary, in which invasion of the CNS occurs through direct invasion by the pathogen, or secondary, post-infectious or para-infectious, which represents a complication of the primary infection on an immunologically mediated basis and is sometimes caused by reactivation of a latent virus. Secondary encephalitis primarily affects the white matter, and a previous history of infection or immunization can often be identified (poxviruses, varicella-zoster virus).

The etiological classification allows for a broader evaluation of different clinical presentations and differentiates encephalitis based on the infecting agent (viral, bacterial, fungal, parasitic, immune-mediated forms).

25.5 Viral encephalitis

25.5.1 Herpes virus encephalitis

Herpes simplex type 1 and type 2 (HSV1 and HSV2)

Herpes encephalitis is the most common cause of viral encephalitis in Italy and worldwide, with an incidence of approximately 1 case per 250,000-500,000 people per year. About 90% of cases are caused by Herpes simplex virus type 1 (HSV1), while the remaining 10% is caused by type 2 (HSV2). Most cases of encephalitis are associated with reactivation of a latent infection. Prior to the introduction of specific antiviral therapy, the mortality rate exceeded 70%, and only 2.5% of patients had no neurological sequelae. It is believed that during primary infection, the virus infects neurons in the olfactory bulb and reaches the CNS via retrograde spread, while in cases of virus reactivation (herpes labialis), the spread occurs from the trigeminal ganglia through the tentorium to the frontal and temporal lobes.

Recent studies suggest that herpes encephalitis may develop in individuals with a genetic predisposition. Mutations in genes involved in innate immunity against HSV-1, such as UNC-93B and Toll-like receptor 3 (TLR3), as well as genes encoding STAT-1 and NEMO transcription factors, have been identified in some children with herpes encephalitis. These mutations affect proteins involved in the IFN pathways induced by TLR3 receptor stimulation, impeding the production of IFN-α/β e IFN-λ in fibroblasts and virus-infected neurons, thereby rendering these cells more susceptible to the virus. However, these mutations exhibit incomplete penetrance, suggesting the involvement of other factors such as age and viral load in the pathogenesis of the disease.

The most common clinical manifestations are alterations in consciousness, fever, and headache, sometimes associated with aphasia and personality disorders. MRI shows involvement of the temporal lobes (Figure 25.1), while EEG is characterized by the presence of periodic patterns occurring at regular intervals of 2 to 3 seconds. CSF may show mild to moderate lymphocytic pleocytosis of 5-500 cells/mm3, a slight increase in protein levels, and normal or slightly decreased glucose levels. In approximately 5% of patients, CSF examination is normal.

HSV2 is among the infectious agents responsible for neonatal encephalitis and more commonly causes lymphocytic meningitis and myelitis in adults. Unlike HSV1, HSV2 typically results in a diffuse encephalitic picture and is generally not localized to the temporal and frontal lobes.

Varicella zoster virus

Varicella-zoster virus (VZV) infection is responsible for varicella (primary infection) and herpes zoster (secondary reactivation of the virus). Neurological involvement is rare, especially after the introduction of vaccination. In non-immunized individuals, primary infection can involve the cerebellum and present with cerebellar symptoms (ataxia, nystagmus) without alteration of consciousness. Following primary infection, VZV remains latent in spinal ganglia but can reactivate, causing the characteristic vesicular rash of herpes zoster. CNS involvement is rare and more commonly occurs in immunocompromised individuals. Similar to HSV infections, the diagnosis of VZV encephalitis relies on PCR to identify viral antigens in the cerebrospinal fluid.

Epstein-barr virus (EBV) and other herpes virus

EBV is an ubiquitous virus that selectively infects B lymphocytes in the most of individuals, and its most frequent clinical manifestation is mononucleosis. Like other herpes viruses, EBV can establish latent infection with the potential for reactivation. Neurological complications during primary infection are very rare (1-5%) and more commonly develop in pediatric patients, even in the absence of

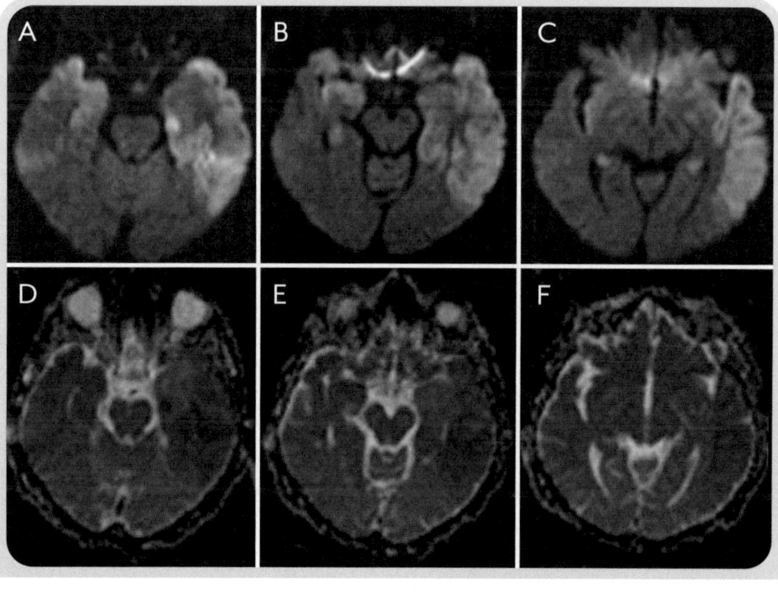

Figure 25.1

Herpetic encephalitis. Diffusion-weighted MRI (A-C) shows a left temporal alteration.

typical mononucleosis symptoms. Diagnosis is made using a combination of serological and molecular analysis. Given the widespread of the virus, infecting B lymphocytes (present in inflammatory states), positive PCR results in the cerebrospinal fluid are frequently observed as an incidental finding of latent virus detection. PCR should always be accompanied by serological evaluation for the detection of antibodies against viral capsid and nuclear antigen.

Cytomegalovirus (CMV) is another virus that can cause encephalitis, although rarely, affecting immunocompromised individuals or neonates through transplacental infection. Human herpesvirus 6 has also been identified as a cause of encephalitis in immunocompromised patients, particularly those undergoing organ transplantation, but its pathogenic role in healthy individuals has not been confirmed.

25.5.2 Arbovirus encephalitis

West Nile virus (WNV)

West Nile virus (WNV), an RNA virus of the Flavivirus family, is transmitted through mosquito bites serving as the reservoir of infection. As with other arbovirus infections, only a minority of infected individuals develop symptoms; approximately 20% of infected individuals experience a flu-like illness (West Nile fever), and less than 1% exhibit CNS involvement. Elderly individuals and immunocompromised patients are more likely to present with severe neurological symptoms and have a higher risk of mortality and long-term disability. Diagnosis is made by examining cerebrospinal fluid, which typically shows lymphocytic pleocytosis, although neutrophil predominance may be present in approximately 40% of cases. The "gold standard" for diagnosing WNV infection is the detection of IgM antibodies in the cerebrospinal fluid, which can be observed in approximately 90% of patients with WNV encephalitis, 8-10 days after symptom onset. Peripheral nervous system involvement is also a useful feature for differential diagnosis.

Other arboviruses

In addition to WNV, other arboviruses have been associated with cases of encephalitis, although they generally cause sporadic infections with limited geographic distribution. These include the La Crosse virus, St. Louis encephalitis virus, and Eastern equine encephalitis virus, which represent endemic and occasionally epidemic causes of encephalitis.

25.5.3 Enterovirus Encephalitis (EV)

More than 68 serotypes of enteroviruses have been identified, associated with a heterogeneous group of clinical syndromes. EV are well known as a cause of aseptic meningitis, and only recently have they been identified as the cause of encephalitis, primarily in children. Many of these viruses, however, cause infections with mild symptoms.

25.5.4 (Tick Borne Encephalitis TBE)

Tick-borne encephalitis is an infection caused by a flavivirus and primarily transmitted through tick bites. It includes three subtypes: the European subtype, transmitted by the *ixodes ricinus*, tick, endemic in rural areas and forests of Central, Eastern, and Northern Europe; the Far Eastern subtype, primarily transmitted by the *I. persulcatus tick*, endemic in eastern regions of Russia, forests in China, and Japan; and the Siberian subtype, also transmitted by I. persulcatus tick, endemic in the Ural region, Siberia, eastern regions of Russia, and some areas of northeastern Europe.

Transmission through the ingestion of unpasteurized raw milk from infected animals (goats, sheep, cattle) has also been described. TBE has been known in Europe since the beginning of the century and is currently endemic in 27 European countries, with more than 10,000 hospitalizations annually. TBE is becoming an increasingly relevant public health issue, and national surveillance plans are implemented every year. At the European level, the disease has been notifiable since 2012, and the latest data published by the European Centre for Disease Prevention and Control (ECDC) indicate that endemic areas are expanding. In 2015, 1,908 cases were reported, with an incidence of 0.4 per 100,000 population, which tends to be higher in the Czech Republic and Lithuania.

In total, from 2000 to 2016, 456 confirmed TBE cases were reported in Italy, primarily located in the alpine and subalpine regions of northeastern regions. Individuals exposed and at higher risk of infection are those who, for professional or recreational reasons, frequent tick-infested areas, particularly wooded or uncultivated areas below 1,000-1,300 meters above sea level.

After tick bites, there is an incubation period of approximately 8 days (range 4-28 days), but if the infection is acquired through food, the incubation period is generally shorter, about 4 days. The symptoms vary widely: approximately two-thirds of human infections are asymptomatic, while in the remaining third, mild febrile (60-70%) or flu-like febrile forms with a biphasic course of fever, myalgia, nausea, vomiting, and potential CNS involvement (5-30% with meningoencephalitis) can occur.

Diagnosis relies on serological tests to detect specific antibodies in the cerebrospinal fluid and molecular diagnostic tools (RT-PCR).

25.5.5 Measles virus encephalitis (Subacute Sclerosing Panencephalitis, SSPE)

SSPE is a subacute infection caused by the measles virus. It primarily affects children, with an average age at onset at 7 years and an incidence of 1 in 1,000,000.

The clinical course is highly variable, but initial symptoms often include psychiatric disorders and signs of cognitive impairment. Subsequently, motor deficits, dysarthria, coordination disorders, and tremors may appear. Myoclonus and epileptic seizures are common. The disease has a rapidly progressive course with a high mortality rate.

25.5.6 Rabies virus encephalitis

Rabies is caused by a rhabdovirus and is generally contracted through the bite of an infected animal. The introduction of vaccinations for domestic dogs and strict control over stray dogs has resulted in the almost complete disappearance of this infection in Western Europe and Italy. Following virus inoculation, there is a relatively long incubation period during which the vaccine can be administered, in the absence of which the prognosis is poor. The disease can present with typical encephalitis symptoms, such as agitation, dysarthria, and dysphagia. However, clinical diagnosis can be complicated by a generally nonspecific clinical presentation (fever, sore throat, chills, malaise, cough, weakness), especially when symptoms are exclusively psychiatric and the patient has not been bitten by dogs.

25.5.7 Progressive multifocal leukoencephalopathy (PML)

Progressive multifocal leukoencephalopathy is caused by the reactivation of the JC virus (JC stands for the initials of the patient from whom JCV was first isolated in 1971), a common polyomavirus that infects 75% of the general population, with asymptomatic seroconversion usually occurring in childhood. The virus remains latent in lymphoid organs and kidneys. The encephalitis affects patients with AIDS (in 5% of cases), lymphoproliferative disorders, individuals with sarcoidosis (or other chronic diseases such as cirrhosis and pulmonary fibrosis), or those treated with immunosuppressive drugs (e.g., monoclonal antibodies such as natalizumab used in the treatment of multiple sclerosis). Apart from age (over 66 years), there are no other predisposing conditions. Viremia is present in 60-80% of cases. The clinical presentation is characterized by subacute encephalitis with altered cognitive function associated with focal neurological deficits (hemiparesis, hemianopsia, or ataxia). Lesions can occur in any areas of the nervous system, except for the optic nerves and spinal cord. Generally, the lesions are bilateral, asymmetric, involving the subcortical *U fibers*, as well as the basal ganglia and cortical gray matter (seizures can occur in 18% of cases).

25.5.8 HIV encephalitis

HIV reaches the CNS early in the infection through a mechanism that is still highly debated. It is believed that the virus reaches the CNS by crossing the blood-brain barrier through infected macrophages from the peripheral circulation. Within the CNS, the infection primarily localizes in microglia and macrophages originating from peripheral blood monocytes, while neurons are not infected, although neuronal degeneration is a fundamental neuropathological aspect in HIV-associated dementia forms.

The introduction of antiretroviral therapy in the last 10 years has led to a drastic reduction in morbidity and mortality associated with HIV infection, including a decrease in the prevalence of opportunistic infections resulting from immunosuppression. Despite these therapeutic advancements, HIV-associated neurocognitive disorders (HAND) characterized by cognitive impairments remain common. In 2007, a consensus panel redefined the diagnostic characterization of HAND, identifying different degrees of severity. HIV-associated dementia (HAD) represents the most severe form, while mild neurocognitive disorders (MND) represent the more moderate form with an impact on daily life activities.

In general, cognitive impairments are often associated with apathy and depression, while motor disturbances are more frequent in HAND cases in older individuals.

From a diagnostic perspective, CSF analysis may reveal mild lymphocytic pleocytosis, increased protein levels, and the presence of oligoclonal bands. However, due to immunosuppression, individuals with meningitis or encephalitis may have normal CSF findings. Brain computed tomography (CT) is often normal or may show mild atrophy associated with subtle hypodensity. In the focal form of encephalopathy, MRI may reveal small, single or multiple lesions in the white matter of the cerebral hemispheres without enhancement after contrast administration.

25.5.9 SARS-CoV-2 encephalitis

Although COVID-19 primarily affects the respiratory tract, recent studies have shown that involvement of the central nervous system is among the severe complications of the virus.

Three different pathophysiological mechanisms have been hypothesized for COVID-19 encephalitis: direct entry into the central nervous system through the olfactory bulb expressing receptors (ACE2) to which the virus can bind; hematogenous spread across the blood-brain barrier; or molecular mimicry. However, the available data on the pathophysiology of COVID-19 encephalitis are still limited and unclear.

Clinically, the most common symptoms are typical of COVID-19 infection, such as shortness of breath and fever, accompanied by altered consciousness, seizures, headache, and fatigue. Other less common symptoms include aphasia, ataxia, and myoclonus. Approximately 25% of cases were reported to be asymptomatic.

Brain magnetic resonance imaging reveals diffuse hyperintensity of the white matter and hemorrhagic lesions.

In some cases, a neuroimaging pattern characterized by cerebral edema and venous sinus thrombosis has been described.

25.6 Bacterial encephalitis

Bacterial encephalitis is much rarer than viral forms and generally occurs as a consequence of meningitis, with shared etiological agents (refer to the chapter on meningitis). Tick-borne encephalitis caused by tick bites, such as Rocky Mountain spotted fever, is a particular condition prevalent mainly in the United States. The infection is characterized by a febrile syndrome associated with headache, rarely resulting in altered consciousness (20%). Rash is present in 90% of cases, which tends to worsen after the onset of fever. Laboratory tests may reveal thrombocytopenia and elevated liver transaminases, while CSF pleocytosis, when present, is usually less than 100 cells/mm^3, with a predominance of lymphocytes. The detection of an increased antibody titer is useful for diagnosis.

25.7 Autoimmune encephalitis

Autoimmune encephalitis encompasses a heterogeneous group of diseases characterized by an immune system reaction against antigens expressed by neurons in the central nervous system (intracellular or extracellular antigens such as cell surface proteins, ion channels, or receptors). The involvement of the immune system is demonstrated by the presence of specific antibodies (anti-neuronal antibodies) detectable in the serum and CSF. In antibody-mediated forms (immune response against extracellular antigens), the antibodies are not directly responsible for the neurological damage, but their presence represents as an important diagnostic marker, enabling early identification for timely administration of immunomodulatory therapies, positively affecting the prognosis. In forms with antibodies directed against intracellular antigens, the immune response is cell-mediated, resulting in direct neuronal damage and a worse prognosis. Most of these forms are paraneoplastic.

Since autoimmune encephalitis develops in otherwise healthy individuals without other autoimmune conditions, a genetic predisposition has been hypothesized, and some studies have suggested a possible association with certain genes of the major histocompatibility complex HLA II.

The incidence is 1-5 cases per million population, and the most common form in adults is anti-LGI1 antibody-mediated encephalitis. Approximately 60% of patients experience nonspecific prodromal syndromes such as fever, malaise, or headache. The clinical symptoms are primarily characterized by behavioral changes, psychosis, epileptic seizures, memory and cognitive impairments, presence of involuntary movements, dysautonomia, and altered consciousness. The symptoms evolve over days or weeks, except in rare cases where the progression is slower (forms with anti-CASPR2 or anti-LGI1 antibodies) (Figure 25.2). In most patients, the neuroimaging findings and CSF examination overlap with those of viral encephalitis cases. A recent position paper attempted to define the diagnostic criteria for autoimmune encephalitis by combining clinical and instrumental features (Table 25.2).

25.8 Limbic Encephalitis

Limbic encephalitis, a fairly common form of autoimmune encephalitis, is generally paraneoplastic and has been described in association with small cell lung cancer (50%), testicular tumors (> 20%), and breast cancer (> 13%). Rare associations include Hodgkin's lymphoma (4%), thymoma (2%), teratoma (4%), bladder, colon, and kidney tumors.

Recent studies tend to classify limbic encephalitis into subtypes based on the following immunological aspects:

- Type of anti-neuronal antibodies: forms with anti-Hu or ANNA1 antibodies in small cell lung cancer; forms with anti-Ma2 (anti-Ta) antibodies in testicular tumors; forms with CRMP5/(anti-CV2) antibodies in lymphomas, thymomas, and small cell lung cancer; forms with ANNA3 antibodies in small cell lung cancer and VGCC (N-type) antibodies in small cell lung cancer and breast cancer.
- Localization of the primary target antigen of the antibodies: forms with antibodies directed against intracellular antigens (Hu, CV2, amphiphysin, Ri, Yo, and Ma2) and forms with antibodies directed against surface antigens (VGKC potassium channels, NMDA, AMPA, GABA, and glycine receptors). In forms with antibodies against surface antigens, where antibodies seem to play a significant pathogenic role, there is a greater likelihood of response to immunomodulatory treatments aimed at their removal.

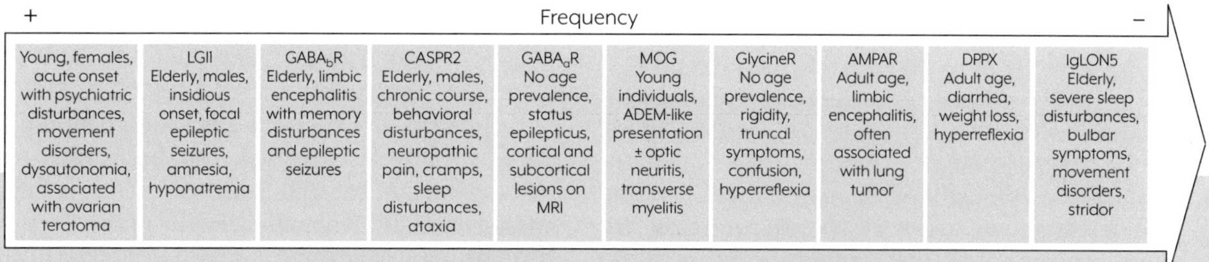

Figure 25.2

Clinical features of encephalitis due to antibodies directed against surface antigens of neuronal cells.

Table 25.2 DIAGNOSTIC CRITERIA FOR AUTOIMMUNE ENCEPHALITIS

Clinical Presentation
Subacute onset (rapid progression in less than 3 months) characterized by memory deficits (short-term memory loss), reduced or altered consciousness, psychiatric disturbances
Associated with at least 2 of the following criteria
New focal lesions in the central nervous system
Pleocytosis on cerebrospinal fluid examination (number of cells > 5 for mm^3)
Brain MRI (FLAIR sequences) revealing lesions in one or both temporal lobes or multifocal lesions involving gray matter, white matter, or both, compatible with demyelination or inflammation

Limbic encephalitis is clinically characterized by impairments of short-term memory, alterations in consciousness, confusion, and psychiatric disorders, including anxiety, depression, agitation, and visual and auditory hallucinations, progressing to defined psychosis. Epileptic seizures, generally complex partial seizures originating from the temporal lobe, are also common. Seizures are characteristic in a form of encephalitis that predominantly affects females with an early onset (around the second decade) and is associated with anti-glutamic acid decarboxylase (GAD) antibodies without evidence of tumor.

In Morvan syndrome, associated with anti-VGKC antibodies in over 70% of cases, psychiatric symptoms manifest in association with neuromyotonia, autonomic dysfunction, and neuropathic pain.

In limbic encephalitis, in addition to neurological symptoms, symptoms related to the underlying neoplasm may also be present. Movement disorders, such as chorea, can occur in forms associated with anti-CV2 antibodies. EEG generally reveals epileptic activity in one or both temporal lobes or may show diffuse slow activity. CSF analysis is abnormal in approximately 80% of cases and shows mild pleocytosis, increased protein levels, normal glucose levels, increased IgG index, and the presence of oligoclonal bands. The detection of anti-neuronal antibodies in serum and/or CSF is positive in only 50-60% of cases. Brain CT is generally normal, and hypodensity areas in one or both temporal lobes are rarely detectable. MRI reveals signal abnormalities without contrast enhancement in the mesial regions of the temporal lobes in 70-80% of cases. In some cases, such as Ophelia syndrome (a limbic encephalitis that occurs in patients with Hodgkin's lymphoma associated with antibodies against the glutamate receptor subunit 5), visible MRI abnormalities tend to assume a diffuse appearance. Functional imaging studies are extremely useful and often identify bilateral abnormalities complementary to conventional neuroimaging. Positron emission tomography with fluorodeoxyglucose (FDG-PET) can show early alterations, indicating increased metabolism. In approximately 60% of cases, the neurological syndrome precedes the diagnosis of neoplasm. Therefore, in suspected limbic encephalitis, all diagnostic investigations should be performed to search for an associated tumor (chest and abdominal CT or CT-PET).

The definitive diagnosis of paraneoplastic limbic encephalitis requires clinical and morphological evidence of limbic system involvement and the presence of antibodies or a tumor within 5 years of symptom onset.

In paraneoplastic forms, tumor removal and appropriate treatment can lead to rapid improvement in neurological symptoms. Currently, plasmapheresis and intravenous immunoglobulins represent the most effective treatments, in addition to high-dose intravenous corticosteroids.

25.9 Rare forms: Bickerstaff's encephalitis, anti-NMDAR encephalitis, and Rasmussen's encephalitis

Bickerstaff's encephalitis is an encephalitis that selectively involves the brainstem and is described in one-third of patients with paraneoplastic encephalitis. It presents with impairment of several cranial nerves, resulting in dysphagia, dysphonia, dysarthria, and deafness. The clinical picture is complicated by the onset of dizziness, ataxia, and nystagmus due to involvement of the olivary system and cerebellar projections. Progressive bulbar palsy can rarely develop. In advanced stages, respiratory disturbances with central hypoventilation and movement disorders such as akinetic-rigid syndrome (involvement of the mesencephalic substantia nigra) or hyperkinetic disorders such as chorea and dystonia (involvement of the subthalamic nucleus) may occur. Some patients may also present with Guillain-Barré syndrome, and the same type of antibodies (anti-GQ1b) described in Miller Fisher syndrome, a variant of Guillain-Barré syndrome, have been identified in the serum. This suggests the possibility of a common immune mechanism in which the two conditions represent different aspects of the same pathology. In the first weeks, CSF examination may show a normal protein concentration with pleocytosis, followed by an increase in protein levels. Approximately one-third of patients may show white matter alterations in the brainstem, thalamus, cerebellum, and cerebral hemispheres on T2-weighted MRI images.

Rasmussen's encephalitis is a progressive disorder that affects a single cerebral hemisphere. The inflammatory process appears to be cell-mediated, but the role of autoantibodies is not yet well defined. It typically begins in childhood, but cases with later onset in adolescence or young adulthood have been described. Clinically, it is characterized by a form of simple or complex partial epilepsy and continuous partial epilepsy (present in over half of the cases), recurrent status epilepticus, neurological deficits secondary to involvement of the affected hemisphere, and cognitive deterioration. Hemiparesis and hemianopsia are common. MRI reveals focal cortical atrophy involving a single hemisphere, atrophy of the head of the caudate nucleus, and white matter alterations.

25.10 Transmissible spongiform encephalopathies

Transmissible spongiform encephalopathies, also known as prion diseases, are neurodegenerative disorders that can occur in both animals and humans. The most well-known animal forms are bovine spongiform encephalopathy (BSE) and scrapie in sheep and goats. In humans, the most common form (with an average annual incidence rate slightly higher than 1 case per million) is Creutzfeldt-Jakob disease. Rarer forms include Kuru, a disease associated with cannibalistic rituals practiced by certain tribes in Papua New Guinea and nearly eradicated, Gerstmann-Sträussler-Sheinker syndrome, fatal familial insomnia, and the variant form of Creutzfeldt-Jakob disease linked to the bovine spongiform encephalopathy epidemic.

Prion diseases are characterized by extremely long incubation periods, often insidious onset, and a poor prognosis. From an anatomopathological perspective, the lesions exclusively affect the central nervous system and are characterized by neuronal loss, spongiosis of the neuropil, hyperplasia, and hypertrophy of glial cells.

The common pathogenic feature of all prion diseases is the conformational change of a cellular protein called PrPC (cellular prion protein) into a pathological isoform called PrPSc (scrapie-associated prion protein). PrPC and PrPSc share the same primary structure, but while the physiological protein predominates in a helical structure, the pathological isoform has a beta-sheet structure that confers distinctive features such as partial resistance to proteases, insolubility, tendency to deposit as amyloid fibrils in the central nervous system, and the ability to replicate through an autocatalytic mechanism using endogenous molecules of PrPC. This last property gives prion diseases their transmissibility characteristic. Approximately one-third of patients generally present with nonspecific prodromal symptoms such as weight loss, sleep disturbances, malaise, and diffuse pain, followed by progressive impairment of higher cortical functions leading to dementia. In the early stages of the disease, patients may experience behavioral disturbances, lack of coordination, and visual impairments. In advanced stages, extrapyramidal disorders such as involuntary movements may appear. Myoclonus develops in approximately 90% of patients during the course of the disease. The most of Creutzfeldt-Jakob disease cases are of "sporadic" type with unknown etiology and clinically manifest as rapidly progressive dementia associated with focal neurological signs (myoclonus, cerebellar, visual, pyramidal, and extrapyramidal impairment).

The presence of homozygosity (methionine/methionine or valine/valine) at codon 129 in the PRNP gene is a risk factor for sporadic forms.

Approximately 10-15% of cases are of "genetic" type caused by point mutations in the PRNP gene, while only a very small percentage is of "iatrogenic" origin, caused by person-to-person transmission during medical procedures such as the use of intracerebral electrodes for EEG recordings, dura mater grafts following neurosurgical procedures, corneal transplants, or pituitary hormone replacement therapy. There is also a recently described "variant" form, which has been causally linked to the consumption of beef contaminated with the agent of bovine spongiform encephalopathy. In these forms, the onset is generally characterized by behavioral disorders, anxiety, depression, psychosis, visual hallucinations, and ataxia, with cognitive deterioration occurring only at a later stage.

In the early stages of the disease, EEG is generally normal, while in advanced stages, periodic sharp or polyphasic waves may be present, which, although not pathognomonic, are an important diagnostic sign. Cerebrospinal fluid is usually normal, or there may be a high level of 14-3-3 proteins, which are highly sensitive and specific markers for sporadic forms. CT scans may be normal or show cortical atrophy, while MRI can reveal hyperintensity on T2-weighted images localized in the basal ganglia, thalamus, and brainstem. Despite the presence of clinical signs, the definitive diagnosis can only be made through autopsy or by identifying PrPSc in brain biopsy tissue or olfactory mucosa. Currently, there are no drugs that can alter the course of the disease, and therapy remains symptomatic, although recent data on protein translation activation offer some hope for effective treatments.

25.10.1 General therapy

One of the most important phases of encephalitis treatment is supportive care. All patients with encephalitis should be hospitalized in facilities with intensive care units. Cardiac and respiratory activity, as well as hydroelectrolyte balance, should be closely monitored. Seizures should be treated with intravenous antiepileptic drugs (phenytoin). Mild intracranial hypertension does not require pharmacological treatment. However, when the condition becomes severe, with associated papilledema and rapid cognitive impairment, administration of mannitol and/or intravenous steroids is indicated. In rare cases of inadequate response to drug therapy, neurosurgical treatment of intracranial hypertension may be necessary. Isolation is only required for individuals with severe immunodeficiency, patients with rabies encephalitis, viral exanthematous diseases, and hemorrhagic fever forms. Rehabilitation, especially in the post-hospitalization phase, is of significant importance.

25.10.2 Specific therapy

In most cases of encephalitis caused by bacteria, fungi, or parasites, the same therapies used for systemic infections are administered. However, for viral encephalitis, there are proven effective therapies only for herpes simplex and herpes zoster infections. The main pharmacological treatment in these cases involves the use of acyclovir, which, if administered in the early stages of the disease before the onset of altered consciousness, can reduce mortality and morbidity. As acyclovir is excreted renally, patients with renal insufficiency require dose adjustments based on renal clearance values. Renal function should be monitored in all patients during treatment. Clinical relapses, occurring weeks or months later, have been reported in cases where treatment was shorter or equal to 10 days. Therefore, according to guidelines, treatment should be extended for approximately 3 weeks. If the drug is administered upon admission and brain MRI is normal, treatment should be continued until PCR becomes negative. In cases of acyclovir resistance, slow infusion of foscarnet for 3 weeks is recommended.

CMV encephalitis shows a poorer response to antiviral drugs. An initial induction therapy with combination therapy of ganciclovir and foscarnet is generally recommended, followed by maintenance therapy with ganciclovir or foscarnet. Treatment should be continued for 3 weeks in immunocompetent patients and 6 weeks in immunocompromised individuals.

In cases of HHV6 infection, treatment with foscarnet is indicated for both variant A and variant B, while ganciclovir can be used as an alternative only for variant B infections.

For other viral agents, particularly arboviruses, there is currently no clear scientific evidence regarding the efficacy of specific therapies. New antiviral drugs such as valacyclovir appear to be potentially effective for HSV and VZV infections, while pleconaril seems potentially useful in the treatment of enterovirus infections.

The administration of corticosteroids (high-dose dexamethasone or cycles of methylprednisolone) in the treatment of acute viral encephalitis is controversial. Their use is reserved exclusively for individuals with progressive alteration of consciousness and a poor prognosis. The combination of acyclovir and steroids can be used in immunocompetent individuals with severe VZV encephalitis and signs of severe cerebral edema.

In paraneoplastic autoimmune forms, treatment is directly related to tumor removal and follows the general criteria for all autoimmune diseases. Preferred treatments include plasmapheresis and intravenous immunoglobulins, possibly combined with high-dose methylprednisolone. In severe cases that do not respond to the aforementioned therapies, treatment with cyclophosphamide or rituximab is indicated.

Bibliography

Antinori A., Arendt G., Becker J.T., Brew B.J., Byrd D.A., Cherner M. et al., Updated research nosology for HIV-associated neurocognitive disorders. Neurology; 69(18):1789-99, 2007.

Dalmau J., Graus F. Antibody-Mediated Encephalitis. N Engl J Med; 378(9):840-851, 2018.

Granerod J., Crowcroft N.S., The epidemiology of acute encephalitis. Neuropsychological Rehabilitation; 17(4):406-428, 2007.

Graus F., Titulaer M.J., Balu R., Benseler S., Bien C.G., Cellucci T., Cortese I., Dale R.C., Gelfand J.M., Geschwind M., Glaser C.A., Honnorat J., Höftberger R., Iizuka T., Irani S.R., Lancaster E., Leypoldt F., Prüss H., Rae-Grant A., Reindl M., Rosenfeld M.R., Rostásy K., Saiz A., Venkatesan A., Vincent A., Wandinger K.P., Waters P., Dalmau J. A clinical approach to diagnosis of autoimmune encephalitis. Lancet Neurol; 15(4):391-404,2016.

Johnson R.T. Acute encephalitis. Clinical Infectious Diseases; 23:219-226, 1996.

Kumar R. Understanding and managing acute encephalitis. F1000Res. 2020 Jan 29;9:F1000 Faculty Rev-60.

Lindl K.A., Marks D.R,. Kolson D.L., Jordan Sciutto K.L. HIV-associated neurocognitive disorder: pathogenesis and therapeutic opportunities. J Neuroimmune Pharmacol; 5(3): 294-309, 2010.

Siow I, Lee KS, Zhang JJY, Saffari SE, Ng A. Encephalitis as a neurological complication of COVID-19: A systematic review and meta-analysis of incidence, outcomes, and predictors. Eur J Neurol. 2021;28(10):3491-3502. doi:10.1111/ene.14913.

Solomon T., Michael B.D., Smith P.E., Sanderson F., Davies N.W., Hart I.J., Holland M., Easton A., Buckley C., Kneen R., Beeching N.J.; National Encephalitis Guidelines Development and Stakeholder Groups. Management of suspected viral encephalitis in adults--Association of British Neurologists and British Infection Association National Guidelines. J Infect. 2012;64(4):347-73.

Steinera I., Budkac H., Chaudhurid A., Koskiniemie M., Sainiof K., Saloneng O. Kennedyh PGE. Viral meningoencephalitis: a review of diagnostic methods and guidelines for management. European Journal of Neurology; 17:999-1009, 2010.

Venkatesan A., Tunkel A.R., Bloch K.C., Lauring A.S., Sejvar J., Bitnun A., Stahl J.P., Mailles A., Drebot M., Rupprecht C.E., Yoder J., Cope J.R., Wilson M.R., Whitley R.J., Sullivan J., Granerod J., Jones C., Eastwood K., Ward K.N., Durrheim D.N., Solbrig M.V., Guo-Dong L., Glaser C.A.; International Encephalitis Consortium. Case definitions, diagnostic algorithms, and priorities in encephalitis: consensus statement of the international encephalitis consortium. Clin Infect Dis. 2013;57(8):1114-28.

Vitaliani R., Zoccarato M., Vianello M., Giometto B., Clinical, immunological and therapeutic aspects of autoimmune encephalitis. Recent Pat CNS Drug Discov; 3(1):16-22, 2008.

White M.K., Khalili K., Pathogenesis of progressive multifocal leukoencephalopathy-revisited. J Infect Dis; 203(5):578-86, 2011.

Zhang S.Y., Abel L., Casanova J.L. Mendelian predisposition to herpes simplex encephalitis. Handb Clin Neurol; 112:1091-7, 2013.

Zuliani L, Marangoni S, De Gaspari P, Rosellini I, Nosadini M, Fleming JM, De Riva V, Galloni E, Perini F, Frigo AC, Sartori S, Zoccarato M, Giometto B. Epidemiology of neuronal surface antibody-mediated autoimmune encephalitis and antibody-based diagnostics. J Neuroimmunol.; 357:577-598, 2021.

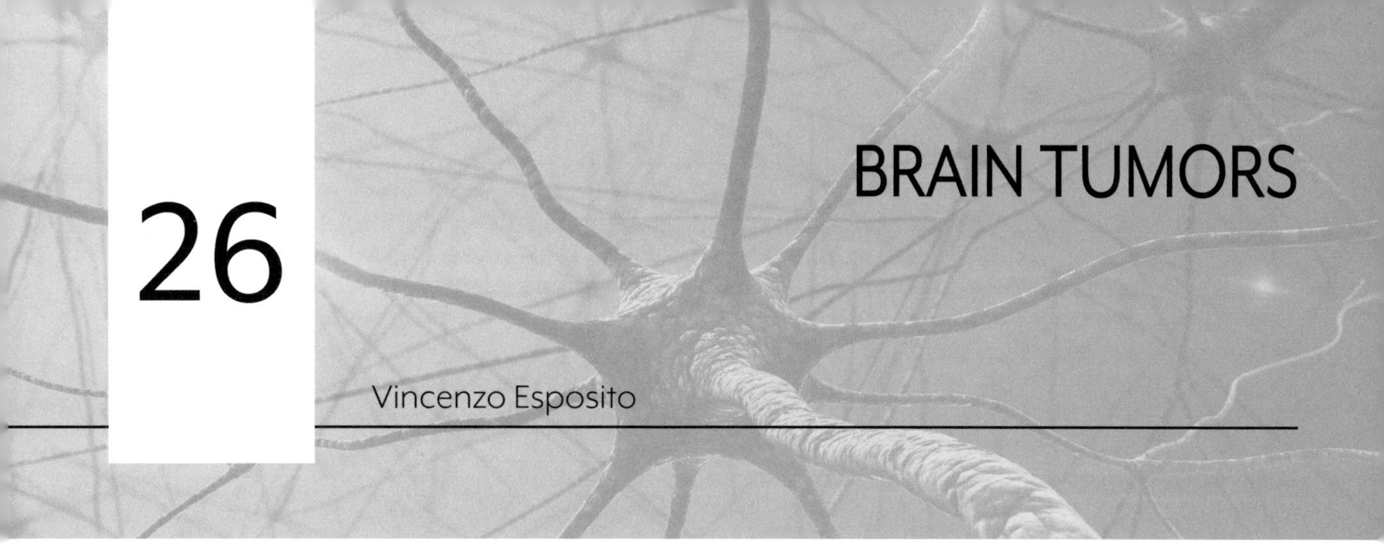

26 BRAIN TUMORS

Vincenzo Esposito

Brain tumors are classified into primary tumors, which originate from the transformation of brain cells, and secondary tumors, which result from the intracranial metastasis of neoplasms originating in other parts of the body. Primary tumors can be benign or malignant. Due to the enormous variety of cell types present within the skull, the classification of intracranial tumors is very complex. There is a fundamental distinction between *intrinsic tumors (or intracerebral tumors)*, which originate within the brain parenchyma, and *extrinsic tumors* (*or extracerebral tumors*), which originate from the covering tissues or from nervous structures external to the brain (such as cranial nerves). In general, intrinsic tumors have infiltrative growth with progressive invasion of healthy brain tissue; they are not clearly separable from the normal parenchyma and cannot be surgically removed in their entirety. In contrast, extrinsic tumors come from outside the brain mass and compress it without invading it; thus, it is possible to identify a clear plane of separation between the brain tissue and the tumor, allowing for the complete removal of the neoplasm. However, these general rules have various exceptions.

26.1 Epidemiology and etiology

The incidence of primary brain tumors, both benign and malignant, in industrialized countries ranges from 15 to 19 cases per 100,000 people per year. Of these, a percentage ranging from half to two-thirds is histologically benign. Among pediatric neoplasms, brain tumors are the second most frequent after leukemias, with an incidence of 4.8 cases per 100,000 children per year. In the United States, the prevalence of individuals with a brain tumor was 221.8 per 100,000 in 2010. The prevalence is higher in women (264.8 per 100,000) compared to men (158.7 per 100,000), likely due to the higher frequency of meningiomas in females, which have significantly higher survival rates. The average prevalence of malignant tumors (42.5 per 100,000) is lower than that of non-malignant tumors (166.5 per 100,000). The incidence of metastases varies in different epidemiological studies, ranging from approximately equal to double that of primary tumors. In autopsies, the incidence is even higher due to the presence of many asymptomatic cases that do not result in clinical effects and remain undiagnosed during the patient's lifetime. The primary malignancies that most commonly metastasize to the brain are lung, kidney, breast tumors, and melanomas. Regarding primary brain tumors, malignant tumors more frequently affect men, while women have a higher incidence of non-malignant neoplasms, mainly meningiomas. The incidence also varies depending on age: in pediatric patients (under 15 years old), the most common tumors are medulloblastomas (23.5%) and low-grade gliomas (31.7%), while in adults, high-grade gliomas (30.5%) and meningiomas (29.4%) are more prevalent. In most histological types, age at diagnosis influences survival, which decreases as age increases. In terms of environmental risk factors, ionizing radiation plays an important role, especially for high-grade gliomas and meningiomas. However, the statistically significant association between the use of cell phones, which has been the subject of numerous studies, and brain tumorigenesis has not been proven. Some genetic syndromes, such as neurofibromatosis, tuberous sclerosis, Von Hippel-Lindau syndrome, and Turcot syndrome, are characterized by a higher incidence of various types of brain tumors. In AIDS patients, there is an increased incidence of primary cerebral lymphomas, but not other types of neoplasms.

26.2 Symptoms

The presence of a tumor inside the skull causes symptoms related to both the irritative effect on the cerebral cortex and the progressive compression of the parenchyma, resulting in general effects (intracranial hypertension and cerebral hernias) and local dysfunction related to the compression or destruction of functional brain tissue. It should be noted that even a benign tumor, if not removed, can lead to death or serious disability because it grows within the rigid and closed space of the intracranial compartment. Three different categories of symptoms can be distinguished: irritative symptoms (seizures), symptoms of intracranial hypertension, and neurological syndromes based on the location of the neoplasm.

26.3 Irritative symptoms

Tumors located in the cortex of the cerebral hemispheres can cause epileptic seizures. These seizures can be focal or partial with secondary generalization and, less frequently, they can be primarily generalized. Epileptic seizures never occur in infratentorial tumors, which are located in the cerebellum and brainstem. Epilepsy is a common initial symptom of a brain tumor. Therefore, the first occurrence of an epileptic seizure in a person of any age requires an endocranial Magnetic Resonance Imaging (MRI) with contrast enhancement.

26.4 Intracranial hypertension

The cranial vault can be considered a rigid container that contains three components in equilibrium: the brain parenchyma, which constitutes about 80% of the total volume, blood, and cerebrospinal fluid (CSF), both accounting for approximately 10%. When there is an increase in one or more of these elements, due to the rigidity of the container, the inevitable effect is an increase in intracranial pressure, which brings various consequences.

Pathophysiology of intracranial hypertension

A growing mass within the skull leads to a series of consequences that ultimately result in an increase in all three intracranial components and intracranial pressure itself (Figure 26.1). A tumor primarily increases brain mass, both directly and by inducing cerebral edema. Cerebral edema is the swelling of brain tissue due to an increase in its fluid content. In the case of tumors, the edema is typically vasogenic, meaning that substances produced by the neoplasms cause the opening of endothelial *tight junctions* that constitute the blood-brain barrier. As a result, proteins and plasma fluids, which are normally excluded from the brain parenchyma, enter the extracellular space, attracting additional fluid and progressively extending the edema. The tendency to cause edema depends on the type of tumor, generally being greater in malignant tumors (metastases, glioblastomas) and cerebral abscesses. The presence of edema amplifies the effect of the tumor; the tumor mass itself may be much smaller than the total volume of edema. This is why anti-edema treatments can provide significant benefits to patients with brain tumors. An expansive intracranial process also affects blood and CSF circulation. In particular, even a slight increase in intracranial pressure causes compression or collapse of the low-pressure venous circulation while having minimal effects on the high-pressure arterial supply. This leads to venous stasis, increased intracranial blood volume, and further elevation of intracranial pressure. CSF circulation also occurs at low pressure. CSF is formed in the choroid plexuses of the cerebral ventricles (lateral ventricles, third and fourth ventricles) through both filtration and active transport processes performed by ependymal cells lining the plexuses. From the lateral ventricles, CSF passes through the foramina of Monro and reaches the third ventricle. From there, it crosses the Sylvian aqueduct and enters

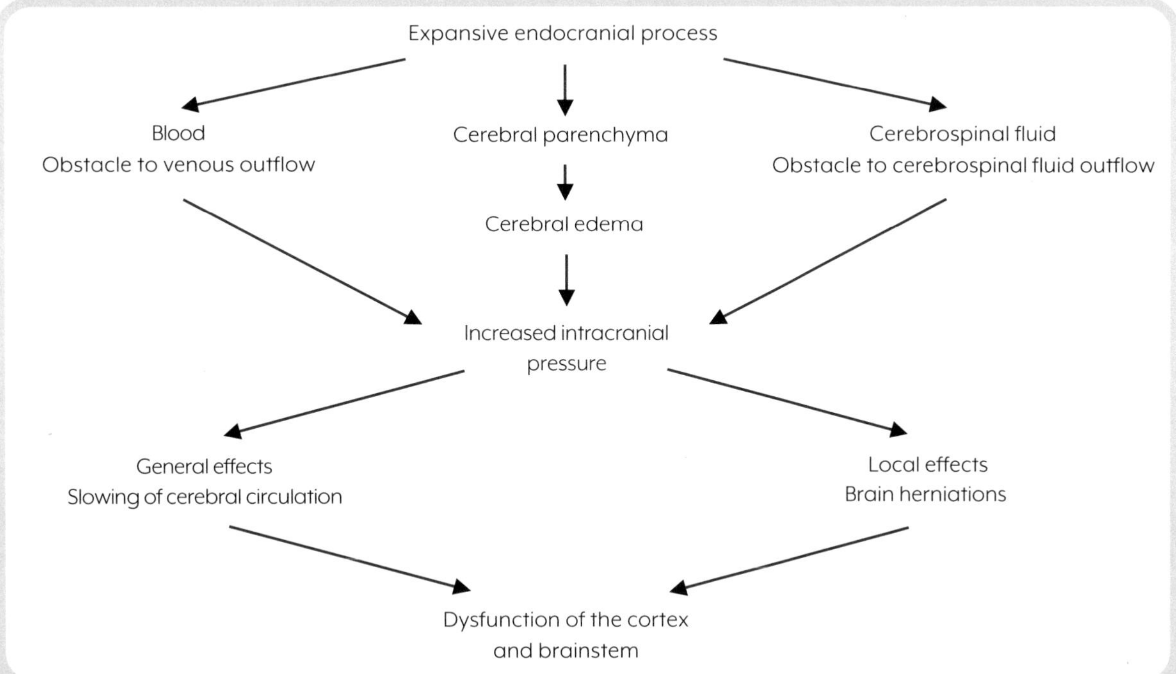

Figure 26.1

Pathophysiology of intracranial hypertension.

the fourth ventricle. It exits the ventricular system through the foramina of Luschka and Magendie, flowing into the subarachnoid space at the base of the brain. Finally, it traverses this space upward along the cerebral convexity and is reabsorbed into the bloodstream through the arachnoid granulations of Pacchioni located in the superior sagittal sinus. The daily production of CSF is approximately 500 ml (or 20 ml/hour). CSF is propelled along the neuraxis by the pulsations of the cerebral arteries. The CSF pressure, measured through a lumbar puncture with the patient in the lateral decubitus position, is between 10 and 18 cmH_2O, equivalent to 8-15 mmHg. Even a slight increase in local pressure due to the presence of a neoplasm can cause a slowdown or blockage of circulation, leading to CSF accumulation in the ventricular cavities, which can dilate (hydrocephalus). The increase in intracranial CSF content contributes to further intracranial pressure elevation. As mentioned earlier, the entire CSF flow passes through narrow-caliber regions that are particularly susceptible to closure by adjacent neoplasms, such as the foramina of Monro, the third ventricle, the Sylvian aqueduct, and the foramina of Luschka and Magendie. Various forms of hydrocephalus result from the obstruction of these regions: monoventricular hydrocephalus (closure of a foramen of Monro with dilation of the corresponding lateral ventricle), biventricular hydrocephalus (closure of both foramina of Monro or the third ventricle with dilation of both lateral ventricles), triventricular hydrocephalus (closure of the Sylvian aqueduct with dilation of the lateral ventricles and the third ventricle), and tetraventricular hydrocephalus (closure of the foramina of Luschka and Magendie with dilation of the lateral ventricles, the third ventricle, and the fourth ventricle).

The increase in intracranial pressure produces general and local effects. The general effects are related to the reduction of blood circulation due to the slowing of venous circulation. Since the brain lacks energy reserves, it is highly sensitive to continuous nutrient supply from the blood flow. Any reduction in blood flow leads to a decrease in cerebral functions, especially higher cognitive functions (reasoning, attention, ideation), and subsequently, a decrease in consciousness.

Brain herniations | The local effects of intracranial hypertension are the consequences of displacements of brain tissue caused by pressure exerted by the expanding process in its immediate vicinity. The interior of the cranial vault is divided into compartments by rigid dural membranes: the tentorium, which separates the infratentorial space from the supratentorial space, and the falx cerebri, which separates the supratentorial space into two halves, each containing a cerebral hemisphere. The division into compartments is incomplete to allow for the passage of the brainstem and the corpus callosum, connecting the two cerebral hemispheres, and their respective blood vessels. As a result, there are several orifices within the skull, delimited by dural membranes. An important orifice is the foramen magnum, which represents the largest opening at the base of the skull. The increase in brain mass due to the action of the neoplasm, cerebral edema, and blockage of CSF circulation leads to the herniation of brain tissue through points of least resistance represented by these various orifices. This is a serious clinical condition that often precedes death if not promptly treated. One of the most common brain hernias is the herniation of the uncal region of the temporal lobe beneath the tentorium, with possible compression of the third cranial nerve and the brainstem. In addition to signs of brainstem dysfunction, fixed mydriasis (dilated pupil) occurs on the side of the compression due to third cranial nerve paralysis, while the pupil on the opposite side maintains a normal diameter, resulting in a condition called anisocoria (difference in pupil size). The presence of anisocoria in a patient with intracranial hypertension is a sign of severe brain injury and imminent life-threatening danger, requiring immediate treatment; the midriatic pupil indicates the side of the compression. Another frequent herniation is that of the cerebellar tonsils through the foramen magnum, with compression of the medulla. The most common clinical signs include neck pain, with the head tilted toward the side of the herniation, and subsequent signs of brainstem dysfunction, including severe disturbances of consciousness, respiratory rhythm, and heart rate that immediately precede death.

Infratentorial tumors have potentially earlier and more severe effects compared to supratentorial tumors because the infratentorial compartment is significantly smaller than the supratentorial one and contains the brainstem, a vital structure for maintaining vegetative activity and consciousness.

The final effects of intracranial hypertension are alterations in cortical and brainstem functions, with progressive disturbances of consciousness, respiratory and cardiac rhythm, ultimately leading to death.

Signs and symptoms of intracranial hypertension | The clinical syndrome of intracranial hypertension manifests quite uniformly regardless of its causes. It is characterized by the following clinical signs and symptoms.

- *Headache*: it can manifest in various ways and with varying intensity and may sometimes be absent.
- *Vomiting*: typically projectile, sudden, and unrelated to meals. Sometimes, especially in tumors of the posterior cranial fossa, vomiting is so significant and predominant that the patient is mistakenly diagnosed with a gastrointestinal problem.
- *Edema of the optic papilla (papilledema)*: It is swelling of the optic disc or papilla, which is visible upon examination of the fundus of the eye. Typically, it is bilateral. The appearance of this sign depends on the fact that the intracranial subarachnoid space, filled with CSF, is continuous with a similar space surrounding the optic nerve within the orbit, contained within the optic nerve sheath. The increase in intracranial pressure is transmitted through CSF to the optic nerve sheath, exerting compression around the nerve itself. The first consequence of this phenomenon is venous stasis in the central retinal vein, which runs inside the optic nerve and drains venous blood from the retina. In the initial stage, there is swelling of the papilla, with elevated and blurred papillary margins. Subsequently, venous stasis in the papillary veins becomes evident, possibly leading to papillary hemorrhages in severe

cases. Chronic papilledema can result in the atrophy of the optic disc, causing severe visual disturbances.

- *Psycho-organic symptoms and alterations in consciousness*: Patients with intracranial hypertension may experience mental impairment and altered consciousness, starting with slowed ideation and reduced initiative in the early stages and progressing to confusion and a tendency to somnolence. As intracranial hypertension worsens, there is progressive dysfunction of the brainstem, particularly the reticular activating system, leading to increasingly altered consciousness, ultimately resulting in coma.
- *Disturbances in cardiac and respiratory rhythm and blood pressure*: Arterial hypertension and bradycardia are the first autonomic symptoms related to alterations in brainstem function. Subsequently, respiratory rhythm disturbances occur, which precede the patient's death.

Brain herniation signs often appear during the course of intracranial hypertension. If left untreated, they accelerate clinical deterioration and rapidly lead to the patient's death. The manifestation of intracranial hypertension depends on its rate of progression. Tumors that grow very slowly do not cause intracranial hypertension for a long time but only manifest with irritative signs (seizures) and possibly focal signs. The brain has time to adapt to the presence of a slowly expanding mass within the skull. In contrast, in rapidly growing tumors, especially those complicated by cerebral edema and/or blockage of CSF circulation, the clinical picture of intracranial hypertension is predominant.

26.5 Neurological syndromes by location (focal signs)

These signs are related to the compression or destruction of brain tissue hosting or adjacent to the tumor. These signs vary greatly from each other, as they are an expression of the different functions of the various cerebral lobes affected by the neoplasms. Below is a brief description:

Tumors of the frontal lobe | Typical signs include euphoria (tendency to be frivolous, joke without reason, etc.) or, conversely, depression. Furthermore, given the importance of the frontal lobes in higher functions, there may be difficulties in reasoning abilities, attention, and initiative, with a tendency toward apathy and inertia. In the dominant hemisphere, involvement of the posterior part of the third frontal gyrus, the location of Broca's area, can lead to motor aphasia. Anosmia is also possible due to bilateral compression/destruction of the olfactory bulbs and tracts.

Tumors of the rolandic region | Tumors in this location cause motor disturbances with contralateral hemiparesis and disturbances in discriminative somatosensory functions of the contralateral body side.

Tumors of the temporal lobe | These tumors cause disturbances in recent memory, verbal memory (dominant hemisphere), and visuospatial memory (non-dominant hemisphere). In the dominant hemisphere, language impairments result from impairment of the posterior part of the first temporal gyrus (Wernicke's area), leading to sensory aphasia. Finally, a superior homonymous quadrantanopia may occur on the opposite side of the tumor due to involvement of the optic radiations surrounding the temporal horn.

Tumors of the parietal lobe | Involvement of this region causes symptoms related to discriminative sensory deficits, apraxia, and disturbances in body schema. An inferior homonymous quadrantanopia may occur on the opposite side due to involvement of the optic radiations. Language disturbances of a sensory nature (Wernicke's area) are also possible in the dominant hemisphere.

Tumors of the occipital lobe | These tumors typically manifest as visual disturbances with contralateral homonymous lateral hemianopia.

Tumors of the basal nuclei | The most frequent disturbances are contralateral hemiparesis and hypoesthesia of the contralateral body side due to involvement of the pyramidal motor pathway in the posterior limb of the internal capsule and the sensory pathways in the thalamus.

Tumors of the sellar-suprasellar region | This category includes various types of tumors, with pituitary adenoma being the most common, followed by meningioma and craniopharyngioma. The presence of diencephalo-hypophyseal axis structures in this region explains the significant endocrine aspects of the clinical picture caused by tumors developing in this area. There are two types of symptoms:

1) *Hormonal syndrome*, associated with:
   a) Compression/destruction of the pituitary gland parenchyma, leading to pituitary insufficiency;
   b) Compression/destruction of the pituitary stalk, resulting in the so-called stalk effect characterized by increased blood levels of prolactin (PRL) and decreased secretion of antidiuretic hormone (ADH). PRL secretion is normally inhibited by dopamine produced by the hypothalamus, which is released into the hypothalamo-hypophyseal portal vessels in the median eminence and reaches the pituitary gland through the pituitary stalk. Severing the stalk leads to hyperprolactinemia. In women, this can cause menstrual cycle alterations and sometimes galactorrhea, while in men, it can lead to impotence and decreased libido. ADH is synthesized by osmoreceptor hypothalamic neurons in the supraoptic and paraventricular nuclei. It travels within their axons in the pituitary stalk and is released at the neurohypophysis; a decrease in ADH causes diabetes insipidus, characterized by increased urine volume with low specific gravity and increased thirst;
   c) In the case of secreting adenomas, there is hyperproduction of specific hormones.
2) *Neurological syndrome*, resulting from tumor growth beyond the sellar boundaries, with compression of the optic pathways (chiasm and optic nerves). As the tumor continues to grow, it can compress the third ventricle and cause biventricular hydrocephalus. Symptoms of this syndrome include headache related to compression of the diaphragma sellae and visual disturbances, often prominent, with progressive unilateral or bilateral decrease in visual acuity and visual field alterations such as bitemporal hemianopia due to symmetric compression of the chiasm. Compression of the cavernous sinus can cause disorders of extraocular movements with diplopia and ptosis. Lastly, extension to the third ventricle and the development of hydrocephalus can lead to even more severe disorders such as stupor or coma.

The sequence and importance of the two syndromes vary due to the different growth patterns of these tumors. In adenomas that primarily grow within the pituitary gland, the hormonal syndrome precedes the neurological syndrome, especially in secreting adenomas. In craniopharyngiomas, which originate from remnants of the craniopharyngeal duct in the pituitary stalk, diabetes insipidus is an early symptom (while it is extremely rare in pituitary adenomas), followed immediately by visual disturbances. In meningiomas (tuberculum sellae, diaphragma sellae, clinoidal, and the third inner wing of the sphenoid), the neurological syndrome with visual disturbances occurs early.

Tumors of the pineal region | These tumors give rise to a syndrome characterized by upward gaze paralysis (Parinaud's syndrome), possibly associated with pupillary or oculomotor paresis, due to impairment of the superior colliculi, as well as triventricular hydrocephalus due to aqueductal obstruction and intracranial hypertension. The most frequent tumors in this region are pinealomas, germinomas, midbrain tectal plate astrocytomas, and teratomas. In children, precocious pseudopuberty can occur due to beta-HCG secretion by a germinoma.

Tumors of the posterior cranial fossa | Cerebellar tumors result in a cerebellar syndrome characterized by motor coordination disturbances. A particular syndrome is the cerebellopontine angle syndrome, specific to extrinsic tumors located between the cerebellum and brainstem, the most typical being acoustic neuroma. Symptoms initially involve various combinations of cranial nerves (8th, 5th, and 7th), followed by cerebellar and brainstem disturbances. Tumors in the brainstem cause complex symptoms, with multiple cranial nerve and long tract involvements.

26.6 Instrumental diagnosis

The diagnostic imaging method of choice for the anatomical study of intracranial tumors is brain Magnetic Resonance Imaging (MRI), complemented by the administration of a contrast agent, gadolinium (■ Figure 26.2). This examination allows for rapid diagnosis with very precise anatomical delineation. Brain parenchyma and neoplasms are visualized with significantly higher resolution compared to Computed Tomography (CT). Specific MRI sequences such as perfusion, spectroscopy, and diffusion provide information on vascularity and the presence of certain chemical compounds, often allowing for a presumptive diagnosis of the tumor type. MR angiography provides information on the displacement of intracranial vessels caused by neoplasms. In special cases, functional MRI based on the Blood Oxygenation Level Dependent (BOLD) effect provides indications of the cerebral localization of relevant functions, particularly motor activity and language. Diffusion Tensor Imaging (DTI) tractography allows for the delineation of major white matter tracts, such as the corticospinal tract or arcuate fasciculus, and their spatial relationships with the neoplasm (■ Figure 26.3). The information derived from these latter two studies can be very useful for planning potential surgical approaches and assessing their risks. Brain CT scan with contrast enhancement should be reserved for cases where MRI is not feasible or in specific situations such as the examination of calcifications and bone lesions. Positron Emission Tomography (PET) is a non-invasive functional imaging technique primarily used in the diagnosis and grading of brain gliomas and differentiation between tumor recurrence and radiation necrosis.

26.7 Classification of brain tumors

Due to the considerable variety of cell types present within the skull, the classification of brain tumors is extremely complex. The World Health Organization (WHO) classifies Central Nervous System (CNS) tumors into specific histotypes and 4 grades of malignancy, according to criteria subject to periodic revisions. In 2016, for the first time, many tumor entities, particularly brain gliomas, were defined using genetic and molecular parameters in addition to classical histology, with the aim of improving prognostic reliability. The most recent revision in 2021,

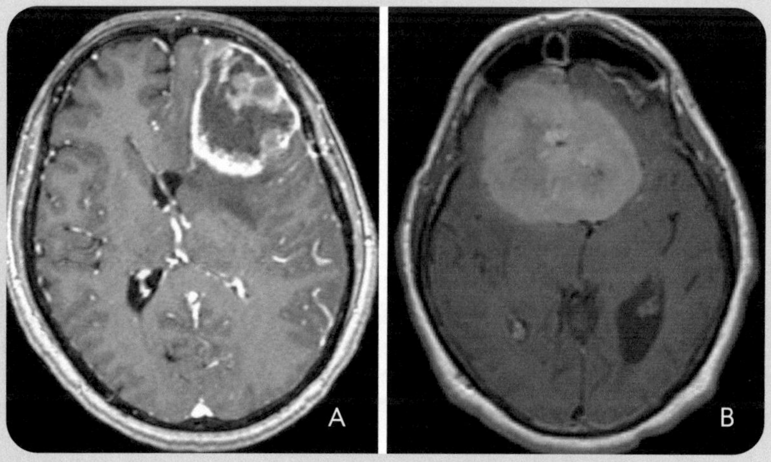

Figure 26.2

Cerebral MRI, T1 sequences after contrast agent administration. A) Glioblastoma: Note the heterogeneous appearance of the neoplasm, with a "ring-enhancing" contrast uptake area (white in this sequence) surrounding a predominantly hypodense (black) central area, representing necrosis. Around the neoplastic mass, the brain parenchyma appears hypodense due to edema. The resulting mass effect is significant, with brain displacement and ventricular deformation. B) Meningioma: Note the intense and homogeneous contrast uptake, with almost complete absence of peritumoral edema.

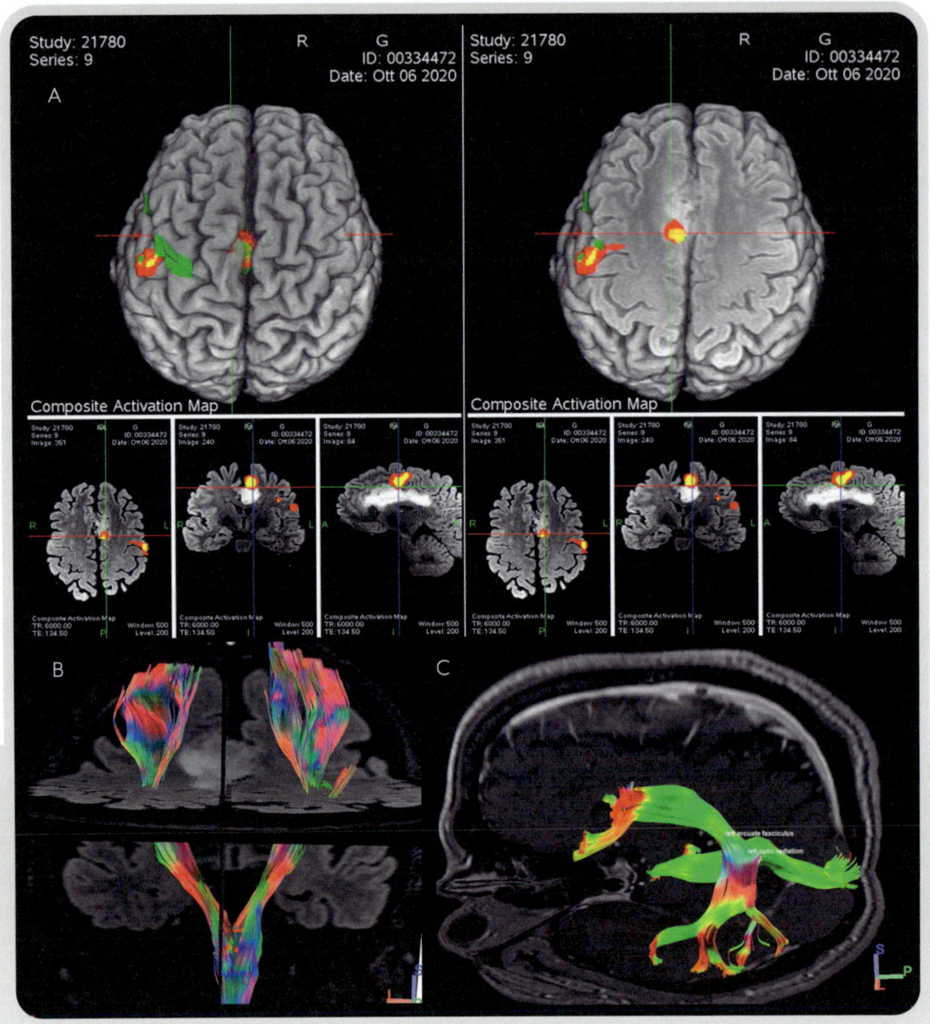

Figure 26.3

Functional MRI and DTI tractography: a) cortical activations for language; b) reconstruction of the pyramidal tracts; c) reconstruction of the arcuate fasciculus and optic radiations.

shown in Table 26.1, introduced further innovations, emphasizing the importance of an integrated diagnosis. These innovations have been particularly relevant in defining adult brain gliomas. Regarding these tumors, the most important molecular biomarkers currently identified are the genetic mutation of isocitrate dehydrogenase 1 or 2 (IDH1/IDH2), 1p/19q codeletion, and methylation of the promoter of 06-Methylguanine-DNA-Methyltransferase (MGMT). However, many other markers have been studied for their role in tumorigenesis and prognosis, such as TERT promoter mutation, ATRX gene mutation, TP53 mutation, CDKN2A/B deletion, EGFR gene amplification, and +7/-10 chromosomal alterations. In addition to the different WHO grades of malignancy, the presence of these alterations can stratify tumors into entities characterized by specific clinical behaviors, different susceptibility to treatments, and prognosis.

26.8 Grades of malignancy

From a prognostic perspective, there are four grades of progressive malignancy based on the presence of nuclear atypia, mitosis, endothelial proliferation, and necrosis (Table 26.2).

Grade I tumors have low proliferative potential, and complete surgical removal can lead to cure without the need for additional therapies. The cells have a typical appearance.

CLASSIFICATION OF CENTRAL NERVOUS SYSTEM TUMORS ACCORDING TO THE WORLD HEALTH ORGANIZATION (LOUIS ET AL., NEURO-ONCOLOGY 2021)

Table 26.1 ABBREVIATIONS: CNS, CENTRAL NERVOUS SYSTEM; IDH, ISOCITRATE DEHYDROGENASE; NK, NATURAL KILLER; PITNET, PITUITARY

GLIOMAS
Adult-type diffuse gliomas
Astrocytoma, IDH-mutant
Oligodendroglioma, IDH-mutant, and 1p/19q-codeleted
Glioblastoma, IDH-wildtype
Pediatric-type diffuse low-grade gliomas
Diffuse astrocytoma, MYB- or MYBL1-altered
Angiocentric glioma
Polymorphous low-grade neuroepithelial tumor of the young
Diffuse low-grade glioma, MAPK pathway-altered
Pediatric-type diffuse high-grade gliomas
Diffuse midline glioma, H3 K27-altered
Diffuse hemispheric glioma, H3 G34-mutant
Diffuse pediatric-type high-grade glioma, H3-wildtype and IDH-wildtype
Infant-type hemispheric glioma
Circumscribed astrocytic gliomas
Pilocytic astrocytoma
High-grade astrocytoma with piloid features
Pleomorphic xanthoastrocytoma
Subependymal giant cell astrocytoma
Chordoid glioma
Astroblastoma, MN1-altered

GLIONEURONAL AND NEURONAL TUMORS
Ganglioglioma
Desmoplastic infantile ganglioglioma desmoplastic infantile astrocytoma
Dysembryoplastic neuroepithelial tumor
Diffuse glioneuronal tumor with oligodendroglioma-like features and nuclear clusters
Papillary glioneuronal tumor
Rosette-forming glioneuronal tumor
Myxoid glioneuronal tumor
Diffuse leptomeningeal glioneuronal tumor
Gangliocytoma
Multinodular and vacuolating neuronal tumor
Dysplastic cerebellar gangliocytoma (Lhermitte-Duclos disease)
Central neurocytoma
Extraventricular neurocytoma
Cerebellar liponeurocytoma

EPENDYMAL TUMORS
Supratentorial ependymoma
Supratentorial ependymoma, ZFTA fusion-positive
Supratentorial ependymoma, YAP1 fusion-positive
Posterior fossa ependymoma
Posterior fossa ependymoma, group PFA
Posterior fossa ependymoma, group PFB
Spinal ependymoma
Spinal ependymoma, MYCN-amplified
Myxopapillary ependymoma
Subependymoma

CHOROID PLEXUS TUMORS
Choroid plexus papilloma
Atypical choroid plexus papilloma
Choroid plexus carcinoma

EMBRYONAL TUMORS
Medulloblastoma
Medulloblastomas, molecularly defined
Medulloblastoma, WNT-activated
Medulloblastoma, SHH-activated and TP53-wildtype
Medulloblastoma, SHH-activated and TP53-mutant
Medulloblastoma, non-WNT/non-SHH
Medulloblastomas, histologically defined
Other CNS embryonal tumors
Atypical teratoid/rhabdoid tumor
Cribriform neuroepithelial tumor
Embryonal tumor with multilayered rosettes
CNS neuroblastoma, FOXR2-activated
CNS tumor with BCOR internal tandem duplication
CNS embryonal tumor

PINEAL TUMORS
Pineocytoma
Pineal parenchymal tumor of intermediate differentiation
Pineoblastoma
Papillary tumor of the pineal region
Desmoplastic myxoid tumor of the pineal region, SMARCB1-mutant

CRANIAL AND PARASPINAL NERVE TUMORS
Schwannoma
Neurofibroma
Perineurioma
Hybrid nerve sheath tumor
Malignant melanotic nerve sheath tumor
Malignant peripheral nerve sheath tumor
Paraganglioma

MENINGIOMAS
Meningioma

MESENCHYMAL, NON-MENINGOTHELIAL TUMORS
Soft tissue tumors
Fibroblastic and myofibroblastic tumors
Solitary fibrous tumor
Vascular tumors
Hemangiomas and vascular malformations
Hemangioblastoma
Skeletal muscle tumors
Rhabdomyosarcoma
Uncertain differentiation
Intracranial mesenchymal tumor, FET-CREB fusion-positive
CIC-rearranged sarcoma
Primary intracranial sarcoma, DICER1-mutant
Ewing sarcoma

Chondro-osseous tumors
Chondrogenic tumors
Mesenchymal chondrosarcoma
Chondrosarcoma

NOTOCHORDAL TUMORS
Chordoma (including poorly differentiated chordoma)

MELANOCYTIC TUMORS
Diffuse meningeal melanocytic neoplasms
Meningeal melanocytosis and meningeal melanomatosis
Circumscribed meningeal melanocytic neoplasms
Meningeal melanocytoma and meningeal melanoma

HEMATOLYMPHOID TUMORS
Lymphomas
CNS lymphomas
Primary diffuse large B-cell lymphoma of the CNS
Immunodeficiency-associated CNS lymphoma
Lymphomatoid granulomatosis
Intravascular large B-cell lymphoma
Miscellaneous rare lymphomas in the CNS
MALT lymphoma of the dura
Other low-grade B-cell lymphomas of the CNS
Anaplastic large cell lymphoma (ALK+/ALK-)
T-cell and NK/T-cell lymphomas
Histiocytic tumors
Erdheim-Chester disease
Rosai-Dorfman disease
Juvenile xanthogranuloma
Langerhans cell histiocytosis
Histiocytic sarcoma

GERM CELL TUMORS
Mature teratoma
Immature teratoma
Teratoma with somatic-type malignancy
Germinoma
Embryonal carcinoma
Yolk sac tumor
Choriocarcinoma
Mixed germ cell tumor

TUMORS OF THE SELLAR REGION
Adamantinomatous craniopharyngioma
Papillary craniopharyngioma
Pituicytoma, granular cell tumor of the sellar region, and spindle cell oncocytoma
Pituitary adenoma/PitNET
Pituitary blastoma

METASTASES TO THE CNS
Metastases to the brain and spinal cord parenchyma
Metastases to the meninges

Grade II tumors have high cellularity without cellular or nuclear atypia or mitosis. They generally exhibit infiltrative behavior and, despite low proliferative activity, often recur. Grade II tumors can progress to higher grades of malignancy; for example, low-grade diffuse astrocytomas can transform into anaplastic astrocytomas and then into glioblastomas. Similar transformations can occur in oligodendrogliomas and oligoastrocytomas.

Grade III tumors show histological evidence of malignancy, with nuclear atypia and mitosis. In the majority of cases, treatment requires not only surgery but also radiotherapy and/or chemotherapy.

Grade IV tumors are cytologically malignant, with high mitotic activity, endothelial/vascular proliferation, and/or areas of tumor necrosis. These neoplasms have rapid progression and often have a fatal course. Examples of Grade IV tumors include glioblastomas, medulloblastomas, and many sarcomas. Some tumors of this type are characterized by widespread infiltration of the surrounding brain parenchyma and a propensity for craniospinal dissemination.

26.9 Tumor types

Intracranial tumors can grow outside the brain and compress it (*extracerebral tumors*) or originate and develop within the brain parenchyma (*intracerebral tumors*) or within the ventricles (*intraventricular tumors*).

26.10 Extracerebral tumors

26.10.1 Meningiomas

Meningiomas are very common tumors and represent 13-24% of primary brain tumors. They originate from the meninges, particularly the arachnoid membrane. In the majority of cases, they present as histologically benign tumors. They are more common in women (two-thirds of cases) and in middle-aged to older individuals. They grow more rapidly during pregnancy and are somewhat associated with breast carcinoma. These circumstances suggest that hormonal factors are involved in their pathogenesis. Indeed, meningiomas often express progesterone receptors, although their

Table 26.2 CNS WHO GRADES OF SELECTED TYPES, COVERING ENTITIES FOR WHICH THERE IS A NEW APPROACH TO GRADING, AN UPDATED GRADE, OR A NEWLY RECOGNIZED TUMOR THAT HAS AN ACCEPTED GRADE

Selected Typesof Tumors	CNS WHO Grades
Astrocytoma, IDH-mutant	2, 3, 4
Oligodendroglioma, IDH-mutant, and 1p/19q-codeleted	2, 3
Glioblastoma, IDH-wildtype	4
Diffuse astrocytoma, MYB- or MYBL1-altered	1
Polymorphous low-grade neuroepithelial tumor of the young	1
Diffuse hemispheric glioma, H3 G34-mutant	4
Pleomorphic xanthoastrocytoma	2, 3
Multinodular and vacuolating neuronal tumor	1
Supratentorial ependymoma	2, 3
Posterior fossa ependymoma	2, 3
Myxopapillary ependymoma	2
Meningioma	1, 2, 3
Solitary fibrous tumor	1, 2, 3

role is not yet well-defined. Previous head trauma and cranial irradiation may also play a role in meningioma formation. Sometimes, meningiomas are associated with hyperostosis of the adjacent cranial bone, which seems to be a bone reaction resulting from neoplastic invasion. Meningioma growth is often slow, allowing the brain to adapt to their presence. As a result, compressive symptoms often occur late when the meningioma has reached significant size. They are usually highly vascularized through the meningeal arteries, branches of the external carotid artery circulation. In the initial stages of growth, the meningioma deforms the brain but does not extend beyond the pia mater, so a separation plane can be found between the tumor and the parenchyma. The onset of cerebral edema often indicates breach of the pial plane, which can occur in very large tumors or those with more aggressive behavior. Brain MRI with gadolinium allows for diagnosis by showing the dural attachment of the neoplasm, its extracerebral location, and brain compression. CT can reveal reactive hyperostosis areas and calcifications that are sometimes present in meningiomas. In most cases, complete surgical removal is possible, including the dural attachment and infiltrated bone. However, exceeding the pial plane with involvement of vessels or nerves can preclude total resection.

Meningiomatosis | Is a disease characterized by a tendency to form multiple meningiomas, both intracranial and spinal. In these cases, treatment is determined by clinical symptoms and directed towards those meningiomas causing symptoms. These patients require lifelong clinical and neuroradiological follow-up to monitor the growth and clinical expression of the various tumors.

26.10.2 Pituitary adenomas

Pituitary adenomas are usually biologically benign tumors originating from the cells of the adenohypophysis. They are distinguished based on size into microadenomas (with a diameter up to 10 mm) and macroadenomas (with a diameter exceeding 10 mm). As sellar tumors, they cause two different types of symptoms: endocrine symptoms first, followed by neurological symptoms. During the *endocrine phase*, symptoms can be caused by *hormone hypersecretion* (in adenomas that abnormally secrete pituitary hormones), leading to typical endocrine syndromes, and/or by *hypopituitarism*, related to progressive compression and destruction of healthy pituitary tissue by the tumor. The *neurological phase* is associated with further tumor growth, extending beyond the sellar boundaries and compressing the overlying optic pathways (chiasm and optic nerves). As the tumor continues to grow, it can compress the third ventricle and cause biventricular hydrocephalus.

Pituitary adenomas | Are usually classified based on their secretory capacity into Prolactin-secreting adenomas, Growth Hormone (GH)-secreting adenomas, Adrenocorticotropic Hormone (ACTH)-secreting adenomas, Thyroid-Stimulating Hormone (TSH)-secreting adenomas, Gonadotropin-secreting adenomas, and non-secreting adenomas.

Prolactin-secreting adenomas cause an endocrine syndrome that differs between sexes. In women, who are more commonly affected, they cause amenorrhea often associated with galactorrhea. In men, they cause impotence and decreased libido. It is important to note that medical treatment options are highly effective for Prolactin-secreting adenomas. Dopamine agonist drugs can normalize or significantly reduce hyperprolactinemia and can also shrink the tumor in many cases, avoiding the need for surgery.

GH-secreting adenomas | Cause the disease known as acromegaly. In adults, whose skeletal growth has concluded, excessive GH production causes enlargement of the extremities (hands, feet, nose), increased tongue size (macroglossia), deepening of the voice due to vocal cord hypertrophy, hypertrophy of various internal organs such as the heart and liver, and may also lead to diabetes and hypertension. Before puberty, GH excess causes gigantism.

ACTH-secreting adenomas | Cause Cushing's disease, characterized by hyper-cortisolism due to stimulation of corticosteroid production by ACTH. Patients exhibit typical features such as moon facies, centripetal obesity (concentrated in the trunk and abdomen, while the limbs remain thin due to muscle atrophy), striae on the abdomen, muscle atrophy, increased susceptibility to osteoporotic fractures and infections in general, and psychiatric disturbances. The disease is severe due to the associated diabetes and hypertension. Differential diagnosis should be made with other possible causes of hypercortisolism, such as adrenal diseases, tumors, and paraneoplastic syndromes.

TSH-secreting adenomas | Are very rare and cause hyperthyroidism.

Gonadotropin-secreting adenomas | Produce LH and FSH, hormones that do not cause a well-characterized endocrine hypersecretion syndrome. Consequently, symptoms are similar to those of non-secreting adenomas.

Non-secreting adenomas | Do not produce hormones. In this type of adenoma, symptoms related to hypopituitarism predominate, which is clinically more relevant in the context of corticosteroid and thyroid function. In men, hypogonadism with impotence and decreased libido is not uncommon. Often, these tumors are not recognized during the hypopituitarism phase, and the diagnosis is made only when neurological symptoms arise.

Pituitary apoplexy | Some adenomas can present with macroscopic hemorrhages within them, leading to a sudden and massive increase in volume. The resulting syndrome is usually severe, with sudden pituitary insufficiency, rapid decrease in vision, and cavernous sinus syndrome, including sometimes complete ophthalmoplegia in one or both eyes. The diagnosis can be made using MRI. The treatment is urgent and involves both medical management with hormone replacement therapy, especially corticosteroids for severe pituitary insufficiency, and surgical intervention with transsphenoidal decompression of the sellar contents to alleviate neurological symptoms.

26.10.3 Craniopharyngiomas

They originate from remnants of the craniopharyngeal duct and are located in the sella turcica or, more commonly, just above it. They can be solid, cystic, or mixed and often occur in children or adolescents but are not uncommon in adults. Diabetes insipidus is an early symptom, and in children, compression of the diencephalic-hypothalamic region leads to a syndrome characterized by stunted growth and sexual development, often associated with obesity and visual disturbances. In contrast, visual disturbances are more prominent in adults who have already reached sexual maturation. They are biologically benign, but their surgical removal is often challenging due to strong adherence to the diencephalic region. Postoperative disturbances in fluid and electrolyte balance are particularly concerning.

26.10.4 Vestibular Schwannomas (or acoustic neuromas)

They originate from the vestibular branch of the vestibulocochlear nerve deep within the internal acoustic canal. As they grow, they cause early hearing loss and subsequent unilateral deafness. When they extend beyond the internal acoustic canal, they grow in the cerebellopontine angle, leading to cranial nerve disorders (trigeminal, facial, glossopharyngeal, and vagus nerves), compression of the cerebellum and brainstem. They are biologically benign tumors but surgically challenging due to the depth of the operative field, the adherence of the facial nerve to the tumor surface (posing a risk of permanent damage), and their proximity to the brainstem. Intraoperative monitoring of the facial nerve is crucial in reducing the risk of injury. Preserving hearing on the affected side is more difficult to achieve surgically, especially in patients who still have hearing function. Due to the surgical difficulties, radiation therapy (stereotactic radiosurgery) can be a valid alternative treatment option, although it is not without side effects. Vestibular schwannomas can also occur in the context of neurofibromatosis type 2 (NF-2), where they are often bilateral. In these cases, treatment decisions are delicate because both the natural progression of the disease and its possible treatments (surgery and radiosurgery) carry the risk of bilateral deafness.

26.10.5 Chordomas

Chordomas arise within the bone from remnants of the embryonic notochord. They are located along the midline, with a preferential intracranial location in the clivus. They originate within the bone and initially grow extradurally. However, due to their invasive nature, they can penetrate the dura mater. They clinically present with cranial nerve disorders, especially involving the oculomotor nerves. Chordomas frequently recur after surgical removal, leading to a poor long-term prognosis.

26.10.6 Glomus tumors (chemodectomas)

Glomus tumors are very rare, usually benign tumors that develop in the jugular glomus, located in the jugular foramen at the base of the skull. They are highly vascularized and grow slowly. They invade the temporal bone and can extend to the middle ear, causing erosion of the petrous bone, as well as to the cerebellopontine region, exerting compression on the brainstem and affecting the cranial nerves in that area (glossopharyngeal, vagus, and accessory nerves). Due to their significant vascularity, they can present with pulsatile tinnitus. Subsequent symptoms include hearing loss and difficulties with speech and swallowing due to compression of the cranial nerves in the jugular foramen. Surgical removal is complex due to the tumor's location in the skull base, involvement of cranial nerves, and rich vascularity. Preoperative endovascular embolization is useful in reducing intraoperative bleeding. Radiation therapy is employed in cases where complete removal is not possible.

26.10.7 Malignant tumors of the skull base

These tumors invade the bones of the skull base and can include metastases, lymphomas, sarcomas, or carcinomas originating from nearby tissues. Initial symptoms typically involve cranial nerves. Complete radical resection is often impossible due to the invasive nature of the tumor, involvement of cranial nerves, and challenging surgical access.

26.10.8 Arachnoid cysts (or leptomeningeal cysts)

These are not neoplasms but can behave like them. They are cysts containing cerebrospinal fluid located in the subarachnoid space. The cyst walls consist of a duplication of the arachnoid membrane, creating a closed compartment where cerebrospinal fluid is trapped. They are usually found in children and young adults, predominantly males. The most common locations are the Sylvian fissure, the cisterna magna, the cerebellopontine angle, and the suprasellar region. It can be challenging to differentiate them from ex vacuo cerebrospinal fluid collections that occur in partial cerebral atrophies. In these cases, a portion of the brain has not developed during fetal life, often without causing any symptoms, and the space left empty by the parenchyma is filled with cerebrospinal fluid. Ex vacuo collections are generally harmless and do not increase in size over time. Arachnoid cysts require periodic clinical and radiological monitoring using MRI. Surgical treatment is indicated when symptoms appear and/or when there is evidence of cyst enlargement.

26.11 Intracerebral tumors

26.11.1 Gliomas

Gliomas are tumors that originate from glial cells within the brain parenchyma. They grow by infiltrating the nervous tissue and tend to become increasingly aggressive over time. Grade I and II WHO tumors are *low-grade gliomas*, which are well-differentiated histologically and have slow growth. They most commonly occur in young adults and present with epileptic seizures, which often remain the only symptoms for a long time. If left untreated, these tumors tend to progress to high-grade gliomas. Grade III and IV tumors are called *high-grade gliomas*, which have aggressive behavior, rapid growth, greater infiltrative tendency, and a worse prognosis compared to low-grade gliomas. Due to their rapid growth and the presence of edema, increased intracranial pressure is common, with headaches being the most common symptom, often associated with neurological deficits.

Astrocytomas, derived from astrocytes, constitute the most frequent type of glioma. They can be recognized immunohistochemically because they are positive for glial fibrillary acidic protein (GFAP).

Grade I astrocytomas are well-circumscribed tumors that are very rare in adults. In children, pilocytic astrocytoma of the cerebellum is quite common (25% of pediatric brain tumors). They often have cystic components and have an excellent surgical prognosis when completely removed. In children, particularly those with neurofibromatosis type 1, grade I astrocytomas can also be found in the chiasm and optic nerves. Due to the risk of vision loss associated with surgical treatment of this type of neoplasm, surgical removal is performed in cases with clear progression and complete monocular or binocular blindness. Subependymal giant cell astrocytoma is a slow-growing tumor often associated with tuberous sclerosis, originating from the walls of the ventricles. Complete surgical removal results in a good prognosis.

Among grade II astrocytomas, the most common type is diffuse astrocytoma. They are typically located in the cerebral hemispheres and grow slowly. Usually, cerebral edema is absent or minimal, and these tumors generally do not show contrast enhancement on CT or MRI. The initial manifestation is commonly an epileptic seizure, and for years there may be no other symptoms. These tumors tend to become more aggressive over time and transform into anaplastic astrocytomas. Radical surgical resection can delay this progression.

Pleomorphic xanthoastrocytoma is a tumor located on the surface of the cerebral hemisphere, often consisting of a cyst with a mural nodule on the wall. The tumor enhances with contrast on neuroimaging examinations. It is usually well-circumscribed, and complete surgical removal significantly improves prognosis.

Anaplastic astrocytomas (grade III) are more aggressive both histologically and behaviorally, showing nuclear atypia and mitosis in the absence of vascular proliferation and necrosis. They often enhance with contrast on MRI and cause cerebral edema. In addition to surgery, they require radiation therapy and chemotherapy.

Grade IV astrocytomas, or glioblastoma multiforme, are among the most common brain tumors. They most commonly occur in males over 50 years of age and almost always in supratentorial regions. Histologically, they are characterized by high cellularity, nuclear atypia, nuclear polymorphism, as well as vascular or endothelial proliferation and necrosis. Despite multimodal treatment, including surgery, radiation therapy, and chemotherapy (temozolomide) as the standard approach, the median survival is around 12 to 14 months. Neoplastic recurrences are mostly local, with a tendency to spread further within the nervous tissue and become less responsive to therapy. It is very rare for glioblastomas to metastasize outside the central nervous system. *Primary glioblastomas* arise as such from the beginning, distinguishing them from *secondary glioblastomas*, which are rarer and arise from malignant transformation of lower-grade gliomas. Secondary glioblastomas generally have a better prognosis and are characterized by the presence of a somatic mutation in the isocitrate dehydrogenase 1 (IDH1) gene, also present in the majority of grade II and III gliomas. Primary and secondary glioblastomas are morphologically indistinguishable, but the use of a monoclonal antibody for IDH1 allows for important prognostic distinction. In glioblastomas, unlike low-grade gliomas, symptoms often involve neurological deficits and rapidly evolving increased intracranial pressure due to their fast growth, accompanied by cerebral edema. Neuroradiologically, they appear as a heterogeneous mass with peripheral ring enhancement, representing the intensely vascularized portion of the tumor where the blood-brain barrier is disrupted, with a hypointense core in the center due to necrosis. The mass is usually surrounded by peritumoral edema (■ Figure 26.2A). Standard treatment includes management of cerebral edema (corticosteroids and/or osmotic diuretics), surgical resection, radiation therapy, and chemotherapy with temozolomide for at least 6 months. The combination of the latter two complementary treatments has been shown to significantly extend patient survival (Stupp protocol). Recently, a subtype of glioblastoma characterized by methylation of the O-6-methylguanine-DNA methyltransferase (MGMT) gene promoter has been identified. Patients with methylated MGMT respond better to temozolomide chemotherapy and have a better prognosis. Younger patients (below 50 years old), those with better functional status (Karnofsky performance status between 80 and 100), and those in whom surgical removal of at least 98% of the tumor is achieved have a better prognosis than the average. Despite the overall poor prognosis, a percentage of patients (approximately 20-30%) have a survival exceeding two years.

Oligodendrogliomas derive from oligodendrocytes. They are less frequent compared to astrocytomas and usually have a more benign course, respond better to chemotherapy and have a better prognosis. Intratumoral calcifications are often present. They also have a preferential localization in the cerebral hemispheres. Oligodendrogliomas are characterized by typical genetic alterations, such as loss of heterozygosity related to translocation or deletion of the chromosomal arms 1p and 19q. Oligodendrogliomas are classified into low-grade tumors and anaplastic tumors. Grade II oligodendrogliomas occur in young adults, and epileptic seizures are the presenting symptom. On MRI, they appear hyperintense on T2 and FLAIR sequences and usually do not enhance with contrast. Calcifications appear as signal void areas. Their behavior is initially indolent, and they are often observed without any treatment other than antiepileptic medication. The risk of anaplastic transformation and the adoption of more refined surgical techniques, which allow for better functional preservation, lead to preferential initial treatment with surgical removal. In case of incomplete resection, radiotherapy can be combined with chemotherapy using temozolomide. In the case of anaplastic oligodendrogliomas (grade III), in addition to surgical removal, radiotherapy and chemotherapy are indicated.

26.11.2 Ependymomas

They originate from the ependyma that lines the ventricular walls. In children and young adults, they are more frequently located in the posterior fossa (ependymoma of the fourth ventricle), while in adults, they are more common in the supratentorial region. They are classified into grade I (subependymoma, very slow-growing tumors of the ventricular walls, where complete surgical removal leads to cure), grade II, and grade III (anaplastic). Grade II and III ependymomas can spread through the leptomeninges. Complete removal of a low-grade ependymoma can ensure cure. In cases of incomplete resection and anaplastic ependymomas, combination with radiotherapy is indicated.

26.11.3 Cerebral gliomatosis

It is characterized by diffuse infiltration of gliomatous cells into the brain parenchyma, often astrocytic, frequently involving multiple cerebral lobes without the formation of distinct tumor nodules. The usually extensive involvement makes radical surgery and radiotherapy (the latter due to the risk of toxicity) impractical. The usual treatment is chemotherapy with temozolomide. The prognosis is not good due to the tendency of the lesion to spread and progress anaplastically.

26.11.4 Multiple gliomas

They are gliomas that originate from different points in the brain. In multifocal gliomas, the various locations result from dissemination or growth of the glioma along established routes (such as the corpus callosum or fornix) or through cerebrospinal fluid dissemination or local metastasis. Multicentric gliomas, on the other hand, are separate lesions that arise in different lobes or hemispheres, not attributable to the aforementioned routes. They can also occur at different times. Due to the multiple locations, the prognosis for multiple gliomas is not good, and survival is limited to a few months in most cases. Survival is better in patients who can have complete removal of the various lesions.

26.11.5 Neuronal and glioneuronal tumors

These are rare tumors with low proliferative potential, typical in children and young adults, often associated with drug-resistant epilepsy. They generally have a good prognosis, but despite their indolent course, the importance of complete removal is recognized to prevent possible, albeit rare, malignant transformation. They are frequently associated with foci of *cortical dysplasia*, which is a developmental malformation of the cortex, also epileptogenic, where the normal laminar organization of the cerebral cortex is lost, with the possible presence of abnormal neurons. The association with cortical dysplasia suggests that these tumors may represent a neoplastic transformation of the dysplasia itself or a benign tumor originating from an embryogenic disorder. Epilepsy caused by these tumors has a favorable prognosis after surgical removal of the neoplasm and any associated dysplasia. This group includes ganglioglioma/gangliocytoma, central neurocytoma, often located endoventricularly, and dysembryoplastic neuroepithelial tumors (DNET).

26.11.6 Germinoma

It is a tumor of adolescence that originates from germ cells that did not migrate correctly during embryonic development. It is localized in the pineal region or, more rarely, in the sellar region. Histologically, it is identical to testicular seminoma. Metastatic spread through the cerebrospinal fluid is possible. Cytological examination of the cerebrospinal fluid can detect the presence of neoplastic cells. High levels of HCG, placental alkaline phosphatase, and alpha-fetoprotein in the blood and cerebrospinal fluid can confirm the diagnosis. These molecules, therefore, constitute true tumor markers and can also be used to monitor the effectiveness of therapy. Germinoma is a highly radiosensitive tumor, and complete disappearance is common after radiotherapy.

26.11.7 Medulloblastoma

It is a malignant tumor that originates from primitive embryonic cells, probably located in the external granular layer of the cerebellum. It belongs to the group of primitive neuroectodermal tumors (PNETs). It is common in children, accounting for 25% of all intracranial tumors, and is second in incidence only to astrocytomas. However, it can also occur, albeit less frequently, in young adults. It predominantly occurs in the cerebellum, more often in the vermis than in the cerebellar hemispheres. The early invasion of the fourth ventricle causes obstruction of the cerebrospinal fluid circulation, leading to hydrocephalus and intracranial hypertension, in addition to more specific cerebellar symptoms. Leptomeningeal dissemination is common, detectable in approximately 40% of cases. Gadolinium-enhanced MRI is the diagnostic imaging modality of choice. It typically shows a contrast-enhancing mass in the posterior fossa, often associated with hydrocephalus. Surgical removal is the main treatment, aiming to achieve complete removal of the lesion and resolve any obstruction of the cerebrospinal fluid circulation. Once histological confirmation of medulloblastoma is obtained, the possible presence of spinal dissemination must be verified. Surgical treatment is combined with craniospinal irradiation and chemotherapy. In younger children, irradiation can be associated with neurocognitive and endocrine deficits, affecting growth. Due to therapeutic advances, a significant proportion of patients achieve prolonged survival or cure.

26.11.8 Hemangioblastoma (or Angioreticuloma)

It is a rare, benign intra-axial vascular tumor, most commonly located in the cerebellum and spinal cord. It is more common in males. In the majority of cases, hemangioblastoma is a solitary lesion. In about a quarter of cases, it occurs within the context of an autosomal dominant genetic disorder, von Hippel-Lindau syndrome, where these patients tend to develop multiple tumors in the cerebellum and spinal cord. Hemangioblastomas can present as solid or cystic lesions. In the latter case, a usually large cystic wall contains a much smaller mural nodule that contains the actual neoplastic tissue. It grows within the neural tissue but is often in contact with the pia mater, and its rich vascularization is supplied by pial vessels. Clinical presentation may involve a combination of cerebellar symptoms and increased intracranial pressure due to cerebrospinal fluid obstruction. Gadolinium-enhanced MRI is the imaging modality of choice. In case of a suspected hemangioblastoma, spinal MRI is also recommended to exclude the presence of other hemangioblastomas, and screening for von Hippel-Lindau disease is performed. This includes spinal MRI, fundoscopy to detect retinal hemangioblastomas, and abdominal radiological examinations to identify any renal, adrenal, or pancreatic neoplasms or cysts. Complete surgical removal guarantees cure in sporadic cases not associated with von Hippel-Lindau syndrome. In cases of incomplete resection, hemangioblastoma can recur. Hemangioblastoma can produce substances similar to erythropoietin, leading to polycythemia.

26.11.9 Epidermoid and dermoid cysts

An epidermoid cyst is a benign tumor originating from ectodermal cells that remain trapped in the nervous system due to an embryonic developmental error. These cells give rise to the cyst, whose wall is composed of a stratified squamous epithelium, similar to the epidermis, that grows and sheds inward, resulting in the formation and accumulation of keratinaceous and cholesterol-rich material that fills and progressively expands the cyst. Dermoid cysts, which are rarer, form similarly but differ from epidermoid cysts as they consist of both epidermal and dermal elements, including sweat glands and hair follicles. The cysts grow slowly and are filled with flaky material. In rare cases, they can rupture, releasing cholesterol material into the subarachnoid space, causing chemical meningitis due to its irritant effect. The most frequent intracranial locations are the posterior fossa, particularly the ponto-cerebellar angle, the suprasellar region, and the temporal lobe. Although they are congenital, symptoms usually appear between the ages of 20 and 40 due to their slow growth. The diagnosis is aided by MRI, where the tissue appears isointense to cerebrospinal fluid in all sequences, making it difficult to distinguish from arachnoid cysts. The only MRI sequence capable of differentiating epidermoid cysts from cerebrospinal fluid is *Diffusion Weighted Imaging* (DWI), in which the keratin appears hyperintense. Surgical removal is the treatment of choice. Since the cystic wall is often intimately adherent to the brain tissue, complete removal is not always possible. In these cases, recurrence is quite common; however, cyst growth is slow, and many years may pass before it becomes symptomatic again. Operated patients, especially those with incomplete resection, should be monitored with MRI for a long period.

26.11.10 Brain metastases

Brain metastases are the most common intracranial neoplasms in adults. Their incidence surpasses that of all other intracranial tumors and is progressively increasing due to improved efficacy of therapies for the primary tumor. The most common primary tumors that metastasize to the brain are lung, breast, kidney, colorectal carcinomas, and melanomas. Lung carcinomas are the most frequent source in men, while breast carcinoma is the most frequent in women. The incidence of brain metastases peaks in the fifth and sixth decades of life but is much lower in pediatric age. The imaging modality of choice for radiological diagnosis is contrast-enhanced brain MRI, as it can detect even very small metastases that may not be visible on contrast-enhanced CT. Metastases are often surrounded by edema. It is not uncommon for the diagnosis of brain metastasis to be the first evidence of an existing malignancy in the body. If neuroimaging shows a suspected metastasis in a patient without a previous diagnosis of malignancy, further radiological imaging of the entire body, such as CT or PET-CT, combined with a skeletal scintigraphy, is indicated to identify the primary tumor and the possible presence of other metastases. Treatment involves a combination of medical therapy (anti-edema, antiepileptic, and chemotherapy), surgical intervention (in cases of solitary lesions in accessible brain regions with low risk), and radiation therapy. Prognosis varies and depends on the type of primary cancer, patient age (it is less unfavorable in younger patients), the presence or absence of extracranial metastases, and the number of brain metastases.

26.11.11 Cavernous angioma

It is a vascular malformation, not a true neoplasm, but it can behave like one. It consists of a collection of dilated capillary vessels, delimited by a single layer of endothelial cells, resembling sinusoidal cavities filled with blood circulating at low flow. The vessels are closely packed together without interposition of nervous tissue. The walls of the capillaries are thinner than normal and easily rupture. It is believed that cavernous angiomas grow as blood, leaked from repeated microscopic hemorrhages, organizes and forms new dilated cavernous capillaries within them. It is commonly believed that these malformations are congenital, but ex novo formation has also been observed. They can appear sporadically or in hereditary conditions. Microscopic hemorrhages are asymptomatic. Macroscopic hemorrhages can also occur with symptoms such as headache, neurological deficits, and radiological evidence of fresh blood. The most appropriate examination for diagnosis is MRI; on FLAIR and T2 sequences, cavernous angiomas appear as a heterogeneous core consisting of blood in various stages of evolution, surrounded by a hypointense ring of hemosiderin. Cavernous angiomas can be solitary or sometimes multiple (*cavernomatosis*), with the latter being more frequently associated with hereditary forms. Cavernous angiomas have a highly variable clinical expression. They can be completely asymptomatic, be associated with epileptic seizures, or manifest with neurological deterioration related to macroscopic hemorrhages or volumetric growth. The possibility of surgical treatment should be considered in cases of recurrent macroscopic hemorrhages, progressive neurological deterioration, or pharmacologically intractable epilepsy.

26.12 Intraventricular tumors

They are characterized by the prevalence of symptoms of cerebrospinal fluid hypertension due to the blockage of cerebrospinal fluid circulation, leading to hydrocephalus. They are usually represented by ependymomas, gliomas, and neurocytomas, less frequently by meningiomas, choroid plexus papillomas (rare, highly vascularized tumors causing hydrocephalus due to excessive production of cerebrospinal fluid), and colloid cysts.

26.12.1 Colloid cysts

They are benign tumors located in the anterior portion of the third ventricle, immediately behind the foramina of Monro. They consist of a cyst with an epithelial wall containing viscous fluid. Their location carries the risk of obstructive biventricular hydrocephalus, which can also lead to severe morbidity or sudden death. Although they are believed to be congenital, clinical manifestations usually occur between the ages of 20 and 50, with increased intracranial pressure. Surgical intervention, either transcranial or endoscopic, allows for the drainage and removal of the cyst, restoring normal cerebrospinal fluid circulation in the vast majority of cases.

26.13 Genetic disorders with associated tumors

In the past, they were grouped under the common name of phakomatoses or neuro-cutaneous syndromes. Recent genetic studies have shown that they are actually distinct entities.

26.13.1 Neurofibromatosis

Neurofibromatoses are a group of three genetically distinct neurocutaneous diseases with autosomal dominant inheritance that cause tumors in the nervous system. Approximately half of the cases are due to ex novo mutations, and there are no other affected family members. The diseases are *neurofibromatosis type 1* (NF1, or von Recklinghausen disease), *neurofibromatosis type 2* (NF2), and *schwannomatosis*, previously considered a variant of NF2. The diseases affect both sexes, all races, and ethnic groups. All cells derived from neural crest cells are involved (Schwann cells, melanocytes, and endoneurial fibroblasts). The most common tumors in NF1 are neurofibromas of peripheral nerves, sometimes located on the skin, while schwannomas are more common in NF2 and schwannomatosis. The tumors are mostly benign, although they can occasionally become malignant. The uncontrolled proliferation of melanocytes causes a disorder of skin pigmentation, with the presence of café-au-lait spots, a typical sign of neurofibromatoses.

NF1 is the most common type (over 90% of cases) and is characterized by the presence of various manifestations occurring in varying combinations: cutaneous or subcutaneous neurofibromas, plexiform neurofibromas (a cluster of tumors involving multiple nerves), inguinal or axillary freckling, café-au-lait spots (pigmented skin spots with indistinct borders), skeletal abnormalities or deformities, Lisch nodules (iris hamartomas), freckling in the iris, optic gliomas, macrocephaly, epilepsy, and juvenile cataracts. NF1 is associated with an increased incidence of other tumors, such as meningiomas, gliomas, and pheochromocytomas.

NF2, less common than NF1 (about 10% of cases), also known as central neurofibromatosis, is characterized by bilateral acoustic neuromas with frequent early-onset hearing loss around the age of 20. Schwannomas can occur in any nerve in the body, including cranial, spinal, and peripheral nerves. In *schwannomatosis* multiple schwannomas occur in cranial, spinal, and peripheral nerves, but the vestibulocochlear nerve is not affected, resulting in no hearing loss. Patients have an increased incidence of epilepsy and leukemia; learning difficulties and cognitive deficits are common, but severe mental retardation is not. They often require multiple surgical interventions. A delicate and unresolved issue is the prevention of deafness in NF2. Genetic testing is available for families with documented cases of NF1 and NF2, but not yet for schwannomatosis.

26.13.2 Sturge-Weber syndrome

Sturge-Weber syndrome, or encephalo-trigeminal angiomatosis, is a congenital neurocutaneous disease characterized by the presence of angiomas involving the leptomeninges (leptomeningeal angiomas) and the facial skin, typically in the distribution areas of the trigeminal nerve, especially the first (forehead and upper eyelid) and second branch (lower eyelid and jaw). The facial angiomas have a wine-colored appearance and are present at birth. Leptomeningeal angiomas are usually unilateral and located in the parietal or occipital region. The mechanism of vascular steal, caused by the angiomas, is responsible for ischemic phenomena in the adjacent cortical cerebral territory, resulting in neurological manifestations such as epilepsy, often refractory, focal deficits, usually transient, such as hemiparesis and hemianopsia, developmental disorders, learning difficulties, and mental retardation (more common with bilateral angiomas). Complications in the eye on the same side as the facial angioma are possible, with glaucoma and potential blindness being the most feared. Psychomotor impairment varies, partly depending on the success of controlling epileptic seizures. During the course of the disease, ipsilateral cerebral atrophy and calcifications on the cortical surface can be observed. This syndrome is not an inherited disease, and the etiology is unknown.

26.13.3 Von Hippel-Lindau disease

Von Hippel-Lindau disease (VHL) is a rare autosomal dominant inherited disease associated with an alteration in chromosome 3. It is characterized by the presence of multiple hemangioblastomas in the cerebellum, spinal cord, kidneys, and retina. Other conditions that can occur include renal angioma, pheochromocytoma, renal carcinoma, and pancreatic cysts. The diagnosis is established by finding a single hemangioblastoma in a patient with a positive family history. In the absence of a family history, the presence of at least two cerebellar hemangioblastomas or one hemangioblastoma plus a visceral tumor justifies the diagnosis.

26.13.4 Tuberous sclerosis

Tuberous sclerosis is a rare autosomal dominant genetic disease, multisystemic, characterized by the growth of non-malignant tumors in the brain and other organs such as the kidneys, heart, eyes, lungs, and skin. Cutaneous abnormalities are present in almost all patients and help establish the diagnosis. The most typical is the adenoma sebaceum, which appears as reddish patches or raised areas on the nose and cheeks with a butterfly distribution. Hypomelanotic macules, consisting of hypopigmented skin areas, are also common. Symptoms include epilepsy, varying combinations of psychomotor developmental delay, behavioral and learning problems, mental retardation, skin abnormalities, and lung and kidney diseases. It is caused by a mutation in either the TSC1 or TSC2 genes, which encode the proteins hamartin and tuberin, respectively. These proteins act as tumor growth suppressors and regulate cell proliferation and differentiation. The mutation is sporadic in most cases, occurring ex novo in families without any previous cases. There are three types of cerebral lesions:

Cortical and subcortical tubers, pale-looking clusters believed to be foci of abnormal neuronal migration that can calcify over time, *subependymal nodules*, located in the ventricular walls, consisting of swollen glial cells and bizarre multinucleated cells with uncertain glial or neuronal origin; and *giant cell astrocytoma*, derived from neoplastic transformation of subependymal nodules, often forming in the region of the foramen of Monro and causing blockage of cerebrospinal fluid circulation with hydrocephalus.

26.13.5 Benign intracranial hypertension or idiopathic intracranial hypertension (pseudotumor cerebri)

It is a condition characterized by a chronic increase in intracranial pressure in the absence of hydrocephalus, intracranial neoplasms, or infectious or inflammatory processes. It is predominantly found in obese women of childbearing age, particularly if there has been a significant and recent weight gain. The most clinically relevant issue is the presence of papilledema, which can lead to progressive optic atrophy and blindness over time. The pathogenesis is not well understood, but the most widely accepted hypothesis suggests an increase in resistance to cerebrospinal fluid reabsorption through the arachnoid granulations located in the dural venous sinuses. This situation could be due to increased cerebral venous pressure, which may result from stenosis of the cerebral venous sinuses (superior sagittal sinus or transverse sinuses) or partial occlusion of these sinuses due to venous thrombosis. Typical symptoms include progressively worsening headache and initially transient visual disturbances (such as episodes of blurred vision lasting a few seconds) associated with papilledema. With the chronicity of papilledema, these symptoms can become more severe and permanent due to progressive optic atrophy, leading to a gradual concentric narrowing of the visual field, starting from the lower nasal quadrants and progressing to blindness. Brain MRI with gadolinium, along with venous MR angiography, is used to exclude the presence of brain neoplasms and other causes of intracranial hypertension and to identify any stenosis or thrombosis of the venous sinuses. Often, the examination shows an empty sella, which refers to a situation where an arachnoid diverticulum filled with cerebrospinal fluid herniates into the sella turcica, compressing the pituitary gland. After excluding the presence of brain neoplasms on MRI, the definitive diagnosis requires measurement of cerebrospinal fluid pressure through lumbar puncture. Treatment options include weight loss, which can improve the clinical picture, and medical treatment with acetazolamide, a carbonic anhydrase inhibitor diuretic that reduces cerebrospinal fluid production. In cases that do not respond to these treatments, surgical intervention may be indicated. The most commonly performed surgical treatment is a lumboperitoneal shunt, in which a silicone catheter is implanted between the spinal subarachnoid space and the peritoneum, allowing cerebrospinal fluid drainage into the peritoneal cavity. This procedure can globally reduce intracranial hypertension, improving headache and vision. Another possible surgical intervention is optic nerve sheath fenestration, where cerebrospinal fluid surrounding the optic nerve is allowed to escape into the orbit, where it is reabsorbed, resulting in improved vision but not headache. Recently, venous sinus stenting has been proposed for cases where MRI has demonstrated stenosis.

26.14 Treatment

The treatment is aimed not only at the neoplasms themselves but also at the effects they cause. Therefore, the treatment of intracranial hypertension and epilepsy is discussed first, followed by surgical removal and other treatments directed against the neoplasms.

Treatment of intracranial hypertension

Cerebral edema plays a significant role in the development of intracranial hypertension caused by brain neoplasms. Some neoplasms, such as malignant intrinsic neoplasms (high-grade gliomas, medulloblastomas, metastases), and sometimes meningiomas, are associated with significant edema, which greatly amplifies the mass effect related to the neoplasm volume alone. The treatment of cerebral edema can significantly benefit the patient. In the *acute treatment* of cerebral edema, intravenous osmotic therapy with diuretics such as mannitol or hypertonic saline solutions is important. Osmotic therapy reduces intracranial hypertension within a few minutes since the increased blood osmolarity quickly draws fluids from the brain parenchyma. In particular, the rapid intravenous administration of mannitol can rapidly reverse a life-threatening condition, reducing intracranial hypertension within 1-5 minutes, reaching its maximum effect between 20 and 60 minutes, and lasting from 1.5 to 6 hours after administration. However, a rebound phenomenon can occur, with increased edema after the cessation of the anti-edematous effect. Therefore, the administration of osmotic diuretics should be performed periodically, every 4-6 hours, and gradually tapered. Additionally, their efficacy tends to decrease over time. For *chronic treatment* of cerebral edema, corticosteroids are more suitable. They act by reducing the permeability of the endothelial tight junctions, facilitating the restoration of normal blood-brain barrier properties, which is the cause of vasogenic edema in brain tumors. Their effect gradually develops over a few hours, reaching its peak in a few days, and persists over time, making them suitable for prolonged treatment of cerebral edema.

If intracranial hypertension is caused by *hydrocephalus*, cerebrospinal fluid diversion surgery can rapidly reduce intracranial pressure. In cases of triventricular hydrocephalus, which is associated with obstruction of the Sylvian aqueduct, endoscopic third ventriculostomy can be performed by creating a new pathway for cerebrospinal fluid to flow into the basal cisterns through the floor of the third ventricle. In other cases, a ventriculoperitoneal shunt is performed, in which one end of a silicone tube, placed under the skin, is inserted into a lateral ventricle, and the other end is introduced into the abdominal cavity, allowing cerebrospinal fluid to be absorbed through the peritoneal membrane. In emergency cases, an external cerebrospinal fluid diversion is performed, in which a silicone catheter is inserted into the lateral ventricle through a burr hole in the skull and connected to an external drainage bag. Due to the risk of infection, the external diversion should be converted to an internal diversion, such as a ventriculoperitoneal shunt, within a few days.

Certain intensive care procedures, such as *hyperventilation* in intubated and mechanically ventilated patients, also affect intracranial pressure. Hyperventilation reduces the partial pressure of CO_2, causing alkalization of the cerebrospinal fluid, leading to arterial vasoconstriction and consequent reduction in cerebral blood volume and intracranial pressure. However, this effect lasts only a few hours because the cerebrospinal fluid quickly adapts to the new levels of CO_2, and the arteries dilate again.

In cases where intracranial hypertension does not respond satisfactorily to the aforementioned treatments, *decompressive craniectomy* may be useful. This procedure involves removing a large portion of the skull, converting the closed intracranial compartment to an open one. It significantly facilitates the control of intracranial pressure, and the adequately preserved bone can be re-implanted once the emergency situation has resolved.

Treatment of epilepsy | Supratentorial brain tumors can cause epileptic seizures. In certain types of neoplasms, such as low-grade gliomas, epilepsy is frequently the first and, for a long time, the only symptom. In patients with these tumors, seizures and antiepileptic therapy, with their side effects (especially cognitive disturbances), are the most important factors affecting the deterioration of quality of life. Pharmacological antiepileptic treatment is indicated in patients with brain tumors and epilepsy. First-generation antiepileptic drugs (carbamazepine, phenobarbital, phenytoin) are no longer considered first-line treatments due to significant drug interactions with many chemotherapeutic agents, leading to reduced effectiveness of both categories of drugs (reduced antitumor and antiepileptic efficacy) and increased occurrence of adverse events. Therefore, the administration of second-generation antiepileptic drugs (levetiracetam, oxcarbazepine, lamotrigine, topiramate) is preferred. It should be noted that radical tumor removal represents the most effective treatment for tumor-related epilepsy. However, surgical intervention itself can have epileptogenic potential, as it can cause cortical irritation due to ischemic damage, hemorrhage, or infection. Regarding prophylaxis, antiepileptic drugs should not be routinely used in non-epileptic patients with newly diagnosed brain tumors to prevent the occurrence of epileptic seizures. Antiepileptic drugs are not effective in preventing seizures and have multiple adverse effects in this specific patient population. However, since surgical intervention carries epileptogenic potential, the possibility of prophylaxis in the first few days after surgery can be considered. Early seizures, defined as those occurring within the first 7 days after surgery, are particularly alarming due to the potentially deleterious effects of repeated epileptic activity on a recently operated brain. However, the clinical usefulness of antiepileptic prophylaxis for early seizures is uncertain, with scientific evidence on this matter being inconclusive and conflicting. In these patients, it is appropriate to discontinue antiepileptic drugs after the first postoperative week. It should be emphasized that the appearance of epileptic seizures in a patient with a brain neoplasm can indicate tumor progression or recurrence.

Surgical treatment | Surgical treatment of brain neoplasms has several objectives: the removal or reduction of the neoplastic mass, the preservation or improvement of neurological function, including symptoms related to intracranial hypertension, histological diagnosis necessary for planning additional treatments such as radiotherapy and chemotherapy, scheduling postoperative clinical follow-ups, and obtaining prognostic information, as well as the performance of other local antitumor treatments (chemotherapy, radiotherapy, immunotherapy) in certain cases. In benign tumors (meningiomas, schwannomas, etc.), total removal is theoretically always the primary goal due to the presence of a cleavage plane between the tumor and the brain parenchyma. However, achieving this goal is not always possible due to infiltration of arterial vessels, venous sinuses, or important cranial nerves. Gliomas, due to their infiltrative nature, generally cannot be completely resected except in specific cases (cystic astrocytoma, ventricular ependymoma). Since brain regions infiltrated by or adjacent to the neoplasm may have important functions, it is necessary to monitor and map these functions before and during surgical intervention. The brain regions with the most relevant functions for social life include the Rolandic region, primary language areas such as Broca's area (the posterior part of the third frontal gyrus in the dominant hemisphere) and Wernicke's area (the area between the posterior part of the first temporal gyrus and the lower part of the parietal lobe in the dominant hemisphere), the insula, basal nuclei, and the brainstem. Important functions such as language and motor control can be preoperatively located using radiological examinations such as functional MRI. The currently most commonly used method is electrical stimulation of the cerebral cortex. Since the brain itself is insensitive, patients can undergo surgery while awake, under local anesthesia (awake surgery), allowing direct assessment of neurological responses to stimulation of the brain areas to be removed. Alternatively, with the patient under general anesthesia, neurophysiological monitoring can be performed, assessing motor responses to cortical electrical stimulation using electromyography. Some surgical complications can lead to the onset of new neurological deficits or exacerbation of pre-existing deficits, including violation of highly functional tissue, ischemic or hemorrhagic damage, cerebral edema, disturbances of cerebrospinal fluid circulation, alterations in fluid and electrolyte balance, and postoperative infections. The occurrence of adverse events is more frequent in the first 48 hours, and in many cases, a period of monitoring in intensive care is warranted in the postoperative course. Cerebral neurosurgery is constantly evolving, with improvements in surgical techniques, surgical instrumentation, anatomical and physiological knowledge, leading to a significant reduction in postoperative morbidity and mortality.

Brain biopsy | It is a surgical procedure aimed at obtaining a limited sample of a brain lesion to obtain a histological diagnosis when radical removal surgery carries high risks or is not indicated. As previously mentioned, histological diagnosis of a brain tumor is essential for guiding treatment decisions, such as planning radiotherapy and/or chemotherapy, and for prognostic purposes. Biopsy can be performed using various surgical techniques, either open through craniotomy or less invasive procedures such as stereotactic[1] or neuronavigation-guided biopsy[2], where a thin instrument is directed to the lesion through a burr hole in the skull. It should be noted that obtaining a reliable diagnosis is not always possible, especially in lesions that do not enhance with contrast medium. Additionally, since many tumors consist of heterogeneous masses, limited sampling of one or a few fragments may not be representative of the actual behavior of the neoplasm, leading to sampling error. Despite being less invasive than radical resection, brain biopsy is not without potential complications, with hemorrhage being the most frequent. Advancements in surgical techniques have made brain biopsy less necessary in many cases.

Other treatments | In the case of malignant neoplasms, non-resectable remnants of benign neoplasms, or tumors where radical surgery is not feasible or not indicated, other treatments such as radiotherapy and chemotherapy can be performed. In recent decades, there has been significant technological advancement in the field of radiotherapy. Current techniques are no longer limited to conventional external beam radiotherapy but include numerous other methods such as stereotactic radiosurgery, conformal radiotherapy, and particle therapy. These techniques aim to increase the energy delivered to tumor cells while minimizing irradiation of healthy tissue. As a result, outcomes have improved, and complications have decreased. The radiosensitivity of intracranial tumors is usually proportional to their mitotic activity, with higher sensitivity observed in malignant tumors. High radiosensitivity is seen in medulloblastomas, germinomas, pinealoblastomas, anaplastic ependymomas, and lymphomas; moderate sensitivity in glioblastomas, astrocytomas, and anaplastic oligodendrogliomas; and low sensitivity in low-grade astrocytomas and oligodendrogliomas. Chemotherapy has also seen advancements with the introduction of new drugs such as temozolomide, which are more tolerable and easier to administer. Radiotherapy and chemotherapy are part of the standard postoperative treatment for high-grade gliomas (grade III and IV). Other treatments currently under study and experimentation include immunotherapies and vaccines. The choice of diagnostic and treatment modalities involves complex considerations that are not easily standardized. The experience and preferences of individual practitioners still remain the

---

[1] *Stereotaxis*: A method of brain localization based on the attachment of a rigid reference system (stereotactic frame) to the skull. By performing radiological exams (ventriculography, angiography, CT, or MRI) with this system, the coordinates of any point within the skull can be determined relative to the frame. In the operating room, the frame serves as a guide to reach the predetermined points with submillimeter precision.

[2] *Neuronavigation*: A method of brain localization that, while following the principles of stereotaxis, does not require the attachment of rigid frames. Instead, it involves the application of adhesive reference points (fiducials) on the skin, which are used during the MRI scan. The acquired MRI data is then input into a computer in the operating room, which is equipped with a camera capable of "seeing" the skin fiducials on the patient. The computer establishes a correlation between the actual skull and the virtual skull derived from the radiological exams, mapping each point from one to the other and vice versa. By using surgical instruments that also have fiducials, it is possible to project the position of the instruments onto the patient's MRI images and accurately determine their location.

primary criteria for decision-making. In the case of higher-grade tumors, it is necessary to decide on the appropriateness of multimodal treatment (surgery, radiotherapy, and chemotherapy). Therefore, the establishment of multidisciplinary neuro-oncology teams that oversee treatment decisions and patient follow-up is advisable.

Bibliography

Buckner J.C., Brown P.D., O'Neill B.P., Meyer F.B., Wetmore C.J., Uhm J.H., Central Nervous System Tumors. Mayo Clinic Proceedings; 82(10):1271-1286, 2007.

Carapella C.M., Jandolo B., Maschio M., Mauro A., Riva M., Rudà R., Scerrati M., Soffietti R., Certezze e controversie nella gestione dell'epilessia tumorale. Raccomandazioni dell'Associazione Italiana di Neuro-Oncologia (www.neuro-oncologia.eu/sites/default/files/news/raccomandazioni_Epi_tumorale_1-2008.pdf). Elsevier Masson, 2008.

Glantz M., Cole B.F., Forsyth P.A., Recht L.D., Wen P.Y., Chamberlain M.C., Grossman S.A., Cairncross J.G., Practice parameter: anticonvulsant prophylaxis in patients with newly diagnosed brain tumors. Report of the Quality Standards Subcommittee of the American Academy of Neurology. Neurology; 54:1886-93, 2000.

Louis D.N., Perry A., Reifenberger G., von Deimling A., Figarella-Branger D., Cavenee W.K., Ohgaki H., Wiestler O.D., Kleihues P., Ellison D.W. The 2016 World Health Organization Classification of Tumors of the Central Nervous System: a summary. Acta Neuropathologica 131:803-820, 2016.

Louis D.N., Perry A., Wesseling P., Brat D.J., Cree I.A., Figarella-Branger D., Hawkins C., Ng H.K., Pfister S.M., Reifenberger G., Soffietti R., von Deimling A., Ellison D.W. The 2021 WHO Classification of Tumors of the Central Nervous System: a summary. Neuro-Oncology 23(8): 1231-1251, 2021.

Porter K.R., McCarthy B.J., Freels S., Kim Y., Davis F.G., Prevalence estimates for primary brain tumors in the United States by age, gender, behavior, and histology. Neuro-Oncology; 12(6):520-527, 2010.

Stupp R., Mason W.P., van den Bent M.J., Weller M., Fisher B., Taphoorn M.J.B., Belanger K., Brandes A.A., Marosi C., Bogdahn U., Curschmann J., Janzer R.C., Ludwin S.K., Gorlia T., Allgeier A., Lacombe D., Cairncross J.G., Eisenhauer E., Mirimanoff R.O., Radiotherapy plus Concomitant and Adjuvant Temozolomide for Glioblastoma. New England Journal of Medicine 352(10); 987-996, 2005.

Yan H., Parsons D.W., Jin G., McLendon R., Rasheed B.A., Yuan W., Kos I., Batinic-Haberle I., Jones S., Riggins G.J., Friedman H., Friedman A., Reardon D., Herndon J., Kinzler K.W., Velculescu V.E., Vogelstein B., Bigner D.D., IDH1 and IDH2 Mutations in Gliomas. New England Journal of Medicine; 360:765-73, 2009.

27 TRAUMATIC BRAIN INJURY

Luca D'Angelo, Roberto Delfini, Antonio Santoro

Traumatic brain injury is the result of linear and rotational forces acting on the brain tissue, leading to structural damage associated with functional alterations of different types of brain cells. Approximately 2% of the population experiences a traumatic brain injury each year. Although most cases are mild, traumatic brain injury is among the leading causes of death and severe disability among young people in Europe, with approximately 100,000 individuals undergoing neurosurgical intervention annually. Half of the cases of traumatic brain injury involve individuals under the age of 15, with males being twice as likely as females to be affected. The speed at which medical or surgical treatment is administered determines the prognosis of these patients.

27.1 Types of traumatic brain injury

Traumatic brain injuries can be classified as *closed, open,* or *penetrating*. Closed injuries can be as severe as open injuries. In open injuries, part of the energy released during the trauma is not transmitted to the nervous tissues and is dissipated in the laceration of extracerebral tissues or in a fracture. In closed injuries, however, all the energy is transferred to the brain. Penetrating injuries are specific forms of open trauma in which a foreign object penetrates into deeper layers of the tissues.

A traumatic brain injury can cause primary damage (cortical contusions, lacerations, bone fragmentations, diffuse axonal injury, brainstem contusions) and secondary damage, represented by a series of events that occur after the trauma (edema, metabolic disturbances, oxidative stress, excitotoxicity, hypoxia, vasospasm, and ischemia). While primary damage can be reduced through preventive measures (such as wearing protective helmets, fastening seat belts, etc.), secondary damage can be limited by the rapid application of medical and surgical treatments. It is, therefore, crucial to recognize the etiology of all clinical signs and symptoms upon the patient's arrival. It should be noted that hypotension is rarely attributable to a cranial lesion, except in hemodynamically unstable patients (due to thoracic, cardiac, or profuse bleeding causes), patients in terminal stages (due to brainstem dysfunction and cardiovascular collapse), and pediatric patients (blood loss caused by intracranial or even subgaleal hematomas can result in hypovolemia).

Issues concerning cerebral edema are particularly delicate (■ Figure 27.1), with three recognized types that often overlap and combine with each other (distinguishable on Magnetic Resonance Imaging using diffusion-weighted imaging sequences).

1) Cytotoxic edema: extracellular space reduces as fluids accumulate inside the cells due to membrane exchange dysfunction. Depending on the extent of cellular swelling, this phase is reversible (cells can return to normal). The blood-brain barrier is intact, and therefore, there is no contrast medium uptake in MRI/CT. This is the typical edema seen in cranial traumas.
2) Vasogenic edema: caused by increased permeability of endothelial capillary cells, allowing plasma to escape into the extracellular spaces. It is limited to the

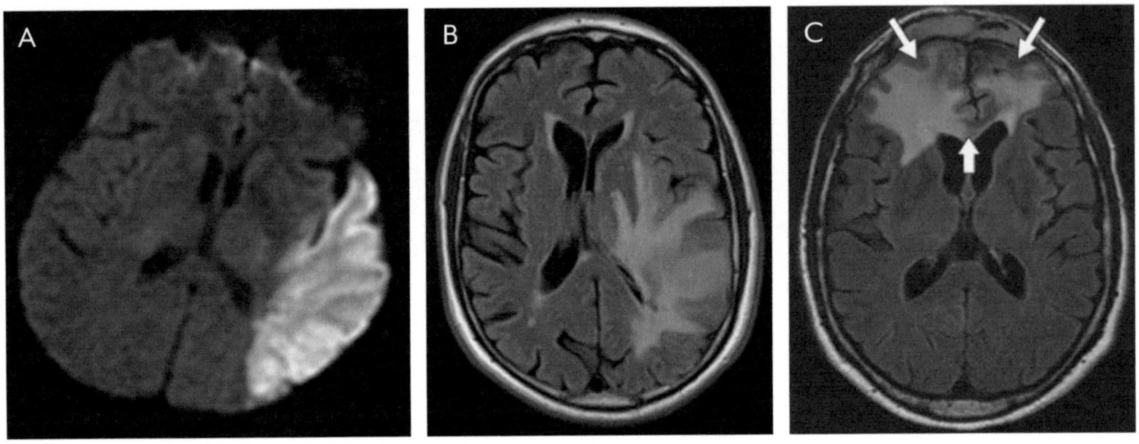

Figure 27.1

Different types of cerebral edema on MRI: A) The diffusion-weighted imaging (DWI) sequence shows the characteristic pattern of cytotoxic edema with the presence of a hyperintense area in the temporo-parietal region. B) T2-FLAIR sequence shows the characteristic finger-like appearance (limited to the white matter) of vasogenic edema in a patient with metastatic breast carcinoma. C) Ischemic edema shows hybrid features between the previous entities, involving both the subcortical white matter and cerebral cortex.

cerebral white matter and is more frequently present in oncological conditions.

3) Ischemic edema: caused by hypoxia, resulting from the combination of the pathophysiological mechanisms underlying the previous types of edema. Extracellular space reduces (cytotoxic phase) and then expands (vasogenic phase). Due to its complex temporal progression, ischemic edema is most likely to cause delayed clinical deterioration following a previous traumatic injury.

Edema tends to generate intracranial hypertension, which is compensated for by the mechanisms described in the Monro-Kellie doctrine. In adults, the skull is a fixed, rigid, and non-expandable structure with a constant volume composed of brain parenchyma (approximately 1400 cc), circulating blood (approximately 150 cc among arteries, capillaries, and veins), and cerebrospinal fluid (approximately 150 cc). An increase in total volume (e.g., due to hematoma or edema) therefore occurs at the expense of the normal components within the cranial cavity: to maintain constant pressure, the cerebrospinal fluid, venous blood, and arterial blood decrease in that order. Once these compensatory mechanisms are exhausted, intracranial pressure (ICP) increases exponentially (Figure 27.2). Subacute situations of intracranial hypertension also lead to irreversible reduction in brain parenchyma.

The method for measuring ICP (intracranial pressure) involves the insertion of a specialized probe that not only records the average value of intracranial pressure but also produces a graph representing its real-time variations in relation to the cardiac cycle (Figure 27.3). These pieces of information, along with the monitoring of arterial pressure and, in certain cases, venous pressure, allow for the extraction of all the parameters used by neuro-anesthesiologists for optimal management of cerebral metabolic values (cerebral perfusion pressure, cerebral blood flow, cerebral blood volume, oxygen extraction fraction). Although ICP monitoring is an invasive procedure, it should be performed for all patients with a Glasgow Coma Scale (GCS) ≤ 8. Maintaining an intracranial pressure below 20 mmHg and a cerebral perfusion pressure between 60 and 70 mmHg is crucial for improving the prognosis of patients with cranial trauma. In cases where it is not possible to control ICP with anesthetic/pharmacological measures

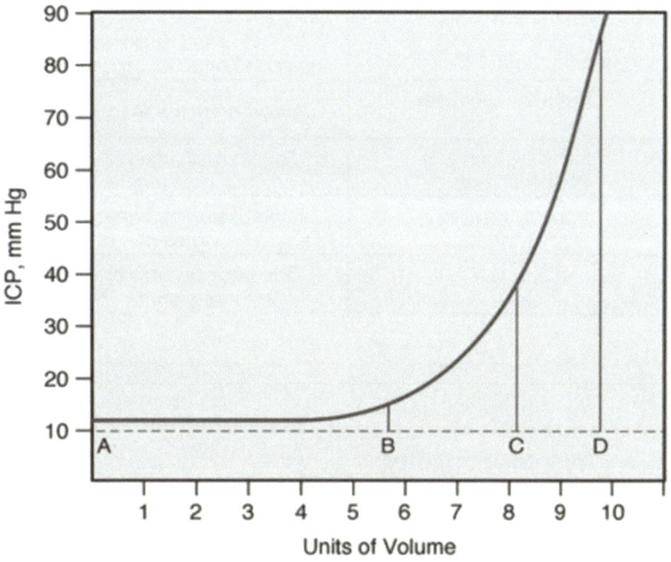

Figure 27.2

The Monro-Kellie curve or pressure-volume curve describes a hyperbola. According to this theory, there is no linear correlation between an increase in volume (neoplasm, hematoma, hydrocephalus) and an increase in intracranial pressure. This indicates that in the initial phase of the curve, the trend is approximately horizontal, meaning that up to certain volume values, there is no significant increase in intracranial pressure (ICP). However, above these values, even minimal increases in volume can cause significant increments in ICP.

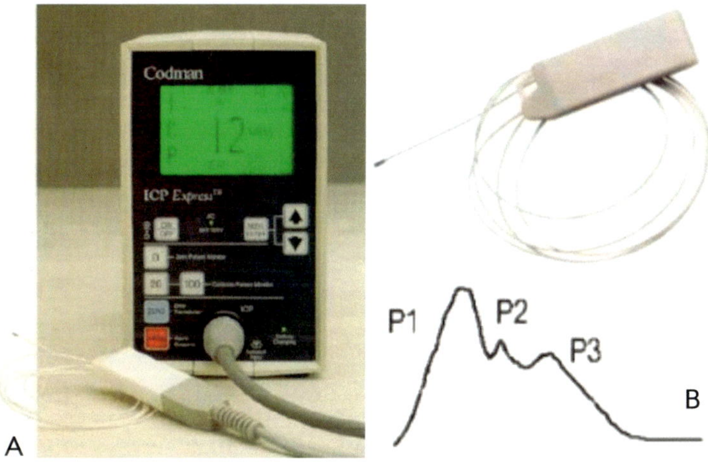

Figure 27.3

A) Monitor and sensor necessary for intracranial pressure (ICP) monitoring.
B) ICP wave: There are three characteristic peaks in the wave that describes the ICP trend. PI is the so-called percussion wave caused by arterial pressure transmitted from the choroid plexus to the ventricle. P2 is the current curve associated with the elastic compensation (compliance) of the brain tissue, and finally P3 is due to the closure of the aortic valve.

(> 20mmHg for 6 consecutive hours or less if the cause of intracranial hypertension is not expected to be resolved), surgical intervention is necessary. In cases where there is no specific surgical target (such as diffuse axonal injury or other unilateral/bi-hemispheric brain edemas), surgical decompression of the cranial vault with a craniotomy of approximately 100 cm^2, is indicated, typically involving the frontotemporal region to the floor of the middle cranial fossa, or with bifrontal craniectomies to the floor of the anterior cranial fossa.

27.2 Evaluation of the severity of cranial trauma

The neurological examination represents the first essential tool for the proper assessment of patients with cranial trauma. It serves as the reference point for subsequent neurological evaluations, which determine the stability of the clinical picture and the need for radiological examinations. Based on this principle, there is a need to develop an assessment tool for

Table 27.1 GLASGOW COMA SCALE

	Eye response	Verbal response	Motor response
1	Doesn't open the eyes	No verbal response no sound or intubated patient	No movement
2	Opens the eyes with painful stimulus	Incomprehensible sounds	Extension to pain (decerebrate response)
3	Opens the eyes with verbal stimulus	Speaks and utters words, but incoherently	Flexion to pain (decorticate response)
4	Opens the eyes spontaneously	Confusion, disconnected phrases	Withdrawal from pain (withdraws quickly when a painful stimulus is applied)
5		Oriented and appropriate response	Localizes pain (attempts to locate the area where the painful stimulus is applied)
6			Able to obey commands

cranial trauma patients that is easily codifiable and less prone to ambiguity.

The most effective assessment tool for traumatized patients is the Glasgow Coma Scale (GCS), which is based on responses to stimuli (eye, verbal, and motor) and is summarized by a number that represents the sum of individual function evaluations (Table 27.1).

Patients are classified into 2 groups and 5 fundamental classes:

Minor cranial trauma

- Minimal: GCS = 15, no loss of consciousness, no amnesia;
- Mild: GCS = 14 or GCS = 15 with brief loss of consciousness (< 5 minutes) or amnesia or drowsiness or disturbances in concentration/attention/spatial-temporal-personal orientation;

Major cranial trauma

- Moderate: GCS = 9-13 or loss of consciousness > 5 minutes or focal neurological deficit;
- Severe: GCS = 5-8;
- In critical condition: GCS = 3-4.

27.3 Cranial trauma imaging techniques

Computed Tomography (CT) of the skull is the primary imaging modality for evaluating traumatized patients. It allows for a rapid assessment of the type, location, and extent of the trauma-related injury. The main features that should be evaluated on cranial CT include:

- Presence of intracranial hematomas;
- Appearance of the cranial base cisterns at the mesencephalic level (compression and/or obliteration of which is associated with increased intracranial pressure);
- Possible subarachnoid hemorrhage.

Approximately 15% of cranial CT scans in patients with severe cranial trauma do not show significant abnormalities in the initial stages. The most commonly associated risk factors for the delayed development of brain damage in the presence of initially negative CT findings are the initial neurological status assessed by the Glasgow Coma Scale (GCS), the need for cardiopulmonary resuscitation at the time of trauma, and the presence of coagulopathies or the use of antiplatelet and/or anticoagulant medications.

A cranial CT scan should also be performed in cases of suspected cranial fracture if the traumatic event was significant and if symptoms are persistent or progressive. Additionally, it is necessary to evaluate the presence of any damage to other organs in the body (which is present in over half of patients with severe cranial trauma). The patient should be observed for at least 6 hours in cases of minimal cranial trauma, at least 12 hours in cases of mild cranial trauma, and should be hospitalized in the presence of neurological deficits or persistent symptoms. Neurosurgical evaluation is necessary if the cranial CT shows lesions or if the patient has neurological deficits. The caregiver of a patient with minor cranial trauma should be informed, at the time of discharge, about any symptoms that require careful medical observation through a reminder containing a series of instructions (appropriate informational sheets are generally available in the hospital).

27.4 Main pathological entities resulting from cranial trauma

Depressed cranial fractures | This type of fracture occurs in 65% of patients with epidural hematoma, 18% of patients with subdural hematomas, and 40% of patients with intraparenchymal hematomas. These fractures can be linear or compound (Figure 27.4). In such cases, the choice between conservative treatment and surgical treatment should consider the geometry of the fracture, involvement of anatomical structures near the fracture (skin and galea), and associated clinical conditions. In most cases of linear fractures of the cranial vault, conservative treatment is recommended, as well as for fractures that are only mildly depressed below the level of the cranial vault. Depressed fractures of the cranial vault (Figure 27.5 and 6), on the other hand, should be surgically treated when they present: depression of the fractured fragment greater than the thickness of the adjacent bone; an intraparenchymal hematoma that requires surgical treatment; and finally, when there is a discontinuity in the galea and overlying skin at the site of the fracture (in this case, in addition

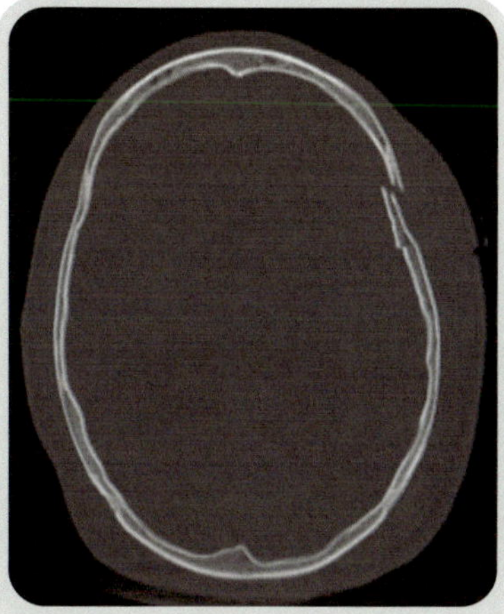

Figure 27.4

Linear fracture of the cranial vault with slight separation of the bone segments.

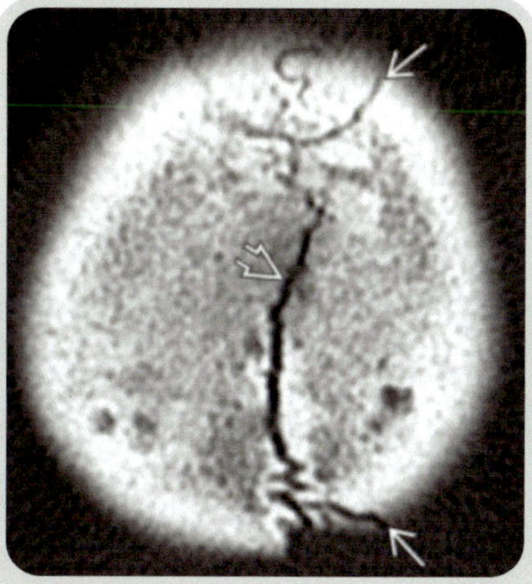

Figure 27.5

Sequence for cranial bone in a CT scan showing a depressed fracture of the cranial vault.

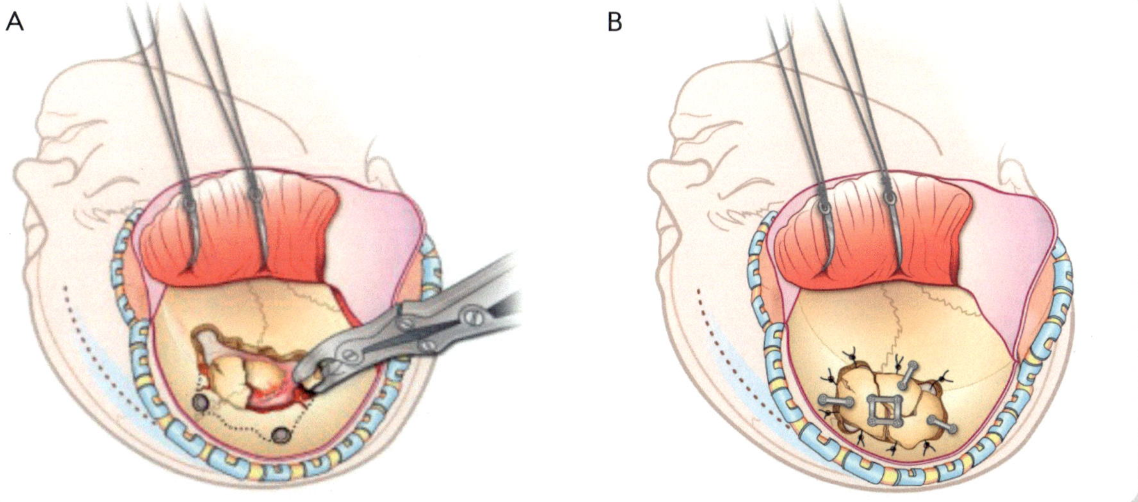

Figure 27.6

A) Surgical approach to a depressed fracture. The fracture is delimited by a wide craniotomy, and the fracture fragments are removed and repositioned. Opening of the dura mater is necessary when the CT scan shows the presence of a subdural hematoma component. B) At the end of the procedure, the different fragments are reassembled, allowing the fractured fragment to be restored to the same level as the cranial vault.

to performing a craniotomy and elevating the bone flap, proper treatment of the scalp wound is also necessary). In cases where surgical intervention is indicated, the surgery should be performed as soon as possible to avoid the development of infections by pathogens that may spread deeply from the wound.

Fractures of the cranial base | Most of these fractures are the result of fractures in the cranial vault that transfer energy along the physiological force pillars present in the skull (petrous ridge, clivus and occipital condyle, maxillary and ethmoid bones). They are diagnosed using CT scans based on clinical evaluation (presence of dural fractures, cerebrospinal fluid rhinorrhea/otorrhea, periauricular or periorbital ecchymosis, or lesions of cranial nerves I, II, VI, or VII). The majority of these fractures do not require surgical reduction or fixation. However, some may lead to complications that require specific treatments, such as post-traumatic aneurysms, carotid-cavernous fistulas, cerebrospinal fluid fistulas, meningitis or brain abscesses, deformities, and paralysis of affected nerves.

Fractures of the frontal sinus | The presence of a fracture of the frontal sinus (Figure 27.7) with pneumocephalus (presence of air bubbles in the neurocranium), even without clinical evidence of cerebrospinal fluid fistula, should raise suspicion of associated dural laceration. Complications of frontal sinus opening into the anterior cranial fossa are often delayed and include cerebral abscess, cerebrospinal fluid fistula with meningitis, and mucocele formation (due to traumatic obstruction of mucous drainage from the frontal sinus, resulting in chronic sinusitis). Most post-traumatic fistulas spontaneously close after a period of bed rest or conservative therapy (carbonic anhydrase inhibitors, lumbar drainage). Prophylactic antibiotic therapy (without clinical/radiological and laboratory evidence of infection) is not necessary. Administration of Pneumovax 23 is indicated for pneumocephalus to prevent pneumococcal meningitis. Surgical repair of the frontal sinus involves cranialization (removal of the posterior sinus wall and obliteration of any cells or recesses), removal of the frontal mucosa up to the nasofrontal duct, multilayer closure with the placement of temporal fascia/muscle, biological adhesives, and possibly autologous fat on the cranialized sinus to provide a barrier between the paranasal cavities and the anterior cranial fossa.

Concussion and cerebral contusion | Concussion is characterized by altered consciousness without structural damage, resulting from a non-penetrating head injury. The symptoms are short-lived, transient, and characterized by immediate loss of consciousness, rapid resolution, confusion

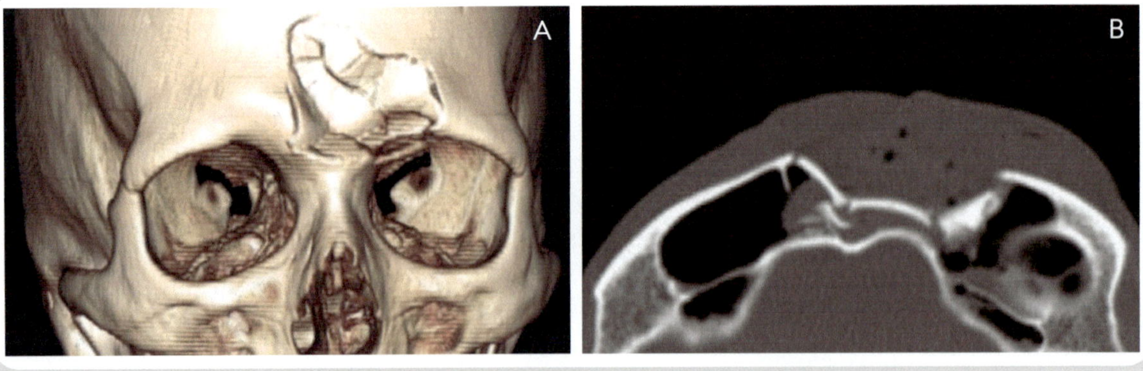

Figure 27.7

A) 3D Reconstruction of a cranial CT scan showing the outcomes of a trauma in the frontal region. B) Axial sequence in the same patient revealing the presence of a fracture in both the anterior and posterior walls of the frontal sinus, requiring a frontal sinus cranialization intervention.

or clouding of sensorium, amnesia, and incongruous behaviors. All patients who have experienced a concussive head injury should undergo Level I imaging studies (brain CT) and careful clinical monitoring. In the 7-10 days following the injury, the brain is more vulnerable, and therefore, a second traumatic event could have disproportionately more severe consequences than normal. Cerebral contusion, on the other hand, refers to a non-penetrating head injury that causes detectable structural damage on CT or MRI scans (edema, petechial hemorrhages).

Diffuse axonal injury | Diffuse axonal injury is the second most frequent parenchymal brain injury caused by a head trauma. It is secondary to closed traumas that result in abrupt rotational accelerations and decelerations due to the difference in velocity between the motion of the cerebral cortex and that of the subcortical white matter. The initial CT scan is generally negative in the early stages after trauma (which contrasts with the patient's clinical condition, typically in a coma). Subsequent CT scans may reveal the presence of multiple small "petechiae" hemorrhages located at the interface between gray and white matter and at the genu of the corpus callosum. Each of these small hemorrhagic areas can continue to expand, leading to an edematous reaction and an increase in intracranial pressure. The most useful imaging technique for evaluating Diffuse Axonal Injury is MRI, which can detect small hyperintense foci in T2-weighted sequences, indicative of microbleeds that are not visible in the early stages on CT scans. Most patients with Diffuse Axonal Injury present in the Emergency Department already in a coma that is difficult to reverse; a percentage of patients, around 5-10%, who awaken from the coma have a highly disabling impairment of neurological functions (Figure 27.8).

Hemorrhagic contusions | These are blood collections larger than one centimeter that are visible on CT scans. They occur in areas where the brain impacts bony prominences due to a direct blow or secondary impact from the sudden deceleration of the head during the trauma (cerebral poles are particularly susceptible). They can evolve and progress over time, for more than 48 hours, or they can manifest within 72 hours of the trauma. Neurological conditions deteriorate at the time of their formation or progression. Predisposing factors for the worsening of a hematoma include coagulopathies, pre-existing necrotic and/or mushy brain tissue, and the presence of petechial hemorrhagic extravasations. After the acute phase, once intraparenchymal hematomas are absorbed, a mild degeneration of brain tissue may remain. Surgical indications for the removal of these hematomas include progressive neurological deterioration associated with the hematoma, a hematoma volume larger than 50 cc, a GCS (Glasgow Coma Scale) score < 8 with a >5mm midline shift or compression of the basal cisterns (Figure 27.9).

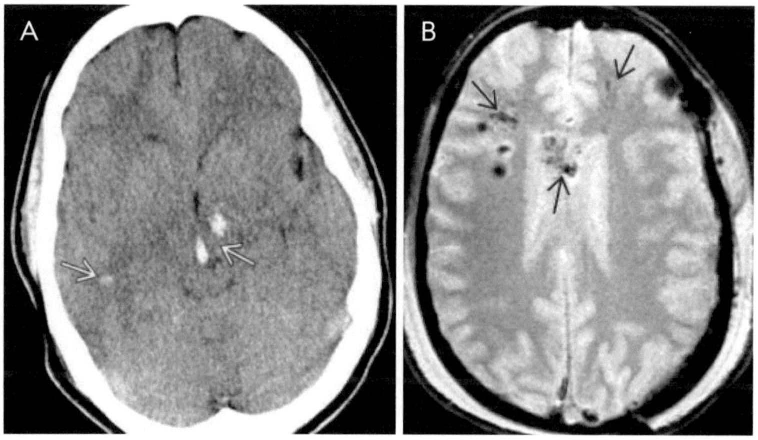

Figure 27.8

A) CT scan of a patient involved in a severe car accident. The characteristic signs of intracranial hypertension are evident (flattening of the sulci and reduction in ventricular size), along with the presence of subcortical hemorrhagic petechiae consistent with Diffuse Axonal Injury. B) MRI with T2 GRE sequence in a patient with severe head trauma shows the presence of multiple signal restriction areas in the subcortical frontal region and along the corpus callosum, also consistent with a diagnosis of Diffuse Axonal Injury.

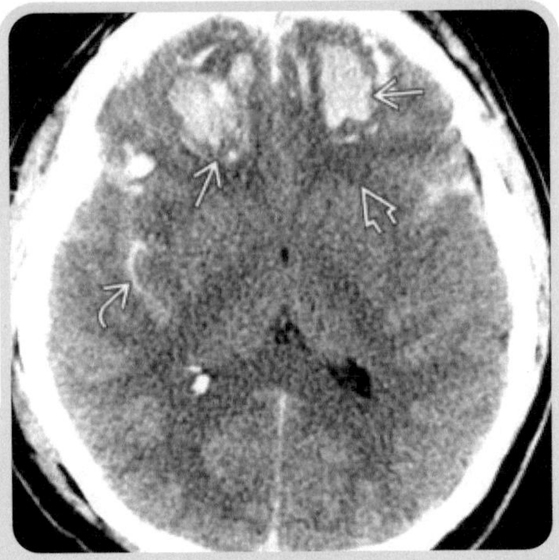

Figure 27.9

Bifrontal cerebral contusions (linear arrows) surrounded by reactive edema (large arrow) and associated with post-traumatic subarachnoid hemorrhage (curved arrow).

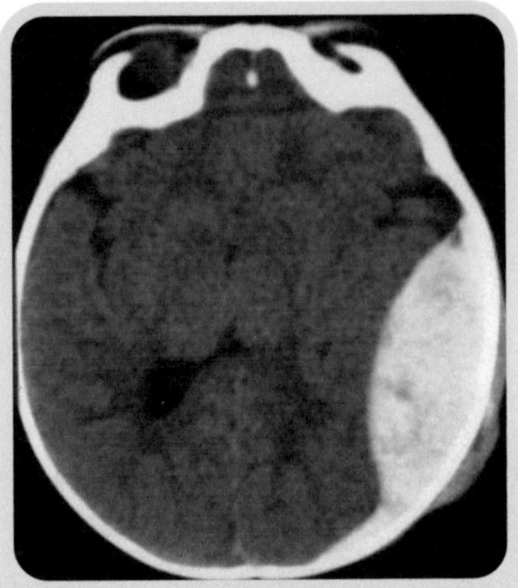

Figure 27.10

The cranial CT scan shows a large acute left temporal epidural hematoma (the characteristic hyperdense biconvex lens-shaped form of the hematoma can be appreciated).

Epidural hematomas | Epidural hematomas are blood collections that develop between the inner portion of the skull and the outer surface of the dura mater. They represent a rare but potentially lethal complication of head trauma. They occur in approximately 2.5-5% of head injuries, with a male-to-female ratio of 4:1, and can affect patients of varying ages. Depending on the cause of bleeding, they can be classified as arterial epidural hematomas (by far the most common) or venous epidural hematomas. Over 90% of these hematomas are located in the supratentorial space and are caused by a fracture of the cranial vault that extends along one of the branches of the middle meningeal artery, tearing it. In less frequent cases, the fracture may cause venous extravasation or lacerate a venous sinus. In about a quarter of patients, there is the classical temporal triad characterized by a brief loss of consciousness, a "lucid interval" of a few hours without symptoms (a period free from cognitive disturbances and alterations in consciousness during which the hematoma forms and produces symptoms), and an altered level of consciousness with contralateral hemiparesis and anisocoria with homolateral mydriasis (in cases with uncal herniation through the free edge of the tentorium into the posterior cranial fossa, resulting in compression of the third cranial nerve, the posterior cerebral artery, and the midbrain). Less common presenting symptoms include vomiting and epileptic seizures. In pediatric patients, a cranial CT scan is mandatory in case of doubt.

The CT scan typically shows a hyperdense lenticular-shaped epidural collection (Figure 27.10). The mortality rate for patients with this type of hematoma ranges from 20 to 55%, but rapid diagnosis and optimal treatment can limit it to 5-10%. Negative prognostic factors include the presence of decerebrate posturing and the association of an epidural hematoma with subarachnoid hemorrhage (present in 20% of cases). The main cause of death is respiratory arrest caused by uncal herniation and subsequent midbrain injury.

The treatment of epidural hematomas depends on various factors, including the patient's neurological status, the size of the hematoma, and any initial signs of herniation.

In the early stages, if the hematoma is small, the patient undergoes close clinical monitoring with repeated neurological evaluations and serial CT scans to assess the growth or radiological stability of the hematoma. Factors indicating hematoma growth include the use of oral anticoagulants or the presence of coagulopathies.

It is advisable to perform an evacuative craniotomy for hematomas larger than 30 cc, regardless of the GCS score, and in cases that do not meet the criteria for conservative treatment. Pediatric patients tolerate a sudden increase in intracranial volume (due to the hematoma)

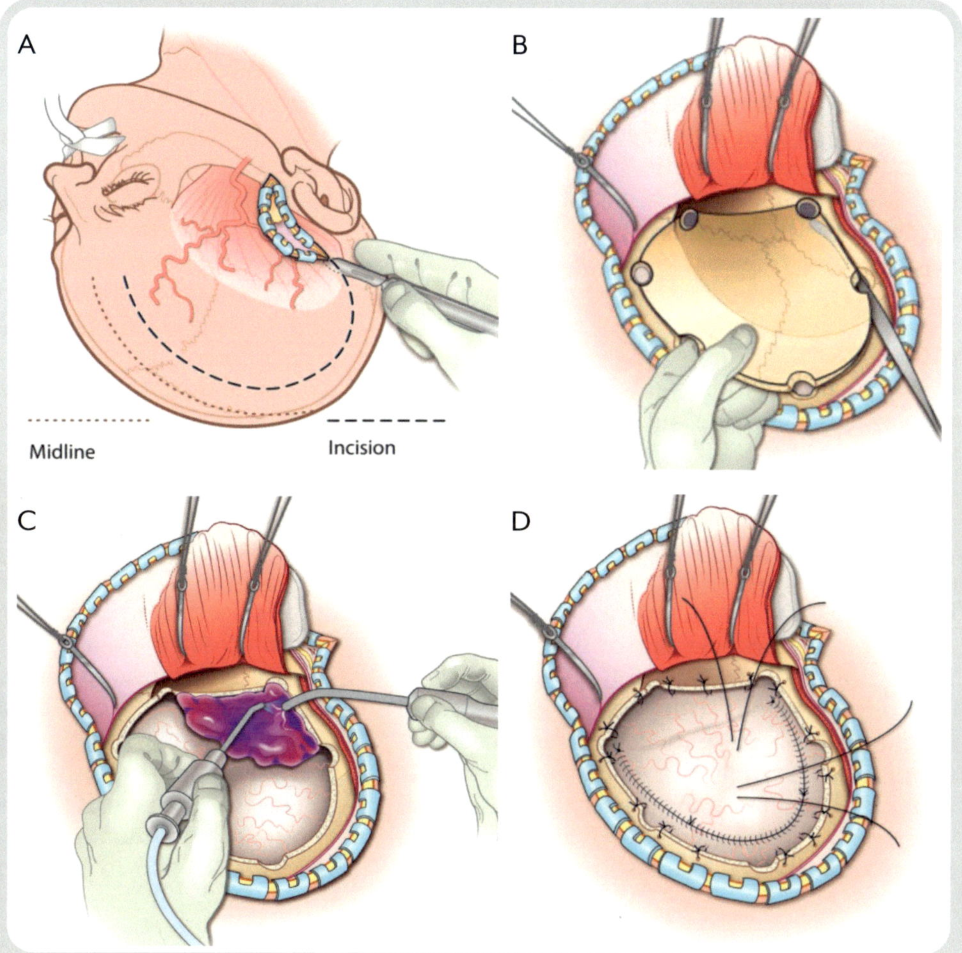

Figure 27.11

Sequential schematic sequence of the different phases of epidural hematoma removal: A) wide incision in a “question mark” shape. B) wide craniotomy flap. C) removal of the epidural hematoma with abundant irrigation and aspiration. D) dural closure with central and peripheral suspensions.

less well, so the previous indications are not applicable, and the choice of treatment should be tailored to the specific case. During the procedure, it is important to create a craniotomy that matches the extent of the hematoma (generally performed as a question mark-shaped incision in cases of temporal and/or parietal epidural hematomas). The clot is then removed, the cause(s) of bleeding are identified, hemostasis is achieved, and measures are taken to prevent further bleeding by suturing the dural suspension points both centrally and at the edges of the craniotomy (Figure 27.11).

Acute subdural hematomas | Acute subdural hematomas are collections of blood that form between the inner layer of the dura mater and the outer surface of the brain, usually resulting from high-intensity head trauma with a rotational component that causes stretching and subsequent rupture of bridging veins as they traverse the subdural space to drain into the venous sinuses. They represent the second most frequent extracranial hemorrhage, preceded only by subarachnoid hemorrhage. These types of hematomas can affect any age group (with a higher incidence in elderly individuals undergoing anticoagulant treatment) without a gender predominance.

The severity of the primary damage is generally greater in this type of hematoma compared to epidural hematoma (where secondary damage plays a fundamental role). Acute subdural hematomas often coexist with injuries to the brain parenchyma. Based on the causes, two types of acute subdural hematoma are distinguished. The first type is caused by an accumulation of blood around parenchymal lacerations due to rupture of the cortex-pia-arachnoid barrier. It is generally caused by violent primary injury, often accompanied by immediate neurological symptoms. The blood spreads into the subdural and subarachnoid compartments due to parenchymal lacerations (Figure 27.12). The second type is formed by the laceration of cortical vessels (or veins) that are stretched and distended by the rapid alternating acceleration and deceleration resulting from trauma. In these cases, the trauma is generally less severe, and there may be an interval free of clinical symptoms followed by subsequent rapid clinical deterioration. The blood remains within the subdural compartment without invading the subarachnoid space (if the arachnoid barrier remains intact), and the hematoma has a prognosis similar to that of an epidural hematoma (Figure 27.13).

In both types of hematomas, the symptoms are caused by the compression of underlying brain structures, brain damage and/or edema, and possible displacement of brain structures from the midline, indicating compression of central brain structures. Patients with coagulopathies or undergoing anticoagulant therapy are at high risk of developing acute subdural hematomas even after minor trauma. The computed tomography (CT) scan shows a semilunar hyperdense lesion adjacent to the inner table of the skull, with corresponding brain edema. Unlike epidural hematoma, the subdural hematoma is usually located at the convexity and appears more diffuse and less hyperdense. The hyperdense lesion tends to gradually become isodense (in about 2 weeks) and subsequently hypodense.

The criteria for surgical intervention include hematoma thickness (>1 cm), lateral displacement of midline structures, rapidity of clinical deterioration, pupil status (an indirect sign of uncal herniation), intracranial pressure trends, and hematoma location. Therapy with anticoagulants or antiplatelet agents does not delay surgical treatment. It is necessary to restore normal hematological factors in patients in good neurological condition and proceed with surgery in patients with neurological deterioration. Acute subdural hematomas are surgically treated by performing an extensive decompressive craniotomy that exposes the frontal and temporal poles. Therefore, a wide "question mark" skin incision is necessary to expose an adequate cranial surface. Once the craniotomy is performed, the dura mater is opened, and the acute blood clot is evacuated using aspiration and multiple irrigations (Figure 27.14). At the end of the procedure,

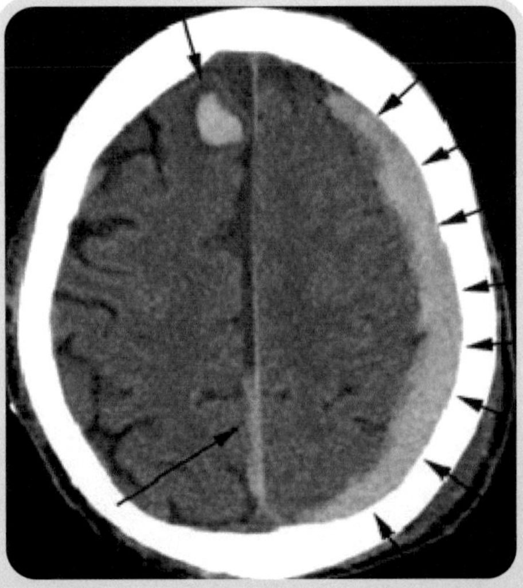

Figure 27.12

Acute left subdural hematoma associated with a contralateral frontal hemorrhagic focus.

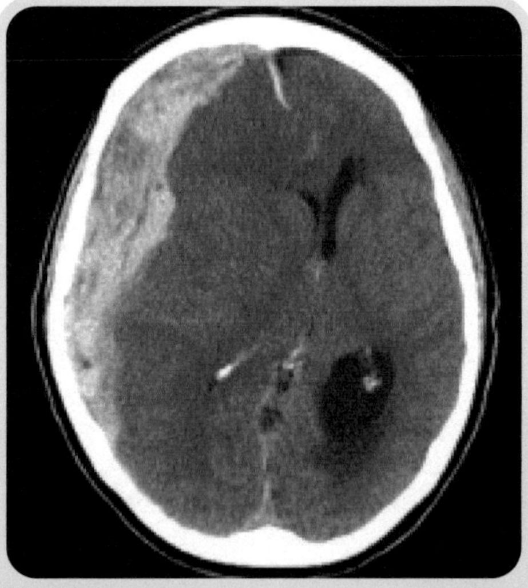

Figure 27.13

CT image of a large acute subdural hemorrhage (without evident signs of cerebral contusion) that displaces the brain structures, causing a shift of >1 cm and significant compressive effects on the supratentorial ventricular system.

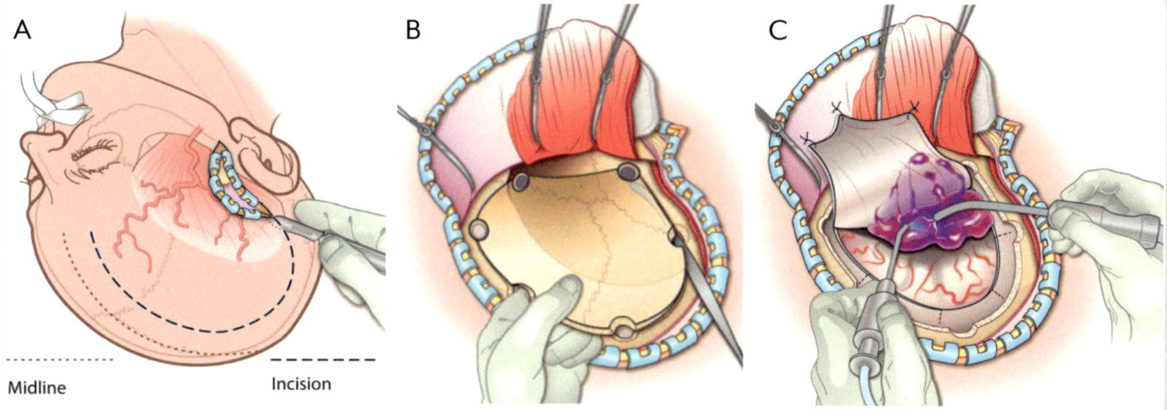

Figure 27.14

Surgical steps necessary for the evacuation of an acute subdural hematoma: A) Skin incision in the shape of a "question mark". B) Large craniotomy flap. C) Dural opening and removal of the blood clot with abundant irrigation and gentle aspiration.

in cases of significant brain swelling, the dura mater is closed using bovine pericardium patches. It is necessary to consider not replacing the autologous bone flap during the closure phase, allowing the brain parenchyma to expand beyond the limits of the cranial opening during the initial stages. The bone flap will be repositioned during a second surgical procedure (cranioplasty) when the neuroimaging findings appear stable (Figure 27.15 and 16) In these cases, it is necessary to ensure that the craniectomy is tangential to the affected skull base (anterior or middle) to significantly increase cerebral compliance and prevent uncal herniation. The bleeding site is not always easily identifiable during surgery, also due to the presence of minor sources of bleeding, usually venous in nature.

The mortality rate of patients with this type of hematoma ranges from 50-90%, depending on concurrent primary brain injuries (such as contusions and diffuse axonal injury), the presence of coagulopathies, and the patient's age (> 60 years have a worse prognosis). The time interval between the traumatic event and intervention or the timing of the surgery (within 4 hours of trauma) plays a crucial role in the patient's prognosis. Motorcycle accidents represent the traumatic mechanism associated with a poorer prognosis.

Chronic subdural hematomas | Are one of the most common post-traumatic neurosurgical conditions. The elderly population is often affected (with an average age of 63 years), with a clear predominance in males compared to females (Figure 27.17). A quarter of cases present with bilateral hematomas, showing the classic "butterfly" appearance on brain CT, caused by chronic bilateral compression of the cerebral hemispheres, which are flattened toward the midline and resemble butterfly wings. A history of head trauma can be identified in less than 50% of cases. Alcohol abuse, epilepsy, fistulas or CSF shunts, coagulopathies (including anticoagulant treatments), and patients at risk of falls are predisposing factors for chronic subdural hematoma.

Chronic subdural hematomas can develop approximately 3-4 weeks after previous acute subdural hematomas that were not properly resorbed. Even a small acute subdural hematoma that is difficult to visualize on CT or only indirectly visible on MRI (due to dural layer separation and/or thickening) can evolve into chronic subdural hematoma, as a result of hypertrophy of the inner dural layer as an inflammatory response to the initial bleeding. Due to the presence of inflammatory processes, chronic subdural hematomas are not static entities but can gradually increase

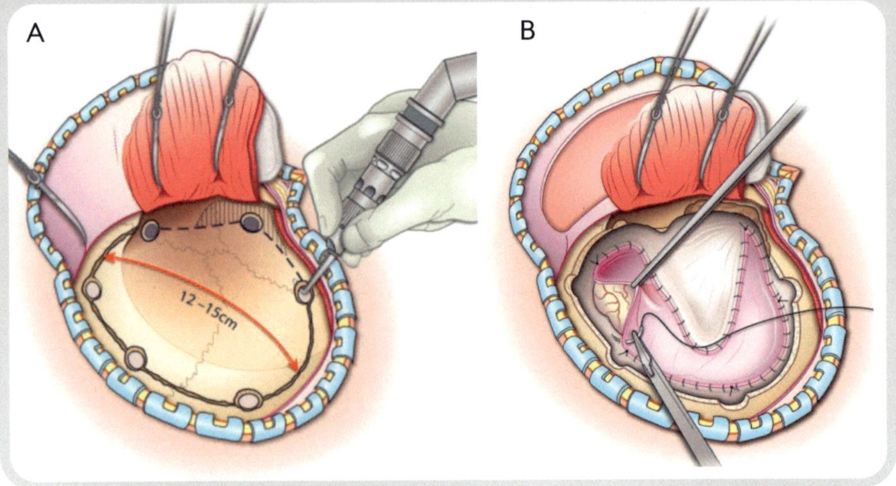

Figure 27.15

A) Bone flap used to perform decompressive craniectomy in case of significant increase in intracranial volume. The cranial bone flap must measure at least 12 cm in diameter to ensure adequate decompression of the underlying brain tissue. B) Dural patch made from bovine pericardium used for closure of the dura mater in cases of brain tissue swelling (due to edematous processes).

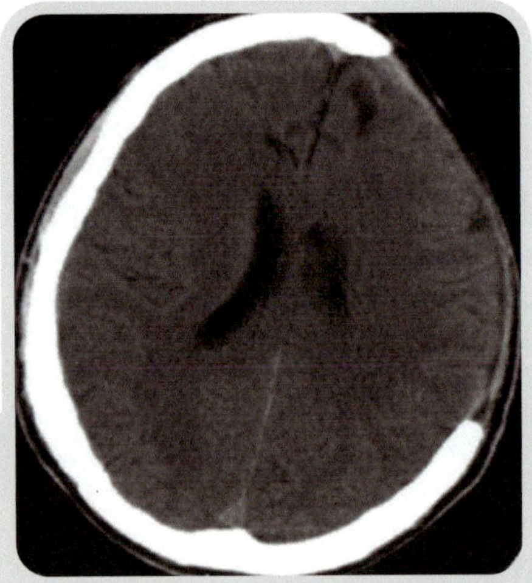

Figure 27.16

Postoperative CT showing the results of a decompressive craniectomy.

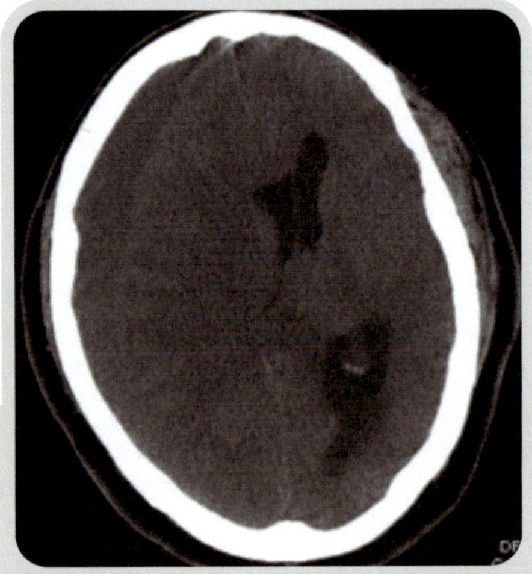

Figure 27.17

CT image of a chronic subdural hematoma (hypodense blood collection) with significant brain shift.

or spontaneously resorb, sometimes with steroid therapy. Patients may present with mild symptoms (headache, confusion, language difficulties) or symptoms simulating a transient ischemic attack, or severe alterations in consciousness, weakness, and seizures. Surgical evacuation of chronic subdural hematomas (Figure 27.18) can be performed under local anesthesia or, less commonly, general anesthesia. Through a cranial hole and subsequent incision of the dura mater, the hematoma is released under variable pressure, appearing as a liquid with a dark brown/coffee-like color. The subdural compartment is then washed with saline solution, and a subdural drainage is inserted into the space previously occupied by the hematoma. The drainage is removed on the first or second postoperative day. Optimal hydration of the patient in the weeks following the procedure promotes brain tissue expansion, reducing the recurrence rate. Equally valid surgical techniques for the treatment of chronic subdural hematomas include creating a small cranial flap and subsequently opening the dura mater (especially useful in cases where the hematoma has multiple septa and clots inside) or performing two cranial holes, one located just anterior to the coronal suture and the other located on the parietal bone, with subsequent

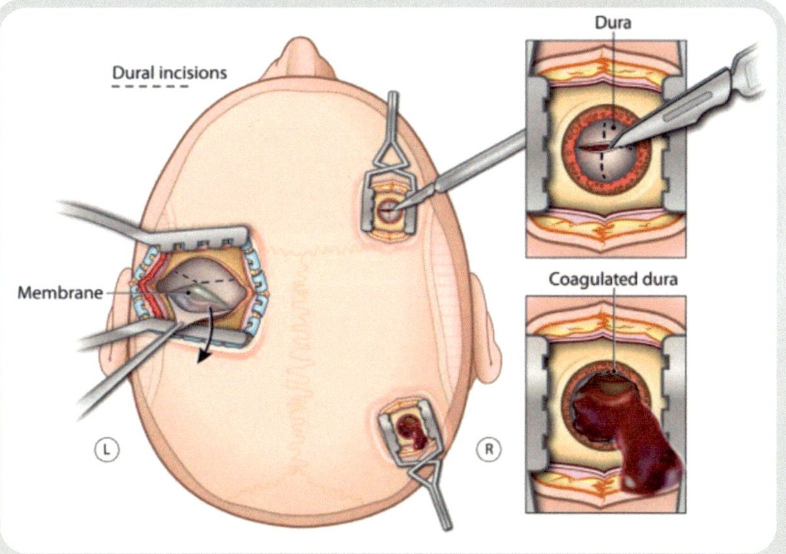

Figure 27.18

Illustration of the various techniques for the evacuation of a chronic subdural hematoma, including mini-craniotomy, double burr hole craniotomy, and single burr hole craniotomy.

placement of a subdural drainage (which is also removed within 24-48 hours of surgery).

Clinical improvement, resulting from the reduction of intracranial pressure, is evident after the removal of 20% of the hematoma. The presence of residual hematoma portions after treatment is common (up to 78% of cases). Therefore, continued observation of patients with residual hematoma detected on CT is necessary, especially in the first 20 days. Clinical deterioration is possible (in about 4% of cases), and complications such as seizures (including drug-resistant status epilepticus) and cerebral hemorrhages (1-5%), often devastating, can occur in a small percentage of cases. The overall mortality associated with surgical treatment of these hematomas ranges from 1% to 8%.

Post-traumatic subarachnoid hemorrhage (SAH) | Is the collection of blood in the arachnoid cisterns, which are normally filled with cerebrospinal fluid, due to the rupture of usually arterial vessels or the invasion of this compartment by hemorrhages from other adjacent structures (intraparenchymal hematomas, subdural hematomas, epidural hematomas, penetrating fractures). Post-traumatic SAH is the most frequent cause of SAH.

Although not clearly demonstrated, the continuous intravenous administration of nimodipine (10 ml/h) may improve the prognosis in patients with SAH visible on CT scans, reducing the risk of arterial vasospasm and protecting, to a certain extent, the nervous tissue from consequent hypoxia. Nimodipine also has a systemic vasodilatory action, therefore blood pressure should be monitored, and if it drops below critical values (80/60 mmHg), blood volume should be expanded with crystalloids administered intravenously.

Traumatic injuries in the posterior cranial fossa | Involve less than 3% of traumatic brain injuries, mostly epidural hematomas caused by bleeding into one of the two transverse sinuses. In such cases, in addition to the risk of mechanical compression by the primary lesion, there is also a risk of acute hydrocephalus due to compression of the fourth ventricle or the Sylvian aqueduct. Most cerebellar hemorrhages $<$ 3 cm do not require surgical intervention. A rare entity of posterior cranial fossa hematomas is represented by clival epidural hematomas, which are rare lesions generally secondary to hyperflexion or hyperextension injuries in adults. The main symptoms of posterior cranial fossa hematomas include nausea, vomiting, and neurological deterioration (Figure 27.19). However, all symptomatic lesions or those causing mass effect should be surgically treated as an emergency, through a suboccipital craniotomy (median, paramedian, or, more rarely, lateral).

Post-traumatic hygroma | Is the collection of cerebrospinal fluid that forms in the subdural space. The mechanism of formation is likely secondary to a laceration of the arachnoid barrier within the subdural compartment. Clinically, it is indistinguishable from a chronic subdural hematoma, and the diagnosis is radiological. Asymptomatic patients do not require any treatment. Recurrences after drainage through a cranial opening are frequent. In these cases, where the presence of a valve mechanism causing a new accumulation of cerebrospinal fluid shortly after drainage is likely, a permanent subdural-peritoneal shunt is recommended.

Post-traumatic hydrocephalus | Develops in a significant percentage of cases with significant head trauma, usually 1-2 months after the trauma. Signs indicating the presence of hydrocephalus include papilledema on fundoscopy, evidence of transependymal resorption on CT or T2-weighted MRI, cessation/deterioration of the patient's clinical condition or a clinical picture worse than expected. Timely implementation of ventriculoperitoneal shunt treatment is necessary to prevent irreversible brain damage caused by increased intracranial pressure due to hydrocephalus.

27.5 General aspects of therapy useful in patients with severe head trauma or critical conditions

Early tracheostomy reduces the number of days on mechanical ventilation but does not affect mortality or the incidence of pneumonia.

Early extubation does not increase the risk of pneumonia, allows for closer clinical monitoring, but may not allow for optimal control of metabolic and neurophysiological parameters (especially intracranial pressure (ICP) and cerebral perfusion pressure (CPP)).

To reduce the risk of deep vein thrombosis, the patient should be provided with elastic stockings or intermittent compression until awakening and active mobilization. In patients with intracranial hemorrhage, the use of low-molecular-weight heparin or low-dose unfractionated heparin is not recommended for the first 15 days, as these drugs increase the risk of hematomas or intracranial hemorrhages, despite lowering the risk of deep vein thrombosis. Nutrition should be restored after 72 hours of trauma. A normocaloric diet should be administered enterally/parenterally from the seventh day after trauma.

Intracranial pressure (ICP) monitoring | The factors regulating ICP (10-15 mmHg, 13-20 cm H_2O) are: brain parenchyma (1400 cc), blood (150cc), and cerebrospinal fluid (150 cc). An increase in volume of one of these three constituents must necessarily be compensated by the other two to maintain constant pressure (Monro-Kellie doctrine). When these compensatory mechanisms are exhausted, ICP increases, and cerebral perfusion pressure (CPP) decreases (normal value > 60 mmHg).

The main causes of intracranial hypertension are: cerebral edema, hyperemia

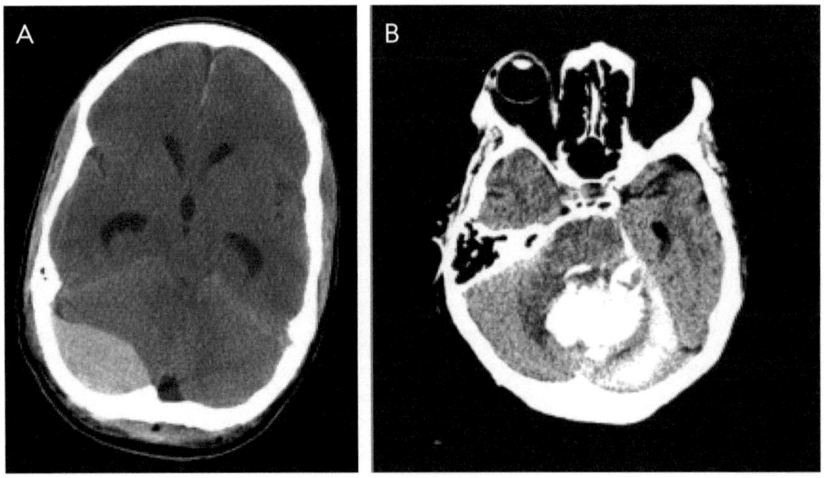

Figure 27.19

A) Epidural hematoma of the posterior cranial fossa. B) Intraparenchymal cerebellar hematoma.

(due to response to head trauma), hematomas, hydrocephalus, hypoventilation (due to hypercapnia causing vasodilation and therefore hyperemia), hypertension, venous sinus thrombosis, status epilepticus, and Valsalva maneuvers (due to psychomotor agitation or concurrent thoracic and/or abdominal issues).

ICP can be monitored by inserting a probe subdurally, intraparenchymally, or intraventricularly. The latter option, in addition to being more accurate, allows for cerebrospinal fluid drainage to rebalance ICP. ICP monitoring is advisable in patients with a Glasgow Coma Scale (GCS) ≤ 8.

General measures to lower ICP include positioning the patient's head at 30° while maintaining a neutral position (to avoid venous congestion), mild sedation, avoiding hyperventilation (maintain $pCO_2 \geq 35$ mmHg) and hypotension (systolic > 90 mmHg), controlling hypertension and hyperthermia, preventing hyperglycemia (which worsens cerebral edema), intubating the patient if GCS < 8 or if respiratory distress is present. If, despite pharmacological therapy, ICP remains above 20 mmHg and/or CPP is below 60 mmHg, the surgical cause of intracranial hypertension should be addressed.

To control ICP, cerebrospinal fluid can be drained from the lateral ventricles using an external ventricular drain (Figure 27.20). There are commercially available external ventricular drains with integrated ICP catheters in the tip (while standard ICP catheters can be inserted directly in the emergency room or intensive care unit, this special intraventricular type must be inserted in the operating room).

In the management of external ventricular drains, it is essential to keep in mind that the external auditory meatus corresponds to the projection of the foramina of Monro, where the tip of the ventricular catheter should be positioned, representing the "zero" of the system (which follows the physics of communicating vessels). Therefore, the drainage catheter outlet into the cerebrospinal fluid collection bag should initially be placed 8-15 cm above the external auditory meatus to maintain intracranial pressure within the normal range.

Prognosis of patients with head trauma

Recovery from closed head trauma is better in children. In adults, the presence of decerebrate posture or flaccidity with loss of pupillary reflex or oculovestibular reflexes is associated with a poor prognosis. In closed head trauma, negative prognostic factors include persistent ICP > 20 mmHg, age, absence of eye movements, absence or sluggishness of the pupillary light reflex, hypotension (< 90 mmHg), hypercapnia, hypoxia, anemia, and partial or total obliteration of perimesencephalic cisterns.

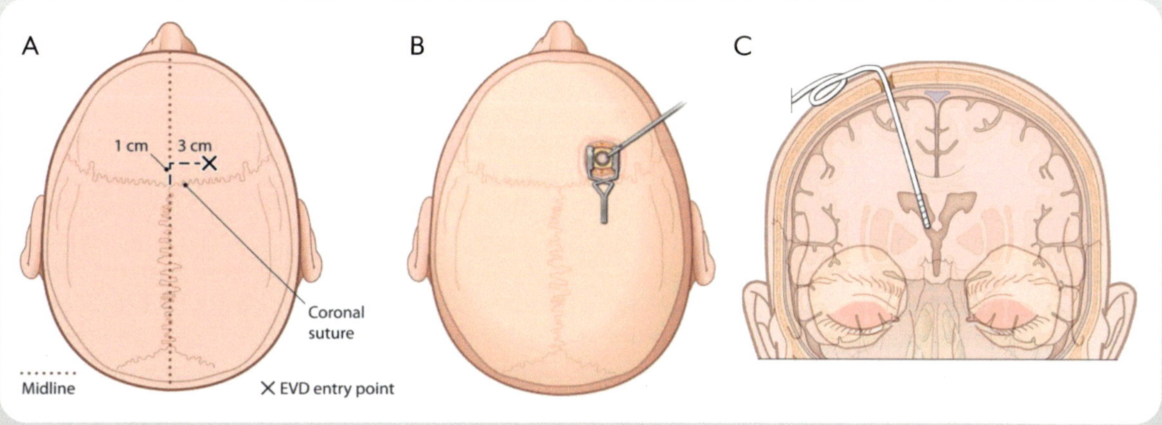

Figure 27.20

A) Kocher's point (located 1 cm anterior to the coronal suture and 3 cm laterally to the midline) represents the insertion point of the ventricular catheter. B) Skin incision and craniotomy hole at the site of insertion for the external ventricular drain. C) The ventricular drain is correctly positioned at the frontal horn of the right lateral ventricle.

Late complications of cranial trauma | Include post-traumatic epilepsy, communicating hydrocephalus, hypogonadotropic hypogonadism, and Alzheimer's disease (due to amyloid deposition favored by severe cranial trauma). Post-traumatic syndrome is a potential consequence of any cranial trauma. It is characterized by general disturbances such as headache, attention and memory deficits, dizziness, anosmia, tinnitus, loss of libido, alterations in the sleep-wake cycle, photophobia, asthenia, and mood alterations. Patients affected by early post-traumatic syndrome often recover quickly, while those in whom symptoms develop over time tend to have a more prolonged course.

Chronic traumatic encephalopathy is often present in boxers and is referred to as "punch-drunk syndrome." It should be distinguished from post-traumatic dementia (which follows a single traumatic event) and post-traumatic Alzheimer's.

27.6 Special types of cranial trauma

Firearm injuries | Firearm injuries represent a significant percentage of penetrating traumas. In the USA, they account for over one-third of deaths due to cranial trauma in patients under 45 years old. These are lethal cranial injuries: two-thirds of cases die before reaching the hospital, and the overall mortality rate is over 90%. The primary damage is caused by soft tissue damage, *comminuted fractures*, and direct brain injury. The impact velocity (distinct from the muzzle velocity and always lower than the latter) is correlated with the primary damage, and a high impact velocity (> 100 m/s) causes an explosive trauma that is invariably fatal. Additional damage from penetrating body shockwaves, brain injuries from coup or contrecoup, secondary damage from cerebral edema and hemorrhage leading to a sudden increase in intracranial pressure (ICP), even within a few minutes, can also occur.

Potential late complications include cerebral abscesses, post-traumatic aneurysms, epilepsy, and intraventricular migration of fragments with possible obstructive hydrocephalus. Therefore, removal of the penetrating object is necessary.

In general, the goal of surgical treatment is debridement of necrotic tissue, which may be hidden by cerebral edema, removal of accessible hematomas and bone fragments, retrieval of the projectile, including for medicolegal purposes, suturing the dura mater in a "water-tight" manner (i.e., hermetically sealed to prevent the passage of cerebrospinal fluid), and potential repair of the paranasal sinuses.

Penetrating injuries from edged weapons | Penetrating injuries from edged weapons (pointed, bladed, or blunt weapons) have an impact velocity that does not exceed 58 m/s (approximately 200 km/h). The foreign body should never be removed before the patient arrives in the operating room. On the contrary, the weapon or its fragment should be stabilized to prevent movement or rotation within the cranial cavity.

27.7 Pediatric cranial trauma

Cranial trauma is one of the most common reasons for emergency department visits in pediatric patients. 90% of pediatric patients are admitted for clinical observation of minor injuries, and cranial trauma is the leading cause of death in the first 12 years of life. The overall mortality rate for all hospitalized cranial traumas is 10-13%, while severe cranial trauma presenting with decerebrate posture has a mortality rate of 71%.

In the case of the pediatric population, neurological evaluation, similar to adults, is crucial in assessing the injured individual. However, it is necessary to consider significant differences, especially in the age group between 0 and 12 months. Therefore, a modified neurological assessment system called the Pediatric Glasgow Coma Scale (GCS) has been developed for these patients. The main difference from the classic GCS lies in the verbal response, which is evaluated based on crying characteristics in this age group (Table 27.2).

The pediatric age group has unique characteristics. There are birth-related injuries (subgaleal, subperiosteal, epidural, subdural, intraparenchymal hemorrhages, fractures),

Table 27.2 PEDIATRIC GLASGOW COMA SCALE

	Eye response	Verbal response	Motor response
1	Doesn't open the eyes	Absent	Absent motor response
2	Opens the eyes with painful stimulus	Inconsolable moaning	Extension to pain (decerebrate response)
3	Opens the eyes with verbal stimulus	Inconsolable crying	Flexion to pain (decorticate response)
4	Opens the eyes spontaneously	Consolable crying	Withdrawal from pain (withdraws quickly when a painful stimulus is applied)
5		Interacts - follows with gaze	Localization of pain (attempts to localize the area where the painful stimulus is applied)
6			Spontaneous movements

shaken baby syndrome (due to child abuse), and injuries resulting from children's games (playground accidents, darts, etc.). Children are more prone than adults to develop "malignant cerebral edema," which can occur acutely after a major cranial trauma (likely due to hyperemia). There is also a higher incidence of post-traumatic epilepsy, especially during the first day after the trauma.

It is always advisable to perform a cranial CT scan in pediatric patients with minor cranial trauma when there is evidence of neurological abnormalities or suspicion of a linear or depressed fracture. In children under one year old who appear agitated and meet the aforementioned criteria but raise doubts about the need for sedation, performing a cranial X-ray in the appropriate projections (anterolateral, lateral, oblique, open-mouth for craniospinal junction assessment) is acceptable.

In reality, 10% of children under 10 years old brought to the emergency department for suspected accidents are victims of abuse, a percentage that increases in children under 3 years old. Signs that raise suspicion of possible abuse include retinal hemorrhages, chronic subdural hematomas (bilateral in 80% of cases) in children under 2 years old, multiple cranial fractures or fractures associated with deeper intracranial injuries (e.g., subarachnoid hemorrhages), and significant neurological deficits with minimal external signs of trauma. Vigorous shaking of the child produces an angular acceleration-deceleration similar to that seen in cervical whiplash injuries (due to an accelerative-decelerative transfer of energy to the neck resulting from anterior-posterior or lateral impacts). This syndrome occurs because the child's head is relatively large in proportion to the body, and the neck muscles are relatively weak. There are generally no external signs of trauma, although sometimes there may be finger marks on the chest, multiple rib fractures, and/or lung compressions with hematomas in the lung parenchyma. Differential diagnosis should always exclude the presence of craniospinal junction injuries using CT or, alternatively, an open-mouth cranial X-ray. In these cases, deaths are almost always caused by the development of increased intracranial pressure.

Bibliography

A.A.V.V., "ATLS: advanced trauma life support for doctors" IX edition, American College of Surgeons Committee on Trauma, Chicago, Illinois, 2013.

Greenberg M.S., Handbook of Neurosurgery. VII edition, Thieme, Lakeland Florida, 2010.

Randolph W. Evans M.D., Neurology and trauma. II edition, Oxford University Press, New York, 2006.

Suarez J.I., Critical Care Neurology and Neurosurgery, Humana Press, Totowa, New Jersey, 2004.

Whitfield P.C., Thomas E.O., Summers F., Whyte M., Hutchinson P.J., Head injury: A multidisciplinary approach. Cambridge Medicine Press, Cambridge UK, 2009.

Ullman J.S. Raksin P.B., Atlas of Emergency Neurosurgery, Thieme, 2018.

Osborn A.G., Brain, Piccin 2014.

Quinones-Hinojosa A., Shmidek e Sweet Operative Neurosurgical Techniques Vol.2, Elselvier, 2006.

Goodrich J.T., Pediatric Neurosurgery, Thieme, 2008.

28 ARTHRITIC, TRAUMATIC AND ONCOLOGICAL PATHOLOGY OF THE SPINE

Francesco Marzetti, Luigi Valentino Berra, Luca D'Angelo, Antonio Santoro

28.1 Spinal osteoarthritis

Congenital or acquired conditions that cause narrowing of lumbar spinal canal diameters result in incongruity between containing structures and contained structures, leading to characteristic symptoms (painful and/or deficitary) that are typical of such pathologies.

The degenerative process involving the vertebral column has intervertebral discopathy as its first event, which is the progressive loss of its water content, fissuring of annulus fibrosus, and the protrusion of nucleus pulposus into the spinal canal. This phase, which constitutes the initial step of the so-called "degenerative cascade," forms the pathological picture known as a herniated disc. Disc degeneration causes a change in the biomechanical alignment of the spine, resulting in an increased segmental movement of each motion segment. This phase is known as the "instability phase" of degenerative cascade, which characterizes the pathological condition of spondylolisthesis. The consequence is thickening of ligamentous and osteoarticular structures, leading to a considerable increase in volume at the expense of diameter of the spinal canal. This phase, known as the "reactive phase" of degenerative cascade, forms the pathological picture of stenosis. In other words, disc herniation is only the first step of a progressive degenerative disease that will inevitably result in stenosis. This disease is known as spondyloarthrosis.

28.1.1 Lumbar-sacral disc herniation

Disc herniation is caused by the protrusion of the nucleus pulposus of the intervertebral disc through the fibers of annulus and its potential migration outside of them. The migration of nucleus pulposus results in both mechanical compression of neural structures and an inflammatory reaction with the release of various biochemical factors.

Classification

Lumbar disc herniations are classified based on level of the herniated disc's nucleus (e.g., L4-L5), the position of herniation within the spinal canal (central/median, slightly shifted to one side/paramedian, etc.), extent of disc material escaping beyond the limits of the annulus (extruded) or not (contained), rupture of the posterior longitudinal ligament, and migration in a caudal (downward) or cranial (upward) direction. Migration of a lumbar disc herniation is a common occurrence. Expelled disc fragment can migrate in various directions, with caudal migration being the most frequent. The position assumed by herniation within the vertebral canal has significant clinical significance because it determines both the presentation of pathology and the potential surgical approach. A lateral herniation (intraforaminal or extraforaminal) compresses the emerging nerve root at the level of herniated disc, while a central (median) herniation can compress the roots that will emerge from the levels below the herniated disc.

The clinical picture varies depending on the type of herniation. Often, symptoms present with classic clinical features that not only allow for a clinical diagnosis of disc herniation but also provide its precise localization. Very rarely a lumbar disc herniation represents a clinical emergency requiring immediate discectomy. Disc herniations at L4-L5 and L5-S1 are by far the most common.

Typically, patients with lumbar disc herniation complain of unilateral lumbosciatica (L4-L5, L5-S1) or lumbocruralgia (L2-L3, L3-L4). Although bilateral involvement is possible (e.g., with large median disc herniations), it is rather rare. Some patients only experience sciatic or crural pain and do not report any component of low back pain except as a feeling of tenderness or muscle tightness.

Sciatica refers to radiating pain in the lower limb along the course of the sciatic nerve, composed of the L4 (partially), L5, and S1 nerve roots. Femoral neuralgia, on the other hand, refers to radiating pain in the anterior or anteromedial thigh extending to the knee (involving L2, L3, and part of L4). Sciatic or femoral pain can be described as either continuous radiation originating from the lumbar spine along the dermatome of affected root or as isolated pain localized in a specific area without spatial continuity with the lumbar spine. Sometimes, only low back pain is reported. This is the case with contained or subligamentous median or paramedian disc herniations, where there is no involvement of nerve root structures. Low back pain sometimes represents the initial clinical presentation, followed by radicular pain. Pain is typically exacerbated by spinal movements, coughing, sneezing, straining, and the Valsalva maneuver. Some patients may experience "paralyzing sciatica," where the predominant sign is difficulty in walking due to muscle weakness. Finally, the symptomatology may begin with "cauda equina syndrome," a multiradicular involvement associated with severe sphincter compromise (inability to retain urine and feces) and saddle anesthesia.

Disc herniation can compress the nerve structures and cause both motor and sensory deficits. Motor deficits can range from a simple reduction in the strength of a single muscle in the lower limb to complete paralysis of multiple muscles. Sensory deficits affect the dermatome of the herniated root.

Clinical evaluation

Following criteria of radicular distribution of the muscles in the lower limbs, the strength of individual muscles should be evaluated. Patient is asked to perform a specific movement (e.g., dorsiflexion of the foot) and then perform the same movement against resistance.

Superficial sensitivity can be evaluated in its tactile, painful, and thermal components in various dermatomal areas. Deep sensitivity is evaluated using a tuning fork that produces perceivable vibrations in the absence of radicular compression. Evaluation of cutaneous sensitivity in the perianal area is particularly important in patients with possible cauda equina syndrome. Radicular compression results in a reduction (compared to the reflex of the contralateral limb) or absence of osteotendinous reflex through the compressed root (Table 28.1). In reality, research and evaluation of osteotendinous reflexes do not always provide the expected results. Difficulty in evoking a reflex can be due to multiple causes: a constitutional hypoexcitability state of the patient, their conditions (pain, difficulty in relaxation), and previous pathologies.

Table 28.1 SYMPTOMS AND SIGNS OF LUMBAR DISC HERNIATION

L5-S1 herniation
Involved root: S1 *Motor deficit:* plantar flexion of the foot *Involved reflex:* achilles reflex *Radiation area:* gluteal region, posterior aspect of the thigh and leg, Achilles tendon, heel, sole of the foot, and lateral aspect of the fifth toe
L4-L5 herniation
Involved root: L5 *Motor deficit:* dorsiflexion of the foot and toes (especially of the big toe) *Radiation area:* Gluteal region, posterior-lateral aspect of the thigh, anterior tibial region and lateral malleolus, instep, big toe and second toe
L3-L4 herniation
Involved root: L4 *Motor deficit:* extension of the leg at the thigh (quadriceps) and, to a lesser extent, dorsiflexion of the foot *Involved reflex:* patellar *Radiation area:* Lateral aspect of the buttock, anterior and anterolateral thigh region, inguinal region, inner aspect of the knee, medial aspect of the leg

Other clinical assessments

Lasègue maneuver (L4-L5-S1) | The patient lies in a supine position. The operator lifts the lower limb with the knee extended, which elicits or exacerbates the patient's radicular pain (sciatica). The operator then repeats the maneuver with the knee flexed, increasing hip flexion. In this case, a patient with radicular pain will experience a reduction in pain, while a patient with coxalgia will complain of increased pain due to increased hip flexion.

Wasserman test (L2-L3-L4) | The patient lies prone; the operator flexes the patient's knee until the onset or exacerbation of femoral neuralgia. This test is accentuated by simultaneous extension of the hip.

Instrumental examinations | Radiograph of lumbosacral spine in standard projections (anteroposterior and lateral)represents the initial examination, which can be followed by functional or dynamic studies (flexion and extension of the spine) in lateral projection. The main examination to be performed in cases of suspected disc herniation is magnetic resonance imaging (MRI), which provides a qualitative evaluation of the spinal structures, including the disc, and visualizes large segments of the spine simultaneously (Figure 28.1). Computed tomography (CT) of lumbosacral spine is now less commonly used, although it is a sensitive and specific examination. Other instrumental examinations are used for differential diagnosis with other pathologies (bone scintigraphy, lower limb or abdominal Doppler ultrasound, laboratory tests, abdominal CT, etc.). Electromyography and electroneurography (EMG, ENG) play a fundamental role in assessing the involvement and functionality of the affected roots. In particular, electromyographic demonstration of signs of denervation is an important prognostic factor in the therapeutic evaluation of the patient.

Surgical indications | Disc herniations tend to regress spontaneously in 98% of cases, so surgical indication should be carefully evaluated. Indications for discectomy surgery can be absolute (necessity of the intervention) or relative. *Absolute indication*: presence of neurological deficits affecting multiple roots or a single root with electromyography (EMG) showing signs of denervation. In such cases, early decompression leads to resolution, at least partially, of the neurological deficit in a significant percentage of patients. *Relative indications*: presence of pain or the presence of associated pathologies. Disc herniation pain is often intolerable for patient. If pain does not respond well to supportive therapy (anti-inflammatory drugs, analgesics, etc.), patient may request surgery. In this case, surgical indication is clearly discussed, explaining the risk-benefit ratio of intervention to the patient.

Surgical treatment | Microdiscectomy with interlaminar approach remains the surgical

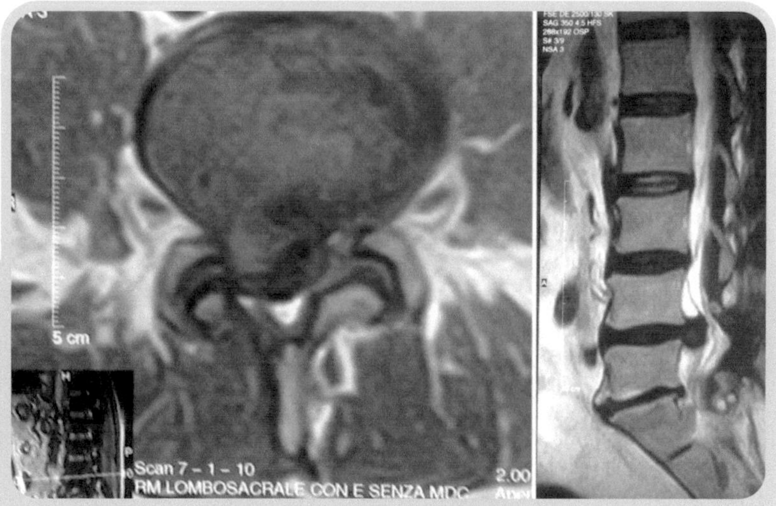

Figure 28.1

Axial and sagittal T2-weighted MRI examination: evidence of a right paramedian disc herniation at the L4-L5 level with compression of the ipsilateral L5 nerve root and almost complete obliteration of the spinal canal.

intervention for lumbar disc herniation that provides the best clinical and functional outcomes. It is performed with the patient in the prone position, with a minimal skin incision (approximately 3 cm), through which unilateral access is gained to the affected disc space, with limited removal of the yellow ligament (flavectomy) and partial removal of the upper lamina (interlaminectomy). After flavectomy, the microsurgical field provides access to the vertebral canal where dural sac and nerve root are located, beneath which the herniation is found. Following hernia removal, discectomy is performed, which involves using specific instruments to clean the nucleus pulposus in order to minimize the risk of recurrence as much as possible. The procedure concludes with opening of the neural foramen (foraminotomy). Additional techniques that can be used include endoscopic discectomy and percutaneous discectomy with tubular dilators, which provide good results in treating herniations with hydrated disc fragments but are still inferior to the classical microdiscectomy for selective indications of the hernia type to be treated. Other percutaneous techniques include nucleoaspiration, nucleoplasty, ozone therapy, radiofrequency, and others, but they are characterized by a high recurrence rate of painful symptoms, especially in herniations with expelled disc fragments.

28.1.2 Lumbar stenosis

Lumbar stenosis represents the so-called reactive phase of the degenerative cascade, in which the excessive movement of the spinal structures resulting from disc degeneration is countered by the hypertrophy of osteo-ligamentous structures.

Symptoms are characterized by localized pain (low back pain) and pain secondary to the compression of spinal roots, felt in the corresponding territories (radiating pain). The characteristic symptom of lumbar spinal canal stenosis is called "neurogenic claudication." It refers to an increase in pain, radiating to the lower limbs, experienced by the patient during walking, which forces the individual to stop to find relief. Claudication is caused by a reduction in blood flow in the perivertebral plexus, thus primarily being a symptom of a vascular nature.

Diagnosis

The diagnosis of lumbar stenosis is primarily clinical. However, it is necessary to confirm diagnosis through instrumental diagnostic investigations. Among these, in addition to radiographic examination (the first test that can provide only indirect signs), CT scans (Figure 28.2), MRI, and neurophysiological assessments, particularly electromyography (EMG), should be considered. Dynamic X-ray studies aimed at identifying vertebral instability associated with stenosis can be useful. Magnetic Resonance Imaging (MRI) provides direct images not only about content (the dural sac) but also of surrounding tissues, especially disc ligamentous system. Figure 28.3 describes a classification of 4 degrees of stenosis based on detection, by lumbar-sacral MRI examination in axial T2 sequences, of a quantitative decrease in cerebrospinal fluid that is normally present in the absence of stenosis. CT is capable of demonstrating, with greater accuracy than MRI, bony structures whose hypertrophy can cause narrowing of the intervertebral foramina through which the spinal roots exit. EMG highlights the involvement of the affected nerve roots.

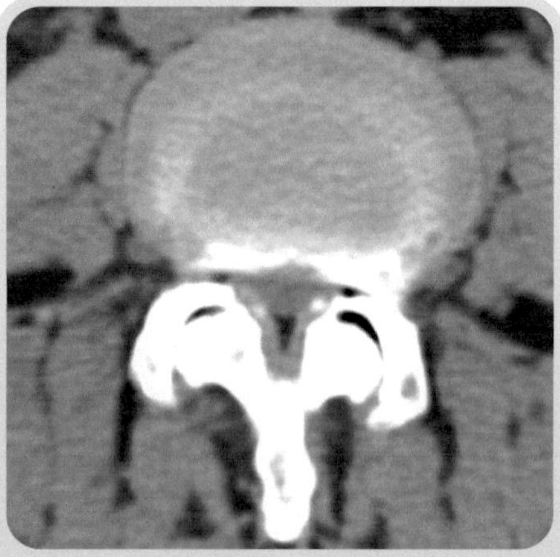

Figure 28.2

Lumbo-sacral CT without contrast medium: axial plane sequences showing marked osteo-ligamentous hypertrophy with consequent canal and neuroforaminal stenosis.

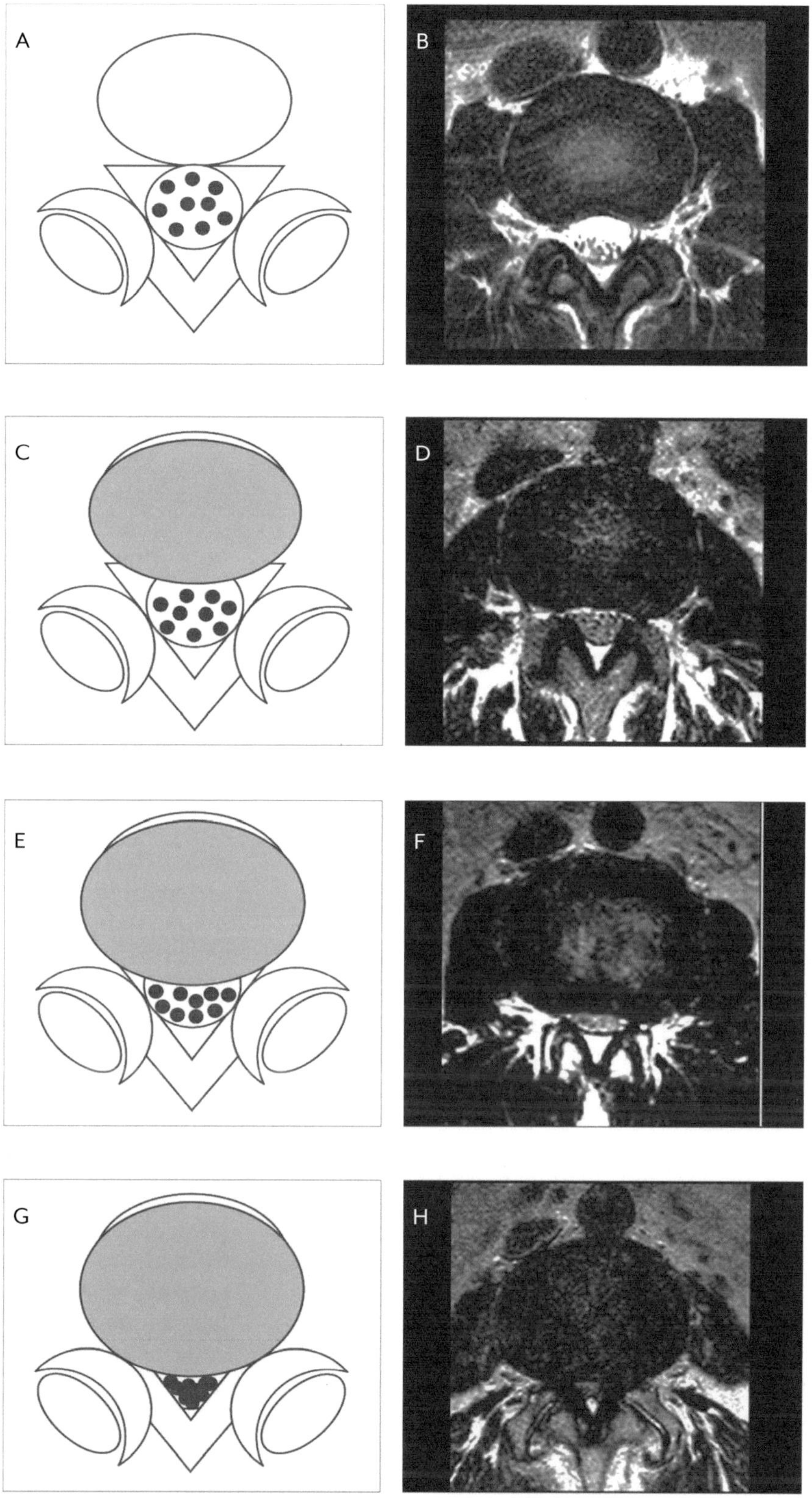

Figure 28.3

Classification of stenosis degree based on visualization method inside the lumbar canal of cerebrospinal fluid on MRI examination with axial T2-weighted sequences: A-B: normal presence of cerebrospinal fluid in the canal - grade 0; C-D: absence of cerebrospinal fluid in the anterior component of the canal - grade 1; E-F: limited presence of cerebrospinal fluid throughout the canal diameter with moderate to severe radicular compression - grade 2; G-H: absence of cerebrospinal fluid with marked osteo-ligamentous hypertrophy and severe radicular compression - grade 3.

Surgical treatment

Surgical treatment is necessary if conservative treatments do not yield satisfactory results. The goal of surgical treatment for lumbar spinal canal stenosis is the decompression of the spinal roots. To achieve this goal, a posterior surgical approach and a targeted and not overly extensive removal of structures (laminae, zygapophysis, yellow ligaments, joint capsules) that are responsible for compression due to hypertrophy or congenital alteration are indicated. It is important to remember that the removal of anatomical structures from the motion segment (this term refers to the combination of two adjacent vertebrae with all the disc ligamentous apparatus that binds them together) can lead to increased intervertebral movements (instability) and, therefore, to a new pathological condition. In some cases, based on the "instability" of the spine diagnosed by radiographic examination in flexion-extension, vertebral stabilization can be associated with the decompression procedure using instrumentation (screws and metal rods) and posterior-lateral or interbody fusion with cages made of osteoinductive materials. This therapeutic choice is undertaken both to restore stability to a spinal segment that has lost the properties and limits of physiological movement due to degenerative-arthritic changes and to prevent the development of pathological mobility related to the necessary decompression of compressed nerve structures.

28.1.3 Cauda equina syndrome

The terminal portion of the spinal cord is called conus medullaris and includes nine pairs of nerve roots (from L2 to S5) known as the cauda equina (CE) roots. The cauda equina roots are responsible for motor innervation of all muscles of the lower limbs, as well as the external anal and urethral sphincters, sensory innervation of the lower limbs and the saddle region, and parasympathetic innervation of the bladder and distal portion of the intestine. The conus medullaris also contains the spinal reflex center for micturition, defecation, and sexual function. Compression of these nerves can cause a syndrome known as Cauda Equina Syndrome (CES), which represents a neurological disorder requiring immediate treatment.

CES can be caused by numerous pathologies, including massive herniation of a lumbar disc, predominantly in the central position. The incidence of CES caused by lumbar herniation is estimated to be less than 1 in 2,000 patients with severe low back pain. However, CES is found in 1-16% of all lumbar disc herniations and in 2-3% of all patients with disc herniation requiring surgery. About 70% of cases have a clinical history of low back pain, with or without sciatica. The remaining 30% have an acute onset without previous clinical symptoms. Disc herniation causing CES is often a massive herniation that can occur on a predisposing condition of preexisting lumbar canal stenosis, or on a tethered cord condition or in the presence of arachnoid adhesions.

The failure to diagnose CES can lead to severe morbidity such as loss of bladder, bowel, and sexual function, as well as varying degrees of muscle weakness, with potential medicolegal consequences.

CES, to be defined as such, must include at least one of the following symptoms: urinary and/or fecal dysfunction, saddle anesthesia, sexual dysfunction, accompanied by symptoms of lower limb radiculopathy (sensory and/or motor deficits, hypo-reflexia), and possibly accompanied by low back pain. If all of the previously described symptoms are present at the same time, the syndrome is referred to as "complete," meaning that all the roots that make up the cauda equina are affected. However, if not all symptoms are present, but only some, the syndrome is referred to as "incomplete."

CES is characterized by a highly variable clinical presentation, which is why it can be difficult to diagnose. It is characterized by sensory disturbances in the corresponding dermatomes (radicular-type hypoesthesia or anesthesia of the lower limbs, buttocks, perineum, and genitals), motor deficits in all the muscles of the lower limbs innervated by the spinal cord segments below L1 (peripheral-type weakness or paralysis), and autonomic dysfunctions (disturbances in sphincter functions, sexual dysfunction). The most significant symptom is urinary retention, which has an incidence of 90%. A crucial factor for defining urinary retention is the post-void residual volume, which is measured by catheterizing the patient after voluntary urination and is considered positive when the volume exceeds 200 ml (normal range: 50-100 ml). Urinary incontinence may also be present as the opposite symptom. Fecal retention or incontinence may also occur, with decreased sphincter tone observed in 50-75% of patients. Saddle anesthesia has been observed in 75% of CES patients and may involve the loss of sensation in the anal sphincter, lower genitals, perineum, buttocks, and sometimes the posterior aspect of the thigh. Motor deficits can also be severe and usually involve more than one nerve root. These disturbances can be bilateral but are rarely symmetrical (usually, one side is more affected than the other). If not promptly treated, these deficits can become very severe, progressing to complete paralysis. Reflexes are usually hypoactive or absent. Sexual dysfunction may include erectile or ejaculatory dysfunction and impotence in males, as well as alterations in vaginal lubrication or decreased pleasure sensation in females.

Diagnosis

Magnetic resonance imaging (MRI) | MRI represents the gold standard examination for the diagnosis of CES. It is now the diagnostic test of choice that allows optimal visualization of the capsulo-ligamentous structures and the intervertebral disc. Axial T2-weighted scans are particularly useful for differentiating intervertebral disc from any osteophytes and for assessing the relationship between herniated disc material and hypointense posterior longitudinal ligament.

Computed tomography (CT) | CT is a fast, reliable, and easily accessible examination with good sensitivity. It is minimally invasive and generally does not have contraindications, except for concerns regarding the use of X-rays (such as during pregnancy). CT is especially useful for visualizing osteophytes and determining the actual consistency of the herniation itself. This is crucial in the diagnostic and therapeutic process for selecting the appropriate treatment. Other tests that may be useful in the diagnosis of CES include urodynamic testing, electromyography of the perineal floor, and assessment of sexual function.

Treatment of CES

If temporary conservative treatment is required, it would consist exclusively of bladder catheterization and pharmacological therapy. Laxatives can be administered if fecal retention is present, along with painkillers and corticosteroids (with appropriate gastrointestinal protection).

Surgical treatment

The choice between laminectomy or hemilaminectomy mainly depends on herniation's size, but most clinicians prefer to perform a laminectomy with discectomy. Adequate mobilization of dural sac is important in the removal of a herniation causing CES to optimally decompress both sac and nerve roots. Therefore, laminectomy represents the ideal surgical approach.

Surgical procedure is microdiscectomy with a posterior approach. The gold standard for performing this type of intervention is the microsurgical technique, using operating microscope. After the procedure, the affected nerve roots should appear well mobilizable. In the immediate postoperative period, radicular pain disappears, while regression of other symptoms can occur gradually. Improvement can be observed in both hypoesthesia and muscle weakness. However, complete recovery of motor function can be slow and may require supportive physiotherapy.

Prognosis

In general, motor and/or sensory deficits, unless complete, tend to improve due to reinnervation processes. Typically, patients experience improvement that can be further enhanced with the help of physiotherapy. Recovery of sphincter deficits and sexual dysfunction depends on the degree of pre-surgical impairment: the greater the impairment, the worse the outcome. Reflexes tend to normalize in the immediate postoperative period.

28.1.4 Degenerative dorso-lumbar spondylolisthesis

Degenerative spondylolisthesis is a common condition in individuals over 50 years of age, particularly in women. It originates as a result of vertebral arthritis and occurs during the phase of degenerative cascade of the vertebral metamere known as the "unstable phase." In this case, spondylolisthesis occurs due to the wear and tear of the articular masses and the vertebral disc, which progressively become hypermobile, leading to reduced resistance in articulation of the vertebrae and thus instability. Degenerative spondylolisthesis is not associated with isthmic lysis and is almost always accompanied by arthritic compression of neural structures, resulting in disc herniation, canal stenosis, and spondyloarthrosis.

The most commonly affected vertebra by slippage (listhesis) is L4, followed by L3. Spondylolisthesis, regardless of its nature, is classified based on the percentage of vertebral body slippage according to the Mayerding classification: Grade I (< 25%), Grade II (25-50%), Grade III (50-75%), and Grade IV (> 75%). The degree of vertebral slippage varies widely but rarely exceeds Grade 2, meaning a slippage of 25%-50% compared to the underlying vertebra.

In degenerative spondylolisthesis, when posterior arch remains intact and slides along with the vertebral body, it always leads to spinal canal narrowing. Patients often present with a clinical picture of chronic mechanical low back pain, which worsens with prolonged standing and walking but tends to alleviate in a supine position. In presence of concurrent central or lateral stenosis, radicular symptoms, either unilateral or bilateral, are often associated, as previously described into degenerative lumbar stenosis's section.

Diagnosis

Instrumental diagnosis primarily relies on radiographic imaging, including standard and dynamic lateral projections. CT scans (Figure 28.4) are also useful to identify associated lumbar stenosis and for differential diagnosis from isthmic spondylolisthesis. MRI (Figure 28.5) plays an important role as well, as it can reveal associated disc herniations or degenerative synovial pathologies of the posterior joints.

Surgical treatment

The suggested surgical treatment of degenerative spondylolisthesis, in presence of chronic, intense, and continuous low back pain, consists of instrumented postero-lateral fusion (using transpedicular screws connected by titanium rods), possibly in combination with interbody fusion using cages (Figure 28.6).

In patients with radicular symptoms, i.e., with a combination of spondylolisthesis and symptomatic lumbar stenosis, it is

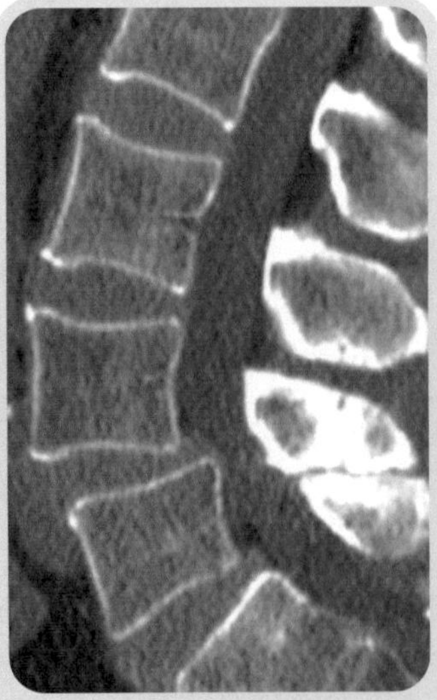

Figure 28.4

Lumbo-sacral TC without significant pathological findings: sagittal plane sequences showing grade I anterolisthesis of L4 on L5 and reduction in the dimensions of the canal at that level.

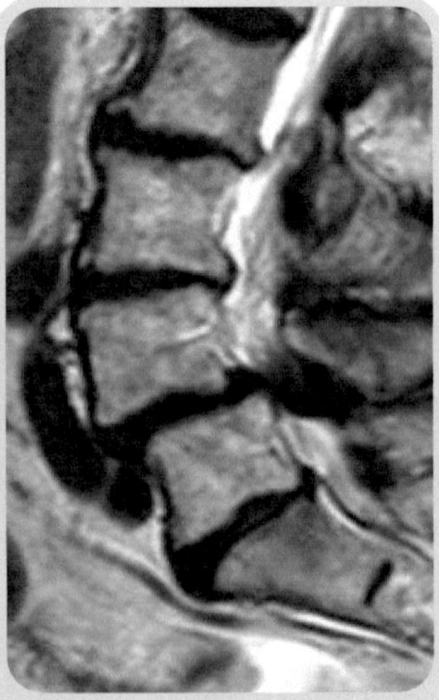

Figure 28.5

Lumbo-sacral MRI without contrast medium: T2 sequences on the sagittal plane showing Grade I anterolisthesis of L4 on L5 with consequent compensatory osteo-ligamentous hypertrophy due to instability and stenosis of the canal at that level.

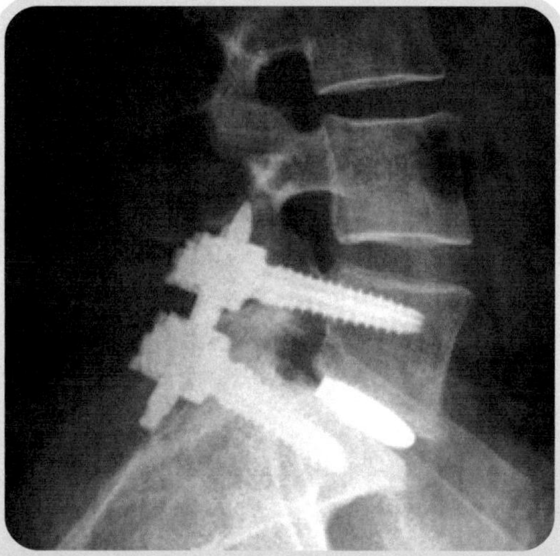

Figure 28.6

Lateral view lumbosacral X-ray showing the outcomes of transpedicular stabilization with titanium screws and rods and placement of TLIF.

always preferable to perform a bilateral decompressive laminectomy after stabilizing the vertebral slippage with pedicular screws and rods. Reducing the slippage of the affected vertebra, although possible with current surgical techniques, does not seem necessary to achieve better clinical recovery compared to simple stabilization.

Approaches for fusion | In the treatment of the aforementioned conditions (single or multilevel discopathy), various vertebral fusion techniques with different approaches have been developed in recent years, based on the symptoms and radiological findings. Anterior vertebral fusion (A-lif) aims to remove the compromised intervertebral disc(s) (discectomy) and replace them with a rigid insert filled with synthetic bone (called cage), which promotes the growth of "natural" bone over time. Thus, over time, the treated vertebrae fuse together, forming a single bone, gaining stability, resolving neurological and painful symptoms, and preventing degeneration progression in the treated area.

To access the spine, the surgeon experienced in this technique makes a few centimeters incision on the patient's abdomen, proceeding to create a passage by moving the abdominal muscles, organs, and blood vessels without severing them, including the peritoneum. In practice, an existing but virtual space called the retroperitoneal space is utilized, which is only "expanded" and returns to its original condition at the end of the procedure. By not cutting through tissues or detaching muscles from bone structures, a less painful and faster surgical course is achieved compared to a more invasive procedure. Complications associated with this type of surgical approach are related to the risk of vascular and upper hypogastric plexus injuries, leading to the possibility of retrograde ejaculation in male patients.

Intervertebral fusion using a lateral approach (X-lif, Figure 28.7) is used when fusion involves vertebral spaces from T12/L1 to L4/L5, as the L5/S1 level is laterally inaccessible due to the presence of the iliac crest. With the patient in a lateral position, after a skin incision, a guide wire is inserted into the disc space, and through this, a specific tissue retractor is positioned, allowing for the creation of a corridor through which the surgeon can work, while simultaneously protecting nerve plexus and peritoneum by the presence of psoas muscle, and an interbody cage is inserted.

Fusion through a posterior (P-lif, Figure 28.8) or postero-lateral approach (T-lif, Figure 28.9) is predominantly used in open or minimally invasive approaches when there is stenosis of the lumbar canal or neuroforamen due to the disc-ligament complex, and often involves posterior pedicular stabilization or interspinous devices. Various types of cages are applied following flavectomy and discectomy, as illustrated in the figures.

A-lif approach, especially in cases of single-level discopathy, allows for the placement of a larger cage compared to other approaches, due to the characteristics of the approach, thereby providing greater opportunities to restore proper postoperative lordosis.

28.1.5 Cervical hernia and stenosis

At level of cervical spine, the content of the canal is represented by spinal cord. For this reason, symptoms can be caused by both nerve roots (radiculopathy) and spinal cord compression (with clinical signs of irritation or deficit, involving the sensory-motor

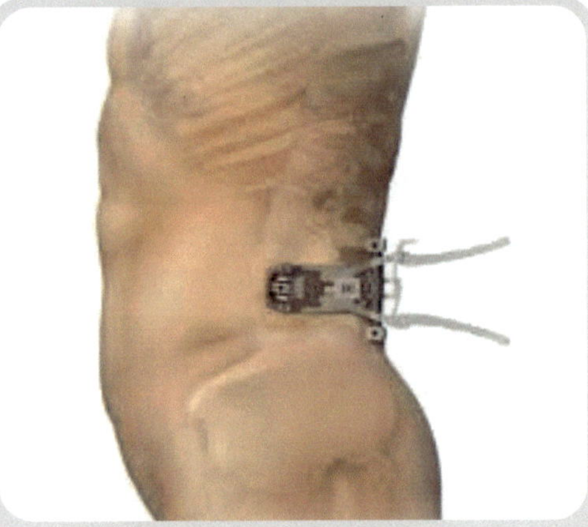

Figure 28.7

Graphic reconstruction of XLIF positioning on the sagittal plane.

pathways). In these cases, it is referred to as cervical myelopathy or involvement of both components, myeloradiculopathy.

The symptoms reported by patients with cervical herniation or stenosis consist of neck pain and radiating pain (radicular) (■ Table 28.2). In case of spinal cord involvement (myelopathy), there are signs of hypertonia in the muscles of the lower limbs (spasticity), leading to worsening quadriparesis. Although the narrowing of the cervical spinal canal occurs slowly and progressively over time, with consequent adaptation of the structures within, clinical symptoms are initially represented by pain and paresthesia, followed by deficits in strength and sensation (radicular), and subsequently by more complex symptoms (related to the spinal cord).

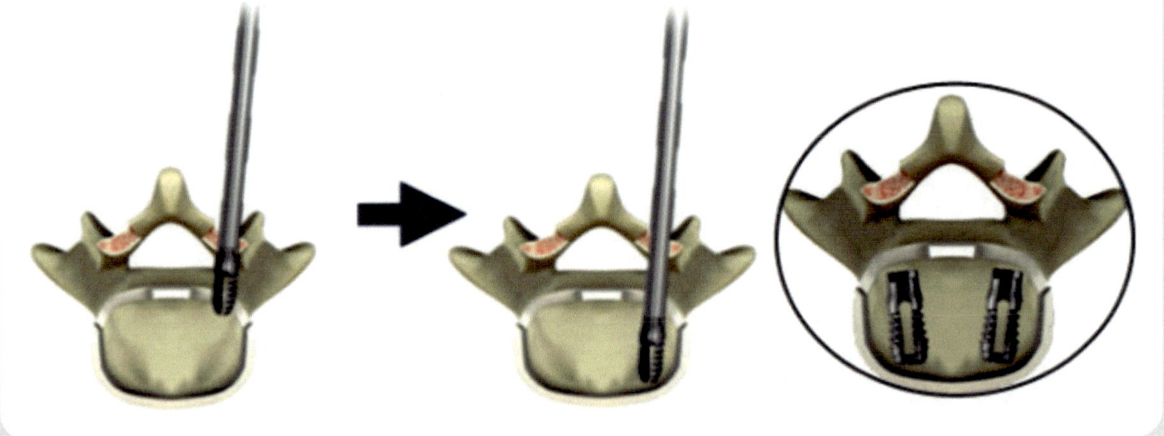

Figure 28.8

Graphical reconstruction of PLIF positioning on the axial plane.

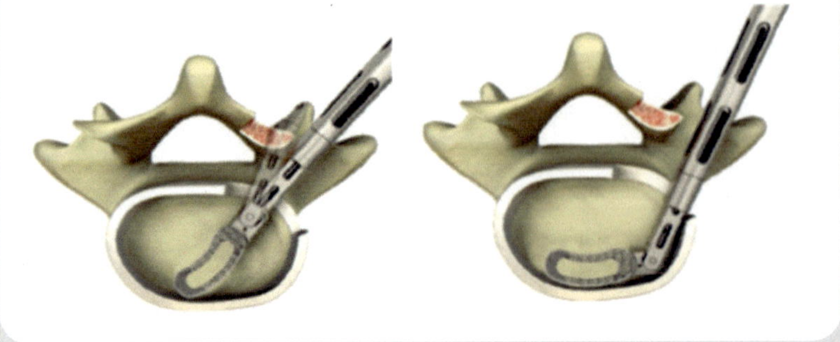

Figure 28.9

Graphic reconstruction of TLIF positioning on the axial plane.

Table 28.2 SYMPTOMS AND SIGNS OF CERVICAL DISC HERNIATION

C3-C4 herniation
Involved root: C4 *Motor deficit:* deltoid weakness *Radiation area:* anterior and upper surface of the shoulder up to the insertion of the deltoid on the arm, posterior surface of the trapezius
C4-C5 herniation
Involved root: C5 *Motor deficit:* biceps brachii weakness *Involved reflex:* biceps reflex *Radiation area:* lateral aspect of the arm (skin surface over the deltoid muscle)
C5-C6 herniation
Involved root: C6 *Motor deficit:* biceps brachii weakness *Involved reflex:* biceps reflex *Radiation area:* anterior surface of the biceps muscle, forearm, and palm of the first and second fingers
C6-C7 herniation
Involved root: C7 *Motor deficit:* triceps weakness *Involved reflex:* triceps reflex *Radiation area:* posterior surface of the triceps, dorsal surface of the third finger
C7-T1 herniation
Involved root: C8 *Motor deficit:* intrinsic hand muscles (dorsal interossei) *Involved reflex:* finger flexor reflex *Radiation area:* dorsal and volar surfaces of the last two fingers

Diagnosis

It is primarily clinical, but it is necessary to confirm the diagnosis with diagnostic imaging investigations, including radiographic examination (the first test that can provide only indirect but important signs), CT scan, MRI (Figure 28.10), and neurophysiological assessments (EMG, Somatosensory and Motor Evoked Potentials).

The most representative clinical scenarios are constituted by herniations at C5-C6, C6-C7, and C7-T1. Involvement of the remaining cervical segments is not characterized by a detailed clinical picture but rather nonspecific.

Surgical treatment

If there are significant clinical signs (spinal cord compression) and conservative treatment (pharmacological and orthopedic immobilization) does not yield the desired results, patient is directed towards

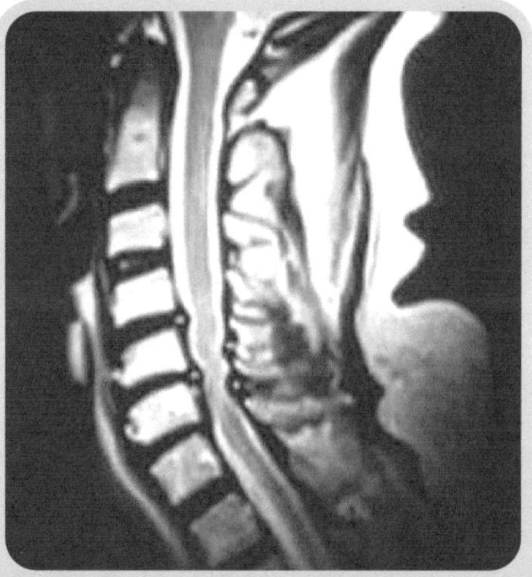

Figure 28.10

Cervical Stenosis: MRI examination with T2-weighted sequences reveals evidence of stenosis of the cervical canal involving the C4-C5, C5-C6, and C6-C7 levels with a significant reduction in the diameter of the spinal canal, most notably at C5-C6.

surgical treatment, which aims at cervical decompression. This can be achieved through an anterior surgical approach, via discectomy and intersomatic arthrodesis with a mono or multilevel cage, or a posterior approach, through laminectomy or laminoplasty.

In some cases, due to congenital laxity of the anterior longitudinal ligament (ALL) or posterior longitudinal ligament (PLL), or due to previous cervical traumas, cervical spondylodiscopathy may also present with instability, characterized by appearance of listhesis (i.e., anterior or posterior vertebral slippage) at the same level of degenerative pathology. In such cases, at the surgical level, anterior stabilization plate placement is associated with discectomy and arthrodesis, or in extreme cases, posterior fixation of instability using cervical screws placed at the level of the articular masses.

28.1.6 Herniated discs

Compared to cervical and lumbar hernias, dorsal hernia is less common and only requires surgery in rare cases. This condition is, on average, more frequent between the ages of 55 and 60 and can be differentially diagnosed from other conditions that can cause muscle or joint pain, such as rheumatoid arthritis, osteoarthritis, or cardiovascular and gastrointestinal disorders. Thoracic spine is composed of two regions:

- Upper thoracic spine, from T1 to T9, is considered the fixed thoracic spine. Its biomechanical characteristics are regulated by the rib cage, which originates dorsally from the costotransverse joint and runs anteriorly to join with the sternum;
- Lower thoracic spine extends from T10 to T12 and is much more mobile. This lower segment of thoracic spine bridges the gap between anterior thoracic spine and lumbar spine, both structurally and functionally. Ribs from T10 to T12 do not have a fixed ventral sternal attachment point and are therefore more mobile. This transitional zone bears the majority of the mechanical stress on thoracic spine.

The rarity of thoracic hernias is therefore secondary to the relative immobility of thoracic spine. However, as the mobility of thoracic spine increases in rostrocaudal direction, it becomes progressively more susceptible to degeneration and disc herniation. In fact, 75% of thoracic hernias occur below T8, and hernias at the T11 and T12 levels are the most frequent.

In many cases, dorsal hernias are asymptomatic (up to 40% of patients do not report any specific symptoms). When symptoms do occur, they may include:

- Lateral chest pain (referred to as "belt-like" pain);
- Thoracoabdominal hypoesthesia with sensory level referred to two upper vertebral segments above the level of the dorsal hernia;
- Stiffness in the lower limbs with osteotendinous hyperreflexia, which manifests as an early sign of spasticity;
- Varying degrees of spastic paraparesis sometimes associated with sphincter disturbances.

Radicular symptoms are due to nerve root's compression by laterally herniated disc material or osteophytic foraminal stenosis. Myelopathic symptoms are caused by spinal cord dysfunction due to extradural compression by herniated disc material or the formation of calcified osteophytes.

Instrumental examinations

The diagnosis of a dorsal hernia is based on an initial examination of the patient's medical history and a subsequent medical evaluation. To confirm the diagnosis, the following tests are typically performed (Figure 28.11):

- Dorsal MRI without contrast medium injection: a diagnostic examination to assess the extent and spinal compression associated with the intracanal disc component of the hernia, as well as to identify any signs of intramedullary suffering;
- Dorsal CT scan: a useful examination for quantifying the hernia's calcified component;
- Motor and somatosensory evoked potentials (MEP and SSEP): these are important preoperative tests to diagnose any conduction disorders affecting the spinal cord stimulus.

Surgical treatment

In comparison to cervical and lumbar herniations, disc herniations affecting the thoracic region require surgical treatment only in clinically selected cases due to the challenges associated with various approaches related to the thoracic region and the impossibility of posterior removal due to the anterior hernia's location relative to the spinal cord. Surgical procedure is performed using a microsurgical or endoscopic postero-lateral approach, laterally achievable through a transpedicular or costotransverse approach, depending on the median hernia's extension. This approach avoids any traction on spinal cord. Depending on type of approach and lateral osteo-articular extension, in addition to the risks of worsening motor-sensory disturbances, which require the use of intraoperative neurophysiological monitoring for control, there is also a risk of instability. This may necessitate transpedicular stabilization associated with the upper and lower vertebral levels relative to the hernia site.

28.2 Spinal traumatology

Spinal trauma can cause injuries to the vertebral osteo-ligamentous system, involving spinal cord. In some cases, spinal cord injury resulting from trauma is so severe that it precludes any possibility of functional recovery. In other cases, it is possible to

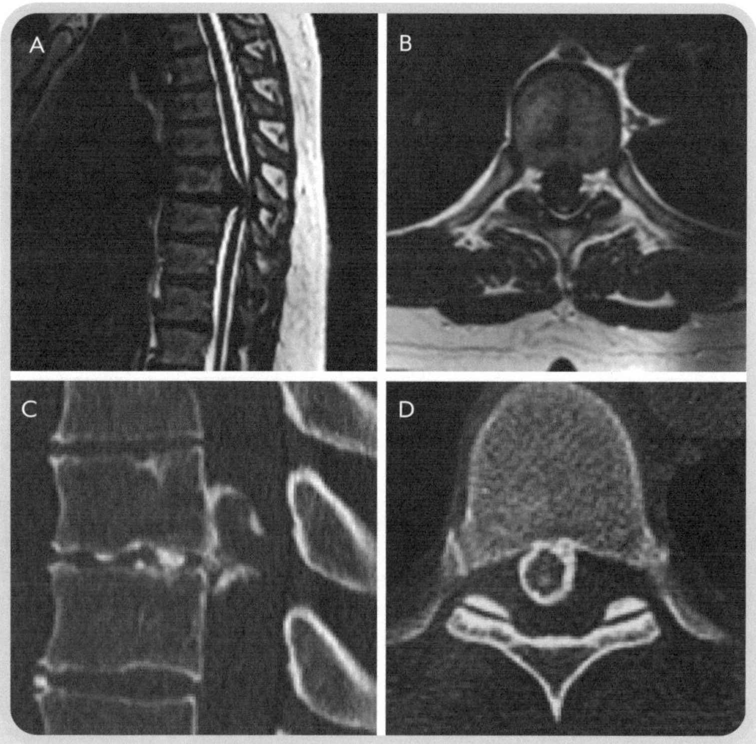

Figure 28.11

Dorsal hernia visualized through sagittal T2-weighted MRI sequences with compression and intramedullary signal distress (A-B), sagittal and axial CT sequences to evaluate the calcified component of the hernia (C-D).

improve functional prognosis by intervening early, decompressing the nervous tissue, and stabilizing vertebral fractures. Several factors need to be evaluated, including mode and location of the trauma, fracture's type, evolution of neurological damage, and associated clinical picture. In particular, osteo-ligamentous injuries of the spine generally involve fractures and dislocations, but they differ biomechanically and anatomopathologically depending on the segments involved.

It is important to consider that trauma capable of causing vertebral and spinal cord osteoligamentous injuries is characterized by energy sufficient to also damage other tissues and organs. Therefore, the approach to a polytraumatized patient should always be multidisciplinary.

The clinical picture is primarily characterized by pain, antalgic contraction, and functional limitation. Focal neurological signs may also be present, indicating myeloradicular involvement, such as paresis, paralysis, hyperexcitability of reflexes, sphincter disturbances, gait disorders, and hypoesthesia. A thorough neurological examination allows for the correct localization and assessment of extent of the lesion. Traumatic spinal injuries can involve spinal roots or the spinal cord when the injury affects cervical and dorsal spinal cord down to the first lumbar vertebra. Spinal cord injuries can be classified as complete, characterized by the absence of sensory-motor function in the segments caudal to the lesion, or incomplete, presenting with characteristic syndromes.

Incomplete spinal syndromes | Incomplete spinal *spinal cord syndromes* are commonly associated with hyperextension cervical injuries in patients with degenerative canal stenosis. Clinically, they are characterized by a predominant motor deficit in the upper limbs compared to the lower limbs and burning pain in the hands. *Anterior spinal syndrome* is generally associated with ischemic infarction in the territory of anterior spinal artery and is clinically characterized by tetraplegia (in cranial lesions at the C7 level) or paraplegia and dissociated sensory deficit below the lesion with loss of thermo-dolorific sensitivity (due to spinothalamic tract's damage) and sparing of discriminative, deep, and proprioceptive sensitivity. *Brown-*

Sequard syndrome, or hemisection of spinal cord syndrome, is characterized by ipsilateral and contralateral symptoms to the lesion. Ipsilaterally, there is motor paralysis below the lesion and loss of proprioceptive and vibratory sensation. Contralaterally, there is dissociated anesthesia characterized by loss of thermo-dolorific sensitivity (2-3 segments below the lesion due to interruption of the spinothalamic tract) and preserved tactile sensitivity. *Posterior spinal syndrome*, which is rather rare, is characterized by neck and trunk pain and paresthesia, as well as mild paresis in the lower limbs.

Radiological diagnosis

Standard spine X-rays, to be performed on entire spine or at the suspected site of injury, are essential. In presence of a demonstrated bone lesion or changes in the physiological alignment of the spine, a targeted CT scan is advisable. However, an MRI is imperative for evaluating integrity of nervous structures and capsuloligamentous structures. In selected cases, dynamic X-rays can highlight instabilities that may escape standard examinations.

Treatment

In case of spinal trauma, a first approach to the patient directly at trauma site is fundamental, correctly applying the first aid protocol. Immobilization with a cervical collar and transportation on a spinal board is imperative until arrival at hospital in order to avoid dislocations of any bone segments resulting from fractures. In case of high-impact polytrauma, upon arrival at emergency department, it is essential to stabilize the patient from a circulatory and internal medicine perspective and rule out multiorgan involvement before undertaking urgent neurosurgical treatments, to be performed urgently once the cardiovascular stability is achieved. Additionally, if a spinal cord injury is suspected, high-dose cortisone treatment may be recommended in the acute phase. The treatment of the injury, whether medical or surgical, should always have three main objectives: reduction of any dislocation (traction, manual or surgical reduction), spinal canal decompression (in the event that spinal cord or roots are compressed by disc material, bone, or blood), and stabilization of lesion (with surgical internal fixation or rigid external orthosis).

28.2.1 Cervical trauma

Cervical spine is characterized by significant mobility in both flexion-extension and axial rotation, as well as lateral inclination. In particular, the occipital condyles and the first two cervical vertebrae, atlas and axis, form the so-called occipito-cervical hinge, which experiences the highest percentage of axial rotation movements of head and neck. Considerable degree of mobility of cervical spine is the basis for the high percentage of observed traumas at this level (35% of spinal traumas), with automobile accidents being the main cause.

Traumatic injuries to the occipito-cervical hinge (C1-C2) constitute 25% of cervical traumatic injuries. At this level, atlanto-occipital dislocation and fractures of the occipital condyles are rare events, occasionally lethal, which can be observed in high-energy traumas. The most frequently observed fractures are those of C1 and C2. Fractures of C1 are generally considered stable as long as they are not associated with C2 fractures and typically occur as a result of axial trauma (diving accidents). They are characterized by a disruption of anterior and posterior arches of the atlas and lateral masses displacement. Fractures of C2 can take various forms, but the most common condition is a fracture of odontoid process (dens of the axis) (▪ Figure 28.12). Fractures of odontoid process can involve the base of dens or extend into vertebral body. Fractures of the pedicles of C2, or hangman's fractures, can exclusively involve bony structures or more often be associated with C2-C3 disc-ligamentous injuries.

Mechanisms that can cause fractures between C3 and C7 include compression, flexion-distraction, or rotation. Fractures can exclusively affect bony segments (vertebral bodies, lateral masses, pedicles, laminae, transverse or spinous processes) or involve disc-ligamentous structures (intervertebral discs, longitudinal ligaments). Often, multiple types of injuries are present in the same patient (▪ Figure 28.13 and 28.14 show preoperative images and treatment of post-traumatic cervical fracture-dislocation). At level of C7, flexion-extension traumas are very common. The most common symptomatology resulting from cervical trauma is whiplash, caused by a sudden flexion-extension movement of cervical spine, usually as a consequence of automobile accidents. The symptoms consist of neck pain, antalgic muscle contracture, functional limitation, often associated with sensory disturbances in the upper limbs, dizziness, and postural instability. Generally, there are no signs of myelopathy or radiculopathy.

Neurological signs appearance such as segmental deficits, paraparesis, tetraparesis, bladder and bowel dysfunction, hypo-hyperreflexia, spasticity, etc., suggests probable myeloradiculopathy involvement. In case of cervical trauma, patient should always be immobilized with a cervical collar until specific radiological investigations are performed. Cervical X-ray should always be the first investigation, including transoral projection. CT is recommended in high-energy traumas and in cases where a bone injury is demonstrated to properly characterize the fracture. MRI should be performed to assess the capsuloligamentous system and detect any post-traumatic hematomas.

Treatment

In cases of neurological compromise, spinal surgical decompression is imperative. This procedure should be combined with stabilization techniques aimed at restoring stability to the affected area. In absence of neurological compromise, the decision for surgical or conservative treatment depends on nature and type of trauma-related injury. The treatment for occipito-cervical junction injuries can be either conservative or surgical. Generally, isolated fractures of atlas are treated conservatively with immobilization using a rigid collar (such as a Halo-Vest) to be worn for at least 3 months. In cases of fractures of

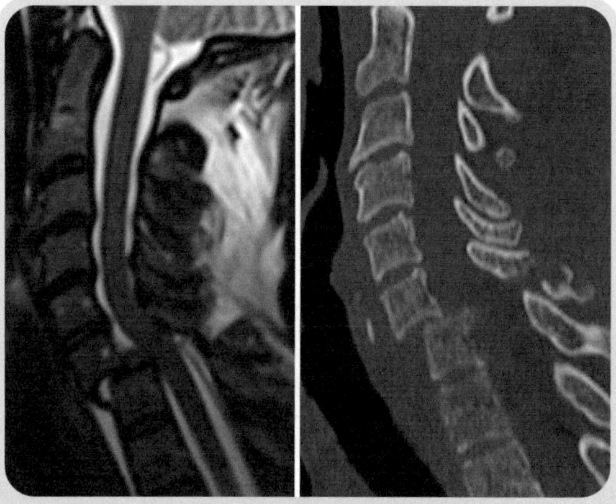

Figure 28.13

Sagittal MRI and CT images of a complex fracture with high instability and bilateral C6-C7 dislocation in a patient with trauma from a road accident.

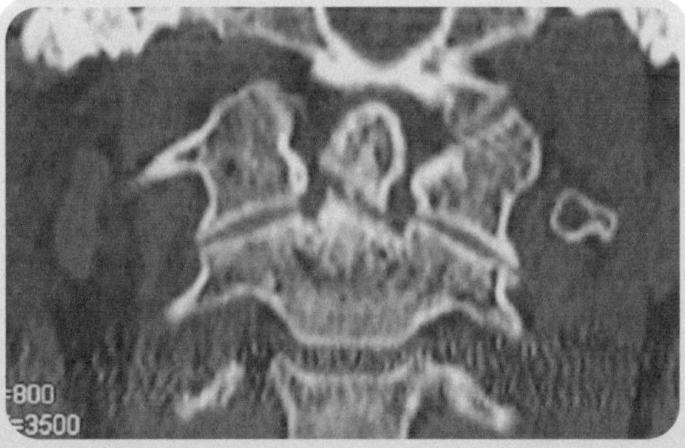

Figure 28.12

Fracture of the odontoid process: CT reconstructions in coronal sections of the craniospinal junction. Evidence of a fracture at the base of the C2 tooth with an oblique course, classifiable as an Anderson type II fracture.

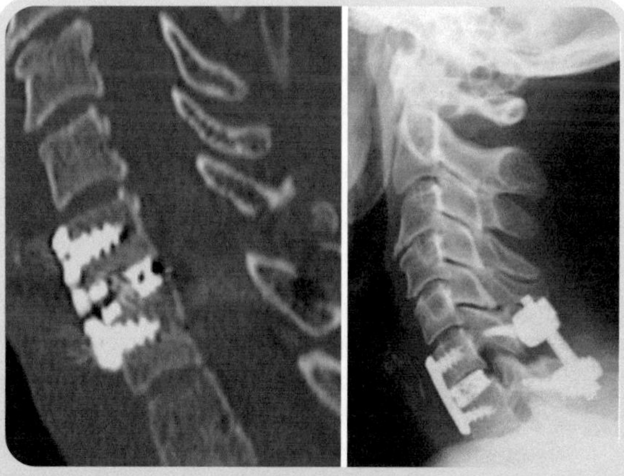

Figure 28.14

The postoperative CT and cervical X-ray results show correct realignment following the double anterior and posterior stabilization surgery.

axis (C2), the decision for surgery depends on anatomical integrity of the transverse ligament of atlas and type of fracture. In some cases, it is advisable to first attempt conservative treatment with immobilization using a collar and then proceed with surgical treatment if fracture does not heal.

Regarding treatment of C3-C7 injuries, anterior approach with vertebral body replacement and fixation using an anterior plate and screws is reserved for fractures with a high degree of fragment comminution, but with intact posterior ligamentous structures as demonstrated by MRI. On the other hand, this approach is associated with a subsequent posterior approach involving laminectomy and fixation with screws and rods in fractures that involve rupture of the posterior ligaments, aiming to restore the correct physiological curvature and ensure adequate spinal stability.

28.2.2 Dorsolumbar trauma

Dorsolumbar traumas constitute approximately 80% of all spinal traumas. Fractures involving these segments are the most common, mostly affecting T12, L1, and L2, which represent the thoracolumbar junction. They are more frequent in males and in adults. Mechanisms involved are similar to cervical fractures, including compression, flexion-distraction, and rotation.

Clinical symptoms are characterized by local, spontaneous pain caused by pressure on corresponding spinous process of the fracture site, as well as stiffness of the lumbar spine associated with antalgic muscle contractions. In cases of spinal cord involvement, segmental or cord-related neurological signs may be present. Diagnostic tests to be performed include X-ray of the thoracolumbar spine, CT scan with bone sequences, and MRI.

Most thoracolumbar vertebral fractures can be classified into four main types:

1) Compression fractures: These occur as a result of flexion-compression injuries, where anterior part of the vertebral body is crushed and deformed into a wedge shape.
2) Burst fractures: In these fractures, the vertebral body is compressed with a direction perpendicular to the vertebra, and fragments are pushed in all directions, potentially causing bone fragments to enter the spinal canal
3) Fracture-dislocations: These occur when severe ligamentous injury accompanies the bony lesion, causing a segment of spine to separate and move in any direction. These injuries are unstable and are often caused by compression, torsion, or severe tension.
4) Seatbelt fractures: These result from anterior flexion with an anterior fulcrum and are characterized by compression of anterior portion of the spine and distraction of intermediate and posterior portions. The injuries can involve bone or ligaments.

Treatment

Accurate classification of a vertebral fracture and identification of stable and unstable fractures are crucial factors in determining the appropriate treatment plan. A classic method for determining stability of thoracolumbar fractures is the theory of the three columns (Figure 28.15). Anterior column consists of anterior longitudinal ligament and anterior half of the vertebral body, disc, and annulus. Middle column consists of posterior half of the vertebral body, disc, and annulus, as well as posterior longitudinal ligament. Posterior column consists of facet joints, yellow ligament, interspinous ligaments, and supraspinous ligaments. Generally, a fracture is considered stable if only anterior column is involved, as is the case with most wedge fractures. When anterior and middle columns are involved, this type of fracture is considered more unstable. When all three columns are involved, this type of fracture is by definition considered unstable due to loss of integrity of the posterior stabilizing ligaments.

In fractures without spinal cord involvement, treatment can be either conservative or surgical, depending on type of injury and the pathogenetic mechanism. Generally, fractures defined as stable can benefit from conservative treatment with immobilization using a rigid orthosis; a valid alternative may be posterior surgical stabilization with a percutaneous technique. Other fractures, based on extensive involvement of capsuloligamentous and disc-articular structures, are considered unstable and require surgical treatment. In cases of spinal cord involvement, partial compromise requires urgent surgical decompression, to be performed within 12-24 hours of the trauma. Complete neurological compromise can be surgically treated depending on stabilization of the patient's general condition.

28.2.3 Vertebral-spinal cord tumors

Vertebral-spinal cord tumors are expansive processes of various origins that, during their development within spinal canal, exert compression on spinal cord and roots, generating a syndrome of spinal cord and/or radicular compression. The tumor can originate from the "container," namely the bone tissue, ligaments, tendons, and spinal joints, or from the "content," namely meningeal coverings, roots, and spinal cord. Therefore, spinal tumors are classified based on their location in relation to the spinal cord.

28.2.4 Spinal tumors

Spinal tumors are classified, based on their origin, into *primary* and *secondary* (metastatic), tumors. From the perspective of their tendency to proliferate and invade surrounding structures, they are further categorized into *benign* and *malignant bone tumors*. They represent approximately 10% of all skeletal neoplasms.

The classification adopted for primary spinal tumors is based on the histogenesis and the tumor's tendency to differentiate into different tissues during its growth. Therefore, they are categorized as benign forms, low malignancy forms, and malignant lesions.

Benign spinal tumors can be latent, active, or aggressive. They are further divided into three subgroups: *Stage I* (encapsulated tumors with minimal or no growth capacity); *Stage II* (benign tumors with slow growth and a pseudocapsule that tends to compress adjacent bone structures); and *Stage III* (tumors with an extremely thin capsule and a thick reactive pseudocapsule that tend to extend beyond the vertebral profiles).

Malignant tumors are divided into three major groups based on cell proliferation rate, each with two subgroups (A and B). Group IA describes neoplasms that border the vertebral structures without invading them, while group IB includes formations that invade paravertebral structures.

Groups II and III describe malignant neoplasms with a high cell turnover rate and a strong tendency to invade surrounding healthy tissues. Group III differs from Group II only in presence of metastasis.

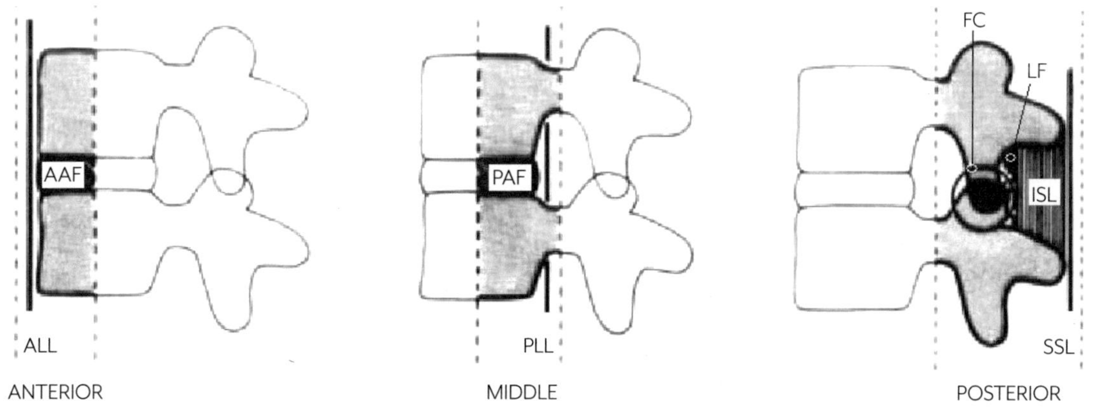

Figure 28.15

The concept of the three columns in the thoracolumbar spine. Generally, a lesion involving two columns (anterior and middle or middle and posterior) is considered unstable.

The majority of bone tumors are malignant, particularly in adults, while the pediatric population has a higher number of benign neoplasms.

Regarding primary malignant forms, the most frequent histotype is represented by chordoma. This neoplasm, which is itself rare (1-4% of all primary bone tumors), embryologically originates from remnants of the fetal dorsal notochordal tissue. Chordomas are typical in young adults, have a slow progression, and can cause a slowly progressive myeloradicular compression with insidious and gradual onset of spastic paraparesis or tetraparesis. They may have a tendency to transform into malignant forms. They are mainly localized at the cervical level of vertebral column, particularly at second vertebral metamere (C2). Microscopically, these neoplasms consist of filamentous cells surrounded by a gelatinous matrix produced by cells themselves.

The diagnosis is based on contrast-enhanced MRI. Additionally, they exhibit significant resistance to radiation therapy and chemotherapy. For this reason, the goal of surgical removal remains complete excision with clear margins, although this is not always feasible.

Among primary malignant spinal lesions, multiple myeloma is one that predominantly affects males and manifests when systemic disease is in an advanced stage. The typical symptoms of multiple myeloma include back pain (rachialgia) and neurological disorders resulting from compression of spinal nerves or vertebral fractures that may occur as a consequence. Treatment should involve decompression of nerve structures, as radical removal of lesion as possible, and subsequent specific medical therapy to control the underlying disease. Ewing's sarcoma, chondrosarcomas, and osteosarcomas cause progressively worsening symptoms, characterized by deep, dull, poorly localized pain typically referred to midline, which worsens at night. This is followed by sudden onset of paraparesis or tetraparesis with sphincter disturbances. These lesions are radiosensitive but exhibit relentlessly progressive evolution.

Skeletal tissue, particularly the vertebral segments, represents the most common site of metastasis development after the lungs and liver. Vertebral metastases are more frequent compared to primary tumors. The tumors that most frequently metastasize to vertebral level, in descending order, are prostate, breast, kidney, lung, and thyroid. The age group most affected is between 50 and 70 years, with a male predominance. Thoracic region is the most frequently involved segment, followed by lumbosacral and cervical regions. The most frequent anatomical site is the vertebral body, which is rich in red marrow.

Radiologically, vertebral metastases can be divided into lytic, sclerotic, or mixed lesions. Osteolytic forms demonstrate aggressive behavior with variable growth rates and early vertebral collapse. Sclerotic forms are mainly secondary to dissemination of carcinomatous cells originating from the prostate or gastrointestinal tract. The use of contrast-enhanced MRI allows for early detection of edematous phenomena and replacement of intraspongious marrow with highly cellular neoplastic tissue (■ Figure 28.16). In cases of vertebral collapse with subsequent spinal cord compression, early decompressive spinal cord surgery is necessary through a posterior approach (decompressive laminectomy) to prevent spinal cord injury that could lead to irreversible neurological deficits.

Among benign vertebral tumors, the most common histotype is osteoid osteoma, characterized by the presence of unique osteoid tissue surrounded by an inflammatory-exudative reaction of peritumoral soft tissues. It is relatively frequent (10% of all benign bone neoplasms) and is mainly located in the lumbar spine, typically originating from laminae in most cases. The most characteristic and nearly constant symptom of these neoplasms is pain (usually nocturnal) that responds to use of nonsteroidal anti-inflammatory drugs (NSAIDs). Histologically, these lesions consist of closely packed trabeculae immersed in a densely cellular tissue containing osteoblasts, osteoclasts, and numerous interposed capillaries. Primary angiomas in the vertebral bodies, generally in thoracolumbar region, are rare and typical in young individuals. They are generally asymptomatic as they remain confined to vertebral body but can cause local or radicular pain when extending into the

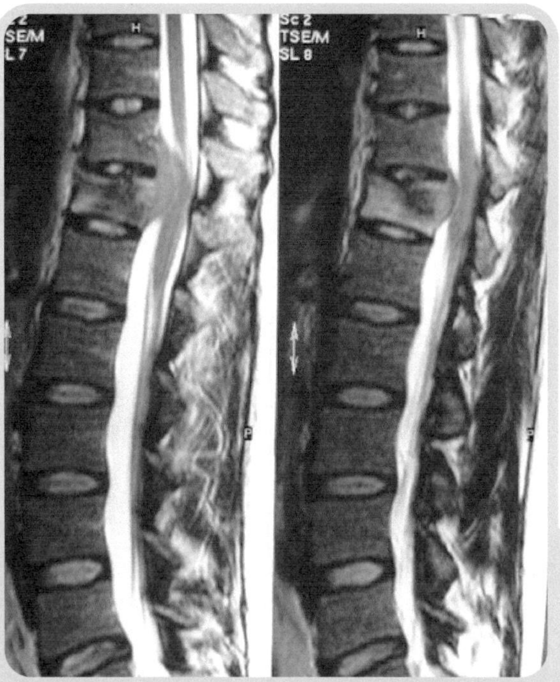

Figure 28.16

Dorsal metastasis: MRI examination with sagittal T2 sequences; evidence of T12 fracture due to substitutive lesion from breast cancer with protruding material occupying the spinal canal, causing compression on the neurological structures.

endospecular region. The diagnosis is primarily based on MRI and CT scans, which reveal erosive bone lesions and invasion into the spinal canal. If symptomatic, they are treated with radiotherapy and possible surgical excision.

28.2.5 Intradural extramedullary tumors

These are the most commonly observed spinal cord tumors, accounting for approximately 51% of all spinal tumors. They originate and develop within the dural sac but outside the spinal cord. They are generally benign tumors that compress and displace spinal cord without invading it. They consist of 70-80% meningiomas and schwannomas, while the remaining 20-30% includes amartomas, neuroblastomas, metastases, melanocytomas, teratomas, and chordomas. Most patients experience a slowly progressive course characterized initially by the onset of pain, followed by the emergence of radicular symptoms, and finally myelopathy with appearance of sphincter disturbances. Occurrence of hydrocephalus as the first symptom of these neoplasms is an extremely rare condition but described in literature, and it is due to an obstruction of normal cerebrospinal fluid outflow pathways. Generally, intradural extramedullary neoplasms (particularly meningiomas) develop in the thoracic spine (47%), cervical spine (26%), lumbar spine (23%), and sacral spine (4%).

Meningiomas | Are benign tumors and represent the most common intradural extramedullary lesions. They can occur as solitary or multiple lesions (in the context of syndromic diseases such as neurofibromatosis type II). They have a peak incidence after the age of 50 and are more prevalent in females than males (M : F = 1 : 3). They are generally located in the dorsal portion of spinal cord (▯ Figure 28.17). They typically appear as a round mass with a smooth surface that diffusely and homogeneously enhances with contrast on MRI, exhibiting endoscapular extrusion. Infiltrative forms within the spinal cord are extremely rare. The histological variants are the same as those found in intracranial forms. Surgical therapy is necessary, involving tumor removal along with its base of attachment and subsequent dural reconstruction. Complete removal of lesion has an excellent prognosis.

Neurinomas | Also known as "schwannomas," are benign tumors that originate from the sheath surrounding the spinal root after it emerges from spinal cord (▯ Figure 28.18). They mostly derive from sensory root, although forms originating from motor root are not uncommon. Their growth is non-infiltrative and generally results in compression and displacement of adjacent structures, spinal cord, or roots. They have the highest incidence between the ages of 30 and 60 and can have a genetic predisposition, as they are typical of neurofibromatosis type II. Symptomatically, they cause localized radicular pain at one or multiple levels, depending on the extent within the canal and the number of roots affected by compression. Symptoms of spinal cord compromise appear later. If diagnosis is not promptly made, there

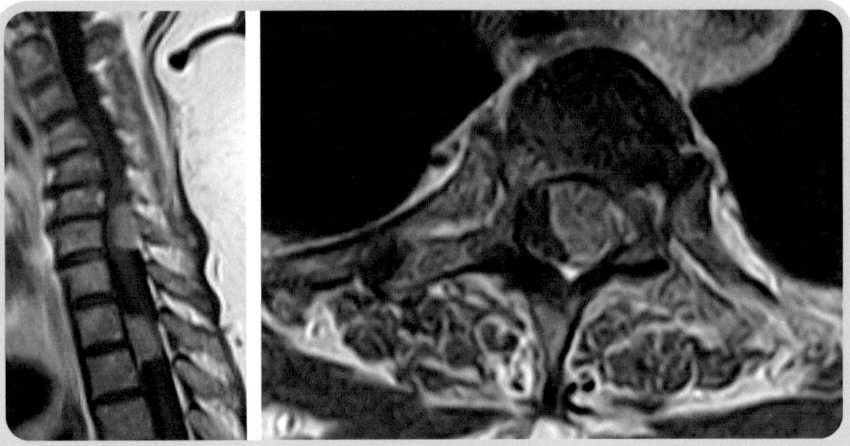

Figure 28.17

Cervico-dorsal MRI with gadolinium administration shows the presence of two meningiomas at the C6-C7 and D2-D3 levels in a patient with severe spastic paraparesis affecting the lower limbs. The axial sequence reveals marked intradural extramedullary compression caused by the meningioma at the D2-D3 level, with rightward displacement of the spinal cord.

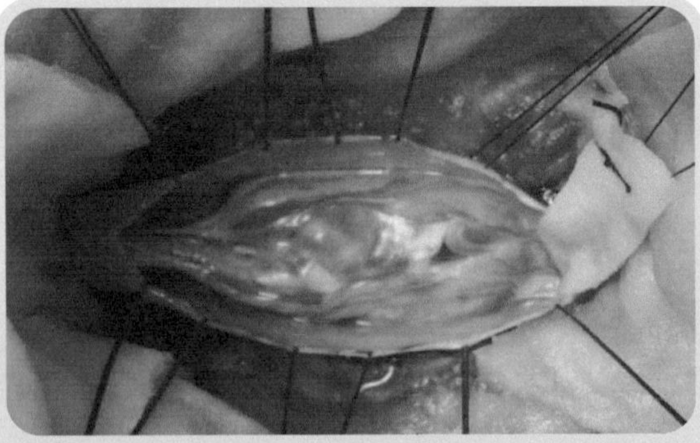

Figure 28.18

Intradural tumor; Intradural extramedullary lesion; Histological examination: Schwannoma.

is a progressive worsening of symptoms that can lead to complete paralysis with total anesthesia. Other, though rarer forms, are represented by lipomas, mostly located at the cervical level.

28.2.6 Intradural intramedullary tumors

Intradural intramedullary tumors represent approximately 20% of all intradural tumors and about 2-4% of Central Nervous System tumors. Epidemiologically, ependymomas are the most common neoplasms, followed by astrocytomas, angioblastomas, hamartomas, glioependymal cysts, and metastases, which represent the rarest type of intramedullary tumor (Table 28.3).

Table 28.3 INCIDENCE OF INTRAMEDULLARY TUMORS

Tumor	Incidence
Ependymoma	30-40%
Astrocytoma	25-30%
Hemangioblastoma	2-15%
Ependymal cyst	2-5%
Metastasis	1-2%

They develop within the spinal cord, meaning they are intrinsic to the spinal cord. Clinical presentation of these neoplasms is deeply influenced by various factors such as size and location of the tumor, rate of growth, and histological grading. The clinical picture has a subtle onset, with pain localized to middle region of the back, without radiation, followed by appearance of cord symptoms characterized by paresthesia, pain, and sensory disturbances below the level of the lesion. Motor deficits only appear later.

Approximately 36% of intramedullary lesions are located in the cervical spine, 50% in the thoracic region, and 14% in the conus medullaris. The peak incidence occurs approximately in the fourth decade of life. The onset of symptoms is characterized by a slow and progressive development of neurological symptoms without remission phases.

Ependymomas | Can be found at all levels of the spinal cord, usually extending over a single spinal segment, although they can reach multiple segments in size. The tumor has an intramedullary extrusion, with a well-defined macroscopic appearance compared to surrounding spinal cord, but without a distinct capsule separating it from surrounding healthy tissue (to which they tend to be firmly adhered). However, some forms have a notable infiltrative tendency. Those located at the level of the filum terminale are particular forms that can reach significant sizes, giving rise to cauda equina syndrome, but they are obviously extramedullary. Macroscopically, they appear as reddish-colored lesions. Microscopically, the cells of an ependymoma tend to form cell clusters (pseudo-rosettes) surrounded by blood vessels. Four main subgroups of ependymoma are distinguished: cellular, clear cell, papillary, and tanycytic.

Astrocytomas | Are less common and present the same histological characteristics as their cerebral counterparts and similar malignant features. They tend to localize more frequently at cervical spine and thoracic region. The peak incidence is between 10 and 30 years of age, with a higher incidence in males (M:F = 2:1). The most common histological variants are pilocytic astrocytoma (WHO grade I-II) and anaplastic astrocytoma (WHO grade III). Intradural glioblastomas are very rare.

The therapeutic goal remains surgical removal, especially in cases of low-grade ependymomas and astrocytomas. For high-grade forms, current guidelines recommend biopsy, followed by chemotherapy and radiotherapy. High-grade malignant forms have an unfavorable prognosis.

Diagnosis

The diagnosis is primarily clinical and instrumental, as specific symptoms should always be followed by a detailed analysis of radiological examinations. Regarding ependymomas, execution of contrast-enhanced MRI is crucial, which in most cases reveals homogeneously enhancing, well-circumscribed lesions, within which cystic cavities and intralesional hemorrhages may develop (Figure 28.19). Sometimes these neoplasms can be associated with dilations of the ependymal canal (hydromyelia) or true intramedullary cavities called "syrinxes" (syringomyelia) that are not delimited by ependymal cells. In T1-weighted sequences without contrast, these neoplasms present an isointense signal compared to healthy spinal cord tissue, while in T2-weighted sequences, they generally appear hyperintense. The role of contrast-enhanced CT is limited to bony lesions. Another important examination to perform is motor and somatosensory evoked potentials in order to assess the functionality of central motor and somatosensory pathways preoperatively and intraoperatively.

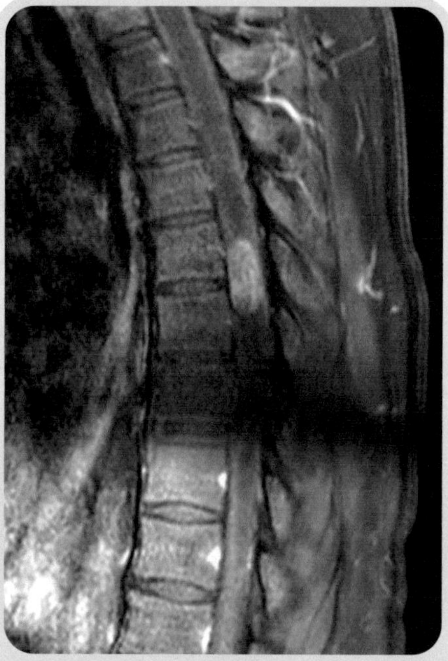

Figure 28.19

Intramidullary MRI with contrast medium showing the presence of a uniformly enhancing oval neoformation (radiological suspicion of intramedullary ependymoma).

Surgical treatment of intramedullary lesions and reduction of surgical risks

The surgical treatment of intramedullary lesions is exclusively performed through a posterior approach with patient in a prone position. Once patient's positioning is completed, the level of lesion is identified intraoperatively through fluoroscopic control. After making a midline linear skin incision, the paravertebral muscles are "skeletonized" subperiosteally to achieve proper exposure of vertebral laminae, which are subsequently removed to ensure adequate exposure of spinal cord. Once the dura mater is incised and its flaps are suspended to prevent epidural bleeding, intraoperative neurophysiological monitoring is used to identify the midline raphe of spinal cord (the point where SSEPs [somatosensory evoked potentials] exhibit equivalent voltage and symmetric graphical pattern) to avoid damaging the gracile and cuneate fasciculi (important ascending pathways for transmitting peripheral sensory information). The identification of the neoplasm can be facilitated by the use of intraoperative ultrasound, which identifies ependymomas as circumscribed areas of endomedullary hyperechogenicity. Subsequently, a cleavage plane of lesion is identified in relation to the surrounding spinal cord parenchyma, avoiding damage to the latter during surgical procedure with excessive traction (■ Figure 28.20).

Neurophysiological monitoring is necessary during surgical resection, particularly using SSEPs (somatosensory evoked potentials) and MEPs (motor evoked potentials), with D wave intraoperative monitoring evoked by motor pathway stimulation. The latter, recorded by placing an epidural electrode downstream from the lesion, represents the only currently known prognostic factor for motor function in surgery for intramedullary neoplasms. A reduction in voltage, equal to or greater than 50% of the intraoperatively recorded D wave, is associated with a low probability of postoperative motor function recovery. Conversely, if intraoperative voltage variations of the D wave are less than 50%, the chances of motor function recovery in the postoperative course are quite high, even in cases of missed MEP registration.

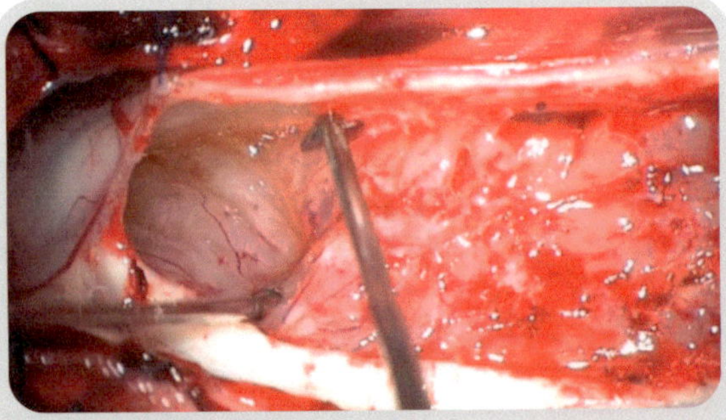

Figure 28.20

Intramedullary ependymoma resection, the lesion appears firmly adhered to the surrounding healthy tissue.

Therapy

Treatment of spinal cord and vertebral lesions differs in cases of benign or malignant lesions. In most cases, surgical treatment remains the main approach, which can be followed by radiation therapy and chemotherapy.

Benign lesions | Benign bone lesions are generally treated with pharmacological therapies for pain reduction. Surgical excision is reserved for lesions that do not respond to medical therapy. Benign intradural extramedullary or intramedullary lesions require total surgical excision, as complete removal leads to complete patient recovery. In cases of intramedullary lesions, the surgical risk of neurological deficits is quite high, as is the incidence of local disease recurrence.

Malignant lesions | Surgical treatment should involve complete removal of lesion to avoid the risk of recurrence. Regarding intramedullary glial tumors, complete removal is often not possible. In many cases, surgical cytoreduction is preferred, followed by dural reconstruction and subsequent radiation therapy and chemotherapy. Even in patients where surgical removal appears to be microscopically total, radiation therapy and chemotherapy should be performed to prevent or control local disease recurrence as much as possible. However, prognosis for these lesions is generally poor.

Bibliography

Benzel E., Spine Surgery: Techniques, Complication Avoidance, and Management, 2 Vol. Elsevier, 2004.

Dal Pozzo G., Risonanza Magnetica-Cranio e Rachide, UTET, 2007.

Deletis V., Shils J., Neurophysiology in Neurosurgery, Academic Press, 2002.

Delfini R., Cantore G.P.: Appropriatezza della diagnosi e del trattamento chirurgico dell'ernia del disco lombare sintomatica: linee guida regione Lazio- PNLG9, 2005 (agg. Ottobre 2008).

Delfini R., Landi A., Manuale pratico di terapia dell'ernia del disco, Esculapio, 2014.

Fessler RG, Atlas of Neurosurgical techniques, 2006.

Klekamp J., Samii M., Surgery of spinal tumours, Springer, 2007.

Winn H. et al., Youmans Neurological Surgery - Manual, Saunders, 2011.

Vaccaro AR, Spine surgery, 2008.

Vaccaro AR et al. Lumbar spinal stenosis: how is it classified? J Am Acad Orthop Surg, 2016.

29 CEREBROSPINAL FLUID CIRCULATION DISORDERS

Sergio Paolini, Paolo Missori

29.1 Brief overview of cerebrospinal fluid physiology

Cerebrospinal fluid (CSF), also known as "liquor" permeates the entire subarachnoid space, filling the void between the brain and the meninges. The main function of CSF is to dissipate energy and provide protection to the intracranial structures during sudden accelerations, such as in head trauma. In addition to its mechanical functions, CSF also plays trophic and immunological roles.

CSF is continuously produced (approximately 400 to 500 ml every 24 hours) by the choroid plexuses located within the ventricles. Considering that the total CSF volume in the intracranial and spinal spaces is approximately 140 ml, it is evident that this volume can only be maintained through a continuous process of CSF reabsorption. This reabsorption occurs at the cranial convexity, where specialized structures called arachnoid granulations or villi are located within the dura mater. Through a complex and not yet fully understood process of filtration, the arachnoid villi channel the absorbed CSF into the veins of the dura mater and, ultimately, into the superior sagittal sinus. Thus, there is a correlation between central venous pressure, CSF volume, and intracranial pressure.

The "CSF circulation" is the pathway that CSF takes from its site of production to its site of reabsorption. Simplifying, CSF produced in a lateral ventricle reaches the third ventricle by passing through the respective foramen of Monro, then reaches the fourth ventricle through the Sylvian aqueduct, and traverses the basal subarachnoid spaces through the foramina of Luschka and Magendie; It diffusely flows through the subarachnoid spaces of the convexity and reaches the arachnoid granulations. Part of the CSF is displaced into the spinal canal at the perimedullary level. The transfer of CSF from the intracranial compartment to the spinal compartment is one of the body's earliest and most effective mechanisms to counteract increases in intracranial pressure. However, it should be noted that the basic model of CSF circulation has been repeatedly challenged in favor of the theory that suggests the diffusion of cerebrospinal fluid from production sites (choroid plexuses) and its reabsorption in other anatomical locations (Pacchionian granulations, lumbar perispinal space, cribriform plate of the frontal base). CSF movement is generated only by the cardiac cycle during systole/diastole, transmitting pressure waves into the cerebral circulation. The secondary effect is a continuous pulsatility on the CSF, which "beats" synchronously with cardiac action. Systole and diastole indirectly generate the rapid movement of CSF through narrower anatomical passages such as the foramen of Monro, Sylvian aqueduct, and foramina of Luschka and Magendie.

29.2 Hydrocephalus

The term hydrocephalus generally refers to an abnormal accumulation of cerebrospinal fluid within the intracranial space. The site of accumulation is almost always intraventricular, which is why it is customary to identify hydrocephalus with intraventricular dilation. However, there is also an "external" hydrocephalus, where the accumulation of CSF occurs in the subarachnoid spaces, resulting in equally pathological effects.

Hydrocephalus can be caused by a disturbance in CSF production, circulation, or reabsorption. There are conditions in which the increase in intracranial CSF content does not reflect a circulation disorder but rather an accumulation of CSF or ventricular dilation, which is passively favored by various types of parenchymal agenesis or malacia (resulting from hemorrhages, ischemia, or surgical cavities). The term "ex vacuo hydrocephalus" historically referred to these cases, although it is inappropriate.

Hydrocephalus can be classically classified as *communicating* or *non-communicating*, with the terminology referring to the presence of communication between the ventricles and the subarachnoid space. Another distinction can be made based on a morphological criterion, namely the number of ventricles affected by dilation: tetraventricular, triventricular, biventricular, monoventricular. Both criteria are widely used in clinical practice to synthetically define the type of hydrocephalus, but it is evident that the optimal treatment always derives from a precise understanding of the etiological aspect of hydrocephalus.

Causes of hydrocephalus

The mechanisms by which hydrocephalus can occur are always associated with a pathology of CSF circulation. The possibilities are easy to remember and have therapeutic implications:

- Circulation defect (obstructive hydrocephalus)
- Reabsorption blockage (aresorptive hydrocephalus)
- Excessive production (hypersecretory hydrocephalus)

29.2.1 Obstructive hydrocephalus

Many cases of hydrocephalus observed in clinical practice are due to obstacles in CSF circulation. Blockage of CSF circulation most commonly occurs at certain anatomical narrowings: the foramina of Monro, Sylvian aqueduct, and the foramina of Luschka and Magendie. The caliber of these passages is inherently small, and any compromise can easily result in blockage of CSF circulation. The narrowing of a foramen or the Sylvian aqueduct may be due to:

a) True "obstruction" (reduction in caliber due to endoluminal masses). An example is

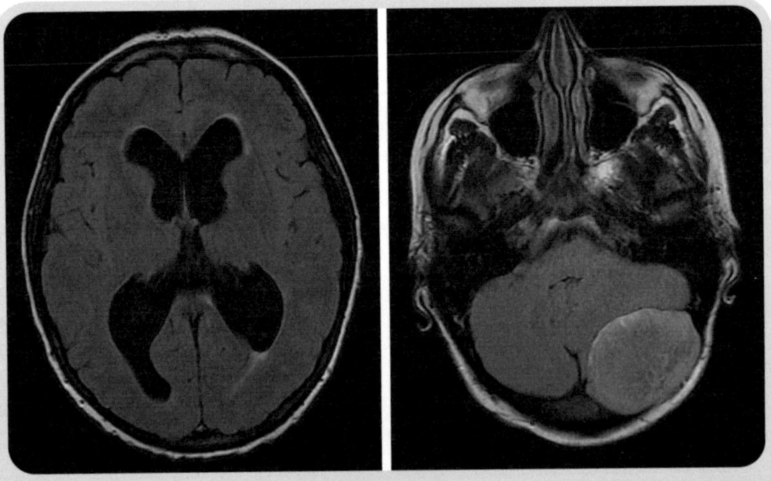

Figure 29.1

48-year-old woman in whom axial MRI (left panel) shows marked dilation of the supratentorial ventricular system, with flattening of the cerebral convolutions and initial subependymal periventricular frontal alteration. In the posterior cranial fossa (right panel), there is a large mass that compresses and displaces the fourth ventricle, resulting in triventricular obstructive hydrocephalus from the previous scan.

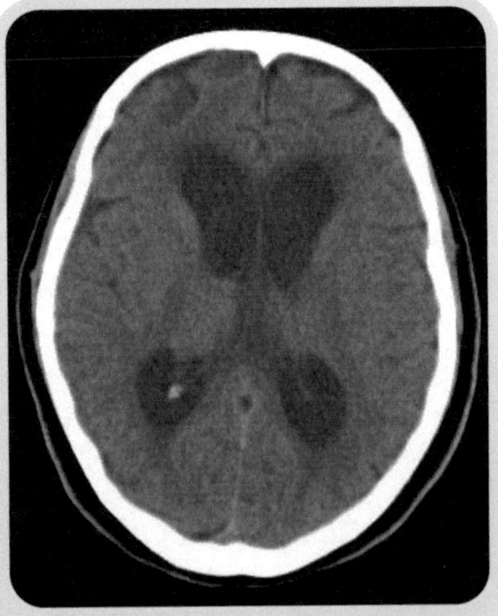

Figure 29.2

CT scan of a 53-year-old patient six weeks after a subarachnoid hemorrhage due to rupture of a basilar apex aneurysm. Hydrocephalus is secondary to the obstruction of cerebrospinal fluid reabsorption pathways.

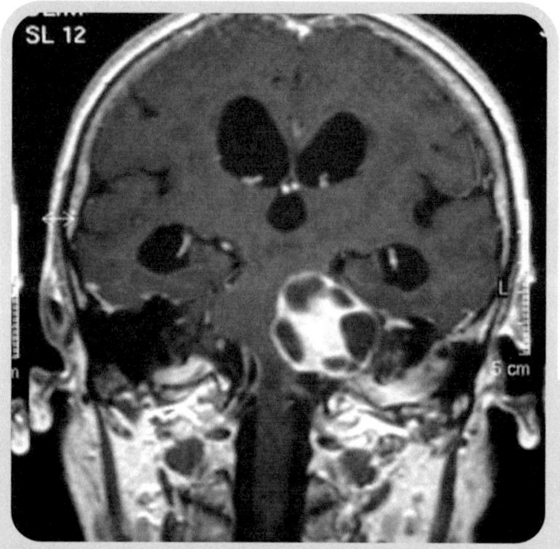

Figure 29.3

RM, coronal scan. Extrinsic mass (vestibular schwannoma) in the posterior cranial fossa, causing compression of the brainstem and secondary ventricular dilation.

hydrocephalus resulting from the presence of expansive lesions (tumors, infectious or other types of embryonic cysts) or hematomas within the ventricles (Figure 29.1 and 29.2);

b) Compressions (reduction in caliber due to extrinsic compression on the luminal walls). The most typical and frequent example is tri- or tetraventricular hydrocephalus resulting from compression on the brainstem by extrinsic masses located infratentorially (e.g., acoustic neuroma) (Figure 29.3);
c) Stenosis (intrinsic reduction in caliber). Rare and mostly pediatric cases involve idiopathic stenosis of the Sylvian aqueduct. In adults, stenosis of the foramina can occur as a consequence of scarring processes following subarachnoid hemorrhages or meningitis.

29.2.2 Aresorptive hydrocephalus

The most typical form of hydrocephalus resulting from compromised CSF reabsorption is the one that can follow subarachnoid hemorrhage. In these cases, it is believed that subarachnoid blood, upon reaching the cranial convexity, causes micro-obstruction and progressive fibrosis of the arachnoid villi, compromising their function. Subarachnoid hemorrhage, one of the most frequent causes of hydrocephalus, can, therefore, lead to ventricular dilation with multiple and often concurrent mechanisms, including acute ventricular cavity obstruction, stenosis of the ventricular cavities, basal subarachnoid adhesions, and fibrosis of the arachnoid villi.

There are at least three other less frequent but equally important forms of aresorptive hydrocephalus:

a) Hydrocephalus due to venous hypertension: Arachnoid villi drain into the superior sagittal sinus. Thus, a significant increase in pressure within the sinus, resulting from thrombotic events or venous hypertension of various origins (e.g., jugular foramen stenosis), can lead to impaired functioning of the villi and subsequent hydrocephalus.
b) Post-irradiation hydrocephalus: In some cases, radiation therapy to the brain can cause fibrosis of the arachnoid villi.
c) Hydrocephalus condition implied in the concept of "shunt dependency": It is known that chronic drainage of a ventricular cavity (e.g., ventriculoperitoneal shunting) not only bypasses the defective CSF outflow system but also renders the arachnoid granulations' reabsorption system inactive. This phenomenon tends to generate progressive fibrosis of the villi and becomes irreversible over time (months or years) after shunt implantation. Consequently, patients generally become dependent on the shunt, regardless of the reason for its placement.

29.2.3 Hypersecretory hydrocephalus

Excessive production of cerebrospinal fluid (CSF) occurs in the presence of a papilloma, a functioning tumor of the choroid plexus. This is an extremely rare occurrence.

Diagnosis

The diagnosis of hydrocephalus is essential through neuroimaging. Both CT and MRI show ventricular dilation, which initially primarily affects the frontal horns. To differentiate ventriculomegaly (enlargement of the ventricular cavities) from hydrocephalus, the measurement of the Evans index is a fundamental radiological criterion for a possible diagnosis of hydrocephalus. Therefore, it is necessary to measure the ratio of the maximum width of the frontal horns at the level of the foramen of Monro to the maximum width of the inner table of the skull (Figure 29.4). Often, an alteration in the signal of the periventricular brain parenchyma coexists (hypodensity on CT and hyperintensity on T2-weighted sequences and hypointensity on T1-weighted sequences of MRI), reflecting the so-called "transependymal resorption".

However, it should be noted that although radiological investigations are necessary, they are not always sufficient for the diagnosis and treatment of hydrocephalus. Many individuals in good health may have idiopathic ventricular dilation, congenital ventricular dilation, or dilation associated with ex vacuo phenomena. Furthermore, ventricles that have undergone hydrocephalic dilation may maintain increased sizes regardless of the actual pressure of CSF within them. Therefore, it is always essential to correlate the radiological findings with clinical data. In the absence of convincing correlation, ventricular dilation should be considered suspicious, especially if it is of recent onset and if the dilation has occurred rapidly.

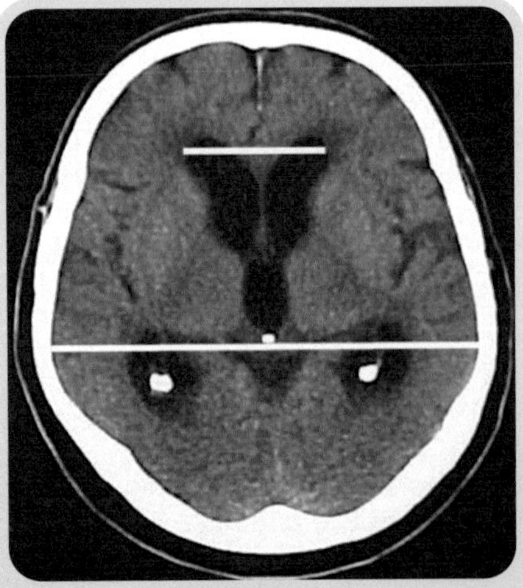

Figure 29.4

The Evans Index is calculated by dividing the measurement of the maximum dilation of the frontal horns at the level of the foramen of Monro by the maximum width of the inner table of the skull: 4.1/12.9 = 0.31. A value greater than 0.30 indicates the radiological diagnosis of hydrocephalus.

Clinical presentation

Acute hydrocephalus | Untreated hydrocephalus (except for rare "compensated" forms) can be fatal. Based on simple considerations of CSF physiology, the human body produces between 400 and 500 ml of CSF daily, while the normal CSF volume in the central nervous system is approximately 140 ml. Consequently, CSF is substantially replaced more than three times a day, and the mechanism by which this occurs does not tolerate inefficiencies. The slightest imbalance between CSF inflow and outflow results in an excess of volume and, therefore, intolerable intracranial pressure.

For this reason, the symptoms of acute hydrocephalus are essentially those of intracranial hypertension. Unlike other cases of intracranial hypertension, in the absence of specific lesions, there may be no focal neurological symptoms. Patients with hydrocephalus may experience headache, lethargy, disorientation, diplopia, vomiting, and alterations in consciousness ranging from drowsiness to coma.

The timing and progression of symptoms can vary. Acute hydrocephalus resulting from a significant blockage of CSF circulation is a true neurosurgical emergency, and clinical manifestations can worsen within minutes. In such cases, neurosurgeons urgently apply an external CSF diversion to immediately decompress the severely compressed brain parenchyma. In other cases, patients go through phases of relative compensation, allowing symptoms to remain stable for several weeks. Unlike other cases of intracranial hypertension, in the absence of specific lesions, there may be no focal neurological symptoms.

Chronic hydrocephalus | In cases where a patient develops slowly progressing hydrocephalus, the symptoms can be highly variable, going unnoticed or misinterpreted for a long time. These symptoms may include behavioral disturbances, a possible frontal syndrome (disinhibition), aggressiveness, short-term memory deficits, gait disturbances, drowsiness, frequent urination, and even urgent or urinary incontinence, constipation, and parkinsonism.

Treatment

The treatment for hydrocephalus is surgical. Some diuretics, particularly acetazolamide, are occasionally used to reduce intracranial CSF volume but have limited efficacy and purely palliative value. Whenever possible, etiological therapy is the preferred choice. The removal of a posterior fossa tumor is the most effective and definitive method for resolving hydrocephalus secondary to the tumor itself. Similarly, the removal of an intraventricular clot can be the definitive solution for hemorrhagic hydrocephalus. When etiological therapy is not possible or fails to produce immediate effects, CSF diversion becomes necessary. CSF, continuously produced by the choroid plexus even under conditions of intracranial hypertension, needs to be redirected elsewhere. In emergency cases or whenever permanent CSF diversion is not feasible or advisable, diversion is carried out externally through the insertion of a drainage system into a lateral ventricle.

When hydrocephalus is considered irreversible, and the patient's clinical conditions allow for it, internal diversion is performed. The ventricular CSF is redirected, using a subcutaneous draining system with appropriate pressure calibration, to a strictly sterile body cavity where it can be gradually absorbed by the tissues. The peritoneal cavity is usually the first choice, followed by the atrial cavity.

A particularly advantageous form of CSF diversion, when feasible, is the application of a *by-pass* obtained by endoscopically fenestrating the anterior part of the floor of the third ventricle. In this way, CSF can bypass the fourth ventricle, directly reach the subarachnoid space at the interpeduncular cistern, and proceed to the cranial convexity. This procedure is very beneficial because it allows for the treatment of hydrocephalus without leaving foreign bodies (such as internal drainage systems). However, it is evident that the only suitable condition with reasonable chances of success for endoscopic ventriculostomy is obstructive triventricular or tetraventricular hydrocephalus.

29.2.4 "Normal pressure" hydrocephalus

"Normal pressure" hydrocephalus is a clinical condition with debated characteristics and still partly unknown aspects. It is typical of advanced age and is characterized by tetraventricular dilation that communicates and manifests with chronic symptoms. The ventricular dilation in question, although potentially suitable for surgical treatment, needs to be investigated without the need for urgent drainage, as in the majority of hydrocephalus cases. The symptoms of "normal pressure" hydrocephalus are summarized in Hakim's classic triad:

- *Gait disturbance.* Typically, this is the earliest symptom. The gait is typically bradykinetic with a broad base.
- *Urinary incontinence.* It can range in severity from urgency to complete incontinence.
- *Cognitive decline.* It usually begins with decreased attention and memory, sluggishness, and decreased initiative. It gradually progresses to frank dementia.

These symptoms can vary in combination, appear in a variable sequence, and do not exhaust the clinical picture of "normal pressure" hydrocephalus. In male patients, a frequent and relatively underrecognized symptom is decreased libido, resulting in sexual dysfunction.

Diagnosis

The correct diagnostic classification of "normal pressure" hydrocephalus poses difficulties. Even in the presence of symptomatic hydrocephalus, the radiological and clinical pictures are rather nonspecific. Ventricular dilation is a result that remains within certain physiological limits in the average elderly population due to normal brain atrophy. Urinary incontinence, motor impairment, and cognitive decline enter the differential diagnosis with various conditions typical of advanced age (urological dysfunctions, cervical myelopathy, encephalovasculopathy, other types of dementia). Although the presence of ventriculomegaly with transependymal resorption and Hakim's classic triad are suggestive of the diagnosis, instrumental confirmation is necessary. Various techniques have been used over time, including CSF infusion tests, myelo-CT with study of CSF dynamics, radionuclide cisternography, and CSF depletion tests. The intrathecal infusion test (Katzman test) is performed by introducing a saline solution into the lumbar subarachnoid space at a constant speed and simultaneously measuring the cerebrospinal fluid pressure. Patients with a resistance to outflow ranging from 12 to 19 mm Hg/ml/min may show clinical improvement after surgery. This method requires extensive and prolonged experience and the use of computer systems. Currently, the most sensitive and specific test for diagnosing hydrocephalus is CSF depletion through lumbar puncture, the so-called tap test. Since "normal pressure" hydrocephalus is a communicative condition, the removal of 30-50 ml of CSF via lumbar puncture temporarily simulates the effects of a ventriculoperitoneal shunt. The test is considered positive when the patient shows a significant and objective improvement in symptoms in the hours following lumbar puncture.

Differential diagnosis

There are many conditions in which ventricular dilation (secondary hydrocephalus) can be present concomitantly with degenerative neurological diseases (Table 29.1). This condition is often complicated by a clinical-neurological picture that is frequently similar to that of primary hydrocephalus. Specialized expertise and preoperative tests contribute to guiding the clinician, with greater likelihood, towards a correct diagnosis. However, diagnostic certainty can only be guaranteed during follow-up, where the definitive determination between primary hydrocephalus and secondary hydrocephalus in degenerative disease can be established.

Table 29.1 NEUROLOGICAL DISEASES ASSOCIATED WITH VENTRICULAR SYSTEM DILATION: SECONDARY DEGENERATIVE HYDROCEPHALUS

- Alzheimer's Syndrome
- Parkinson's Syndrome
- Multi-Infarct Encephalopathy
- Lewy Body Disease
- Huntington's Disease
- Binswanger's Disease
- Progressive Supranuclear Palsy
- Neurosarcoidosis
- Amyloid Angiopathy

Treatment

The treatment of choice for "normal pressure" hydrocephalus is ventriculoperitoneal shunting. In selected cases, ventriculoatrial shunting can be considered with results similar to ventriculoperitoneal shunting. Although extensively studied and debated, endoscopic third ventriculostomy does not appear to be effective in the treatment of "normal pressure" hydrocephalus.

Despite being technically straightforward, ventriculoperitoneal shunting is not without risks. In the presence of appropriate preoperative selection, "normal pressure" hydrocephalus can have an excellent response to surgical therapy, especially concerning gait disturbances and urinary incontinence. Dementia, particularly if well-established for years, tends to remain unchanged.

29.3 Chiari Malformation

Also known as Arnold-Chiari syndrome, Chiari malformation encompasses a series of malformative conditions characterized by the presence of cerebellar tonsillar descent below the margin of the foramen magnum.

Among the various described forms, the most common and clinically relevant is Type I, which is identified by cerebellar descent alone (Figure 29.5).

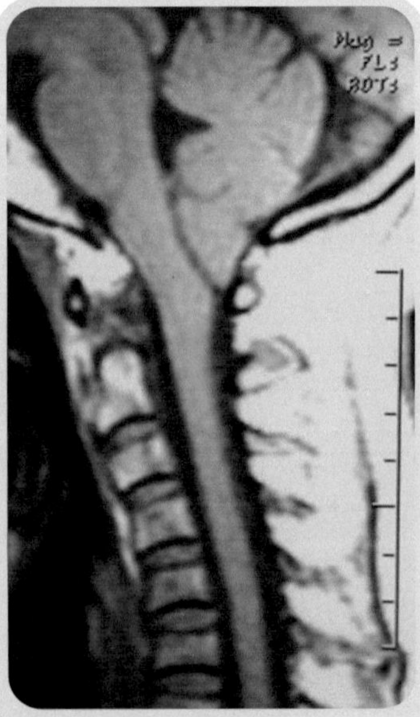

Figure 29.5

Sagittal MRI scan. Chiari I syndrome. Descend of cerebellar tonsils. The cerebello-medullary cistern is clearly absent.

Chiari Type II malformation is rarer. In this case, cerebellar descent is pronounced and always associated with myelomeningocele. The symptoms are typically due to compression of the brainstem and lower cranial nerves or the often associated hydrocephalus.

There are other forms of Chiari malformation (Type 0, Type III, Type IV), but their actual relevance to a single malformation disorder is debatable.

29.3.1 Causes of Chiari I malformation

The descent of the cerebellar tonsils below the margin of the foramen magnum is characteristic of Chiari I malformation. However, it is only the most evident aspect of a malformative disorder, with a probable genetic basis, whose main feature is hypoplasia of the posterior cranial fossa. The cerebellum, therefore, being larger than its bony container, tends to herniate caudally through the spinal foramen during development. While in Type II malformation, cerebellar herniation is often severe and causes symptoms of brainstem compression, this is less frequent in Chiari I. The symptoms, when present, depend on the absence of the cerebellomedullary cistern (the subarachnoid space through which cerebrospinal fluid exits the fourth ventricle), which is obliterated by the cerebellum itself. The resulting cerebrospinal fluid blockage is the main problem of the malformation and the target of surgical therapy. For this reason, although Chiari I is a malformative condition, it can be considered, from a semiotic point of view, among disorders of cerebrospinal fluid circulation.

29.3.2 Clinical presentation

Chiari malformation is not always symptomatic. The widespread use of Magnetic Resonance Imaging (MRI) has led to incidental findings of the malformation. It has been found that the actual prevalence of the malformation in the population is higher (0.1-0.5%) than previously believed.

In clinically evident forms, the main symptom of Chiari I is headache. It is a particular headache, localized in the nuchal region or less commonly supraorbital, typically worsened by exertion or in cases of increased abdominal pressure (coughing, sneezing, straining). Typically, since the cerebellum and brainstem are relatively compressed in a small space (foramen magnum), both structures can show signs of dysfunction: pyramidal symptoms, cranial nerve dysfunction, ataxia, nystagmus, or others. Chiari I malformation can be associated with the development of syringomyelia. In these cases, the clinical picture becomes more complex and may include manifestations typically more severe and related to syringomyelia.

29.3.3 Diagnosis

The diagnosis of Chiari malformation is made using MRI. It can be an incidental finding or discovered during investigations for headaches. The imaging does not pose diagnostic problems. Sagittal sequences allow for the simple and unequivocal identification of tonsillar descent. However, it is essential to differentiate true Chiari malformation from acquired tonsillar descent, which is related to cerebrospinal fluid hypotension (a less frequent occurrence). Cerebrospinal fluid hypotension can be spontaneous, post-traumatic, or iatrogenic, and the common denominator is the presence, usually at the spinal level, of a cerebrospinal fluid leak (leakage of cerebrospinal fluid outside the dural sac) that lowers intradural pressure and causes apparent herniation of the cerebellum through the foramen magnum, indistinguishable from Chiari I. Cerebrospinal fluid hypotension is also associated with headaches, but the characteristics are distinct from those of Chiari I. In Chiari I, the headache is typically exertional, while in cerebrospinal fluid hypotension, the headache is typically orthostatic (headache worsens in an upright position). The diagnosis of cerebrospinal fluid hypotension should be suspected based on the patient's medical history, and confirmation can be obtained through contrast-enhanced MRI, which shows characteristic enhancement of the dural structures.

29.3.4 Treatment of Chiari I malformation

The surgical treatment of Chiari malformation involves suboccipital decompression, aiming to restore the cerebellomedullary cistern and the flow of cerebrospinal fluid within it. This is achieved by removing the lower part of the occipital bone and the posterior arch of the atlas and enlarging the size of the dural sac using a patch of dura mater. Surgical experience has shown that Chiari malformation is often accompanied by pathological thickening of the basal arachnoid. Therefore, it is customary, once the dura mater is opened, to perform lysis of arachnoid adhesions until there is a good outflow of cerebrospinal fluid from the openings of the fourth ventricle. Surgical therapy carries minimal risks and is usually effective in the majority of cases.

29.4 Syringomyelia

The term syringomyelia refers to the dilation of the central spinal cord canal. It is more commonly found in the cervical region, although in specific cases and depending on the etiology, it can affect the entire spinal cord. The clinical presentation of syringomyelia resembles that of an intramedullary tumor. Motor symptoms consist of a combination of upper and lower motor neuron signs. A characteristic sensory feature is the so-called "suspended anesthesia": compression of the central gray matter of the spinal cord results in segmental hypoesthesia to temperature and pain (with relative preservation of epicritic tactile sensation), typically localized between the clavicle and the nipple line, including the upper limbs. Sensory symptoms also often include difficult-to-treat cornual-type pain radiating to one or both upper limbs. Syringomyelia has a chronic course and can potentially cause significant disability.

Regarding etiology, syringomyelia can be post-traumatic, peritumoral, associated with hydrocephalus, associated with Chiari malformation, or idiopathic. Additionally, although rare, an association has been documented between syringomyelia and common conditions such as disc herniation or spinal canal stenosis. Although the details are not fully understood, the central moment in the development of syringomyelia, common to all the aforementioned cases, appears to coincide with the alteration of normal cerebrospinal fluid circulation. It is plausible that changes in pressure gradients resulting from obstruction of the perimedullary subarachnoid spaces may trigger the formation of the syrinx cavity.

The diagnosis is obtained through MRI. In rare cases where there is an absolute contraindication to MRI, myelo-CT may be used if clinically justified. Contrast-enhanced MRI without contrast has a diagnostic sensitivity close to 100%. In cases of apparently isolated syringomyelia, it is always important to search for the coexistence of Chiari malformation or, in doubtful cases, supplement the examination with contrast to exclude satellite expansive lesions.

29.4.1 Post-traumatic syringomyelia

It can develop at the site of spinal cord trauma or hemorrhage. Sometimes it represents a morphological finding, such as an accumulation of cerebrospinal fluid in relation to spinal cord softening (malacia). Other times, it results from an alteration in local cerebrospinal fluid dynamics in response to scar tissue formation. In these cases, syringomyelia may have an evolving nature and cause symptoms. These are the few cases of syringomyelia in which direct drainage of the cavity can provide clinical benefit to the patient.

29.4.2 Peritumoral syringomyelia

Despite the established terminology, these are not true syringomyelia but satellite cavities associated with intramedullary tumors. They are relatively common, for example, in cases of ependymomas or hemangioblastomas. They are preferentially located at the poles of the tumor mass and can be multiloculated. They contain products of tumor secretion, and their walls are non-neoplastic. They usually regress after tumor removal.

29.4.3 Syringomyelia associated with hydrocephalus

Rarely, typically within the context of broader malformative disorders, syringomyelia can be associated with tetraventricular hydrocephalus. These are "communicating" syringomyelia cases with a good prognosis, even with drainage of the hydrocephalus alone.

29.4.4 Syringomyelia associated with Chiari malformation

This is the most frequent form of syringomyelia (Figure 29.6). In the past, these Chiari-associated syringomyelia cases were considered idiopathic or "degenerative" and therefore essentially incurable. It has been established that, in Chiari-associated syringomyelia, the dilation of the central spinal canal is a long-term consequence of the pathological diversion of cerebrospinal fluid that occurs at the craniospinal junction. The treatment of syringomyelia, regardless of its extent and caudal extension, coincides with that of Chiari malformation and involves suboccipital decompression. The clinical and radiological improvement of syringomyelia following treatment of the craniospinal junction pathology is consistent, although the extent of recovery cannot be predicted with certainty, it is often remarkable (Figure 29.7).

Surgical treatment is indicated in symptomatic cases, while the therapeutic approach for asymptomatic cases is highly controversial.

29.4.5 Idiopathic syringomyelia

It is not uncommon to find a circumscribed dilation of the spinal canal on MRI without any other diagnostic indications. These are typically incidental findings that are clinically silent and only require clinical observation. Less commonly, significant and symptomatic idiopathic syringomyelia can be identified, meaning it is not associated with any of the aforementioned conditions. The optimal treatment for these cases is controversial.

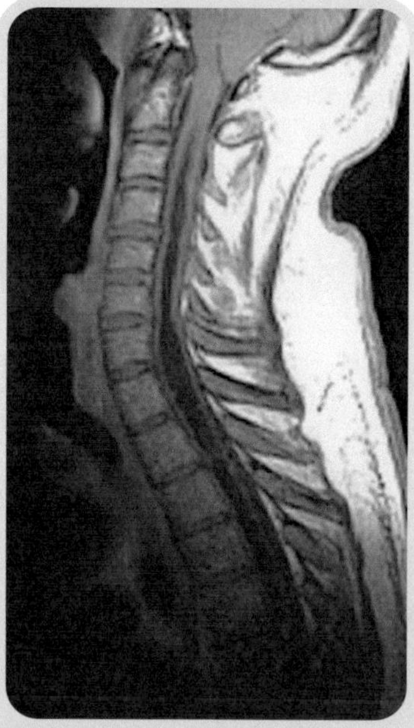

Figure 29.6

Sagittal MRI scan: There is evident extensive cervicodorsal syringomyelia, with associated Chiari malformation.

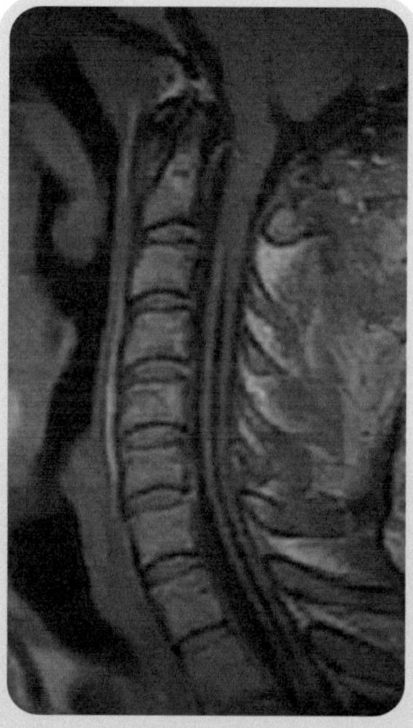

Figure 29.7

Post-operative examination (same patient as in Figure 29.6). The surgical treatment has restored the cerebello-medullary cistern, resulting in a drastic reduction of syringomyelia.

Even in the absence of evident signs of Chiari malformation, basal arachnoiditis may be suspected. In such cases, surgical decompression with lysis of arachnoid adhesions can yield unexpected results.

Bibliography

Heiss J.D., Patronas N., DeVroom H.L., Shawker T., Ennis R., Kammerer W., Eidsath A., Talbot T., Morris J., Eskioglu E., Oldfield E.H., Elucidating the pathophysiology of syringomyelia. J Neurosurg; 91(4):553-62, 1999.

Lu J., Ji N., Yang Z., Zhao X., Prognosis and treatment of acute hydrocephalus following aneurysmal subarachnoid haemorrhage. J Clin Neurosci; 19(5):669-72, 2012.

Milhorat T.H., Nishikawa M., Kula R.W., Dlugacz Y.D., Mechanisms of cerebellar tonsil herniation in patients with Chiari malformations as guide to clinical management. Acta Neurochir; 152(7):1117-27, 2010.

Mori K., Management of idiopathic normalpressure hydrocephalus: a multiinstitutional study conducted in Japan. J Neurosurg; 95(6):970-3, 2001.

Roy A.K., Slimack N.P., Ganju A., Idiopathic syringomyelia: retrospective case series, comprehensive review, and update on management. Neurosurg Focus; 31(6), 2011.

30

BRAIN DEATH

Oriano Mecarelli, Patrizia Pulitano, Edoardo Vicenzini

Death, from a conceptual and natural standpoint, is considered an event that definitively terminates an individual's life and is caused by permanent and irreversible damage to the brain, which will inevitably lead to the degeneration of the body.

On the other hand, brain death represents a clinical condition characterized by the primitive and irreversible loss of all cerebral functions, which will result in cardiac circulatory arrest upon the suspension of artificial ventilatory support. Therefore, it is an unnatural condition, somewhat dependent on the development of resuscitative techniques, and persists as long as those techniques are maintained.

In 1968, the first guidelines for determining brain death in a resuscitated individual were published in the United States by the Harvard Medical School. The Harvard criteria, which are still substantially valid half a century after their definition, have been further updated over the years. In 1995, the American Academy of Neurology published the first Guidelines, stating that the diagnosis of brain death is primarily clinical and must be based on the following fundamental requirements:

- The etiology of the coma must be known.
- Confounding concomitant conditions that can produce clinical signs similar to those of brain death must be excluded.
- Brain death must be documented by a state of unconsciousness with unresponsiveness to stimulation, absence of brainstem reflexes, and absence of spontaneous respiration.

Brain death is the outcome of a coma, which is a transient condition that can evolve into the following:

- Recovery of consciousness;
- Persistent vegetative state or minimally conscious state (conditions different from coma);
- Brain death.

Table 30.1 CLINICAL AND ELECTROENCEPHALOGRAPHIC CHARACTERISTICS OF CONSCIOUSNESS DISORDERS

Clinical condition	Consciousness	Alertness	Vegetative functions	Motor responses	EEG patterns
Minimally conscious state	Partial impairment	Preserved	Preserved	Variable/finalistic movements	Nonspecific alterations; reactivity ±
Vegetative state	Absent	Preserved	Preserved	Present but non-finalistic	Nonspecific alterations; reactivity ±
Coma	Absent	Absent	Partially compromised	Reflexes/postural responses	Distinct patterns; reactivity ±
Brain death	Absent	Absent	Absent	Absent brainstem reflexes	Electrocerebral inactivity
Locked-in Syndrome	Preserved	Preserved/partially compromised	Preserved/partially compromised	Tetraplegia, pseudobulbar palsy	Normal EEG

The clinical and neurophysiological characteristics of these different conditions are illustrated in ■ Table 30.1.

The diagnosis of brain death is defined by the its declaration while the patient is still under cardio-respiratory support, and it is based on clinical criteria (coma, absence of brainstem reflexes, absence of spontaneous breathing confirmed by the apnea test) and on the base of the anamnestic data (certainty of etiology and irreversibility of coma, exclusion of confounding clinical and pharmacological factors). Some instrumental investigations, solely aimed at diagnostic confirmation, assist in the clinical examination. These investigations include neurophysiological tests to confirm the absence of cerebral bioelectrical activity (EEG, evoked potentials) and techniques to demonstrate the absence of cerebral blood flow (conventional angiography, SPECT, CT and MRI angiography, transcranial Doppler ultrasonography).

30.1 Clinical diagnosis

The necessary prerequisites for the diagnosis of brain death include:

- Knowledge of the most immediate cause of coma and confirmation of its irreversibility. The patient's clinical history, physical examination, neuroimaging, and laboratory tests will help determine this more definitively.
- Exclusion of confounding factors that may compromise the patient's level of consciousness and that are potentially reversible (electrolyte and acid-base imbalances, endocrine disorders).
- Exclusion of significant alterations in body temperature, especially hypothermia. Body temperature should be normal or nearly normal (> 35-36 °C).
- Exclusion of major alterations in blood pressure. Systolic blood pressure should be ≥ 100 mmHg (normotension, euvolemia).
- Exclusion of drug intoxication or poisoning (assessing plasma concentrations of drugs acting on the central nervous system).

The clinical and neurological examination must verify the presence of three cardinal elements:

1) Comatose state or unresponsiveness. This condition must be clinically demonstrated by the absence of eye movements and motor responses to noxious stimuli. Spinal reflexes to painful stimuli, which can sometimes mimic complex movements (triple flexion of the lower limbs, Lazarus sign, etc.), should not be considered as motor responses.
2) Absence of brainstem reflexes. The neurological examination should confirm the absence of the following reflexes:
   - Pupillary reflex: In the condition of brain death, the pupils are fixed in an intermediate or dilated position (4-9 mm), unresponsive to light (a mydriasis may be possible if the insult responsible for coma partially spares the cervical sympathetic system, while miosis may result from drug intoxication). It is important to note that drugs taken in toxic doses alter pupil diameter but rarely significantly affect pupillary responsiveness to light.
   - Corneal reflex: Stimulation of the cornea with a wisp of cotton will not elicit any blink response.
   - Oculocephalic reflex: Passive rotation of the patient's head to the right and left and in flexion/extension will not result in any eye movement in the opposite direction.
   - Oculovestibular reflex: Irrigation of the patient's ear with 50 cc of cold water will not cause any deviation of gaze toward the irrigated side.
   - Painful reflexes in the territory of the trigeminal and facial nerves (painful pressure over the supraorbital region, at the temporomandibular joint, etc.).
   - Pharyngeal and tracheal (or carinal) reflexes: These reflexes, elicited by stimulation of the posterior pharynx ("gag reflex") and the trachea above the carina ("cough reflex"), should be absent.
3) Absence of spontaneous respiration, which can be documented using the apnea test. The test is performed by interrupting artificial ventilation for 5-10 minutes and administering pure oxygen at a rate of 6 L/min. Apnea should be documented by

blood gas analysis, showing a blood pH below 7.40, a $pCO_2 \geq 60$ mmHg and the absence of spontaneous respiratory efforts, which indicates the lack of compensation by the brainstem respiratory centers for hypercapnia and thus their irreversibly impaired functioning.

In theory, if all the above conditions are verified, the diagnosis of brain death could be made without further tests or prolongation of the observation period. In fact, the determination of brain death is based on the evaluation of purely clinical criteria.

30.2 Instrumental examinations and legislative-procedural tools

For the determination of brain death, most countries require confirmatory instrumental tests (mandatory or optional), which can also be used in specific clinical situations. In Italy, according to the current legislation (Ministerial Decree of 11/04/2008 published in the Official Gazette No. 136 of 12/06/2008, updating Ministerial Decree No. 582 of 22/08/1994), besides documenting the absence of wakefulness and consciousness, absence of brainstem reflexes, and absence of spontaneous respiration, it is mandatory to verify the state of "cerebral electrical silence" through prolonged scalp electroencephalographic recording (EEG) for 30 minutes, performed at the beginning and end of the at least 6 hours observation period.

Cerebral electrical silence (better defined as electro-cerebral inactivity) refers to the absence of electrically recorded brain activity from the scalp using surface electrodes and large signal amplification (20 μV/cm). The absence of electrical activity should be tested both under spontaneous conditions and during and after the application of standardized stimuli of different natures, mainly acoustic and noxious stimuli. EEG is the most sensitive, widespread, and commonly used neurophysiological test to confirm the clinical diagnosis of brain death. EEG changes appear in close correlation with the reduction of cerebral blood flow. When this parameter is persistently lower than 10 ml/100 g/min, cellular death is inevitable, and the EEG shows an isoelectric ("flat") pattern. Within 20-30 seconds after cardiac arrest, electrocerebral inactivity can already be observed on the EEG, which will remain persistent/permanent if the cardio-circulatory conditions are not restored.

In cases of brain death, EEG should be performed according to the parameters established by the relevant legislation by an experienced neurophysiology technician under medical supervision. A sufficient number of electrodes should be applied to explore the frontal, temporal, parietal, and occipital cortical areas, and the recorded signal should be amplified five times more than the routine amplification (Figure 30.1). The technician should also minimize artifact activity and verify the absence of reactivity of the EEG to

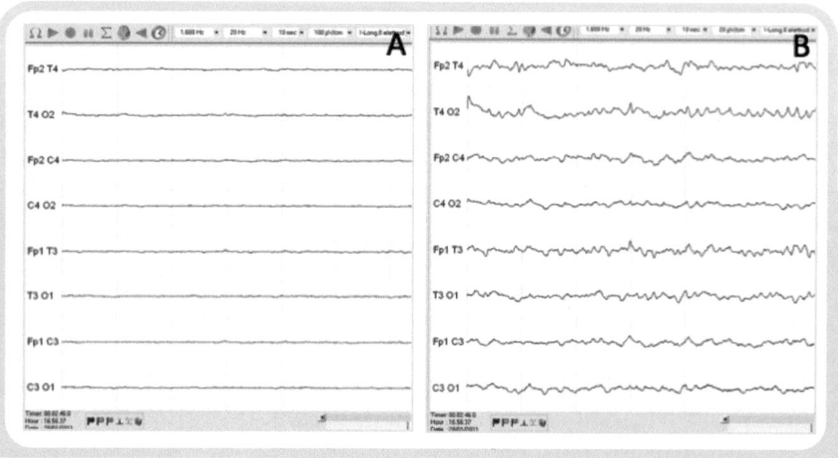

Figure 30.1

A) At standard amplification (100 μV/cm) the tracing appears isoelectric. B) At higher amplification (20 μV/cm)), the persistence of cortical bioelectrical activity is instead observed.

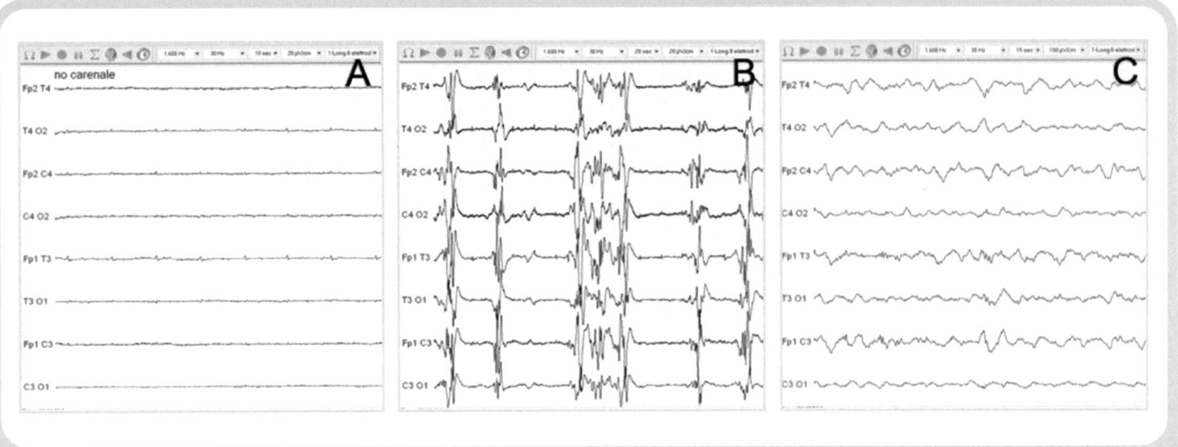

Figure 30.2

A) "Flat" EEG pattern in a comatose patient treated with high doses of thiopental for several days. B) After 24 hours of sedative discontinuation, the EEG shows a burst-suppression pattern. C) After an additional 48 hours, an EEG pattern characterized by widespread slow waves, predominantly in the mid-anterior region, is observed.

visual, acoustic, and noxious stimuli. However, the appearance of electrocerebral inactivity can also be caused by iatrogenic factors. EEG is particularly sensitive to the effects of hypothermia and/or certain drugs acting on the central nervous system (benzodiazepines, barbiturates, anesthetics, etc.), posing a risk of false positives (Figure 30.2). Therefore, all possible physiopathological variables potentially capable of causing evaluation errors in the EEG (drugs, body temperature, blood pressure, oxygen saturation) must be known and reported.

Among the neurophysiological techniques that can be used to demonstrate electrocerebral inactivity (although not legally required), it is worth mentioning short-latency evoked potentials, which allow testing the functionality of both the brainstem and the cerebral cortex and are not affected by sedative drugs and hypothermia, unlike EEG. Specifically, somatosensory evoked potentials (SSEPs) are capable of assessing the integrity of the medial lemniscus, thalamus, and somatosensory cortex. The absence of the main cortical wave (N20) bilaterally represents a marker of cortical inactivity.

In our country, the evaluation, both clinical and electroencephalographic, must be performed at least twice, at a 6-hour interval, regardless of the individual's age. In neonates, the determination of death can only be performed if the birth occurred at term (after the 38th week of gestation) and after 7 days of extrauterine life.

In the case of an anoxic nature of the cerebral insult (resulting from cardiac arrest), the observation period should begin at least 24 hours after the anoxic insult (unless cerebral blood flow is absent).

The medical panel authorized to declare death is appointed by the Hospital Health Management and consists of three physicians (a forensic physician or a physician from the Health Management or a pathologist, an anesthesiologist-intensivist, a neurophysiologist, or in their absence, an experienced EEG neurologist or neurosurgeon), and all the three professionals must be present during both observations.

Italian law also mandates the obligatory determination of the absence of cerebral blood flow in the following situations:

- Children under 1 year of age.
- Situations that do not allow for a definite etiopathogenic diagnosis or special clinical conditions in which clinical and EEG evaluations are not feasible (e.g., significant craniofacial trauma that hinders the evaluation of brainstem reflexes and/or

EEG recording).
- Inability to establish the essential prerequisites for clinical-instrumental evaluation (hypothermia, central nervous system depressant drugs, severe systemic hypotension, endocrine-metabolic disturbances, electrolyte imbalances, etc.).

The presence or absence of cerebral blood flow can be assessed using various instrumental investigations: cerebral angiography, cerebral scintigraphy (SPECT), angio-CT, angio-MRI, and transcranial Doppler (TCD). Conventional cerebral angiography is considered the "gold standard" for evaluating cerebral blood flow and allows for documenting the absence of filling in the intracranial arteries (petrous portion for the internal carotid arteries and the level of the foramen ovale for the vertebral arteries). It is performed through intrafemoral arterial catheterization, where the catheter is advanced to the supra-aortic trunks, and then iodinated contrast medium is injected using an automatic pump. Although theoretically the best examination for evaluating cerebral blood flow, it is an invasive procedure that cannot be performed at the patient's bedside. Additionally, catheterization may damage the vessels, and the contrast agent used could compromise renal function, which is detrimental in cases of organ donation. Cerebral scintigraphy (SPECT) involves the use of a radiopharmaceutical (technetium 99mTC HMPAO or 99mTC ECD) that crosses the blood-brain barrier and is retained by brain cells after an initial perfusion phase, indicating not only the presence of perfusion but also any cerebral activity. The technique is 100% specific and highly sensitive but is costly, cannot be performed at the bedside, and is available in only a few facilities. Other neuroimaging techniques (angio-CT and angio-MRI) are still insufficiently validated in this context. Transcranial Doppler (TCD) is a highly specific and sensitive method for evaluating intracerebral blood flow. It is easily performed at the bedside, non-invasive, and cost-effective requiring skilled sonographers. However, it is operator-dependent, limited by the temporal window's adequacy, and influenced by hemodynamic parameters and any interventions for decompression. In cases of brain death, circulatory arrest on TCD is characterized by the following patterns:
- Inversion of the signal direction in diastole compared to systole
- Presence of only systolic spikes without any diastolic signal
- Absence of signal both during systole and diastole.

30.3 Conclusion

The neurological standard for determining death, starting from the Harvard criteria, is scientifically and legally recognized as reliable for certifying an individual's death by the majority of countries worldwide. The neurological and neurophysiological evaluation criteria also allow for clearly and unequivocally identifying clinical situations entirely different from brain death, such as vegetative state, minimally conscious state, complete locked-in syndrome, toxic states, etc.

Italian legislative norms require a clinical and medico-legal procedure involving multiple specialists to ensure completeness, accuracy, and certainty in determining death. It should be noted that the determination of death according to neurological standards is a due process that must be clearly separated from any other purpose, such as organ donation, even though the individual's death is an obvious prerequisite for organ donation.

Figure 30.3 summarizes the process that starts with the determination of brain death and leads either to organ retrieval, in the case of a donor subject, or the withdrawal of ventilatory support.

Bibliography

Beecher H. A definition of irreversible coma. Report of the Ad Hoc Committee. A definition of irreversible coma. Report of the Ad Hoc Committee of the Harvard Medical School to Examine the Definition of Brain Death. JAMA. 1968; 205: 337-340.

National Transplant Center. Guidelines. Application of instrumental investigations of cerebral blood flow. Updated version as of

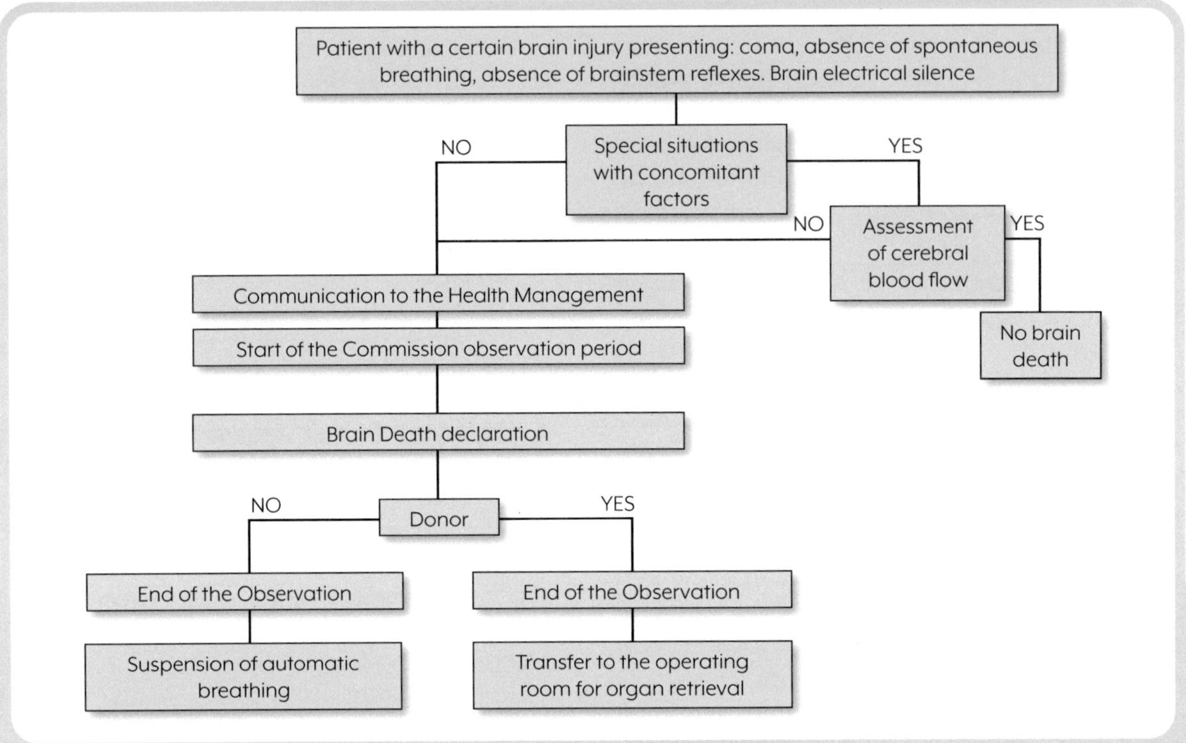

Figure 30.3

February 20, 2009. http://www.trapianti.salute.gov.it.

Ministry of Health Decree, April 11, 2008. Amendment of the Decree of August 22, 1994, No. 582 concerning the Regulations for the determination and certification of death. Official Gazette No. 136 of June 12, 2008.

Mecarelli O. Coma e Morte cerebrale. In Mecarelli O., Manuale Teorico-Pratico di Elettroencefalografia. Springer Healthcare Italia, 2009.

Mecarelli O, Vicenzini E. Brain Death. In: Clinical Electroencephalography. O. Mecarelli Ed, Springer, 2019, pp 767-787.

Practice parameters for determining brain death in adults (summary statement). Report of the Quality Standards Subcommittee of the American Academy of Neurology. Neurology. 1995; 45: 1012-1014.

Vicenzini E., Pro S., Randi F., et al. Transcranial Doppler for brain death after decompressive craniectomy: persistence of cerebral blood flow with flat EEG. Intensive Care Med. 2010; 36:2163-2164.

Vicenzini E., Pro S., Pulitano P., et al. Current practice of brain death determination and use of confirmatory tests in an Italian University hospital: a report of 66 cases. Minerva Anestesiol. 2013; 79:485-491.

Wijdicks EFM., Varelas P.N., Gronseth G.S., Greer D.M. Evidence-based guideline update: determining brain death in adults. Report of the Quality Standards Subcommittee of the American Academy of Neurology. Neurology. 2010; 74:1911-1918.

Wijdicks EFM. The case against confirmatory tests for determining brain death in adults. Neurology. 2010; 75: 77-83.

31 NEUROREHABILITATION

Michelangelo Bartolo, Mariano Serrao,
Stefano Filippo Castiglia, Francesco Pierelli

In the broader context of Rehabilitation, which deals with the recovery of lost or unacquired abilities due to various pathological processes, Neurorehabilitation is identified as a discipline that studies the reorganizational capacities of the nervous system after an injury and is concerned with the recovery and/or functional maintenance of individuals affected by neurological disorders.

Neurorehabilitation is based on the assumption that different types of interventions, such as motor exercises, modulation of sensory input, and stimulation with physical means (transcranial electrical currents, transcranial magnetic stimulation), can modulate neuroplasticity processes. In clinical practice, a series of interventions are performed with the aim of reducing disability through the recovery of functional deficits and the optimal utilization of remaining abilities. There is now a widespread consensus that various pathological and non-pathological conditions can modify the distribution of different functional modules through which the nervous system operates. This modulation represents an intrinsic property of the nervous system, closely dependent on the activities performed, and defines the so-called activity-dependent plasticity. In recent decades, this concept has provided the theoretical basis for explaining the effectiveness of neurorehabilitation treatment. Numerous studies have indeed shown how rehabilitative exercise can lead to structural reorganization of the nervous system (plasticity) and promote functional recovery. Moreover, experimental and clinical data support the hypothesis that motor representations are closely dependent on the characteristics of motor activity, with evident differences between individuals and even within the same individual as the characteristics and intensity of motor tasks vary. Numerous studies using functional neuroimaging techniques have demonstrated how the functional organization of the cerebral cortex undergoes structural and functional changes at the cortical level before and after motor training. Rehabilitation, therefore, should be regarded as a process that, through a wide range of interventions, aims to enable individuals to achieve the highest possible degree of autonomy and independence, and consequently, the best possible quality of life in physical, cognitive, and social domains. To ensure a good level of effectiveness, any rehabilitation pathway must be personalized and targeted at achieving meaningful goals for the individual and/or their caregivers, with the main objective of reintegrating the individual into their family and social environment.

This approach is based on the bio-psycho-social model proposed by the International Classification of Functioning, Disability, and Health (ICF) of the World Health Organization in 2001, in which health is assessed comprehensively along three dimensions: biological, individual, and social, integrating the medical and social concepts of disability.

31.1 Rehabilitation team

Rehabilitative interventions, tailored to the individual's needs, require the interactive contribution of a multidisciplinary team (medical specialists, physiotherapists, speech therapists, occupational therapists, nurses, psychologists/neuropsychologists, bioengineers, social workers, etc.) coordinated by a rehabilitation physician. Following an objective clinical and functional evaluation conducted by each team member, with the support of validated scales and scores, the rehabilitation team identifies the biological damage, the level of autonomy, the remaining abilities, and the patient's medical, functional, psychological, and social needs. Based on the identified issues, the team determines the prognosis, defines the objectives of the rehabilitation project, and outlines the implementation methods through an individualized program aimed at achieving maximum functional independence.

31.2 Rehabilitation plan

The "Individual Rehabilitation Plan" refers to the set of provisions developed by the multidisciplinary team coordinated by the responsible physician. This project must consider not only the individual's disabilities but also contextual environmental factors. It must define expectations, priorities, and anticipated outcomes. Furthermore, it should establish short, medium, and long-term goals and outline the actions and conditions necessary to achieve them.

31.3 Rehabilitation program

Within the rehabilitation project, the "rehabilitation program" defines specific areas of intervention, the involved professionals, the methods and timing of individual services, and the evaluation of achieved results. Based on complexity, quantity, and quality of resources required, rehabilitation activities can be classified as follows:

a) *Intensive rehabilitation activities* aim to treat severe but modifiable disabilities that require a high level of rehabilitative effort in terms of complexity and duration of intervention. According to current regulations in Italy, these activities must be performed for at least three hours per day and involve specific therapy provided by rehabilitation healthcare professionals (physiotherapists, speech therapists, occupational therapists, nurses, psychologists/neuropsychologists, etc.).
b) *Extensive rehabilitation activities* are characterized by a moderate therapeutic effort coupled with significant support and assistance. Although the clinical and therapeutic commitment is less intensive, it still requires specifically rehabilitative work. Therapy sessions can vary in duration from one to three hours per day.

31.4 Assessment scales and scores

Assessment scales and scores are used as tools to support evaluation and as indicators of outcomes. They can be categorized into three main types:

1) Clinical scales based on analysis of general clinical problems, specific neurological conditions, and resulting disability levels.
2) Scales related to individual well-being and quality of life.
3) Scales related to patient satisfaction with the interventions performed and the outcomes achieved.

Table 31.1 presents some examples of scales and scores used in Neurorehabilitation.

31.5 Neurorehabilitation methods

Since the 1960s, many methods for motor recovery in neurological rehabilitation have been developed. Despite the abundance of proposals and the evident effectiveness of stroke rehabilitation, there are no comparative studies documenting the superiority of one technique over another. Some methods are primarily based on motor exercises involving active, passive, and/or assisted movement repetitions, while others focus on sensory stimulation. Still, others combine both aspects using different modalities. However, it is widely demonstrated that any motor exercise is most effective when it is meaningful to the patient, motivating, and incorporates cognitive and functional components. The common goal of different approaches is to facilitate the recovery of absent or partially recoverable motor patterns. The following are the main methodologies and techniques, with a general description of their underlying theoretical principles.

Table 31.1 EXAMPLES OF ASSESSMENT SCALES IN THE FIELD OF NEUROLOGICAL REHABILITATION

Scale*	Evaluated function	Items	Score	Administration time	Use
Barthel Index	Independence/disability	10	0-100	10-20 minutes	General
Functional Independence Measure (FIM)	Independence/disability	18	18- 126	40 minutes	General
Motricity Index	Motor Function	15		5 minutes	General
Modified ashworth scale	Spasticity	5	0-4	5 minutes	General
SF-36	Quality of life	36	0-100**	30-40 minutes	General
Extended Activities of Daily Living (ADL)	Activities of daily living (ADL)	22			General
Beck Depression Inventory	Depression	21	0-3**	10 minutes	General
Montgomery Asberg Depression Rating Scale (MADRS)	Depression	10	0-6**	15 minutes	General
Modified Rankin Scale	Global disability	7	0-6	5 minutes	Cerebral stroke
Fugl-Meyer Assessment	Motor function	155	0-100	30-40 minutes	Cerebral stroke
Rivermead Mobility Index	Motor function	15	0-15	5 minutes	Cerebral stroke
Unified Parkinson's Disease Rating Scale (UPDRS) Part III	Independence/disability	14	0-56	5-10 minutes	Parkinson's Disease
Unified Parkinson's Disease Rating Scale (UPDRS) Part II - ADL	Independence/disability	13	0-52	5-10 minutes	Parkinson's Disease
Hoen-Yahr Scale	Clinical Stage	5	0-5	5 minutes	Parkinson's Disease
Parkinson's Disease Questionnaire (PDQ-39)	Quality of life	39	0-100	10 minutes	Parkinson's Disease
Freezing of Gait Questionnaire (FOGQ)	Freezing of gait	6	0-24	5 minutes	Parkinson's Disease
Modified Parkinson Activities Scale (MPAS)	Activity of Daily Living (ADL)	7	---	20-30 minutes	Parkinson's Disease
Extended Disability Status Scale (EDSS)	Independence/Disability	8	0-10	15-30 minutes	Multiple sclerosis
Glasgow Coma Scale	Neurological Status/Level of Consciousness	3	0-15	5-10 minutes	Traumatic brain Injuries
ASIA (American Spinal Injury Association)	Functional Deficit (Strength and Sensation)	18			Spinal cord injuries
Quadriplegia Index of Function (QIF)	Functional Status/ADL	30	0-4**	35-40 minutes	Spinal cord injuries
Spinal Cord Independence Measure (SCIM)	Functional Status/ADL	---	100	30 minutes	Spinal cord injuries
ICARS (International Cooperative Ataxia Rating Scale)	Functional Status	4	100	20 minutes	Ataxias

* In the case of a cerebral stroke, certain clinical assessment scales (such as the National Institute of Health Stroke Scale-NIHSS and the Canadian Neurological Scale-CNS) have shown varying degrees of correlation with different outcome scales in various studies. Therefore, they can be considered as supplementary tools for functional assessment with prognostic and developmental purposes. ** Score per individual item.

31.5.1 Vojta method

The method was initially developed in the pediatric field and later found application in adults with neurological disorders. Vojta observed that the use of repeated sensory stimulation in children with cerebral palsy counteracts the structuring of altered motor patterns. The restoration of patterns can be achieved through stimulation of the three components (postural, righting, and motor) that constitute the building blocks of voluntary movement.

The technique represents the first rehabilitative approach strongly characterized by the concept of prevention, based on early diagnosis (neurological screening of the child) and a therapeutic approach aimed at preventing secondary effects resulting from the primary damage (central nervous system lesion). According to Vojta, sensory deprivation resulting from neurological damage and reduced function leads to a slowdown in developmental progression and a gradual loss of even the most basic cerebral functions.

31.5.2 Kabat method (proprioceptive neuromuscular facilitation, PNF)

The method considers two basic principles of neurophysiology for motor control: temporal facilitation and spatial facilitation.

The first principle refers to the phenomenon in which a stimulus applied to a neural system facilitates the passage of subsequent stimuli. The second principle refers to the neurobiological property in which the response to a stimulus can be strengthened or inhibited by other stimuli converging on the same nerve cells.

These cellular communication mechanisms allow the restoration of sensory-motor functions through the induction of control activities by intact cells. Activities guided by the physical therapist act as a multisensory stimulation, leading to hyperactivity and involvement of all still functioning nerve cells. The repetition of stimuli determines sensorimotor responses fundamental for learning, which can be verbally reinforced, directing the organization of motor behavior.

The technique is based on observations conducted in the sports and dance fields, noting that most movements performed by athletes and dancers follow diagonal lines relative to the body's sagittal axis and involve rotation. Subsequent studies highlighted that the muscles of the limbs and trunk are functionally grouped into motor patterns composed of diagonal-spiral movements and a combination of flexion-extension, abduction-adduction, and rotation movements. From this technique, a number of motor patterns are derived, configured into therapeutic diagonal-spiral patterns classified as base patterns.

In Italy, the Kabat concept has been further developed and updated Progressive Modular Rebalancing (RMP) system. The RMP system emphasizes the exercise of bi-articular muscles, postural exercises, and postural transitions, with the trunk playing a central role as the basis for the recovery of functional motor patterns and synergies, and the key center of the entire locomotor system. All exercises are combined in a progression from least to most demanding, based on the patient's functional level achieved. The foundation of RMP is to restore the structural and postural alignment of the skeletal and neuromuscular systems of the body, invoking "global" motor patterns that repeat and reconstruct the evolutionary stages of vertical motor control.

31.5.3 Bobath method

The method, developed based on empirical observations, is based on the assumption that the Central Nervous System (CNS), functions more as a "reaction" organ than an "action" organ in response to various stimuli from the external and internal environment. According to Bobath, only a portion of actions is entirely free, while the majority of motor activities occur in an "automatic" manner, being modulated by pre-existing facilitated circuits. The CNS coordinates and programs motor responses, which are products of the integration of stimuli and sensory information.

In the case of CNS lesions, the abilities of perception and processing are greater than those of production, creating an imbalance that can be remodeled through a relearning process guided by rehabilitation work.

31.5.4 Perfetti method (cognitive therapeutic exercise, action comparison, or neurocognitive rehabilitation)

The method is based on the principle that any movement has a "cognitive meaning" as it connects a person with the surrounding environment. Recovery from a neurological injury is therefore seen as a learning process under pathological conditions, also known as "Cognitive Therapeutic Exercise" (CTE), emphasizing the awareness of different sensorimotor experiences by the individual. The method aims to observe and address the relationships between higher organizational levels (CNS) and the peripheral level, relating the effectors of movement (muscles, bones, joints) to control and coordination systems. Movement is considered the result of processes carried out by a system that interacts with the environment according to its needs, establishing a close relationship between movement and information processing.

31.5.5 Grimaldi method

The method is based on the *distretch-shortening techniques* that include passive mobilization of various body areas. Muscle responses are believed to generate recovery of strength: sudden muscle shortening following passive stretching prevents the development of altered neuromuscular modulation, resulting in permanent adaptive adjustment (learning) of descending control signals.

31.5.6 Hydrokinesitherapy

Functional rehabilitation in water is a therapy based on facilitating movement through exercises performed in heated pools with water temperature close to body temperature (31°-35° Celsius). This therapy takes advantage of the physical properties of water, such as partial abolition of the effects of gravity and the modest resistance provided during movement, allowing for sensory and proprioceptive stimulation.

31.5.7 Action observation therapy

The method is based on the assumption that observing a gesture performed by others activates the same neural structures required for performing the same action in the observer. The areas involved in this observation-action mechanism are defined as the mirror neuron system. L'*Action Observation Therapy* (AOT) uses this mechanism to recover motor skills. The application of the method involves having the subject observe a specific activity (usually related to daily life activities) through video recordings or digital media and then perform the same activity immediately after observation.

31.6 Main pathologies undergoing neurorehabilitation

31.6.1 Stroke

The primary element in defining the rehabilitation plan for a patient with recent stroke is the comprehensive functional assessment, aiming to determine the overall clinical status, motor conditions, sensory and cognitive functions, psychological conditions, communication abilities, social and environmental factors, characteristics of external support, and autonomy in activities of daily living. The use of validated and standardized clinical scales allows for quantifying the initial conditions and monitoring the degree of recovery achieved by the patient over time, thereby assessing the effectiveness of the intervention. The data collected through the assessment help identify possible objectives within the rehabilitation plan, initially focusing on regaining autonomy in major activities of daily living (short-term objectives) and subsequently aiming for social reintegration (long-term objectives).

Clinical assessment should be conducted within the first few days following a stroke, according to agreed protocols within the healthcare team. Some basic functions should be assessed within the first 24-48 hours of the acute event, including consciousness and swallowing capacity, general characteristics of cognitive abilities, patient needs related to immobilization and loss of manipulation capacity. Early assessment of nutritional status and the risk of pressure ulcers is also crucial to activate nursing care for the patient.

It is widely accepted that rehabilitative treatment should preferably begin within the first week of admission to the acute care facility, if the patient's general condition allows. In this initial phase, specific rehabilitative proposals may not be possible, but preventive measures can be taken to avoid tertiary damage and facilitate the emergence of any residual potential. As long as the patient's clinical condition is stable, intensive treatment is recommended to promote neural plasticity processes that are active from the early stages of cerebral damage.

The complexity of the patient's needs requires the collaboration of multiple professionals (physicians, physiotherapists, nurses, speech therapists, neuropsychologists, psychologists, occupational therapists, orthopedic technicians, social workers) in the rehabilitation process. In recent years, the use of technological systems for assessment and rehabilitation has introduced additional team members, such as engineers and neurophysiology technicians. Therefore, professional autonomy should be integrated into a team where the contributions of different skills are most valuable when coordinated and synergistic.

Early mobilization is indicated in the early stages after a stroke to avoid joint stiffness development and prevent "learned non-use" of the affected limbs. Early mobilization also contributes to the prevention of pressure injuries, bronchial stasis, postural malalignment, and other severe complications of bed rest. The timeliness of patient mobilization and training is the main factor related to returning home within six weeks of a stroke. The possibility of training for walking depends on the acquisition of adequate trunk control and posture, especially in patients with severe lower limb weakness who are unable to support body weight during gait. Therefore, early administration of rehabilitative exercises aimed at trunk control and the use of tools for progressive weight-bearing and early walking exercise is desirable. Although there is no definitive evidence, several studies provide indications for the correct and safe application of these devices, supported by the use of anthropometric tables and principles of bioengineering.

Cognitive impairments, along with sensory and motor disorders, are common outcomes of stroke, leading to morbidity, disability, and reduced quality of life. Cognitive rehabilitation aims to recover and/or compensate for compromised cognitive and behavioral skills, aiming to achieve the highest possible level of independence and autonomy for the individual. Traditionally, cognitive rehabilitation has been carried out with pencil-and-paper exercises, but today it also utilizes computerized tools and, less commonly, virtual reality technology. An important aspect of the rehabilitation process is the assessment and treatment of language and swallowing disorders. Verbal communication is often assessed using standardized batteries, including brief and quick administration. In patients with severe language impairments, the presence of a speech therapist in the rehabilitation team allows for the adoption of alternative communication tools. Additionally, the speech therapist evaluates the presence of dysphagia, which is considered crucial for the improvement of stroke patients. Dysphagia has the potential to cause severe respiratory complications. Therefore, patients should undergo fiberoptic endoscopic evaluation of swallowing (FEES) to early assess the degree of swallowing dysfunction.

Occupational therapy plays an important role in stroke rehabilitation. The activities carried out by occupational therapists aim to employ strategies to promote residual functionality and retrain patients in self-management and performance of daily activities. A recent systematic review documents small but significant benefits achieved with occupational therapy in basic activities of daily living (self-care, mobility), some additional activities (household chores and leisure), and participation in social activities.

In recent years, in addition to traditional physiotherapy techniques, other rehabilitative approaches have emerged, including:

1) *Constraint-Induced Movement Therapy (CIMT)*, a method based on immobilizing the healthy limb to force the patient to use the affected limb. The underlying idea is that the affected limb, affected by a "*learned non-use*" phenomenon, needs to be forced (*forced use*) to move again to facilitate functional recovery.
2) *Motor imagery*, based on functional neuroimaging studies showing that mental representation of motor events (*motor imagery*) involves the same cortical areas activated during the execution of voluntary movements. This observation suggests that "thinking" about movement can promote activation and recovery of neural structures involved in the necessary motor patterns.
3) *Mirror therapy*, which recreates the illusion of bilateral movement synchronization by having the patient perform voluntary

movements with the unaffected limb while observing the reflected image in a sagittal. The false perception of bilateral movement is believed to facilitate the activation of premotor areas.

Instrumental methods have also undergone significant development in recent years, and numerous studies have been dedicated to their use and effectiveness. Among these, transcranial electrical stimulation (tDCS) and transcranial magnetic stimulation (TMS), techniques are used to promote cortical excitability changes with long-term effects. Particularly, tDCS has a neuromodulatory effect, while TMS has a neurostimulatory effect. It is believed that these techniques, possibly through mechanisms of neural plasticity, facilitate motor recovery, especially when combined with traditional physiotherapy techniques.

The use of robots in rehabilitative practice for patients with stroke sequelae (*robot-assisted therapy*) is a new and promising field in continuous development, primarily used in the rehabilitation of the paretic upper limb (*target reaching task*) and passive walking. There are several advantages compared to traditional rehabilitation, including the possibility for the patient to engage in intensive training (*repetitive task training*), recording of kinematic and dynamic parameters to track recovery progress and adapt exercises, impose controlled perturbations, and provide prosthetic assistance when movement does not follow predefined trajectories or parameters, ensuring a high level of repeatability of the movement.

There are various studies supporting the use of the aforementioned approaches, although there is still no definitive evidence of their complete efficacy.

Organizational models for stroke management

Patients with stroke benefit from an organized management model within dedicated facilities. A literature review, analyzing 23 randomized controlled clinical trials (including 4911 patients), has shown a reduction in mortality, disability, and institutionalization when patients are treated in dedicated stroke management units (Stroke Units) rather than internal medicine departments. A European survey highlighted different organizational modalities for Stroke Units (SU): acute-phase SU, admitting patients with acute stroke for less than a week; Comprehensive SU, admitting patients with acute stroke and providing several weeks of treatment and rehabilitation if needed; combined acute and rehabilitation SU, admitting patients 1-2 weeks after the acute event and providing treatment and rehabilitation for several weeks or months. Among the proposed organizational models, there is also the Mobile Stroke Team, a group of professionals assisting patients in different departments. Among these different intervention modalities, it has been demonstrated that the combined acute and rehabilitation SU and the rehabilitative SU are more effective in reducing mortality and disability.

31.6.2 Parkinson's disease

Patients with Parkinson's disease (PD) experience motor impairment, gait alterations, and postural abnormalities. They also have difficulty performing motor tasks that are part of daily life, such as initiating walking, changing direction, stopping, rising from a chair, or transfers. All of these dysfunctions can profoundly affect quality of life and participation in social activities. Rehabilitation for motor disorders in PD is based on three fundamental principles. The first involves teaching patients how to move more easily and maintain good postural stability through the development of strategies to compensate for motor dysfunctions related to basal ganglia pathology. The second focuses on treating complications involving the musculoskeletal system and the cardiorespiratory system, which can result from reduced physical activity and advanced age. The third aims to promote permanent lifestyle changes through exercises and physical activities aimed at fall prevention. Rehabilitative intervention strategies differ based on the severity stage of the disease, typically defined by the Hoehn and Yahr disease stage classification (HY). In this regard, rehabilitative objectives for patients with mild disability (HY 1-2.5) focus on preventing inactivity and maintaining motor capacity through the promotion of active lifestyles and social activities. For patients with moderate disability (HY 3-4), rehabilitative goals shift towards fall prevention and reducing limitations in transfer abilities, postural attitudes, manual skills, balance, and gait through individual exercises based on specific rehabilitation strategies. For patients with severe disability (HY 5), rehabilitation focuses on maintaining vital functions and preventing the consequences of immobilization.

Rehabilitation strategies

Patients with PD can improve their gait performance through the use of visual or auditory cues. For example, they can follow colored lines arranged on the ground to form visual pathways or listen to rhythmic beats like those of a metronome or a musical piece. These sensory cues techniques can positively contribute to step length and cadence. Other strategies involve the patient mentally "imagining" taking long steps and mentally rehearsing the desired movement before executing it. It is also helpful to have the patient break down complex motor sequences into simpler parts. This model is based on the theory that the ability to perform learned movements is not lost in patients with PD but that there is an activation problem that can be overcome through targeted physiotherapy. In the early stages of the disease, patients still have good motor learning ability. During this phase, repeated exercise of the upper limb leads to increased speed and precision of voluntary movements. Similarly, simple walking exercises performed for approximately 30 minutes a day for at least three weeks improve walking speed and step length. Therefore, the rehabilitation plan and program should be tailored based on the stage of the disease. For patients in the early stage, physiotherapy should be more intense and focused on motor learning. For patients in the advanced stage or those with compromised cognitive functions, physiotherapy should focus on compensatory strategies, avoiding multitasking, and instead segmenting actions into simpler components. In addition to a lower degree of disability, greater walking speed, step length, and trunk rotation capacity during gait are predictors of successful rehabilitation.

Treatment of musculoskeletal consequences

Patients with PD may experience complications related to their underlying neurological condition, further impairing their ability to perform common daily activities. Muscle weakness, reduced joint range of motion, and increased muscle rigidity (*stiffness*) should be considered as significant treatment targets in rehabilitation. Increased attention to these pathological aspects can improve gait, balance, and overall motor function. Patients with PD often exhibit abnormal postures with trunk flexion and/or lateral inclination. Dysfunction in axial mobility can contribute to the loss of postural control, balance, and motor function decline. Rehabilitation aimed at improving trunk control should, therefore, be considered a primary objective. Combining exercises for trunk mobility, stretching, and muscle recruitment with gait training using sensory cues enhances the effectiveness of cognitive strategies on improving gait kinematic parameters (▪ Table 31.2).

Promotion of physical activity and fall prevention

PD is a progressive disorder. Therefore, therapeutic exercise should be sustained over time to maintain benefits and prevent deterioration. It is important for patients with PD to engage in regular and consistent physical exercise immediately after diagnosis and throughout the course of the disease, even independently, with regular check-ups to monitor the clinical situation.

Regular participation in dance represents an appealing option for some individuals and can improve balance in patients with PD. Non-motor disturbances, such as depression with apathy and loss of initiative, have a significant impact on many patients. These disturbances can affect the ability to engage in regular physical activity, making it important for clinicians to pay attention to the non-motor symptoms of their patients and address them pharmacologically.

In the advanced stages of the disease, frequent falls, mostly occurring during the execution of complex or prolonged motor tasks, are a major inconvenience associated with the motor disorder and should be prevented.

To this end, the rehabilitation team should adequately inform the patient and their family about the risk of falls and identify situations with the highest risk.

31.6.3 Multiple sclerosis

In Multiple Sclerosis (MS), the complexity of the disease, the difficulty in determining appropriate treatment, and the wide range of associated disorders require a comprehensive approach to patient care, including pharmacological and rehabilitative interventions. The functional domains to consider in rehabilitation treatment are multiple and related to the different involvement of anatomical systems. These include motor function (strength, endurance, balance, coordination, muscle fatigue), visual and oculomotor function, somatosensory function, neurovegetative functions (genitourinary dysfunction), cognitive function, and emotional-behavioral aspects. Each functional domain should be treated specifically and effectively, considering the severity and temporal course of the disease.

During the acute phase of the disease, immobilization should be avoided, and its secondary effects prevented. Neuro-motor therapy during bed rest involves frequent changes in posture, passive mobilization exercises, and respiratory exercises to prevent complications (pressure sores, muscle-tendon retractions, joint contractures, respiratory infections, etc.). In general, the rehabilitation

Table 31.2 EXAMPLES OF EXERCISES FOR PARKINSON'S DISEASE ACCORDING TO THE PROGRESSIVE MODULAR REBALANCE SYSTEM (MODIFIED FROM SERRAO ET AL., 2019)*

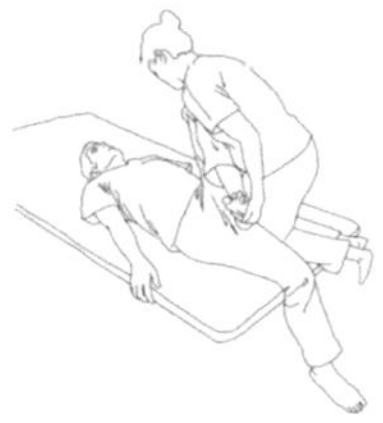	**Stretching of the middle gluteal muscle** The therapist flexes, adducts, and externally rotates the limb to be stretched. The contralateral leg is extended, adducted, externally rotated, and the knee flexed. The therapist asks to extend, abduct, and internally rotate the hip being stretched against their body and, after the release, gains range of motion. Repetitions: from 3 to 5 times..	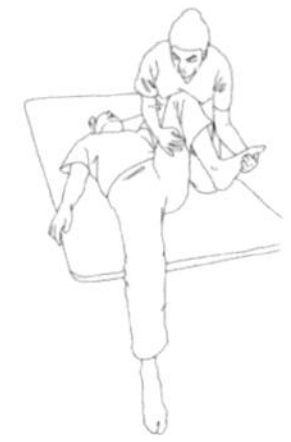	**Stretching of the gluteus maximus and adductor magnus muscles** The therapist flexes, abducts, and internally rotates the hip to be stretched. The contralateral hip is extended, abducted, and internally rotated, with the knee flexed. The therapist asks to extend, adduct, and externally rotate the hip being stretched against their resistance, to maintain the contraction, and, after the release, gains range of motion. Repetitions: 3-5 times.
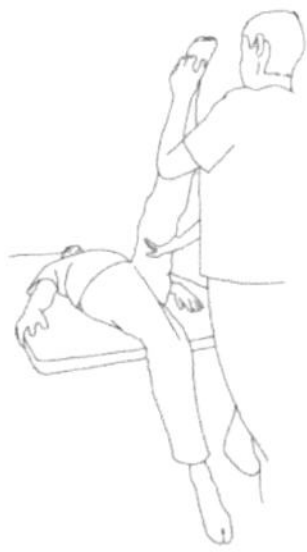	**Hamstring muscle stretch** The therapist flexes, adducts, and externally rotates the leg to be stretched with a straight knee. The contralateral leg is extended, adducted, and externally rotated, with the knee flexed. The therapist asks to extend, abduct, and internally rotate the hip being stretched against their body and, after the release, gains range of motion. Repetitions: from 3 to 5 times.	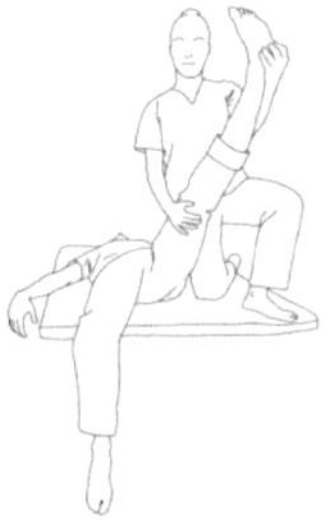	**Stretching of the semitendinosus and semimembranosus muscles** The therapist flexes, abducts, and internally rotates the leg to be stretched with a straight knee. The contralateral hip is extended, abducted, and internally rotated, with the knee flexed. The therapist asks to extend, adduct, and externally rotate the hip being stretched against their resistance, to maintain the contraction, and, after the release, gains range of motion. Repetitions: 3-5 times.
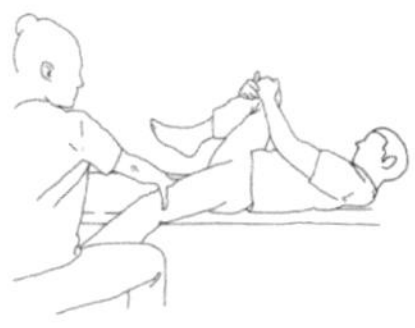	**Iliopsoas muscle stretch** The therapist extends, abducts, and internally rotates the hip to be stretched, with the knee extended. The contralateral leg is flexed, abducted, and internally rotated. The therapist asks to flex, adduct, and externally rotate the hip against their resistance, maintain the contraction, and, after the release, gains range of motion. Repetitions: 3-5 times.	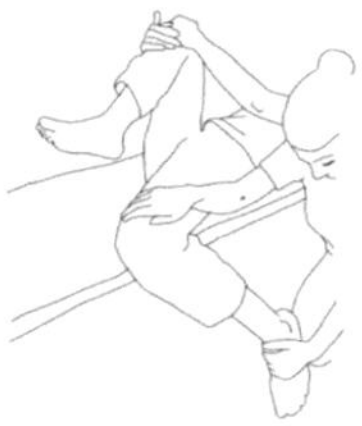	**Stretching of the quadriceps femoris muscle** The therapist extends, abducts, and internally rotates the hip to be stretched and flexes the knee. The contralateral leg is flexed, abducted, and internally rotated. The therapist asks to flex, adduct, and externally rotate the hip and extend the knee being stretched against their resistance, to maintain the contraction, and, after the release, gains range of motion in knee flexion. Repetitions: 3-5 times.

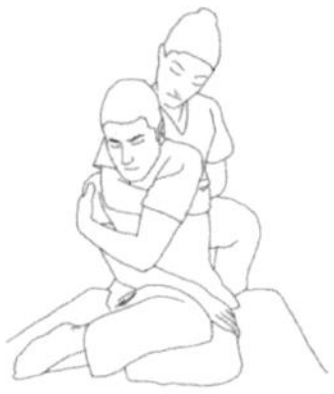

Trunk rotator muscles stretch

The patient is seated sideways, with the therapist positioned behind them, rotating the torso and asking the patient to resist the rotation while maintaining contraction. After relaxation, the therapist gains range of motion towards the concave side. Repetitions: 3-5 times.

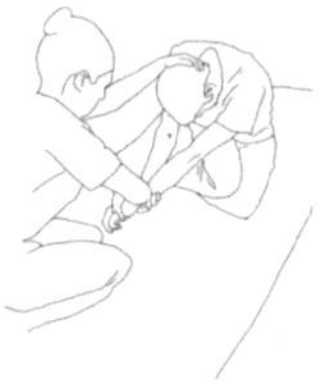

Trunk extensor muscles stretch

The patient is seated sideways, with the therapist facing them, flexing the torso, bending the head, and extending the arms. The therapist asks the patient to raise their arms against resistance, maintain the contraction, and then, after relaxation, achieve range of motion towards the concave side. Repetitions: 3-5 times.

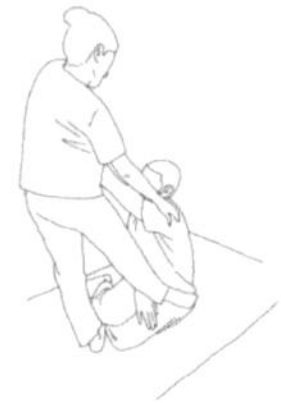

Trunk inclinator muscles stretch

The patient is seated sideways. The therapist stands in front of them, raising the patient's arm while tilting the torso towards the concave side. The therapist asks the patient to extend, abduct, and internally rotate their arm, then maintain the contraction. After relaxation, the therapist further inclines the torso towards the concave side. Repetitions: 3-5 times.

Trunk postural alignment exercises

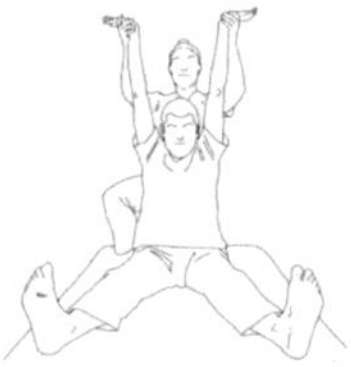

Exercises for recruiting the erector spinae muscles

The patient is seated with legs extended, and the therapist is behind them, asking them to maintain an isometric contraction against their resistance at the end of a bilateral pattern of flexion-abduction-external rotation for at least five seconds.

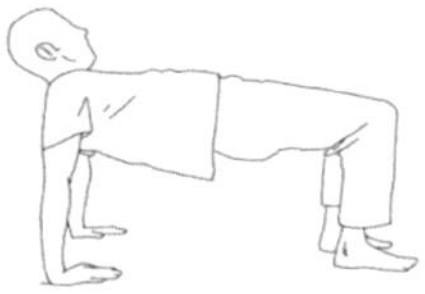

Upside-down table exercise

After stretching the muscles of the shoulder, arm, and lower limbs and performing the supine bridge exercise, the goal is to reach and maintain this position with extended knees and knees flexed at 90°, the head flexed, and the shoulder blades well adducted.

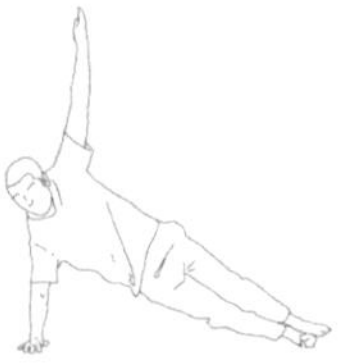

Side bridge exercise

After stretching the oblique muscles on the inclined side and recruiting those on the weaker side, perform this exercise on the weaker side. The goal for patients with the Tower of Pisa Syndrome is to execute the exercise by leaning on the elbow or even flexing the knee.

Path training

Rhythmic stimulation of scapulohumeral girdle movements

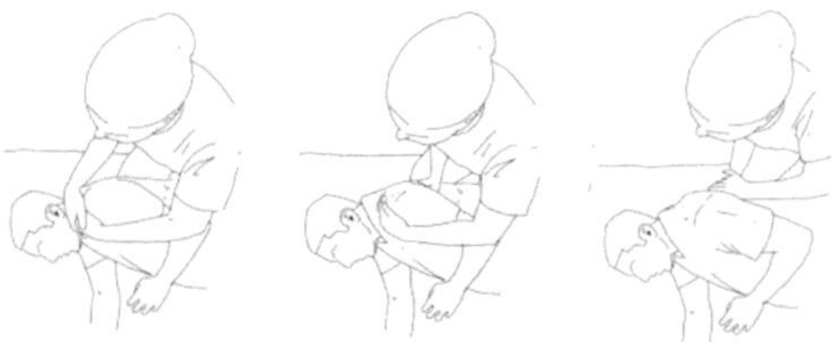

Therapists rhythmically instruct the patient to raise the shoulder anteriorly toward the nose or lower it posteriorly by bringing the scapula closer to the spine. Initially, the patient must perceive the passive movement performed by the therapist and then execute it actively against resistance. Once the patient can perform both movements, the therapist asks them to activate anterior elevation and posterior depression reciprocally.

Rhythmic stimulation of pelvic girdle movements

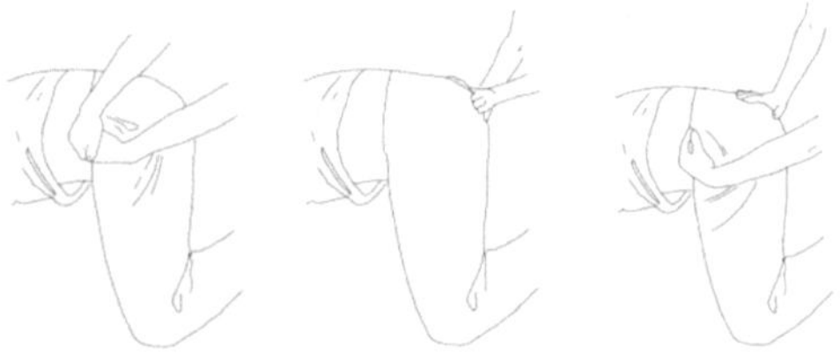

Therapists rhythmically instruct the patient to anteriorly elevate the pelvis toward it or posteriorly depress it. Initially, the patient must perceive the passive movement executed by the therapist and then execute it actively against resistance. When the patient can perform the two movements separately, the therapist asks them to activate anterior elevation and posterior depression reciprocally.

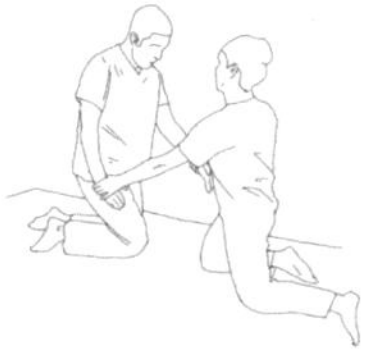

Guided knee walking

Therapists guide patients in walking on their knees by alternately stimulating a flexion-adduction-external rotation pattern of the upper limb on the weight-bearing side and an extension-abduction-internal rotation pattern of the upper limb on the swinging side.

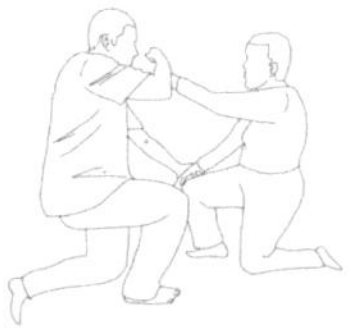

Postural transition into Half-Kneeling

The patient must transition from a kneeling position to a half-kneeling position. The therapist facilitates this transition using two upper limb patterns: flexion-adduction-external rotation of the upper limb on the weight-bearing side and extension-abduction-internal rotation pattern of the upper limb on the swinging side.

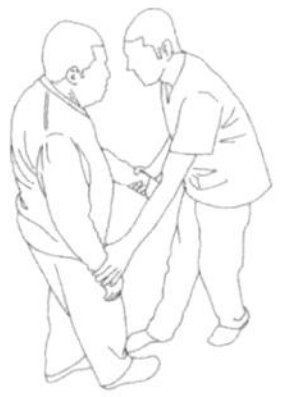

Guided distal walking

The therapist facilitates the patient's walking using two upper limb patterns: flexion-adduction-external rotation of the upper limb on the weight-bearing side and extension-internal rotation-abduction pattern of the upper limb on the swinging side.

* Exercises proposed in Serrao et al., 2019. In conjunction with gait training using visual cueing, the group performing these exercises showed significantly greater improvements in motor function, dynamic balance parameters, and trunk control compared to subjects undergoing conventional rehabilitation with visual cueing.

program is often hindered by the fatigue associated with the disease, which limits not only the patient's ability to move but also cognitive and behavioral functions.

The main objectives in the management of patients with MS include improving motor abilities by increasing muscle strength and normalizing muscle tone, maintaining or increasing joint range of motion, improving coordination and balance, managing and controlling urinary incontinence, improving respiratory function, and muscle stretching and relaxation. The continuity of the rehabilitation process should involve exercises that address the specific problems associated with the disease.

Various rehabilitation approaches and techniques have been proposed in the literature in recent years. Some of these methods are aimed at recovering impaired function, while others focus on improving specific motor tasks (*task-oriented*).

Balance and coordination

Balance and coordination problems are common symptoms of MS that cause movement difficulties. Therefore, including balance and coordination exercises in therapy is crucial. These exercises enhance stability during walking, prevent falls, and improve postural control. Coordination exercises consist of motor acts of specific and gradual complexity, which improve movement coherence and reduce energy consumption due to coordination deficits.

Balance and proprioceptive exercises in patients with upright stability can also be performed using biofeedback – based stabilometric platforms based. Several studies have shown that examinations conducted with these devices can improve postural control. Coordination and balance exercises can be combined with proprioceptive exercises, which can be performed in both seated and standing positions. In addition to conventional physiotherapy with coordination and static and dynamic balance exercises, several techniques have been proposed, including hippotherapy, dance therapy, virtual reality, and robot-assisted therapy. Among the different options, hippotherapy has been extensively studied and is an alternative form of exercise that improves balance and stability in patients with MS.

Gait disorders

Gait disturbances in patients with MS can be caused by various neurological deficits, such as balance and coordination impairments, resulting in ataxic gait, or by spasticity and weakness, resulting in para- or hemiparetic gait. Gait impairment is one of the most disabling symptoms for patients, significantly limiting their independence and quality of life. Gait rehabilitation should be preceded by a thorough analysis that evaluates the gait disturbance at different stages and compares it with that of a healthy individual. Several task-oriented methodologies have been proposed for gait rehabilitation. These include the use of treadmills with or without body weight support systems, as well as the use of robotic exoskeletons such as LOKOMAT, especially in the advanced stages of the disease. Hydrotherapy is another comprehensive physiotherapy approach that acts on the patient's entire body. The physical properties of water, such as hydrostatic pressure, hydrodynamic pressure, viscosity, and buoyancy (reducing body weight), allow for a greater range of motion and reduction of pain. Some evidence shows that hydrotherapy significantly improves independence, mobility, and reduces symptoms such as depression and fatigue.

Spasticity

Spasticity is one of the many symptoms associated with MS, affecting approximately 40-60% of patients and further complicating treatment and rehabilitation efforts. Spastic paresis affects both the lower and upper limbs, with greater severity in distal regions. High levels of spasticity (grade 3 or 4 on the Ashworth scale) can lead to contractures, joint deformities, and pressure sores.

Physiotherapy with standing and active stretching exercises is still essential in the treatment of spasticity. However, various physical methods have been proposed to reduce spasticity, although not all have clear scientific evidence. Cryotherapy, for example, aims to reduce spasticity by decreasing afferent input and also has an analgesic effect by alleviating fatigue syndrome. A recent systematic review and meta-analysis have concluded that some physical methods, such as electrotherapy and vibratory therapy, are valid options for reducing spasticity. Electrical stimulation of the neuromuscular system (NMES), transcutaneous electrical nerve stimulation (TENS), and functional electrical stimulation (FES) are among the electrotherapy applications useful for treating spasticity in patients with MS. Vibratory therapy, using high-frequency mechanical stimulation, has been shown to be effective when applied both locally and to the whole body.

Urinary disorders

The rehabilitation program should also include pelvic floor muscle exercises aimed at countering the neurogenic damage that causes bladder dysfunction, which occurs in approximately 78% of patients. Sphincteric disorders manifest as urinary incontinence or retention. Urinary disturbances often limit the participation of patients in daily and social activities. Pelvic floor muscle exercises involve isometric exercises that target specific muscle groups, aiming to increase muscle mass, strengthen and improve resting tension in these muscles. These exercises allow for prolonged muscle contraction, improving neuro-muscular control and the elasticity of connective tissue, stabilizing the pelvis, and improving the mechanism of urination. Training the pelvic floor muscles should be combined with training of deep muscles, such as the transversus abdominis, to enhance the synergistic action of these structures. Generally, since co-activation of pelvic muscles is reduced or absent in patients with urinary incontinence, pelvic floor rehabilitation should include strengthening and improved motor control of gluteal muscles, adductors, and hamstrings. Additionally, in conjunction with physiotherapeutic rehabilitation, the use of EMG biofeedback and electrical stimulation are valuable methods that have produced encouraging results.

31.6.4 Amyotrophic lateral sclerosis

Despite the lack of curative treatments for Amyotrophic Lateral Sclerosis (ALS), rehabilitation can help patients maintain functional independence in the early stages of the disease and manage symptoms in the advanced stages.

The development of new technologies, such as robotics and brain-computer interfaces, holds promise for delaying the effects of disease progression, allowing for greater interaction with the environment and improving quality of life.

The American Academy of Neurology recommends early referral of patients to multidisciplinary clinical facilities, which provide an ideal environment for evaluating and coordinating rehabilitation needs and interventions at all stages of the disease. In specialized clinics, the rehabilitation team is often supported by other specialists (nutritionists, orthopedic technicians, assistive technology experts, environmental modification/design experts, palliative care specialists) to ensure a comprehensive approach that optimizes healthcare by consolidating different areas of expertise and providing continuity and consistency of care.

Multidisciplinary care has been associated with increased survival time, improved quality of life, increased use of riluzole, non-invasive positive pressure ventilation, and enteral feeding devices.

It is crucial to regularly reassess rehabilitation strategies and modify them based on changes in the disease state. For example, in the early stages of the disease, physiotherapists can educate patients on energy conservation techniques and managing muscle fatigue through intermittent rest during strenuous activities. Subsequently, based on clinical and functional context, patients may be trained in the use of adaptive equipment and mobility aids to adapt to evolving weakness. Instead of providing generic therapy prescriptions, it is better to address specific issues that arise (e.g., gait training, transfer training, wheelchair evaluation, etc.). Due to the progressive nature of ALS, the rehabilitation paradigm is distinct from other diseases and requires the involvement of professionals familiar with the complexity of the condition.

The role of physiotherapy in ALS has been a topic of inquiry. When patients inquire about physical exercise, most of them refer to aerobic training and strength programs. However, evidence regarding the risks and benefits of aerobic or strength exercises in ALS is limited. In murine models of ALS, moderate exercise appears to delay disease onset and increase survival, while high-intensity training seems to be detrimental. Generally, current studies suggest that physiotherapy and moderate-intensity exercise can reduce decline and promote better functionality without adverse effects. However, excessive effort leading to prolonged post-exercise fatigue, muscle soreness, or discomfort should be avoided, as these symptoms may indicate muscle damage induced by excessive workload. Stretching and mobility exercises should be encouraged early in the course of the disease as part of a gentle daily physical activity routine aimed at well-being. Clinical experience suggests that performing simple targeted stretching exercises for major joints helps prevent the development of painful contractures. Working with a physiotherapist to develop an appropriate exercise routine and periodically modify the program as the disease progresses are recommended.

Upper limbs

The involvement of the upper limbs ranges from proximal weakness of the shoulder muscles to distal weakness involving the wrist and intrinsic hand muscles. Hand weakness interferes with activities requiring motor skills such as grasping and manipulating objects. Patients may have difficulty with activities of daily living and instrumental activities such as using handles, buttons, zippers, writing, cutting food, and opening cans and jars. A wide variety of tools are available to assist with activities of daily living, with the goal of prolonging independence for as long as possible. In this regard, the guidance of an occupational therapist experienced in treating patients with ALS is crucial to ensure the selection of the most appropriate devices. Hand orthoses (splints) can also be considered as aids in activities particularly affected by hand muscle weakness. In recent years, various robotic systems, both active and passive, have been developed with both rehabilitative and assistive functions. In the near future, these systems could be controlled through the activation of remaining functioning muscles or segments (shoulder movements, tongue movements, eye movements) or through brain-computer interfaces, which read brain signals.

Lower limbs

The rehabilitation evaluation should include a thorough initial assessment of gait, balance, range of motion, muscle tone of the lower limbs, and fall risk to optimize remaining function. Daily functional activities are reviewed to identify areas for intervention. Assessment and modification of home and work environments (such as removing carpets and installing night lights) can improve safety and promote independence. It is important to note that in the case of falls, resulting injuries and subsequent periods of immobilization can be associated with significant functional decline, making fall prevention a high priority in ALS care.

Fatigue can be addressed by recommending energy conservation techniques, rest breaks, and the use of reinforcement and adaptive equipment. A variety of lower limb orthoses are available. Ankle-foot orthoses (AFOs) assist individuals with ankle dorsiflexion weakness. The involvement of physiotherapists and orthopedic technicians experienced in ALS care is essential to identify the brace that best suits the individual patient's needs. It is important to note that the brace may require adjustments over time as the patient's functional status evolves.

Respiratory dysfunction

The majority of deaths in ALS are due to respiratory failure resulting from weakness of the respiratory muscles. For this reason, the diagnosis and management of respiratory symptoms are extremely important in this disease. It is crucial to discuss breathing options, including tracheostomy and ventilatory support, early on, well before they are clinically indicated, to allow for advance planning.

Respiratory function should be assessed at least every three months from the time of diagnosis. Initial management may include respiratory physiotherapy and postural drainage, especially if the patient has difficulty clearing secretions. The use of suction devices is often recommended for this purpose.

Preventing respiratory infections is a primary goal, and the use of influenza vaccines should always be considered to prevent potential risks. Respiratory muscle exercise can be initiated early and may delay the onset of ventilatory failure. Non-invasive ventilation (NIV) should be considered, particularly when respiratory dysfunction becomes symptomatic during nighttime hours. NIV has been shown to significantly improve quality of life and can prolong survival in patients with normal or moderately reduced bulbar function, especially when used for at least 4 hours per day.

Invasive ventilation should be considered when long-term survival is the primary goal. Counseling is necessary regarding benefits and costs (expenses, intensive physical support with suctioning and nursing care, high caregiver burden) when home management of the patient is not feasible, and referral to specialized centers is preferred.

Language and communication

Dysarthria is a very common symptom due to bulbar involvement and is often a significant source of frustration for patients and their families. Early changes include hypernasality and reduced vocal volume (hypophonia). As the weakness and spasticity of the tongue and laryngeal muscles increase, there will be hypernasality of sounds, harshness of voice, alteration of speech and breath rhythm, reduced sound volume, and impaired intelligibility. Speech and language therapists can address these aspects through techniques aimed at slowing down the rate, exaggerating speech articulation, and improving respiratory efficiency through phrasing. The use of palatal lift prostheses and palatal augmentation can be helpful in reducing the hypernasal aspect of dysarthria.

When communication is compromised, augmentative and alternative communication (AAC) tools can be used, ranging from low-technology options (gestural techniques, communication boards) to high-technology options (electronic communication devices with voice output such as Light-WRITER word generators). These devices can be used as long as there is residual voluntary motor movement (usually eye movements). The specific access method to the device depends on the patient's ability, such as indicating with a body part or a pointer, but adapted mice, joysticks, switches, and scanning technologies can also be used. For patients without residual voluntary motor control, brain-computer interface systems appear to be the most promising.

Swallowing and nutrition

Dysphagia affects one-third of people with ALS at onset, reaching nearly all patients in advanced stages. Dysphagia increases the risk of malnutrition with suboptimal calorie and fluid intake and can contribute to worsening muscle weakness and fatigue. Aspiration pneumonia (13%) is a respiratory complication associated with increased mortality. Difficulties in the oral preparatory phase of swallowing are very common, with symptoms characterized by jaw weakness, fatigue, drooling, slow chewing, and choking. Swallowing function can be evaluated by a speech and language therapist through direct observation or by a physician using instrumental methods such as fiber-optic laryngoscopy or videofluoroscopy. Management of dysphagia involves specific interventions such as adaptations to food consistencies (pureed, thickeners, etc.), modifications of the bolus (smaller sizes), adoption of facilitating and protective postures (vertical positioning, chin-tuck for liquids, etc.) and the use of supportive head aids. Monitoring nutritional status through body weight, percentage of weight loss, and body mass index is important. In these cases, appropriate diets (high-calorie) and nutritional supplements are indicated. Special attention should be given to preventing dehydration, which contributes to a sense of fatigue and promotes thickening of respiratory secretions. In advanced stages, when the progression of dysphagia no longer allows for adequate and safe nutrition, percutaneous endoscopic gastrostomy (PEG) should be considered. PEG is indicated to supplement oral intake and ensure adequate weight maintenance, thereby prolonging survival. Currently, there is limited evidence regarding the impact of PEG on quality of life.

Drooling can be a significant problem in ALS, generally not related to increased saliva production but rather due to reduced ability to swallow saliva, combined with weakness of facial muscles, lip incompetence, and weakness of neck muscles. Optimal management of posture, use of aids (cervical collar), and performance of exercises for the orolingual area can be helpful, in addition to the use of medications (anticholinergics, botulinum toxin, etc.).

31.6.5 Ataxia

Numerous nerve structures contribute, in various ways, to the coordination of voluntary movements and the maintenance of normal postural balance, both static and dynamic (cerebellum, visual system, peripheral and central proprioceptive pathways, vestibular system). The term "ataxia" refers to a neurological condition characterized by incoordination and dysfunction of balance. Three categories of ataxia can be distinguished: sensory (due to proprioceptive information deficit), cerebellar, and vestibular. Mixed forms include symptoms of at least two of the basic forms. For this reason, various neurological disorders can lead to a clinical picture of ataxia (multiple sclerosis, cerebrovascular accidents, cranial trauma, peripheral neuropathies, etc.).

The primary goal of rehabilitation is to stimulate the functional recovery of the patient and, if not possible, help them develop compensatory strategies. The rehabilitation process, aimed at functional recovery, pursues the following objectives: improve balance and postural reactions to external stimuli in different levels of gravity; improve joint stabilization and, consequently, posture; improve upper limb functions. In the rehabilitation process, exercises should initially be performed consciously, with the aim of later automating movements as much as possible. It is necessary to start with simple exercises and then progress to more complex ones; begin with exercises with eyes open (assisted by visual control), then perform them with eyes closed; initially work on tone and stabilization of proximal segments, and then focus on improving coordination of distal segments; use compensatory strategies and aids when it is not possible to further increase functional recovery; plan appropriate home treatments and supportive sports activities. Every rehabilitation program must take into account that the proprioceptive, visual, vestibular systems, and cerebellum are closely functionally interconnected, and the overall balance of the patient is established in relation to this functional unit. To intervene on proprioception, it is necessary to increase proprioceptive stimuli through mechanical stimulation of joints, muscles, and tendons (proprioceptive neuromuscular facilitation, rhythmic stabilization, walking exercises on different surfaces, vibratory stimuli). To improve static and dynamic balance of the patient, the primary objective is trunk stabilization. For this purpose, PNF techniques can be used. The patient can be stimulated to improve static and dynamic stability, initially in supine, lateral, and prone positions, then leaning on elbows, knees, and in a sitting position. Stabilization can be further stimulated through external perturbations (pushes and pulls in various directions). Subsequently, the patient can perform exercises with progressively reduced base of support and variations in the center of gravity (lifting a limb while kneeling). Once the orthostatic posture is achieved, the patient can shift body weight forward or backward or to the sides, further reducing the base of support (tandem position). Recently, stabilometric platforms have been used to improve balance and postural control. Patients can perform exercises on the platforms in static and dynamic modes. The static mode, commonly called stabilometry, aims to assess the patient's postural control in a static situation. Patients can evaluate and control the oscillations of their center of pressure (COP) in different directions (anteroposterior and mediolateral), as well as the area and perimeter of the COP. The dynamic mode is used to facilitate global proprioceptive control (postural destabilization). In this case, the subject can control trunk movements (recorded with an inertial sensor) through an avatar projected on the monitor, even in gaming reconstructions (e.g., skiing, running, etc.). This allows the patient to globally manage instability through trunk control and interaction of forces with the platforms.

31.6.6 Severe acquired brain injuries: traumatic brain injury

In about two-thirds of cases, severely traumatized patients in the cranioencephalic region present associated injuries to other organs and systems, which can significantly influence recovery. For this reason, it is necessary to establish an individualized rehabilitation program from the beginning and adapt it over time in relation to the evolution of the clinical picture. The three main phases of rehabilitation treatment in patients with traumatic brain injury are: the acute phase (or resuscitation-neurosurgical phase), the post-acute phase (or rehabilitation phase), and the phase of outcome management.

Acute phase

The acute phase extends from the moment of trauma until the resolution of resuscitation issues. The areas of rehabilitation intervention in the acute phase consist of maintaining adequate respiratory function, facilitating the return to contact with the external environment, and preventing and treating immobilization-related complications. Regarding the latter aspect, it is important to prevent muscle-tendon retractions and the development of intra-articular calcifications due to prolonged maintenance of certain postures through periodic changes in bed position (alternate lateral decubitus, prone position, sitting) and through passive multi-joint mobilization.

Post-acute phase

In the early post-acute phase, interventions focus on definitive internal stabilization (metabolic-nutritional, cardio-circulatory, respiratory balance, resolution of intercurrent complications), treatment of major disabilities, and restoration of autonomy in the simplest activities of daily life (eating, drinking, grasping, and manipulating objects, etc.). In this phase, the patient should be admitted to specialized facilities capable of providing intensive rehabilitation treatment. In the late post-acute phase, interventions are mainly oriented towards regaining autonomy in "complex" activities of daily life, such as managing the home, using means of transportation, reintegrating into school and work. In this phase, typically, interventions aimed at the gradual reintegration of the patient into the non-hospital environment (home, protected facilities, "transition" facilities) begin. Rehabilitative interventions on specific impairments or disabilities, if possible, can continue on a day-hospital or outpatient basis.

Outcome management phase

In this phase, the rehabilitation treatment must mainly aim to maintain the acquired recovery and the social reintegration of the patient. The individual undergoes a long and complex process of processing their own experience, which leads to a conscious acceptance of their residual disability and the reorganization of their life based on real resources.

Cognitive rehabilitation

Cognitive deficits are a determining condition for the social and occupational reintegration of the patient. Approaches to cognitive treatment can be categorized into two categories: recovery techniques and compensatory techniques. The recovery approach focuses on reinforcing the damaged function that remains partially intact, while the compensatory approach aims to teach patients strategies that compensate for the lost function.

Treatments aimed at recovering cognitive function are designed to treat specific components such as selective attention or memory, for example. Compensatory methods are based on the performance of activities of daily living, such as remembering sequences of motor tasks required to perform a specific job. Compensatory techniques may involve the use of electronic memories, alarms, calendars, or post-it notes.

A prerequisite for any action is knowledge of the spatial coordinates of one's own body and the surrounding space. Patients with traumatic brain injury may present different combinations of visuospatial deficits (object localization in space, perception of spatial depth, object, and shape recognition). It is necessary, as soon as possible, to teach patients to increase visual attention in areas of space where there is even minimal residual function. A common problem is hemineglect, a consequence of right hemisphere injuries. This disorder needs to be taken seriously and requires specific treatment because, if present, it limits motor recovery. Daily visual training of the affected side (*visual scanning*), combined with optokinetic stimulation, represents the most suitable treatment.

Assistive memory devices

Particularly interesting are computerized "paging" systems that facilitate mnemonic performance and planning, which are useful in daily activities. Paging systems can be divided into two types: manual or automatic. In the manual system, a message is sent to the operator through a phone call. The operator then sends the message to the medical personnel's pager through a network. In automatic systems, there are continuous incoming requests that are automatically processed by the terminal and sent to the pager. The types of messages that can be sent include alert tones, voice messages, or text messages. The architecture of paging systems consists of six basic elements: end-user equipment (e.g., cellphone or computer), the calling terminal, the operation center, the control station, the base station, and the pager.

Communication (verbal and non-verbal) is often severely compromised in patients with traumatic brain injuries. The treatment involves training through pragmatic language tasks such as *listening* and *initiating* a conversation or participating in activities that involve appropriate social interaction (cooking, playing board games, writing, reading, etc.).

31.6.7 Spinal cord injuries

The clinical course of a patient with spinal cord injury largely depends on the level and severity of the lesion (complete/incomplete). For this reason, rehabilitation programs need to be flexibly adjusted to adapt to changes in the patient's neurological condition. In addition to the typical clinical monitoring in this phase, a series of rehabilitation procedures can be initiated, mainly aimed at preventing respiratory complications, pressure ulcers, muscle-tendon retractions, and intra-articular calcifications.

Respiratory function is particularly compromised in cases of cervical injury with tetraplegia or high dorsal injuries, due to the combined deficit of the intercostal and abdominal muscles. In these cases, techniques such as postural drainage with mechanical assistance (abdominal compression) should be used to facilitate expectoration. To increase the patient's vital capacity, exercises aimed at diaphragm and accessory respiratory muscle strengthening are recommended early on. It is also important to strive for early sitting posture and ensure regular bowel evacuation, conditions that improve diaphragmatic motility.

Patients in supine or lateral decubitus positions should be frequently repositioned. The use of anti-decubitus mattresses and cushions (air, water, etc.), especially in cases of tetraplegia, should always be encouraged. Correct positioning of the trunk and limbs of bedridden patients and early mobilization are the main interventions to be performed in order to avoid the development of joint stiffness.

Joint movements should be performed slowly and repeatedly, avoiding the evocation of pain as much as possible.

The patient with spinal cord injury should be stimulated early on to regain a minimum level of autonomy. It is important to provide suitable tools to involve the tetraparetic patient in everyday life as soon as possible. For example, tools such as a bell, a reading stand, suitable utensils, or a television with a remote control can provide the patient with the motivational drive to interact with the surrounding environment even in the early stages of spinal cord trauma. Additionally, simple activities such as washing hands and face, combing hair, brushing teeth, eating, and drinking independently should be initiated.

The evolution of spinal cord damage leads, after a phase of spinal shock characterized by flaccidity, to the phase of hypertonic spasticity. The main objective of rehabilitation treatment is therefore to counteract spasticity from the early stages through inhibiting postures and active and passive muscle stretching exercises. By reducing spastic hypertonia, the phenomenon of irradiation (involuntary contraction of synergistic and/or antagonistic muscles to the voluntarily activated muscle) is reduced, allowing for more effective performance of all rehabilitation exercises aimed at recovering trunk and limb function.

In patients with cervical lesions and severe tetraparesis, it is important to ensure the maintenance of joint excursions, including sternoclavicular, costoclavicular, costo-vertebral, and scapulo-costal joints, which are important for respiration. Furthermore, particular attention should be paid to the reinforcement of the abdominal muscles for trunk control, an essential prerequisite for wheelchair transfers. The next step is verticalization, which involves providing weight-bearing to strengthen antigravity muscles and recondition them to the body's weight. This helps prevent bone changes, improve functions related to peristalsis, and recondition the cardio-circulatory system. Verticalization is achievable using a static bed and should be sought with promptness, gradualness, and constant monitoring of blood pressure and heart rate.

Cervical injuries are associated with clinical pictures characterized by spastic tetraparesis, which greatly limits hand manipulation function. Even in patients where minimal distal motor activity is preserved relative to the extent of the spinal cord injury, the loss or limitation of elbow extension (spasticity, joint stiffness) implies significant restriction of the working area and the ability to reach and move objects. The first step in the process of recovering hand functionality is the correct positioning of the upper limb to avoid capsular shoulder strains and maintain unloading of the upper limb. Usually, a soft wedge is used with the lower part placed under the shoulder. The position should be changed periodically, alternating between external/internal rotation and supination/pronation of the forearm, while avoiding the hand closing in flexion. The use of orthoses (splints, hand braces) can help prevent finger and wrist deformities. As soon as the clinical picture allows, the recovery of grip and release control of objects should be considered a fundamental outcome to achieve. Even minimal improvements in this function can translate into significant progress in daily life functions such as eating, drinking, brushing teeth, writing, handling money from a wallet, etc. Similar to patients with post-stroke hemiparesis, spinal cord injury patients can benefit from functional electrical prosthetics to facilitate hand opening and closing.

When and if the patient's neurological conditions allow it, the exercise program should be integrated into the patient's rehabilitation plan based on the milestones achieved. The training includes exercises aimed at bed mobility, such as turning from one side to another, prone-supine movements, and upward or downward shifting. This is followed by exercises targeted at basic transfers, such as from the wheelchair to the bed, toilet, shower, or bathtub. Finally, advanced transfers, such as getting in and out of a car with wheelchair positioning, are addressed. Learning to use a wheelchair is a fundamental step because it represents the first level of independence in mobility. In cases of high-level tetraplegia, an electric wheelchair is the only tool that allows for mobility and self-sufficiency.

In the initial stages, an indwelling catheter should be used to ensure bladder emptying, avoiding bladder overdistension. The duration of indwelling catheterization depends on the progression of the neurological condition. Subsequently, intermittent catheterization should be performed by nursing staff and, if possible, by the patient themselves (self-catheterization). In cases of incomplete injury and significant functional recovery, patients can regain good urinary autonomy by using abdominal pressure to empty the bladder.

Activities of daily living (ADL)

Activities of daily living (ADL) testing and training are crucial for assessing and addressing various aspects of a patient's functional abilities. These activities include personal care (eating, washing, dressing, personal hygiene), sphincter control (bladder and bowel), mobility (transfers from bed to wheelchair, toilet, bathtub, shower, or car; walking or wheelchair use).

In patients with paraparesis secondary to dorsal lesions, walking may remain the primary means of movement in the surrounding environment or serve as an occasional alternative to the wheelchair. The recovery of walking ability, through aids and orthoses, can help prevent joint, bone, cardiopulmonary, and vegetative complications resulting from prolonged wheelchair use. Orthoses and walking aids include mechanical orthoses, functional electrical stimulation (FES) or neuromuscular stimulation (FNS), and hybrid systems that combine mechanical orthoses with FES.

Mechanical orthoses stabilize the distal segments, allowing the preserved proximal functions to be utilized. Functional electrical stimulation systems induce contractions of paralyzed muscles to achieve functional synergies (e.g., activation of ankle plantar flexors during the push-off phase of walking).

In addition to conventional neuromotor treatment, recent years have seen the implementation of tools such as mobile platforms combined with body weight support (BWS) systems and robotic exoskeletons (e.g., Lokomat). These devices aim to facilitate the functioning of the spinal central pattern generator (CPG) and, consequently, the reprogramming of walking.

31.6.8 Peripheral nervous system injuries

Damage to peripheral nervous system structures can occur as a result of various etiological conditions. Depending on the etiology (inflammatory, compressive, autoimmune, traumatic, metabolic, toxic), different clinical pictures can be identified, classified according to topographic characteristics (asymmetric or symmetric polyneuropathies, distal and/or proximal, mononeuropathies, multineuropathies, plexopathies, radiculopathies) and based on the severity of the anatomical compromise of the involved nerves (neuropraxia, axonotmesis, neurotmesis). In addition to the clinical examination, which is essential for prognosis, including rehabilitation prognosis, neurophysiological evaluation is of fundamental importance. This involves studying the conduction of peripheral nerves (nerve conduction studies, NCS) and recording the electrical activity of muscles (electromyography, EMG). These tests can confirm the anatomical structure of the involved nerve, determine the distribution pattern, define the pathophysiological process, and assess the severity and progression of the damage.

Rehabilitation in this group of pathologies must consider several factors. The rehabilitative goals in this group of clinical conditions differ based on the extent of the damage, the predominant symptoms (motor or sensory), and the physiological recovery time of the peripheral nerve. In cases of neuropraxia or grade II axonotmesis according to Sunderland classification (axon damage with intact endoneurium), the rehabilitative intervention will mainly focus on muscle recruitment exercises aimed at restoring the impaired functions. In more severe axonotmesis or neurotmesis, the rehabilitation intervention will be more focused on developing compensatory strategies for the functions innervated by preserved structures. In cases where postural instability and hypoesthesia with proprioceptive deficit occur, such as in distal symmetric polyneuropathies, the rehabilitative intervention will be similar to that for ataxias, based on exercises aimed at improving postural balance.

The most commonly used rehabilitation strategies in peripheral nervous system injuries include classical passive and active-assisted kinesiotherapy techniques, which are necessary in the acute denervation phase to maintain joint mobility and muscle elasticity; proprioceptive neuromuscular facilitation (PNF-RMP) techniques, which generate movement in denervated structures through the diffusion of stimuli from remaining connected structures in kinesiological patterns of motor activation; electromyographic biofeedback; neurocognitive methodologies such as Cognitive-Action Therapy (ETC-CTA); and Action Observation Therapy, aimed at enhancing effector system activation through increased central nervous system activation.

From the perspective of instrumental physical therapies, low-frequency stimulation electrotherapy seems to have an enhancing effect on nerve regeneration when combined with active recruitment exercises of the denervated area to prevent the possibility of aberrant regeneration. In an occupational context, the use of both static and dynamic orthoses represents a useful means of preventing secondary damage, such as the development of joint deformities, substituting for the impaired function when there is no residual recruitment capacity, or enhancing the impaired function when contractile capacity is partially preserved. Both static and dynamic orthoses should be tailored to the specific injuries of the individual.

Although evidence is still lacking, robotic therapy appears to have a positive impact on the functional recovery of individuals with peripheral nervous system injuries.

31.7 New frontiers in neurorehabilitation

In recent decades, neurorehabilitation has evolved from an empirical approach to a more objective and reliable one, based on evidence-based medicine. This has allowed for a deeper understanding of the pathophysiological mechanisms underlying neurological deficits and the central mechanisms involved in functional recovery (neuronal plasticity). Innovative technologies have been developed in recent years to significantly contribute to rehabilitation interventions (Table 31.3).

31.7.1 Quantitative movement analysis

Quantitative movement analysis is a method that allows for the quantification of motor deficits and the objective assessment of the complex relationship between the primary deficit, motor adaptations, and compensations. It integrates three disciplines: kinematics, dynamics, and electromyography. Kinematics describes the motion of objects and provides information on the displacements, velocities, and linear and angular accelerations of body segments and joints. Dynamics studies the forces that modify the motion of bodies, including the interactions between the subject and the ground and the development of internal joint moments. Surface electromyography (EMG) enables the study of the electrical signals generated by skeletal muscle activity, detectable on the skin surface. EMG provides simple information about muscle activation intervals (on-off periods) and more complex information about the neural control strategies of voluntary movement.

Optoelectronic systems and miniaturized inertial devices integrating accelerometers and gyroscopes are widely used for human movement analysis. Optoelectronic systems are considered the gold standard for laboratory-based kinematic analysis, capturing the instantaneous positions of reflective markers placed on specific anatomical landmarks (Figure 31.1a). Because of the enormous potential of quantitative movement analysis, the use of modern motion analysis systems is considered of paramount importance for research in the field of neurorehabilitation. The pattern of gait or pathological motor gesture has been extensively studied in many neurological diseases. In some of these diseases, the improvement induced by physiotherapy has been objectified through the monitoring of spatiotemporal, kinematic, kinetic, and electromyographic parameters, providing a greater quantity and quality of information than what can be obtained with traditional clinical scales.

In recent years, there has been increasing interest in the use of magneto-inertial sensors for movement analysis (Figure 31.1b). These devices, with their portability and ease of use, provide reliable information on spatiotemporal

Table 31.3 INNOVATIVE METHODS IN NEUROREHABILITATION

In the field of neurorehabilitation, some innovative methods have recently been developed that can facilitate neuronal plasticity and functional recovery. However, their translation into clinical practice still needs to be fully demonstrated.

ROBOTIC THERAPY		
Function to rehabilitate	Type of system	Type of robot
Gait training	End-effector Exoskeleton	E.g., Gait trainer, Geo system E.g., Lokomat, Ekso
Upper limb mobility	End-effector Exoskeleton	E.g., MIME, MIT-MANUS, Amadeo, Reharob, Rupert, Gentle E.g., ARM-Guide, Armeo, Pneu-WREX, Diego, ARMin, L-exos, Exo7, Medarm
Hand function	End-effector Exoskeleton	PneuGlove, Amadeo, PabloX2 HAWARD, Hand Mentor
VIRTUAL REALITY		
Function to rehabilitate	Type of system	Type of device
Posture and balance Gait training Upper limb mobility	Feedback-centered interaction Gesture-based interaction Haptic stimuli-based interaction Cave automatic virtual environment	Es. Wii, Peripheral nunchuks-balance board (Nintendo) Es. Sistemi "Head mounted displays" Es. PlayStation 2 Eye Toy, Move (Sony) Es. Kinetic (Microsoft)
NON-INVASIVE BRAIN STIMULATION		
Function to rehabilitate	Type of stimulator	Type of stimulus
Upper limb mobility Gait training	Transcranial magnetic stimulation (TMS)	Single-pulse Double-pulse Repetitive stimulation Complex stimulation
	Transcranial electrical stimulation	Direct stimulation Alternate stimulation Random-noise stimulation
BRAIN-COMPUTER INTERFACE (BCI)		
Function to rehabilitate	Type of BCI	Paradigm
Sensory (vision, hearing) Communication - Writing - Reading - Making phone calls - Alarming - Information retrieval Motor - Grasping - Assisted mobility - Motor recovery Entertainment - Gaming - Music browsing - Photo browsing - Motor Recovery	BCI-driven spelling devices BCI control of web browsers BCI and assistive technology Motor Substitution	Motor Imagery P300 Component of Event-Related Potentials Slow Cortical Potentials Visual Evoked Potentials

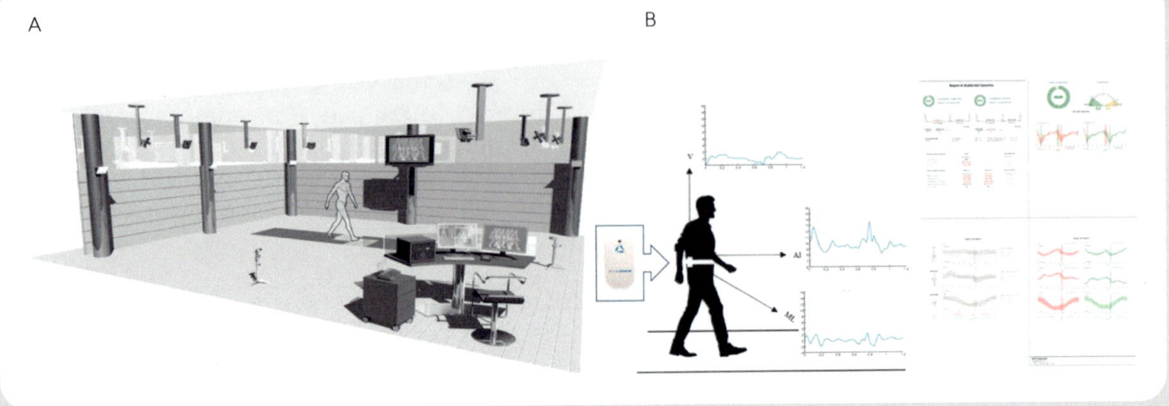

Figure 31.1

parameters and some kinematic parameters of movement.

31.7.2 Robotic rehabilitation

The use of robotics and technology to support rehabilitation programs is a more recent development, primarily used in patients with stroke, traumatic brain injury, or spinal cord injury. Robots are equipped with sensors to record joint positions, velocities, and forces. They embed actuators that can move and/or assist the movement of affected limbs at different speeds and amplitudes. Unlike conventional therapies, robots can deliver highly individualized rehabilitation interventions without limitations in frequency and daily treatment intensity.

Upper extremity robots

Currently, upper extremity robotic systems can be grouped into two types: end-effectors (MIT/IMT-Manus, MIME, GENTLE/s) and exoskeletons (ARMin, Pneu-WREX, RUPERT, REHAROB). With end-effectors, subjects grasp a manipulandum controlled by a robot, allowing for complete adaptation to individual patient characteristics. Exoskeleton systems involve the limb being enclosed within a robot, which, due to its mechanical flexibility, allows for full specification of the limb's configuration (ARM Guide). Exoskeletal systems have the advantage of being able to independently apply and measure forces at each joint. However, the question of whether learning a single movement can translate into effective improvement in overall limb function remains open. For this reason, the motor task should be as extensive as possible, increasing degrees of freedom, the number of tasks, workspace, applied force, and limb geometric configuration.

Lower extremity robots

Lower extremity robots are primarily used for the recovery of upright posture and walking in severe motor disabilities (Erigo, Lokomat, GaitTrainer, Geo-System). Some systems are used early on in patients with spinal cord injuries or stroke to recover trunk control in an upright posture and prevent muscle-tendon contractures and joint stiffness in the lower limbs. Static beds with a robotic stepping system are used for passive mobilization of the lower limbs in an upright position. For gait rehabilitation, electrically operated walking orthoses are used to assist lower limb movement through sophisticated software. These systems provide support, connected to a computer, which can partially or fully unload the patient's weight, assist their walking motion by varying parameters (speed, frequency, step length, knee, and hip joint range of motion), and provide differentiated assistance to one limb compared to the contralateral limb. These methods also allow for online and offline measurement of various movement parameters (joint angles, muscle strength, spasticity).

In recent years, considerable interest has been directed towards wearable exoskeletons. These exoskeletons, initially designed for military purposes, are now used in the rehabilitation of individuals with walking difficulties (spinal cord injuries, post-stroke hemiplegia, multiple sclerosis). Such systems allow patients to move with greater freedom compared to static robotic systems, facilitating their interaction with the environment (participation). Wearable exoskeletal systems are used for both therapist-guided therapeutic exercises and as directly operated assistive devices by the patient.

31.7.3 Virtual reality

Virtual reality refers to a simulation of the real environment generated by dedicated software and experienced through a human-machine interface. In exercises performed in this type of environment, subjects can monitor their own movements as they attempt to imitate optimal movement patterns indicated in real-time in the virtual scenario, with the possibility of receiving visual, auditory, or somatosensory feedback. Overall, this approach promotes "learning by imitation," and the complexity of the required motor tasks can be progressively increased to facilitate the transfer of learned motor patterns to the real world. Virtual reality is a relatively new tool in neurorehabilitation, as it is flexible and easily adaptable to individual patient needs. Several virtual reality systems have been developed, including game-based systems (rehabilitation gaming system), imitation-based learning systems that utilize a virtual instructor whose movements are replicated by the patient, systems with haptic feedback, and combinations of virtual reality with robotic training.

31.7.4 Tele-rehabilitation

Tele-rehabilitation involves the application of computer and telecommunication technologies to support remote rehabilitation services. In this context, tele-rehabilitation enables the monitoring of functional status and the provision of remote rehabilitation exercises, allowing patients to continue their rehabilitation outside of healthcare facilities. The use of tele-rehabilitation experienced rapid growth during the SARS-COV2 pandemic in 2020-21, often serving as the only means for patients to continue their rehabilitation journey. The technologies most commonly used for tele-rehabilitation include video conferencing via smartphones or personal computers, digital personal assistants, sensors provided in patients' homes, robotics, and virtual reality. The development of specific computer applications and technological supports designed for tele-rehabilitation is a rising area of interest in the field of rehabilitation. However, the cost-effectiveness of tele-rehabilitation compared to traditional rehabilitation is still to be confirmed.

Bibliography

Bartolo M., De Luca D., Serrao M., Sinforiani E., Zucchella C., Sandrini G., Caregivers' feeling of burden and needs in community neurorehabilitation. J Rehabil Med; 42:818-822, 2010.

Bartolo M., Zucchella C., Tortola P., Spicciato F., Sandrini G., Pierelli F. Clinical scales for measuring stroke rehabilitation promote functional recovery by supporting teamwork. Eur J Phys Rehabil Med; Apr;52(2):195-202, 2016.

Cicerone K.D., Langenbahn D.M., Braden C. et al., Evidence-based cognitive rehabilitation: updated review of the literature from 2003 through 2008. Arch Phys Med Rehabil; 92:519-30, 2011.

Etoom M., Khraiwesh Y., Lena F., Hawamdeh M., Hawamdeh Z., Centonze D. & Foti C. Effectiveness of Physiotherapy Interventions on Spasticity in People with Multiple Sclerosis. A Systematic Review and Meta-Analysis. Am J Phys Med Rehabil; 97(11):793-807, 2018.

Gensini G.F., Zaninelli A. (Eds), SPREAD – Stroke PRevention and Educational Awareness Diffusion. Linee Guida italiane di prevenzione e trattamento dell'ictus cerebrale (VI Ed.), 2010.

Intercollegiate Stroke Working Party. National clinical guideline for stroke, 3rd edition. London: Royal College of Physicians, 2008.

Iocco M. Trattamento riabilitativo delle lesioni nervose periferiche, Minerva Medica, Torino, 2021.

Khan F., Amatya B. Rehabilitation in Multiple Sclerosis: A Systematic Review of Systematic Reviews. Arch Phys Med Rehabil 98(2):353-367, 2017.

Marsden J., Harris C. Cerebellar ataxia: pathophysiology and rehabilitation. Clin Rehabil. 25(3):195-216, 2011.

Majmudar Wu J., Paganoni S. Rehabilitation in amyotrophic lateral sclerosis: why it matters. Muscle Nerve. 50(1):4-13; 2014.

Monari G. Riequilibrio Modulare Progressivo. Elaborazione Del Concetto Di Kabat. Edi-Ermes. 2013.

Serrao M, Pierelli F, Sinibaldi E, Chini G, Castiglia SF, Priori M, Gimma D, Sellitto G, Ranavolo A, Conte C, Bartolo M, Monari G. Progressive Modular Rebalancing System and Visual Cueing for Gait Rehabilitation in Parkinson's Disease: A Pilot, Randomized, Controlled Trial With Crossover. Front Neurol. 2019 Aug 29;10:902.

Serrao M, Chini G, Caramanico G, Bartolo M, Castiglia SF, Ranavolo A, Conte C, Venditto T, Coppola G, di Lorenzo C, Cardinali P, Pierelli F. Prediction of Responsiveness of Gait Variables to Rehabilitation Training in Parkinson's Disease. Front Neurol. 2019 Aug 2;10:826.

Van Criekinge T, Truijen S, Schröder J, Maebe Z, Blanckaert K, van der Waal C, Vink M, Saeys W. The effectiveness of trunk training on trunk control, sitting and standing balance and mobility post-stroke: a systematic review and meta-analysis. Clin Rehabil. 2019 Jun;33(6):992-1002.

Van Peppen R.P., Kwakkel G., Wood-Dauphinee S., Hendriks H.J., Van der Wees P.J., Dekker J., The impact of physical therapy on functional outcomes after stroke: what's the evidence? Clin Rehabil. 18:833-862, 2004.

32 PEDIATRIC NEUROLOGY

Francesca Nardecchia, Serena Galosi, Mario Mastrangelo,
Francesco Pisani, Vincenzo Leuzzi

Pediatric neurology is characterized by some clinical peculiarities compared to adult neurology. The first pertains to the specific relationship between disease occurrence and the neurodevelopment level of brain structure and functions.

Consequently, the clinical picture is the overall result of the deficit in the functions related to the affected structures, phenomena of anatomical and functional vicariance of the remaining structures, and, finally, the asynchrony between the development processes of functionally connected areas.

In the nosographic aspect, many neurological diseases in children stem from alterations in the biological mechanisms that regulate neurological and mental development. Their deficits lead to qualitative alterations (such as autism) or global quantitative impairments (such as intellectual disabilities) or focal impairments (communication disorders, developmental coordination disorders, specific learning disorders, etc.) in the development of higher cortical functions. This wide range of conditions, which is highly relevant in terms of epidemiology and clinical practice, has now found a specific classification within the Diagnostic and Statistical Manual of Mental Disorders (DSM-5 and DSM-5-TR) under the category of "neurodevelopmental disorders." This group of conditions is defined by early onset (often before entering primary school) and an impairment in the emergence and development of essential human-specific competencies necessary for normal personal, social, academic, and occupational functioning. The extent of the deficit varies, including specific disabilities in certain areas of competence up to global impairment of cognitive or social skills. Often, different disorders coexist (such as autism spectrum disorder and intellectual disabilities, attention deficit/hyperactivity disorder, and specific learning disorder) or follow a sequential pattern (e.g., autism spectrum disorder as an initial symptom and later intellectual disability).

Furthermore, there is a wide range of congenital brain malformations due to anatomical developmental anomalies (focal or generalized) of the brain (e.g., disorders of neuronal migration and cortical development, cerebellar and brainstem malformations, etc.) and/or the spinal cord (e.g., failure of neural tube closure) caused by genetic or acquired factors (infectious diseases, vascular disorders, etc.) that impair anatomical differentiation at a very early embryonic or fetal stage. In all major syndromic areas (from epilepsy to movement disorders), there are conditions that manifest exclusively in childhood or assume a phenotype entirely distinct from that observed in adults.

Finally, in terms of aetiology, inherited or de novo monogenic genetic diseases and chromosomal abnormalities prevail in children compared to the complex or multifactorial alterations that characterise adult neurology (e.g., Parkinson's disease, multiple sclerosis, Alzheimer's disease, etc.). Even in the field of acquired conditions (infectious diseases, trauma, neoplasms, etc.), specific etiologies or lesion patterns characterize the pediatric CNS differently from the adult CNS (e.g., infectious fetopathies, HIV-1 encephalitis, CNS tumors, clinical consequences of repeated head trauma or shaken baby syndrome in abused children, etc.).

Therefore, the neurological examination of children inherently possesses a multidimensional nature, requiring the integration of different levels of *nervous system dysfunction*, including:

a) *Developmental examination*, which explores the child's functioning based on the timing of emergence and level of expected competencies and skills for their age, implying knowledge of normal and pathological development at different ages.
b) *The assessment of the impaired function/skill*, in relation to the expected level of complexity for the patient's age, involving knowledge of the internal organization and development of the specific function/skill.
c) *Localizing anatomic lesion*, based on the patient's symptoms.

A systematic treatment of pediatric neurological conditions is beyond the scope of this chapter. We will focus on some key symptoms that characterize pediatric presentation of neurological diseases and their most frequently associated conditions. We will not discuss neurological disorders that have a clinical presentation in children similar to that in adults.

32.1 Neurodevelopmental disorders

Global developmental delay (previously referred to as psychomotor retardation), intellectual disabilities (intellectual developmental disorder), and autism spectrum disorders (ASD) are three closely related conditions that emerge in the first months or years of life and often coexist or describe successive trajectories of the child's pathological development.

The term "psychomotor retardation", which essentially corresponds to the global developmental delay in the DSM-5, is reserved for conditions where the *timing* of the expected competencies based on the child's chronological age during the first 5 years of life is delayed. Sometimes the delay may involve specific functions (e.g., delay in walking or phonological development) or be associated with typical syndromic features (e.g. Down syndrome). In any case, the term constitutes only a provisional diagnosis that implies subsequent clinical and etiological reassessment. Over time, additional symptoms may become evident, and the condition of delayed development can evolve into qualitative or quantitative alterations in mental functioning and neurological development. This term should not be used when a more appropriate clinical diagnosis is possible or when an etiological diagnosis is available. In these cases, the term assumes a descriptive rather than diagnostic meaning. Furthermore, the term should not be used when clinical history and observation are consistent with the suspicion of a degenerative disease that is disrupting the biological processes underlying psychomotor development (psychomotor delay vs. neurological deterioration).

Global developmental delay, especially when isolated during the observed period has limited localizing value and may result from many acquired, idiopathic, and genetic conditions that emerge in the early years of life. Neuroimaging investigations (Magnetic Resonance Imaging-MRI, Computed Tomography-CT, etc.), in the absence of other associated neurological deficits, provide limited information, leading clinicians to consider this condition as an expression of a maturational gap or the outcome of a fixed encephalopathy, sometimes relying on inconsistent anamnestic elements.

The term "intellectual disability" (ID) refers to a permanent, non-progressive condition (as opposed to mental deterioration) of reduced intellectual functioning emerging in the first 18 years of life. The prevalence of severe presentations of ID is approximately 4 cases per 1,000, with 4 cases per 100 for the mildest forms. Severe ID are often associated with macroscopic structural brain abnormalities acquired or genetic in origin (outcomes of fetal pathologies or severe perinatal distress, chromosomal aberrations, disorders of CNS migration or morphogenesis), and they manifest early with delayed or lack of psychomotor acquisitions preceding a general impairment of higher cortical skills. Over 60% of cases of ID are caused by genetic and genetic-metabolic diseases. This percentage is higher in cohorts with prevalent severe presentations. It is destined to increase as functions of the further refinement of genetic diagnostic techniques.

Acquired conditions (e.g., fetal alcohol syndrome, fetal, neonatal of infantile infectious pathologies, etc.) contribute still significantly to the prevalence of ID. Based on the presence or absence of specific anatomical CNS peculiarities (e.g., microcephaly, cerebellar hypoplasia, agenesis of the corpus callosum, etc.) or other systemic features (poor somatic growth, distinctive facial features, associated visceral malformations), ID is classified into syndromic or non-syndromic forms.

Down syndrome is certainly the most frequent paradigm of a syndromic form of ID. Mild forms of ID are less frequently associated with structural brain abnormalities and may become evident at a later age due to the increased complexity of environmental demands. This group also includes conditions in which social disadvantage (sensory deprivation, understimulation, social/cultural marginalization) plays an important pathogenic role. While ID is a common symptom in pediatric neurology, the conditions causing it can be extremely heterogeneous (and sometimes exceptionally rare). In the *syndromic forms* the phenotype may help the diagnostic process. In *non-syndromic forms*, the peculiar behavioral phenotype may sometimes suggest a specific disorder (for example hyperverbalism in Williams syndrome or the difficulty in social interaction in X-fragile syndrome) suggesting diagnostic hypotheses and laboratory investigations. The clear distinction between syndromic and non-syndromic forms may be overly simplistic and depends on the specific sensitivity and experience of the clinician, as well as the patient's age (e.g., fragile X syndrome does not manifest as a syndromic form in childhood but assumes those characteristics during puberty). Finally, there is no widely accepted and conventional classification of cognitive and behavioral traits, as is the case for somatic traits. However, some behavioral phenotypes demonstrate the same consistency as somatic phenotypes (e.g., Rett syndrome, Angelman syndrome, Williams syndrome, Down syndrome, etc.).

Table 32.1 summarizes the most frequent conditions that present early with intellectual disabilities. Trisomy 21 (Down syndrome) is the most common among the syndromic forms not mentioned in the table.

Another important developmental disorder is *autism*, which is now included in the broader category of autism spectrum disorders (ASD). The first description of this condition dates back to Leo Kanner (1943), who defined it as an "innate inability to develop normal affective relationships with people". Recent estimates indicate a prevalence higher than 1 in 100 children. The male-to-female ratio is approximately 4:1. Autism spectrum disorder is often associated with epilepsy (30% of cases) and intellectual disability (70-80% of cases). Based on aetiology, autism spectrum disorder can be idiopathic or symptomatic (or syndromic). Idiopathic autism exhibits a high non-Mendelian heritability (high concordance among monozygotic twins, increased recurrence risk for siblings, and mild and subclinical autistic traits in family members: "broad autistic phenotype").

Autism spectrum disorders are considered pervasive developmental disorders (pervasive because they involve multiple areas of mental development: communication, language, motivation, and interests). ASD emerge in late infancy and early childhood, determining a typical and persistent profile of mental functioning.

On a clinical ground, autism is characterized by qualitative alterations in social interaction (absence or extreme limitation of social sharing abilities, indifference or avoidance of eye contact, lack of imitation, lack of social motivation and interest in relevant aspects of social behavior, facial expressions, and gaze), communication (delayed acquisition or absence of indicative gestures, absence of language or atypical and bizarre language; speaking in the third person), and adaptation to the environment (extreme sensitivity to changes in the context with pathological reactivity, extreme narrowness of interests, repetitive, stereotyped, or ritualistic behaviors depending on the degree of cognitive deficit). The ability to share attention, an important aspect of a child's normal cognitive development, especially for the development of symbolic function, is one of the first social skills that is impaired in ASD. (Table 32.2 shows some important social skills present from the early months of life).

Autism spectrum disorder is a permanent condition with phases of behavioural difficulties,

Table 32.1 SOME OF THE CONDITIONS ASSOCIATED WITH DELAYED PSYCHOMOTOR DEVELOPMENT AND INTELLECTUAL DISABILITY WITH ONSET IN EARLY CHILDHOOD

Condition	Onset age (months)	Diagnostic markers	Possible associated symptoms in the first year of life
Rett syndrome	0-18 months	Genetic mutations in MECP2, CDKL5, FOXC2 genes, FOXG1	Microcephaly, secondary microcephaly, autism, stereotypies, neurological deterioration, epilepsy, absence of language, severe developmental delay
Fragile X syndrome	From early months	CGG repeat expansion in the X-linked FMR1 gene	Macrocephaly, epilepsy or EEG abnormalities, autism, hyperactivity
Angelman syndrome	0-12 months	Methylation test of the 15q11-q13 region; UB3A gene analysis	Typical facial features, microcephaly, epilepsy, absence of language
Williams syndrome		In situ hybridization (FISH) of chromosome 7q11.23	Typical facial features, dysphagia, somatic hypoevolutism, psychomotor delay, disinhibited and friendly behavior, hoarse voice, small and spaced teeth, hypercalcemia, and cardiovascular abnormalities, including supravalvular aortic stenosis
Phenylketonuria (phenylalanine hydroxylase deficiency)	3-12 months	Hyperphenylalaninemia	Epilepsy (infantile spasms), autism
Creatine synthesis and transport deficiency	3-6 months	Cerebral Cr deficiency, mutations in AGAT, GAMT, SLC8A6 genes	Epilepsy, autism
Homocystinuria	1-12 months	Elevated methionine and homocysteine levels	Lens subluxation
Biotinidase deficiency	3-12 months	Dicarboxylic aciduria	Alopecia, skin rashes, ketoacidosis, lactic acidemia
Adenylosuccinate deficiency/ dihydropyrimidinase deficiency	1-12 months	Increased SAICAR	Autism, hypotonia, feeding difficulties, somatic hypoevolutism
4-Hydroxybutyric Aciduria (Succinic Semialdehyde Dehydrogenase Deficiency)	1-12 months	4-Hydroxybutyric aciduria	Hypotonia, trunk and limb ataxia, oculomotor apraxia, macro/microcephaly, involuntary movements, drowsiness, epilepsy, autism
Mevalonic Aciduria (Mild Form)	1-12 months	Mevalonic aciduria	Hypotonia, muscle hypotrophy, ataxia

especially during periods of developmental transitions (school age, adolescence) that are sometimes associated with self-aggressive or hetero-aggressive behaviours, often disruptive, or (especially in adolescence) with phases of extreme hypo-/bradykinesia bordering on catatonia. The prognosis is influenced by the severity of intellectual disability, often associated with this disorder, the development or absence of language, neurological comorbidities (e.g., epilepsy), and psychiatric comorbidities (e.g., hyperactivity and attentional instability), as well as the timing and quality of rehabilitative interventions.

The current classification of Autism Spectrum Disorders, according to DSM-5, has narrowed down the spectrum of clinical conditions that fall under this diagnostic category, eliminating some diseases with early alterations in neurodevelopmental processes leading to dementia rather than ASD (e.g., Rett syndrome).

ASD is now considered a network disorder, resulting from multifactorial derangement of the complex neuronal pathways implied in the development of social interaction. Like other clinical conditions, currently lacking any diagnostic biomarker, ASD poses challenging

Table 32.2 EARLY SOCIAL/COMMUNICATIVE BEHAVIORS IN INFANTS

- Social Smile: The infant smiles at faces.
- Visual Attention to Faces: The infant's gaze is directed towards the examiner's face.
- Visual Attention to Objects: The infant's gaze is directed towards an object that the examiner shows him.
- Shared Attention: The infant orients his attention to what the adult is observing.
- Non-Verbal Vocalizations: The infant uses non-verbal sounds, vocalizations, or babbling to communicate.
- Alternating Babbling/Vocalizations: The infant interrupts their own babbling when the adult speaks to them.
- Production of Single Words/Word Combinations for Interactive Purposes.

difficulties in diagnostic classification and prognostic anticipation, mainly in relation to two problems: the relationship with intellectual disability (ID) and with some monogenic diseases exhibiting a marked autistic diathesis. While the diagnosis of ASD is alternative to that of ID, it is well known that in children with severe intellectual disabilities, the emergence of autistic behaviours or traits is frequent. In the most severe forms, clear differentiation between autism and ID can be difficult or impossible. On the other hand, the prognosis for many children with Autism Spectrum Disorder who have not developed adequate language and communication skills, given the limited nature of their social relational abilities, is marked by a progressive impoverishment (or lack of enrichment) of cognitive functioning, resulting in intellectual disability in adolescence or adulthood.

In approximately 10% of cases, ASDs are associated with known neurogenetic syndromes (*syndromic autism*, tuberous sclerosis, Fragile X syndrome, Down syndrome, etc.) (Table 32.3). In some of these conditions (such as Duchenne muscular dystrophy), the occurrence of the disorder is significantly higher than in the general population. These conditions, which almost always involve ID, have suggested the hypothesis of the existence of multiple autisms rather than a single entity. Currently, the prevailing approach is to consider these syndromic forms of autism spectrum disorder (in contrast to idiopathic forms) as conditions in which cognitive disability, due to the underlying disease, clinically manifest an independently transmitted autistic vulnerability that would not have been expressed or would have been expressed to a lesser extent otherwise. In other diseases (e.g., Fragile X syndrome), biological functions and/or neuronal networks underlying neural plasticity that are part of or important components of the *social brain* appear to be directly affected. In these cases, the biological relationship with the autistic disorder is more direct.

New genomic analysis have identified a number of genes and genetic alterations associated with primary (idiopathic) autism spectrum disorder. Multiple genes and environmental factors are likely involved in the development and modulation of the complex network of neurons implicated in the development of social behaviour.

32.2 Dementia and mental deterioration

A wide range of metabolic and degenerative alterations manifest in children with a slowdown in psychomotor development and/or cognitive and neurological deterioration. In some cases, the disorder emerges in a syndromic context (coarse facial features, skeletal deformities, bone lesions, hepatosplenomegaly, hirsutism, corneal opacities, joint deformities, micro- or macrocephaly, etc.) that may suggest the diagnostic *work-up* (e.g., mucopolysaccharidoses, Gaucher disease type II, other lysosomal storage diseases). Cognitive deterioration is frequently accompanied by other signs of neurological impairment following a pattern of subcortical dementia. Clinical deterioration may be preceded by a delay in psychomotor development in the early years of life and other neurological signs such as pyramidal deficits, ataxia, epilepsy, visual disturbances, etc. Along with the age of onset, especially in the initial stages, the symptoms associated with mental deterioration may have localizing significance. The presence of epilepsy suggests a predominant involvement of the cerebral cortex (ceroidolipofuscinoses, Lafora disease, MERRF, subacute sclerosing panencephalitis, etc.); the presence of

Table 32.3 MOST COMMON GENETIC CONDITIONS ASSOCIATED WITH AUTISM (> 60 DISEASES; < 10% OF ALL AUTISTIC INDIVIDUALS)

Disease	Gene/locus	Clinical phenotype
PKU	PAH Cr. 12q24.1	Psychomotor delay, intellectual disability, autism, epilepsy, ataxia, depigmented skin and appendages, somatic hypoevolution
Tuberous Sclerosis	TSC1 Cr. 9p TSC2Cr. 16q	Epilepsy, intellectual disability, autism, sebaceous adenomas, nail fibromas, cutaneous, central nervous system, heart, and kidney hamartomas
Neurofibromatosis Type 1	NF1 Cr. 17 q11.2	Seizures, intellectual disability, café-au-lait spots, neurofibromas, hypertension, short stature, autistic traits
Fragile X Syndrome	FMR1 Cr. Xq27.3	Macrocephaly, prominent frontal bossing, macrosomia, epilepsy or EEG abnormalities, autistic traits, hyperactivity, intellectual disability
Rett syndrome	MECP2 Cr. Xq28 CDKL5 Cr. Xp22	Secondary microcephaly, epilepsy, stereotypical hand movements, autism, apraxia of gait
Duchenne muscular dystrophy	DMD Cr. Xp21	Difficulty in walking, waddling gait, calf pseudohypertrophy, skeletal deformities, cardiorespiratory insufficiency, autistic traits
Williams syndrome	Cr.7q11.23	Distinctive facial features, intellectual disability, pragmatic, phonological, and syntactic difficulties, autism, aortic valve stenosis
Prader-Willi syndrome	Cr. 15q11-q13	Short stature, intellectual disability, autism, obesity, hypotonia, characteristic facial features, hypogonadism
Velo-cardio-facial syndrome	Cr. 22q11.2	Thymus and parathyroid hypoplasia, cardiac defects, facial anomalies, and autistic traits
Down syndrome	Trisomy Cr.21 Translocation Cr. 14/Cr.21	Microcephaly, intellectual disability, autistic traits, epicanthal folds, retrognathic neck fat pad, hypotonia, palmar crease, congenital heart disease
Turner syndrome	Cr X0	Intellectual disability, autism, epicanthal folds, ptosis, webbed neck, hypogonadism
Smith-Lemli-Opitz syndrome	Deficit DHCR7 Cr. 11q12-13	Microcephaly, intellectual disability, language disorder, autism, sleep disturbance, self/other-aggression, irritability, *opisthotonos*
Timothy syndrome	CACNA1C	Autism, intellectual disability, lethal arrhythmias, congenital heart disease, immunodeficiency
Phelan-McDermid syndrome	SHANK3 Del Cr.22q13	Hypotonia, developmental delay, absent or severely delayed language, ADD regression, catatonic episodes, dysmorphic features, and autism

movement disorders usually indicates an alteration of the basal ganglia (Wilson disease, pantothenate kinase-associated neurodegeneration, GM1 gangliosidosis, mitochondrial encephalopathies, late-onset forms of ceroidolipofuscinoses, some organic acidurias, etc.); the coexistence of ataxia points to cerebellar involvement (e.g., Niemann-Pick disease); the presence of supranuclear gaze palsy suggests a mesencephalic lesion (e.g., Niemann-Pick disease, Gaucher disease, etc.); neurosensory hearing loss indicates a lesion of the acoustic nerve or its nuclei (e.g., some mitochondrial encephalopathies).

Table 32.4 lists the forms in which the decline of higher cortical functions is a predominant symptom, at least at the onset of the disease, based on the most common age of onset. Within the first months or years of life, the condition that most closely resembles the picture of dementia in adults is Rett syndrome, a progressive and relatively common disease that almost exclusively affects girls (prevalence of approximately 1 in 10,000). It is characterised by a diminished cranial growth (usually in the second half of the first year of life) and secondary microcephaly, neurological regression with progressive loss of social interaction, loss of purposeful hand movements without frank paralysis, loss of language, sometimes loss of gait, and stereotypies. Epilepsy usually begins early, while ataxia,

Table 32.4 METABOLIC AND/OR DEGENERATIVE DISEASES WITH MENTAL DETERIORATION AND BEHAVIORAL DISTURBANCES AS A PREVALENT SYMPTOM

Disease	Onset age (years)	Possible associated signs/symptoms
Hagberg-Santavuori (NCL1, NCL2)	> 0,5	Hypotonia, ataxia, myoclonus, early flattening of EEG tracing, blindness
Rett syndrome	1-2	Secondary microcephaly, epilepsy, stereotypies, autism, apraxia of gait
Jansky Bielschowsky Disease	2-4	Myoclonic epilepsy, polymyoclonus, cerebellar ataxia, retinitis pigmentosa, typical EEG reactivity to low-frequency intermittent photic stimulation (SLI); vacuolated lymphocytes
Schindler disease	0.5-2	Myoclonic epilepsy, hypotonia, spasticity, corneal opacity, optic atrophy, osteoporosis
Sanfilippo syndrome	4-6	Hirsutism, psychomotor agitation, autism
Metachromatic leukodystrophy	> 1 year	Progressive spastic paraparesis → tetraparesis, ataxia, choreoathetosis, peripheral neuropathy, proteinorrhachia, sulfatiduria
Krabbe disease	15 months-10 years	Spastic paraparesis, ataxia, polyneuropathy, optic atrophy, blindness, proteinorrhachia
Adrenoleukodystrophy	3 10 years	Attention disturbances, loss of interest, hyperactivity, apraxia, hemianopsia, central blindness, deafness, pyramidal signs
Pantothenate kinase-associated neurodegeneration (PKAN) (Hallervorden-Spatz disease)	2-15	Dystonia, parkinsonism, dysarthria, spastic paraparesis, retinitis pigmentosa
GM1 gangliosidosis (late infantile variant)	12-18 months	Spastic tetraparesis with pseudobulbar signs, epilepsy, anterosuperior hypoplasia of thoracolumbar vertebral bodies
Spielmeyer-Vogt Disease (NCL3)	5-12	Loss of vision, retinopathy, polymyoclonus, ataxia, dyskinesias, vacuolated lymphocytes
Wilson disease	See Table 32.8	
Huntington's disease	See Table 32.8	
Ornithine transcarbamylase deficiency (OCT)	From infancy to adulthood	Vomiting, lethargy, progressive drowsiness, irritability, agitation, oppositional behavior, disorientation, ataxia, amblyopia. Often: epilepsy, somatic growth retardation, psychomotor delay
Niemann-Pick type C disease	See Table 32.8	
Leigh syndrome	See Table 32.6	
Methylenetetrahydrofolate reductase deficiency	Early years of life	Psychomotor delay, microcephaly, epilepsy, motor disturbances, Marfanoid habitus, homocystinuria, hyperhomocysteinemia, normal-low methionine levels
Subacute sclerosing panencephalitis	> 3 years	Mental deterioration, behavioral disturbances, myoclonus associated with bilateral rhythmic spike-wave complexes; periodic delta wave discharges; anti-measles antibodies (IgG) in blood and cerebrospinal fluid in the absence of ongoing rash

parkinsonism, severe hypokinesia, tremor, and pyramidal signs appear later during the second decade of life. The disease leads to a severe rigid-hypokinetic syndrome. The diagnosis is based on the clinical features and is confirmed by genetic-molecular testing: the MECP2 gene is responsible for the typical form, while other genes (e.g., CDKL5, FOXG1, IQSEC2) have been associated with atypical forms.

Some metabolic alterations with primary involvement of the white matter (leukodystrophies) can present with a predominant deficit in cognitive functions and behavioral disturbances. Among these, particularly noteworthy, are metachromatic leukodystrophy, Krabbe disease, and adrenoleukodystrophy. Especially in the first two conditions, the phenotype characterized by deficits in higher cortical functions and behavioral disorders, is influenced by the age of onset and clinical features are worse in later-onset forms. Adrenoleukodystrophy manifests during school age with initially nonspecific symptoms such as declining school performance, restlessness, and attentional instability preceding more significant neurological deficits (cortical blindness, frank mental deterioration, spasticity, Addisonian syndrome, etc.). In leukodystrophies, brain MRI showing typical white matter lesions, the occurrence of pyramidal and/or peripheral deficits, and the absence or rarity of epileptic manifestations, address the correct nosographic classification, and specific etiology is determined through specific enzymatic and/or genetic investigations.

32.3 Movement disorders in early childhood

In children, central movement disorders can be characterized by an excess of movement activity (hyperkinetic movement disorders as: chorea, athetosis, dystonia, tremor, myoclonus), a reduction of voluntary movements in motor activity (brady-hypokinesia, infantile parkinsonism), or by a disorganization of motor activity due to incoordination (ataxia). These symptoms are variably associated with alterations in postural control, encompassing a wide range of functional impairments, from complete absence of antigravity control to subtle difficulties in motor adaptation that become evident only under conditions of particular postural instability effort. Collectively, they indicate disruptions in neuronal connectivity at different hierarchical levels of the executive motor functions. Other disorders (stereotypies, tics, mannerisms) have a different origin and nature, stemming from impairments in higher levels of motor processing related to intentionality, planning, and purposefulness of motor activity.

The phenomenology of movement disorders may vary depending on the level of central nervous system (CNS) maturation at the onset of symptoms.

However, the clinical definition of symptoms is similar to that used in adults.

Dystonia | Characterized by persistent or intermittent muscle contractions that result in abnormal movements and/or postures, due to the co-contraction of agonist and antagonist muscles, often repetitive in nature.

Athetosis | Refers to slow, continuous, sinuous, often rotational involuntary movements, primarily affecting the limbs, which hinder stable posture maintenance.

Myoclonus | Refers to a rapid, focal, segmental, or generalised jerky movement generated by a sudden muscular contraction of brief duration or an equally sudden and rapid loss of muscle tone and innervation (negative myoclonus), sometimes repetitive but non-rhythmic.

Tremor | Rhythmic movement causing oscillation of a limb or body segment around a joint axis.

Chorea | Manifests as rapid, abrupt, irregular, and arrhythmic involuntary movements, (non-stereotyped), purposeless, spontaneous, and occurring at rest. Choreic movements interfere with voluntary movements, which become irregular, accompanied by grotesque posturing, and leading to alterations in daily activities such as handwriting, feeding, phonation, swallowing, and facial expression, without emotional correspondence.

The term *dyskinesia(s)* is used as an inclusive term for all hyperkinesias in children, especially when their characteristics do not fit into a single defined category or when multiple hyperkinetic movement disorders are present.

Oculogyric crises | Oculogyric crises are characterized by tonic upward deviation of the eyes for variable durations, typically even lasting several seconds, and are not associated with changes in the levels of vigilance (differential diagnosis with epilepsy is mandatory) unlike tonic deviations of the gaze associated with epilepsy.

Frequently in the first year of life movement disorders are often characterized by mixed types of movement disorders and different clinical features with dystonic postures affecting the trunk and limbs, atetoid movements of the limbs, orofacial dyskinesias, sialorrhea due to difficulty in controlling saliva and hypersalivation due to dysautonomia, movements of the mouth. These symptoms are often associated with or preceded by hypokinesia and hypotonia. After the first 3-4 years of life, the phenomenology of movement disorders gradually become similar to those observed in adults.

On an etiological level, movement disorders can be caused by primary genetic alterations affecting the motor network, especially the nigrostriatal system, at multiple levels: synapse homeostasis (energy metabolism disorders, neurotoxic metabolites accumulation), neurodevelopment of cerebral connectivity, neurotransmitter production, impaired presynaptic or postsynaptic signaling, components essential for transmission in motor pathways, especially the nigrostriatal system. Alternatively, numerous acquired causes (pre-perinatal hypoxic damage, encephalitis, autoimmune encephalopathies, tumors, neurotoxic metabolites generated by genetic metabolic disorders) can result in secondary deficits due to acquired lesions or genetic or metabolic diseases that compromise their integrity. Certain symptoms suggest specific etiologies: hypokinesia (including hypomimia), with limb hypotonia or rigidity, and trunk hypotonia, suggest secondary infantile parkinsonism due to congenital or acquired deficits in dopaminergic transmission. Rhythmic limb or more generalized gross oscillations may be present in the first two years of life. The presence of dystonia suggests specific important metabolic disorders (Lesch-Nyhan disease) or degenerative conditions such as conditions associated with basal ganglia iron accumulation (NBIA). The presence of impaired development of antigravity motor functions or their deterioration, as well as signs of involvement at multiple levels of the nervous system (ataxia, spasticity, cranial nerve deficits, retinitis pigmentosa, peripheral neuropathy), indicate symptomatic rather than idiopathic forms, with the former being much more common in children.

The most common acquired movement disorder in children is Sydenham's chorea (rheumatic chorea), which manifests in predisposed individuals, typically 2-6 months after an infection with group A β-hemolytic streptococcal (GABHS) infection (which sometimes can be difficult to individuate in the clinical history but is usually characterized by the high Antistreptolysin O titer with laboratory tests). The onset is acute or subacute, often preceded by subtle psychiatric symptoms such as irritability and obsessive-compulsive behaviors. The course is benign, but recurrent forms are known (following new infections, use of progestins or dopaminergic drugs agonists, or during pregnancies), as well as forms with persistent expression. A reliable biological marker is the presence of echocardiographic abnormalities (some degree of valve damage reported in over 80% of cases), which necessitates long-term antistreptococcal prophylaxis.

Some movement disorders, such as tics and stereotypies, are closely associated with an immature central nervous system and consistent with this may represent the motor correlate of certain neurodevelopmental disorders such as Tourette Syndrome, Autism Spectrum Disorders, and Developmental Coordination Disorder.

Tics | Tics are the most common movement disorder in childhood (up to 20% of the pediatric population), often transient but sometimes chronic (Tourette syndrome). They can be described as fragments of normal motor acts or phonetic productions that are incongruous with the context, easily mimicked by the patient, and occasionally confused with purposeful acts. Their stereotyped and repetitive nature together with suppressibility of the movement or vocal production are the fundamental diagnostic clues. The repertoire of motor and vocal tics is extremely broad, ranging from simple tics (*blinking, sniffing*) to complex tics (coordinated motor sequences, copropraxia, coprolalia, palilalia, echolalia). Their involuntary nature is questioned due to the almost constant presence of premonitory sensations (*urges*). The clinical characteristics vary (often clonic, but sometimes dystonic or tonic), the phenomenology tends to change over time, and the frequency fluctuates significantly with periods of exacerbation interspersed with periods of remission (both on a daily basis and in the short and long term). The onset occurs between 4 and 8 years of age, with the peak of clinical expression reached in the prepubertal phase, followed by stabilization and attenuation in late adolescence.

Comorbidity with psychiatric disorders is highly relevant, especially in terms of psychosocial *impairment*. In 40-80% of cases, there is comorbidity with attention-deficit/hyperactivity disorder (ADHD, either subclinical or clinically apparent) and/or obsessive-compulsive disorder (OCD). Self-injury behaviors (SIBs), impulse control disorders (rage attacks), mood disorders, and personality disorders become clinically significant, particularly during adolescence.

Despite the familial nature of the disorder and the identification of dysfunction in the striato-thalamo-cortical circuits as the pathophysiological basis, the diagnosis is based on clinical grounds, as there is no specific biomarker or consistent genetic findings beyond a limited number of mutations in a small number of families. Even with genetic studies, the diagnosis remains purely clinical.

The association of some tic and/or OCD cases with rheumatic chorea has prompted research into possible relationships with streptococcal infections, leading to the definition of a subtype known as PANDAS (*pediatric autoimmune neuropsychiatric disorders associated with streptococcal infections*). However, its validity remains to be confirmed, and it currently lacks diagnostic tools and shared therapeutic options. More recently, the term PANS has been coined to indicate acute or subacute neuropsychiatric conditions, with or without movement disorders (tics, stereotypies, chorea, mannerisms), in which an infectious trigger and subsequent immune dysregulation are present but not specifically attributable to streptococcus. One agent that seems to be involved in these conditions is Mycoplasma pneumoniae.

Stereotypies | These are semi-voluntary movements that commonly emerge during the first two years of life and are characterized by the repetitive performance of coordinated gestures that are themselves normal but incongruous within the context in which they are activated and repeated. Unlike tics, they tend to have constant characteristics within the same patient, can be facilitated by specific situations (such as boredom or excitement), and can be interrupted if the child is distracted.

Stereotypies are a consistent clinical marker of Rett syndrome and Atypical Rett disorders; however, they are also common in autism spectrum disorders (especially in individuals with severe intellectual impairment), in many individuals with profound intellectual disabilities, and in children with selective developmental disorders (dyspraxia). They are rarely observed in typically developing children. In the latter cases, the prognosis of the disorder is favorable, and there is an attenuation of symptoms or exclusive expression in private settings during preadolescence. Subacute onset of stereotypies and mannerisms, together with other red flags symptoms (epilepsy, psychiatric symptoms, sleep disorder, dysautonomia, etc.) are frequently observed in autoimmune encephalitis such as anti-NMDAR encephalitis.

In some cases, the dyskinesias are transient and have a favorable prognosis. Recognizing them avoids unnecessary and potentially invasive investigations. Table 32.5 presents the most common forms, such as Sandifer syndrome (paroxysmal torticollis associated with gastroesophageal reflux), transient oculogyric crises in infants (conjugate upward gaze deviations of an intermittent nature), *spasmus nutans* (combination of torticollis, head oscillation, and pendular nystagmus), and benign infantile chorea.

Table 32.5 SOME IDIOPATHIC AND TRANSIENT MOVEMENT DISORDERS IN CHILDREN

Disease	Onset age (months)	Clinical features	Progression
Benign idiopathic dystonia	> 5	Presence of dystonic postures with hemisomic, segmental, or focal distribution, occasional or permanent, which disappear with intentional movement	Spontaneous resolution within 18 months of life
Transient paroxysmal dystonia	1-5	Episodes (a few minutes - 2 hours) of opisthotonus or symmetric/asymmetric dystonic postures of the limbs	8-22 months
Benign infantile myoclonus	1-12 months (average 5.6)	Myoclonus of the head, neck, or limbs, "shuddering" of the head and/or neck and/or upper limbs, spasms of the head and/or limbs, negative myoclonus	Resolution between 6-30 months
Paroxysmal Tonic Upgaze (PTU)	< 12	Paroxysmal upward gaze deviation of short or long (up to 3 hours) duration. Downbeat nystagmus when trying to look in this direction, diurnal fluctuation of symptoms, improvement with sleep, exacerbation with fever, ataxia	1-4 years after onset
Spasmus nutans	> 12	Nystagmus, head nodding, torticollis	Resolution within 3-6 years
Sandifer syndrome	> 2	Gastroesophageal reflux, irritability, spasmodic torticollis, trunk dystonia (also paroxysmal)	Dependent on reflux treatment
Benign paroxysmal torticollis	0.5-5	Attacks of torticollis (5-10 days), associated with irritability, dystonia of the upper limbs, vomiting, pallor	Resolution between 5 and 24 months of age

32.3.1 Cerebral palsy (CP)

Cerebral palsy is the most common movement disorder in children. It results from an early non-progressive injury (pre-peri and postnatal, within the first 12 months of life) to the central nervous system (CNS). The incidence is 2-3 per 1000 live births. Clinically, CP is described based on its topography (monoparesis, hemiparesis, diplegia/paraplegia, tetraparesis, disequilibrium syndrome) and the quality of the motor disorder (spastic CP, choreoathetotic-dyskinetic CP, dystonic CP, ataxic CP, mixed CP). Postural disturbance is of great importance and is crucial for the prognosis of the disease. The prevalence of extensor head and trunk posture, reduced threshold for *startle reactions*, and persistence of asymmetric and symmetric tonic neck reflexes are negative prognostic signs regarding the acquisition of effective postural control. Severe postural pattern is often associated with severe dysarthria and dysphagia. Prematurity is the main risk factor on the etiological level, while perinatal asphyxia is present in only 20% of children. Twinning is found in 10% of cases. Pregnancy, delivery, and the perinatal period are normal in a significant number of cases: in approximately 70% of individuals with congenital hemiplegia, 30% with spastic diplegia, 20% with dyskinetic forms, many individuals with ataxic diplegia, and all individuals with non-progressive congenital cerebellar ataxia. Other conditions without anamnestic evidence in the prenatal period can be the cause of CP, such as genetic or acquired cerebral/cerebellar malformations, nutritional deficiencies, vascular and coagulation disorders, and maternal-fetal autoimmune reactions. The most frequent postnatal causes include encephalitis/meningitis, head trauma, tumors, neurological complications of systemic diseases, etc. Some clinical patterns can be attributed to specific etiologies: ataxic forms of CP, almost always associated with severe intellectual disability, are secondary to cerebellar and brainstem malformations; dyskinetic forms, occurring in children often with intact cognitive function, are secondary to selective basal ganglia damage, classically caused by neonatal jaundice (*kernicterus*) or vascular conditions; hemiplegic forms are mainly associated with vascular damage. The prognosis of CP as a motor dysfunction is certainly related to the severity and distribution of the motor disorder. In many cases, additional neurological deficits coexist with the movement disorder and influence the prognosis of the disease, including intellectual disability, epilepsy, nuclear and supranuclear oculomotor deficits with strabismus and amblyopia, hearing impairment, dysphagia, etc. This constellation of symptoms is often encountered in acquired or genetic CNS malformations. By definition, CP is a fixed encephalopathy. Nevertheless, some patients, for unknown reasons, develop very disabling late-onset dyskinesias/dystonias, predominantly affecting the trunk and limbs. Occasionally, they involve the less affected hemisphere compared to the previous paralysis.

Neuroradiological investigations (MRI and CT) of the brain show lesions in approximately 87% of patients with CP. The most frequent lesions include periventricular white matter injuries (in 20% of patients), predominantly cortical lesions (approximately 15%), cortico-subcortical lesions with a vascular pattern (about 12%), and brain malformations (approximately 12%). Nonspecific neuroradiological alterations are found in 18% of patients, and the examination is normal in about 13% of cases. The most severe forms of CP are associated with cortical or basal ganglia damage, hemiplegic forms are associated with vascular injury, dyskinetic forms show a normal or nonspecific neuroradiological pattern, and ataxic forms are related to malformations in the posterior cranial fossa

32.3.2 Other movement disorders in children

Table 32.6 presents some of the most frequent metabolic or degenerative conditions that begin in the first year of life with a predominant motor involvement. In most cases, the clinical progression suggests a degenerative condition and guides the subsequent diagnostic approach. For some metabolic disorders, early diagnosis is crucial due to the availability of etiological therapies, the timeliness of which impacts the prognosis. Among these, disorders of biogenic amine metabolism and transport is the most representative group. In practical terms, they can be classified on the presence or absence of hyperphenylalaninemia, pointing to a concomitant deficiency of the hepatic enzyme phenylalanine hydroxylase. The former (GTP-CH deficiency – autosomal recessive form, 6-PTS deficiency, DHPR deficiency, *DNAJC12* deficiency) can be early identified through neonatal screening for phenylketonuria, which detects increased blood phenylalanine levels. The latter (autosomal dominant GTP-CH deficiency, certain autosomal recessive forms of GTP-CH deficiency, tyrosine hydroxylase deficiency, aromatic amino acid decarboxylase deficiency, sepiapterin reductase deficiency, dopamine transporter deficiency, DAT, vesicular monoamine transporter-2 deficiency) can only be diagnosed based on specific suspicion and targeted metabolic and/or genetic investigations. In some cases, an increase in plasma prolactin levels may indicate a dopamine synthesis disorder. More recently, severe early-onset dyskinesias secondary to postsynaptic signal transduction deficits have been identified. Some of these conditions (autosomal dominant *GNAO1* gene deficiency) present with severe developmental delay (with or without epilepsy) and progressive choreic dyskinesias, with worsening during fever and partial recovery afterward. Other conditions (autosomal dominant - *ADCY5* deficiency) manifest early with orolingual and periorbital dyskinesias, cervical and limb dystonias, and hyperreflexia or, alternatively, chorea and hypotonia.

Early-onset neurological conditions characterized by significant rigidity (with heightened spasmodic component triggered by sensory stimuli) and reduced threshold for startle reactions are observed in GABA synthesis disorders (glutamic acid decarboxylase deficiency) and glycine receptor deficiencies, an inhibitory neurotransmitter at the spinal level (*stiff baby syndrome*).

Table 32.7 summarizes the conditions most frequently associated with movement disorders that begin after the first year of life. During the early months of life, it is

Table 32.6 METABOLIC DISORDERS EMERGING DURING THE FIRST YEAR OF LIFE WITH A PREVALENT MOVEMENT DISORDER

Disease	Age of onset (months)	Prevalent motor disorder	Possible associated signs/symptoms
Deficiency of enzymes involved in the synthesis or regeneration of the cofactor tetrahydrobiopterin (GTP-CH [autosomal recessive form], PTPS, SR, DHPR)	Early months	Axial hypotonia, limb rigidity, dystonia, myoclonus, hypokinesia, oculogyric crises, imbalance syndrome with a tendency for opisthotonus	Epilepsy, mental retardation, somatic hypoevolutism. Intracranial calcifications (DHPR deficiency)
Tyrosine hydroxylase deficiency	Early months	Hypotonia, hypokinesia, limb choreoathetosis, trunk dystonia, oculogyric crises	Somatic hypoevolutism, diurnal fluctuation of symptoms, psychomotor delay
Aromatic amino acid decarboxylase deficiency	1-12	Oculogyric crises, hypotonia, eyelid ptosis	Irritability, psychomotor delay, thermoregulation disorders, drooling, hyperhidrosis, pallor
Dopamine transporter deficiency (DAT)	First months	Significant akinesia-bradykinesia, rigidity, oculogyric crises, severe postural instability	Somatic hypoevolutism
Vesicular amine transporter 2 deficiency (VAMT2)	First months	Hypotonia, loss of head control, prolonged oculogyric crises with crying, akinesia and hypomimia, paroxysmal dystonia with diurnal fluctuations, psychomotor delay	
Glutamate dehydrogenase deficiency (GABA synthesis deficit - *Stiff-baby syndrome*)	Neonatal	Hypertonia, hyperreflexia, severe rigidity, and hypokinesia, reduced startle reflex threshold	Apnea
Glutaric aciduria Type I	First year of life	Generalized dystonia with spastic component, choreoathetosis of limbs, hypotonia, opisthotonus, lingual and facial dyskinesias	Macrocephaly, metabolic acidosis, psychomotor delay, epilepsy. Hepatomegaly. Reye syndrome
Methylmalonic aciduria	Neonatal	Choreoathetosis	Ketoacidosis, feeding difficulties, somatic hypoevolutism, epilepsy; MRI: bilateral pallidal abnormalities
3-methylglutaconic aciduria	5-11	Hypotonia/spasticity	Neonatal hyperammonemia, severe psychomotor delay, microcephaly, optic atrophy, neurological deterioration
4-hydroxybutyric aciduria (succinic semialdehyde dehydrogenase deficiency)	1-12	Hypotonia, truncal and limb ataxia, oculomotor apraxia, involuntary movements	Mental retardation, autism, epilepsy, comatose state, and possible pallidal alterations on MRI
Lesch-Nyhan disease	3-6	Hypotonia, spasticity, dystonia with a tendency towards opisthotonus and spasmodic dystonia of the limbs	Psychomotor delay, recurrent vomiting, early emergence of self-injurious behaviors
Pelizaeus-Merzbacher disease	Neonatal	Pendular nystagmus	MRI: leukodystrophy
Creatine synthesis deficiency (GAMT deficiency)	3-12	Chorea, dystonia	Psychomotor delay, epilepsy, autism. MRI: bilateral pallidal alteration
Leigh syndrome (complex I deficiency, PDHc deficiency, COX deficiency, ATPase deficiency)	0-12	Hypotonia, choreoathetosis, spasticity, dystonia	Ophthalmoplegia, lactic acidemia, hyperpnea, ataxia, bilateral striatal lesions (MRI), mental retardation, behavioral disturbances
Molybdenum cofactor deficiency (sulfite oxidase deficiency)	Neonatal	Axial hypotonia, limb hypertonia, dystonia, athetosis, choreoathetosis, myoclonus	Early feeding difficulties, drug-resistant epilepsy, lens subluxation, severe psychomotor delay. MRI shows diffuse white matter abnormalities
Metachromatic leukodystrophy (arylsulfatase A deficiency)	4-12	Spastic paraparesis → tetraplegia	Dysphagia, dysarthria, cognitive deterioration, peripheral neuropathy
Krabbe disease (galactosylceramidase deficiency)	4-12	Spastic paraparesis → tetraplegia	Dysphagia, dysarthria, peripheral neuropathy, cognitive deterioration
Cytochrome-b5-reductase deficiency	0-12	Athetosis, limb hypertonia, ophthalmoplegia	Severe intellectual disability

Table 32.7 NEUROMETABOLIC AND NEURODEGENERATIVE DISEASES WITH ONSET AFTER THE FIRST YEAR OF LIFE WITH MOVEMENT DISORDERS (DYSTONIA, CHOREA, ATHETOSIS, BALLISM, PARKINSONISM, TREMORS, MYOCLONUS)

Disease	Age of onset	Other associated clinical signs
Familial dopa-responsive dystonia (TH)	After the first year of life in some cases	See Table 32.6
Glutaric Aciduria Type I	1-3 years	See Table 32.6
GM1 Gangliosidosis	> 1 years	Ataxia, mental deterioration, skeletal abnormalities, pyramidal signs, pseudobulbar palsy, epilepsy, strabismus
Familial dopa-responsive dystonia (GTP-CH1)	> 2 years	Psychomotor delay in the first months of life; spastic paraparesis
Sepiapterin reductase deficiency	> 2 years	Mental retardation, microcephaly, hypotonia, oculogyric crises, behavioral disorder, pyramidal deficits, ataxia
Pantothenate kinase-associated neurodegeneration (formerly Hallervorden-Spatz disease)	2-15 years	Dysarthria, pyramidal signs (spastic paraparesis), mental deterioration, retinitis pigmentosa; typical pallidal lesions on MRI
Leigh's sydrome	> 2 years	See Table 32.6
Bilateral striatal necrosis	> 1 year	Pyramidal signs and dystonia
Leber's hereditary optic neuropathy (LHON) and familial striatal necrosis	> 2 years	Leber's optic neuropathy (in some cases)
Huntington's disease	> 2 years	Rigidity and parkinsonism, drug-resistant epilepsy, ophthalmoplegia, dysarthria, dementia
Ataxia-telangiectasia	> 2 years	See Table 32.12
Non-progressive benign familial chorea	1-4 years to adolescence	Recurrent respiratory infections, thyroid deficiency, postural tremor
Neuronal Ceroid lipofuscinosis type 3 (NCL3)	4-7	Dementia, retinitis pigmentosa, dysarthria, epilepsy
GM2 Gangliosidosis	3-6 years	Neurological deterioration, dysarthria, spastic paraparesis, ataxia, myoclonic epilepsy, irritability, aggression, behavioral disturbances, optic atrophy, retinitis pigmentosa
Niemann-Pick type C disease	> 2 years	See Table 32.12
Wilson's disease	> 8 years	Chronic progressive hepatopathy, dysarthria, mental deterioration, Kayser-Fleischer ring
Chorea-acanthocytosis	> 8 years	Acanthocytosis, dementia, behavioral disorders
Deforming muscular dystonia (Primary dystonia)	9-11 years	Pure dystonia not associated with other neurological deficits
Intranuclear neuronal inclusion disease	1-13 years	Parkinsonism, progrèssive ataxia, dysarthria, neuroaxonal neuropathy, cranial nerve deficits, ophthalmoplegia, nystagmus, oculogyric crises, mental deterioration, heteroaggressive behavior

often challenging to establish a differential diagnosis between fixed and progressive encephalopathies. For example, it is not uncommon for a dyskinetic type of cerebral palsy to present with significant hypotonia in the absence of perinatal distress and with a normal brain MRI. Only later, starting from 8-10 months of age, dyskinesias and significant postural development abnormalities will become evident. On the other hand, certain metabolic diseases can be the cause of prematurity (e.g., PTPS deficiency, see Table 32.6), a risk factor for cerebral palsy, or render the CNS more vulnerable to birth-related stressors (e.g., creatine synthesis deficiency, other disorders of energy metabolism), making them not easily identifiable except through the incongruity between anamnestic data and clinical progression.

For an increasing number of metabolic diseases presenting with movement disorders, causative treatment is now available, and its effectiveness depends on the timeliness of treatment initiation (e.g., glutaric aciduria type I, methylmalonic aciduria, deficiencies of biogenic amine synthesis, Wilson's disease, manganese metabolism disorders, etc.). In other cases, early diagnosis may allow for the detection of presymptomatic effects that require prompt management.

The location, distribution, and nature of abnormalities revealed by brain magnetic resonance imaging (MRI) are helpful in establishing the diagnostic workup. A normal brain MRI may point toward non-degenerative idiopathic conditions, such as genetic dystonia or disorders of biogenic amine synthesis, GABA metabolism, or glycine receptors, among others. These diseases require specific, less common investigations, including neuroimaging (SPECT, PET), metabolic assays (measurement of biogenic amine and pterin metabolites in the cerebrospinal fluid), or genetic testing.

Calcifications of the basal ganglia merit special consideration. Calcium deposits in the basal ganglia and other brain structures characterize some inherited metabolic or degenerative encephalopathies, such as Cockayne syndrome, Fahr's disease, mitochondrial encephalopathies like MELAS, and tetrahydrobiopterin regeneration defects. In these conditions, neuroimaging (CT scan) shows that calcium deposits are primarily located in perivascular regions, with minimal involvement of the cerebral cortex. In Aicardi-Goutières syndrome, calcifications of the basal ganglia (alongside progressive cerebral atrophy and white matter involvement) are associated with persistent lymphocytosis. This autosomal recessive disease manifests in the first weeks of life with delayed neurological development, marked hypotonia, opisthotonic spasms, and intellectual disability. HIV encephalopathy can also lead to calcifications of the basal ganglia (accompanied by cerebrospinal fluid pleocytosis).

32.3.3 Hereditary spastic paraplegia

Hereditary spastic paraplegia (HSP) refers to degenerative disorders characterized by progressive spasticity and weakness of the lower limbs. It encompasses a heterogeneous group of conditions, some of which present in childhood. HSP can be inherited in an autosomal dominant, recessive, or X-linked manner. There is considerable variability in their clinical presentation, which can hinder their identification. They are classified into pure forms, which are typically late-onset and nearly monosymptomatic, and *complicated forms*, which are variably associated with intellectual disability, ataxia, hearing loss, peripheral neuropathy, abnormal brain MRI (e.g., white matter changes, cerebellar atrophy, hypoplasia/atrophy of the corpus callosum, etc.), and can manifest as distinct syndromic patterns such as MASA (*Mental retardation, aphasia, shuffling gait, adducted thumbs*) and CRASH (*Corpus callosum hypoplasia, retardation, adducted thumbs, spastic paraparesis, hydrocephalus*). The latter condition often have an earlier onset and pose challenges in differential diagnosis. Several genes have been identified for many of these forms. Family history and observation of the clinical course, along with the results of instrumental examinations, particularly MRI, are helpful to guide diagnosis.

Certain metabolic and neurodegenerative conditions (■ Table 32.8) can either present or develop spastic paraplegia during the disease course. However, in most cases, other symptoms are present, such as upper limb involvement, cerebellar ataxia, dysarthria, dystonia, peripheral neuropathy, or intellectual disability. In some conditions, however, paraplegia is the initial or dominant symptom, as seen in the early stages of metachromatic leukodystrophy, globoid cell leukodystrophy, adrenoleukodystrophy, adrenomyeloneuropathy, HHH syndrome, arginase deficiency, and primary lateral sclerosis.

Table 32.8 NEUROMETABOLIC AND NEURODEGENERATIVE DISEASES THAT ONSET AFTER THE FIRST YEAR OF LIFE WITH SPASTIC PARAPARESIS AS THE PREVALENT OR EARLIEST SYMPTOM

Disease	Age of onset	Other associated symptoms
Spastic paraparesis 1 (SPG1) L1CAM (X-linked)	From early months to adulthood	Hydrocephalus, MASA, CRASH (see text)
Spastic paraparesis 2 (SPG2) PLP (X-linked)	2-8 years	Pure or complicated form: intellectual disability, ataxia, optic atrophy, white matter abnormalities on MRI
Spastic paraparesis 3 (SPG3) SPG3A/atlastin, autosomal dominant	> 2-50 years	Pure form; peripheral neuropathy
Spastic paraparesis 4 (SPG4) spastin, autosomal dominant	From early months of life to adulthood	Pure and complicated form: mental deterioration
Spastic paraparesis 5 (SPG5) autosomal recessive	From early months of life to adulthood	Pure form, peripheral neuropathy, distal amyotrophy
Spastic paraparesis 10 (SPG10) autosomal dominant	From 2 years to adulthood	Pure form, peripheral neuropathy, distal amyotrophy
Spastic paraparesis 11 (SPG11) autosomal recessive	From early months to adulthood	Pure or complicated form: spasticity of the upper limbs, movement disorders, intellectual disability, epilepsy, dysarthria, nystagmus, hypoplasia of the corpus callosum, white matter alterations
Spastic paraparesis 12 (SPG12) reticulon 2, atuosomal dominant	From early months to young adulthood	Pure form
Spastic paraparesis 16 (SPG16) (X-linked)	< 3 years	Expressive aphasia, optic atrophy, mild intellectual disability
Primary lateral sclerosis (ALS2)	3-10 years	Slow progression, ascending course resulting in tetraparesis, dysarthria, pseudobulbar palsy, dysphagia. Brain MRI normal
Arginase deficiency	Early months of life	Mental deterioration, hyperactivity, somatic hypo-evolutism, choreoathetosis (sporadic), vomiting, psychomotor delay, intellectual disability, irritability, epilepsy, hyperammonemia with possible hyperammonemic coma
Hyperornithinemia, Hyperammonemia, Homocitrullinuria	Neonatal, late-onset forms starting in adulthood	Neonatal hyperammonemia (*lethargy, hypotonia, epilepsy, coma*), coagulopathy (*factors VII and X*), ataxia (*late-onset forms*), learning and behavioral disorders (*late-onset forms*)
Sjögren-Larsson Syndrome	Early years of life	Congenital ichthyosis, macular degeneration of the retina, intellectual disability, dysarthria, epilepsy, kyphosis, short stature
Austin disease (multiple sulfatase deficiency)	12-18 months	Mental deterioration, loss of language, generalized or myoclonic epilepsy, optic atrophy, cherry-red spot and pigmentary degeneration of the retina, dysmorphisms (narrow and prominent forehead, flattened nasal bridge, bushy eyebrows, long eyelashes)
Metachromatic leukodystrophy	See table 32.6	
Krabbe disease	See table 32.6	
Hereditary spastic paraplegia (Strümpell-Lorrain type)	> 5 years	Late involvement of the upper limbs, peripheral neuropathy in advanced stages, sphincter disturbances, pigmentary degeneration of the retina
Pantothenate kinase-associated neurodegeneration	See table 32.7	
X-linked adrenoleukodystrophy (adrenomyeloneuropathy)	>15 years	Very slow progression, loss of vibratory and somatosensory sensation, urinary system disorders, sexual dysfunction, increased plasma VLCFAs, Addison's disease

Table 32.9 CLASSIFICATION OF HEREDITARY ATAXIAS

Mitochondrial
- Nuclear DNA (Friedreich's Ataxia, MIRAS, IOSCA) - Mitochondrial DNA (MERFF, NARP, KSS)
Metabolic
- Urea metabolism disorders - Amino acid metabolism disorders - Pyruvate metabolism disorders - Vitamin E deficiency - Lipid metabolism disorders - Storage diseases - Peroxisomal metabolism disorders
DNA repair deficiency
- Ataxia telangiectasia (AT) - Ataxia telangiectasia-like disorder - Ataxia with oculomotor apraxia 1 (AOA1) - Ataxia with oculomotor apraxia 2 (AOA2) - Spinocerebellar ataxia with axonal neuropathy 1 (SCAN 1) - Xeroderma pigmentosum - Cockayne syndrome
Protein assembly and degradation abnormalities
- Autosomal recessive spastic ataxia of Charlevoix-Saguenay (ARSACS) - Polyglutamine ataxias (SCA 1, 2, 3, 6, 7, 12, 17, DRPLA; SCA8 combined mechanism) - Prion diseases (GSS) - Marinesco-Sjogren syndrome
Channelopathies
- Episodic ataxia type 1 (AE-1) - Episodic ataxia type 2 (AE-2)
Others
- Congenital ataxias (Joubert; CAMOS) - Early-onset cerebellar ataxia (EOCA) - Cerebellar ataxia with hypogonadism - Progressive myoclonic ataxia - Dominant ataxias (SCA 4, 5, 10, 11, 13, 14, 15, 16, 18-36)

Table 32.10 COMMON ACUTE FORMS OF PEDIATRIC ONSET ATAXIA

1. Non-metabolic
- Pure ataxia · Infections/immune reactions • acute infectious cerebellitis • post-infectious cerebellitis • brainstem encephalitis • bacterial meningitis · Paraneoplastic syndrome • neuroblastoma · Drug intoxications • benzodiazepines, barbiturates, phenytoin, phenothiazines • Münchausen syndrome · Trauma • contusions or hemorrhages • posterior fossa hematoma • vertebrobasilar occlusion · Increased intracranial pressure • intracranial tumors • hydrocephalus · Demyelinating disorders - Ataxia and weakness · acute brain injuries · spinal cord diseases · Guillain-Barré syndrome - Paroxysmal ataxia · migraines · epilepsy - Functional ataxia · Conversion disorder
2. Metabolic
- Pyruvate dehydrogenase deficiency - Pyruvate carboxylase deficiency - Mitochondrial fatty acid oxidation disorders - Maple syrup urine disease (Leucinosis) - Urea cycle disorders - Organic acidurias - Biotinidase deficiency - Fructose 1,6-bisphosphatase deficiency - Hartnup disease - Familial episodic ataxia responsive to acetazolamide - Serotonin transporter deficiency (SERT deficiency)

32.3.4 Ataxias

Signs of ataxia can be clearly observed from the end of the first year of life when the child acquires a sitting and upright posture and eye-hand coordination skills. Before this period, a diagnosis of ataxia may be suspected when there is muscular hypotonia, hyporeflexia, and motor developmental delay. In older children, the disorder manifests as in adults.

Table 32.9 provides a classification of inherited forms of infantile-onset ataxias.

Acute or recurrent ataxias | Table 32.10 shows acute forms that manifest in childhood. The most common cause (30-50% of cases) is post-infectious cerebellitis associated with viral infections (enteroviruses, Epstein-Barr virus, varicella virus, measles virus, mumps virus, herpes simplex virus, etc.). It is a self-limiting disorder that usually occurs 1-3 weeks after the viral infection. Opsoclonus-myoclonus syndrome or Kinsbourne syndrome is an acute form of motor incoordination typically presenting in the first three years of life characterized by massive myoclonus of the limbs, erratic and movement-triggered, and chaotic, sudden, jerky eye movements (opsoclonus) intensified by changes in gaze shifting, and often accompanied by rapid eyelid flickering (eyelid myoclonus). The motor disturbance has a self-limiting course, with exacerbations during concurrent febrile illnesses. Prognosis depends on the persistence of behavioral disturbances, language impairments, intellectual disability, and the underlying etiology. In approximately 50% of cases, the syndrome is associated with neuroblastoma, sometimes small and localized in the chest, abdomen, or pelvis. In the remaining cases, the etiology is likely autoimmune, induced by concurrent infectious diseases (an association with varicella has been demonstrated). Treatment involves surgical removal of the neoplasm if present and administration of high-dose corticosteroids, immunoglobulins, cyclophosphamide, azathioprine, and rituximab. Plasmapheresis can be a therapeutic option.

Acute ataxia can also result from drug intoxication (with benzodiazepines, carbamazepine, phenytoin, phenothiazines, phenobarbital, valproate, lamotrigine) and can be associated with nystagmus, drowsiness, and vomiting, and jerky movements. In Munchausen syndrome, recurrent episodes of ataxia and drowsiness stem from the intentional administration of drugs by a caregiver to induce symptoms requiring medical attention.

The occurrence of acute or recurrent ataxia as an initial or dominant symptom of a neurometabolic or hereditary ataxia is much rarer. Acute ataxia often associated with lethargy and vomiting, reflects metabolic decompensation induced by concurrent febrile illnesses or catabolic status. Usually, these are milder phenotypic variants of metabolic diseases (e.g., nonketotic hyperglycinemia, pyruvate dehydrogenase deficiency, urea cycle defects, maple syrup urine disease, thiamine metabolism defects) that only manifest under metabolic stress conditions due to increased residual enzymatic activity. In the recurrent ataxia, the disorder can be a manifestation of one of the autosomal dominant episodic ataxias, typically due to channellopathies, in which multiple triggers (e.g.,fever, exertion, physical exercise, fasting, stress, vestibular changes, or stimulating substances such as alcohol or caffeine such as caffeine) can trigger ataxic spells attacks lasting from 15 minutes (EA1) to days (EA2). Interictal examination can reveal associated symptoms such as myokymia in EA1, nystagmus in EA2/EA5/EA8 and seizures and migraine in EA6. These conditions often pose challenges in differential diagnosis, particularly during the early stages and in the absence of neuroimaging abnormalities.

Progressive ataxias | A slowly progressive cerebellar ataxia with insidious onset can be caused by numerous pathological conditions. The possibility of a posterior fossa tumor should be considered, as it can manifest with isolated ataxia for a prolonged period before signs of increased intracranial pressure (papilledema, headache, vomiting, etc.) emerge. In these cases, ataxia often has a focal character, predominantly affecting one hemisphere. Brainstem gliomas typically present with other focal signs such as cranial nerve deficits, pyramidal signs, nystagmus, and other oculomotor deficits. A subacute progressive encephalopathy with ataxia can be associated with measles and rubella virus infection, enterovirus infection in individuals with hypogammaglobulinemia, and HIV infection.

Table 32.11 shows the most common neurometabolic and neurodegenerative diseases in which ataxia is or can be the main clinical sign, based on the age of onset of the disorder. Two conditions can be considered paradigmatic of this group of disorders and are also the most frequent forms: Friedreich's ataxia (incidence of 1-2 cases per 100,000 live births) and Ataxia-Telangiectasia. Friedreich's ataxia typically begins between the ages of 8 and 15 with gait ataxia. Within the first 5 years from onset, progressive dysarthria, peripheral neuropathy with areflexia, hyposthenia, loss of limb position sense, and vibratory sensation, as well as scoliosis, gradually manifest. Hypertrophic cardiomyopathy, detectable by ultrasound in the early stages of the disease, can become symptomatic later on. Approximately 15% of patients develop diabetes mellitus. The disease is caused by abnormal expansion of GAA triplets within the FXN gene, which encodes a protein called frataxin that is

Table 32.11 MAIN PROGRESSIVE ATAXIAS ASSOCIATED WITH NEUROMETABOLIC OR NEURODEGENERATIVE CONDITIONS IN RELATION TO AGE OF ONSET

Disease	Onset age	Other associated clinical signs
	WITHIN THE FIRST YEAR OF LIFE	
Carbohydrate-deficient glycoprotein syndrome (CDG1A)	First year of life	Psychomotor delay, hypotonia, hyporeflexia, respiratory difficulties, characteristic somatic stigmata, retinitis pigmentosa, peripheral neuropathy, spinal atrophy, intellectual disability, kyphoscoliosis, stroke
Semialdehyde succinic dehydrogenase deficiency (SSADH)	First few months of life	Psychomotor delay, hypotonia, hyporeflexia, aggressive behavior, autistic traits, choreoathetosis, epilepsy
Ataxia, megalencephaly, demyelination	First year of life	Macrocephaly, motor delay, epilepsy, lower limb spasticity, mental deterioration; Brain MRI: swelling of the hemispheric white matter, subcortical cysts, normal periventricular white matter
Cockayne syndrome	1 year (type 1-2) 1 year and onwards (type 3)	Cranial and facial dysmorphic features, poor growth. Ataxia, deafness, neuropathy
Abetalipoproteinemia	First year of life	Low levels of cholesterol, triglycerides, vitamins A, D, E. Acanthocytosis, cerebellar atrophy
	1-5 YEARS	
Ataxia-telangiectasia	12-18 months	Teleangiectasias, choreoathetosis, myoclonus, supranuclear ophthalmoplegia, immune deficiency, pronounced tumor diathesis
Early-onset ataxia with preserved oculomotor-trigger reflexes	18 months-20 years	No cardiopathy, intact oculomotor-trigger reflexes, no scoliosis, lower limb ataxia, dysarthria, Babinski sign, no tabetic signs, no peripheral neuropathy
GM2 gangliosidosis	3-6 years	Dysarthria, spastic paraparesis, dystonia, epilepsy, behavior disorders, spinal muscular atrophy
Niemann-Pick disease type C	3-8 years	Supranuclear ophthalmoplegia, dystonia, hepatosplenomegaly, cerebellar atrophy (MRI)
Metachromatic leukodystrophy	> 12 months	Peripheral neuropathy, spastic paraparesis, dementia, leukodystrophy (MRI)
CACH (childhood ataxia and diffuse central nervous system hypomyelination)	> 2 years	Neuromotor deterioration, lower limb spasticity, late-onset optic atrophy, facial and lingual hypotonia, no mental deterioration, mild delay; Brain MRI: diffuse white matter alterations, cortical atrophy, ventricular dilatation, no cysts
Coenzyme Q deficiency	Early years of life (1-4)	Psychomotor delay, intellectual disability, epilepsy, cerebellar atrophy (MRI), epilepsy, chorea, hypotonia, muscular atrophy, high arches, peripheral neuropathy, scoliosis
Marinesco-Sjogren syndrome	Childhood	Ataxia, intellectual disability, and congenital cataracts. Other characteristic features: facial dysmorphisms, short stature, hypergonadotropic hypogonadism, skeletal deformities. Involvement of muscle tissue with muscular atrophy. Sometimes microcephaly, hypoacusia
Ataxia-deafness-leukodystrophy	>2 years	Leukodystrophy (MRI), deafness, cardiopathy
L-2OH Glutaric Acidemia	18 months-10 years	Dysarthria, intellectual disability, epilepsy, pyramidal signs, dystonia
Krabbe leukodystrophy	15 months-10 years	Spastic paraparesis, peripheral neuropathy, spastic tetraparesis, dystonia, visual deficits, leukodystrophy (MRI)
Ceroid lipofuscinosis (late-infantile form)	2-4 years	Epilepsy, myoclonus, polymyoclonus, neurological regression, loss of vision
Ataxia with oculomotor apraxia type I (AOA1)	2-6 years	Gait ataxia, dysarthria, distal muscle weakness, mild impairment of vibratory and proprioceptive sensation. Oculomotor apraxia
Xeroderma pigmentosum	1-2 years	Ataxia, choreoathetosis, spasticity, photosensitivity, early-onset cutaneous neoplasms, keratitis
ARSACS	12-18 months	Spastic paraparesis followed by spastic ataxia, neuropathy, hypertrophy of myelin fibers, cerebellar atrophy

Disease	Onset age	Other associated clinical signs
	5- 10 YEARS	
Friedreich's ataxia (FA)	Around 10 years	Tabetic signs (loss of position sense and vibratory sensation), dysarthria, kyphoscoliosis, high-arched feet, sensory axonal neuropathy, cardiomyopathy, diabetes mellitus
Abetalipoproteinemia	5-10 years	Similar to FA + retinitis pigmentosa, acanthocytosis
Gaucher disease type III	6-15 years	Epilepsy, splenomegaly, supranuclear ophthalmoplegia, Gaucher cells (in bone marrow)
Lafora disease	9-20 years	Polymyoclonus, epilepsy, rapidly progressing dementia
Unverricht-Lundborg myoclonic epilepsy	6-16 years	Myoclonic epilepsy, polymyoclonus
Ataxia with Oculomotor Apraxia Type II (AOA2)	10-22 years	Ataxia, peripheral neuropathy, and oculomotor apraxia
Spinocerebellar Ataxia with Axonal Neuropathy (SCAN1)	10- 19 years	Similar to AT without oculomotor apraxia
	ABOVE 10 YEARS OF AGE AND VARIABLE AGE	
Ataxia with vitamin E deficiency	<20 years	Similar to FA
MERRF	< 20 years	Myoclonic epilepsy, action myoclonus
Ataxia with Oculomotor Apraxia Type II (AOA2)	10- 22 years	Ataxia, peripheral neuropathy, and oculomotor apraxia
Spinocerebellar Ataxia with Axonal Neuropathy (SCAN1)	10- 19 years	Similar to AT without oculomotor apraxia
A-T like disorder	Variable	Ataxia, oculomotor apraxia
Refsum disease	Variable 7 months - 50 years	Peripheral neuropathy, cerebellar degeneration, retinitis pigmentosa, elevated blood and urine levels of phytanic acid

involved in regulating iron ion homeostasis within mitochondria. Deficiency of frataxin triggers a cascade of events leading to apoptosis and neurodegeneration. A clinical picture similar to Friedreich's ataxia is observed in four other conditions: early onset cerebellar ataxia with retained reflexes, abetalipoproteinemia, hypobetalipoproteinemia, and ataxia with selective vitamin E deficiency.

Progressive ataxias can be associated with oculomotor apraxia, pyramidal signs, polyneuropathy, myoclonus, and epilepsy.

Ataxias associated with oculomotor apraxia

The term "oculomotor apraxia" refers to a specific supranuclear disorder of eye movements caused by impairment of both the saccadic and smooth pursuit systems (frontal and occipito-mesencephalic, respectively), resulting in ophthalmoplegia with an altered suppression of the vestibulo-ocular reflex. As a compensatory adaptation, patients often rely on this reflex (activated by head movements) to orient their gaze and avert it. Ataxia-telangiectasia (A-T) is the most common inherited form of ataxia in children under 10 years of age (1 in 40,000 live births, with an incidence of 1 in 7,090 in Italy). It is a multisystemic disease including neurological deterioration, primary immunodeficiency (IgG, IgA, IgE, T-cell) and cancer susceptibility. The disease, in his typical presentation, starts in early childhood with slowly progressive truncal ataxia, often initially indistinguishable from simple postural delay. Ataxia tends to generalise and is often associated with choreoathetosis, while oculomotor apraxia progresses towards severe ophthalmoplegia during the first decade of life. By puberty, the patient loses independent ambulation. Telangiectasias in the conjunctiva, skinfolds behind the ears, and at the elbow or popliteal fossa represent the somatic marker of the disease. In the second decade of life, other symptoms of the disease manifest, including peripheral neuropathy (axonopathy), progeric changes, primarily affecting the skin, and a predisposition to cancer, which, along with bronchopulmonary infections, are the main causes of death, partially expressed in heterozygotes as well. An increase in serum alpha-fetoprotein is found in approximately 90% of individuals and serves as a useful biological marker of the disease. A-T is caused by a genetically based deficiency of a protein called ATM, which is involved in DNA damage signaling and repair mechanisms, as well as cell cycle checkpoints and oxidative stress regulation. Oculomotor apraxia with similar characteristics is also reported in ataxia with oculomotor apraxia type 1 (AOA1) and type 2 (AOA2). Regarding AOA2, some researchers have proposed classifying the condition as SCAN2 (Spinocerebellar Ataxia with Axonal Neuropathy Type 2) because the association of ataxia with neuropathy (present in 90% of patients) seems to be more representative of the clinical picture than the association of ataxia with oculomotor apraxia (present in 47% of patients). Differential diagnosis between these two disorders and A-T is based on the presence of hypoalbuminemia and hypercholesterolemia in AOA1, as well as normal alpha-fetoprotein levels, while telangiectasias are absent, and creatine kinase (CPK) levels are modestly elevated in AOA2. Neuroimaging findings of cerebellar atrophy can provide important diagnostic clues in all these forms. Another condition in which oculomotor apraxia is a characteristic feature is Joubert syndrome, a complex constellation of conditions with an atypical malformation of the brainstem-cerebellar junction.

Ataxia with pyramidal signs | Early-onset ataxia associated with spastic paraparesis and peripheral neuropathy characterizes *autosomal recessive spastic ataxia of Charlevoix-Saguenay* (ARSACS), an autosomal recessive inherited condition.

Symptoms typically begin in early childhood, usually within 12-18 months, and initially involve the lower limbs, causing spasticity accompanied by instability in walking and frequent falls. Other early signs include nystagmus, reduced saccadic velocity, and hypermyelinated retinal fibers that radiate from the optic disc to the papillomacular bundle. The disease has a progressive course due to axonal degeneration of the corticospinal and spinocerebellar tracts of the lateral spinal cord. ARSACS is an autosomal recessive condition caused by pathogenetic variants in the SACS gene (13q11), which encodes sacsin, a large protein whose functions are not yet fully understood. Neuroimaging findings (revealing atrophy of the upper cerebellar vermis and cervical spinal cord) and neurophysiological examination (detecting signs of axonal and demyelinating neuropathy) may support the diagnosis. Retinal alterations, when present, may further support the diagnosis of the disease, which has been improved in the last decade by the diffusion of NGS panel for genetic ataxia, including SACS. Differential diagnosis is necessary with other forms of autosomal recessive ataxia, such as Friedreich's ataxia and ataxia with vitamin E deficiency (AVED), as well as hereditary spastic paraplegia, particularly spastic paraplegia 20 (SPG20, Troyer syndrome).

Ataxia associated with polyneuropathy | Areflexia and loss of deep sensation are present in various forms of hereditary ataxia and in patients with ataxia due to vitamin E deficiency and abetalipoproteinemia (both with a Friedreich-like phenotype) and spinocerebellar ataxia with axonal neuropathy (SCAN1, which presents an AT-like phenotype without oculomotor apraxia).

Ataxia with myoclonus and epilepsy | A group of progressive autosomal recessive cerebellar ataxias is characterized by the presence of myoclonus and epilepsy, which, in most cases, precede ataxia. This group includes Unverricht-Lundborg disease, Lafora disease, ceroid lipofuscinoses, sialidosis, Gaucher disease type III, dentatorubral-pallidoluysian atrophy (DRPLA, classified as spinocerebellar ataxia), and myoclonic epilepsy with ragged-red fibers (MERRF). The most common form is Unverricht-Lundborg disease which is the most common among these rare disease (frequency: 1 in 20,000 in Finland where the disease occurs most frequently). Between 6 and 16 years of age, children with this disorder experience episodes of involuntary muscle jerking or twitching (myoclonus) that increase in frequency and severity over time. Episodes of myoclonus may be brought on by physical exertion, stress, light, or other stimuli. Within 5 to 10 years, the myoclonic episodes may become severe enough to interfere with walking and other everyday activities.

The disease is characterized by onset typically between 6 and 16 years of age, with myoclonus, epilepsy (generalized tonic-clonic seizures). Subsequently, ataxia, dysarthria, and tremor appear. The disease follows an autosomal recessive transmission pattern and is caused by a deficiency of cystatin B. Its pathogenesis is not fully understood, but recent studies have linked cystatin B to lysosomal cathepsin activity.

Non-progressive ataxias | Outside of the ataxic forms of inherited cerebellar degenerative diseases, numerous other acquired (cytomegalovirus infection, less commonly rubella virus) or more frequently congenital conditions result in a syndromic presentation in which ataxia is an integral part (Table 32.11). Malformations of the posterior cranial fossa (mainly involving the cerebellum) are almost always associated with global developmental delay, intellectual disability and hypotonia. They may be multisystemic diseases, involving other tissues (retina, liver, kidney). The most representative syndrome of this group is Joubert syndrome, characterized by a congenital malformation of the brainstem and agenesis or hypoplasia of the cerebellar vermis, leading to central respiratory disorders, nystagmus, hypotonia, ataxia, and global developmental delay and/or intellectual disability. The prevalence is approximately 1 in 100,000.

Cognitive functions can vary in their involvement. When present, intellectual disability is often associated with behavioural alterations such as restlessness, psychomotor instability, and attention deficits. Oculomotor apraxia is frequently observed. Other possible ocular manifestations include retinitis pigmentosa and other progressive retinopathies, Leber congenital amaurosis, and retinal coloboma. Juvenile nephronophthisis, a progressive renal pathology characterized by tubular atrophy, interstitial fibrosis, and cysts predominantly localized at the corticomedullary junction, is found in 30% of cases. The pathognomonic diagnostic marker of Joubert syndrome is a malformation pattern of the posterior cranial fossa, referred to as the *molar tooth sign*, namely a deep interpeduncular fossa, prominent and elongated superior cerebellar peduncles with an anomalous orientation (giving the midbrain the appearance of an inverted molar tooth).

Cerebellar malformation is not synonimous of fixed/non progressive disease. Some cerebellar malformations are associated with rare or ultra-rare metabolic diseases/ degenerative conditions with a progressive clinical course (e.g., protein glycosylation disorders or olivopontocerebellar atrophy) requiring specific diagnostic work-up.

32.4 Epilepsy and epileptic syndromes

Epilepsy is a brain disorder characterized by a predisposition to recurrent paroxysmal episodes ("epileptic seizures") and various neurobiological, cognitive, psychological, and social sequelae.

Epilepsy is the most common neurological disorder in childhood, affecting 0.5-1% of children, with an annual incidence of 5-7 new cases per 10,000 individuals in the age range from birth to 15 years (accounting for 25% of the total global epileptic population of all ages). In approximately 80% of adults with epilepsy, the disease onset occurred before the age of 20.

According to the International League Against Epilepsy (ILAE), the diagnosis of epilepsy implies the presence of at least one of the following conditions:

1) At least two unprovoked (or reflex) epileptic seizures occurring at least 24 hours apart.
2) At least one unprovoked (or reflex) epileptic seizure and a probability of recurrence higher than 60%.
3) Diagnosis of a specific epileptic syndrome.

In the field of epilepsy and epileptic syndromes, classification based on clinical, electroencephalographic, and neuroradiological criteria integrate factors such as age of onset and etiology.

The ILAE identified six etiological classes in their 2017 classification: structural, genetic, infectious, metabolic, autoimmune, and forms of unknown etiology.

Epileptic seizures are classified, according to the same ILAE 2017 classification, as generalized (motor and non-motor), focal (with or without loss of consciousness), and seizures with unknown onset semiology.

The main pediatric epileptic syndromes are summarized in Figure 32.1 and Tables 32.12, 32.13, 32.14.

The diagnostic approach to a child with epilepsy follows, in some ways, the models and methods used in adult patients but also differs significantly. The presence of age-related specific diseases, the importance of genetic and metabolic determinants, disease-causing factors, the impact of pregnancy and birth events and related pathologies, and the issue of differential diagnosis with non-epileptic paroxysmal manifestations (breath holding spells and other anoxic-syncopal forms, tetany, non-epileptic myoclonus, paroxysmal sleep disorders, benign paroxysmal vertigo, etc.; see Table 32.15), make pediatric neurology unique.

A detailed medical history is a central cornerstone for a correct diagnostic approach. The medical history needs to focus on the age of onset and characteristic features of the critical episodes to define their semiology and duration, the presence of triggering factors (e.g., photic stimulation, stimulus-sensitive or noise-sensitive epilepsies, etc.), the mode of termination (spontaneous or pharmacologically induced), and the characteristics of the postictal phase (immediate recovery, postictal drowsiness, Todd's paresis, etc.). In terms of etiological assessment, both genetic and genetic-metabolic causal factors and the role and impact of diseases and adverse events

Table 32.12 EPILEPTIC SYNDROMES WITH ONSET IN THE AGE-RANGE 0-2 YEARS

Epileptic syndrome	Semeiological features	EEG	Therapeutic options
Early Infantile Epileptic and Developmental Encephalopathy (formerly Ohtahara syndrome; Early Myoclonic encephalopathy)	Tonic spasms (isolated or in clusters), myoclonic seizures, focal motor seizures, hemiclonic seizures, tonic seizures	Slowing background, suppression burst pattern, plurifocal abnormalities, ictal desynchronized trace	Vigabatrin, zonisamide, Vitamin B6, valproic acid, benzodiazepiness, ACTH, steroids, immunoglobulines, ketogenic dayt, surgery
Infantile Spasms Syndrome (formerly West syndrome)	Flexor or extension spasms	Hypsarrhythmia	ACTH, steroids, vigabatrin, topiramate
Benign myoclonic epilepsy	Myoclonic seizures (predominant during sleeping)	Normal interictal trace, diffuse epileptiform abnormalities in the ictal phases	Only in recurrent seizures: phenobarbital (first choice under the age of 2), valproic acid (first choice after the age of 2)
Dravet syndrome	Initial febrile seiures, myoclonc seizures, tonic clonic seizures, focal motor seizures, atypical absences, photosensitivity	Normal interictal trace at the onset, diffuse paroxysmal burst including spikes, polyspikes and waves or spikes and slow waves with slowing of background activity	Valproic acid, phenobarbital, topiramate, carbamazepine, stiripentole, levetiracetam, benzodiazepines, ethosuximide, zonisamide, rufinamide, ketogenic dayt
Genetic epilepsy with febrile seizures plus (GEFS+)	Simple or complex recurring febrile seizures, tonic seizures, myoclonic seizures, tonic-clonic seizures, atypical absences	Normal trace at the onset, focal or diffuse epileptiform abnormalities in the subsequent phases	Valproic acid, phenobarbital, topiramate, carbamazepine, levetiracetam, benzodiazepines, ethosuximide, zonisamide, rufinamide, ketogenic dayt

ELECTROCLINICAL SYNDROMES

Neonatal
- Benign neonatal seizures
- Benign familial neonatal epilepsy (BFNE)
- Ohtahara syndrome (early epileptic encephalopathy with suppression-burst)
- Early myoclonic encephalopathy (EME)

Early childhood syndromes
- Febrile seizures and febrile seizures plus
- Benign childhood epilepsy
- Benign familial infantile epilepsy (BFIE)
- West syndrome (infantile spasms)
- Dravet syndrome
- Myoclonic epilepsy in infancy (MEI)
- Myoclonic epilepsy in non-progressive encephalopathy
- Epilepsy with migrating partial seizures in infancy

Late childhood syndromes
- Febrile seizures and febrile seizures plus
- Benign early-onset occipital epilepsy (Panayiotopoulos syndrome)
- Epilepsy with myoclonic-atonic seizures (myoclonic-astatic)
- Childhood absence epilepsy (CAE)
- Benign epilepsy of childhood with centrotemporal spikes (BECTS)
- Autosomal dominant nocturnal frontal lobe epilepsy (ADNFLE)
- Benign epilepsy with occipital paroxysms (Gastaut type)
- Epilepsy with myoclonic absences
- Lennox-Gastaut syndrome (LGS)
- Epileptic encephalopathy with continuous spike and wave during sleep (CSWS)
- Landau-Kleffner syndrome (LKS)

Adolescence and adulthood
- Juvenile myoclonic epilepsy (JME)
- Epilepsy with only generalized tonic-clonic seizures
- Autosomal dominant epilepsy with auditory features (ADEAF)
- Other familial temporal lobe epilepsies

Onset with variable presentation
- Familial focal epilepsies (with variable focal manifestations)
- Progressive myoclonic epilepsy (PME)
- Reflex epilepsies

Figure 32.1

The classification of childhood epilepsies based on the age of onset.

Table 32.13 EPILEPTIC SYNDROMES WITH ONSET IN THE AGE-RANGE 2 YEARS-SCHOOL AGE

Epileptic syndrome	Semeiological features	EEG	Therapeutic options
Lennox Gastaut syndrome	Tonic seizures (mandatory), Atypical absences, Atonic seizures), myoclonic seizures (late onset forms)	Background slowing with diffuse spike and slow waves at 1,5-2,5 Hz, predominant in the anterior regions. Paroxysmal fast activity during sleeping	Valproic acid, rufinamide, felbamato, lamotrigine, topiramate, zonisamide, levetiracetam, benzodiazepines, ethosuximide, ketogenic dayt
Landau-Kleffner syndrome	Progressive aphasia. Possible focal, generalized tonic-clonic, myoclonic seizures or atypical absences	Spikes and spine and waves discharges with a subcontinous trend (in some case involvement of more than 80-85% of slow sleep (Electrical Status Epilepticus during slow sleep - ESES). During the wake focal abnormalities in the fronto-temporal regions.	Valproic acid, phenobarbital, topiramate, carbamazepine, lamotrigine, levetiracetam, benzodiazepines, ethosuximide, zonisamide, rufinamide, ketogenic dayt
Myoclonic astatic epilepsy	Myoclonic seizures, atonic seizures, generalized tonic-clonic seizures	Normal trace at the onset, subsequent disorganization of background activity and diffuse spike and waves discharges during the ictal phases	Valproic acid, ethosuximide, lamotrigine, levetiracetam, benzodiazepines
Absence Epilepsy of Infancy	Staring with possible eyelid myoclonia, automatisms	Diffuse 3-4Hz spike and waves discharges, facilitated by hyperventilation and Intermittent Photo Stimulation	Valproic acid, ethosuximide, lamotrigine, levetiracetam, benzodiazepines
Benign Occipital Epilepsy (Panayiotopoulos Syndrome)	Nocturnal autonomic seizures following lateral deviation of gaze and subsequent hemifacial clonias, myoclonic seizures and automatisms. Seizures often end with episodes of vomiting.	High voltage spike and slow waves discharges during sleeping with a focus that may be in all cerebral regions (with a predominance in the occipital ones)	Valproic acid, topiramate, benzodiazepines, carbamazepine, levetiracetam, benzodiazepines, lamotrigine
Self-limited epilepsy with centrotemporal spikes	Focal seizures predominant during the first phases of sleeping or the awakening with oro-pharingeal phenomena (dysarhtria, oral parahestesias, deglution disturbances), hemifacial myoclonias, tonic or clonic seizures involving one side of the body	Spikes in the centro-temporal regions	No treatment in most of cases. In rare cases: valproic acid, topiramate, carbamazepine o levetiracetam
Childhood occipital lobe epilepsy (gastaut-type)	Visual seizures (illusions, elementary hallucinations, ictal blindness) evolving either to hemiclonic or focal seizures with impaired awareness, with or without secondary generalization. Migraine-type postictal headache was reported in about 25% of the cases	Normal background activity, with high amplitude, unilateral or bilateral, synchronous or asynchronous, occipital spike-and-wave discharges, facilitated by eye closure.	Valproic acid, topiramate, carbamazepine o levetiracetam

Table 32.14 EPILEPSIES AND EPILEPTIC SYNDROMES WITH ONSET DURING THE ADOLESCENCE

Epilepsy/Epileptic syndrome	Semeiological features	EEG	Therapeutic options
Juvenile Absence Epilepsy	Seizures are typical absences in 100% of the patients longer and less frequent than in childhood absence epilepsy (CAE), generalized tonic-clonic seizures (GTCS) in 80% and sporadic myoclonic jerks in 20%.	Diffuse 3-4Hz spike and waves discharges, facilitated by hyperventilation and Intermittent Photo Stimulation	Valproic acid, ethosuximide, lamotrigine, levetiracetam, benzodiazepines
Juvenile myoclonic epilepsy	Myoclonic seizures, generalized tonic-clonic seizures	Rapid, generalized, often irregular spike-waves and polyspike-waves; there is no close phase correlation between EEG spikes and jerks. Photosensitivity.	Valproic acid, lamotrigine, levetiracetam, topiramate, phenobarbital, benzodiazepines
Generalized tonic-clonic epilepsy	Generalized tonic-clonic seizures	Generalized spike/polyspike-and-wave discharges that are increased upon awakening	Valproic acid, lamotrigine, levetiracetam, topiramate, phenobarbital

Table 32.15 PAROXYSMAL NON-EPILEPTIC DISORDERS

- Pseudoseizures
- Migraine
- Parasomnias
- Breath holding spells
- Syncope
- Sandifer syndrome
- Paroxysmal dyskinesia
- Benign Infantile Myoclonus

Table 32.16 DOSAGES, LEVELS FOR THERAPEUTIC DRUG MONITORING AND MAIN SIDE EFFECTS OF ANTISEIZURE MEDICATIONS IN PAEDIATRIC AGE

Antiseizure medication	Dosage	Therapeutic blood level (Toxic Level)	Main side effects
Phenobarbital	Oral: 3-5mg/kg/day; Intravenous (Status epilepticus): 15-20mg/kg poi 5 mg/Kg every 20 minutes (Max 30mg/Kg or 600 mg)	15-40 μg/ml (≥ 40 μg/ml)	Respiratory distress, hypotension, paradoxicol hyperactivity, somnolence, begavioral disturbances, cognitive impairment
Primidone	15-20 mg/kg/day	5-10 μg/ml (≥ 10 μg/ml)	Aggressivesness, nausea, nystagmus, ataxia, vertigo
Phenytoin	Oral: 5-8 mg/kg/day;Intravenous (Status epilepticus): 15-20mg/kg (max=0,5mg/Kg/min and 1 gr/24h)	10-20 μg/ml (≥ 30 μg/ml)	Gengival hyperplasia, vertigo, ataxia, arrhythmias, hypotension, nystagmus, hirsutism, nausea, vomiting, ataxia
Valproic Acid	Oral: 10-30 mg/kg/day; Intravenous: (Status epilepticus) 15-20mg/Kg in 3 min poi 1-2 mg/Kg/hour	40 –100μg/ml (≥ 130 μg/ml)	Tremor, weight gain, alopecia, liver toxicity, coagulation disorders, hyperammoniemia, nausea, vomiting, anorexia, amenorrhea, sedation, vertigo
Ethosuximide	20 -30 mg/kg/day	40-80 μg/ml	Vertigo, behavioral disturbances, rash, liver toxicity, leucopenia, nausea, vomiting
Lamotrigine	1-5 mg/kg/day (with valproic acid); 5-15 mg/Kg/day (without valproic acid)	4-12 μg/ml	Rash, vertigo, headache, ataxia, diplopia, nausea, vomiting
Carbamazepine	10 -20 mg/Kg/day	4-12μg/ml (≥15 μg/ml)	Leucopenia, rash, arrhythmias, vertigo, hyponatriemia, anemia, diplopia, liver toxicity
Oxcarbazepine	10 -20 mg/Kg/day	Not defined	Leucopenia, rash, arrhythmias,, vertigo, hyponatriemia, anemia, diplopia, liver toxicity
Levetiracetam	Oral: 20-50 mg/Kg; Intravenous: 30-60 mg/Kg in 5 minutes	Not defined	Somnolence, vertigo, fatigue, behavioral disturbances
Topiramate	1-9 mg/Kg/day	2-25 μg/ml	Kidney stones, weight loss, hypohidrosis, hypothermia, sleep disorders, fatigue, cognitive impairment
Tiagabine	0,1 mg/Kg/day	Not defined	Stupor, fatigue, vertigo, tremor, attention impairment
Vigabatrin	40-100 mg/Kg/day	Not defined	Sedation, weight gain, visual disturbances, hyperactivity
Felbamate	15-45 mg/Kg/day	Not defined	Liver toxicity, nausea, vomiting, headache, insomnia, aplastic anaemia
Gabapentin	10-30 mg/Kg/day	Not defined	Somnolence, vertigo, ataxia, diplopia, weight gain, vomiting
Zonisamide	200-400 mg/Kg/day	Not defined	Rash, kidney stones,
Acetazolamide	250-750 mg/day	Not defined	Metabolic acidosis, electrolyte dysregulation, gastrointestinal disorders, somnolence, paraesthesia, fever, rash, pancytopenia, liver toxicity, renal toxicity
Clonazepam	0,1-0,2 mg/Kg/day	Not defined	Vertigo, fatigue, behavioral disorders, weight gain, respiratory distress, ataxia
Clobazam	0,25-1 mg/Kg/day	Not defined	Vertigo, fatigue, behavioral disorders, weight gain, respiratory distress, ataxia
Diazepam	Oral: 0,33mg/Kg/dose every 8 hours or 1,5 drop/Kg/day; Intravenous: 0,3 mg/kg in 2-3 minutes, every 15-30 min (max. 10 mg)	Not defined	Vertigo, fatigue, behavioral disorders, weight gain, respiratory distress, ataxia
Lorazepam	Intravenous (Status epilepticus): 0,05-0,1 mg/kg	Not defined	Vertigo, fatigue, behavioral disorders, weight gain, respiratory distress, ataxia
Midazolam	Intravenous (Status epilepticus): 0,1-0,2mg/kg; Intramuscular, Intranasal, or intraosseous (if no intravenous access is available): 0,2 mg/Kg	Not defined	Vertigo, fatigue, behavioral disorders, weight gain, respiratory distress, ataxia
Nitrazepam	2,5-5 mg/day	Not defined	Vertigo, fatigue, behavioral disorders, weight gain, respiratory distress, ataxia
Rufinamide	< 30 Kg without VPA = 200-1000 mg/day; < 30 Kg with VPA = 200-600 mg/day; 30-50 Kg = max 1800 mg/day; 50-70Kg = max 2400 mg/day;	Not defined	Headache, vertigo, somnolence, fatigue, nausea, vomiting
Lacosamide	Oral: 5 mg/Kg; Intravenous (Status epilepticus): 8mg/Kg	Not defined	Vertigo, nausea, diplopia, ataxia, psychiatric symptoms, jaundice, arrhythmias
Perampanel	4-12 mg/day	Not defined	Psychiatric symptoms, vertigo, somnolence, fatigue, nausea, weight gain, balance impairment, ataxia, seizure worsening
Brivaracetam	1-5 mg/Kg/day	Not defined	Psychiatric symptoms, vertigo, somnolence, astenia, nausea, vomiting
Stiripentol	20-50 mg/Kg/day	Not defined	Haematological dysfunctions, liver toxicity
Cannabidiol	5-20 mg/Kg/day	Not defined	Gastrointestinal disorders, liver toxicity

occurring in the pre- and perinatal period (extreme prematurity, congenital infections, perinatal hypoxia-ischemia, congenital malformations) should be evaluated.

Electroencephalography (EEG) remains a fundamental examination for the diagnostic assessment and follow-up of epilepsy in children. The interpretation of the EEG trace in developmental age requires knowledge of non-pathological elements that reflect age-related cerebral maturation and major age-dependent pathological patterns.

The uniqueness of developmental neurophysiology and the transformative diversity characterizing neurotransmission and receptor subtypes in pediatric age also have therapeutic implications.

Antiseizure medications used in pediatric age are fundamentally the same as those used in adults, although issues regarding dosage/body weight ratio and the increased relevance of side effects (e.g., the effect of phenobarbital on cognitive development, topiramate's impact on appetite and thus on growth) mark significant differences in clinical practice. Recent research advances in neurotransmitter physiology and the acquisition of knowledges regarding age-dependent receptor subtypes seem to open up new targeted therapeutic perspectives based on etiology (precision medicine).

Table 32.16 outlines the main medications used in the treatment of epilepsy in developmental age, their dosages, and the most common side effects.

In individuals with drug-resistant epilepsy (defined as a failure in the response to optimal pharmacotherapy with at least two adequate medications for the type of seizures and the child's age for a period of at least two years), possible alternatives to pharmacological treatment, such as surgical removal of the epileptogenic focus, the ketogenic diet, or vagal nerve stimulation, require highly specialized interventions.

Like adult epilepsy, periodic clinical and electroencephalographic monitoring is essential for the proper long-term control of epilepsy treatment in children. Additionally, attention must be paid to evaluating the effects of seizures and their sequelae, as well as the pharmacological therapy, on psychomotor development.

32.4.1 Epileptic and developmental encephalopathies (DEE)

In 2010, the International League Against Epilepsy (ILAE) coined the diagnostic category of epileptic encephalopathy, defined as a condition in which developmental arrest, regression, or more generally, observable cognitive deficits are a direct consequence of epileptic activity itself, exceeding what is expected from the underlying pathology alone (e.g., cortical malformation). Subsequently, the expansion of diagnostic possibilities, especially in the genetic field has shown the limitation of this definition for conditions in which genetic alterations cause both neurodevelopmental disorders and frequent epileptic activity.

All these considerations led to a revision of the classification of epilepsies by the ILAE, which concluded in 2017 with the introduction of the concept of "epileptic and developmental encephalopathies" (DEE) aiming to highlight both the genetic cause and epilepsy itself in the final clinical picture. Often, the distinction between the contribution of genetic alterations and that of epileptic activity on the clinical picture proves to be extremely difficult, and therefore, the use of this new category DEE is recommended.

32.4.2 Most common epileptic syndromes in pediatric age

Tables 32.12-32.14 summarize the semiological and electroencephalographic characteristics, as well as general treatment guidelines, for the main forms of epilepsy with onset in the first 2 years of life and from 2 years of age to school and adolescence. In this paragraph, we will summarize the general characteristics of the major epileptic and developmental encephalopathies with infantile onset.

Infantile Spasms syndrome (formerly West Syndrome) or Infantile Spasms or Salaam Tic Syndrome | It falls within the generalized cryptogenic or symptomatic syndromes and represents an early-onset syndrome

(4-7 months), often severe, characterized by the electroclinical triad: flexion or extensor spasms, hypsarrhythmia on EEG, and developmental delay, regression, or arrest. The spasms, in flexion or extension, sometimes mixed (flexion-extension), are sudden and occur in clusters of 20-40 up to 100 spasms, with a frequency of 1-10 clusters per day. The hypsarrhythmic pattern may be absent, and the history of previous psychomotor development can be either normal or already compromised. From an etiopathogenetic viewpoint, 50-90% of cases involve pre- or perinatal brain damage, and in a limited number of cases, a specific genetic etiology is identified (currently described in at least 37 monogenic forms). Evolution often progresses to other forms of epilepsy, particularly Lennox-Gastaut syndrome (50-60% of cases), and is associated with developmental impairment and intellectual disability (70-80% of cases).

Lennox-Gastaut Syndrome | Is an epileptic and developmental encephalopathy characterized by polymorphic seizures (the presence of tonic seizures is mandatory but also, atonic, atypical absence, and myoclonic seizures may be observed), mostly drug-resistant, often activated during sleep, cognitive impairment, and behavioral disturbances associated with a generalized EEG pattern of slow spike-and-wave or polyspike-and-wave at 2-3 Hz and paroxysmal fast activity during sleeping. It generally starts between the onset of seizures is usually between the first and seventh year of life, often representing the evolution of a previous West syndrome in about 25% of the cases. The etiology is variable and often associated with monogenic or malformative conditions. The prognosis is negative due to the persistence and drug resistance of seizures and the impairment of psychomotor development.

Landau-Kleffner Syndrome | Is characterized by the association of acquired aphasia and epilepsy, representing a specific form of epilepsy in childhood. It usually starts around the age of 6, with a subacute and fluctuating course. This condition remains clinically and pathogenetically controversial and presents numerous differential diagnostic challenges concerning autistic spectrum disorders and the genesis of the "aphasia" phenomenon. The seizures, when present, are polymorphic, and the EEG typically shows a predominant pattern of focal posterior temporal spikes or waves, either unilateral or bilateral, often activated during deep sleep. The prognosis is marked by the disappearance of seizures, if present, and normalization of the EEG around the age of 15, while language and cognitive impairments tend to commonly persist in the majority of patients (70-80% of cases).

32.4.3 Febrile seizures

Febrile seizures are convulsive episodes that occur in children with fever, without signs of acute central nervous system infections, and no previous history of febrile seizures. They represent the most common convulsive disorder and affect 2-5% of the pediatric population between 6 months and 5 years of age, with a uniformly benign prognosis. Febrile seizures are classified as simple or complex. Simple febrile seizures are characterized by a duration of less than 15 minutes, generalized tonic or tonic-clonic seizures that typically do not recur during the same febrile episode, and the absence of postictal neurological deficits. On the other hand, complex febrile seizures have a duration longer than 15 minutes, often have focal features, may be associated with focal neurological deficits, and can recur during the same febrile episode.

Simple febrile seizures do not require an electroencephalogram (EEG) or neuro-imaging investigations. However, such investigations should always be considered in cases of complex febrile seizures. The development of epilepsy in individuals with a history of febrile seizures may be correlated with genetic factors or specific epileptic syndromes (e.g., GEFS+ or Dravet syndrome). This occurrence is observed in 1-1.5% of simple febrile seizures (comparable to the risk in the general population) and 4-15% of cases of complex febrile seizures. Specific risk factors include a positive family history of epilepsy, onset of febrile seizures before the age of 9 months, presence of delayed psychomotor development, or altered neurological examination.

The treatment of ongoing febrile seizures is limited to supportive measures and the administration of rectal diazepam microclism (5 mg below 3 years of age and 10 mg above 3 years of age). In a hospital setting, the treatment of an ongoing seizure should be administered intravenously following the same sequence indicated for status epilepticus. Antipyretics have no effect on febrile seizures but are useful in reducing fever. Intermittent prophylaxis with oral diazepam and continuous prophylaxis with antiseizure medications such as valproic acid or phenobarbital are not recommended due to possible side effects in an otherwise benign condition that, in the majority of cases, has a benign nature. Hospital admission for diagnostic investigations should be reserved for children under the age of 18 months of age in whom central nervous system infection needs to be ruled out, cases with clinical instability, complex febrile seizures, or comorbidity with other conditions suggesting the necessity of treatment and observation in a protected setting.

32.4.4 Genetic-metabolic epilepsies

With the widespread use of next-generation sequencing techniques, it has become possible to determine the genetic-molecular basis of at least 40% of severe epilepsy cases, with or without pharmaco resistance. A clear genotype-phenotype correlation has been established for 210 genes and 400 chromosomal alterations. The most severe conditions are those in which epileptic manifestations begin in the first year of life (Table 32.17).

Inborn errors of metabolism, although responsible for a limited number of epilepsies, have a variable incidence ranging from 0.1 to 300 cases per 100,000 live births, indicating inadequate knowledge due to variability and the lack of diagnostic and epidemiological monitoring in different countries. The influence of genetic factors appears to be more significant. Mono- and polygenic causes are believed to account for approximately 20-40% of epileptic syndromes. Recent advances in the field of neurobiology demonstrate the importance of alterations in synaptogenesis, dendritic pruning, neuronal migration and differentiation, neurotransmitter synthesis and release, as well as the structural and functional integrity of enzymes, receptors, and neuronal transporters as causal factors underlying seizure disorders. The multiplicity and overlapping of clinical phenotypes associated with different genetic and genetic-metabolic conditions make it challenging to develop a categorical model to guide clinical approaches.

Genetic-metabolic early-onset epileptic and developmental encephalopathies can be classified, based on associated symptoms, into:

1) Forms in which epilepsy is the sole or defining clinical symptom.
2) Forms in which epilepsy is associated with several symptoms within a complex phenotype that may include:
   a) Typical somatic features (dysmorphism or micro/macrocephaly).
   b) Acute multiorgan involvement.
   c) Chronic multiorgan involvement.
   d) Movement disorders.

In the field of early epilepsies, some genetic-metabolic diseases have particular relevance due to their diagnostic and therapeutic implications. In the following paragraphs, we outline the essential characteristics of some of these diseases.

Table 32.17 GENETIC-METABOLIC EPILEPTIC ENCEPHALOPATHIES ONSET IN THE FIRST YEAR OF LIFE

Disease		Pathophysiology
EPILEPTIC AND DEVELOPMENTAL ENCEPHALOPATHIES PRESENTING WITH SEIZURES AS PREDOMINANT/ISOLATED SYMPTOM		
Pyridoxine dependent seizure Folinic acid responsive seizure Pyridoxal-5'-phosphate responsive seizure		Vitamin or enzymatic cofactor dependency
Dravet and Dravet-like syndrome		Channellopathy
Ohtahara syndrome (EIEE) Early myoclonic encaphalopathy (EME)		Unknown / multiple etiology
Protocadherin 19 related epileptic encephalopathy Mitochondrial transporters deficiencies (GC1, AGC1) Phospholipase C beta-1 deficiency		Single enzyme or protein dysfunction
Hyperprolinemia type II		Disorders of amino acids metabolism
GABA transaminase deficiency		Neurotransmitters disorders
ENCEPHALOPATHIES PRESENTING WITH SEIZURES ASSOCIATED WITH A SYNDROMIC PHENOTYPE INCLUDING		
Suggestive somatic features (i.e. dysmorphic features and/or alterations of head circumference)	Phenylketonuria and hyperphanylalaninemias	Disorders of amino acids metabolism
	Sulfite oxidase deficiency Molybdenum cofactor deficiency Menkes' disease	Vitamin or enzymatic cofactor dependency
	Early infantile epileptic encephalopathy type I (EIEE1-LISX2)	Cerebral malformations associated disorders
	Angelman syndrome Rett syndrome	Single enzyme or protein dysfunction
	Adenilosuccinate lyase deficiency Dihydropyriminidase and Dihydropyrimidine dehydrogenase deficiency	Purine and pyrimidine metabolism disorders
Acute multiorgan impairment	Urea cycle disorders Organic acidurias Congenital disorders of glycosilation Glutathione synthetase deficiency Mitochondrial disorders (SUCLA2, SUCLG1)	Endogenous toxicity
	Biotin metabolism disorders	Vitamin or enzymatic cofactor dependency
	Congenital glutamine deficiency	Neurotransmitter disorders
	Developmental delay, Epilepsy and Neonatal Diabetes (DEND syndrome)	Channellopathy
	Hyperinsulinism/Hyperammoniemia (HI/HA)	Single enzyme or protein dysfunction
Chronic multiorgan impairment	Mitochondrial disorders (Leigh syndrome, multiple deletion syndrome or Alpers disease, pyruvate dehydrogenase complex deficiency)	Energetic failure
	Lysosomal disorder (Krabbe disease) Peroxisomal disorder (Neonatal adrenoleukodystrophy, Zellweger syndrome, Infantile Refsum disease, punctuate rhyzomelic chondrodysplasia) Niemann-Pick disease type A and C Neuronal ceroid lipofuscinosis	Storage disorders
	MAGI2 deletion syndrome	Single enzyme or protein dysfunction
	Serine byosynthesis disorders	Disorders of amino acids metabolism
	Nesidioblastosis	Unknown
Movement disorders	GLUT1 deficiency syndrome Creatine deficiency syndromes (AGAT, GAMT and X-linked creatine transporter deficiency)	Energetic failure
	EIEE1 (ARX related epileptic encephalopathy)	Cerebral malformations associated disorders
	4-hydroxybutyric aciduria (SSADH)	Neurotransmitter disorders

32.4.5 Epilepsies related to pyridoxine metabolism dysfunctions

This is an autosomal recessive disorder caused by a mutation in the ALDH7A1 gene located on chromosome 5q31, which encodes for antiquitin, a mitochondrially localized aldehyde dehydrogenase that closely resembles the prototype of vitamin-responsive epileptic and developmental encephalopathies. Pyridoxine (vitamin B6) serves as a cofactor in over 140 metabolic pathways, particularly those involved in amino acid and neurotransmitter metabolism. Clinically, a classic or typical variant of the disease can be distinguished from one or more atypical variants. The classic variant is characterized by early-onset seizures, occurring hours or days after birth. Atypical variants include late-onset forms (up to 2 years of age) or those with atypical therapeutic response (latency, pyridoxine dosage, temporary response to conventional antiseizure medications). Additionally, they are associated with symptoms such as neonatal jaundice, hypothermia, dystonia, microcephaly, as well as peripartum asphyxia, feeding difficulties, alterations in ocular motility, and pre-ictal symptoms of restlessness, irritability, and vomiting. Seizures in this syndromic context may present with variable semiology, often manifesting as status epilepticus leading to generalized or partial epilepsy. For practical purposes, a diagnostic hypothesis seems justified in cases where neonatal-onset epilepsy, often in the form of drug-resistant prolonged seizures, occurs in a patient with negative gestational and perinatal history, predominantly myoclonic epilepsy, and a burst-suppression EEG pattern. An allelic variant of pyridoxine-dependent epilepsy is folinic acid deficiency epilepsy. The common responsiveness to pyridoxine, clinical and biochemical parallels, lead to considering these forms as two variants of the same disease.

Another syndromic variant of pyridoxine-dependent epilepsy is pyridoxal-5'-phosphate (PLP)-responsive epilepsy. This form is linked to mutations in the gene encoding for pyridox(am)ine 5'-phosphate oxidase (PNPO), located on chromosome 17q21.2. The enzyme is responsible for synthesizing the biologically active form of vitamin B6 from vitamers obtained through diet. The characteristic symptoms of this epileptic and developmental encephalopathy include polymorphic seizures starting within a few hours of birth, associated with prematurity, respiratory distress, growth deficits, metabolic acidosis, anemia, hypoglycemia, and hypotonia. Patients do not respond to conventional antiseizure medications but may be responsive to pyridoxine as well as pyridoxal-5'-phosphate.

Other forms responsive to pyridoxine include PLP-binding protein (PLP-BP) deficiency and milder forms such as type 2 hyperprolinemia.

32.4.6 Epilepsy due to glucose transporter deficiency (GLUT1 deficiency)

This epileptic and developmental encephalopathy presents with a variable clinical phenotype in terms of age of onset and clinical presentation and is associated with mutations in the SLC2A1 gene. It can manifest as neonatal or infantile myoclonic epilepsy early-onset absence epilepsy, developmental delay, or fluctuating ataxia. The disease can be classified into a classic variant, an atypical variant, a carbohydrate-responsive phenotype (neurological symptoms correlate with feeding: motor and mental performance worsen with fasting and improve with a carbohydrate-rich diet), and a phenotype with epilepsy associated with paroxysmal exertional dyskinesia (dystonic, choreoathetoid, or ballistic movements induced by prolonged physical effort affecting the affected body parts). The impression is that the phenotypic spectrum of the disease is likely to expand further with advancing knowledge and the number of diagnosed cases. The association of early-onset polymorphic epilepsy with ocular movement abnormalities and the occurrence of paroxysmal movement disorders should raise suspicion of this condition. A cerebrospinal fluid (CSF) glucose-to-blood glucose ratio below 0.35 or an absolute low CSF glucose level is highly suggestive and should guide genetic-molecular confirmation of the disease. The ketogenic diet, commonly used in other drug-resistant epilepsies, represents a specific and mandatory therapy in this case, as in pyruvate dehydrogenase complex deficiency epilepsy.

32.4.7 Epilepsy due to biotin metabolism disorders

Biotin metabolism disorders include two pathological entities: biotinidase deficiency and multiple carboxylase deficiency (or holocarboxylase synthetase deficiency). Clinically, they present with an early-onset syndromic picture (1-3 months of age) characterized by lethargy or coma, lactic acidosis and ketosis, conjunctivitis, and cutaneous signs (erythematous dermatitis, blistering eruptions, alopecia, and dermatosis). Other symptoms include respiratory disorders, progressive optic atrophy, early-onset drug-resistant epilepsy, global developmental delay, movement disorders, and sensorineural hearing loss. Both forms are caused by a biotin deficiency resulting from either the inability to hydrolyze biocytin (biotinyl-lysine) introduced through the diet (biotinidase deficiency, 3p25) or the function of holocarboxylase synthetase, the enzyme responsible for the covalent binding of biotin to five different carboxylases (multiple carboxylase deficiency, 21q22.1). The quantitative or functional deficiency of biotin leads to altered metabolism of fatty acids, amino acids, and glucose. The precise mechanism through which this deficiency contributes to epilepsy remains uncertain, given the wide range of biotin functions, including gene expression control and cellular mitotic activity. An acute metabolic picture associated with drug-resistant epilepsy should always raise suspicion of this condition.

32.4.8 Serine metabolism deficiency

Serine biosynthesis disorders include three variants: classical variant or phosphoglycerate dehydrogenase deficiency (*PHGDH*, 1q12), atypical variant or 3-phosphoserine phosphatase deficiency (*PSPH*, 7p15.2), and variant due to phosphoserine aminotransferase deficiency (*PAST1*, 9q21.2). The syndrome is characterized by a congenital microcephaly, global developmental delay, and drug-resistant epilepsy, along with other progressively emerging symptoms. Neonatal-onset forms present with intrauterine growth retardation, dysmorphic features, skeletal abnormalities, ichthyosis, sometimes leading to neonatal lethality. Infantile-onset forms are characterized by congenital microcephaly, feeding difficulties, drug-resistant epilepsy, and developmental delay. Late-onset forms present with epilepsy, intellectual disability, and progressive sensorimotor polyneuropathy. Additional reported symptoms include megaloblastic anemia, cataracts, hypogonadism, delayed puberty, and spastic quadriplegia. The pathogenesis is still unknown but seems to be secondary to a deficiency in serine synthesis, which becomes an essential amino acid. L-serine plays vital roles in the cell beyond protein synthesis, as it is a precursor for important compounds such as cysteine, phosphatidylserine (a phospholipid constituent of cellular membranes), sphingomyelin, D-serine, and glycine, the latter two being important neurotransmitters. It also serves as a source of methylene-tetrahydrofolate, essential for purine and thymidine synthesis.

32.4.9 Status epilepticus

It is useful to provide a brief overview of status epilepticus (SE) in pediatric patients, given the frequency with which this emergency occurs during childhood. SE is a severe complication characterized by prolonged or recurrent seizures without recovery of functions during interictal periods and is classified as convulsive and non convulsive status epilepticus based on the presence or absence of motor manifestations. It represents a condition in which all physiological mechanisms responsible for down-regulating neuronal excitability and consequently terminating any epileptogenic event fail.

SE is often associated with febrile episodes (febrile SE, approximately 25% of cases) or a history of central nervous system (CNS) injury (25-35% of cases) or is caused by acute events (hypoxia, hemorrhage, infections, and trauma in 25% of cases). In many cases, the cause remains unidentified (25% of cases). More rarely, it is a symptom of progressive encephalopathy (3-4% of cases).

The high incidence of secondary neurological complications and irreversible neurological damage justifies the growing attention from neurologists and pediatric intensive care physicians, leading to the development of national and international guidelines for treatment. Figure 32.2 suggests a therapeutic algorithm for the management of status epilepticus in pediatric patients. The activation of this therapeutic algorithm should be timed according to the definitions established by the International League Against Epilepsy (ILAE) in the recent redefinition of status epilepticus in 2015:

a) time t1 = the time at which a seizure is less likely to resolve spontaneously (the time at which pharmacological treatment should be initiated);
b) time t2 = the time beyond which a seizure is more likely to cause clinically significant sequelae (the time by which pharmacological treatment should have resolved the seizure).

32.5 Hypotonia and neuroperipheral pathology

Hypotonia in children is a common and relatively nonspecific symptom in terms of etiology. It is defined as reduced muscle tone relative to the child's age and is assessed, especially in the first few months of life, based on joint angles. Achieving the required condition of relaxation for assessing the muscle tones is challenging in children. Therefore, other aspects are considered, such as age-related joint angles, possible postural abnormalities indicating muscle weakness (as in myopathies and peripheral neuropathies), presence of osteotendinous reflexes. In some conditions, hypotonia is accompanied by ligamentous laxity, making it difficult to distinguish between the two.

Among the non-neurological causes of hypotonia in children are endocrine disorders (hypothyroidism), cardiac conditions, primary connective tissue disorders (such as Ehlers-Danlos syndrome), electrolyte imbalances, vitamin deficiencies (rickets), renal disorders (renal tubular acidosis), and food intolerances (celiac disease).

Central hypotonia is a common symptom in many neurodevelopmental disorders, intellectual disabilities associated with chromosomal aberrations (e.g., Trisomy 21), and various genetic diseases affecting the central nervous system (such as fragile X syndrome, Angelman syndrome).

Hypotonia of the limbs and trunk can be an initial symptom of dyskinetic and ataxic forms of cerebral palsy and often precedes the emergence of specific motor deficits characteristic of these forms. Other central forms of hypotonia include those associated with ataxia (acquired or genetic) and chorea.

Lower motor neuron lesions (tumors, malformations, inflammation involving the spinal cord) cause hypotonia, weakness, and peripheral paralysis, as in adults.

Degenerative diseases affecting the motor neurons of the anterior horns of the spinal cord are particularly important in children. These diseases present with variable clinical severity depending on the age of onset and the speed of progression and are characterized by hypotonia, hyposthenia, areflexia, and amyotrophy (spinal muscular atrophy, SMA). The responsible gene for these diseases is on chromosome 5 (5q12.2-q13.3) and encodes the survival motor neuron (SMN) protein. In the most severe forms, hypotonia/hyposthenia may be present from birth or the first weeks of life and fall within the differential diagnosis of the floppy infant syndrome. Early recognition of this condition is crucial due to the possibility of a highly promising therapy if administered in the early stages of the disease (genetic or antisense oligonucleotide therapy). For this reason, early diagnosis, ideally in the pre-symptomatic phase, has become a strong requirement that has led to the proposal of introducing genetic neonatal screening for SMA.

Among the acquired forms, the acute post-infectious demyelinating polyneuropathy (Guillain-Barré syndrome, GBS) has a particular epidemiological relevance in children and is the most common cause of acquired peripheral paralysis. It is usually preceded by a bacterial or viral infection (particularly *Campylobacter jejuni*) and manifests as ascending symmetric paralysis with the disappearance of deep tendon reflexes and painful paresthesias in the limbs. In severe cases, it can cause loss of ambulation, cranial nerve deficits, respiratory insufficiency, and autonomic dysfunction.

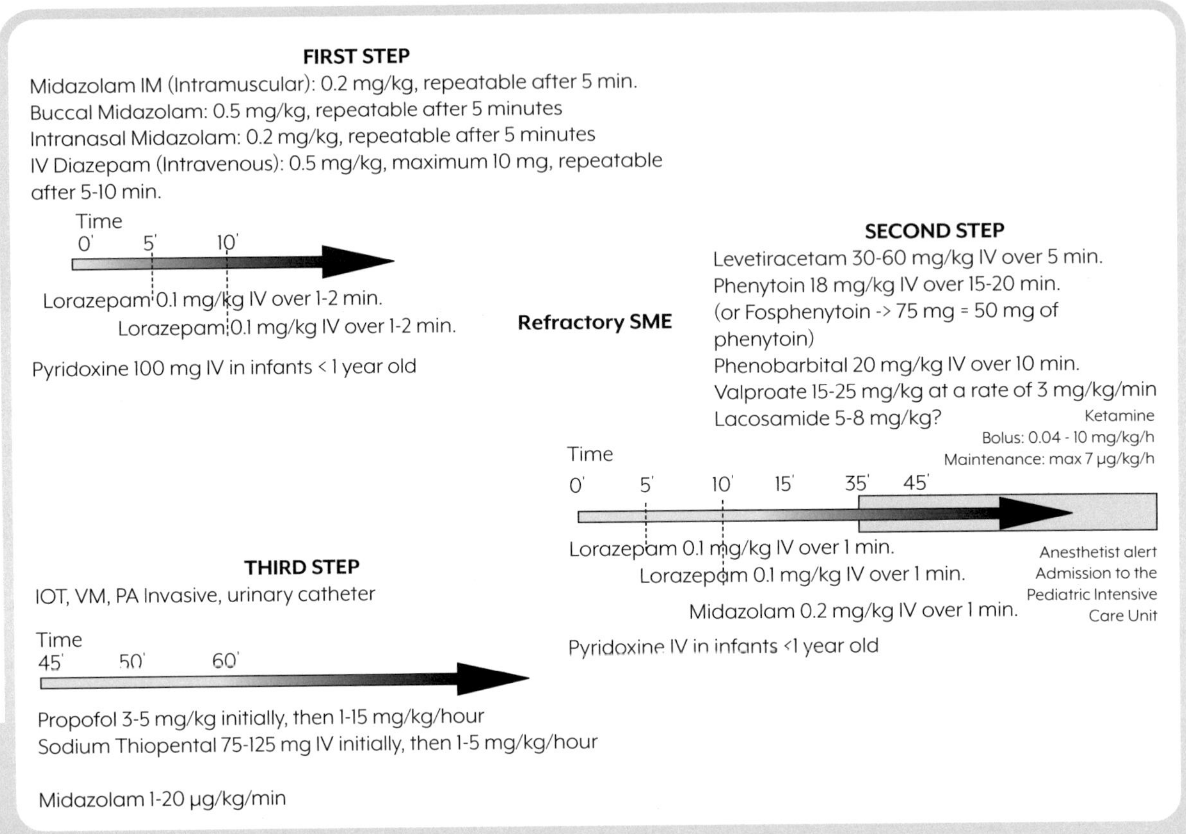

Figure 32.2

Therapeutic Algorithm for the Treatment of Pediatric Status Epilepticus.

Muscle diseases, whether acquired or genetically determined, are a frequent cause of hypotonia in children. Among acquired forms, there are inflammatory muscle diseases, sometimes immune-mediated. Among congenital forms, there is a wide and heterogeneous spectrum of conditions presenting with the typical floppy infant picture. These conditions can be divided into three categories: congenital myopathies, dystrophinopathies, and congenital muscular dystrophies.

The term "*congenital myopathies*" was introduced in the 1950s to describe a group of pathological conditions that cause hypotonia and muscle weakness, with onset at birth or in early childhood. These conditions exhibit typical but not pathognomonic histological and histochemical features on muscle tissue examination, in the absence of signs of dystrophy. This group includes numerous forms, each with multiple responsible genes.

Dystrophinopathies are the most common muscular dystrophies in humans, transmitted with an X-linked pattern and caused by alterations in the *dystrophin gene*. Duchenne muscular dystrophy begins around 2-4 years of age with a gait disturbance secondary to hyposthenia of the pelvic girdle muscles, more evident in anti-gravitational activities. Disease progression leads to loss of ambulation, cardiac problems (dilated cardiomyopathy), and respiratory issues. The course of Becker muscular dystrophy is less severe, with later onset, less pronounced motor impairment, and a longer life expectancy, although there are significant interindividual differences. Congenital muscular dystrophies (CMD) constitute a heterogeneous group of conditions characterized by muscle dystrophy on muscle biopsy. Among them, clinical entities differ in onset, severity, course of muscle impairment, and genetic alterations. Common clinical features include less involvement of facial muscles and less frequent occurrence compared to other congenital myopathies with ophthalmoplegia. This group includes primary merosin/laminin-α2, deficiency, α-dystroglycanopathies, secondary merosin deficiency, glycosylation disorders (CDG) associated with α-dystroglycan glycosylation deficiency, merosin-positive CMD with extracellular matrix deficiency, and other forms of CMD. These conditions are often associated with CNS malformations (lissencephaly, vermian atrophy, white matter abnormalities) and intellectual disabilities, even in the absence of cerebral malformations.

32.6 Isolated cranial nerve deficits in children

Apart from possible acquired causes (such as trauma, iatrogenic factors, oncological conditions, post-infectious factors, etc.), focal neurological deficits in children can sometimes be the only or primary presenting sign of a metabolic or degenerative condition. It is important to emphasize that even an isolated focal neurological symptom should be considered a warning sign for one of these conditions if alternative diagnostic hypotheses have been ruled out. Although the most common etiology of isolated (non-syndromic) hearing loss is genetic rather than metabolic, neurosensory hearing impairment can be an early and significant sign of various neurometabolic or degenerative conditions, such as biotinidase deficiency or mannosidase deficiency (alpha and beta), certain mitochondrial encephalopathies (MELAS, MERRF, Kearns-Sayre syndrome, matrilineal inherited isolated deafness), Refsum disease, Usher syndrome, and Cockayne syndrome.

In some mucopolysaccharidoses (IH, IH-S, II, III), hearing loss causes significant behavioral disturbances that can sometimes lead to the suspicion of a primary psychiatric disorder. In other conditions (Leigh syndrome/disease, Friedreich's ataxia, autosomal dominant spinocerebellar ataxia, adrenoleukodystrophy, Lafora disease, etc.), hearing impairment occurs later and is one of several deficits within a complex clinical picture.

Ocular anomalies and visual deficits are highly prevalent in neurometabolic or neurodegenerative diseases and include ocular motility disorders, retinal abnormalities (involving photoreceptors, pigmented epithelium, ganglion cells, ganglion fibers, and the optic nerve), corneal opacities, and lens abnormalities. Accumulation of phospholipids in ganglion cells of the perimacular region causes the characteristic cherry-red spot (*macular cherry red spot*), mainly observed in neurolipidoses (GM2 gangliosidosis: Tay-Sachs disease, Sandhoff disease; GM1 gangliosidosis) and sialidosis.

Retinal pigment degeneration (tapetoretinal degeneration), characterized by night blindness, photophobia, concentric narrowing of the visual field, and abnormalities in electroretinography (ERG), is a symptom of multiple metabolic and degenerative conditions (Cockayne syndrome, Kearns-Sayre syndrome, maternally inherited Leigh syndrome, hyperornithinemia, ceroid lipofuscinosis, Refsum disease, etc.), as well as isolated non-syndromic forms with different genetic transmission (autosomal dominant, recessive, X-linked), which constitute the most common cause of inherited blindness. It can also occur in non-progressive syndromic forms (associated with deafness), such as Leber congenital amaurosis, Usher syndromes, Laurence-Moon syndrome, and Alstrom syndrome. Optic neuropathy with varying degrees of visual impairment can be a symptom of numerous metabolic conditions affecting the central nervous system (Canavan disease, neuroaxonal dystrophy, juvenile forms of Krabbe leukodystrophy and adrenoleukodystrophy, etc.). Optic atrophy, preceded by typical tortuosity of peripapillary vessels, characterizes Leber optic neuropathy, a condition typically presenting acutely or subacutely in the second decade of life, with progressive but self-limiting evolution once a plateau is reached, usually occurring as the only symptom in isolation. The disease is maternally transmitted and associated with mutations in mitochondrial DNA. A similar form, but with autosomal dominant transmission, is caused by the defect of OPA1 gene.

Blindness or visual agnosia secondary to retrogeniculate visual pathway lesions can be the initial symptom of adrenoleukodystrophy or Krabbe leukodystrophy.

Finally, hemianopsia can result from focal ischemic complications of MELAS, homocystinuria, or Fabry disease.

Oculomotor nuclear palsy is a typical sign of Kearns-Sayre syndrome, characterized by progressive external ophthalmoplegia. Many conditions manifest with supranuclear oculomotor palsy. The most suggestive pathological patterns include horizontal gaze disturbances with saccadic paresis and hyperfunction of the vestibulo-ocular reflex in ataxia-telangiectasia, vertical gaze palsy in Niemann-Pick disease type C, and lateral and vertical gaze palsy in Gaucher disease type III. Early-onset congenital pendular nystagmus is a presenting symptom of Pelizaeus-Merzbacher disease.

Bibliography

Scriver C.R., Beaudet A.L., Sly W.S., Valle D. (Eds), The Molecular & Molecular Bases of Inherited Disease (8th Ed.). McGraw-Hill New York, 2001 (vedi anche l'edizione on line aggiornata sul sito www.ommbid.com).

Fernandez-Alvarez E., Aicardi J., Movement Disorders in Children. MacKeith Press, 2001.

Fernandes J., Saudubray J.M., van den Berghe G., Walter J.H. (Eds), Inborn Metabolic Diseases Diagnosis and Treatment. Springer Medizin Verlag Heidelberg, 2006.

Menkes J.H., Sarnat H.B., Maria B.L. (Eds), Child Neurology. Lippincott Williams & Wilkins, 2005.

Blau N, Duran M, Gibson KM, Dionisi-Vici C Physician's Guide to the Diagnosis, Treatment, and Follow-up of Inherited Metabolic Diseases. Springer-Verlag, Berin, Heidelberg, 2014.

Shorvon S.D., Andermann F., Guerrini R. (Eds), The Causes of Epilepsy: Common and Uncommon Causes in Adults and Children. Cambridge Medicine, 2019.

We thank Dr. Francesco Cardona for his contribution to the chapter in the previous edition.

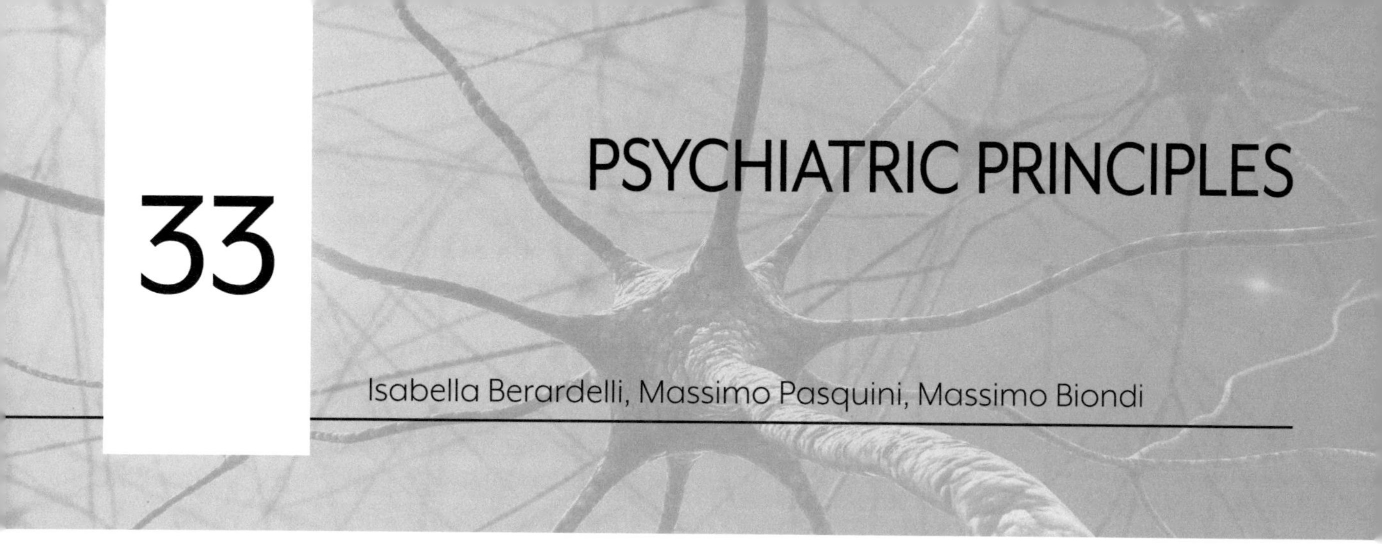

33 PSYCHIATRIC PRINCIPLES

Isabella Berardelli, Massimo Pasquini, Massimo Biondi

In recent years there have been numerous developments in the management and treatment of psychiatric disorders aimed at highlighting the close link between several neurological conditions and psychiatric symptoms. Although there is still a tendency to differentiate Psychiatry from Neurology.

Both neurologists and psychiatrists have recognized the high incidence of psychiatric symptoms or disorders and neurological conditions. Moreover, some psychiatric disorders, such as cognitive disorders, obsessive-compulsive disorder, and mood disorders, can arise as a consequence of structural brain injuries.

The term "neuropsychiatry" is currently used to refer to the branch of medicine that "studies the psychiatric manifestations of neurological diseases and the neurobiological bases of psychiatric disorders" in a perspective that considers the brain as the "organ of the mind," once again bringing psychiatry closer to neurology. Current knowledge about the neurobiology of cognitive and emotional processes, as well as the observation of the influence of organic disturbances on human behavior, led to the identification of common behavioral substrates in "primary" psychiatric disorders and "secondary" neurological disorders. Psychiatry, like other medical disciplines, generally operates using a paradigm evolving from the evaluation and definition of symptoms, signs, and syndromes reported by patients and leading to the understanding of the pathophysiological and pathogenetic mechanisms underlying the disorder. While the application of this paradigm is straightforward for most neurological syndromes, for some psychiatric disorders, despite the numerous advances in methodological and diagnostic techniques, the identification of pathophysiological mechanisms remains controversial.

The classification of mental illnesses has undergone continuous changes over the past two centuries. To partially overcome a lack of agreement on diagnostic definitions, the American Psychiatric Association introduced in 1952 the Diagnostic and Statistical Manual of Mental Disorders (DSM) as a nosographic tool. The current fifth revised edition (DSM-5), includes more than 300 mental disorders described on the basis of the prevalence of specific symptom clusters. The framework of DSM-5 is essentially similar to the original DSM-III, primarily based on observable phenomena, interchangeable criteria lists, conventionally chosen timeframes, and the creation of Not Otherwise Specified (NOS) categories. The main innovations introduced in DSM-5 include the elimination of the "multi-axial" evaluation and the introduction of the more sophisticated World Health Organization Disability Assessment Schedule (WHODAS) 2.0 instead of the Global Assessment of Functioning (GAF). This change indicates a strong common purpose between the DSM-5 and the emerging ICD-11.

The main purpose of this chapter is to familiarize the reader with concepts and terms of modern psychiatry and to provide the basic elements of psychopathological observation for the recognition and management of major psychiatric disorders.

33.1 Psychopathological evaluation

Clinical medicine clearly distinguishes signs from symptoms; in the case of psychiatric disorders this differentiation is not straight forward. The patient's description of a mental phenomenon is usually referred to as a symptom, whether they complain about something that causes them distress or simply describe their mental experience, which appears pathological to an observer. The collection of symptoms in psychiatric disorders, crucial for formulating an accurate diagnosis, includes both a comprehensive observation of the patient's behavior and listening to the description of their internal state and personal suffering (reason for consultation, current symptoms, family history, personal history, and assessment of premorbid personality). During a psychiatric interview, which is the primary semiotic tool for understanding and assessing a person's mental state, the clinician must observe the patient as a whole evaluating the main mental functions including *consciousness, memory, attention, perception, thought, mood* and *affectivity, will* and *psychomotor activity, experience,* and *self-awareness.*

Consciousness | Consciousness is defined as the ability to be aware of oneself and the world. Alterations of consciousness can be divided into *quantitative*, changes such as clouding, drowsiness, stupor, coma, and qualitative, changes such as delirium, fluctuations of consciousness, confusion, twilight state, hypnoid state, oneiric state, and stupor. The observation of the patient's level of consciousness must be accompanied by the evaluation of attention, concentration, and orientation to time, space, and people.

Memory | Memory disturbances include alterations in *registration* (acute confusional psychosis), *retention* (retrograde amnesia from brain trauma), *recollection* or simple recall defects and reconstruction (acute anxiety states). In association with organic-origin amnesia, *confabulation* may often occur, which is the falsification of memory that occurs in a lucid state of consciousness. During confabulation the patient tries to cover the evidence of a memory gap with adventurous experiences, usually of a fantastic nature. In some personality disorders (histrionic or antisocial personality disorders), *selective forgetfulness* and *falsification of reality*, known as pseudologia fantastica, can be observed; in this case the patient verbalizes plausible and unrestrained lies.

Perceptions | Disorders of perception (sensory distortions) are divided into distortions of perceptual quality, intensity, and associated feeling, as well as false perceptions (*hallucinations and illusions*). *Hallucinations*, defined by Esquirol in 1817 as "perceptions without an object," can occur within any of the five senses.

Auditory hallucinations scan take the form of elementary hallucinations (ringing and tinkling) as seen in acute organic states, or complex hallucinations, which are typical symptoms of schizophrenia, chronic alcoholic hallucinosis, and certain affective psychoses. In auditory hallucinations, voices can be single or multiple, female or male, familiar or unfamiliar, and are experienced as coming from outside the mind or self. Furthermore, the patient believes that it is a normal perception. Particularly significant in schizophrenia are commenting, imperative, and derogatory voices; sometimes, there are voices that loudly express the patient's thoughts, argue with each other, or discuss things.

Visual hallucinations occur more characteristically in organic states rather than functional psychoses and schizophrenia. *Pseudo-hallucinations* are more common in schizophrenia and are experiences located within the patient's subjective space. Visual hallucinations can be observed in the following neurological disorders: metabolic and/or toxic encephalopathy, alcohol or hypnotic withdrawal, LSD and methamphetamine intoxication, Lewy body disease, Parkinson's Disease treated with dopamine agonists, and temporal lobe epilepsy.

Somatic hallucinations are frequently present in patients with schizophrenia and are usually connected to delusions They can be divided into superficial, cenesthetic, and visceral hallucinations.

Olfactory hallucinations occur in schizophrenia, epilepsy, migraines, and other organic conditions, taking the form of smells, either pleasant or unpleasant, to which the patient attributes a special personal meaning.

Gustatory hallucinations are generally associated with delusions as persistent tastes, mostly unpleasant, or changes in the taste of drinks or food. They can also be observed in temporal lobe epilepsy.

Thought | Thought is a complex psychic activity that allows the evaluation of reality and the formulation of judgments through processes of association, correlation, integration, abstraction, and symbolization of informational data derived from perceptions. Thought disorders can be divided into disorders of thought content and disorders of thought form. Among the disorders of thought content *prevailing ideas* and *delusional ideation*. Prevailing ideas are acceptable, comprehensible ideas that, due to their intense affective charge, dominate over other ideational content, temporarily or permanently characterizing the individual's personality. Delusion is an idea, a belief, a thought that varies in content and does not correspond to objective reality. Jasper considered delusion as a "distorted vision of reality supported by an unusual conviction not reducible to logic". The absurdity or falseness of their content is evident to others and cannot be attributed to the individual's cultural or educational background. Based on the different content of delusional ideation, we can *identify persecutory delusions, jealous delusions, megalomaniacal delusions, and depressive delusions*. *Persecutory delusions* are the most common type and manifest in the patient's mind as persecution or malevolent intentions from external individuals. This type of delusion occurs in different conditions: in schizophrenia, affective psychoses of manic or depressive type, and some organic conditions. The affectivity associated with delusional belief can manifest as inappropriate indifference and apathy or as a profound sense of anguish and terror. *Jealous delusions* are common in alcoholics and some organic conditions. *Grandiose delusions* are typical of manic episodes and involve the belief of possessing special qualities to the extent of stable identification with famous figures. *Guilt, unworthiness, and poverty delusions* are typical of depressed patients: the patient feels responsible for ruining the family, guilty of very serious crimes, and senses that the world is about to end. In *nihilistic delusion*, the individual denies having visible or, more often, "internal" body parts (*Cotard's syndrome*). *Hypochondriacal delusion*, also typical of depressed patients, involves the firm belief that there is something severely dysfunctional in one's own body, reaching the certainty of being afflicted by an incurable illness.

Delusions have not been associated with specific brain alterations; however, the most consistent neurobiological model predicts dysfunction in the temporal lobes and the caudate nucleus. In the case of brain injuries, delusions may be associated with bilateral lesions in the temporal lobes and the caudate nucleus. Among neurological disorders, a particular type of delusion observed in post-traumatic encephalopathies and cerebrovascular lesions is reduplicative paramnesia. It is a condition in which the patient believes that a place or scene has been duplicated, existing in two or more locations simultaneously or that they have been transported to another place. Reduplicative paramnesia has been associated with lesions involving the right parietal cortex and bilateral frontal alterations. Other forms of delusions are frequently observed in the following neurological conditions: delirium, dementia, temporal epilepsy, multiple sclerosis, post-traumatic encephalopathies, and Wilson's disease.

Formal thought disorders encompass two distinct categories: intrinsic thought disorder and language and speech disorder. The first category includes concrete thinking, which involves the subject's tendency to focus on a quality of a concept or thing at the expense of the overall meaning; *overinclusion*, characterized by the inclusion of false or irrelevant aspects in a concept or category; and *illogical thinking* which entails offering bizarre explanations completely contrary to any form of logic. As for language and speech disorders, *both quantitative* and *qualitative disturbances* can be observed. Quantitative disorders range from *logorrhoea* and *flight of ideas*, which are present in manic patients and involve an acceleration and jumbling of thoughts, to the *slowing of speech* and complete mutism in depressed patients. Qualitative disturbances include *rumination*, which consists of the subject persistently dwelling on the same theme without reaching a conclusion (typically corresponds to a dominant idea); *verbigeration*, which is the frequent repetition of words and entire phrases; *circumstantiality*, which involves getting lost in irrelevant details; *tangentiality*, which entails responding in an irrelevant manner; *derailment*, typical of confusional psychosis, leading to a complete loss of the thread of discourse; *incoherence*, where the lack of continuity extends within individual sentences, rendering the speech entirely incomprehensible, and even reaching a state of "*word salad*"; and neologisms, typically present in schizophrenia (individual words coined by the subject without generally recognized meaning).

Anankastic thinking or *obsessive ideation* is characterized by an idea or thought that persistently recurs in the subject's mind. These thoughts are recognized as abnormal and illogical, but the patient is unable to eliminate them from consciousness ("*parasitic psyche*" and "*defense psyche*"). Obsessive ideation is often accompanied by an urgent urge to engage in unintentional actions (*compulsions*), from which the subject is unable to free themselves.

Mood | Mood is generally defined as the overall emotional state with which the world is perceived. The main alterations of mood tone include depressed mood, manic state, and dysphoria. In the case of depressed mood, feelings of sadness, unhappiness, melancholy, guilt, and discouragement prevail, usually accompanied by inhibition and slowing down of all psychic life, apathy, and anhedonia. Manic mood is characterized by an abnormal and stable elevation of mood tone in a euphoric and sometimes irritable sense, accompanied by motor hyperactivity, distractibility, accelerated ideation, and possible alterations in thought content. The definition of dysphoria lacks consensus in descriptive psychopathology. Therefore, dysphoric mood, or unpleasant mood, can be attributed to individuals affected by mixed states or to temperamental traits that characterize the person and their way of suffering, unrelated to mood disorders.

Affectivity | Affectivity is a subjective and variable emotional-sentimental condition; it is the ability to experience emotions in changing environmental and relational conditions in terms of significance. Its alterations include *states of anxiety, anguish, fear, affective ambivalence, apathy, anhedonia, blunted affect, alexithymia, affective dissociation, and perplexity*. Affective ambivalence manifests as a mood state in which feelings and attitudes of opposite polarity (love-hate) are present simultaneously. Apathy presents as a lack of response to external or internal stimuli that would normally provoke a response. Anhedonia is a decrease in the capacity to experience pleasure from any type of life experience. Blunted affect is a significant reduction in affective expression, typical in schizophrenia. Alexithymia refers to the inability to recognize and verbalize emotions and is accompanied by a poverty of the capacity to fantasize and difficulty in distinguishing physical sensations from feelings. Affective dissociation, typical of schizophrenia, involves the disconnection between stimuli and the emotional resonance displayed by the individual. Perplexity is a prolonged state of doubt and anguish in which the individual is unable to express judgments about the meaning of what is happening in their inner world and the external world.

Self-awareness | Disturbances in self-awareness (feelings of estrangement) include *depersonalization* and *derealization*. Depersonalization is a term used to describe a peculiar change in self-awareness during which the person has the unpleasant sensation of being unreal; derealization indicates a similar change in awareness of the external world. These symptoms can be associated with Dissociative Disorders as well as with organic conditions such as temporal lobe epilepsy, alcohol and substance abuse, and the onset of neurotic and psychotic syndromes. Generally, they occur in a circumscribed manner and are of short duration, even in healthy individuals.

33.2 Psychiatric disorders in neurological diseases

This section illustrates psychiatric disorders commonly observed in major neurological syndromes. It should be noted that some psychopathological phenomena occur indiscriminately in neurological diseases with different etiopathogenesis. In cerebrovascular diseases, in addition to varying degrees of cognitive impairment, including dementia, it is common to observe depressive states, manic states, anxiety disorders, pathological laughter and crying. In Parkinson's Disease, various forms of depression can be observed, ranging from atypical depression to major depression, with a frequency of about 40-50%. Generalized anxiety disorder is observed with the same frequency, while panic disorder develops in 25% of cases. Visual hallucinations and impaired impulse control are generally attributed to therapy with dopamine agonists. Regarding other movement disorders, depressive and adjustment disorders are more prevalent in dystonias and essential tremor, while obsessive-compulsive disorder and ADHD are often associated with Tourette's Syndrome. In Alzheimer's Disease, depressive states with a prevalent abulic-apathetic component are integral to the disease, while hallucinations and delusions are observed in 40% of patients. In Multiple Sclerosis, the most frequent disorders are depressive disorders, manic episodes, and conversion disorders. Furthermore, over 50% of patients with epilepsy manifest psychiatric disorders, particularly affective disorders and less frequently psychotic disorders, whose characteristics vary depending on the type of epilepsy and the brain region involved. These disorders can precede seizure episodes but often occur in the interictal period.

33.2.1 Mood disorders

Mood disorders are a group of psychiatric pathologies where the alteration of mood dominates the clinical picture. The alteration is disproportionate to any stressor and/or contingent condition; it manifests with symptoms that can last from a few weeks to several months and significantly impair the individual's normal lifestyle. In the DSM-5, Bipolar Disorders have been separated from Depressive Disorders. The latter include Major Depressive Disorder, Persistent Depressive Disorder or Dysthymia, Depressive Disorder due to a medical condition or substance, Disruptive Mood Dysregulation Disorder, and Premenstrual Dysphoric Disorder.

Depression

The term "*depression*" derives from the Latin word "depressio" and refers to a state of low mood experienced by the individual with extreme suffering and discomfort. Historically, the term "melancholia" was used to describe this condition, introduced by Hippocrates in the treatise *"On the Nature of Man"*. In the 19th century, Kraepelin described manic-depressive psychosis, which included "periodic circular insanities," "mania," and "melancholia." The term "melancholia" was used to indicate endogenous depression, which could manifest with different clinical facets, but its central symptoms consisted of a lowered mood and a slowing down of physical and mental processes. According to the DSM-5, based on the duration and severity of depressive symptoms reported by patients and the degree of impairment in social and occupational functioning, depressive disorders are classified as *Major Depressive Disorder (MDD)*, *Dysthymia* and *Depressive Disorder Not Otherwise Specified (NOS)*. Epidemiological studies show that depressive syndromes are currently the leading cause of dysfunction in individuals between the ages of 14 and 44, with a one-year prevalence ranging from 5% to 9% for women and 2% to 3% for men.

Among the five necessary symptoms for the diagnosis of *Major Depressive Episode*, the DSM-5 highlights *depressed mood* and *loss of pleasure* or *interest*, listing a series of other symptoms frequently associated with the core symptoms, which must be present for at least 2 weeks. In addition to the primary symptoms in the affective-emotional domain, there are alterations in psychomotor activity, cognitive functioning, and somatic-vegetative functions. Patients with depressive disorders often describe a feeling of sadness, hopelessness, guilt, worthlessness, and inadequacy, sometimes accompanied by a pervasive state of worry, irritability, loss of appetite, weight loss, and insomnia. On the motor level, the syndrome can present with fatigue, agitation, or psychomotor retardation (mutism-stupor), while on the cognitive level, there may be memory gaps and difficulties with concentration. Severe depression may involve recurrent thoughts of death and suicide. It is not uncommon for patients to report a loss of the ability to experience emotions and hope for recovery; in some cases, these beliefs can take on a delusional character, especially nihilistic delusions (delusion of guilt, ruin, bodily denial, Cotard syndrome) or hypochondriacal delusions. Hallucinations may also be present, in the form of accusing voices or visions of deceased individuals, accompanied by a strong sense of guilt. If present, both delusions and hallucinations are usually congruent with the mood, meaning their content is in line with the patient's mood. The DSM-5 introduced the subtype "with mixed features," which encompasses patients with Major Depression and at least three manic/hypomanic symptoms. This allows for maintaining the diagnosis of Major Depression in patients who, despite presenting symptoms of excitement, have never met the diagnostic criteria for a manic/hypomanic episode. According to the DSM-5, bereavement is not sufficient to exclude a diagnosis of Major Depression, even beyond the first 2 months following the loss. A decrease in mood within this range was considered to be within the normal range in the DSM-IV.

The average age of onset for *Major Depressive Disorder* is approximately 25 years, and the course varies. About 60% of patients who have experienced a Major Depressive Episode may have a second episode during their lifetime. In about two-thirds of cases, these episodes can resolve completely, partially, or not at all (in about one-third of cases).

Persistent Depressive Disorder, or *Dysthymia,* is characterized by chronically depressed mood that persists for most of the day for at least 2 years. The onset is often early, and the course is chronic.

Mood Disorder Due to a *General Medical Condition* or *Substance-Induced Mood Disorder* is a significant and persistent alteration in mood characterized by either depressed mood and anhedonia, and/or expansive or irritable mood. From the patient's history, physical examination, and laboratory data, it is clear that the alteration is a direct physiological consequence of a general medical condition. It is distinguished from the patient's "depressive reaction" to an illness (classifiable as an Adjustment Disorder with Depressed Mood).

The category known as *Unspecified Depressive Disorder* includes disorders with depressive manifestations that do not fit into previously described depressive disorders (including Depressive Disorder Due to Another Medical Condition, such as an adjustment disorder with depressive mood).

Within the field of neurological conditions, depressive disorders manifest in approximately 30% of patients affected by cerebrovascular diseases, Parkinson's disease, Huntington's chorea, brain traumas, multiple sclerosis, and dementia. Specifically, in Parkinson's disease, depressive symptoms can precede the onset of motor disturbances by several months.

Neurobiological hypotheses | In the 1960s, the first neurophysiopathological hypothesis of depressive disorders was formulated based on alterations in the neurotransmitters norepinephrine, serotonin, and dopamine. However, in the genesis of depressive symptoms, in addition to the main neurotransmitters, multiple interconnected cerebral systems are implicated. These include acetylcholine, gamma-aminobutyric acid (GABA), glutamate, the hypothalamic-pituitary-adrenal axis (HPA), the hypothalamic-pituitary-thyroid axis, growth hormone, sex hormones, certain neuropeptides, Brain-Derived Neurotrophic Factor (BDNF), proteins involved in signal transduction and second messengers, as well as alterations in enzymatic systems and neural networks. From a neuroanatomical perspective, it has been hypothesized that the pathophysiology of mood disorders involves dysfunction in two important neural circuits, namely the limbic-thalamo-cortical circuit and the limbic-striato-pallido-thalamic circuit. Tractography studies using brain magnetic resonance imaging have revealed alterations in the anterior cingulate cortex, orbitofrontal and dorsolateral prefrontal cortices.

Bipolar disorder

Bipolar disorder is a recurrent disorder characterized by alternating polar states of excitement (mania) and inhibition of psychic activity (depression). This functional dysregulation leads to imbalances in mood, ideation processes, motor function, behavioral initiative, and neurovegetative manifestations. The DSM-IV-TR identifies four different forms of bipolar disorders: *bipolar disorder I, bipolar disorder II, cyclothymic disorder, mixed state*, and the category referred to as *"Not Otherwise Specified"* bipolar disorder. The lifetime prevalence of bipolar disorder is approximately 1%. Onset typically occurs during adolescence, around 18 years for bipolar disorder I and 22 years for bipolar disorder II.

Based on the severity of the symptoms, *manic and hypomanic episodes* can be distinguished. The distinctive features of a *manic episode* include elevated mood, increased motor activity, and racing thoughts. Speech is accelerated, sometimes characterized by rhymes, wordplay, and humorous associations. It can become incoherent or lead to mutism due to the extreme difficulty in articulating words at the same speed as thoughts are formulated. The patient experiences an increase in self-esteem, with an exaggerated and unrealistic evaluation of their own resources and abilities, an altered judgment of their own limitations, and a lack of awareness of the illness that limits or completely compromises the patient's willingness to undergo therapeutic treatment. The individual often engages in potentially risky behaviors, convinced that they can accomplish anything, and may undertake impulsive, daring, and sometimes illegal ventures. Cognitive impairments may be present, such as attention and concentration deficits (the individual is constantly distracted by even minimal environmental stimuli) and sleep disturbances (lack of a sense of tiredness), accompanied by increased appetite and sexual desire. Not all manic patients are euphoric; some may be highly irritable. In severe cases, psychotic symptoms may occur, including grandiose and persecution delusions, hallucinations, and ideas of reference. Patients often report having a special relationship with a deity or a famous person, believing they possess extraordinary strength, artistic or scientific talent, or exceptional inventiveness, and that they possess great wealth. Remission of a manic episode occurs within a period ranging from a few days to 3-4 months, but in some cases, it may be followed by a *Major Depressive Episode* or a *Mixed State* (a period during which criteria for both a manic episode and a major depressive episode are met). In *hypomania*, the elevation of mood is modest and accompanied by an increase in energy and activity without a marked impairment of socio-occupational functioning. A *mixed state* represents a clinical condition characterized by the simultaneous presence, in the same individual and during the same period, of symptoms from both poles; this diagnosis is reserved for clinical pictures in which depressive and manic symptoms persist for a sufficiently long period without a clear orientation towards one of the two poles.

Bipolar Disorder I is characterized by the cyclic alternation of depressive phases and manic or mixed phases, or by the sole presence of recurrent manic episodes. Generally, manic and depressive phases follow each other without intervals. In other forms, however, there is a period of stable mood between the phases, and the manic phase is often so severe as to require hospitalization.

Bipolar Disorder II involves cyclic alternation between depressive and hypomanic phases.

Cyclothymic Disorder is characterized by a chronic alteration of mood lasting for at least two years. To diagnose *Cyclothymic Disorder*, the occurrence of hypomanic episodes and depressive symptoms is required, but they should not lead the patient to a diagnosis of major depressive disorder. The main characteristic of this condition is significant mood instability with rapid fluctuations, even within the same day.

In *Bipolar Disorder I* a manic episode is followed, at a variable interval, by new depressive or manic episodes in 90% of cases. The disease-free interval tends to shorten over time, and chronicity is more common in severe forms with psychotic symptoms. *Bipolar Disorder II* and *Cyclothymic Disorder* have a less dramatic onset compared to Bipolar Disorder I. A secondary manic state, i.e., not due to Bipolar Disorder, can be found in the following neurological disorders: acute cerebrovascular diseases, temporal lobe tumors, epilepsy, Parkinson's disease treated with dopamine agonists, frontal lobe lesions, and idiopathic calcification of the basal ganglia.

Neurobiological hypotheses | Currently, there is greater evidence of a hereditary component for Bipolar Disorder compared to Unipolar Depressive Disorders. In monozygotic twins, the probability of developing bipolar disorder if the other twin is affected varies between 33-90%. These data support the hypothesis of an association between bipolar disorders and certain regions of chromosomes 17, 18, 21, 12, 4, 22, X, as well as genes for dopamine D2 receptors and certain subunits of the GABA receptor.

Functional neuroimaging studies have highlighted dysfunctions among circuits involving the prefrontal cortex-hippocampus-amygdala and the orbitofrontal cortex-frontal striatum, the latter being hyperactive, especially on the left, resulting in emotional dysregulation.

33.2.2 Anxiety disorders

Anxiety is s a state of emotional tension frequently accompanied by somatic symptoms such as trembling, sweating, palpitations, increased heart rate, and difficulty breathing. Anxiety physiologically manifests as a defence and alarm reaction to perceived danger, which may come from external or internal sources. Anxiety symptoms are characterized by both physical and psychological components, manifested as feelings of fear and tension, associated with alterations in the neurovegetative system and higher mental functions such as thinking, perception, and learning. An excessively activated state of anxiety relative to the individual's circumstances, or one that interferes with normal life activities, assumes pathological characteristics.

The term "anxiety disorders" refers to a group of pathologies in which the anxious component assumes relevance. The distinction between acute anxiety and chronic anxiety, based on different symptomatic characteristics, variability in course, and treatment response, represents the fundamental framework of the current nosographic interpretation, supported by the presence of different neurophysiological substrates.

DSM-5 includes the following disorders within anxiety disorders: *Panic Disorder with or without Agoraphobia, Phobias, Generalized Anxiety Disorder, and Other Specified Anxiety Disorder.* Some characteristic symptoms of neurological diseases such as epilepsy, neoplasms, multiple sclerosis, and dementias may include anxious states.

Neurobiological hypotheses | The neurobiology of anxiety disorders is based on the neural mechanisms that underlie the conditioned fear response in individuals, involving different neural circuits. These circuits include the subcortical connecting pathway from the dorsal thalamus to the amygdala (*short loop*), and the slower cortical regulatory pathway, which involves the primary somatosensory cortex, insula, and anterior cingulate cortex/prefrontal cortex (*long loop*). The integrated cortical processing of thc sensation of fear involves not only the amygdala but also the hippocampus and the bed nucleus of the stria terminalis (BNST). Since fear is physiologically necessary, several neurotransmitter systems are involved in its mechanism, including the GABA system, noradrenaline and serotonin systems, neurosteroid modifications, vasopressin, neuropeptide Y, cholecystokinin, substance P, and the glutamatergic system.

Panic disorder and agoraphobia

Panic disorder is a symptom that can occur in various anxiety disorders and other mental disorders. It is characterized by the sudden onset of at least four out of a series of symptoms (such as rapid heartbeat, sweating, trembling, shortness of breath or choking sensation, feeling of suffocation, chest pain or discomfort, nausea or abdominal distress, dizziness, lightheadedness or faintness, derealization or depersonalization, fear of losing control or going crazy, fear of dying, tingling sensations, chills or hot flashes) that peak within about 10 minutes and are generally accompanied by behavioral changes and persistent concerns related to the attack. The term *agoraphobia*, which etymologically indicates the fear of open spaces, is currently also used to refer to those anxiety states that occur in situations or places from which the individual would have difficulty escaping or seeking help. *Panic disorder and agoraphobia* can occur both together and separately. *Panic disorder (PD)* is characterized by the simultaneous presence of psychic, neurovegetative, and psychosensory symptoms that occur suddenly and have a variable duration (from a few seconds to an hour). The patient experiences a sense of apprehension, terror, fear, impending death, and loss of control, accompanied by somatic symptoms such as palpitations, chest pain, choking sensation, and sometimes depersonalization and derealization. The frequency of panic attacks in the general population is about 10%. The age of onset has a bimodal distribution: 15-19 years and 25-30 years. The first anxious manifestation generally occurs spontaneously. The persistence of attacks over time leads to a continuous state of tension and fear, prompting the patient to engage in reassurance-seeking or avoidance behaviours.

Phobic disorders

Phobia is defined as an intense but inadequate and disproportionate fear in relation to a specific stimulus. Phobic stimuli can come from specific social situations or from places, objects, and animals. In the presence of the *phobic object*, which is not usually considered dangerous, the individual tends to engage in avoidance behaviors.

Phobic disorders are divided into *social phobia* and *specific phobias*. Social phobia is a marked and persistent fear of one or more social or performance situations. In public contexts, the person is exposed to possible judgment by others and may experience unpleasant sensations of embarrassment and shame. The persons recognize that the fear they feel is excessive and unreasonable but are unable to overcome it. Interpersonal interaction is either avoided or endured with significant discomfort. *Specific phobias*, on the other hand, are fears that are circumscribed to specific situations such as fear of animals, heights, enclosed spaces, blood or injuries, and contracting specific illnesses. In some cases, the phobic fear can escalate into a full-blown *panic attack*, but it can be controlled by the individual by removing themselves from the phobic stimulus.

The prevalence of phobic disorders is approximately 5%. Onset, except for situational phobias related to traumatic events, typically occurs in early childhood.

Generalized anxiety disorder

The main characteristic of *Generalized Anxiety Disorder (GAD)* is the presence of excessive anxiety compared to the circumstances that the individual faces. It is persistent and fluctuates throughout the day and apparently not related to the presence of particular environmental situations. According to DSM-5, in addition to daily persistent worry, at least three out of six groups of physical symptoms should be present (restlessness, easy fatigue, difficulty concentrating or mind going blank, irritability, muscle tension, sleep disturbances). GAD typically has an early onset, ranging from the second decade to the end of the third decade of life. The course is chronic but fluctuating and may worsen during periods of stress.

33.2.3 Trauma and stressor-related disorders

DSM-5 has collected *Acute Stress Disorder, Post-Traumatic Stress Disorder (PTSD), Adjustment Disorder, and Reactive Attachment Disorder into a single chapter.*

Acute Stress Disorder is a clinical condition that develops in response to an exceptionally severe physical and/or mental stress and generally regresses within a few hours or days. The response is characterized by intense fear, feelings of horror and helplessness, a sense of numbness or emotional detachment, derealization, and depersonalization symptoms.

Post-Traumatic Stress Disorder (PTSD) is an intense, prolonged, and sometimes delayed reaction to a highly stressful event. It typically occurs in victims of rape, violence, survivors of natural disasters, and war veterans. The associated triggering event must be of a threatening or catastrophic nature, causing widespread distress in almost all individuals. The clinical picture is dominated by three main groups of symptoms: *intrusive symptoms*, where the patient persistently relives the event (unpleasant memories, recurrent nightmares, a sense of re-experiencing the traumatic event), *avoidance symptoms* and *emotional numbing*, and *hyperarousal symptoms* (insomnia, irritability, poor concentration, hypervigilance, and exaggerated startle response). Approximately two-thirds of individuals exposed to trauma do not develop pathological responses. The majority of the remaining one-third present with pure PTSD or comorbid depression; 50% of these individuals develop a chronic and persistent form.

Adjustment Disorder (AD) is, in most cases, a transient disorder caused by one or more identifiable psychosocial stressors. It is characterized by intense subjective distress and impairment in occupational, relational, and social functioning. According to DSM-5 criteria, in order to make a diagnosis of AD, the state of distress must occur within three months of the onset of the traumatic event and should not last longer than six months. In AD, there is a close interaction between the event and the individual's psychological response. Traumatic events, even significant ones, may not produce any pathogenic effect in certain individuals, while seemingly more modest everyday life events can result in clinically significant emotional or behavioral symptoms. Based on the predominant symptomatology, DSM-5 recognizes different subtypes of AD: *With Depressed Mood, With Anxiety, With Mixed Anxiety* and *Depressed Mood, With Disturbance of Conduct, With Mixed Disturbance of Emotions* and *Conduct, Not Specified*. AD can occur at any age; the prevalence ranges from 2% to 8% of the population, while it may reach 12% in hospitalized patients. By definition, the disorder presents within 3 months of the onset of a stress-inducing factor.

33.2.4 Obsessive-compulsive disorder and its correlates

DSM-5 finally excludes obsessive-compulsive disorder from the chapter on anxiety disorders, after long-standing criticism and evidence in favor of a distinct diagnostic entity, and includes in a dedicated chapter the *Body Dysmorphic Disorder*, previously classified under somatic symptom disorders, *Hoarding Disorder, Excoriation (Skin-Picking) Disorder, Trichotillomania*, and *other spectrum disorders*.

Obsessive-compulsive disorder (OCD) is a syndrome characterized by the presence of two distinct phenomena: obsessions and compulsions. Obsessive thoughts are recurrent and persistent ideas, images, or impulses experienced as intrusive, causing significant anxiety and distress in the individual. Patients recognize these obsessions as products of their own minds and understand their abnormality compared to their normal thinking. *Compulsive acts* or rituals are repetitive stereotyped behaviors that the person feels compelled to perform in response to an obsession or to comply with rigid rules. These behaviors serve the individual to prevent and reduce the distress caused by obsessive thoughts or to prevent feared events. Compulsions create a high level of suffering and are not always realistically connected to what they are intended to prevent. In severe cases, there may be a complete lack of insight, meaning the person does not recognize that the obsessions and compulsions are excessive or unreasonable. The content of obsessions and compulsions can vary over time and can, in certain circumstances, significantly interfere with school and work activities. OCD can present with different clinical manifestations and be related to the content of obsessions and/or compulsions. The course of the disorder is mostly chronic, but there are forms where the disorder has a fluctuating course. In chronic forms, the different types of obsessions and compulsions are not necessarily stable over time, meaning that the same individual may unknowingly replace the content of them throughout their life.

The most common obsessions are those related to dirt and *contamination*: patients fear the consequences of contact with an object they consider contaminated and tend to both avoid exposure to the object and engage in cleaning rituals. Obsessive thoughts also include ideation with *aggressive content* (both self-directed and other-directed): patients fear causing harm to themselves or others and tend to control this fear with checking rituals, confessions, or seeking reassurance. *Doubting obsessions* mainly concern daily activities (locks, faucets, light switches, etc.): patients fear that their carelessness may cause disasters or terrible events and, driven by excessive responsibility, may spend a significant amount of time in checking rituals. The *need for symmetry* describes the impulse to order or arrange objects symmetrically, sometimes connected to the presence of "magical thinking." The prevalence of this disorder is 2.5-3% in adults and 1-2% in children and adolescents. The typical onset age is between 6 and 15 years for male patients and between 20 and 29 years for female patients. Two-thirds of patients experience onset before the age of 25, and less than 15% of patients experience symptom onset after the age of 35.

Different neurological pathologies or damage to the cerebral cortex and/or basal ganglia can manifest with obsessive-compulsive symptoms. Injuries to certain structures in the fronto-striatal-pallido-thalamo-cortical circuit can stimulate excitatory activity in the cortex, leading to the emergence of obsessive-compulsive manifestations. Repetitive and compulsive behaviors have been observed in cases of reduced orbitofrontal metabolic activity, in some cases of dementia secondary to frontal lobe degeneration and Pick's disease. The association between anankastic symptoms and epileptic phenomena is well-documented, with reported cases in the literature involving frontal focal partial seizures, temporal epilepsy, and epilepsy originating from the cingulate gyrus. The first descriptions of obsessive-compulsive disorder (OCD) associated with parkinsonism involved patients with post-encephalitic parkinsonism caused by von Economo's encephalitis, progressive supranuclear palsy, Huntington's chorea, and Sydenham's chorea. Modern neuroimaging techniques have allowed the documentation of focal basal ganglia lesions in several patients presenting with obsessive-compulsive symptoms. In Gilles de la Tourette syndrome (GTS), affective disturbances, aggressive and impulsive behaviors, learning deficits, and, above all, obsessive-compulsive symptoms are present in 47-63% of cases. There appears to be a close relationship between tics and OCD. Recent studies indeed seem to confirm the observations made by Janet in 1903, according to which GTS and OCD are etiologically linked and tics, obsessions, and compulsions are due to the same pathophysiological mechanism. The phenomenology of obsessive-compulsive manifestations in GTS seems, in some aspects, different from that of idiopathic OCD; in patients with GTS, aggressive self- and hetero-injurious obsessions prevail, as well as violent ideas or images, including sexual content, fear of committing obscene acts, and compulsions to touch oneself and others.

In 1998, Swedo described a pediatric autoimmune neuropsychiatric disorder associated with streptococcal infections (PANDAS), which presented as obsessive-compulsive symptoms in children following a streptococcal infection. The current diagnostic criteria for PANDAS are: the presence of OCD and tics, prepubertal onset, sudden and explosive symptom onset with a course characterized by exacerbations and remissions, the presence of neurological abnormalities characterized by tics, hyperactivity, and choreiform movements, and a temporal relationship between symptom onset/exacerbations and streptococcal infection. This condition represents an important area of research aimed at studying the actual role of streptococcus in the pathophysiology of obsessive-compulsive disorders and other symptoms within the OCD spectrum. According to the autoimmune hypothesis, the similarity between streptococcus amino acid sequences and certain epitopes on brain membranes would activate an abnormal immune response, resulting in inflammatory alterations in the basal ganglia.

Pathophysiological model of OCD | Since the 1980s, various pathogenetic models have been developed as references for understanding the genesis of obsessive-compulsive disorder (OCD). These models include alterations within the fronto-subcortical circuit, which connects the prefrontal cortex, orbitofrontal cortex, cingulate cortex, basal ganglia/limbic system/striatum complex, and medial thalamic nuclei. It has been hypothesized that the underlying pathogenetic mechanism of obsessive symptoms is characterized by excessive disinhibition of the dorsomedial thalamic nucleus. The presence of two inhibitory circuits in a serial position (striato-pallidal and pallido-thalamic) suggests the possibility that, at the basis of thalamic disinhibition, there is a process of "*inhibition of inhibition*": an increase in inhibitory inputs from the caudate nucleus and limbic striatum onto the globus pallidus may result in the latter exerting less inhibitory action on the thalamus. In addition to this pathogenetic hypothesis, another one can be added, which suggests that the frontal cortex, responsible for generating internal stimulus signals to initiate, program, and monitor behaviors, produces these signals excessively in patients with OCD, due to frontal hyperactivity. The neurotransmission in these structures is modulated by serotonin, dopamine, glutamate, GABA, and acetylcholine. Pharmacological research has, for several years, focused on substances that modulate the release of glutamate, whose excess in certain structures causes not only alterations in inhibitory circuits but also irreversible neurotoxicity.

Body dysmorphic disorder

Body dysmorphic disorder is considered a subtype of obsessive-compulsive disorder, characterized by excessive preoccupation with one's appearance, believing that one is ugly or deformed, particularly in a specific part of the body. Often, the perceived defect is related to the face (nose, mouth, asymmetries), which, although present, appears completely disproportionate to the distress expressed. Patients spend a significant amount of time observing themselves in the mirror and evaluating their physical appearance. Due to the fear of being judged by others because of the presumed deformity, they tend to avoid social interactions. This can lead to significant social withdrawal and, at times, prompt the patient to attempt various methods to improve their body image, including resorting to plastic surgery. The onset of the disorder usually occurs during adolescence, and the course of the illness is chronic. It is not uncommon for these patients to have other psychiatric disorders.

33.2.5 Schizophrenia

Towards the end of the century, Emil Kraepelin used the term *dementia praecox* to indicate a psychosis with onset in adolescence, characterized by a highly heterogeneous presentation and featuring delusions, hallucinations, cognitive impairments, and emotional disturbances that led to a progressive decline in affective and intellectual functioning. The term *schizophrenia* was coined by Eugen Bleuler in 1908 to describe a disorder characterized by spaltung or "splitting of the mind," which manifested as fragmentation of associative processes and thinking. According to Bleuler, the fundamental psychopathological manifestations of schizophrenia involved disturbances of associations (now referred to as "formal thought disorders"), disturbances of affectivity (indifference, blunting, dissociation of emotions), ambivalence (simultaneous attraction or repulsion towards thoughts, actions, or feelings), and autism (withdrawal from reality in favor of internal world preoccupations). Only later (by Kurt Schneider) considered delusions and hallucinations characteristic and pathognomonic symptoms of this disorder.

In 1980, T. Crow proposed differentiating schizophrenia based on the presence of positive or negative symptoms: Type I (positive) is characterized by hallucinations, delusions, and disturbances of thought form, while Type II (negative) is characterized by social withdrawal, blunted affect, abulia, and alogia.

According to the DSM-5, a series of diagnostic criteria must be met to diagnose schizophrenia. Criterion A removes the requirement of attributing a peculiar significance to bizarre delusions and Schneiderian hallucinations, stating that only one of these symptoms is not sufficient for diagnosis. This is due to the difficulty in distinguishing between bizarre and non-bizarre delusions. To make the diagnosis, at least two symptoms from Criterion A and at least one of the following are required: delusions, hallucinations, and disorganized speech.

Criterion A: Presence of characteristic symptoms such as delusions, hallucinations, disorganized speech (derailment and incoherence), grossly disorganized or catatonic behavior, negative symptoms, including blunted affect, alogia (reduced thought and speech productivity), and abulia (reduced ability to initiate goal-directed behavior).

Criterion B: Major areas of functioning, such as work, interpersonal relationships, or self-care, are significantly below the level achieved prior to the illness. If onset occurs in childhood or adolescence, there is an inability to achieve expected levels of interpersonal, academic, or occupational functioning.

In DSM-5, diagnostic subtypes have been eliminated due to their reduced diagnostic stability and poor predictive value regarding clinical evolution and treatment response. They have been replaced by a dimensional approach focusing on symptom severity. In DSM-IV, the following subtypes were recognized:

Paranoid-type schizophrenia (which accounts for over half of the cases and presents a highly heterogeneous clinical profile) is characterized by the presence of delusions, typically structured and persecutory in nature, and auditory hallucinations (in the form of whispered voices making derogatory and imperative remarks). Both delusions and hallucinations tend to influence the patient's behavior, sometimes in an incongruous manner. Affective flattening or discordance with delusional ideation is common, while impulse control, intellectual functioning, and psychomotor abilities are generally preserved.

Catatonic-type schizophrenia is characterized by prominent psychomotor symptoms that can rapidly shift between catatonic stupor and catatonic excitement.

Disorganized-type schizophrenia, which closely corresponds to Kraepelin's hebephrenic form, is characterized by disorganized thinking, incomprehensible speech, disorganized behavior, and disturbances in affect and attention. The patient has poor contact with reality, and delusions and hallucinations, if present, are poorly structured.

Undifferentiated-type schizophrenia includes cases that do not fit into the previously described forms, while residual-type schizophrenia primarily involves the outcomes of the schizophrenic process, with minimal or absent productive symptoms and persistence of negative symptoms.

The prevalence of the disorder ranges from 0.5% to 1.5% of the overall adult population. Onset age is unimodal for men (between 18 and 25 years) and bimodal for women (25-35 years / 49-59 years). Epidemiological data indicate a male-to-female ratio of approximately 1.4. Over the years, several psychosocial risk factors have been identified (such as the theory of the double bind and the schizophrenogenic mother), including traumatic events in early childhood and environmental risk factors (such as viral infections during pregnancy). There is some supporting evidence for a genetic hypothesis involving genes encoding dysbindin (DTNBP1) and neuroregulin (NRG1), but robust evidence is currently lacking.

Delusional ideation can be observed in the early and intermediate stages of the following conditions: dementia, temporal lobe epilepsy, Huntington's chorea, viral encephalitis, Parkinson's disease treated with dopaminergic agonists, acute cerebral vascular diseases, and temporal lobe tumors.

Neurobiological hypotheses | The main pathophysiological model of schizophrenia is the dopaminergic dysregulation, according to which the hyperactivity of the mesolimbic dopaminergic pathway (projecting from the ventral tegmentum of the brainstem to limbic areas) determines positive symptoms. Negative symptoms, on the other hand, are attributed to a dopaminergic deficit in the projection areas of the mesocortical dopaminergic pathway, such as the dorsolateral prefrontal area (DLPFC). In general, an excess of dopamine leads to the attribution of specific meanings to neutral stimuli. Studies using Magnetic Resonance Imaging have highlighted neuronal losses in the temporal lobes, prefrontal lobes, and connecting structures such as the uncinate fasciculus, corpus callosum, and internal capsule.

Schizoaffective disorder

In the 1930s, Kasanin used the term "*schizoaffective*" to define those acute psychoses with sudden onset, characterized by strong emotional turmoil, sensory distortions, and remissions within a few weeks or months. In the following years, the Norwegian Langfeld distinguished from the group of schizophrenias a 'schizophreniform' group characterized by a good prognosis. Associated with this new diagnosis, he identified a series of factors such as well-adapted premorbid personality, identifiable precipitating factors, sudden onset, presence of a mood disorder, clouding of consciousness, and absence of blunted affect. The reference criteria for the diagnosis of schizoaffective disorder require the presence of a *Major Depressive Episode* or a *Mixed Episode*, along with symptoms that meet Criterion A of schizophrenia. In the DSM-5, it is prescribed that, for the diagnosis, there must be a major alteration of mood sustained throughout the entire observation period. In this way, the disorder assumes the status of an independent longitudinal diagnosis, rather than being between schizophrenia, bipolar disorders, and major depression.

Regarding the frequency of *schizoaffective disorder*, the currently available scientific data are contradictory but indicate, nonetheless, a lower frequency compared to schizophrenia. The typical onset age is in early adulthood, and the prognosis appears to be more favorable than schizophrenia.

Delusional disorder

The term *Delusional Disorder* is the successor of the more well-known term "paranoia." The fundamental aspect of the disorder is the presence of a persistent, systematized delusion focused around a non-bizarre theme, such as being pursued, controlled, poisoned, loved from afar, or betrayed. It is not associated with schizophrenia, is not secondary to a mood disorder, and must last for more than a month. Kraepelin designated this term for a specific pathology, distinct from paranoid schizophrenia, described as a "psychosis characterized by the slow development of a chronic delusional system, accompanied by perfect preservation of sensorial lucidity and order of thought, will, and affectivity." The content of delusions is persecutory-assertive in nature, sometimes assuming the configuration of inventive delusion, genealogical delusion, or mystical-prophetic delusion. In 40% of patients, especially males, there is jealousy delusion, while erotomanic delusions are more common in females. In a small percentage, it presents as body dysmorphic delusion, olfactory delusional disorder, delusional parasitosis, or hypochondriacal delusion. Delusional ideation adheres to real facts, experienced with intense emotional involvement, and coherent in its themes. Sometimes, the convictions are so well-organized in their logic and staunchly defended that they are shared by others (religious sects and political groups). Differential diagnosis should be made with paranoid schizophrenia, where the delusion appears disconnected and implausible, and hallucinations and signs of ideational-affective dissociation are present.

The peak incidence of delusional disorder is in the fifth decade of life, and the prognosis is variable. In approximately half of the cases, the symptomatology completely resolves, while in the other half, the disorder becomes chronic.

33.2.6 Somatic symptoms and related disorders

This diagnostic category brings together different syndromes but united by a clinical presentation based on predominantly somatic symptoms (in the absence of demonstrable organic alterations and known pathophysiological mechanisms). The symptoms are not secondary to a general medical condition or another psychiatric disorder. In DSM-5, the number of disorders and their subcategories is reduced, and the boundaries between various somatoform disorders are better defined. Although lacking identifiable organic causes through common clinical and instrumental investigations, somatic symptom and related disorders create significant distress for the patient, both physically and psychologically, as the difficulty in identifying a reason for their discomfort generates stress and anxiety. Additionally, there is the sensation of not being evaluated and treated optimally. If not managed and compensated for, over time, the concern for one's health can become persistent, causing considerable psychoemotional suffering and eventually becoming disabling. Some diagnostic entities have been removed: undifferentiated somatoform disorder, hypochondria, somatization disorder, and pain disorder. DSM-5 establishes maladaptive experience as a diagnostic criterion in terms of thought and feelings, as well as relevant behaviors related to somatic symptoms, thus overcoming the distinction between somatization and undifferentiated somatoform disorder and the numerical criterion. The DSM-5 redefines Illness Anxiety Disorder or Hypochondria and introduces *Medically Unexplained Symptoms*. While DSM-IV emphasized the absence of a medical diagnosis, widening the mind-body dualism, DSM-5 prefers to assess the positive dimension of physical symptoms caused by psychological stress, highlighting their association with maladaptive experiences.

Somatic symptom disorder

Somatic Symptom Disorder is characterized by multiple and recurrent somatic complaints that show a chronic fluctuating course, leading the patient to frequently seek medical visits, diagnostic tests, and hospitalizations. The reported symptoms are mostly nonspecific, subjective, not justifiable by an organic pathology or substance abuse, and disproportionate to any potential organic substrate.

According to the criteria proposed by DSM-5, the typical symptoms for a diagnosis of somatic symptom disorder include eight types: four painful, two gastrointestinal, one sexual, and one pseudoneurological. In 75% of cases, patients with this disorder have comorbidity with depressive disorder, anxiety disorder, or substance abuse. Comorbidity with Axis II disorders is more frequently observed, ranging from personality traits to a true disorder, particularly histrionic, paranoid, and dependent types.

Conversion disorder

Conversion Disorder, along with dissociative disorders, is the new designation for the classic "hysterical" condition. The term "hysterical conversion" was adopted by Freud to describe a process in which, following the repression of ideas or thoughts unacceptable to the individual's moral sensitivity, the subject manifests pseudo-neurological symptoms. The psychoanalytic model implies that, in conversion disorder, the somatic symptom replaces an unconscious conflict that is repressed. In somatization, on the other hand, in the absence of conflicts, the symptom directly replaces psychic activity. According to psychodynamic theories, the patient has a dual advantage from expressing a syndromic presentation: the removal of a conflict and assuming the role of a patient. The diagnosis of *Conversion Disorder* requires the presence of one or more neurological signs or deficits, affecting sensory and motor areas, in the absence of a general medical condition, substance abuse, and a correspondence between the anatomy of nerve pathways and the reported symptom.

Conversion Disorder: the new criteria emphasize the importance of neurological examination and the possibility that triggering psychological factors may not be detectable upon the initial examination of the patient. Among the most frequently reported disorders are: anesthesia, paresthesia, motor paralysis, atonia, aphonia, diplopia, dizziness, pseudo-seizures, and dysphagia. DSM-5 includes the presence of stressful life events preceding and contributing to the onset or exacerbation of the disorder as diagnostic criteria. The disorder would predominantly affect females, typically appearing during adolescence or early adulthood. There is also evidence of a cause-effect relationship between traumatic events experienced in childhood, particularly physical and sexual violence, and the subsequent development of the disorder. Generally, these episodes are of short duration and resolve rapidly, but there are cases where the disorder can have a chronic course. Conversion disorders are common in patients with epilepsy and multiple sclerosis, with similar manifestations that are difficult to distinguish from primary symptoms and signs. Psychogenic movement disorders, such as dystonia, parkinsonism, dyskinesias, and tremors, are widely described.

33.2.7 Dissociative disorders

In the current classification, dissociation is defined as the disconnection of usually integrated functions of consciousness, affectivity, memory, identity, or perception of the environment. In dissociative disorders, consciousness is the most compromised function. Both Freud and Janet believed that traumatic emotional memories play a fundamental role in the genesis of dissociative disorders. According to these authors, dissociation would be a defense mechanism of the mind in the face of traumatic events, a psychological escape that makes these events less intense through dissociative alterations of perceptions (depersonalization and derealization) or dissociative alterations of memory (dissociative amnesia).

Dissociative symptoms include *Depersonalization/Derealization Disorder*, Dissociative amnesia including Dissociative Fugue, and Dissociative Identity Disorder.

Clinically, primary and secondary forms are differentiated, with the latter being able to appear in the course of other pathologies such as epilepsy and head trauma or as a result of drug and substance use.

Dissociative Identity Disorder (formerly known as Multiple Personality Disorder) is characterized, according to the criteria of DSM-5, by the presence of two or more distinct identities or personality states that take control of the individual's behavior. The disorder is also characterized by amnesia for significant personal information. It has a higher incidence in women. Among all dissociative disorders, DID is the one most strongly associated with traumatic events (approximately 90% of individuals have experienced physical or sexual abuse). The number of different personalities that can alternate varies from two to over a hundred. The transition from the dominant personality (the host) to an alter (subordinate personality) is often sudden and worsens in the presence of psychosocial stress, hypnosis, or drug use. The return to the dominant personality is marked often by a severe headache and amnesia for the actions, words, and thoughts of the alter, which usually presents with characteristics different from the dominant personality (e.g., name, age, ethnicity). The different personalities manifest in the individual with differences in voice, accent, handwriting, visual acuity, and EEG patterns compared to the dominant personality. The permeability, or the degree of mutual awareness between different personalities, can vary over time.

Dissociative fugue

Dissociative fugue manifests as the sudden departure of the individual from their home or workplace, with an inability to remember their past and a state of confusion about their personal identity. Dissociative fugue shares stress factors, such as significant psychosocial stressors, with dissociative amnesia, and its incidence increases in cases of conflicts and natural disasters. The onset is often sudden. The duration and extent of the fugue can vary. Both the onset and resolution frequently occur during altered states of consciousness, such as upon waking from sleep. Unlike dissociative amnesia, the patient is not aware of the amnesia, and when the episode resolves, they do not remember what they did during the fugue.

Depersonalization/derealization disorder

Depersonalization is the persistent or recurrent experience of feeling like an external observer of one's own mental processes or body (autoscopy or somatoscopy). Reality testing remains intact, meaning there are no psychotic symptoms present. Individuals with this disorder report the sudden onset of feelings of detachment and alienation from oneself (feeling like living in a dream and being an observer of one's own actions). Paresthesia and other somatic sensations are often associated with this condition. Depersonalization is frequently present in other psychiatric disorders such as panic disorder, schizophrenia, and depression. Transient experiences of depersonalization appear to be quite common (around 50% of the population) and are often triggered by psychophysical stress and the use of substances such as cannabinoids. The disorder has a similar prevalence in both sexes and typically begins in youth.

Dissociative identity disorder

Dissociative Identity Disorder is an alteration of identity characterized by the presence of two or more distinct identities or personalities within an individual. In this disorder, the person rapidly switches between different identity states (or personalities) and unknowingly alters their way of acting, thinking, and relating to others. The identities appear to be completely separate, with an amnesic barrier preventing communication between them. As a result, when the person is in one identity state, they do not remember what they did in the other state. The disorder is characterized by the extensive use of *dissociation* as a mental mechanism by the individual. Dissociation is a normal human response to traumatic and stressful situations, as it is a mental process that protects one from the overwhelming amount of distressing information contained in these events. Dissociation can be described as an "alteration of consciousness" or a trance-like state that involves analgesia and amnesia for events occurring during that state.

33.2.8 Eating disorders

Eating disorders refer to the presence of abnormal eating behaviors. According to the DSM-5, the two main categories of eating disorders are Anorexia Nervosa and Bulimia Nervosa, with Binge Eating Disorder being an additional category.

Anorexia nervosa

Anorexia nervosa is characterized by a complex symptom profile involving psychological and physical symptoms, with a high mortality rate, suicidal risk, and medical complications. The onset of the disorder is often gradual and progressive, facilitated by family denial. The course of the disorder varies over time, with frequent relapses. The disorder is characterized by a general dissatisfaction with one's body image, accompanied by sudden behavioral changes such as an excessive focus on calorie content, recipes, and diets, highly selective and sometimes eccentric food choices, and discomfort with social aspects of eating. The disorder becomes evident when the individual loses control over their eating behavior, adopting severe dietary restrictions or engaging in binge-eating episodes and purging behaviors (self-induced vomiting, diuretics, laxatives, appetite suppressant medications), leading to significant weight loss and pervasive fear of gaining weight (delusional symptoms are common). These behaviors are associated with medical complications such as amenorrhea (absence of menstruation for at least 3 months), cutaneous dehydration, loss of subcutaneous adipose tissue, yellowish skin coloration, alterations in the hematopoietic system (nutritional anemias), and other symptoms affecting the gastrointestinal, musculoskeletal (bone demineralization, osteoporosis), cardiovascular (bradycardia, orthostatic hypotension), and renal systems..

Bulimia nervosa

According to the DSM-5 criteria, symptoms of bulimia nervosa include a preoccupation with thinness and recurrent episodes of binge eating, followed by inappropriate compensatory behaviors (at least once a week for a minimum of three months) to prevent weight gain (such as self-induced vomiting, strict dieting, misuse of laxatives and diuretics, and excessive exercise). Binge eating refers to the consumption of a significant amount of food within a discrete period of time, accompanied by a sense of loss of control during the episode (i.e., the inability to stop eating or control what or how much is being eaten, sometimes accompanied by a sense of detachment). Bulimic episodes are characterized by the consumption of excessive amounts of food, initially hypercaloric and appealing, but later also unpleasant; over time, these episodes become secretive and solitary. Additionally, individuals with bulimia nervosa excessively base their self-esteem on body shape and weight. The disorder tends to fluctuate over time and is accompanied by mood swings: patients experience tension due to the need to overeat and feelings of guilt and anger after binge eating episodes. Although patients with bulimia nervosa may fall within the normal weight range or be overweight (body mass index BMI > 18.5 and < 30), the consequences can be clinically serious. The frequent use of laxatives or diuretics can lead to severe electrolyte imbalances, renal complications, and arrhythmias. Rarely, esophageal tears, gastric rupture, and significant gastrointestinal symptoms, as well as rectal prolapse in cases of chronic laxative abuse, can occur.

33.2.9 Personality disorders

Personality is defined as a stable organization of coherent patterns of inner experience, thinking, and behavior, while *temperament* refers to the biological disposition derived from a genetic substrate that determines an individual's particular way of responding to external stimuli. *Character* primarily relates to behavioral aspects determined by experience.

Abnormal variants of personality have been recognized since ancient times, and the term *"personality disorders"* is used by the DSM to define a "enduring pattern of inner experience and behavior that deviates markedly from the expectations of the individual's culture." This pattern manifests in the cognitive, affective, relational, and impulse control areas, significantly impairing the individual's long-term functioning in the intrapsychic and interpersonal dimensions from early adulthood onward.

In DSM-5, personality disorders are found in both Section II, which includes the same diagnostic categories as DSM-IV-TR, and Section III, which introduces the new "hybrid" model. The purpose is to familiarize clinicians with the new classification, which is dimensional and trait-specific, and to guide research in this direction.

Before making an actual diagnosis, the experienced clinician must follow a series of guidelines that lead to assessing the severity of the presented disorder and the patient's interpersonal functioning. Essentially, there are three levels to evaluate: general functioning, pathology, and traits/domains. Firstly, a dimensional assessment of the level of impairment of the self and interpersonal relationships is performed, using a severity continuum expressed with 5 levels (Self and Interpersonal Functioning Continuum). Subsequently, the clinician must determine if there is a pathological personality disorder present (borderline, avoidant, etc.). In the case where there is no pathology but only a general impairment resulting from the initial assessment, the evaluation moves on to assessing the personality traits/domains, which is an initial evaluative step aiming to define different levels of personality organization. The Personality Functioning Level Scale allows for the identification of dimensions that are divided into disturbances of the self and interpersonal functioning. Regarding disturbances of the self, there are two areas to evaluate along a severity continuum:

1) Identity, understood as the experience of oneself as a unique individual with defined boundaries, the stability of one's self-esteem, the accuracy of self-evaluation, and the ability to regulate a wide range of emotions.
2) Self-direction, understood as the ability to pursue short-term goals and coherent and meaningful life purposes, the utilization of constructive and prosocial internal behavioral standards, and the capacity for productive self-reflection.

Interpersonal functioning, on the other hand, is assessed taking into account two dimensions:

1) Empathy, understood as the understanding of others' experiences and motivations, tolerance for different perspectives, and understanding the effects of one's behavior on others.
2) Intimacy, understood as the depth and duration of positive relationships with others, the desire and capacity for intimacy and mutual respect.

After defining this general part, the actual diagnostic phase, the second step, follows. There are six personality disorders that can be diagnosed: schizotypal, antisocial, borderline, narcissistic, avoidant, and obsessive-compulsive. The schizoid, histrionic, paranoid, and dependent personality disorders are absent and will not be reintegrated. Each of these personality disorders is presented in a more detailed manner compared to the DSM-IV-TR, as they are characterized by, on one hand, general functioning, and on the other hand, relatively stable pathological personality traits that cannot be attributed to the individual's sociocultural conditions or general medical condition or substance use. In essence, the following criteria must be met for a diagnosis of a personality disorder:

- *Criterion A*: Significant impairments in self and interpersonal functioning (empathy or intimacy).
- *Criterion B*: One or more domains of pathological personality traits or facets/ aspects of the trait.
- *Criterion C*: Impairment in personality functioning and expression of the individual's personality trait are relatively stable over time and consistent across situations.
- *Criterion D*: Impairment in personality functioning and expression of the individual's personality trait is not

considered normative for the individual's developmental phase or sociocultural environment.
- *Criterion E*: Impairment in personality functioning and expression of the individual's personality trait is not attributable to the direct physiological effects of a substance or general medical condition.

Once this is done, we move on to the next part, which is the identification of 5 major traits/domains: Negative Affectivity (NA), Detachment (D), Antagonism (A), Disinhibition vs. Compulsivity (DS vs. C), and Psychoticism (P). These 5 domains, also evaluated on a dimensional scale (0-4), can be further broken down into a total of 28 subdomains or trait facets. Therefore, if a patient meets the criteria for pathological functioning but not for any of the 6 personality disorders, the clinician is encouraged to evaluate them according to the 5 major domains listed above. Through these domains, a series of Personality Disorders Trait Specified (PDTs) are described, replacing the well-known Not Otherwise Specified personality disorders from the DSM-IV-TR. Each trait domain can be further evaluated dimensionally using a 4-point scale (from 0 to 3). This description can be further explored by considering the 28 trait facets associated with the various domains. The information derived from the domains and subdomains can then be used for case formulation, even if none of the criteria for personality disorders are met.

Personality disorders include paranoid, schizoid, and schizotypal personality disorders, which are characterized by eccentric and odd behavior. s Histrionic, narcissistic, antisocial, and borderline personality disorders, which are characterized by dramatic and emotional behavior. Finally, avoidant, dependent, and obsessive-compulsive personality disorders, which are characterized by anxious and insecure behavior.

Paranoid personality disorder

Individuals with *paranoid personality disorder* may appear reserved and guarded or rigidly arrogant, irritable, and argumentative. They are hyper-vigilant, unable to relax, and constantly searching for hidden meanings that could justify perceived hostility in the environment and interpersonal relationships. They attribute negative meanings to events and malevolent intentions to people. The cognitive style is rigid and inflexible. Ideas of reference and suspicious elaborations towards others are common: "the other" is considered a potential enemy, a source of deceit and manipulation.

Schizoid personality disorder

Schizoid personality disorder is characterized by a serious impairment in relational capacities. Individuals with this disorder show little (or absent) desire to engage in relationships with others and are extremely socially isolated; they prefer to live in solitude and engage in occupations that do not require contact with others. Emotionally, they appear cold, detached, formal, and estranged from deep human relationships.

Schizotypal personality disorder

Individuals with *schizotypal personality disorder* exhibit strange, eccentric behavior associated with perceptual and cognitive distortions such as ideas of reference, bodily illusions, unusual experiences of clairvoyance or telepathy, and magical thinking. This eccentricity leads to significant difficulties in adaptation, relational distress, and impairs the relationship with reality (which can also be altered by transient psychotic episodes). Often, these individuals experience excessive social anxiety characterized by paranoid concerns; affectivity is inhibited and inappropriate.

Antisocial personality disorder

A patient with antisocial *personality disorder* displays socially irresponsible behavioral patterns that can escalate to sadistic and violent actions, reflecting a disregard for the rights of others, a lack of moral rules, loyalty, guilt, and remorse. These patients often engage in behaviors that violate laws, leading to legal proceedings. The main characteristics of the disorder are impulsivity, lack of planning, irritability, aggression, and lack of remorse.

Borderline personality disorder

Borderline personality disorder is characterized by marked instability in affective relationships, impulse control, interpersonal relationships, and self-image. Affective instability is characterized by sudden mood swings and feelings of anger. Impulsivity manifests in potentially dangerous areas for the individual (promiscuous sexuality, impulsive aggression, substance abuse) and also includes suicidal and self-harming behaviors. Interpersonal relationships are unstable, intense, and ambivalent, characterized by fear of abandonment even during temporary separations. In the face of stressful events, dissociative experiences and transient psychotic symptoms may occur.

Histrionic personality disorder

The central features of *histrionic personality disorder* are excessive concern with appearance, excessive seeking of attention, and intensely emotional, dramatic, and theatrical behavior. Interpersonally, histrionic individuals appear seductive and provocative, and all their actions are aimed at seeking attention, admiration, and reassurance. If these desires are frustrated, deep feelings of inadequacy and anguish emerge, leading to self-injurious gestures and demonstrative suicide attempts. Affective expressions are labile, superficial, and exuberant; cognitively, histrionic individuals are easily distracted, unable to maintain concentration for long periods, and analyze events critically. Their language is impressionistic, superficial, and rich in hyperbolic descriptions.

Narcissistic personality disorder

Individuals with *narcissistic personality disorder* exhibit an exaggerated sense of importance and self-worth. They feel unique and special, although maintaining their self-esteem requires constant validation from others. Interpersonal relationships are driven by a constant search for admiration, often through manipulation and exploitation. A key characteristic of this disorder is a lack of empathy and difficulty in recognizing and understanding the needs of others as separate and distinct from their own. There is a low tolerance for frustration, and individuals react to criticism and rejection with intense anger, hatred, and vengefulness. The emotional core of the disorder is thought to involve a marked susceptibility to shame, an inner sense of inadequacy and vulnerability, with fluctuations between excessive and low self-esteem, and a complete lack of self-worth.

Avoidant personality disorder

Avoidant personality disorder is characterized by excessive anxiety and a deep sense of discomfort in social contexts and intimate relationships, driven by a fear of disapproval or rejection from others. Avoidant individuals have low self-esteem and are highly sensitive to (real or imagined) criticism, leading them to avoid any activity that involves exposure to judgment from others. They often appear awkward, embarrassed, and inept in social situations.

Dependent personality disorder

The primary feature of *dependent personality disorder* is a pervasive need for care and nurturing from others, which results in excessively submissive and compliant behavior. Individuals with this disorder are unable to make decisions for themselves, tend to delegate decision-making, avoid taking responsibility, constantly seek reassurance, and fear separation and abandonment. Feelings of weakness and vulnerability undermine any attempt at autonomy. In terms of relationships, individuals tend to form attachments to powerful figures, displaying excessive submissiveness out of fear of being abandoned.

Obsessive-compulsive personality disorder

Individuals with *obsessive-compulsive personality disorder* appear rigid, inflexible, scrupulous, and perfectionistic in emotional, social, and occupational dimensions. They adopt a lifestyle characterized by order, discipline, and rigor, not only for themselves but also for others. They are organized, punctual, and conscientious. However, their level of performance does not always exceed the norm, as this perseverance can become unproductive and reveal maladaptive tendencies in excessive attention to details, loss of sight of the ultimate goal, inflexibility, and perfectionism that interfere with task completion. The dynamics of duty and control are central. In relationships, individuals may seem cold and reluctant to engage in emotional expressions they consider chaotic and illogical.

Treatment of personality disorders

The *treatment of personality disorders* is often challenging due to their poor adaptive capacity and chronic course, which are experienced in an egosyntonic manner and integrated into the individual's lifestyle. For these reasons, patients rarely seek psychiatric consultation spontaneously unless they concurrently suffer from an Axis I disorder. Current guidelines recommend the integration of individual psychotherapies, pharmacological treatments, occupational activities, rehabilitative interventions, and psychosocial and family interventions.

33.3 Therapeutic opportunities

33.3.1 Psychopharmacotherapy

The choice of a pharmacological intervention in psychiatry involves prescribing a molecule for which the technical specifications authorize its use in the specific disorder. However, the selection of one medication over another within the same category is based on scientific evidence and the clinician's experience. Moreover, drugs that were once considered exclusively antipsychotics are now indicated as mood stabilizers, just as drugs initially introduced as antidepressants are used for anxiety disorders or obsessive-compulsive disorder. This is due to the pharmacodynamic properties of the individual drug, which the clinician must thoroughly understand. Furthermore, in recent years, pharmacological interventions have increasingly relied on an integrated dimensional approach rather than a categorical approach. This means that the clinician considers the predominant symptoms exhibited by the patient to choose the most appropriate medication.

Benzodiazepines (BDZ) | Are a class of drugs widely used in clinical practice. They can be administered for acute situations or continuously for anxiety disorders (for sleep-inducing purposes), acute psychomotor agitation, or during the latency phase of antidepressant action. They act through selective facilitation of the inhibitory action of gamma-aminobutyric acid (GABA) in the Central Nervous System, which is normally mediated by two types of receptors, GABAa and GABAb. The interaction between GABA and the GABAa receptor, which surrounds a chloride channel, leads to increased chloride conductance within the neuron and consequently inhibits the neuron's firing rate. Adjacent to the GABA binding site is the benzodiazepine receptor site, capable of modulating chloride conductance through an allosteric modulation mechanism. Based on plasma half-life and metabolism, benzodiazepines are classified into medium-long half-life benzodiazepines, with slow half-life and formation of active metabolites (such as diazepam, flurazepam), and short and ultrashort half-life benzodiazepines (such as alprazolam, oxazepam-like), primarily used for sleep induction and anxiety states. Due to the high potential for inducing pharmacological dependence, withdrawal syndrome, and tolerance in patients, prolonged use of these drugs is generally contraindicated. Commonly reported adverse effects include an exaggeration of the pharmacological properties of these drugs: excessive sedation, asthenia, dizziness, and in elderly individuals, mental confusion, retrograde amnesia, and paradoxical effects such as motor restlessness, agitation, and excitement.

Antidepressants | The mechanism of action of currently available antidepressant drugs consists of modulating the neurotransmitters norepinephrine, serotonin, and dopamine, resulting in enhanced neurotransmission (Table 33.1, 33.2). Selective Serotonin Reuptake Inhibitors (SSRIs) represent a pharmacological class that offers greater tolerability and safety compared to tricyclic antidepressants (TCAs) and monoamine oxidase inhibitors (MAOIs) in the treatment of depressive and anxiety disorders. SSRIs (fluoxetine, paroxetine, fluvoxamine, sertraline, citalopram, escitalopram) inhibit serotonin reuptake, with partial action on other neurotransmitter systems. They have a series of similar side effects largely determined by the enhancement of serotonin transmission, which stimulates 5HT1a, 5HT2, and 5HT3 receptors. These side effects may include nausea, which tends to diminish or resolve with continued

Table 33.1 ANTIDEPRESSANT DRUGS

Class	Active Ingredients
TCA	Imipramine, Amitriptyline, Clomipramine, Doxepin, Dosulepin, Trimipramine, Nortriptyline
IMAO	Tranylcypromine, Phenelzine, Isocarboxazide, Moclobemide
SSRI	Citalopram, Escitalopram, Paroxetine, Fluoxetine, Fluvoxamine, Sertraline
NaRI	Reboxetine
SNRI	Venlafaxine, Duloxetine
NDRI	Bupropion
SMS	Vortioxetine
Others	Mirtazapine, Trazodone, Agomelatine, Tianeptine, Sulpiride/Amisulpride, Mianserin

Table 33.2 MINIMUM EFFECTIVE DOSAGES OF ANTIDEPRESSANTS

Clomipramine 75-150 mg/day
SSRIs
Citalopram 20 mg/day Escitalopram 20 mg/day Fluoxetine 20 mg/day Fluvoxamine 50 mg/day Paroxetine 20 mg/day Sertraline 50 mg/day
Others
Agomelatine 25 mg/day Duloxetine 60 mg/day Mirtazapine 30 mg/day Trazodone 150 mg/day Venlafaxine 75 mg/day Vortioxetine 10 mg/day
Adapted from The Maudsley Prescribing Guidelines in Psychiatry, 13th edition, edited by David M. Taylor, Thomas R. E. Barnes, Allan H. Young.

treatment, occasional insomnia and irritability, and, less commonly, sexual dysfunction such as anorgasmia and delayed ejaculation. Due to their good tolerability, these drugs can also be used in patients for whom other classes of antidepressants are contraindicated.

Among other pharmacological classes currently used in clinical practice are Selective Serotonin and Norepinephrine Reuptake Inhibitors (SNRIs), which include venlafaxine and duloxetine; mirtazapine, belonging to the class of Specific Serotonin and Norepinephrine Antidepressants (NASSAs), which increase noradrenergic and serotoninergic transmission by blocking central presynaptic alpha-adrenergic receptors and 5HT2 and 5HT3 receptors; bupropion, which acts by inhibiting dopamine and norepinephrine reuptake; tricyclic antidepressants (TCAs), which vary in their predominant action on serotonin or norepinephrine; and monoamine oxidase inhibitors (MAOIs). Vortioxetine is an antidepressant drug for the treatment of depressive disorders that falls under the pharmacological category of SMS (Serotonin Modulator and Stimulator) due to its peculiar mechanism of action, characterized by inhibition of serotonin reuptake and antagonism or agonism on serotonin receptors. Vortioxetine has a multimodal action as it combines blocking of the serotonin transporter reuptake with action on multiple serotonin receptors (antagonist of 5-HT3, 5-HT7, and 5-HT1D receptors, agonist of 5-HT1A receptor, and partial agonist of 5-HT1B receptor).

Mood Stabilizers | The term "mood stabilizers" refers to a heterogeneous class of drugs with multiple clinical indications, used in psychiatry for the treatment of acute manic phase and prophylaxis of bipolar disorder, hypomanic episodes, including mixed episodes, and major depressive episodes (Table 33.3).

Lithium carbonate. Lithium is a monovalent cation that belongs to the first group of the Periodic Table of Elements. Through alterations in Na+ and K+ exchange and complex action on various enzymatic systems, particularly

Table 33.3 TREATMENTS FOR MANIC EPISODE

Lithium carbonate 900-1200 mg/day, initial dose 400 mg/day with adjustments based on blood levels
Sodium valproate 250 mg/3 times a day, with adjustments based on plasma levels
Aripiprazole 15-30 mg/day
Asenapine 5-10 mg/day
Olanzapine 10-20 mg/day
Risperidone 2-6 mg/day
Quetiapine 100-800 mg/day
Haloperidol 5–7 mg/day
Lorazepam 4 mg/day
Clonazepam 8 mg/day
Adapted from The Maudsley Prescribing Guidelines in Psychiatry, 13th edition, edited by David M. Taylor, Thomas R. E. Barnes, Allan H. Young.

adenylate cyclase (inhibition of cyclic AMP synthesis) and phosphoinositides (inhibition of phosphoinositide synthesis), lithium is able to modify the physiology of neuronal membranes. The most common side effects include mild diarrhea, polydipsia, polyuria, mild tremor in the upper limbs, edema, weight gain, and dermatological side effects. Renal function can be partially reversible and decline due to lithium. Cardiac effects often include ST segment alterations and inversion or flattening of the T wave, with occasional conduction or rhythm disturbances. Thyroid effects include goiter and sometimes euthyroid goiter and hypothyroidism with increased plasma levels of TSH, occasionally accompanied by primary hyperparathyroidism with increased plasma levels of parathyroid hormone, calcium, and magnesium. Due to its interference with organs and systems, lithium therapy should be monitored through periodic measurement of plasma drug levels (lithium levels).

Carbamazepine. It is an anticonvulsant and analgesic drug that prolongs the inactivation phase of ion channels, particularly potassium and calcium channels, resulting in an increased threshold of neuronal excitability and enhanced inhibitory action of GABA. It possesses mood-stabilizing properties and is used for the prophylaxis of bipolar and unipolar disorders, as well as schizoaffective disorders. The drug is usually well-tolerated, but gastrointestinal, dermatological, neurological, thyroid-related side effects may occur, and less commonly, blood disorders, cholestatic hepatitis, or cardiac conduction abnormalities.

Valproic acid. The anticonvulsant and mood-stabilizing effects of valproic acid are primarily attributed to its enhancement of GABAergic transmission and inhibitory action on the glutamate system. It may also exert a direct stabilizing action on neuronal membranes.

Among other mood stabilizers used in clinical practice, the following are also mentioned: lamotrigine, gabapentin, pregabalin, and some atypical antipsychotics such as olanzapine, quetiapine, and asenapine.

Antipsychotic drugs | Antipsychotic drugs (AP) are divided into typical or first-generation antipsychotics and atypical or second-generation antipsychotics. Typical antipsychotics, also known as neuroleptics, are drugs belonging to different chemical classes that exert their pharmacological effects primarily through blockade of postsynaptic D2 and D1 dopamine receptors, mainly present in the limbic system (Table 33.4). These drugs are particularly effective against the positive symptoms of psychotic disorders. They also act through blockade of serotonin, acetylcholine, histamine, and noradrenaline receptors. They are used for the short-term and long-term treatment of schizophrenia and other psychotic disorders (delusional syndromes, manic states). Even at therapeutic dosages, they can cause adverse effects. During both the acute and maintenance phases of treatment, unwanted effects may occur, including acute extrapyramidal disorders (EPD) such as acute

Table 33.4 MAXIMUM DOSAGES OF ANTIPSYCHOTICS

First-generation oral antipsychotics
Chlorpromazine 1000 mg/day
Flupentixol 18 mg/day
Haloperidol 20 mg/day
Perphenazine 24 mg/day
Pimozide 20 mg/day
Sulpiride 2400 mg/day
Trifluoperazine 30 mg/day
Zuclopenthixol 150 mg/day
Second-generation oral antipsychotics
Amisulpride 1200 mg/day
Aripiprazole 30 mg/day
Asenapine 20 mg/day
Clozapine 900 mg/day
Lurasidone hydrochloride 148 mg/day
Olanzapine 20 mg/day
Paliperidone 12 mg/day
Quetiapine 750 mg/day
Risperidone 8-12 mg/day
Sertindole 24 mg/day
Depot antipsychotic formulations
Aripiprazole depot 400 mg/month
Flupentixol depot 400 mg/week
Fluphenazine depot 100 mg every 2 weeks
Haloperidol depot 300 mg every 4 weeks
Paliperidone depot –150 mg/month
Paliperidone depot – 525 mg every 3 months
Risperidone 50 mg every 2 weeks
Zuclopenthixol depot 600 mg/week

Adapted from The Maudsley Prescribing Guidelines in Psychiatry, 13th edition, edited by David M. Taylor, Thomas R. E. Barnes, Allan H. Young.

dystonias, parkinsonism, and akathisia. After prolonged treatment, tardive dyskinesia, with a high incidence (5%) and prevalence (24%), can occur, which is irreversible in 30% of patients. Other side effects include hyperprolactinemia, weight gain, blood disorders, and metabolic syndromes.

The main pharmacodynamic characteristics of atypical or second-generation antipsychotics include: lower affinity for D2 receptors in the nigrostriatal and tuberoinfundibular systems, higher affinity for D2 receptors in the mesolimbic and mesocortical systems, and for serotonin 5HT2A receptors (Table 33.4). These characteristics result in a low likelihood of inducing secondary negative symptoms, reduced induction of EPS in the short and long term, and a limited and transient induction of hyperprolactinemia (except for risperidone). Some drugs in this class (clozapine, risperidone, olanzapine, quetiapine, aripiprazole) have demonstrated their efficacy in the short-term and long-term treatment of schizophrenia, related psychoses, and mania in bipolar disorder, while ziprasidone and asenapine, which have been recently introduced to the market, await more consistent efficacy evidence. Lurasidone, a relatively new molecule, is an atypical antipsychotic with high affinity for dopamine D2 receptors and serotonin 5HT2A and 5HT7 receptors, used for the treatment of schizophrenia in adult patients. Due to their complex pharmacodynamic mechanisms, these drugs are also used for the long-term treatment of bipolar disorder and in the acute phase of depressive episodes.

33.3.2 Psychotherapy

The term psychotherapy refers to the interpersonal, conscious, and planned process aimed at influencing behavioral disorders and situations of suffering using purely psychological means, mostly verbal but also non-verbal. The objective is to achieve symptom reduction or modification of personality structure through techniques that differ based on different theoretical orientations. Psychotherapies can be divided into therapies based on the patient-therapist relationship and therapies based on experimental technical procedures. The first group includes psychoanalytic-oriented psychologies such as psychoanalysis, individual psychology, analytical psychology, and various forms of psychotherapy that reference different orientations of depth psychology. The second group includes cognitive and behavioral therapies (which propose symptom modification) and biofeedback techniques for treating psychosomatic disorders through learned control of physiological functions. In between these two types of therapy are forms of treatment based on the method of suggestion, such as hypnosis and autogenic training based on the practice of systematic muscle relaxation for reducing emotional tension. Among other psychotherapeutic approaches, systemic and interpersonal family therapy are also included (Table 33.5).

Psychoanalysis

The term “psychoanalysis” was introduced in the late 19th century by Sigmund Freud and refers to a particular method for treating neurotic suffering based on the assumption that psychic life, in all its manifestations, is predominantly characterized by unconscious processes. According to Freud, mental disorders, dreams, and involuntary errors (known as slips) are expressions of latent psychic contents that the process of repression keeps away from consciousness and relegates to the unconscious. The psychoanalytic method consists of allowing the patient, through clinical dialogue with the analyst, to follow free associations of images, ideas, or memories that form in consciousness. These associations, along with the analysis of dream content, gradually bring the repressed content, which already implicitly manifests itself in various symptoms, to consciousness. In this way, the traumatic event that gave rise to the mental illness is reconstructed. Knowledge of the event has the effect of dissolving the pathological symptom that the unconscious imposes on consciousness and leading the patient to healing.

Freud divided the psychic apparatus into three regions: the Superego, the Ego, and the Id. The Id, the unconscious, is the foundation of the psychic person and the psychic expression of instinctual needs originating from the body. The Ego is the most superficial part of the

Table 33.5 TECHNIQUE AND INDICATIONS FOR PSYCHOTHERAPY

NAME	Psychoanalysis	Behavioral therapy	Cognitive psychotherapy	Systemic-relational therapy
TECHNIQUE	Free associations of images, ideas, or memories that form in consciousness, along with the analysis of dream content, gradually may bring to consciousness the repressed content that already implicitly manifests in various symptoms. This way, the traumatic event that gave rise to mental illness will be reconstructed	The S-R (stimulus-response) linear model and the experimental method become analytical tools for understanding behaviors and individuals. All actions are reducible to basic associative mechanisms, whether it involves the association between two stimuli and a response (classical conditioning of Pavlov's studies) or the reinforcement of randomly occurring operant behaviors (operant conditioning by Skinner)	Identification and modification of negative automatic thoughts and dysfunctional cognitive patterns to regulate painful emotions, break vicious cycles that sustain suffering over time, and create conditions for problem resolution	Observation of the relationship patterns between the patient and their family and aims to modify, through a co-construction process between therapist and individual/family, the dysfunctional patterns within the context in which the patient's distress emerged, by stimulating family resources
INDICATIONS	Anxiety Disorders, Depressive Disorders, OCD, Schizophrenia, Personality Disorders, Psychosomatic Disorders, Eating Disorders	Psychopedagogical and rehabilitative interventions applied in cases of intellectual deficits and residual forms of schizophrenia, anxiety disorders, OCD, and eating disorders	Anxiety Disorders, Depressive Disorders, OCD, Schizophrenia, Personality Disorders, Psychosomatic Disorders, Eating Disorders	Anxiety and Phobic Disorders, Eating Disorders, Depression, Couple Issues, Personality Disorders

psychic apparatus and has the task of mediating between the instinctual needs of the Id and the external world. The Superego is the system of censorship that regulates the transition from the instincts of the Id to the Ego and carries out repression by pushing into the unconscious what moral consciousness cannot tolerate. In the more mature elaboration of Freudian thought, the unconscious is not just the product of repression but appears as the original state of psychic activity linked to somatic needs.

In the years following the development of this thought, other authors have developed models that are often very different from the original one but are all based on the fundamental concepts of psychoanalysis described above. Among these authors, we can mention Carl Gustav Jung (1875-1961), Freud's student, who developed analytical psychology after the death of his master, and Alfred Adler (1870-1937), the theorist of individual psychology.

Behavioral therapy

Behavioral therapy is a theoretical approach in social psychology that emerged in the early 20th century with the works of Pavlov, followed by Skinner and Watson. It developed in the socio-cultural climate of the United States to meet the needs of psychological sciences striving to establish themselves as a valid science, on a par with traditional sciences. According to behaviorism, individuals are born as a "tabula rasa" upon which environmental influences (stimuli) can imprint any information, knowledge, and behavior. Departing from the study of elements of psychic life and mentalistic content, behaviorism focuses on objective conditions, the set of stimuli that generate behavior, i.e., the process of learning. Behavior and its acquisition are attributed to a causal chain of external stimuli and observable, measurable responses. Thus, the linear model of S-R (stimulus-response) and the experimental method become analytical tools for understanding behaviors and individuals. Within the behavioral paradigm, all actions can be reduced to basic associative mechanisms, whether it involves the association between two stimuli and a response (classical conditioning, as studied by Pavlov) or reinforcement of operant behaviors (operant conditioning by Skinner). Subsequently, studies by Bandura (social learning theory) and Dollard sought to overcome the criticisms of elementalism inherent in behaviorism, which explained the intersection between psychological processes and social processes without considering feelings, perceptions, and opinions (i.e., emotional and cognitive states). These two authors reconsidered the variables and the individual's mediation in the decoding of stimuli within the stimulus (environment)-organism (O)-response (behavior) connection, redefining the linear model as S-O-R. The main techniques used in behavioral therapy include deconditioning techniques, widely applied in neuroses, and deconditioning techniques, which encompass psychoeducational and rehabilitative interventions in cases of intellectual deficits and residual forms of schizophrenia.

Cognitive psychotherapy

Cognitive psychotherapy is a therapeutic orientation derived from behaviorism that emerged in the United States around the late 1960s with the publication of the clinical work of Aron T. Beck. Beck developed a model of clinical intervention based on conscious reflection on emotions and associated thoughts, aiming to remove thoughts that interfered with a person's emotional equilibrium. The therapy was named "cognitive psychotherapy" by Beck himself because, according to him, thought constituted both the primary psychological problem and its cure.

This therapeutic approach was assuming that the motivations for mental suffering and mechanisms of psychological change are not necessarily rooted in the unconscious but can be understood by analyzing the individual's conscious experience. From this perspective, the experiences a child has with parents (or caregivers) form memories and expectations called "Internal Working Models," which can determine subsequent relationships with significant figures.

According to cognitive psychotherapy, there is a close relationship between thoughts, emotions, and behaviors, and emotional problems are influenced by what we think and do in the present. Our emotional and behavioral reactions are determined by how we interpret various situations, in other words, by the meaning we attribute to events. This explains why the same situation can elicit completely opposite reactions in different individuals or in the same individual at different times. Cognitive therapy therefore focuses on negative automatic thoughts and dysfunctional cognitive patterns to regulate painful emotions, interrupt vicious cycles that maintain suffering over time, and create conditions for problem resolution. Numerous scientific studies have demonstrated the effectiveness of the cognitive-behavioral model and techniques in understanding and treating anxiety disorders and depressive disorders. For this reason, in the guidelines of the American Psychiatric Association, cognitive psychotherapy is indicated as an elective treatment for patients suffering from several psychiatric disorders.

Systemic-relational therapy

Systemic-relational therapy, on the other hand, posits that symptoms and distress experienced by an individual are the result of a complex interplay between subjective experience, the quality of significant interpersonal relationships, and the individual's cognitive abilities to self-evaluate their situation. The basic concepts derive from systems theory and cybernetics. Within the framework of the "family life cycle" definition, a term coined around the 1940s, the evolution of the family system is assumed to encounter certain "nodal events" that, through the disorganization-reorganization of the system itself, involve overcoming certain developmental tasks, thus allowing the transition to a subsequent phase.

A person's symptoms, acquire a specific function within the relational system in which they emerge. Conflicts that tend to disintegrate the family system create an emotional tension that is usually experienced dramatically by the individual carrying the symptom. Through the manifestation of symptoms, they take on the responsibility of diverting family members from openly addressing their own relational difficulties, focusing the attention on themselves. Therefore, the symptom has a dual value: it signals the existence of distress to the family and, at the same time, renders its destructive power harmless by centralizing all concerns on the individual with the symptom. The techniques, through the use of tasks to be implemented both in therapy sessions and at home, revolve around issues of roles, hierarchy, alliances, and the quality of communication.

33.3.3 Physical therapies

Physical therapies include Electroconvulsive Therapy (ECT), Transcranial Magnetic Stimulation (TMS), deep brain stimulation (DBS), and light therapy (Table 33.6). In Italy, following the circular from the Ministry of Health on February 15, 1999, ECT should be administered exclusively in cases of "severe depressive episodes with psychotic symptoms and psychomotor retardation" after obtaining the patient's written informed consent, who must be informed about the risks, benefits of the treatment, and possible alternatives. Such restrictions do not exist in Europe and other countries, as the effectiveness of this treatment is evaluated solely based on scientific evidence and is therefore practiced daily in day hospitals. Currently, the other listed physical therapies are used experimentally for the treatment of atypical or treatment-resistant depression (light therapy and TMS), while deep brain stimulation (DBS) has been approved for refractory obsessive-compulsive disorder.

33.3.4 Treatment of major psychiatric disorders

Treatment of depressive disorder

The main objectives of the therapeutic approach are the resolution of symptoms, functional recovery of the patient, reduction of the risk of relapse, and improvement in quality of life. According to the guidelines of the National Institute for Health and Clinical Excellence (NICE), the treatment for moderate to severe depression involves an integrated pharmacological and psychotherapeutic approach. Pharmacological therapy should involve the use of an antidepressant belonging to the Selective Serotonin Reuptake Inhibitors (SSRI) class, combined with cognitive-behavioral therapy (CBT) or interpersonal therapy (IPT). If the patient experiences acute anxiety and psychomotor agitation, short-term treatment with benzodiazepines may be considered. If, after an adequate period of time, there is no clinical improvement, the antidepressant can be switched to another molecule, still belonging to the SSRI class or other newer pharmacological classes. Only later, less well-tolerated drugs such as venlafaxine, tricyclic antidepressants (TCA), and monoamine oxidase inhibitors (MAOIs) can be administered. If there is no symptomatic efficacy, the use of lithium or other antidepressant drugs such as mirtazapine or mianserin, or an atypical antipsychotic (aripiprazole, olanzapine, quetiapine, or risperidone) should be considered. Pharmacological treatment should be continued for at least six months after the resolution of the acute episode. In cases of severe depression with psychotic symptoms, the addition of an antipsychotic drug is advisable. If the clinical conditions do not improve, electroconvulsive therapy (ECT) and repetitive transcranial magnetic stimulation (TMS) should be considered.

Table 33.6 TECHNIQUE AND INDICATIONS OF PHYSICAL THERAPIES

NAME	Electroconvulsive Therapy (ECT)	Transcranial Magnetic Stimulation (TMS)	Deep Brain Stimulation (DBS)	Light Therapy
TECHNIQUE	Therapeutic technique based on inducing seizures in the patient following the passage of an electric current through brain tissue	Non-invasive technique of electromagnetic stimulation of brain tissue. Through this technique, it is possible to study the functioning of circuits and neuronal connections within the brain	Surgical treatment aimed at reducing debilitating motor symptoms characteristic of movement disorders	Therapeutic technique based on the use of light
INDICATIONS	Severe depressive episodes with psychotic symptoms and psychomotor retardation, after obtaining the patient's informed written consent	Experimentally for the treatment of atypical or treatment-resistant depression	Obsessive-compulsive disorder refractory to treatments	Experimentally for the treatment of atypical or treatment-resistant depression

Treatment of bipolar disorder

The treatment of bipolar disorders is primarily based on pharmacological therapy to reduce the severity of symptoms, stabilize mood, and prevent recurrence of manic and depressive episodes. According to the NICE guidelines, for the treatment of acute manic and hypomanic episodes, the recommended drugs are lithium, olanzapine, quetiapine, risperidone, and valproate. During critical periods, when psychomotor agitation is present, sedative drugs such as benzodiazepines may be used. If the patient is receiving treatment with antidepressant drugs, these should be gradually discontinued. If the patient is receiving valproate, second-generation antipsychotic drugs should be added. In the case of an acute depressive crisis, pharmacological treatment involves the use of an antidepressant drug combined with a mood stabilizer. If there is no clinical efficacy, it is advisable to switch to a different class of antidepressant (venlafaxine, mirtazapine), or introduce an atypical antipsychotic or lithium. If symptoms are persistent and severe, Electroconvulsive Therapy (ECT) should be considered. For long-term treatment and prevention of manic episodes, pharmacological therapy should include the use of lithium, olanzapine, or valproate for at least two years after the acute episode. For the prevention of depressive episodes, long-term treatment includes the use of a mood stabilizer administered at the minimum effective dose, in combination with an atypical antipsychotic and cognitive psychotherapy.

Treatment of anxiety disorders

According to the NICE guidelines, the first-line treatment for Generalized Anxiety Disorder is pharmacological treatment combined with psychological intervention (CBT). SSRIs are the first-choice medications; however, if no clinical benefit is observed, SNRIs or pregabalin may be used. Benzodiazepines are recommended only for the initial period. The preferred therapy for *Panic Disorder* involves brief psychotherapy (usually CBT) along with the use of antidepressant medications (SSRIs and tricyclics). As for PTSD, if symptoms are mild, cognitive-behavioral therapy focusing on the traumatic event is the recommended treatment. If therapy is insufficient, pharmacological treatment should be introduced. Among the medications that have shown efficacy for PTSD symptoms are paroxetine, sertraline, mirtazapine, and amitriptyline.

Treatment of obsessive-compulsive disorder

The NICE guidelines indicate that an integrated treatment approach combining pharmacotherapy and psychotherapy (CBT) is the first-line therapeutic option for patients with OCD. Numerous randomized trials have demonstrated the effectiveness of psycho-pharmacological treatment in OCD. In particular, clomipramine, fluvoxamine, fluoxetine, sertraline, and paroxetine are approved for the treatment of OCD. Although SSRIs and clomipramine have been considered the first-line treatment for OCD for several years, a percentage of patients, ranging from 30% to 60%, show poor or no clinical improvement. The NICE guidelines propose various substitution strategies (SSRIs, Clomipramine, SNRIs) and pharmacological augmentation by adding serotonergic and dopaminergic agents (typical and atypical antipsychotics). In patients resistant to pharmacological treatments, deep brain stimulation of the subthalamic nucleus has been successfully employed, leading to a reduction in prefrontal cortex metabolism.

Treatment of schizophrenia

The treatment of patients with schizophrenia is primarily pharmacological, although the NICE guidelines also suggest the possibility of concurrent psychological treatment (CBT) during maintenance phases. The first-choice medications are atypical and typical antipsychotics, which can also be used in injectable formulations in combination with benzodiazepines during acute phases. For long-term treatment, some antipsychotics can be administered orally or as extended-release formulations. Clozapine is indicated for cases of treatment-resistant schizophrenia.

Compulsory hospital admissionr

According to current legislation, a citizen can be subjected to involuntary health treatment in the following cases: immediate risk to their life, mandatory vaccinations, if affected by sexually transmitted diseases, if drug-dependent, or if suffering from mental disorders.

Regarding mental disorders, in 1978 the "Basaglia Law" (Law 180) initiated a process of transformation of psychiatric care, including psychiatry within the national health service. In particular, it involved organizing psychiatric care on a territorial basis and within general hospitals, as well as establishing teamwork between the hospital structure and the community service to ensure the patient's therapeutic continuity. All this led to the abolition of mental asylums, the establishment of psychiatric diagnosis and treatment services (SPDC) within general hospitals, and the regulation of procedures for compulsory health treatments (CHT) (always to be carried out with respect for the dignity and civil and political rights of the person).

Compulsory hospital admission , in a hospitalization setting, is an act ordered by the mayor under the following conditions:

1) Presence of mental disturbances requiring urgent therapeutic intervention.
2) Patient's refusal to accept the aforementioned interventions.
3) Absence of conditions and circumstances allowing for timely and appropriate extra-hospital health measures (Article 34, Law 833/78).

CHT is structured in the following stages:

1) A qualified physician, after examining the patient and accepting their condition, prepares a motivated proposal stating the clinical condition and the reason for the measure.
2) A second physician belonging to the National Health Service, after reviewing the CHT proposal and verifying the validity of the certified conditions through a thorough examination, may validate the proposal. In both stages, the physician can intervene using the most suitable therapeutic measures (immediate hospitalization or adoption of other health measures) if a state of necessity exists (Article 54, Penal Code).
3) If the physician's proposal is validated, the documents are sent to the mayor of the patient's municipality. Within 48 hours, the mayor issues an ordinance ordering the "CHT in a hospitalization setting".
4) Within 48 hours of admission to the SPDC, the mayor notifies the competent guardianship judge of the hospitalization CHT measure through a municipal officer. After verifying the regularity of the submitted documents, the judge validates the measure and communicates it to the mayor (Execution of the ordinance).
5) The physician at the SPDC, after examining the patient, carries out the admission procedures to the department (admission to the SPDC) and simultaneously informs the mayor of the patient's admission.

The entire healthcare procedure is structured to protect the patient. All parties involved can interrupt the procedure at any time if the criteria that made it necessary are no longer present. CHT must be carried out while respecting the civil and political rights of the individual, guaranteed by the Constitution, and all necessary initiatives must be taken to obtain the patient's consent to the treatment. Its duration is 7 days from the date of the ordinance. In cases where hospitalization needs to be extended, the person in charge of the SPDC must submit a "extension" proposal to the mayor who ordered the hospitalization; subsequent ordinances can be requested without predetermined limits.

Emergencies and suicide risk in psychiatry

Emergency in psychiatry is defined as a condition in which immediate intervention is necessary due to a severe event caused by or impending due to the presence of a psychiatric disorder. However, not all psychiatric emergencies are attributable to a psychiatric disorder, as in the case of delirium, substance intoxication, emotional reactions to psychosocial stressors, or psychiatric symptoms within a medical condition, the existence of which must always be ascertained or excluded in an emergency context and in the process of differential diagnosis.

The most commonly observed urgent clinical conditions in clinical practice are psychomotor agitation, delirium, and suicide risk.

Psychomotor agitation | Psychomotor agitation is a clinical condition characterized mainly by increased motor, mental, and verbal activity with consequences on behavior, emotional sphere, and ideation process. The etiopathology of psychomotor agitation includes both organic conditions and psychiatric disorders. The approach to a patient with psychomotor agitation involves the application of verbal de-escalation techniques and, in severe cases, pharmacological and physical restraint interventions aimed at preventing imminent harm to the patient. Pharmacological treatment involves the administration of medications that lead to rapid symptom resolution (rapid tranquilization). The most frequently used medications are benzodiazepines, atypical and typical antipsychotics, and anticonvulsant drugs. Early intervention is necessary as psychomotor agitation typically follows a progressively worsening course over time. Pharmacological administration can be performed parenterally, preferably intramuscularly. Psychiatric disorders that most commonly co-occur with episodes of psychomotor agitation include psychotic disorders, schizophrenia, bipolar disorder, as well as personality disorders and anxiety disorders.

Delirium | Delirium is an acute, transient, and generally reversible neuropsychiatric syndrome. It typically has an acute onset with fluctuating course throughout the day. Delirium is frequently observed in hospitalized patients and elderly individuals with preexisting cognitive deficits or dementia. The etiopathogenesis is multifactorial, with common risk factors including severe medical conditions, infections, surgical procedures, anesthesia, malnutrition, electrolyte imbalances, use of sedative medications such as benzodiazepines or drugs with anticholinergic effects, abrupt discontinuation of medications or alcohol. The clinical picture is primarily characterized by attention disturbances, alterations in consciousness, spatial-temporal disorientation, memory deficits, sleep-wake cycle disturbances, often insomnia, language disturbances, emotional lability, delusions, illusions, and occasionally hallucinations. Treatment involves identifying and correcting the underlying causes of delirium. Antipsychotics are considered the pharmacological treatment of choice, with haloperidol being the most commonly used medication; scientific evidence also highlights the efficacy of atypical antipsychotics.

Suicide risk | Suicide is a multifactorial phenomenon involving numerous risk factors. Despite the modern position of suicidology considering suicide risk as a construct separate from the presence of a psychiatric disorder, the presence of certain psychiatric conditions is an important risk factor for suicidal behavior. Suicide risk should be carefully assessed in emergency settings through an interview with the patient aimed at evaluating the presence of suicidal ideation, intent, death wishes, or planning of the act. During the interview, a thorough analysis of major suicide risk factors should also be conducted, such as a history of previous suicide attempts, accessibility to means of suicide, presence of psychomotor agitation, insomnia, depressive symptoms, hopelessness, helplessness, substance abuse or alcohol misuse. The clinician should also investigate any triggering factors for the suicidal crisis, such as relational stressors or bereavement. If the clinician perceives and identifies suicide risk, all prevention measures should be implemented, including pharmacological management of the patient, possible hospitalization, and the formulation of a therapeutic pathway that may also include non-pharmacological therapeutic techniques.

Bibliography

American Psychiatric Association, Diagnostic and Statistical Manual of Mental Disorders (DSM-5) 5th ed. Washington, DC, American Psychiatric Association, 2013.

Biondi M. (ed.) Manuale di Psichiatria. Elsevier, 2010.

Cummings J., Trimble M.R., A Concise Guide to Behavioural Neurology and Neuropsychiatry, 2nd ed. Washington, DC, American Psychiatric Association, 2002.

Minkoswki E., La Schizofrenia. Einaudi, 1996.

Pancheri P., Cassano G.B., Pavan L., Pazzagli A., Ravizza L., Smeraldi E., Volterra V. (eds.) Trattato Italiano di Psichaitria. Masson, Milano, 1999.

Rundell J.R., Wise M.G., La Psichiatria nella Pratica Medica. Textbook of Consultation-Liaison Psychiatry. Rovera GG (italian edition ed.). Centro Scientifico Editore, Torino, 1996.

Sims A., Introduzione alla psicopatologia descrittiva. Raffaello Cortina Editore, Milano, 1997.

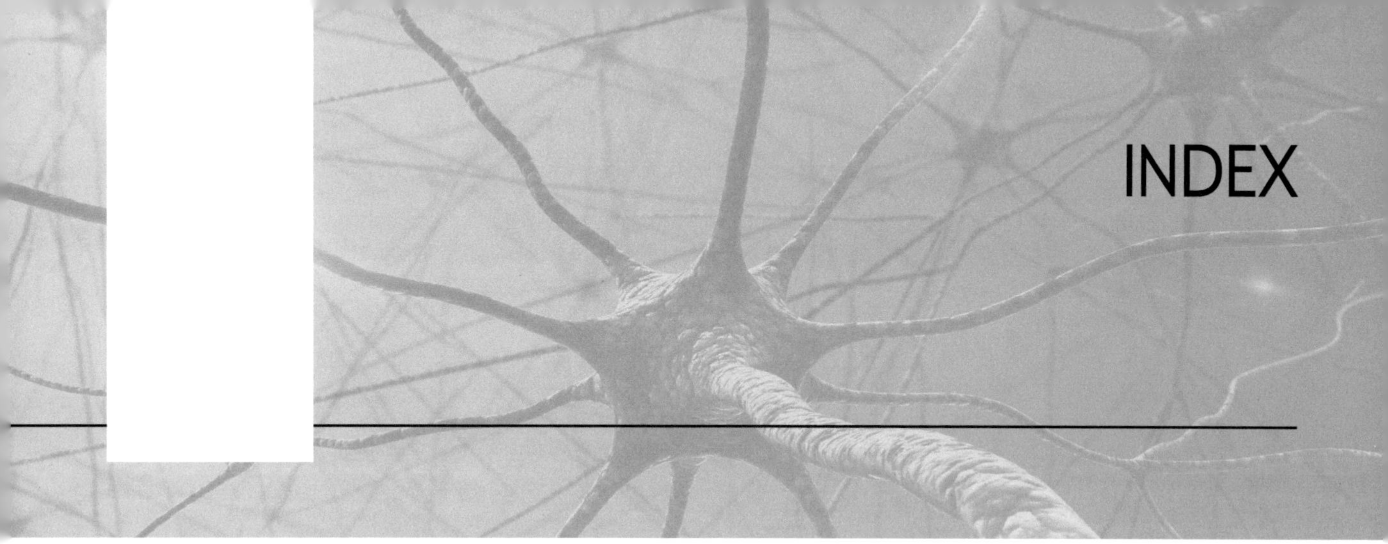

INDEX

Symbols

A

B

C

D

E

F

G

H

I

K

L

M

N

O

P

R

S

T

U

V

W

Made in the USA
Monee, IL
09 October 2026

65307999R00459